*To Mom*
*for her love and joy and strength*

*and*

*In memory of*
*Michael Dixon*
*fellow wordsmith and friend*
*1946–1990*

iii

**CLAUDIA TESSIER, CAE,**
Executive Director
American Association for Medical Transcription
Modesto, California

# THE SURGICAL WORD BOOK

**W.B. SAUNDERS COMPANY**
**A Division of Harcourt Brace & Company**
Philadelphia London Toronto Montreal Sydney Tokyo

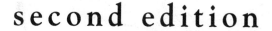

## second edition

**...nders Company**

_. Division of_
_Harcourt Brace & Company_

The Curtis Center
Independence Square West
Philadelphia, Pennsylvania 19106

---

### Library of Congress Cataloging-in-Publication Data

Tessier, Claudia J.
    The surgical word book / Claudia Tessier. — 2nd ed.
       p.    cm.
    ISBN 0-7216-2128-7
    1. Surgery—Nomenclature.    2. Surgical instruments and
apparatus—Nomenclature.  I. Title.
    [DNLM: 1. Surgery—terminology.    WO 15 T339s]
RD16.T47  1991
DNLM/DLC                     91-14966

---

_Editor:_  Margaret Biblis
_Designer:_  Karen O'Keefe
_Production Manager:_  Bill Preston
_Manuscript Editor:_  Rose Marie Klimowicz
_Cover Designer:_  Ellen Bodner-Zanolle

THE SURGICAL WORD BOOK          ISBN 0-7216-2128-7

Last digit is the print number:    9   8   7   6

# Preface

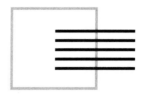

My fascination with medical terminology, in particular surgical terminology, continues, and through the years since the release of the first edition of *The Surgical Word Book*, I have collected new terms and noted corrections to be made. The result is this second edition, which is almost three times the size of the first: 105,000 terms instead of 35,000.

I have sought again to provide a compact, easy-to-use, and comprehensive text at an affordable price. Intended primarily for medical transcriptionists, it will also be useful to teachers, supervisors, students, coders, and other healthcare professionals.

Surgical terminology is more dynamic than ever. New terms, new procedures, new instrumentation, and new materials are developed daily, and preparation of a third edition has already begun. Should you identify additions, inaccuracies, or inconsistencies, please send them to me c/o W. B. Saunders Company, The Curtis Center, Independence Square West, Philadelphia, PA 19106. Your suggestions will be welcomed.

Claudia Tessier, CAE, CMT, RRA
Modesto, California
February 1991

# Acknowledgements

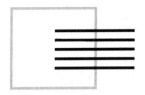

I am grateful to all who have contributed directly or indirectly to the preparation of this expanded list of surgical terms: to my employer and cause, the American Association for Medical Transcription (AAMT), for all it has done for the profession of medical transcription and for encouraging me to prepare this second edition; to the many medical transcriptionists who contributed terms; to my friend and associate Pat Forbis, CMT, for contributing to, reviewing, editing, proofreading, and critiquing the manuscript and galleys, and for being there when I or the book needed her; to my editor Margaret Biblis and other W. B. Saunders staff, in particular Neil Litt and Amy Norwitz, for their assistance and guidance; and most especially, to my husband David Bryon, my family, and my friends for their encouragement, support, and tolerance.

# Notes on Using This Text

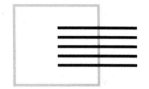

Like the first edition, this edition of *The Surgical Word Book (SWB)* requires no table of contents or index. All entries are in alphabetical order for easy access. Of its more than 400 cross-indexed categories, most are surgical instruments and materials (for example, bandages, forceps, and retractors), but also cross-indexed are categories such as incisions, positions, and sutures.

The cross-indexing feature is of particular value when you are uncertain of a spelling or when an eponym or other modifier is applied to instruments. For example, you can find the entry "Tessier elevator" in alphabetical order under "T" as well as under the category "elevator." If you thought the spelling to be "Teffier," a quick check through the "T" entries under "elevator" would identify "Tessier" as the correct spelling. If the physician dictated "Tessier retractor," you would not find it under "retractor," but by checking the general alphabetical listings you would find "Tessier dislodger," "Tessier elevator," "Tessier operation," etc., and these other entries would support the use of the eponym with retractor as well. Cross-indexing encourages and helps you to explore alternative spellings and uses.

Category lists include only those entries that do not begin with the category term. Entries that begin with the category term are treated as separate entries and are alphabetized accordingly. Thus:

> roller
> > Devonshire roller
> > Unger adenoid pressure roller
> roller bandage
> roller dressing

Consistent with the standard set by the American Association for Medical Transcription (AAMT), the possessive form with eponyms is not used in this text. I encourage you to adopt this usage for consistency and clarity.

Hyphenated terms, including eponyms, are alphabetized as if they were one word. Exception: when a term begins with a single letter followed by a hyphen, it is alphabetized as if the single letter were followed by a space. Thus,

> salpingography
> salpingo-oophorectomy
> salpingo-ovariolysis
> salpingopalatine fold

*and*

> Sachs retractor
> Sachs vein retractor
> Sachs-Cushing retractor

*but*

> D&C...
> D-Tach needle
> Dacomed Omni Phase penile prosthesis

Other punctuation marks (commas, virgules, periods) are ignored in alphabetizing.

Parenthetical entries are ignored in alphabetizing.

Abbreviations are placed alphabetically as if the abbreviations themselves were words; meanings are given in parentheses.

Plurals formed by standard English rules are not included. Those formed by Latin or Greek rules are noted in parentheses; many are cross-referenced.

> falces (*sing.* falx)
> falx (*pl.* falces)

An entry preceded by a numeral is placed at the beginning of the letter section the numeral would be in if the numeral were spelled out. Thus, "3-point chuck" is at the beginning of the T's, along with "3D knee system," "3M drape," etc. Of course, numbers that are written out rather than presented as numerals are in their appropriate alphabetical place.

Subscript and superscript numerals are not used in this text. Use subscripts and superscripts only if your equipment accurately places them as smaller-sized numerals. Otherwise, enter such numerals on the same line as the letters they accompany. In such instances, do not place a hyphen between the letters and numerals within a chemical symbol: $CO_2$; however, separate mass numbers from chemical symbols with a hyphen: I-131.

Physicians commonly mix the Latin and English forms for anatomic terms, dictating, for example, "extensor pollicis brevis muscle." Thus, to assist in identifying the Latin terms for arteries, muscles, nerves, and veins, they are entered not under "arteria," "musculus," "nervus," and "vena" but rather under the specific anatomic term. For example,

> *Dictated*:   extensor pollicis brevis muscle
> *SWB entry:*   extensor pollicis brevis, musculus
> *Transcribe*:   musculus extensor pollicis brevis *(the correct Latin form) or*
> short extensor muscle of thumb *(if you translate) or*
> extensor pollicis brevis muscle *(if you transcribe as dictated)*

# a

à demeure catheter
A&P (anterior and posterior)
A&P colporrhaphy
A&P repair of cervix
A&P repair of cystocele and rectocele
A-a gradient (alveolar-arterial gradient)
à-boule bougie
A-frame orthosis
A-line (arterial line)
A-mode echocardiogram
A-mode echocardiography
A-mode image
A-O minus cylinder Phoroptor
A-O osteotome
A-O plus cylinder Phoroptor
A-O screw
A-scan
A-scan ultrasound
A-Turner prosthesis
A2 (aortic second sound)
AA (ascending aorta)
AA1 single-chamber pacemaker
AAA (abdominal aortic aneurysm)
AAI pacemaker
AAIR pacemaker
AAL (anterior axillary line)
Aaron sign
Aarskog syndrome
AAT pacemaker
ab externo incision
ab externum
Abadie clamp
Abadie enterostomy clamp
Abadie self-retaining retractor
Abadie sign
abarthrosis
abarticular
abarticulation

abate
abatement
Abbé condenser
Abbé flap repair of lip
Abbe intestinal anastomosis
Abbé lip flap
Abbe neurectomy
Abbe operation
Abbe operation for esophageal stricture
Abbé repair
Abbe ring
Abbe small bowel operation
Abbé stage I cheiloplasty
Abbé stage II cheiloplasty
Abbé-Estlander cheiloplasty
Abbé-Estlander flap
Abbé-Estlander operation
Abbey needle holder
Abbé-Zeiss counting chamber
Abbokinase
Abbott approach
Abbott arthrodesis
Abbott arthrodesis of hip
Abbott elevator
Abbott esophagogastrostomy
Abbott gouge
Abbott method
Abbott operation
Abbott PCA pump
Abbott scoop
Abbott table
Abbott table elevator
Abbott tube
Abbott-Carpenter approach
Abbott-Fisher-Lucas hip fusion
Abbott-Lucas approach
Abbott-Lucas operation
Abbott-Lucas shoulder operation
Abbott-Mayfield forceps

Abbott-Miller tube
Abbott-Rawson double-lumen
    gastrointestinal tube
Abbott-Rawson tube
ABC (aneurysmal bone cyst)
ABC (aspiration biopsy cytol-
    ogy)
ABC protocol (airway, breath-
    ing, circulation protocol)
ABCDs of melanoma (asymme-
    try, border, color, diameter)
ABD (abdomen)
ABD dressing
ABD pad
Abderhalden dialysis
abdomen (ABD)
abdominal
abdominal abscess
abdominal aneurysm
abdominal aorta
abdominal aortic aneurysm
    (AAA, triple A)
abdominal aortic aneurysmec-
    tomy
abdominal aortic counterpulsa-
    tion device
abdominal aortic endarterec-
    tomy
abdominal aortogram
abdominal aortography
abdominal ballottement
abdominal bandage
abdominal bruit
abdominal canal
abdominal cavity
abdominal circumference
abdominal colectomy
abdominal contents
abdominal distention
abdominal esophagus
abdominal fat
abdominal fat pad
abdominal fluid wave
abdominal girth
abdominal heart
abdominal hernia
abdominal hysterectomy

abdominal ileitis
abdominal incision
abdominal incision dehiscence
abdominal lap pad
abdominal lavage
abdominal left ventricular assist
    device (ALVAD)
abdominal needle
abdominal nephrectomy
abdominal nephrotomy
abdominal pad
abdominal paracentesis
abdominal peritoneum
abdominal pull-through
    operation
abdominal rectopexy
abdominal reservoir
abdominal respiration
abdominal retractor
abdominal rigidity
abdominal ring
abdominal ring retractor
abdominal scissors
abdominal scoop
abdominal section
abdominal situs inversus
abdominal stoma
abdominal strain gauge
abdominal surgery
abdominal surgery instrument
    set
abdominal tap
abdominal trauma index (ATI)
abdominal ultrasound
abdominal vagotomy
abdominal version
abdominal viscera
abdominal wall
abdominal wall hernia
abdominal wall venous pattern
abdominal-perineal resection
    (APR)
abdominal-vascular retractor
abdominocardiac reflex
abdominocentesis
abdominohysterectomy
abdominoparacentesis

abdominopelvic amputation
abdominoperineal
abdominoperineal resection (APR)
abdominoperineal resection of colon
abdominoperineal resection of rectum
abdominoplasty
abdominoscopy
abdominothoracic arch
abdominothoracic flap
abdominothoracic incision
abdominouterotomy
abducens nerve (cranial nerve VI)
abducens nerve sign
abducens, nervus
abducent nerve
abduction
abduction contraction of hip
abduction exercises
abduction finger splint
abduction pillow
abduction splint
abduction thumb splint
abducto valgus
abducto varus
abductor digiti minimi manus, musculus
abductor digiti minimi pedis, musculus
abductor digiti quinti manus, musculus
abductor digiti quinti pedis, musculus
abductor hallucis, musculus
abductor indicis, musculus
abductor muscle
abductor pollicis brevis, musculus
abductor pollicis longus, musculus
abductory wedge osteotomy
Abée support
Abell hysteropexy
Abell operation
Abell uterine suspension

Abell-Gilliam suspension
Abelson adenotome
Abelson cannula
Abelson cricothyrotomy cannula
Abelson cricothyrotomy trocar
Aberhart disposable urinal bag
Abernethy operation
aberrant
aberrant artery
aberrant AV bypass tract
aberrant breast
aberrant cystic duct
aberrant hepatic duct
aberrant pancreas
aberrant sebaceous glands of anus
aberrant thyroid
aberrant vessel
aberration
ABGs (arterial blood gases)
Abiomed BVAD 5000 (biventricular assist device)
ablate
ablatio
ablatio placentae
ablatio retinae
ablation
ablative hormonal therapy
ablative instrument
ablative laser therapy
Ablaza clamp
Ablaza retractor
Ablaza-Blanco retractor
Ablaza-Morse approximator
abluent
ablution
abnormal lobulation
abortion
abortive
abortive clonus
abortive pneumonia
above-elbow amputation (AE amputation)
above-knee amputation (AK amputation)
abrachia
abrachiocephalia

abrader (see also *dermabrader)*
    cartilage abrader
    corneal abrader
    dermabrader
    diamond dermabrader
    Dingman abrader
    Howard abrader
    Iverson dermabrader
    lid dermabrader
    Lieberman abrader
    Montague abrader
    sandpaper dermabrader
    Stryker dermabrader
abrading instrument
Abraham cannula
Abraham elevator
Abraham enterotome
Abraham iridectomy lens
Abraham knife
Abraham laryngeal cannula
Abraham lens
Abraham tonsil knife
Abramowicz artery
Abrams biopsy punch
Abrams heart reflex
Abrams needle
Abrams pleural biopsy punch
Abrams punch
Abrams reflex
Abrams-Lucas flap heart valve
Abramson catheter
Abramson sump drain
Abramson tube
abrasio corneae
abrasion
abrasion of cornea
abrasive disk
Abrikosov tumor
abruptio placentae
abscess
abscess forceps
abscess knife
abscess lancet
abscise
abscission
abscission needle
absconsio

absence of (organ, organ part, tissue, etc.)
absent bowel sounds
absent breath sounds
absent peristalsis
absent pulmonary valve
absent respiration
absolute cardiac dullness (ACD)
absolute glaucoma
absorb
absorbable
absorbable dressing
absorbable dusting powder
absorbable film
absorbable gauze
absorbable gelatin film
absorbable gelatin sponge
absorbable sponge
absorbable sutures
absorbent
absorbent cotton
absorbent gauze
absorbent sterile towel
absorptiometry
absorption anesthesia
Aburel operation
abut
abutment
AC (acromioclavicular)
AC joint
AC separation
acalculus
acampsia
acantha
acanthesthesia
ACAT (automated computerized axial tomography)
ACBE (air contrast barium enema)
accelerated
acceleration
Ac'cents permanent lash liner
access
access peak flowmeter
accessiflexor
accessories
accessorius, nervus

accessory
accessory adrenal gland
accessory arteriovenous
    connection
accessory AV connection
accessory blood vessels
accessory bone
accessory cephalic vein
accessory cuneate nucleus
accessory duct
accessory hemiazygos vein
accessory hepatic duct
accessory instruments
accessory ligament
accessory maxillary hiatus
accessory navicular bone
accessory nerve (cranial nerve
    XI)
accessory nerve sign
accessory nerves
accessory obturator artery
accessory ovary
accessory pancreas
accessory pancreatic duct
accessory parotid gland
accessory phrenic nerves
accessory placenta
accessory saphenous vein
accessory spleen
accessory structure
accessory thyroid gland
accessory trocar
ACCO orthodontic appliance
accompanying artery of sciatic
    nerve
accompanying vein of hypo-
    glossal nerve
accordion drain
accordion graft
accordion implant
accordion prosthesis
accouchement forcé
accretio
Accucap CO2/O2 monitor
Accucom cardiac output
    monitor
Accu-dyne antiseptic products

Accudynemic adjustable
    damping
Accufix pacemaker
Accufix pacemaker lead
Accuflex punch
Acculith pacemaker
accumulation
accumulative radiation
Accu-Path acetabular cup
Accu-Path acetabular cup
    system
AccuPressure infusion pump
Accurate Surgical and Scientific
    Instruments (ASSI)
AccuSpan tissue expander
Accustaple
Accu-Temp hot wire cautery
Accutorr monitor
Accutracker II ambulatory blood
    pressure monitoring
ACD (absolute cardiac dullness)
Ace adherent bandage
Ace adherent dressing
Ace bandage
Ace cannulated cancellous hip
    screw
Ace cannulated cancellous
    screw
Ace captured hip screw
Ace Colles technique
Ace cortical bone screw
Ace elastic dressing
Ace hip screw
Ace Kyle prosthesis
Ace longitudinal strips dressing
ace of spades sign
Ace pin
Ace pinning
Ace rubber elastic dressing
Ace screw
Ace Unifix fixation system
Ace Unifix fixator
Ace Universal tongs
Ace wrap
Ace-Fischer fixator
Ace-Fischer frame
Ace-Hesive dressing

acellular
acentric
acentric occlusion
acephalobrachia
acephalopodia
acephalorhachia
acetabula (*sing.* acetabulum)
acetabular component
acetabular cup
acetabular cup gauge
acetabular cup positioner
acetabular cup template
acetabular cup trial
acetabular guide
acetabular index
acetabular knife
acetabular notch
acetabular reamer
acetabular rim
acetabular seating hole
acetabulectomy
acetabuloplasty
acetabulum (*pl.* acetabula)
acetazolamide (Diamox)
acetylcholine chloride
    (Miochol)
acetylcholinesterase
ACF (anterior cervical fusion)
achalasia
acheiria
acheiropodia
Achilles bursa
Achilles jerk
Achilles reflex
Achilles tendon
achillodynia
achillorrhaphy
achillotenotomy
achillotomy
achlorhydria
achlorhydria apepsia
achondroplasia
achondroplasty
achroacytosis of lacrimal gland
achromatic lens
achromatic mass
acid
acid peptic ulcer

acidosteophyte
acinar pattern
acinar tissue
acinarization of pancreas
acini (*sing.* acinus)
acinous adenoma
acinous gland
acinus (*pl.* acini)
acircular amputation
ACL (anterior cruciate ligament)
ACL drill
ACL drill guide
ACL guide
ACL repair
Acland clamp
Acland clamp approximator
Acland clip
Acland double-clamp approximator
Acland microvascular clamp
Acland microvascular clamp
    applier
Acland needle
Acland repair
Acland-Banis arteriotomy set
Acland-Buncke counterpressor
aclasia
aclasis
ACLS (advanced cardiac life
    support)
ACMI Alcock catheter
ACMI antroscope
ACMI bag
ACMI battery cord
ACMI biopsy loop electrode
ACMI bronchoscope
ACMI catheter
ACMI cystoscope
ACMI cystoscopic tip
ACMI cystourethroscope
ACMI duodenoscope
ACMI Emmett hemostatic
    catheter
ACMI endoscope
ACMI esophagoscope
ACMI examining gastroscope
ACMI fiberoptic esophagoscope
ACMI fiberoptic light source

ACMI fiberoptic procto-
    sigmoidoscope
ACMI flexible sigmoidoscope
ACMI forceps
ACMI gastroscope
ACMI hysteroscope
ACMI irrigating valve
ACMI laparoscope
ACMI light-carrying bundle
ACMI Martin endoscopy forceps
ACMI Martin forceps
ACMI microlens cystourethro-
    scope
ACMI microlens Foroblique
    telescope
ACMI microlens telescope
ACMI monopolar electrode
ACMI nasopharyngoscope
ACMI operating coloscope
ACMI Owens catheter
ACMI pediatric resectoscope
ACMI Pezzer drain
ACMI positive pressure catheter
ACMI proctoscope
ACMI proctosigmoidoscope
ACMI resectoscope
ACMI resistor
ACMI retrograde electrode
ACMI teaching attachment
ACMI telescope
ACMI ulcer-measuring device
ACMI ureteral catheter
ACMI urethroscope
ACMI Valentine tube
ACMI valve
Acmistat catheter
acne lancet
acorn
acorn cannula
Acorn nebulizer
acorn-shaped implant
acorn-tipped bougie
acorn-tipped catheter
Acosta classification of pelvic
    endometriosis
acoustic, acoustical
acoustic enhancement

acoustic impedance
acoustic interface
acoustic nerve
acoustic nerve sign
acoustic neuroma
acoustic neurotomy
acoustic shadow
acoustic window
acquired harelip
acquired hernia
acquired immunodeficiency
    syndrome (AIDS)
acquired megacolon
acquired ventricular septal
    defect
acquisition time
Acra-Cut cranial perforator
Acrad HS catheter (hystero-
    salpingography catheter)
acral
acral anesthesia
acral-lentiginous melanoma
acrania
Acrax prosthesis
Acrel ganglion
acroagnosis
acrobrachycephaly
acrocephalia
acrocephalopolysyndactyly
acrocephalosyndactyly
acrocontracture
acrodysplasia
acroedema
acromegalic
acromegaly
acromial bone
acromial bursa
acromial process
acromioclavicular articulation
acromioclavicular dislocation
    harness sling
acromioclavicular joint
acromioclavicular ligament
acromioclavicular separation
acromiocoracoid ligament
acromiohumeral
acromion

acromion process
acromion scapulae
acromionectomy
acromioplasty
acromioscapular
acromiothoracic
acromiothoracic artery
acromyotonia
acro-osteolysis
acroparalysis
acroparesthesia
acropathy
acrosclerosis
acrosyndactyly
Acrotorque bur
acrylic ball eye implant
acrylic bar
acrylic bar prosthesis
acrylic bite block
acrylic bone cement
acrylic cap splint
acrylic conformer
acrylic conformer eye implant
acrylic eye implant
acrylic graft
acrylic implant
acrylic lens
acrylic mold
acrylic plastic
acrylic prosthesis
acrylic resin dressing
acrylic resin teeth
acrylic splint
acrylic surgical splint
acryocyanosis
ACS (Alcon Closure System)
ACS angioplasty Y-connector
ACS catheter
ACS exchange guide wire
ACS exchange guiding catheter
ACS exchange wire
ACS floppy-tip guide wire
ACS floppy-tip guiding catheter
ACS gold-standard guide wire
ACS gold-standard wire
ACS guide wire
ACS JL4 catheter
ACS LIMA guide

ACS Mini catheter
ACS needle
ACS RX coronary dilatation
    catheter
ACS SOF-T guide wire
ACS SULP II balloon
ACTH (adrenocorticotropic
    hormone)
actinomycosis
actinotherapy
Action Eyes and Albany eye
    guards
Action OR table pads
Activase
activated balloon expandable
    intravascular stent
activated graft
activation
activator
active bowel sounds
active duodenal ulcer
active length needle
active phase arrest
active range of motion
active-assistive range of motion
actively bleeding varices
Activitrax pacemaker
Activitrax single-chamber
    responsive pacemaker
Activitrax variable rate pace-
    maker
activity-sensing pacemaker
actual cautery
actuation
Acu-Brush
Acu-derm wound dressing
Acu-dyne antiseptic
Acufex arthroscope
Acufex arthroscopic instruments
Acufex curved basket forceps
Acufex drawknife
Acufex duckbill punch
Acufex guide
Acufex linear grasper
Acufex linear punch
Acufex microsurgical instru-
    ments
Acufex power shaver

Acufex rotary basket forceps
Acufex rotary punch
Acufex scissors
Acufex straight basket forceps
Acufex straight forceps
Acuflex intraocular lens implant
acuminatum (*pl.* acuminata)
acupoint
acupressure
acupuncture
acupuncture anesthesia
acupuncture instruments
acupuncture technique
acupuncture treatment
acusection
Acuson cardiovascular system
Acuson computed sonography
acute
acute angle
acute infective endocarditis
    (AIE)
acute myocardial infarction
    (AMI)
acute renal failure (ARF)
acute warning sign
ACUTENS transcutaneous nerve
    stimulator
Acutrol sutures
acyanotic
acyclovir
AD (right ear)
ad lib
Ada dissecting scissors
Ada scissors
adactyly
Adair breast clamp
Adair breast tenaculum
Adair breast tenaculum forceps
Adair clamp
Adair forceps
Adair hemostat
Adair procedure
Adair screw compressor
Adair tenaculum
Adair tenaculum forceps
Adair tissue-holding forceps
Adair uterine forceps

Adair uterine tenaculum
Adair uterine tenaculum forceps
Adair-Allis forceps
Adair-Allis tenaculum
Adair-Allis tissue forceps
Adam and Eve rib belt splint
adamantinoma
Adamkiewicz artery
Adams advancement of round
    ligaments
Adams ankle arthrodesis
Adam's apple
Adams aspirator
Adams clasp
Adams crushing of nasal
    septum
Adams ectropion operation
Adams excision of palmar fascia
Adams hip operation
Adams operation
Adams operation for ectropion
Adams orthodontic clip
Adams otoplasty
Adams position
Adams retractor
Adams rib contractor
Adams saw
Adams tourniquet
Adams-DeWeese vena caval
    clip
Adams-DeWeese vena caval
    serrated clip
Adams-Horwitz ankle fusion
Adams-Stokes disease
Adams-Stokes syncope
Adams-Stokes syndrome
adaptation
adapted instruments
adapter
    Air-Lon adapter
    Alcock conical catheter
        adapter
    B-D adapter
    butterfly adapter
    cannula tubing adapter
    catheter adapter
    catheter tubing adapter

adapter *continued*
    chuck adapter
    Curry hip nail counter-
      bore with Lloyd
      adapter
    cystoscope-urethroscope
      adapter
    ear suction adapter
    fiberoptic cable adapter
    House adapter
    House suction adapter
    House suction tube
      adapter
    Kaufman adapter
    KleenSpec otoscope
      adapter
    Luer suction cannula
      adapter
    resectoscope adapter
    sheath with side-arm
      adapter
    side-arm adapter
    sleeve adapter
    Storz catheter adapter
    Storz fiberoptic cable
      adapter
    suction adapter
    T-adapter
    terminal adapter
      electrode
    terminal electrode
      adapter
    two-way adapter for
      K-Temp thermometer
    Universal T-adapter
    Venturi ventilation
      adapter
    Wullstein chuck adapter
adapter catheter
Adaptic dressing
Adaptic gauze
Adaptic gauze dressing
Adaptic gauze pack
Adaptic gauze packing
Adaptic needle holder
Adasoy procedure
Addison plane

Addison point
additive
Addix needle
Addix tier
adduction
adduction contracture of hip
adduction position
adductor brevis, musculus
adductor canal
adductor hallucis, musculus
adductor hiatus
adductor longus, musculus
adductor magnus, musculus
adductor muscle
adductor pollicis, musculus
adductor pollicis obliquus,
    musculus
adductor tenotomy
adductor tenotomy with total
    hip
adductor tubercle
Adelmann finger disarticulation
Adelmann operation
adenectomy
adenocarcinoma
adenochondroma
adenochondrosarcoma
adenofibroma
adenohypophysectomy
adenoid curet
adenoid forceps
adenoid instruments
adenoid punch
adenoidectomy
adenoids
adenoma (*pl.* adenomas,
    adenomata)
adenomammectomy
adenomata (*sing.* adenoma)
adenomatosis
adenomatous
adenomatous goiter
adenomatous polyp
adenomyofibroma
adenomyosarcoma
adenomyosis
adenopathy

adenotome
- Abelson adenotome
- Box adenotome
- Box-DeJager adenotome
- Breitman adenotome
- Cullom-Mueller adenotome
- direct-vision adenotome
- guillotine adenotome
- Kelly adenotome
- LaForce adenotome
- LaForce adenotome blade
- LaForce-Grieshaber adenotome
- LaForce-Stevenson adenotome
- LaForce-Storz adenotome
- Mueller-LaForce adenotome
- Myles adenotome
- Myles guillotine adenotome
- Shambaugh adenotome
- Sluder adenotome
- St. Clair-Thompson adenotome
- Stevenson-LaForce adenotome
- Storz-LaForce adenotome
- Storz-LaForce-Stevenson adenotome

adenotome blade
adenotomy
adenotonsillectomy
adequacy
adequate
adhere
adherent bandage
adherent cataract
adherent lens
adherent pericardium
adherent placenta
adherent tongue
AD-Hese-Away dressing
adhesiolysis
adhesion

adhesiotomy
adhesive
adhesive absorbent dressing
adhesive aluminum splint
adhesive band
adhesive bandage
adhesive capsulitis
adhesive cement
adhesive colpitis
adhesive drape
adhesive dressing
adhesive dressing board
adhesive gauze
adhesive ileus
adhesive inflammation
adhesive needle holder
adhesive pericarditis
adhesive phlebitis
adhesive plaster
adhesive plastic drape
adhesive pleurisy
adhesive pyelophlebitis
adhesive silicone implant
adhesive tape
adhesive tape strips
adhesive tenosynovitis
adhesive vulvitis
adhesiveness
Adie pupil
Adie syndrome
adipectomy
adipocele
adiponecrosis
adiposa hernia
adipose
adipose capsule of kidney
adipose ligament
adipose renal capsule
adipose tissue
adiposis
aditus
adjacent
adjacent tissue
adjunctive procedure
adjustable breast implant
adjustable cross splint
adjustable cup reamer

adjustable headrest
adjustable leg and ankle
    repositioning mechanism
    (ALARM)
adjustable nail
adjustable splint
adjustable strap arm sling
adjustable vaginal stent
Adjusta-Rak
adjustment
adjustment of cardiac pace-
    maker
adjuvant chemotherapy
adjuvant therapy
Adkins spinal arthrodesis
Adkins spinal fusion
Adkins strut
Adler attic ear punch
Adler bone forceps
Adler forceps
Adler lens loupe
Adler operation
Adler punch
Adler punch forceps
adnexa
adnexa uteri
adnexal area
adnexal mass
adnexal metastasis
adnexal region
adnexal structures
adnexopexy
adolescent cataract
ADR Ultramark ultrasound
ADR ultrasound
adrenal
adrenal cortical hyperfunction
adrenal cortical hypofunction
adrenal gland cyst
adrenal glands
adrenal medullary implants
adrenal veins
adrenalectomize
adrenalectomy
Adrenalin
adrenalorrhaphy
adrenalotomy

adrenergic
adrenoceptor
adrenocorticotropic hormone
    (ACTH)
Adrian-Flat prosthesis
adromia
Adson aneurysm needle
Adson angular hook
Adson artery forceps
Adson bayonet dressing forceps
Adson blunt dissecting hook
Adson blunt hook
Adson blunt knife
Adson bone rongeur
Adson brain clip
Adson brain forceps
Adson brain hook
Adson brain retractor
Adson brain suction tip
Adson brain suction tube
Adson brain-exploring cannula
Adson bur
Adson cannula
Adson cerebellar retractor
Adson chisel
Adson clip
Adson clip-applying forceps
Adson clip-introducing forceps
Adson conductor
Adson cranial rongeur
Adson cranial rongeur forceps
Adson dissecting hook
Adson dissector
Adson dissector hook
Adson drainage cannula
Adson dressing forceps
Adson drill
Adson drill guide
Adson dura protector
Adson dural hook
Adson dural knife
Adson dural scissors
Adson elevator
Adson enlarging bur
Adson exploring cannula
Adson forceps
Adson ganglion scissors

Adson Gigli saw
Adson Gigli-saw guide
Adson headrest
Adson hemostat
Adson hemostatic forceps
Adson hook
Adson hypophyseal forceps
Adson knife
Adson knot tier
Adson knot tier hook
Adson laminectomy chisel
Adson maneuver
Adson microbipolar forceps
Adson microdressing forceps
Adson microtissue forceps
Adson needle
Adson needle holder
Adson perforating bur
Adson periosteal elevator
Adson retractor
Adson rongeur
Adson saw conductor
Adson saw guide
Adson scalp clip
Adson scalp clip-applying
    forceps
Adson scalp hemostasis clips
Adson scalp needle
Adson scissors
Adson sharp hook
Adson sharp knife
Adson sign
Adson speculum
Adson spiral drill
Adson splanchnic retractor
Adson straight suction tube
Adson suction tube
Adson suture needle
Adson test
Adson thumb forceps
Adson tissue forceps
Adson tube
Adson twist drill
Adson Vital tissue forceps
Adson-Beckman retractor
Adson-Brown clamp
Adson-Brown forceps

Adson-Brown tissue forceps
Adson-Coffey scalenectomy
Adson-Mixter forceps
Adson-Mixter neurosurgical
    forceps
Adson-Murphy needle
Adson-Murphy trocar point
    needle
Adson-Rogers cranial bur
Adson-Rogers perforating drill
Adson-Shaefer dural guide
adsorb
adsorbent
adult laryngoscope
adult reverse-bevel laryngo-
    scope
adult sigmoidoscope
advanced cardiac life support
    (ACLS)
advancement
advancement flap
advancement forceps
advancement needle
advancement of muscle
advancement of ocular muscle
advancement of rectal flap
advancement of round ligament
advancement of superior
    oblique muscle
advancement of tendon
advantageous
adventitia
adventitial bed
adventitial cells
adventitial sheath
adventitial tissue
adventitious
adventitious breath sounds
adventitious bursa
adventitious membrane
adventitious sounds
advisable
adynamic
adynamic bladder
adynamic ileus
adynamic intestinal obstruction
AE (above-elbow, aryepiglottic)

AE amputation (above-elbow amputation)
AE fold (aryepiglottic fold)
Aebli corneal scissors
Aebli corneal section scissors
Aebli scissors
Aebli-Manson scissors
Aeby muscle
Aeby plane
AEC pacemaker
AEI button for replacement gastrostomy
Aequitron pacemaker
aerate
aeration
aeration time
aeremia
AeroChamber
aerodermectasia
aeroembolism
aero-flo tip catheter
aerogram
aerography
aerohydrotherapy
Aeroplast dressing
Aeroplasty
aerosol
aerosolize
Aerozoin skin conditioner
Aesculap cast-cutting instruments
Aesculap forceps
Aesculap instruments
Aesculap needle holder
Aesculap saw
aesthetic surgery
AF (anti-fog, anti-fogging)
AF agent (anti-fog agent)
AF solution (anti-fog solution)
AF tube (anti-fog tube)
AFB needle guide (aortofemoral bypass needle guide)
AFBG (aortofemoral bypass graft)
afferent
afferent fibers
afferent limb
afferent loop
afferent loop syndrome

afferent nerve
afferent veins
AFI coaxial headlight system
AFI Micros 5 microscope system
AFO (ankle-foot orthosis)
AFO brace
AFP pacemaker
aftercare
aftereffect
afterload
afterload reduction
afterloading colpostat
afterloading screw
afterloading tandem (AL tandem)
aftertreatment
AG Bovie electrosurgical unit
AGA (appropriate for gestational age)
aganglionic
aganglionic bowel
Agarose gel electrophoresis
AGC knee program implant
AGE (angle of greatest extension)
Agee 4-pin fixation device
Agee fiberoptic carpal tunnel operation
Agee fiberoptic carpal tunnel release
Agee WristJack
agenesis
agenetic fracture
AGF (angle of greatest flexion)
agger (pl. aggares)
agger nasi cells
agglomerated
agglutinant
agglutination
agglutinative
aggravate
aggregate
aggregated human IgG (AHuG)
Aggressor meniscal blade
agility drill
agnathia
Agnew canaliculus knife
Agnew canthoplasty

Agnew keratome
Agnew knife
Agnew needle
Agnew operation
Agnew splint
Agnew tattooing needle
Agnew traction
Agnew-Hunt reduction
Agnew-Verhoeff incision
agnosia
agonal respirations
agonal thrombosis
agonal thrombus
agonist
agonistic muscle
agraffe
agraffe clamp
agraphia
Agrikola (also Agricola)
Agrikola lacrimal sac retractor
Agrikola retractor
AgX antimicrobial Foley
    catheter
AHG (antihemophilic globulin)
AHJ (artificial hip joint)
Ahlfeld method
Ahlfeld sign
Ahlquist-Durham clip
Ahlquist-Durham embolism
    clamp
Ahlquist-Durham vena cava clip
AHuG (aggregated human IgG)
AI (aortic insufficiency)
AI angle
AICA (anterior inferior commu-
    nicating artery)
AICD (automatic implantable
    cardioverter-defibrillator)
AICD (automatic internal
    cardioverter-defibrillator)
AICD device
AICD pacemaker
AID (artificial insemination
    donor)
AID (automatic implantable
    defibrillator)
AID-B defibrillator
AID-B pacemaker

AIDS (acquired immunodefi-
    ciency syndrome)
AIDS-related complex (ARC)
AIE (acute infective endocardi-
    tis)
AIH (artificial insemination
    husband)
AIM CPM (continuous passive
    motion)
Aim retractor
Ainsworth punch
AIO compression plate
air bag
air bed
air block
air bronchogram sign
air bubble
air cannula
air cell casts
air cells
air compressor
air contrast barium enema
    (ACBE)
air cyst
air cystogram
air cystography
air dermatome
air dome sign
air drill
air embolism
air embolus
air exchange
air inflatable tube
air injection cannula
air myelography
Air Plus low-air-loss bed
air pressure dressing
air pyelogram
air saccule
air sacs
air space
air syringe
air trapping
air tube
air velocity index
air-bone gap
Aircast air-stirrup leg brace
Aircast brace

Aircast fracture brace
Aircast pneumatic brace
air-filled loop
airflow limitation
airflow obstruction
airflow resistance
air-fluid level
air-fluidized bed
airfoam splint
AIRLens contact lens
Air-Lon adapter
Air-Lon decannulation plug
Air-Lon inhalation cannula
Air-Lon inhalation catheter
Air-Lon laryngectomy tube
Air-Lon plug
Air-Lon tracheal tube
Air-Lon tracheal tube brush
Air-Lon tube
airplane splint
air-puff tonometer
air-spaced electrode
airsplint
air-stirrup ankle brace
airtight
airtight closure
airway

    Beck mouth tube airway
    Berman airway
    Berman disposable
      airway
    Berman intubating
      pharyngeal airway
    binasal pharyngeal
      airway
    Coburg-Connell airway
    Connell airway
    disposable airway
    esophageal airway
    Foerger airway
    Guedel airway
    Guedel rubber airway
    major airway
    nasal airway
    O'Brien airway needle
    rubber airway
    Safar-S airway

airway, breathing, circulation
  protocol (ABC protocol)
airway pressure
airway resistance
Airy rings
AJ (ankle jerk)
AK amputation (above-knee
  amputation)
AKC varicose vein operation
Aker pusher
Akerlund deformity
Akerlund diaphragm
akidogalvanocautery
Akin bunionectomy
akinesia
akinesis
akinetic
Akiyama prosthesis
Akutsu artificial heart
AL tandem (afterloading
  tandem)
AL-1 catheter
ala (*pl.* alae)
ala auris
ala cerebelli
ala cinerea
ala ilii
ala nasi
ala of ilium
ala of nose
Alabama University forceps
Alabama University utility
  forceps
Alabama-Green needle eye
  holder
Alabama-Green needle holder
alae protector
Alanson amputation
alar
alar bone
alar branch of external maxillary artery
alar cartilage
alar chest
alar flaring
alar folds
alar incision

alar osteotome
alar retractor
alar scapula
alar-columella implant
ALARM (adjustable leg and
    ankle repositioning
    mechanism)
alarplasty
Albarran bridge
Albarran cystoscope
Albarran cystoscope attachment
Albarran gland
Albarran urethroscope
Albee arthrodesis
Albee bone graft
Albee bone graft calipers
Albee bone saw
Albee fracture table
Albee fusion
Albee graft
Albee hip operation
Albee hip reconstruction
Albee operation
Albee osteotomy
Albee saw
Albee shelf procedure
Albee spinal fusion
Albee table
Albee technique
Albee-Compere fracture table
Albee-Delbet operation
Albers-Schoenberg chalk bones
Albers-Schoenberg position
Albert bronchoscope
Albert knee operation
Albert operation
Albert position
Albert slotted bronchoscope
Albert sutures
Albert-Andrews laryngoscope
Albert-Chase procedure
Albert-Smith pessary
albicans
Albion-Ford stethoscope
Albright hip synovectomy
albuginea
albugineotomy

albumin
albumin-coated vascular graft
Alcatel pacemaker
Alcock bag
Alcock bladder syringe
Alcock boots
Alcock canal
Alcock catheter
Alcock catheter plug
Alcock conical catheter adapter
Alcock hemostatic bag
Alcock hemostatic catheter
Alcock lithotrite
Alcock obturator
Alcock plug
Alcock return-flow hemostatic
    catheter
Alcock syringe
Alcock-Hendrickson lithotrite
Alcock-Timberlake obturator
alcohol
alcohol anesthetic agent
alcoholic cirrhosis
alcoholic fatty liver
alcoholic varices
Alcon cautery
Alcon Closure System (ACS)
Alcon cryoextractor
Alcon cryophake
Alcon hand cautery
Alcon I-knife
Alcon intraocular lens
Alcon lens
Alcon microsponge
Alcon surgical knife
Alcon sutures
Alcott catheter
aldehyde-tanned bovine carotid
    artery graft
Alden loop gastric bypass
Alden retractor
Alderkreutz forceps
Aldridge operation
Aldridge urethropexy
Aldridge-Studdefort urethral
    suspension
Alesen tube

Alexander antrostomy punch
Alexander approximator
Alexander biopsy punch
Alexander bone gouge
Alexander chisel
Alexander costal periosteotome
Alexander dressing forceps
Alexander elevator
Alexander gouge
Alexander incision
Alexander mastoid bone
    gouge
Alexander mastoid chisel
Alexander mastoid gouge
Alexander needle
Alexander operation
Alexander osteotome
Alexander otoplasty
Alexander otoplasty knife
Alexander perforating osteo-
    tome
Alexander periosteotome
Alexander prostatectomy
Alexander punch
Alexander raspatory
Alexander retractor
Alexander rib rasp
Alexander rib raspatory
Alexander rib stripper
Alexander shortening of round
    ligaments
Alexander syringe
Alexander tonsil needle
Alexander-Adams hystero-
    pexy
Alexander-Adams operation
Alexander-Adams uterine
    suspension
Alexander-Ballen orbital
    retractor
Alexander-Farabeuf costal
    periosteotome
Alexander-Farabeuf elevator
Alexander-Farabeuf periosteo-
    tome
Alexander-Farabeuf rib rasp
Alexander-Matson retractor

Alexian Brothers overhead
    fracture frame
Alexian Hospital model
    retractor
Alfonso speculum
Alfred M. Large clamp
Alfred M. Large vena cava
    clamp
Alfred snare
algefacient
alignment
alignment cord
aliment
alimentary
alimentary canal
alimentary system
alimentary tract
alimentation
alimentation catheter
aliquot
Alivium prosthesis
Alivium prosthesis cup
Aljan prosthesis
alkali
alkaline battery cautery
Allan bone lengthening
Allan calcaneus procedure
allantoic membrane
Allarton operation
Allconox
All-Cord bench engine
All-Cord surgical engine
Allegist syringe
Allen anastomosis clamp
Allen applicator
Allen arm surgery table
Allen cecostomy trocar
Allen clamp
Allen cyclodialysis
Allen eye implant
Allen eye introducer
Allen fetal stethoscope
Allen forceps
Allen hand surgery table
Allen implant
Allen intestinal clamp
Allen intestinal forceps

Allen maneuver
Allen operation
Allen orbital implant
Allen pliers
Allen retractor
Allen root pliers
Allen saw
Allen screw
Allen shoulder arthroscopy
    traction system
Allen sphere introducer
Allen Supramid implant
Allen trocar
Allen uterine forceps
Allen wire threader
Allen wrench
Allen-Barkan knife
Allen-Brailey intraocular lens
    implant
Allen-Brown prosthesis
Allen-Brown shunt
Allen-Hanbury knife
Allen-headed screwdriver
Allen-Heffernan nasal specu-
    lum
Allen-Kocher clamp
Allen-Schiøtz tonometer
Allen-Thorpe gonioscope
Allerdyce approximator
Allerdyce dissector
Allerdyce elevator
alleviate
alleviating disease
alleviation of pain
alleviation of symptoms
Allgower stitch
alligator cable
alligator crimper forceps
alligator ear forceps
alligator forceps
alligator grasping forceps
alligator nasal forceps
alligator pacing cable
alligator scissors
alligator-type grasping forceps
Allingham colotomy
Allingham excision of rectum
Allingham operation

Allingham rectal speculum
Allingham speculum
Allingham ulcer
Allis catheter
Allis clamp
Allis dissector
Allis dry dissector
Allis forceps
Allis hemostat
Allis inhaler
Allis intestinal forceps
Allis Micro-Line pediatric
    forceps
Allis periosteal elevator
Allis retractor
Allis thoracic forceps
Allis tissue forceps
Allis tissue-holding forceps
Allis-Abramson breast biopsy
    forceps
Allis-Adair forceps
Allis-Adair tissue forceps
Allis-Coakley forceps
Allis-Coakley tonsil forceps
Allis-Coakley tonsil-seizing
    forceps
Allis-Duval forceps
Allis-Ochsner forceps
Allis-Ochsner tonsil forceps
Allison clamp
Allison gastroesophageal reflux
    operation
Allison herniorrhaphy
Allison hiatal hernia repair
Allison lung retractor
Allison sutures
Allis-Willauer forceps
Allis-Willauer tissue forceps
Allman ankle reconstruction
Allman classification of AC joint
all-metal ear syringe
allogeneic
allogeneic graft
allogeneic transplantation
allograft
allograft reaction
allograft survival
allograft tissue transplantation

allokeratoplasty
allometric
alloplast
alloplastic
Allo-Pro prosthesis
allotransplantation
alloy
Allport bur
Allport eustachian bur
Allport gauze packer
Allport hook
Allport incus hook
Allport mastoid searcher
Allport mastoid sound
Allport operation
Allport packer
Allport ptosis correction
    procedure
Allport retractor
Allport searcher
Allport-Babcock mastoid
    searcher
Allport-Babcock retractor
Allport-Babcock searcher
Allport-Babcock sound
Allport-Gifford retractor
all-purpose lamp
all-purpose stretcher
all-purpose transilluminator
Alm minor surgery retractor
Alm retractor
Alm self-retaining retractor
Almoor extrapetrosal drainage
Almoor operation
Alnico magneprobe magnet
aloe
aloe stitch scissors
aloe tape dressing
Aloetherm diathermy
Aloka ultrasound diagnostic
    equipment
Alouette amputation
Alouette operation
Alpar implant
Alpar intraocular lens implant
Alpar lens
Alpha Chymar

alpha loop
alpha loop maneuver
alpha sigmoid loop
alpha-chymotrypsin
alpha-chymotrypsin cannula
alpha-fetoglobulin
alpha-fetoprotein
alphaprodine anesthetic agent
already-threaded sutures
ALRI (anterolateral rotatory
    instability)
Alsus-Knapp eyelid repair
Alsus-Knapp operation
Altemeier operation
Altemeier rectal prolapse
    procedure
Alter lip retractor
alternating
alternating sutures
alternation
alternative approach
alternatives of management
    (AOM)
Altmann needle
Alumafoam splint
aluminum
aluminum alloy fork
aluminum bridge splint
aluminum cortex retractor
aluminum eye shield
aluminum fence splint
aluminum finger cot splint
aluminum foam splint
aluminum mallet
aluminum paste
aluminum splint
aluminum wire sutures
aluminum-bronze wire sutures
ALVAD (abdominal left
    ventricular assist device)
Alvarado orthopedic guide
Alvarado Orthopedic Research
    instruments (AOR instru-
    ments)
Alvarado surgical knee holder
Alvarez prosthesis
Alvarez valve prosthesis

Alvarez-Rodriguez cardiac
    catheter
Alvegniat pump
alveodental suppuration
Alveograf bone-grafting material
alveolabial sulcus
alveolar
alveolar abscess
alveolar arches
alveolar artery
alveolar branch of internal
    maxillary artery
alveolar duct
alveolar nerve
alveolar process
alveolar ridge
alveolares superiores anteriores,
    arteriae
alveolares superiores, nervi
alveolaris inferior, arteria
alveolaris inferior, nervus
alveolaris superior posterior,
    arteria
alveolectomy
alveoli (*sing.* alveolus)
alveolingual sulcus
alveolodental membrane
alveoloplasty
alveoloplasty reparative closure
alveolotomy
alveolus (*pl.* alveoli)
alveoplasty
alvine calculus
Alvis curet
Alvis fixation forceps
Alvis forceps
Alvis foreign body curet
Alvis operation
Alvis ptosis correction proce-
    dure
Alvis spud
Alvis-Lancaster sclerotome
Alwall artificial kidney
Alyea clamp
Alyea vas clamp
AMA-Fab scintigraphy
amalgam

amalgam carrier
amalgam filling
amalgam scraper
Amark perimeter
amber latex catheter
Ambi compression hip screw
Ambi hip screw
ambient air
ambient oxygen
ambiguity
ambiguous
Ambler dilator
amblyopia
Ambrose eye forceps
Ambrose operation
Ambrose ureterovesicoplasty
Ambu bag
Ambu respirator
Ambu resuscitator
ambulant
ambulatory
ambulatory Holter monitor
Ambulift
ambustion
AMC needle
AMC total wrist system
AMC wrist prosthesis
Amcath catheter
AME bone growth stimulator
AME PinSite shield
amelia
amelioration
ameloblastoma
Amenabar capsule forceps
Amenabar knife
Amenabar lens loupe
Amenabar retractor
amenable
amenorrhea
Americaine anesthetic agent
American Bentley cardiopul-
    monary bypass system
American Dilation System
    dilator
American endoscopy dilator
American endoscopy esopha-
    geal dilator

American endoscopy mechanical lithotriptor
American Hamilton stretcher
American intraocular lens
American Lapidus Airfloat system
American Lapidus bed
American laryngectomy
American Medical Optics intraocular lens
American Medical Systems inflatable penile prosthesis
American Optic R-inhibited pacemaker
American Optical Cardiocare pacemaker
American Optical Company instruments
American Optical photocoagulator
American pattern scissors
American pattern umbilical scissors
American tracheotomy tube
American umbilical scissors
American V. Mueller urological instruments
American vascular stapler
Amersham intracavitary radium system
Amerson bone elevator
Ames reflectance meter
Ames shunt
Ames ventriculoperitoneal shunt
amethocaine anesthetic agent
AMI (acute myocardial infarction)
Amici disk
Amici line
Amici striae
Amico chisel
Amico drill
Amico extractor
Amico osteotome
Amicon diafilter
amide-type local anesthesia unit
aminophylline
AMK total knee system

Amko vaginal speculum
AML (anatomic medullary locking)
AML orthopedic prosthesis
AML total hip system
Ammon blepharoplasty
Ammon blue dye
Ammon canthoplasty
Ammon dacryocystotomy
Ammon eyelid repair
Ammon horn
Ammon operation
Ammon scleral prominence
Amnihook perforator
amniocentesis
amniogram
amniography
amnion
amnioscope
amnioscopy
amniotic
amniotic adhesions
amniotic amputation
amniotic cyst
amniotic hernia
amniotic membrane perforator
amniotic sac
amniotic trocar
amniotome
    Baylor amniotome
    Beacham amniotome
amniotomy
AMO intraocular lens implant
AMO laser
amobarbital anesthetic agent
Amoils cryoextractor
Amoils cryopencil
Amoils cryoprobe
Amoils iris retractor
Amoils retractor
Amoils-Keeler cryounit
AMP dialysis
ampere
amphiarthrodial joint
amphiarthrosis
amphiarthrotic pubic symphysis
amphidiarthrodial joint
amphidiarthrosis

Amplatz angiography needle
Amplatz aortography catheter
Amplatz cardiac catheter
Amplatz catheter
Amplatz coronary catheter
Amplatz dilator
Amplatz femoral catheter
Amplatz guide
Amplatz injector
Amplatz needle
Amplatz Super Stiff guide wire
Amplatz torque wire
Amplatz II curve
amplification
amplifier
amplitude
ampule
ampulla (*pl.* ampullae)
ampulla of Vater
ampullaris anterior, nervus
ampullaris lateralis, nervus
ampullaris posterior, nervus
ampullary aneurysm
ampullary nerve
ampullary stenosis
amputating knife
amputating saw
amputation
amputation by transfixion
amputation in contiguity
amputation in continuity
amputation knife
amputation rake
amputation retractor
amputation saw
amputation stump
amputation technique
amputation through surgical
    neck of humerus
amputee
Amreich vaginal extirpation
AMRI (anteromedial rotatory
    instability)
AMS artificial urethral sphincter
AMS Hydroflex penile prosthe-
    sis
AMS inflatable penile prosthesis
AMS malleable penile prosthesis

AMS rasp
AMS semirigid penile prosthesis
AMSI artificial urinary sphincter
Amsler chart marker
Amsler corneal graft operation
Amsler needle
Amsler operation
Amsler scleral marker
Amsterdam stent
Amsterdam tube
Amstutz total hip
Amstutz-Wilson osteotomy
Amtech-Killeen pacemaker
Amussat incision
Amussat operation
Amussat probe
amygdaloid body
amygdaloid fossa
amygdaloidectomy
amygdalotomy
amylase
amyloid
amyotrophy
Amytal anesthetic agent
anabiosis
anabiotic
anaclasis
anaerobe
anaerobic culture tube
anaeroplasty
Anagnostakis operation
anal
anal atresia
anal bulging
anal canal
anal column
anal crypt
anal dilatation
anal dilator
anal fissure
anal fissure excision
anal fistula
anal fistulectomy
anal fistulotomy
anal gland
anal ileostomy with preserva-
    tion of sphincter
anal manometry

anal orifice
anal papillae
anal pit
anal plate
anal prolapse
anal protrusion
anal reflex
anal retractor
anal speculum
anal sphincter
anal sphincter tone
anal sphincterotomy
anal stenosis
anal stretch operation
anal stricture
anal tags
anal tone
anal verge
anal wink
analgesia
analgesic
analog
Analog knee orthosis
analogous
analogous rhythm
analogous tissue
analogue
analyzer
Anametric knee prosthesis
Anametric prosthesis
anaphylactic
anaphylactic crisis
anaphylactic reaction
anaphylactic shock
anaphylactoid crisis
anaphylactoid reaction
anaphylactoid shock
anaphylaxis
anaplastic
anapophysis
anarrhexis
anasarca
anasarca troċar
anastomose
anastomosis
anastomosis apparatus
anastomosis arteriolovenularis
anastomosis arteriovenosa

anastomosis clamp
anastomosis forceps
anastomosis of ascending aorta
    to pulmonary artery
anastomosis of bile duct to
    stomach
anastomosis of epididymis to
    vas
anastomosis of esophagus
anastomosis of internal mam-
    mary artery to coronary
    artery
anastomosis of left pulmonary
    artery to descending aorta
anastomosis of mesenteric
    arteries
anastomosis of nerves
anastomosis of rectum
anastomosis of retinal and
    choroidal vessels
anastomosis of right atrium to
    pulmonary artery
anastomosis of right pulmonary
    artery to ascending aorta
anastomosis of right subclavian
    artery to pulmonary artery
anastomosis of Riolan
anastomosis of small intestine
anastomosis of superior vena
    cava to distal right pulmo-
    nary artery
anastomosis of superior vena
    cava to pulmonary artery
anastomosis of vas deferens
anastomotic
anastomotic branch of artery
anastomotic operation
anastomotic site
anastomotic ulcer
anastomotic ulceration
anastomotic vein
anastomotica inferior, vena
anastomotica superior, vena
anatomic, anatomical
anatomic closure
anatomic medullary locking
    (AML)
anatomic neck

anatomic porous replacement
   (APR)
anatomic position
anatomic snuffbox
anatomically
Anatomique osteal prosthesis
anatomy
Ancap braided-silk sutures
Ancap silk suture
anchor
      fixation anchor
      Lemoine-Searcy anchor
Anchor all-nylon hand brush
anchor band
Anchor brush dispenser
Anchor needle-sterilizing box
anchor plate
anchor splint
Anchor spring-suture needle
   holder
Anchor surgical needle
anchor with suture ligature
anchorage
anchorage procedure
anchoring sutures
anchovy arthroplasty
anchovy procedure
anconeal
anconeus muscle
anconeus, musculus
Andersen triad
Anderson antrum punch
Anderson columella prosthesis
Anderson curet
Anderson flexible suction tube
Anderson nasal strut
Anderson operation
Anderson portoenterostomy
Anderson procedure
Anderson splint
Anderson suction tube
Anderson tibial lengthening
Anderson traction bow
Anderson tractor
Anderson tube
Anderson-Adson retractor
Anderson-Fowler osteotomy

Anderson-Hutchins tibial
   fracture operation
Anderson-Hynes pyeloplasty
Anderson-Neivert osteotome
Andrews applicator
Andrews bottle operation
Andrews chisel
Andrews comedo extractor
Andrews cotton applicator
Andrews decompressor
Andrews ear applicator
Andrews forceps
Andrews frame
Andrews gouge
Andrews hydrocelectomy
Andrews inguinal hernior-
   rhaphy
Andrews knee reconstruction
Andrews laryngoscope
Andrews mastoid gouge
Andrews nasal applicator
Andrews operation
Andrews osteotome
Andrews retractor
Andrews rigid chest support
   holder
Andrews spinal table
Andrews suction tip
Andrews suction tube
Andrews tenodesis
Andrews tongue depressor
Andrews tonsil forceps
Andrews tonsil-seizing forceps
Andrews tracheal retractor
Andrews-Hartmann ear rongeur
Andrews-Hartmann forceps
Andrews-Hartmann rongeur
Andrews-Pynchon decompres-
   sor
Andrews-Pynchon suction tube
Andrews-Pynchon tongue
   depressor
Andrews-Pynchon tube
Andrews-Yankauer suction tube
androgen
androgenous
android pelvis

Andy Gump facies
anechoic
Anectine anesthetic agent
Anel dilation of lacrimal duct
Anel lacrimal dilation
Anel lacrimal probe
Anel lacrimal syringe
Anel method
Anel operation
Anel syringe
aneroid manometry
aneroid sphygmomanometer
Anestacon anesthetic agent
anesthesia
anesthesia block needle
anesthesiologist
anesthesiology
anesthetic
anesthetic agent
anesthetic tube
anesthetist
anesthetist's folding laryngo-
    scope
anesthetist's stool
anesthetist's table
anesthetize
anesthetizing agent
aneuploidy
Aneuroplast hemostatic agent
aneuroplastic kit
aneuroplasty
aneurysm
aneurysm clamp
aneurysm clip
aneurysm clip applier
aneurysm clip case
aneurysm forceps
aneurysm in orbit
aneurysm needle
aneurysm of pancreatic artery
aneurysm of splenic artery
aneurysm wrapping
aneurysmal '
aneurysmal bone cyst (ABC)
aneurysmal varix
aneurysmectomy
aneurysmoid varix

aneurysmoplasty
aneurysmorrhaphy
aneurysmotomy
Angelchik antireflux prosthesis
Angelchik prosthesis
Angell curet
Angell-James dissector
Angell-James hypophysectomy
    forceps
Angell-Shiley bioprosthetic
    valve
Angell-Shiley xenograft pros-
    thetic valve
Angelucci operation
Angelucci ptosis correction
    procedure
Anger camera
angiectomy
angio-aortic arch study
angiocardiogram
angiocardiography
Angiocath PRN catheter
angiocatheter
angioclast
Angiocor prosthetic valve
angiodynagraphic evaluation
angiodysplasia
angiogram
angiographic balloon occlusion
    catheter
angiographic catheter
angiographic guide wire
angiographic series
angiographically occult intracra-
    nial vascular malformation
    (AOIVM)
angiography
angiography needle
Angio-Kit catheter
angiolith
angioma (pl. angiomas,
    angiomata)
angioneurectomy
angioneurotic edema of vessels
angioneurotomy
angiopancreatitis
angiopathy of retina

angiopigtail catheter
angioplasty
angioplasty balloon catheter
angioplasty sheath
angiopressure
angiorrhaphy
angiosclerosis
angioscope
       Mitsubishi angioscope
       Olympus angioscope
       Optiscope angioscope
angioscopy
Angioskop-D
angiospasm
angiospastic
angiospastic anesthesia
angiostomy
angiostrophe
angiostrophy
angiotomy
angiotribe
angiotribe forceps
angiotripsy
Angle arch
angle band
angle board
angle drain
Angle Eager I microprocessor
angle handpiece
angle knife
angle of greatest extension
   (AGE)
angle of greatest flexion (AGF)
angle of His
angle of Louis
angle of Ludwig
angle of Sylvius
angle port pump
Angle splint
angle sutures
Angle vessel hook
angle-closure glaucoma
angled ball-end electrode
angled balloon catheter
angled clamp
angled curet

angled director
angled needle holder
angled peripheral vascular
   clamp
angled probe
angled scissors
angled stone forceps
angled suction tube
angled-vision lens system
Angle-Pezzer drain
angle-tip electrode
angry-looking ulcer
angular acceleration
angular artery
angular displacement
angular elevator
angular forceps
angular frequency
angular gyrus
angular incision
angular knife
angular needle
angular needle holder
angular oval punch
angular rongeur
angular saw
angular scissors
angular tract of cervical fascia
angular vein
angularis, arteria
angularis, vena
angular-tip electrode
angulated catheter
angulated forceps
angulated-blade electrode
angulated-needle holder
angulated-vein hemostat
angulation
angulation of ureter
angulation osteotomy
angulus
Angus-Esterlie recorder
anhaustral colonic gas pattern
Anis corneal forceps
Anis corneoscleral forceps
Anis forceps

Anis microsurgical eye instruments
Anis microsurgical needle holder
Anis microsurgical tying forceps
Anis posterior chamber capsule intraocular lens
Anis Staple implant cataract lens
Anis tying forceps
anisocoria
anisometropia
Anitomic total hip system
Ankeney retractor
Ankeney sternal retractor
ankle air stirrup
ankle air-stirrup brace
ankle bone
ankle jerk (AJ)
ankle joint
ankle mortise
ankle prosthesis
ankle-brachial index
ankle-foot orthosis (AFO)
ankyloproctia
ankylosis
ankylotomy
Ann Arbor clamp
Ann Arbor double towel clamp
Ann Arbor phrenic retractor
Ann Arbor retractor
Annandale knee operation
Annandale operation
anneal
annular
annular adenocarcinoma
annular ligament
annular pulley
annular scleritis
annular stricture
annuli (*sing.* annulus)
annuloplasty
annuloplasty valve
annulorrhaphy
annulus (*pl.* annuli; see also *anulus*)
annulus gouge
annulus of Zinn

annulus tympanicus
anococcygeal body
anococcygeal nerves
anococcygei, nervi
anode tube
anodontia
anomalous
anomalous artery
anomaly
anonychia
anoperineal
anophthalmos
anoplasty
anopouch angle
anorchism
anorectal angle
anorectal dressing
anorectal fistula
anorectal junction
anorectal malformation
anorectal manometry
anorectal orifice
anorectal ring
anorectal sphincter
anorectal stenosis
anorectocolonic
anorectoplasty
anorectum
anoscope
    Bacon anoscope
    Bodenheimer anoscope
    Boehm anoscope
    Brinkerhoff anoscope
    Buie-Hirschman anoscope
    Fansler anoscope
    fiberoptic anoscope
    Goldbacher anoscope
    Goldbacher anoscope speculum
    Hirschman anoscope
    Hirschman anoscope with obturator
    Ives anoscope
    Muer anoscope
    Otis anoscope
    Pratt anoscope

anoscope *continued*
    Pruitt anoscope
    rectoromanoscope
    romanoscope
    rotating anoscope
    rotating speculum
        anoscope
    Sims anoscope
    Sklar anoscope
    Smith anoscope
    speculum anoscope
    Welch Allyn anoscope
anoscope speculum
anoscope with obturator
anoscopic examination
anoscopy
anoscopy with biopsy
anoscopy with excision
anosigmoidoscope
anosigmoidoscopy
anospinal
ansa cervicalis
ansa subclavia
anserine bursa
Anson-McVay femoral herniorrhaphy
Anson-McVay herniorrhaphy
Anson-McVay inguinal herniorrhaphy
Anson-McVay operation
Anspach cement eater
Anspach leg holder
antagonist
antebrachial fascia
antebrachial region
antebrachial vein
antecedent sign
antecolic
antecolic anastomosis
antecolic gastrectomy
antecolic gastrojejunostomy
antecolic jejunostomy
antecolic long-loop isoperistaltic gastrojejunostomy
antecubital
antecubital fossa
anteflexed uterus

anteflexion
antegonial angle
antegonial notch
antegrade aortogram
antegrade biliary drainage
antegrade flow
antegrade pyelography
antegrade urography
antehelical fold
antepartum
antephase
anterior abdominal wall
anterior acute-flexion elbow splint
anterior alveolar branch of maxillary nerve
anterior ampullary nerve
anterior and posterior colporrhaphy (A&P repair)
anterior and posterior repair of cervix (A&P repair)
anterior and posterior repair of cystocele and rectocele (A&P repair)
anterior annular ligament
anterior approach
anterior auricular muscle
anterior auricular nerve
anterior auricular vein
anterior axillary line (AAL)
anterior band of colon
anterior bulbi camera
anterior capsule forceps
anterior cardiac veins
anterior cecal artery
anterior central gyrus
anterior cerebral artery
anterior cerebral vein
anterior cerebrospinal fasciculus
anterior cervical disk interbody fusion instruments
anterior cervical fusion (ACF)
anterior cervical lip
anterior chamber
anterior chamber cannula
anterior chamber depth-measuring equipment

anterior chamber dipstick
anterior chamber intraocular
  lens
anterior chamber irrigating
  cannula
anterior chamber irrigator
anterior choroidal artery
anterior ciliary artery
anterior circumflex humeral
  artery
anterior colon resection
anterior colporrhaphy
anterior column
anterior commissurotomy
anterior commissure
anterior commissure laryngoscope
anterior commissure laryngoscope blade
anterior communicating artery
anterior conjunctival artery
anterior cornu
anterior cruciate ligament (ACL)
anterior crurotomy nipper
anterior drawer sign
anterior drawer test
anterior ethmoid canal
anterior ethmoidal branch of
  ophthalmic artery
anterior ethmoidal nerve
anterior external arcuate fibers
anterior femoral resection guide
anterior forceps
anterior funiculus
anterior fusion operation
anterior gastrectomy
anterior gastrojejunostomy
anterior gray commissure
anterior heel
anterior iliac obturator hernia
anterior inferior cerebellar
  artery
anterior inferior communicating
  artery (AICA)
anterior inferior iliac spine
anterior intercostal veins
anterior interosseous artery
anterior interosseous nerve

anterior interventricular
  groove
anterior iridodialysis
anterior jejunostomy
anterior jugular vein
anterior labial nerve
anterior labial vein
anterior ligament
anterior median fissure
anterior medullary velum
anterior meningeal artery
anterior nephrectomy
anterior nerve roots
anterior palatine nerve
anterior palatine sutures
anterior pelvic exenteration
anterior pillar
anterior pillar incision
anterior polar cataract
anterior Polya operation
anterior process
anterior rectopexy
anterior rectus fascia
anterior rectus sheath
anterior resection clamp
anterior resection of sigmoid
  and rectum
anterior retinal orbital canal
anterior retractor
anterior rhizotomy
anterior sagittal pelvic inlet
anterior sandwich patch closure
  technique
anterior scalene muscle
anterior scrotal nerves
anterior scrotal veins
anterior segment forceps
anterior serratus muscle
anterior spinal artery
anterior splint
anterior superior alveolar artery
anterior synechia
anterior table
anterior talocalcaneal ligament
anterior talofibular ligament
anterior temporal diploic vein
anterior thalamotomy
anterior thoracoplasty

anterior tibial artery
anterior tibial muscle
anterior tibial recurrent artery
anterior tibial sign
anterior tibial tendon
anterior tibial vein
anterior tympanic artery
anterior urethropexy
anterior uterus
anterior vagal trunk
anterior vitrectomy
anterior wall
anterior wall antral ulcer
anterior white commissure
anterior-chamber irrigator
anterior-superior iliac spine
    (ASIS)
anteroapical
anterocolic anastomosis
anterodistal border
anteroinferior
anteroinferior aspect
anterolateral
anterolateral approach
anterolateral aspect
anterolateral displacement
anterolateral infarction
anterolateral region
anterolateral rotatory instability
    (ALRI)
anterolateral sulcus
anterolateral thoracoplasty
anterolateral thoracotomy
    incision
anterolisthesis
anteromedial
anteromedial rotatory instability
    (AMRI)
anteromedian
antero-oblique position
anteroposterior (AP)
anteroposterior x-ray view
anteroseptal
anteroseptal infarct
anteroseptal myocardial
    infarction (AMI)
anterosuperior
anterosuperior iliac spine (ASIS)

anterotransverse diameter
anteroventral
anteversion
anteverted
anteverted position
Anthony compressor
Anthony elevator
Anthony enucleation compres-
    sor
Anthony mastoid suction tube
Anthony mastoid tube
Anthony orbital enucleation
    compressor
Anthony pillar retractor
Anthony retractor
Anthony suction tube
Anthony tube
Anthony-Fisher antrum balloon
Anthony-Fisher balloon
Anthony-Fisher forceps
Anthron heparinized catheter
antibasement membrane
antibiotic irrigation
antibiotic prophylaxis
antibiotics
anticholinesterase anesthetic
    agent
anticoagulants
anticus
antiembolic hose
antiembolism stockings
anti-fog, anti-fogging (AF)
anti-fog solution
anti-fog tube
anti-fogging agent
anti-fogging solution (AF
    solution)
antiglaucoma peripheral
    iridectomy
antihelix
antihemophilic globulin (AHG)
anti-incontinence penile
    prosthesis
anti-infective
anti-inflammatory
antimesenteric
antimesenteric border
antimesenteric fat operation

antimesenteric fat pad
antimesocolic side of cecum
antimicrobial
antineoplastic
antiperistalsis
antiperistaltic
antiperistaltic anastomosis
antiperistaltic gastrojejunostomy
antiperistaltic jejunostomy
antiperistaltic operation
antireflux operation
antireflux prosthesis
Anti-Sept bactericidal scrub
    solution
antiseptic
antiseptic dressing
antiseptic surgery
antishock suit
anti-siphon device
antispasmodic
antispastic
antistriated muscle biopsy
antithymocyte globulin (ATG)
antitragus muscle
antiviral
Antole-Condale elevator
antra (*sing.* antrum)
antral
antral balloon
antral bur
antral cannula
antral chisel
antral curet
antral drain
antral drainage tube
antral edema
antral floor
antral folds
antral forceps
antral gouge
antral irrigator
antral knife
antral mucosa
antral needle
antral perforator
antral punch
antral rasp

antral resection
antral retractor
antral rongeur
antral saw
antral sinus cannula
antral stenosis
antral stoma
antral stricture
antral syringe
antral trephine
antral trocar
antral ulcer
antral wash tube
antral window operation
antrectomy
antro-aural fistula
antroduodenectomy
antrosaucerization
antroscope
    ACMI antroscope
    Reichert antroscope
antroscopy
antrostomy
antrostomy punch
antrotomy
antrum (*pl.* antra)
antrum balloon
antrum instruments (see also
    *antral*)
antrum of Willis
antrum pyloricum
antrum rasp
antrum-exploring needle
antrum-irrigating tube
anuli (*sing.* anulus; see also
    *annulus*)
anuloplasty
anulus (*pl.* anuli)
anulus fibrosus
anulus tympanicus
anulus of Zinn
anuria
anus
anvil
any-angle splint
AO (ankle orthosis)
AO brace

AO clamp
AO compression plate
AO plate
AO Reichert scientific instruments
AO technique
AO/ASIF orthopedic surgical instruments and implants
AOA cervical immobilization brace
AOA-CHICK halo traction
AOC-CHICK ambulatory halo system
AOD (arteriosclerotic occlusive disease)
AOI compression plate
AOIVM (angiographically occult intracranial vascular malformation)
AOM (alternatives of management)
AOO pacemaker (atrial asynchronous)
AOR (Alvarado Orthopedic Research instruments)
AOR collateral ligament retractor
AOR guide
AOR instruments
AOR knee instrumentation system
AOR system
aorta
aorta abdominalis
aorta aneurysm clamp
aorta aneurysm forceps
aorta ascendens
aorta cannulae clamp
aorta clamp
aorta descendens
aorta forceps
aorta occluder
aorta punch
aorta retractor
aorta thoracica
aorta to first obtuse marginal branch bypass

aorta to LAD bypass (aorta to left anterior descending coronary artery bypass)
aorta to marginal branch bypass
aorta to posterior descending coronary artery bypass
aorta to pulmonary artery shunt
aorta valve retractor
aorta vent needle
aorta-and-runoff arteriogram
aortic anastomosis
aortic aneurysm
aortic aneurysm clamp
aortic aneurysm forceps
aortic aneurysm graft
aortic aneurysm repair
aortic arch
aortic arch arteriogram
aortic arch arteriography
aortic arch cannula
aortic balloon pump
aortic cannula
aortic cannula clamp
aortic catheter
aortic clamp
aortic commissure
aortic crossclamp
aortic crossclamp time
aortic cuff
aortic curet
aortic cusp
aortic dilator
aortic dissection
aortic forceps
aortic incompetence
aortic insufficiency
aortic isthmus
aortic knob
aortic knuckle
aortic lymph node
aortic murmur
aortic notch
aortic occluder
aortic occlusion clamp
aortic occlusion forceps
aortic opening
aortic orifice

aortic plexus
aortic pressure
aortic pulmonary window
aortic punch
aortic regurgitation
aortic retractor
aortic ring
aortic root
aortic root perfusion needle
aortic root replacement
aortic runoff
aortic sac
aortic scissors
aortic second sound (A2)
aortic septal defect
aortic sinotubular junction
aortic sound
aortic sulcus
aortic suprarenal artery
aortic thrill
aortic valve
aortic valve brush
aortic valve prosthesis
aortic valve replacement
aortic valve retractor
aortic valve rongeur
aortic valvotomy
aortic valvuloplasty
aortic valvulotomy
aortic vent needle
aortic window
aortic-femoral bypass
aortic-left ventricular tunnel
aorticocoronary bypass
aorticopulmonary anastomosis
aorticopulmonary septal defect
aorticopulmonary shunt
aorticopulmonary window
aorticopulmonary window
    operation
aorticorenal
aortoarteriography
aortobifemoral bypass
aortobi-iliac bypass
aortocarotid bypass
aortocoronary
aortocoronary bypass

aortocoronary bypass graft
aortocoronary snake graft
aortocoronary vein bypass
aortocoronary-saphenous vein
    bypass
aortoduodenal fistula
aortoesophageal fistula
aortofemoral bypass
aortofemoral bypass graft
    (AFBG)
aortofemoral prosthesis
aortogram
aortogram catheter
aortogram needle
aortogram with distal runoff
aortographic catheter
aortographic suction tip
aortography
aortography needle
aortohepatic arterial graft
aortoiliac
aortoiliac bypass
aortoiliac endarterectomy
aortoiliofemoral bypass
aortoiliofemoral endarterectomy
aortoplasty
aortopulmonary
aortopulmonary fenestration
aortopulmonary shunt
aortopulmonary tunnel
aortopulmonary window
aortorenal bypass
aortorrhaphy
aortosigmoid fistula
aorto-subclavian-carotid-
    axilloaxillary bypass
aortotomy
aortotomy incision
aortovein bypass graft
aortoventriculoplasty
AP (anteroposterior)
AP diameter of chest
AP femoral sizer
AP sizer
apatite urinary tract stones
ape hand
ape-hand deformity

apepsia
aperiosteal amputation
aperiosteal supracondylar
    tendoplastic amputation
aperistaltic esophagus
Apert disease
apertognathia
apertognathia repair
aperture
aperture of inguinal hernia
apex (*pl.* apices)
apex cardiogram
apex cardiography
apex of duodenal bulb
apex of external ring
apex of heart
Apgar score
aphagia
aphakia
aphalangia
aphasia
apheresis
aphonic bruit
aphthoid ulcer
aphthous stomatitis
aphthous ulcer
aphthous-type lesion
apical
apical abscess
apical cyst
apical granuloma
apical impulse
apical lordotic x-ray view
apical murmur
apical thoracoplasty
apicectomy
apices (*sing.* apex)
apicoectomy
apicolysis
apicolysis retractor
apicoseptal aneurysmectomy
apicostomy
aplasia
aplastic
Apley grind test
Apley knee test
Apley maneuver

Apley sign
Apley test
Apley traction
apnea monitor
apnea neonatorum
apneustic respirations
apocope
apocoptic
apocrine gland
apocrine metaplasia
aponeurectomy
aponeurorrhaphy
aponeurosis (*pl.* aponeuroses)
aponeurosis of biceps brachii
aponeurosis of external oblique
    muscle
aponeurosis of musculus
    transversus abdominis
aponeurosis of velum
aponeurosis of Zinn
aponeurotic falx
aponeurotic fascia
aponeurotome
aponeurotomy
apophyseal fracture
apophysis
apparatus (see also *suspension
    apparatus, pneumothorax
    apparatus*)
        anastomosis apparatus
        aspiration apparatus
        Bárány alarm apparatus
        Bárány apparatus
        Bárány noise apparatus
        Bárány noise apparatus
            whistle
        Bárány-Larm apparatus
        Belzer apparatus
        biphase Morris fixation
            apparatus
        blow-by apparatus
        Brawley suction appara-
            tus
        cryosurgical apparatus
        Davidson pneumothorax
            apparatus
        Desault apparatus

apparatus *continued*

Deyerle apparatus
Dietrich apparatus
Doppler apparatus
electro-oculogram
apparatus
extension apparatus
Fell-O'Dwyer apparatus
fixation apparatus
fracture-banding
apparatus
Frigitronics nitrous oxide
cryosurgery apparatus
Georgiade visor halo
fixation apparatus
Golgi apparatus
Hodgen apparatus
Howse-Coventry hip
apparatus
ICLH apparatus (Imperial
College, London
Hospital)
Jaquet apparatus
Killian apparatus
Killian suspension
apparatus
Kirschner apparatus
Kirschner traction
apparatus
Kroner apparatus
Küntscher traction
apparatus
lacrimal apparatus
Lewy suspension
apparatus
Light-Veley apparatus
Lynch suspension
apparatus
Malgaigne apparatus
Marstock apparatus
McAtee apparatus
McKesson pneumothorax
apparatus
Naugh os calcis appara-
tus tractor
Osteo-Stim apparatus
Plummer-Vinson
apparatus

apparatus *continued*

pneumothorax apparatus
Potain apparatus
Robinson artificial
apparatus
Roger Anderson appara-
tus
Sayre apparatus
Singer portable appara-
tus
suction apparatus
suspension apparatus
Swenko gastric-cooling
apparatus
Tallerman apparatus
Taylor apparatus
Tobold apparatus
Todd-Wells stereotaxic
apparatus
traction apparatus
vacuum aspiration
apparatus
Venturi apparatus
Volutrol apparatus
Volutrol apparatus for IV
von Petz suturing
apparatus
Wagner apparatus
Waldenberg apparatus
Wangensteen apparatus
Zander apparatus
apparent
apparent death
appendage clamp
appendalgia
appendectomy
appendectomy retractor
appendectomy spoon
appendical
appendiceal
appendiceal abscess
appendiceal base
appendiceal fecalith
appendiceal intussusception
appendiceal mass
appendiceal mesentery
appendiceal stump
appendiceal tissue

appendicealgia
appendicectasis
appendicectomy
appendices (*sing.* appendix)
appendices epiploicae
appendicism
appendicitis by contiguity
appendicitis granulosa
appendicitis larvata
appendicitis obliterans
appendiclausis
appendicocecostomy
appendicocele
appendicoenterostomy
appendicolith
appendicolithiasis
appendicolysis
appendicopathia
appendicopathy
appendicosis
appendicostomy
appendicotomy
appendicular
appendicular artery
appendicular ataxia
appendicular vein
appendicularis, arteria
appendicularis, vena
appendiculoradiogram
appendiculoradiography
appendix (*pl.* appendices, appendixes)
appendix cerebri
appendix inverter
appendix of epididymis
appendix tapes
appendix vermiform
appendix vermiformis
appendolithiasis
appendoroentgenogram
appendoroentgenography
appendotome
appendotome knife
applanation
applanation tonometer
applanation tonometry
applanometer
apple-core lesion

apple-peel bowel
appliance (see also *fracture appliance*)
    ACCO orthodontic appliance
    arch bars facial fracture appliance
    Begg appliance
    Bimler appliance
    Bipro orthodontic appliance
    Bradford fracture appliance
    Buck fracture appliance
    craniofacial appliance
    craniofacial fracture appliance
    Crozat appliance
    Denholtz appliance
    dental appliance
    Dewald halo spinal appliance
    Erich facial fracture appliance
    extraoral appliance
    fixed appliance
    fracture appliance
    Fraenkel appliance
    Gerster fracture appliance
    Goldthwait fracture appliance
    Graber appliance
    Hawley appliance
    Hibbs fracture appliance
    ileostomy appliance
    Janes fracture appliance
    Jewett fracture appliance
    Johnson twin-wire appliance
    Joseph septal fracture appliance
    karaya adhesive appliance
    karaya ring ileostomy appliance
    karaya seal ileostomy appliance

appliance *continued*
  orthodontic appliance
  ostomy appliance
  prosthetic appliance
  removable appliance
  Universal appliance
  Vasocillator fracture appliance
  Whitman fracture appliance
  Wilson fracture appliance
  wire appliance
application
application of apparatus
application of cast
application of obstetric forceps
application of splint
application of therapeutic agent
application of traction device
applicator
  Allen applicator
  Andrews applicator
  Andrews cotton applicator
  Andrews ear applicator
  Andrews nasal applicator
  aural applicator
  Auto-Suture Clip-A-Matic clip applicator
  Barth applicator
  beta irradiation applicator
  beta therapy eye applicator
  Bloedorn applicator
  Brown applicator
  Brown cotton applicator
  Brown nasal applicator
  Buck applicator
  Buck ear applicator
  Buck nasal applicator
  Burnett applicator (sizes A, B, etc.)
  calcium alginate applicator
  Campbell applicator

applicator *continued*
  cesium applicator
  Chaoul applicator
  Clark applicator
  Colpostats applicator
  corneal applicator
  cotton applicator
  cotton ear applicator
  cotton nasal applicator
  cotton-tipped applicator
  Dean applicator
  Dean cotton applicator
  Delclos applicator
  ear applicator
  Edslab applicator
  Ernst applicator
  Ernst radium applicator
  eustachian applicator
  Falope-ring applicator
  Farrell applicator
  Farrell nasal applicator
  Farrior applicator
  Fletcher loading applicator
  Fletcher-Suit afterloading applicator
  Fletcher-Suit applicator
  Gifford applicator
  Gifford corneal applicator
  Holinger applicator
  Hotz ear applicator
  Huzly applicator
  Huzly tampon applicator
  intracavitary gynecologic applicator
  Ivan laryngeal applicator
  Jackson applicator
  Jackson laryngeal applicator
  Jackson laryngeal applicator forceps
  Kumar applicator
  Kyle applicator
  Kyle ear applicator
  laryngeal applicator
  Lathbury applicator

applicator *continued*
Lejeune applicator
loading applicator
Ludwig applicator
Ludwig sinus applicator
metal applicator
Mick applicator
Monel metal radium applicator
nasal applicator
nasopharyngeal applicator
Playfair uterine caustic applicator
Plummer-Vinson applicator
Plummer-Vinson radium applicator
postnasal applicator
Pynchon applicator
radioactive applicator
radioisotope applicator
radium applicator
Ralks applicator
ratchet applicator
Roberts applicator
Sawtell applicator
Sawtell nasal applicator
sealed applicator
sonic applicator
Storz applicator
Syed radium applicator
tampon applicator
Ter-Pogossian applicator
Turnbull applicator
Uebe applicator
Wood applicator
applicator forceps
applicator jar
Appolionio eye implant
Appolionio implant cataract lens
Appolionio lens
Appolito operation
Appolito sutures
Appose disposable skin stapler
Appose skin stapler
apposition

apposition sutures
approach
appropriate for gestational age (AGA)
approximate
approximated
approximation forceps
approximation sutures
approximator (see also *sternal approximator*)
Ablaza-Morse approximator
Acland clamp approximator
Acland double clamp approximator
Alexander approximator
Allerdyce approximator
Bailey rib approximator
Ballenger-Hajek approximator
Ballenger-Hajek elevator
Bunke-Schulz clamp approximator
Henderson approximator
Lalonde tendon approximator
Leksell sternal approximator
Lemmon rib approximator
Lemmon sternal approximator
Link approximator
microanastomosis approximator
microanastomosis clip approximator
Nunez approximator
Pilling Wolvek sternal approximator
sternal approximator
Tamai clamp approximator
Wolvek approximator
Wolvek sternal approximator

appy (appendectomy)
appy tape
APR (abdominoperineal resection)
APR (anatomic porous replacement)
APR hip system
APR reversion total hip system
APR total hip system
APR universal hip system
APRL hooks (Army Prosthetics Research Laboratory hooks)
apron U-shaped incision
apudoma
Aquaflex contact lenses
Aquaflo dressing
Aquamatic dressing
Aquamatic K-Cal calibration well
Aquamatic K-Module
Aquamatic K-Pads
Aquamatic K-Thermia equipment
Aquapad heating pad
Aquaphor gauze dressing
Aquaplast splint
Aquaplast splinting materials
aquapuncture
Aqua-Purator suction device
Aquatech cast padding
Aquavac
aqueduct
aqueduct of Cotunnius
aqueduct of midbrain
aqueduct of Sylvius
aqueduct of vestibule vein
aqueductus vestibuli, vena
aqueous
aqueous glutaraldehyde (Cidex)
aqueous humor
aqueous Zephiran
Aquirre gastrectomy
AR-1 catheter
AR-2 diagnostic catheter
AR-2 guiding catheter
arachnoid

arachnoid granulations
arachnoid knife
arachnoid mater
arachnoid membrane
arachnoid space
arachnoid-shape Beaver blade
arachnoid-shape blade
Arani catheter
Arani double-loop guiding catheter
Arani guide
arborescent cataract
arborization block
arborization heart block
arborization pattern
Arbrook Hemovac
Arbuckle antral knife
Arbuckle antral saw
Arbuckle probe
Arbuckle sinus probe
Arbuckle-Shea trocar
ARC (AIDS-related complex)
arcade
arcade of Frohse
Arcelin view
arch
arch and carotid arteriography
arch angiogram
arch angiography
arch aortogram
arch aortography
arch arteriogram
arch arteriography
arch bar (see also *bar*)
    dental arch bar
    dental arch bar frame
    Erich arch bar
    Erich-Winter arch bar
    fixed arch bar
    Jelenko arch bar
    mandibular arch bar
    Niro arch bar
    retainer arch bar
    Winter arch bar
arch bars facial fracture appliance
arch bars frame

arch of abdominal aorta
arch of aorta
arch of larynx
arch rake retractor
arch support
arch wire
arched palate
Archer forceps
Archer splinter forceps
Archimedean drill
arciform
Arco atomic pacemaker
Arco lithium pacemaker
Arco pacemaker
Arcomax FMA cardiac angiography system
arcuata pedis, arteria
arcuatae renis, arteriae
arcuatae renis, venae
arcuate
arcuate arteries
arcuate arteries of kidney
arcuate artery of foot
arcuate incision
arcuate ligaments
arcuate line
arcuate popliteal ligament
arcuate pubic ligament
arcuate suture
arcuate veins
arcuate veins of kidney
arcus aortae
ARD bandage
areas of innervation
areflexia
Arem retractor
Arem-Madden retractor
Arenberg-Denver inner-ear valve implant
Arenberg-Denver valve
areola (*pl.* areolae)
areolar
areolar gland
areolar incision
areolar tissue
ARF (acute renal failure)
argon laser

argon laser photocoagulator cautery
argon-krypton laser
Argyle catheter
Argyle chest tube
Argyle Medicut R catheter
Argyle Sentinel Seal chest tube
Argyle tube
Argyle-Salem sump pump
Argyle-Salem sump tube
Argyll Robertson operation
Argyll Robertson pupil
Argyll Robertson strap operation for ectropion of eyelid
Argyll Robertson sutures
Aries reductive mammaplasty
Aries space
Aries-Pitanguy breast reduction
Aries-Pitanguy mammaplasty
Aries-Pitanguy mammary ptosis operation
Aries-Pitanguy operation
Arion implant
Arion operation
Arion sling operation
Aristocort
Arizona condylar tibial plateau prosthesis
Arkan sharpening-stone needle
Arlt epicanthus repair
Arlt eyelid repair
Arlt fenestrated lens scoop
Arlt lens loupe
Arlt lens scoop
Arlt loupe
Arlt operation
Arlt pterygium excision
Arlt scoop
Arlt sutures
Arlt-Jaesche operation
Arlt-Jaesche recessus
Arlt-Jaesche sinus
Arlt-Jaesche trachoma
ARM (artificial rupture of membranes)
arm extension position
arm splint

armboard
armed bougie
arm-extension position
Armistead procedure
armored heart
Armour dural knife
Armour endotracheal tube
Armour knife
Armour tube
armpit
armrest
Armsby operation
Armstrong acromionectomy
Armstrong repair
Armstrong tube
Armstrong V-vent tube
Armstrong warmer
Armstrong-Schuknecht stapes
    prosthesis
Army bone gouge
Army osteotome
Army pattern bone gouge
Army pattern chisel
Army pattern osteotome
Army Prosthetics Research
    Laboratory hooks (APRL
    hooks)
Army-Navy retractor
Arndorfer esophageal motility
    probe
Arndorfer pneumocapillary
    infusion pump
Arnold brace
Arnold canal
Arnold ligament
Arnold nerve
Arnold-Chiari deformity
Arnott bed
Arnott dilator
Arnoux sign
Aron Alpha adhesive
Aron Alpha glue
Aronson esophageal retrac-
    tor
Aronson lateral sternomastoid
    retractor
Aronson medial esophageal
    retractor

Aronson-Fletcher antrum
    cannula
array processor
arrector muscles of hair
arrectores pilorum, musculi
arrest
arrest of labor
arrhythmia
Arrhythmia Net arrhythmia
    monitor
arrhythmogenesis
Arrow Hi-flow infusion set
Arrow multilumen catheter
Arrow pulmonary artery
    catheter
Arrow tube
Arrow-Berman balloon
    angioplasty catheter
Arrow-Berman balloon catheter
Arrow-Clarke thoracentesis
    device
Arrowhead canthoplasty
Arrowhead operation
Arrow-Howes multilumen
    catheter
arrow-pin clasp
Arrowsmith electrode
Arrowsmith-Clerf pin-closing
    forceps
Arruga capsule forceps
Arruga cataract extraction
Arruga dacryocystostomy
Arruga encircling suture
Arruga expressor
Arruga eye holder
Arruga eye implant
Arruga eye retractor
Arruga eye speculum
Arruga eye trephine
Arruga forceps
Arruga globe retractor
Arruga implant
Arruga keratoplasty
Arruga lacrimal trephine
Arruga lens expressor
Arruga movable eye implant
Arruga needle holder
Arruga operation

Artegraft

Arruga operation for retinal detachment
Arruga protector
Arruga retractor
Arruga saw
Arruga speculum
Arruga surface electrode
Arruga tenotomy
Arruga tip forceps
Arruga trephine
Arruga-Berens operation
Arruga-Gill forceps
Arruga-McCool capsule forceps
Arruga-McCool forceps
Arruga-Moura-Brazil orbital implant
Arslan fenestration of inner ear
Arslan operation
artefact (see *artifact*)
arteria (*pl.* arteriae) (see specific arteriae)
arterial anastomosis
arterial blood gases (ABGs)
arterial blood needle
arterial cannula
arterial catheter
arterial circle of Willis
arterial cutdown
arterial embolectomy catheter
arterial forceps
arterial graft
arterial line (A-line)
arterial line pressure bag
arterial line transducer
arterial needle
arterial oxygen saturation (SaO2)
arterial prosthesis
arterial puncture
arterial runoff
arterial scissors
arterial sheath
arterial silk sutures
arterial switch
arterial thrombosis
arterial transfusion of blood
arteriectasis
arteriectomy
arteriogram
arteriogram needle
arteriography
arteriolar narrowing
arteriole
arterioles of kidney·
arteriolith
arteriomegaly
arterioplasty
arteriorrhaphy
arteriosclerosis
arteriosclerotic
arteriosclerotic cardiovascular disease (ASCVD)
arteriosclerotic occlusive disease (AOD)
arteriosclerotic peripheral vascular disease (ASPVD)
arteriostrepsis
arteriotomy
arteriotomy incision
arteriotomy scissors
arteriotrepsis
arteriovenostomy
arteriovenous (AV)
arteriovenous anastomosis
arteriovenous aneurysm
arteriovenous angiorrhaphy
arteriovenous fistula (AVF)
arteriovenous Gore-Tex fistula (AV Gore-Tex fistula)
arteriovenous Gore-Tex graft (AV Gore-Tex graft)
arteriovenous malformation (AVM)
arteriovenous oxygen difference (AVDO2)
arteriovenous shunt
arteriovenous shunt site
artery
artery forceps
artery island flap
artery of Adamkiewicz
arthrectomy
arthritides (*sing.* arthritis)
arthritis (*pl.* arthritides)
arthrocentesis
arthroclasia
arthrodesia

arthrodesis
arthrodesis screw
arthrodial joint
ArthroDistractor
arthroendoscopy
arthroereisis
arthrogram
arthrography
arthrogryposis
arthrokatadysis
arthrolith
Arthro-Lok system of Beaver
    blades
arthrolysis
arthrometer
arthrometry
arthrophyte
arthroplastic
arthroplasty
arthroplasty gouge
arthrorisis
arthroscope
    Acufex arthroscope
    Circon arthroscope
    Downs arthroscope
    Dyonics arthroscope
    Dyonics needle-scope
      arthroscope
    Eagle arthroscope
    examining arthroscope
    Flexiscope arthroscope
    Hopkins arthroscope
    lumina rod lens arthro-
      scope
    O'Connor operating
      arthroscope
    Panoview arthroscope
    Richard Wolf arthroscope
    standard arthroscope
    Storz arthroscope
    Storz examining arthro-
      scope
    Takagi arthroscope
    Watanabe arthroscope
arthroscopic instruments
Arthroscopic Screw Installation
    (ASI)

arthroscopic surgery
arthroscopy
arthrosis deformans
arthrostomy
arthrotomy
arthrotomy with drainage
arthrotomy with exploration
arthrotomy with removal
arthroxesis
Arthur Ward planisphere
Arthus reaction
articular capsule
articular cartilage
articular disk
articular fracture
articular muscle
articular osteotome
articular surface
articular system
articularis cubiti, musculus
articularis genus, musculus
articulated optical arm
articulation
articulation osteotome
artifact
artificial ankylosis
artificial anus
artificial blood
artificial gut
artificial heart
artificial hip joint (AHJ)
artificial insemination
artificial insemination donor
    (AID)
artificial insemination husband
    (AIH)
artificial joint implant
artificial kidney
artificial leech
artificial lung
artificial nose
artificial pacemaker
artificial palate
artificial respiration
artificial rupture of membranes
    (ARM)
artificial sphincter

artificial stoma
artificial valve
artificial velum
Artmann chisel
Artmann disarticulation chisel
Artmann elevator
Artmann raspatory
Artus cutting tip
aryepiglottic (AE)
aryepiglottic fold (AE fold)
aryepiglottic muscle
aryepiglotticus, musculus
arytenoid abduction
arytenoid cartilage
arytenoid muscle
arytenoid process
arytenoidectomy
arytenoideus, musculus
arytenoideus obliquus, muscu-
    lus
arytenoideus transversus,
    musculus
arytenoidopexy
arytenoids
Arzco electrode
Arzco pacemaker
AS (Auto-Suture)
asacroliticus
Asai operation
ASC Monorel catheter
ASCAD (atherosclerotic
    coronary artery disease)
ascending aorta (AA)
ascending aorta-to-pulmonary
    artery shunt
ascending cervical artery
ascending colon
ascending lumbar vein
ascending palatine artery
ascending pharyngeal artery
ascending pyelogram
ascending pyelography
ascending ramus
ascending urogram
ascending urography
Asch clamp
Asch forceps

Asch nasal splint
Asch nasal-straightening forceps
Asch operation
Asch septal forceps
Asch septal straightener
Asch septal-straightening
    forceps
Asch splint
Asch straightener
Aschner reflex
Aschoff body
Aschoff cell
Aschoff node
Aschoff nodule
Aschoff-Tawara node
ascites
ascites drainage tube
ascites shunt
ascites suction tube
ascitic fluid
ascribe
ASCVD (arteriosclerotic
    cardiovascular disease)
ASD (atrioseptal defect)
ASE bandage (axilla, shoulder,
    and elbow bandage)
Aselli pancreas
asepsis
aseptic
aseptic fever
aseptic surgery
aseptic technique
aseptic wound
aseptic-antiseptic
asepticism
Asepto aspirating syringe
Asepto bulb syringe
Asepto irrigation syringe
Asepto suction tube
Asepto syringe
ASH (asymmetric septal
    hypertrophy)
Ash catheter
Ash dental forceps
Ashbell hook
Ashby fluoroscopic foreign
    body forceps

Ashby forceps
Ashford mamilliplasty
Ashford mammaplasty
Ashford retracted nipple
    operation
Ashhurst splint
Ashley breast prosthesis
Ashley elevator
Ashley repair
Ashley retractor
Ashman phenomenon
Ashworth arthroplasty
Ashworth Dow Corning
    prosthesis
Ashworth-Blatt implant
ASI (Arthroscopic Screw
    Installation)
ASI ligament repair system
ASI uroplasty TCU dilatation
    catheter
ASIF plate
ASIF screw
ASIF screw and washer
ASIF screw pin
ASIF twist drill
ASIS (anterior-superior iliac
    spine)
askew
Asner screw
Asnis cannulated screw
Asnis guided screw system
Asnis pin
Asnis pinning
Asnis screw
aspermia
aspheric lens implant
Aspiradeps lipodissector
aspirate
aspirating cannula
aspirating curet
aspirating dissector
aspirating needle
aspirating tip
aspirating trocar
aspirating tube
aspiration
aspiration apparatus

aspiration biopsy
aspiration biopsy cytology
    (ABC)
aspiration biopsy needle
aspiration cannula
aspiration curettage
aspiration needle
aspiration of bronchus
aspiration of lung
aspiration of sinuses
aspiration of vitreous
aspiration syringe
aspirator
    Adams aspirator
    blue-tip aspirator
    bronchoscopic aspirator
    Broyles aspirator
    Carabelli aspirator
    Carmody aspirator
    Carmody electric
        aspirator
    cataract aspirator
    Cavitron aspirator
    Cavitron ultrasonic
        aspirator (CUSA)
    clamp-on aspirator
    Clerf aspirator
    Cogsell tip aspirator
    Cook County aspirator
    Cook County Hospital
        aspirator
    CUSA (Cavitron ultra-
        sonic aspirator)
    CUSA aspirator
    DeLee trap aspirator
    DeLee trap meconium
        aspirator
    DeVilbiss Vacu-Aide
        aspirator
    Dia pump aspirator
    Dieulafoy aspirator
    electric aspirator
    faucet aspirator
    Fritz aspirator
    Frye portable aspirator
    gallbladder aspirator
    Gesco aspirator

aspirator *continued*
   Gomco aspirator
   Gomco portable suction
      aspirator
   Gomco suction aspirator
   Gomco uterine aspirator
   Gottschalk aspirator
   Gottschalk middle ear
      aspirator
   Gradwohl sternal bone
      marrow aspirator
   Huzly aspirator
   Hydrojette aspirator
   Leasure aspirator
   Lukens aspirator
   meconium aspirator
   middle ear aspirator
   Nugent aspirator
   Nugent soft cataract
      aspirator
   Penberthy double-action
      aspirator
   phacoemulsifier-aspirator
   portable aspirator
   portable suction aspirator
   Potain aspirator
   red-tip aspirator
   Sklar-Junior Tompkins
      aspirator
   soft cataract aspirator
   Stedman aspirator
   Stedman suction pump
      aspirator
   suction aspirator
   suction pump aspirator
   Taylor aspirator
   Thorek aspirator
   Thorek gallbladder
      aspirator
   Universal aspirator
   uterine aspirator
   Vabra aspirator
   Vabra aspirator dispos-
      able system
   Vabra cervical aspirator
   vacuum aspirator
   yellow-tip aspirator

aspirator cannula
asplenia
asplenic
ASPVD (arteriosclerotic
    peripheral vascular disease)
ASR blade
ASR scalpel
Assal-Javid cerebrospinal shunt
ASSI (Accurate Surgical and
    Scientific Instruments)
ASSI bipolar coagulating forceps
ASSI cranial blades
ASSI dual-ended surgical
    instruments
ASSI forceps
ASSI wire pass drill
assimilation
assimilation pelvis
assisted breech delivery
assisted respiration
assisted ventilation
Asta ligature scissors
asternal rib
Astler-Coller classification of
    Dukes C carcinoma
Astra pacemaker
astragalectomy
astragalonavicular joint
astragalus
astrocytoma
Astropulse cuff
ASVIP pacemaker
asymmetric, asymmetrical
asymmetric septal hypertrophy
    (ASH)
asymmetry
asymptomatic
asymptomatic gallstone
asynchronous bilateral breast
    cancer
asynchronous mode pacemaker
asynchronous pacemaker
asynchronous ventricular VOO
    pacemaker
ataractic
ataraxia
ataxia

atelectasis
atelectatic band
atelectatic rales
ATG (antithymocyte globulin)
Athens forceps
atherectomy
atherectomy cutter
atherectomy device
AtheroCath
AtheroCath spinning blade
    catheter
atheromatosis
atheromatosis cutis
atheromatous
atheromatous plaque
atherosclerosis
atherosclerotic cardiovascular
    disease (ASCVD)
atherosclerotic coronary artery
    disease (ASCAD)
athlete's heart
athyreosis
ATI (abdominal trauma index)
Atkins esophagoscopic tele-
    scope
Atkins knife
Atkins tonsil knife
Atkins-Cannard tube
Atkinson endoprosthesis
Atkinson eye knife
Atkinson keratome
Atkinson lid block
Atkinson needle
Atkinson retrobulbar needle
Atkinson sclerotome
Atkinson silicone rubber tube
Atkinson technique
Atkinson-Walker scissors
Atkins-Tucker laryngoscope
Atkins-Tucker shadow-free
    laryngoscope
ATL real-time NeurosectOR
    scanner'
Atlanta hip brace
Atlanta-Scottish Rite brace
Atlantic ileostomy catheter
atlantoaxial articulation
atlantoaxial joint

atlas
atlas arch
Atlas balloon dilatation
    catheter
Atlas-Storz eye magnet
Atlee bronchus clamp
Atlee clamp
Atlee dilator
Atlee uterine dilator
atomizer
atonia
atonic
atonic labor
atonicity
atony
atony of uterus
Atosoy procedure
Atra-grip clamp
Atra-grip forceps
Atraloc needle
Atraloc sutures
Atraloc-Ethilon sutures
Atraum with Clotstop drain
atraumatic
atraumatic braided silk sutures
atraumatic chromic sutures
atraumatic clamp
atraumatic distending obturator
atraumatic forceps
atraumatic needle
atraumatic suture needle
atraumatic sutures
atraumatic tenaculum
atraumatic tissue forceps
atresia
atretic
atria (*sing.* atrium)
atrial
atrial baffle
atrial balloon septostomy
atrial cannula
atrial cuff
atrial electrode
atrial fibrillation
atrial flutter
atrial instruments
atrial kick
atrial lead

atrial ostium primum defect
atrial pacemaker
atrial pacemaker lead
atrial pacing wire
atrial retractor
atrial septal defect
atrial synchronous ventricular-inhibited pacemaker
atrial tachycardia
atrial tracking pacemaker
atrial triggered ventricular-inhibited pacemaker
atrial-femoral artery bypass
Atricor Cordis pacemaker
Atricor pacemaker
atriocommissuropexy
atriofascicular bypass tract
atrio-His pathway
atrio-His tract
atrio-Hisian bypass tract
atrionodal bypass tract
atrioplasty
atriopressor reflex
atrioseptal defect (ASD)
atrioseptopexy
atrioseptoplasty
atrioseptostomy
atriotomy
atrioventricular (AV)
atrioventricular block (AV block)
atrioventricular bundle (AV bundle)
atrioventricular canal
atrioventricular canal defect
atrioventricular conduction defect (AV conduction defect)
atrioventricular conduction system (AVCS)
atrioventricular dissociation
atrioventricular groove
atrioventricular junction
atrioventricular junctional pacemaker (AV junctional pacemaker)
atrioventricular malformation (AVM)

atrioventricular node
atrioventricular orifice
atrioventricular ring
atrioventricular septal defect
atrioventricular sequential demand pacemaker (AV sequential demand pacemaker)
atrioventricular sequential pacemaker (AV sequential pacemaker)
atrioventricular synchronous pacemaker (AV synchronous pacemaker)
atrioventricular valve
atrioventricular valve replacement
atrioventriculostomy
atrium (*pl.* atria)
atrophic
atrophic fracture
atrophic gastritis
atrophy
atropine
atropine methyl nitrate
attachment
attachment of pacemaker electrodes
attachment of prosthesis
attempted passage of instrument
Attenborough arthroplasty of knee
Attenborough knee prosthesis
attenuated lower uterine segment
attenuation
attic
attic adhesion
attic cannula
attic dissector
attic ear punch
attic hook
atticoantral
atticoantrostomy
atticoantrotomy
atticotomy

atticus punch
atypical
Auchincloss mastectomy
audiography
audiometer
audiometry
auditory artery
auditory canal
auditory nerve
auditory veins
Auenbrugger sign
Auer rod
Auerbach mesenteric plexus
Aufranc approach
Aufranc arthroplasty gouge
Aufranc awl
Aufranc Cobra retractor
Aufranc cup
Aufranc dissector
Aufranc femoral neck retractor
Aufranc finishing ball reamer
Aufranc finishing cup reamer
Aufranc gouge
Aufranc groin apron
Aufranc hip prosthesis
Aufranc hip retractor
Aufranc hook
Aufranc mold for cup arthro-
    plasty
Aufranc offset reamer
Aufranc periosteal elevator
Aufranc psoas retractor
Aufranc push retractor
Aufranc reamer
Aufranc retractor
Aufranc trochanteric awl
Aufranc-Turner acetabular cup
Aufranc-Turner arthroplasty
Aufranc-Turner cemented hip
    prosthesis
Aufranc-Turner hip prosthesis
Aufrecht sign
Aufricht elevator
Aufricht glabellar rasp
Aufricht nasal elevator
Aufricht nasal rasp
Aufricht nasal retractor

Aufricht rasp
Aufricht raspatory
Aufricht retractor
Aufricht retractor-speculum
Aufricht scissors
Aufricht septum speculum
Aufricht speculum
Aufricht-Britetrac nasal retractor
Aufricht-Lipsett nasal rasp
Aufricht-Lipsett rasp
Aufricht-Lipsett raspatory
auger
Augmen bone-grafting material
augmentation
augmentation cystoplasty
augmentation mammaplasty
augmentation of labor
augmentation procedure
augmentation surgery
augmentation with implant
Augustine boat nail
Augustine nail
Ault clamp
Ault intestinal clamp
Ault intestinal occlusion clamp
Aumence eyelid speculum
aural applicator
aural forceps
aural microscope
aural speculum
Aureomycin gauze
Aureomycin gauze dressing
Aureomycin sutures
auricle
auricle clamp
auricular appendage
auricular appendage catheter
auricular appendage clamp
auricular appendage forceps
auricular appendectomy
auricular appendix
auricular artery
auricular artery clamp
auricular fibrillation
auricular ligation
auricular muscle
auricular nerve

auricular premature contraction
auricular standstill
auricular tag
auricular tubercle of Darwin
auricular veins
auriculares anteriores, nervi
auriculares anteriores, venae
auricularis anterior, musculus
auricularis magnus, nervus
auricularis posterior, arteria
auricularis posterior, musculus
auricularis posterior, nervus
auricularis posterior, vena
auricularis profunda, arteria
auricularis superior, musculus
auriculectomy
auriculomastoid
auriculomastoid line
auriculotemporal nerve
auriculotemporalis, nervus
auriculoventricular
auriculoventricular groove
auriculoventricular interval
auriculoventricular orifice
auriculoventricular valve
auriscope
Aurora dual-chamber pace-
    maker
aurotherapy
auscultation
auscultation sites of heart valves
auscultatory findings
auscultatory gap
auscultatory percussion
auscultatory sound
auscultatory triangle
auscultoscope
Ausman microsurgery instru-
    ment
Austin awl
Austin bunionectomy
Austin chisel
Austin clip
Austin dental knife
Austin dental retractor
Austin dissection knife
Austin dissector

Austin duckbill elevator
Austin elevator
Austin excavator
Austin Flint murmur
Austin Flint phenomenon
Austin Flint respiration
Austin gauge
Austin knife
Austin Moore arthroplasty
Austin Moore bone-measuring
    instrument
Austin Moore bone reamer
Austin Moore corkscrew
    femoral head remover
Austin Moore endoprosthetic
    arthroplasty
Austin Moore extractor
Austin Moore hip arthroplasty
Austin Moore hip prosthesis
Austin Moore impactor
Austin Moore inside-outside
    calipers
Austin Moore instruments
Austin Moore mortising chisel
Austin Moore outside calipers
Austin Moore pin
Austin Moore prosthesis
Austin Moore prosthesis rasps
Austin Moore prosthesis-sizing
    set
Austin Moore rasp
Austin Moore reamer
Austin Moore southern ap-
    proach
Austin Moore total hip system
Austin Moore-Murphy bone
    lever
Austin Moore-Murphy bone
    skid
Austin needle
Austin otological microsurgery
    set
Austin pick
Austin retractor
Austin sickle knife
Austin sterilizing storage rack
Austin strut calipers

Austin-Shea tympanoplasty
Autima II dual-chamber cardiac
    pacemaker
Autima II pacemaker
autoamputation
Auto-Band Steri-drape
autochthonous graft
autochthonous stone
autoclavable
autoclave
Autoclip
Autoclip applier
Autoclip remover
autocystoplasty
autodermic
autodermic graft
autodigestion of pancreatic
    tissue
autodrainage
autoepidermic graft
autoerotic rectal trauma
Autoflex II continuous passive
    motion units (CPM units)
autogenic
autogenous bone graft
autogenous graft
autogenous transplant
autogenous vein bypass
autogenous vein graft
autograft
autograft material
autoinfection
autologous
autologous clot
autologous fat graft
autologous graft
autologous patient donor
autologous pericardial patch
autologous transfusion
autologous vein graft
autolysis
autolyzed
automated computerized axial
    tomography (ACAT)
automated intravitreal scissors
automated retractor
automatic catheter

automatic corneal trephine
automatic cranial drill
automatic finger
automatic implantable cardi-
    overter-defibrillator (AICD)
automatic internal cardioverter-
    defibrillator (AICD)
automatic rotating tourniquet
automatic screwdriver
automatic skin retractor
automatic stapling device
automatic suction device
automatic tourniquet
autonomic
auto-ophthalmoscope
auto-ophthalmoscopy
Autophor femoral prosthesis
Autophor hip component
Autophor total hip
autoplastic graft
autoplasty
Autoplot
autopsy
autopsy blade
autopsy blade handle
autoradiographic technique
autoradiography
autoregulation
autoreinfusion
Auto-Suture (AS)
Auto-Suture Clip-A-Matic clip
    applier
Auto-Suture curet
Auto-Suture EEA instrument
Auto-Suture forceps
Auto-Suture GIA stapler
Auto-Suture stapler
Auto-Suture surgical stapler
Auto-Suture Surgiclip
Auto-Suture TA-50 staple gun
Auto-Suture technique
Autosyringe insulin pump
autotome drill
Autotrans system for blood
    recovery
autotransfusion
Autraugrip forceps

Autraugrip tissue forceps
Auvard cranioclast
Auvard speculum
Auvard weighted vaginal
    speculum
Auvard-Remine speculum
Auvard-Remine vaginal specu-
    lum
Auvard-Remine weighted
    speculum
Auvard-Zweifel basiotribe
Auvard-Zweifel forceps
Auvray incision
AV (aortic valve, arteriovenous,
    atrioventricular)
AV aneurysm (arteriovenous
    aneurysm)
AV block (atrioventricular
    block)
AV bundle (atrioventricular
    bundle)
AV conduction defect (atrioven-
    tricular conduction defect)
AV fistula  (arteriovenous
    fistula)
AV Gore-Tex fistula (arterio-
    venous Gore-Tex fistula)
AV Gore-Tex graft (arterio-
    venous Gore-Tex graft)
AV junctional pacemaker
    (atrioventricular junctional
    pacemaker)
AV Miniclinic (atrioventricular
    Miniclinic)
AV node (atrioventricular node)
AV repair (aortic valve repair)
AV sequential demand pace-
    maker (atrioventricular
    sequential demand
    pacemaker)
AV sequential pacemaker
    (atrioventricular sequential
    pacemaker)
AV shunt (arteriovenous shunt)
AV synchronous pacemaker
    (atrioventricular synchro-
    nous pacemaker)

Avalox skin clip
avascular
avascular graft
avascular necrosis
avascular space
avascular tissue
avascularization
AVCO aortic balloon
AVCS (atrioventricular conduc-
    tion system)
AVDO2 (arteriovenous oxygen
    difference)
Aveline Gutierrez parotidec-
    tomy
Averett total hip system
Avertin anesthetic agent
AVF (arteriovenous fistula)
aviator's astragalus
aviator's fracture
Avila approach
Avila operation
Avionics two-channel Holter
    recorder
AVIT vitrectomy handpiece
Avitene hemostatic material
Avitene sandwich
Avius sequential pacemaker
avivement
AVM (arteriovenous malforma-
    tion)
AVM (atrioventricular malforma-
    tion)
avulsed fragment
avulsed laceration
avulsion
avulsion chip fracture
avulsion flap injury
avulsion fracture
avulsion injury
avulsion of epiphysis
avulsion of eyeball
avulsion of nerve
avulsion of optic nerve
awl
    Aufranc awl
    Aufranc trochanteric awl
    Austin awl

awl *continued*
    bone awl
    Carroll awl
    curved awl
    DePuy awl
    reamer awl
    Rochester awl
    Rush pin reamer awl
    sternal perforating awl
    trochanteric awl
    Wangensteen awl
    Wilson awl
    Zuelzer awl
Axenfeld loop
Axenfeld sutures
Axer operation
Axer technique
Axer tendon transfer into talus
axes (*sing.* axis)
Axhausen cleft lip repair
Axhausen needle holder
axial cataract
axial fusiform cataract
axial hiatal hernia
axial myopia
axial plane
axial resolution
axial tractor
axilla (*pl.* axillae)
axilla, shoulder, and elbow
    bandage (ASE bandage)
axillaris, arteria
axillaris, nervus
axillaris, vena
axillary
axillary adenopathy
axillary anesthesia
axillary arch
axillary artery
axillary artery catheterization
axillary block
axillary block anesthesia
axillary bypass
axillary fascia
axillary foramen
axillary fossa

axillary gland
axillary nerve
axillary node
axillary vein
axilloaxillary bypass
axillobifemoral
axillobifemoral bypass
axillofemoral
axillofemoral bypass
axiodistal
axiodistocervical
axiodistoincisal
axiodisto-occlusal
axioincisal
axiolabial
axiolabiogingival
axiolingual
axiolinguogingival
axiolinguo-occlusal
axio-occlusal
Axiom DG balloon angioplasty
Axiom DG balloon angioplasty
    catheter
Axiom double sump pump
Axiom drain
Axiom thoracic trocar
axiomesial
axiomesiocervical
axiomesiodistal
axiomesiogingival
axiomesioincisal
axiomesio-occlusal
axiopulpal
axis (*pl.* axes)
axis deviation
axis ligament
axis traction
axis-traction forceps
axometer
axon
Ayers cardiovascular needle
    holder
Ayers chalazion forceps
Ayers forceps
Ayers needle holder
Ayers sphygmomanometer

Ayers T-piece
Ayerst knife
Ayre brush
Ayre cone knife
Ayre knife
Ayre tube
Ayre-Scott knife
Azar cystitome
Azar flexible-loop anterior
    chamber intraocular lens
Azar forceps
Azar lid speculum
Azar Tripod eye implant

Azar Tripod implant cataract
    lens
Azar Tripod lens
Azar tying forceps
Azar utility forceps
azygogram
azygography
azygoportal interruption
azygos arch
azygos lobe
azygos vein
azygos vein arch
azygos, vena

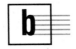

B&D needle
B&S gauge sutures (Brown-Sharp)
B-1 craniotome attachment (also B-2, etc.)
B-12 dental curet
B-B graft
B-chain cystometrogram
B-craniotome
B-curve
B-D (Becton-Dickinson)
B-D adapter
B-D bone marrow biopsy needle
B-D butterfly swab dressing
B-D Fleischer spinal sphygmo-manometer
B-D irrigating tip
B-D Luer-Lok syringe
B-D Multifit control syringe
B-D needle
B-D Potain thoracic trocar
B-D spinal needle
B-D stopcock
B-D Yale syringe
B-H anterior chamber irrigator
B-H forceps
B-H irrigating cannula
B-K dysplastic nevi
B-K moles
B-Line utility cart
B-mode image
B-mode scanning
B-mode ultrasonography
B-mode ultrasound
B-scan
B-scan reflectivity
B-scan ultrasound
B-scan ultrasound machine
B-W graft

Babcock clamp
Babcock empyema trocar
Babcock forceps
Babcock inguinal herniorrhaphy
Babcock intestinal forceps
Babcock jointed vein stripper
Babcock needle
Babcock operation
Babcock plate
Babcock raspatory
Babcock retractor
Babcock stainless suture wire
Babcock suture wire
Babcock thoracic tissue-holding forceps
Babcock tissue clamp
Babcock tissue forceps
Babcock trocar
Babcock tube
Babcock vein stripper
Babcock Vital intestinal forceps
Babcock Vital tissue forceps
Babcock wire sutures
Babcock wire-cutting scissors
Babinski reflex
Babinski sign
baby Adson brain retractor
baby Balfour retractor
baby costal periosteotome
baby dressing forceps
baby hemostatic forceps
baby intestinal tissue forceps
baby Lane bone-holding forceps
baby Metzenbaum scissors
baby needle holder
baby pylorus clamp
baby retractor
baby rib contractor
baby spur crusher

baby tissue forceps
baby Weitlaner retractor
BABYbird respirator
Bachmann bundle
bacitracin dressing
bacitracin ointment
bacitracin solution
bacitracin strips
Baciu-Filibiu ankle arthrodesis
back brace
back manipulation
back table
back vest
backache
back-and-forth motion
back-and-forth sutures
backbiting forceps
backbiting rongeur
backbleed
backbleeding
backbone
backcut incision
backcutting knife
backfire fracture
backflow
backflush
Backhaus clamp
Backhaus clip
Backhaus dilator
Backhaus forceps
Backhaus towel clamp
Backhaus towel forceps
Backhaus-Jones towel clamp
Backhaus-Kocher towel clamp
back-knee
back-stop laser probe
back-stopped laser instruments
backstroke injury
backward-cutting scissors
Bacon anoscope
Bacon bone rongeur
Bacon cranial forceps
Bacon cranial retractor
Bacon cranial rongeur
Bacon cranial rongeur forceps
Bacon forceps
Bacon periosteal raspatory

Bacon proctoscope
Bacon raspatory
Bacon retractor
Bacon rib shears
Bacon rongeur
Bacon thoracic shears
bactericidal
Badal operation
Baden Silastic rod
Badenoch urethroplasty
badger's triangle
Badgley arthrodesis
Badgley hip arthrodesis
Badgley laminectomy retractor
Badgley nail
Badgley operation
Badgley plate
Badgley retractor
Baer bone-cutting forceps
Baer forceps
Baer rib shears
Baer vesicle
Baffe anastomosis
Baffe operation
Baffe transplant
baffle
bag (see also *hemostatic bag*)
    Aberhart disposable
      urinal bag
    ACMI bag
    air bag
    Alcock bag
    Alcock hemostatic bag
    Ambu bag
    arterial line pressure bag
    Bard bag
    Bardex bag
    Bardex hemostatic bag
    Barnes bag
    bile bag
    Bomgart stomal bag
    bowel bag
    Brodney hemostatic bag
    Bunyan bag
    Champetier de Ribes
      obstetrical bag
    Coloplast bag

bag *continued*
> Coloplast colostomy bag
> colostomy bag
> coudé bag
> coudé hemostatic bag
> Davol bag
> dialysate bag
> Douglas bag
> drainage bag
> Duval bag
> Emmet hemostatic bag
> Foley bag
> Foley hemostatic bag
> Foley-Alcock bag
> Foley-Alcock bag
>   catheter
> Foley-Alcock hemostatic
>   bag
> gauze tissue bag
> Greck ileostomy bag
> Hagner bag
> Hagner bag catheter
> Hagner hemostatic bag
> Hagner urethral bag
> hemostatic bag
> Hendrickson bag
> Hendrickson hemostatic
>   bag
> Higgins bag
> Higgins hemostatic bag
> Hofmeister drainage bag
> Hollister bag
> Hollister colostomy bag
> Hollister drainage bag
> Hope bag
> hydrostatic bag
> ice bag
> ileostomy bag
> Incono bag
> inflatable Foley bag
>   catheter
> intestinal bag
> intracervical bag
> karaya seal ileostomy
>   stomal bag
> Kearns bag catheter
> Kern bag

bag *continued*
> Lahey bag
> Lapides collecting bag
> latex bag
> Lyster water bag
> manual resuscitation bag
> Marlen ileostomy bag
> Marlen weightless bag
> Marsan Loop-Loc
>   colostomy bag system
> micturition bag
> millinery bag
> Mosher bag
> Nesbit hemostatic bag
> ostomy bag
> Paul condom bag
> Pearman transurethral
>   hemostatic bag
> pear-shaped fluted bag
> Peel Pak bag
> Perry bag
> Perry ileostomy bag
> Petersen bag
> Petersen rectal bag
> Pilcher bag
> Pilcher bag catheter
> Pilcher hemostatic bag
> Pilcher hemostatic
>   suprapubic bag
> Plummer bag
> pneumatic bag
> pneumatic bag esophag-
>   eal dilatation
> Politzer air bag
> Politzer bag
> prostatectomy bag
> rebreathing bag
> Robertshaw bag resusci-
>   tator
> Robinson bag
> ruptured bag of waters
> sandbag
> severance transurethral
>   bag
> Shea-Anthony bag
> short-tip bag
> short-tip hemostatic bag

bag *continued*

Sones hemostatic bag
stomal bag
suprapubic bag
suprapubic hemostatic
bag
Sur-Fit colostomy bag
Swenko bag
Tassett vaginal cup bag
Thackston retropubic
bag
Travenol bag
two-way bag
two-way hemostatic bag
vaginal bag
Van Hove bag
Voorhees bag
Whitmore bag
Wolf nephrostomy bag
catheter

bag catheter
bag of waters
Bagby compression plate
Bagby plate
bagged
bagging
Baggish hysteroscope
Bagley-Wilmer expressor
Bagolini lens
bagpipe vertebral outgrowth
Bahler elbow arthroplasty
Bahn spud
Bahnson aortic clamp
Bahnson appendage clamp
Bahnson cannula
Bahnson clamp
Bahnson retractor
Bahnson sternal retractor
Bahnson-Brown forceps
Bahnson-Brown tissue forceps
Bailey aortic clamp
Bailey aortic valve-cutting
forceps
Bailey aortic valve rongeur
Bailey baby rib contractor
Bailey bur
Bailey cannula

Bailey catheter
Bailey chalazion forceps
Bailey clamp
Bailey conductor
Bailey contractor
Bailey dilator
Bailey drill
Bailey forceps
Bailey Gigli-saw guide
Bailey leukotome
Bailey operation
Bailey pliers
Bailey punch
Bailey rib approximator
Bailey rib contractor
Bailey rib elevator
Bailey rib spreader
Bailey rod
Bailey rongeur
Bailey saw conductor
Bailey shooter
Bailey skull bur
Bailey spreader
Bailey-Badgley arthrodesis
Bailey-Badgley cervical spine
approach
Bailey-Cowley clamp
Bailey-Dubow femoral shaft
procedure
Bailey-Dubow technique
Bailey-Gibbon contractor
Bailey-Gibbon rib contractor
Bailey-Glover-O'Neill commis-
surotomy knife
Bailey-Glover-O'Neill knife
Bailey-Glover-O'Neill valvulo-
tome
Bailey-Morse clamp
Bailey-Morse knife
Bailey-Williamson forceps
Bailey-Williamson obstetrical
forceps
Bailliart ophthalmodyna-
mometer
Bailliart tonometer
bail-lock brace
bail-lock splint

bailout catheter
bailout valvuloplasty
Baim catheter
Baim-Turi monitor
Baim-Turi pacing
Bainbridge clamp
Bainbridge forceps
Bainbridge hemostatic forceps
Bainbridge intestinal clamp
Bainbridge intestinal forceps
Bainbridge reflex
Bainbridge resection forceps
Bainbridge vessel clamp
Baird chalazion forceps
Baird forceps
Bairnsdale ulcer
Baiter modification of Shirodkar procedure
Bakamjian flap
Bakamjian pedicle flap
Bakamjian tubed flap
Bakelite dental chisel
Bakelite hammer
Bakelite mallet
Bakelite resectoscope sheath
Bakelite retractor
Bakelite spatula
Bakelite-handled osteotome
Baker anastomosis
Baker anchorage
Baker cyst
Baker forceps
Baker intestinal decompression tube
Baker jejunostomy tube
Baker patellar tendon procedure
Baker procedure
Baker syndrome
Baker tissue forceps
Baker tube
Baker velum
Baker-Hill osteotomy
Baker-Lima-Baker mask (BLB mask)
Bakes bile duct dilator
Bakes common duct dilator

Bakes dilator
Bakes probe
Bakes-Pearce dilator
Bakst scissors
Bakst valvulotome
BAL (bronchoalveolar lavage)
Balacescu technique
balanced anesthesia
balanced general anesthesia
balanced salt solution (BSS)
balanced suspension
balanoplasty
bald gastric fundus
bald tongue
Baldwin operation
Baldy operation
Baldy-Webster hysteropexy
Baldy-Webster operation for retrodisplacement of uterus
Baldy-Webster uterine suspension
BALF (bronchoalveolar lavage fluid)
Balfour abdominal retractor
Balfour blade
Balfour center blade
Balfour clamp
Balfour fourth-blade extension
Balfour gastrectomy
Balfour gastric resection
Balfour gastroenterostomy
Balfour pediatric retractor
Balfour retractor
Balfour self-retaining retractor
Balkan bed
Balkan fracture frame
Balkan frame
Balkan splint
Ball coagulator
Ball dissector
ball electrode
ball electrode desiccation
ball heart valve
Ball operation
ball poppet
ball reamer
Ball reusable electrode

ball valve
Ballade needle
Ballance mastoid spoon
Ballance sign
ball-and-cage prosthetic valve
ball-and-cage valve prosthesis
ball-and-socket joint
ball-and-socket osteotomy
Ballantine clamp
Ballantine forceps
Ballantine hemilaminectomy
   retractor
Ballantine hysterectomy forceps
Ballantine uterine curet
Ballantine-Drew coagulator
Ballantine-Peterson forceps
Ballantine-Peterson hysterec-
   tomy forceps
ball-cage prosthesis
ball-cage valve
Ballen eye repair
Ballen-Alexander orbital
   retractor
Ballen-Alexander retractor
ball-end elevator
ball-end hook
Ballenger bur
Ballenger cartilage knife
Ballenger chisel
Ballenger curet
Ballenger electrode
Ballenger elevator
Ballenger ethmoid curet
Ballenger follicle electrode
Ballenger forceps
Ballenger gouge
Ballenger knife
Ballenger mastoid bur
Ballenger mucosa knife
Ballenger nose knife
Ballenger periosteotome
Ballenger raspatory
Ballenger septal elevator
Ballenger septal knife
Ballenger sponge forceps
Ballenger sponge-holding
   forceps

Ballenger swivel knife
Ballenger tonsil forceps
Ballenger tonsil-seizing
   forceps
Ballenger urethroscope
Ballenger-Foerster forceps
Ballenger-Hajek approximator
Ballenger-Hajek chisel
Ballenger-Hajek elevator
Ballenger-Lillie bur
Ballenger-Lillie mastoid bur
Ballenger-Sluder guillotine
Ballenger-Sluder tonometer
Ballenger-Sluder tonsillectome
ballet sign
ballistics
ballistocardiogram
ballistocardiography
Ballobes gastric balloon
balloon
   ACS SULP II balloon
   activated balloon
      expandable intravascu-
      lar stent
   angiographic balloon
      occlusion catheter
   angioplasty balloon
      catheter
   angled balloon catheter
   Anthony-Fisher antrum
      balloon
   Anthony-Fisher balloon
   antral balloon
   aortic balloon pump
   Arrow-Berman balloon
      angioplasty catheter
   Arrow-Berman balloon
      catheter
   Atlas balloon dilatation
      catheter
   atrial balloon septos-
      tomy
   AVCO aortic balloon
   Axiom DG balloon
      angioplasty
   Axiom DG balloon
      angioplasty catheter

balloon *continued*

Ballobes gastric balloon
banana-shaped balloon
Baylor balloon
biliary balloon catheter
biliary balloon probe
Brighton balloon
Brighton epistaxis
    balloon
cardiac balloon pump
catheter balloon
counterpulsation balloon
Critikon balloon ther-
    modilution catheter
Critikon balloon-tipped
    end-hole catheter
Datascope balloon
Datascope intra-aortic
    balloon pump
Datascope intra-aortic
    balloon pump catheter
dilatation balloon
    catheter
dilating pressure balloon
    catheter
Dotter caged-balloon
    catheter
Ducor balloon catheter
epistaxis balloon
esophageal balloon
extrusion balloon
    catheter
FAST balloon catheter
    (flow-assisted, short-
    term balloon catheter)
flow-assisted short-term
    balloon catheter
flow-directed balloon-
    tipped catheter
Fogarty balloon
Fogarty balloon biliary
    catheter
Fogarty balloon catheter
Fogarty biliary balloon
    probe
Fogarty-Chin extrusion
    balloon catheter
Foley balloon catheter
Fox balloon

balloon *continued*

Garner balloon shunt
Garren-Edwards balloon
gastric balloon
Gau gastric balloon
Giesy ureteral dilatation
    balloon
Gilbert balloon catheter
Gilbert pediatric balloon
    catheter
Gruentzig arterial
    balloon catheter
Gruentzig balloon
Gruentzig balloon
    catheter
Gruentzig balloon
    catheter angioplasty
Gruentzig balloon dilator
Hartzler angioplasty
    balloon
Hartzler Micro II balloon
    for coronary
    angioplasty
Heishima balloon
    occluder
Honan balloon
Hunter-Sessions balloon
hydrostatic balloon
hydrostatic balloon
    catheter
inflated balloon
Inoue balloon catheter
intra-aortic balloon
intra-aortic balloon assist
    device
intra-aortic balloon
    catheter
intra-aortic balloon
    counterpulsation
intra-aortic balloon
    pump (IABP)
intra-aortic balloon
    pumping (IABP)
intragastric balloon
Katzin-Long balloon
kissing balloon
kissing balloon tech-
    nique
Kontron balloon

balloon *continued*
    Kontron intra-aortic balloon
    laser balloon
    Lo-Profile balloon catheter
    Lo-Profile II balloon catheter
    LPS balloon
    Mansfield balloon
    Mansfield balloon catheter
    Mansfield dilatation balloon catheter
    Meditech balloon catheter
    Medtronic balloon catheter
    mercury-containing balloon
    microballoon probe
    Microvasic Rigiflex balloon
    occlusive balloon
    Olbert balloon catheter
    Olbert balloon dilatation catheter
    Omniflex balloon catheter
    PE Plus II balloon dilatation catheter
    PE Plus II peripheral balloon catheter
    pediatric balloon catheter
    Percival gastric balloon
    Percor dual-lumen intra-aortic balloon catheter
    Percor-Stat intra-aortic balloon
    pneumatic balloon catheter
    pneumatic balloon dilator
    postnasal balloon
    pulmonary artery balloon pump (PABP)
    pulmonary balloon

balloon *continued*
    QuickFurl double-lumen balloon
    QuickFurl single-lumen balloon
    rapid exchange balloon catheter
    Rashkind balloon
    Rashkind septostomy balloon catheter
    recessed balloon septostomy catheter
    rectal balloon
    RediFurl double-lumen balloon
    RediFurl single-lumen balloon
    RF balloon catheter
    Riepe-Bard gastric balloon
    Rigiflex balloon
    Rigiflex balloon dilator
    Rushkin balloon
    Schwarten balloon-dilatation catheter
    Science-Med balloon catheter
    scintigraphic balloon
    Sengstaken balloon
    Sengstaken-Blakemore balloon
    septostomy balloon catheter
    Shea-Anthony balloon
    Simpson PET balloon atherectomy device
    Simpson Ultra Lo-Profile balloon catheter
    sinus balloon
    Taylor gastric balloon
    thermodilution balloon catheter
    Thruflex PTCA balloon catheter
    TLC Baxter balloon catheter
    transluminal balloon

balloon *continued*

USCI Mini-Profile balloon dilatation catheter
valvuloplasty balloon catheter
Wilson-Cook gastric balloon

balloon angioplasty
balloon aortic valvuloplasty
balloon atrial septotomy
balloon biliary catheter
balloon catheter
balloon cholangiogram
balloon counterpulsation
balloon decompression
balloon dilatation catheter
balloon dilating catheter
balloon embolectomy catheter
balloon expandable intravascular stent
balloon flotation catheter
balloon inflation
balloon mitral valvuloplasty
balloon nasostat
balloon occlusion of aneurysm
balloon pulmonary valvuloplasty
balloon pump
balloon reflex manometry
balloon septostomy
balloon shunt
balloon sickness
balloon tamponade
balloon tuboplasty
balloon valvotomy
balloon valvuloplasty
ballooning
ballooning esophagoscope
balloon-like dilation of artery
balloon-tipped angiographic catheter
ballotable
ballotable patella
ballottement
ballpoint scissors
ball-tip electrode
ball-tip reamer
ball-tipped scissors

ball-type prosthesis
ball-type retractor
ball-type valve
ball-valve prosthesis
ball-valve thrombus
ball-valved
balm
Balmer decompressor
Balmer depressor
Balnetar graft materials
Balnetar implant
Balnetar prosthesis
Baloser hysteroscope
balsa wood block
Baltimore nasal scissors
Bamberger area
Bamberger sign
bamboo spine
Bamby clamp
banana (Beaver blade)
banana knife
banana-shaped balloon
Bancroft-Plenk gastrectomy
Bancroft-Plenk operation

band

adhesive band
anchor band
angle band
anterior band of colon
atelectatic band
Auto-Band Steri-drape
BB band
belly band
Bosworth headband
broad adhesive band
broad band
elastic band ligation
elastic rubber band
encircling band
face shield headband
fracture band
Fraenkel headband
free band of colon
Gleason headband
Good-Lite headband
Hall band intrauterine device
Harris band

*Band-Aid*

band *continued*
- headband
- headband-and-mirror set
- His band
- hymenal band
- iliotibial band (ITB)
- Impala rubber band
- ITB (iliotibial band)
- J&J Band-Aid sterile drape
- Kleinert rubber-band splint
- Ladd band
- Lane band
- lateral band
- latex band
- Magill band
- Marlex band
- Matas band
- matrix band
- MB band
- Meckel band
- Mersilene band
- mesocolic band
- metal band
- metal band sutures
- MM band
- oligoclonal band
- omental adhesive band
- omental band
- orthodontic band
- Parham band
- Parham-Martin band
- Parma band
- peritoneal band
- Pynchol headband
- Q-band
- Ray-Tec band
- Remak band
- rubber-band hemorrhoid ligation
- rubber-band ligation
- scultetus binder band
- sheer spot Band-Aid dressing
- silicone elastomer band
- Simonart band
- Sistrunk band retractor

band *continued*
- Sluder headband
- snap gauge band
- Spray Band dressing
- Storz face-shield headband
- table band
- tension band wiring
- TheraBand
- tissue band
- tooth band
- Uchida tubal banding
- ventricular bands
- vessel band
- Worrall headband

band keratitis

band keratopathy

bandage (see also *dressing*)
- abdominal bandage
- Ace adherent bandage
- Ace bandage
- adhesive bandage
- ARD bandage
- ASE bandage (axilla, shoulder, and elbow bandage)
- barrel bandage
- Barton bandage
- Baynton bandage
- Bennell bandage
- binocular bandage
- Borsch bandage
- Buller bandage
- capeline bandage
- Castmate plaster bandage dressing
- Cellamin bandage
- Cellamin resin plaster-of-Paris bandage
- Cellona bandage
- Cellona resin plaster-of-Paris bandage
- Champ elastic bandage
- circular bandage
- Coban bandage
- compression bandage
- cotton elastic bandage

bandage *continued*

- cotton-wool bandage
- Cover-Roll stretch bandage
- cravat bandage
- crepe bandage
- crucial bandage
- Curad plastic bandage
- demigauntlet bandage
- Desault bandage
- E-cotton bandage
- elastic adhesive bandage
- elastic bandage
- elastic foam bandage
- Elastikon bandage
- Elastomull bandage
- Elastomull elastic gauze bandage
- Elastoplast bandage
- Esmarch bandage
- eye bandage
- figure-of-8 bandage
- figure-of-eight bandage
- fixation bandage
- flat eye bandage
- Flexicon gauze bandage
- Flexilite conforming elastic bandage
- Flexilite gauze bandage
- FoaMTrac traction bandage
- four-tailed bandage
- Fractura Flex bandage
- Fractura Flex elastic bandage
- Fricke bandage
- Galen bandage
- Garretson bandage
- gauntlet bandage
- gauze bandage
- Gauztex bandage
- Genga bandage
- Gibney bandage
- Griffin bandage lens dressing
- Guibor Expo flat eye bandage

bandage *continued*

- Haftelast self-adhering bandage
- Hamilton bandage
- hammock bandage
- Heliodorus bandage
- Hermitex bandage
- Hippocrates bandage
- Hueter bandage
- Hydron burn bandage
- immobilizing bandage
- immovable bandage
- Kerlix bandage
- Kerlix conforming bandage dressing
- Kiwisch bandage
- Kling bandage
- Larrey bandage
- Maisonneuve bandage
- many-tailed bandage
- Marlex bandage
- Martin bandage
- moleskin bandage
- monocular bandage
- Morton bandage
- oblique bandage
- Orthoflex elastic plaster bandage
- Pearlcast polymer plaster bandage
- perineal bandage
- plano T-bandage
- plaster bandage
- plaster-of-Paris bandage
- POP bandage (plaster-of-Paris bandage)
- pressure bandage
- Priessnitz bandage
- protective bandage
- REB rubber-reinforced bandage
- recurrent bandage
- reverse bandage
- reversed bandage
- Ribble bandage
- Richet bandage
- Robert Jones bandage

bandage *continued*
    roller bandage
    Sayre bandage
    scarf bandage
    scultetus bandage
    Seutin bandage
    ShowerSafe cast and
        bandage protector
    Silesian bandage
    sling-and-swathe
        bandage
    spica bandage
    spiral bandage
    spiral reverse bandage
    spray bandage
    starch bandage
    stockinette amputation
        bandage
    stockinette bandage
    Surgiflex bandage
    suspensory bandage
    T-bandage
    T-bandage dressing
    Telfa 4 x 4 bandage
    Theden bandage
    Thermophore bandage
    Thillaye bandage
    triangular bandage
    Tubigrip elastic support
        bandage
    Tubiton tubular band-
        age
    Tuffnell bandage
    Velpeau bandage
    Webril bandage
    wet bandage
    woven elastic bandage
    Y-bandage
    Y-bandage dressing
bandage scissors (see also
    *scissors*)
    Bergman bandage
        scissors
    Braun-Stadler bandage
        scissors
    Burnham bandage
        scissors
    Burnham finger bandage
        scissors

bandage scissors *continued*
    gold-plated bandage
        scissors
    Hi-level bandage scissors
    Kayess bandage scissors
    Knowles bandage
        scissors
    Lister bandage scissors
    Lorenz bandage scissors
    Medi bandage scissors
BandageGuard half-leg
    protector
Band-Aid dressing
bandaletta
bandeau
banded gastroplasty
Bandeloux bed
banding
banding of pulmonary artery
Bandl obstetric ring
Bane bone rongeur
Bane forceps
Bane hook
Bane rongeur
Bane rongeur forceps
Bane-Hartmann bone rongeur
Bangerter forceps
Bangerter muscle forceps
Bangerter operation
Bangerter spatula
Bangs bougie
banjo cast
banjo curet
banjo splint
banjo traction splint
banjo tractor
banjo-string adhesions
Bankart dislocation
Bankart lesion
Bankart operation for shoulder
    dislocation
Bankart repair
Bankart retractor
Bankart shoulder repair
Bankart shoulder retractor
Bankart-Magnuson shoulder
    repair
Banks bone graft
Banks graft

Banks-Laufman approach
Banks-Michel herniorrhaphy
Banner enucleation knife
Banner enucleation snare
Banner snare
Banno catheter
BANS area (back, arm, neck,
   shoulder area)
Bantam Bovie coagulator
Bantam Bovie unit
Bantam coagulator
Bantam wire scissors
Bantam wire-cutting scissors
BAPS (biomechanical ankle
   platform system)
bar (see also *arch bar, crossbar*)
   acrylic bar
   acrylic bar prosthesis
   arch bar
   arch bars facial fracture
     appliance
   arch bars frame
   Bose bar
   Buck extension bar
   Burns prism bar
   clasp bar
   Clevedent crossbar
     elevator
   connector bar
   Cottle crossbar chisel
   Cottle crossbar fishtail
     chisel
   crossbar
   crossbar chisel
   crossbar chisel-osteo-
     tome
   crossbar elevator
   dental arch bar
   dental arch bar frame
   Erich arch bar
   Erich arch malleable  bar
   Erich-Winter arch bar
   Fillauer bar
   fixed arch bar
   fracture bar
   Gerster traction bar
   Goldman bar

bar *continued*
   Goldthwait bar
   intramedullary bar
   Jelenko arch bar
   Jelenko bar
   Jewett bar
   Joseph septal bar
   Kazanjian bar
   Kazanjian T-bar
   Kennedy bar
   labial bar
   lingual bar
   Livingston bar
   lumbrical bar
   major connector bar
   mandibular arch bar
   minor connector bar
   Niro arch bars
   occlusal rest bar
   palatal bar
   Passavant bar
   retainer arch bar
   Roger Anderson fixation
     bar
   spreader bar
   stall bar
   strut bar
   strut bar hook
   T-bar elevator
   tarsal bar
   Tommy hip bar
   torsion bar splint
   traction bar
   trapeze bar
   unilateral bar
   unsegmented bar
   Winter arch bar
Bar incision
Bárány alarm apparatus
Bárány apparatus
Bárány box
Bárány noise apparatus
Bárány noise apparatus whistle
Bárány sign
Bárány-Larm apparatus
barb staple
Barbara needle

Barbara pelvimeter
barbed broach
barber pole sign
barbiturate
barbiturate antagonist
barbotage
Barcelona colon anastomosis
    modification
Bard arterial cannula
Bard bag
Bard balloon-directed pacing
    catheter
Bard biopsy sample system
Bard bioptic gun
Bard cardiopulmonary support
    system
Bard catheter
Bard clamp
Bard coil stent
Bard constant contact cord
Bard cystoscope tip
Bard dilator
Bard electrode
Bard Extra Ileo B pouch
Bard graft
Bard guiding catheter
Bard helical catheter
Bard implant
Bard ostomy pouch
Bard PCA pump
Bard pouch
Bard prosthesis
Bard PTFE graft
Bard resectoscope
Bard soft double-pigtail stent
Bard tip
Bard tube
Bard urethral dilator
Bard urethroscopy system
Bard x-ray ureteral catheter
Bardach modification of
    Obwegeser mandibular
    osteotomy
Bardam catheter
Bardam red rubber catheter
Bard-Apter valve
Bardco catheter

Bardeen pad
Bardeen primitive disk
Bardeleben bone-holding
    forceps
Bardelli operation
Bardenheuer extension
Bardenheuer incision
Bardenheuer ligation
Bardex bag
Bardex catheter
Bardex drain
Bardex Foley catheter
Bardex hemostat
Bardex hemostatic bag
Bardex Lubricath Foley catheter
Bardic cannula
Bardic catheter
Bardic curet
Bardic cutdown catheter
Bardic translucent catheter
Bardic tube
Bardic vein catheter
Bard-Parker autopsy blade
Bard-Parker blade
Bard-Parker dermatome
Bard-Parker disposable scalpel
Bard-Parker forceps
Bard-Parker humidifier
Bard-Parker instrument sterilizer
Bard-Parker knife
Bard-Parker knife handle
Bard-Parker scissors
Bard-Parker sterilizer
Bard-Parker surgical blade
Bard-Parker surgical knife
Bard-Parker transfer forceps
bariatric operation
barium
barium column
barium enema
barium esophagram
barium ingestion
barium meal
barium sediment
barium suspension
barium swallow
barium-impregnated poppet

Barkan cyclodialysis
Barkan forceps
Barkan goniolens
Barkan gonioscope
Barkan goniotomy
Barkan goniotomy knife
Barkan goniotomy lens
Barkan illuminator
Barkan implant
Barkan iris forceps
Barkan knife
Barkan lens
Barkan operation
Barkan scissors
Barker bunionectomy
Barker calipers
Barker needle
Barker operation
Barker point
Barker Vacu-tome knife
Barlow forceps
Barlow syndrome
Barnard mitral valve prosthesis
Barnard operation
Barnes bag
Barnes compressor
Barnes dilator
Barnes internal decompression
    trocar
Barnes nasal suction tube
Barnes scissors
Barnes speculum
Barnes suction tube
Barnes trocar
Barnes-Crile forceps
Barnes-Dormia stone basket
Barnes-Hind lens
Barnes-Hind ophthalmic
    dressing
Barnes-Simpson forceps
Barnes-Simpson obstetrical
    forceps
Barnhill adenoid curet
Barnhill adenoid knife
Barnhill curet
Barnhill-Jones curet
Baron ear knife

Baron ear tube
Baron elevator
Baron forceps
Baron knife
Baron lens
Baron palate elevator
Baron retractor
Baron suction tube
Baron technique
Barr anal speculum
Barr bolt
Barr crypt hook
Barr fistula hook
Barr fistula probe
Barr hook
Barr nail
Barr operation
Barr pin
Barr probe
Barr procedure
Barr rectal retractor
Barr rectal speculum
Barr retractor
Barr self-retaining retractor
Barr speculum
Barraquer brush
Barraquer cannula
Barraquer cilia forceps
Barraquer conjunctiva forceps
Barraquer corneal dissector
Barraquer corneal knife
Barraquer corneal section
    scissors
Barraquer corneal trephine
Barraquer cyclodialysis spatula
Barraquer erysiphake
Barraquer eye shield
Barraquer eye speculum
Barraquer fixation forceps
Barraquer forceps
Barraquer implant
Barraquer iris scissors
Barraquer iris spatula
Barraquer irrigator
Barraquer keratomileusis
Barraquer knife
Barraquer lid retractor

Barraquer microneedle holder
Barraquer mosquito forceps
Barraquer needle
Barraquer needle holder
Barraquer operation
Barraquer scissors
Barraquer section scissors
Barraquer silk sutures
Barraquer spatula
Barraquer speculum
Barraquer suture forceps
Barraquer sutures
Barraquer tonometer
Barraquer trephine
Barraquer wire lid speculum
Barraquer wire speculum
Barraquer zonulolysis
Barraquer-Colibri eye speculum
Barraquer-DeWecker iris
    scissors
Barraquer-DeWecker scissors
Barraquer-Kratz speculum
Barraquer-Krumeich-Swinger
    refractive set
Barraquer-Troutman forceps
Barraquer-Vogt needle
Barraquer-von Mandach clot
    forceps
Barraquer-Zeiss microscope
Barraya forceps
Barraya tissue forceps
Barré pyramidal sign
Barré sign
barred teeth
barrel bandage
barrel cervix
barrel chest
barrel dressing
barrel knot suture
barreling distortion
barrel-shaped chest
barrel-shaped thorax
barrel-type chest
Barrett appendix inverter
Barrett epithelium
Barrett esophagus
Barrett forceps

Barrett hebosteotomy needle
Barrett intestinal forceps
Barrett inverter
Barrett knife
Barrett needle
Barrett placenta forceps
Barrett tenaculum
Barrett tenaculum forceps
Barrett uterine knife
Barrett uterine tenaculum
Barrett uterine tenaculum
    forceps
Barrett-Adson cerebellum
    retractor
Barrett-Adson retractor
Barrett-Allen forceps
Barrett-Allen placenta forceps
Barrett-Allen uterine-elevating
    forceps
Barrett-Murphy forceps
Barrett-Murphy intestinal
    forceps
Barrie-Jones forceps
Barrie-Jones operation
Barrier fenestrated sterile field
Barrier sheet
Barrio operation
Barron hemorrhoid ligation
Barron ligation
Barron pump
Barr-Record clubfoot surgery
Barr-Record operation for
    talipes equinovarus
Barr-Shuford rectal specu-
    lum
Barsky cleft lip repair
Barsky elevator
Barsky forceps
Barsky hook
Barsky method
Barsky operation
Barsky osteotome
Barsky pharyngoplasty
Barsky rasp
Barsky raspatory
Barsky retractor
Barsky scissors

Barsky technique
Barstow stapler
Barth applicator
Barth curet
Barth hernia
Barth mastoid curet
Barth mastoid knife
Bartholin gland catheter
Bartholin glands
Bartholin, Skene, and urethral
    glands (BSU glands)
Bartlett fascia stripper
Bartlett stripper
Bartlett-Edwards profilometer
Bartley anastomosis clamp
Bartley partial-occlusion clamp
Barton bandage
Barton blade
Barton dressing
Barton forceps
Barton fracture
Barton hook
Barton maneuver
Barton obstetrical forceps
Barton operation
Barton operation for ankylosis
Barton tongs
Barton tongs wrench
Barton traction handle
Barton-Cone tongs
Baruch circumcision scissors
Baruch scissors
Barwell operation
basal
basal anesthesia
basal cell carcinoma
basal ganglia
basal ganglia guide
basal hypnotic agents
basal iridectomy
basal lamina of choroid
basal lamina of ciliary body
basal neck fracture
basal ophthalmoplegia
basal rales
basal skull fracture
basal vein
basalis, vena

Baschui pigtail catheter
base of prostate
base of skull
base of stapes
baseball elbow
baseball finger
baseball finger fracture
baseball finger splint
baseball splint
baseball sutures
Basedow paralysis
baseline procedure
baseline study
baseline view
basement membrane
basement tissue
bas-fond
bas-fond formation
basic instrument set
basicervical fracture
basicranial
basicranial flexure
basihyal bone
basilar
basilar artery
basilar bone
basilar fracture
basilar membrane
basilar plexus
basilar process
basilar projection
basilar segment
basilar sutures
basilaris, arteria
Basile hip screw
Basile screw
basilic hiatus
basilic vein
basilica, vena
basin
basioccipital
basiotribe
basiotripsy
basis pontis
basivertebral
basivertebral veins
basivertebrales, venae
Basix pacemaker

basket (see also *stone basket*)
  Acufex curved basket
    forceps
  Acufex rotary basket
    forceps
  Acufex straight basket
    forceps
  Barnes-Dormia stone
    basket
  biliary stone basket
  Browne basket
  Browne stone basket
  Councill basket
  Councill stone basket
  disposable stone basket
  Dormia basket
  Dormia biliary stone
    basket
  Dormia stone basket
  Dormia stone basket
    catheter
  Dormia ureteral basket
  Ellik kidney stone basket
  Ellik stone basket
  Ferguson basket
  Ferguson stone basket
  Glassman basket
  Hook basket forceps
  Howard basket
  Howard stone basket
  Johns Hopkins stone
    basket
  Johnson basket
  Johnson stone basket
  Johnson ureteral basket
  Johnson ureteral stone
    basket
  Levant stone dislodger
    basket
  Mitchell basket
  Mitchell stone basket
  Olympus basket-type
    endoscopic forceps
  parrot-beak basket
  parrot-beak basket biter
  Pfister stone basket
  Pfister-Schwartz basket
    forceps

basket *continued*
  Pfister-Schwartz stone
    basket
  Robinson stone basket
  Rutner stone basket
  Segura stone basket
  Shutt minibasket
  sphincterotomy basket
  stone basket
  stone-holding basket
  three-armed basket
    forceps
  ureteral basket stone
    dislodger
  ureteral stone basket
  Wolf biting basket
    forceps
  Wolf curved basket
    forceps
basket cart
basket forceps
basketball heels
basket-cutting forceps
basket-type crushing forceps
basovertical projection
Basset operation
Bassini herniorrhaphy
Bassini inguinal hernia repair
Bassini operation
Bassini repair
basswood splint
bastard sutures
Basterra operation
basting stitch
basting stitch anastomosis
Bastow laminectomy
  raspatory
Bastow raspatory
Batch knee disarticulation
Batch-Spittler-McFadden
  amputation
Batchelor osteotomy of hip
Batchelor plate
Batchelor technique
Batchelor-Girdlestone disarticu-
  lation
Bateman bipolar cup hip
  prosthesis

Bateman denervation of knee or elbow
Bateman finger joint prosthesis
Bateman operation
Bateman prosthesis
Bateman tendon transfer
Bateman Universal proximal femur prosthesis (UPF prosthesis)
Bateman UPF prosthesis (Universal proximal femur prosthesis)
Bates gastrostomy
Bates operation for urethral stricture
bath
Bath respirator
Batson plexus
Batson vein complex
Batson-Carmody elevator
battery
Battle incision
Battle operation
Battle sign
battledore placenta
Battle-Jalaguier-Kammerer incision
bat-wing catheter
bat-wing configuration
Baudelocque diameter
Baudelocque operation
Baudelocque operation for extrauterine pregnancy
Baudelocque pelvimeter
Baudet-Fontan operation
Bauer air valve
Bauer dissecting forceps
Bauer forceps
Bauer sponge forceps
Bauer technique
Bauer-Black sutures
Bauer-Tondra-Trusler cleft lip repair
Bauer-Tondra-Trusler operation for syndactylism
Bauer-Trusler-Tondra cleft lip repair
Bauhin valve
Baum bumps

Baum needle holder
Baum operation
Baum scissors
Baum tonsil needle holder
Bauman angle
Baumanometer sphygmo-manometer
Baumgard and Schwartz technique
Baumgarten gland
Baumgarten Vital wire twister
Baumgartner forceps
Baumgartner holder
Baumgartner needle holder
Baumgartner punch
Baumgartner Vital needle holder
Baum-Hecht forceps
Baum-Hecht tarsorrhaphy forceps
Baum-Metzenbaum needle holder
Baumrucker incontinence clamp
Baumrucker irrigator
Baumrucker post-TUR irrigation clamp
Baumrucker resectoscope
Bausch-Lomb instruments
Bausch-Lomb lens
Bausch-Lomb loupe
Bavarian splint
Bavrona tube
Baxter dilatation catheter
Baxter disposable blade
Baxter TLC dilatation system
Bayley infant scale
Baylor adjustable cross splint
Baylor amniotic perforator
Baylor amniotome
Baylor autologous transfusion system
Baylor balloon
Baylor cardiovascular sump tube
Baylor hammer
Baylor rapid autologous transfusion system (BRAT system)
Baylor splint

Baylor stump
Baylor sump tube
Baynton bandage
Baynton dressing
Baynton operation
bayonet bipolar electrosurgical forceps
bayonet forceps
bayonet incision
bayonet microscissors
bayonet molar forceps
bayonet needle holder
bayonet osteotome
bayonet rongeur
bayonet saw
bayonet scissors
bayonet separator
bayonet-tip electrode
bayonet-type forceps
BB band
BCD Plus cardioplegic unit
BDH hip prosthesis
BDH total hip system
BE amputation (below-elbow amputation)
B.E. glass abdominal retractor
beach-chair position
Beacham amniotome
bead bed
Bead ethmoid forceps
beaded filaments
beaded hepatic duct
beaded hip pin
beaded-tip scissors
beaded-wires traction bow
beading of arteries
beading of myelin
beading sign
beaked cowhorn forceps
beaked pelvis
beaked sheath
beak-like protrusion of nose
Beale intraocular implant lens
Beale lens
Beall bulldog clamp
Beall circumflex artery scissors
Beall disk valve prosthesis
Beall heart valve

Beall mitral obturator
Beall mitral valve prosthesis
Beall prosthetic valve
Beall valve
Beall-Surgitool ball-cage prosthetic valve
Beall-Surgitool disk prosthetic valve
Beall-Surgitool prosthetic valve
BEAM (brain electrical activity mapping)
beam splitter
beam-hardening artifact
bean forceps
Bear adult-volume ventilator
bear claw ulcer
Bear Cub infant ventilator
Bear respirator
bear track pigmentation
Bear ventilator
Beard cataract knife
Beard cystoscope
Beard cystotome
Beard eye speculum
Beard knife
Beard lid knife
Beard operation
Beard speculum
Beard-Cutler operation
Beardsley aortic dilator
Beardsley cecostomy trocar
Beardsley clamp
Beardsley dilator
Beardsley empyema tube
Beardsley esophageal retractor
Beardsley forceps
Beardsley intestinal clamp
Beardsley trocar
Beardsley tube
Beasley-Babcock forceps
beaten silver appearance
Beath operation
Beatson operation
Beatson ovariotomy
Beatty aluminum finger splint
Beatty decompressor
Beatty pillar retractor
beat-up osteotome
beat-up periosteal elevator

Beaulieu camera
Beaupre cilia forceps
Beaupre epilation forceps
Beaupre forceps
Beaver Arthro-Lok blade
Beaver bent blade
Beaver blade
Beaver blade banana
Beaver blade cataract knife
Beaver blade chuck handle
Beaver blade discission knife
Beaver blade handle
Beaver blade keratome
Beaver blade rosette
Beaver cataract blade
Beaver cataract knife blade
Beaver chuck handle
Beaver cryoextractor
Beaver curet
Beaver cutter
Beaver DeBakey blade
Beaver discission blade
Beaver discission knife blade
Beaver dissector
Beaver electrode
Beaver eye surgery blade
Beaver finger ring saw
Beaver keratome
Beaver keratome blade
Beaver knife
Beaver knife handle
Beaver Mini-Blades
Beaver myringotomy blade
Beaver retractor
Beaver rhinoplasty blade
Beaver saw
Beaver surgical blade
Beaver surgical blade handle
Beaver tonsillectomy blade
Bebax plaster cast
Beccaria sign
Bechert  forceps
Bechert intraocular lens cannula
Bechert intraocular lens implant
Bechert intraocular scissors
Bechert irrigating spatula
Bechert microsurgery instru-
    ments

Bechtol cemented hip pros-
    thesis
Bechtol glenohumeral joint
    prosthesis
Bechtol hip prosthesis
Bechtol implant
Bechtol prosthesis
Bechtol screw
Beck abdominal scoop
Beck aortic clamp
Beck bull's eye lamp
Beck cardiopericardiopexy
Beck clamp
Beck forceps
Beck gastrostomy
Beck gastrostomy scoop
Beck knife
Beck loop
Beck miniature aortic clamp
Beck mouth tube airway
Beck operation
Beck poudrage
Beck rasp
Beck raspatory
Beck scoop
Beck shunt
Beck tonsillectome
Beck triad
Beck vascular clamp
Beck I operation
Beck II operation
Beckenbaugh technique
Becker corneal suture scissors
Becker mammary prosthesis
Becker operation
Becker probe
Becker retractor
Becker scissors
Becker screwdriver
Becker septum scissors
Becker technique
Becker tendon repair
Becker trephine
Becker-Joseph saw
Becker-Park eye speculum
Beck-Jianu gastrostomy
Beck-Jianu operation
Beckman laminectomy retractor

Beckman nasal scissors
Beckman nasal speculum
Beckman probe
Beckman retractor
Beckman self-retaining retractor
Beckman speculum
Beckman-Adson laminectomy
    retractor
Beckman-Adson retractor
Beckman-Colver nasal specu-
    lum
Beckman-Colver speculum
Beckman-Eaton laminectomy
    retractor
Beckman-Eaton retractor
Beckman-Weitlaner laminec-
    tomy retractor
Beckman-Weitlaner retractor
Beck-Mueller tonsillectome
Beck-Potts aorta and pulmonic
    clamp
Beck-Potts clamp
Beck-Satinsky clamp
Beck-Schenck tonsil knife
Beck-Schenck tonsil snare
Beck-Schenck tonsillectome
Beck-Storz tonsil snare
Béclard amputation
Béclard hernia
Béclard sign
Béclard sutures
becquerel (Bq)
Becton technique
Becton-Dickinson Teflon-
    sheathed needle
bed
    adventitial bed
    air bed
    Air Plus low-air-loss bed
    air-fluidized bed
    American Lapidus bed
    Arnott bed
    Balkan bed
    Bandeloux bed
    bead bed
    Biomet bed
    capillary beds
    carotid arterial beds

bed *continued*
    CircOlectric bed
    Clinitron air-fluidized
      bed
    electric bed
    ether bed
    Fisher bed
    Flexicair low-air-loss bed
    Foster bed
    fracture bed
    gallbladder bed
    Gatch bed
    head of bed
    hepatic bed
    Hough bed
    Hoverbed
    hydrostatic bed
    hyperbaric bed
    IC bed
    KinAir bed
    Klondike bed
    Lapidus bed
    liver bed
    Medicus bed
    Mediscus low-air-loss
      bed
    monitored bed
    nail bed
    portal vascular bed
    pulmonary bed
    Rose bed dressing
    Roto Kinetic bed
    Roto-Rest bed
    Sanders bed
    sawdust bed
    scleral bed
    Skytron air-fluidized bed
    Span-aid bed supports
    tissue bed
    ulcer bed
    vascular bed
    venous capacitance bed
    water bed
bed-bound
bedewing of cornea
bedrest
Bedrossian eye speculum
bedside suction tube

bedsore
Beebe binocular loupe
Beebe collar scissors
Beebe forceps
Beebe hemostatic forceps
Beebe lens loupe
Beebe loupe
Beebe scissors
Beebe wire-cutting forceps
beefy red mucosa
beefy tongue
Beer canaliculus knife
Beer cataract flap operation
Beer cataract knife
Beer cilia forceps
Beer forceps
beer heart
Beer knife
Beer operation
beer-can capsulotomy
Beeson plaster spreader
Beeth needle
Beevor phenomenon
Beevor sign
Begg appliance
Behnken unit
Behrend cystic duct forceps
Behrend periosteal elevator
Beird eye catheter
Bekhterev arthritis (also
      Bechterew)
Bekhterev test (also Bechterew)
Bel-Air orthopedic stockinette
Belcher clamp
Belfield operation
Belfield vasotomy
Bell clamp
Bell erysiphake
Bell fracture table
Bell operation
Bell scissors
Bell sutures
Bell tonometer
bellclapper deformity of testis
Bell-Dally dislocation of first
      cervical vertebra
Belleview surgical wadding

Bellevue anesthesia unit
Bellfield wire retractor
Bellini drain
Bellini tube
Bellini tubules
Bellman retractor
Bellocq cannula
Bellocq sound
Bellocq tube
Bellows cryoextractor
Bellows murmur
Bellows pack
Bellows sound
bellows suction
bellows traction
Bell-Tawse technique
Bellucci alligator scissors
Bellucci cannula
Bellucci ear scissors
Bellucci elevator
Bellucci forceps
Bellucci hook
Bellucci knife
Bellucci nasal suction tube
Belucci otolaryngology scissors
Bellucci pick
Bellucci scissors
Bellucci suction tube
Bellucci tube
Bellucci-Paparella scissors
belly band
belly bath intraperitoneal
      chemotherapy
belly tap
Belmas operation
below-elbow amputation (BE
      amputation)
below-knee amputation (BK
      amputation)
Belsey antireflux operation
Belsey esophagoplasty
Belsey herniorrhaphy
Belsey hiatal hernia repair
Belsey Mark II fundoplication
Belsey Mark IV operation
Belsey Mark IV repair
Belsey operation

Belsey partial fundoplication
Belsey perfusor
Belsey repair
Belsey two-thirds wrap fundo-
    plication
belt
    Adam and Eve rib belt
        splint
    control belt
    heavy twill belt
    Hollister belt
    Lapides elastic belt
    lumbosacral belt
    Marlen belt
    Marsan belt
    Mayo sacroiliac belt
    Posey belt
    restraint belt
    rib belt
    Robinson belt
    sacroiliac belt
    safety belt
    seat belt
    Silesian belt
    Velcro belt
    Zim-Zip rib belt splint
Belt hypospadias repair
Belt prostatectomy
belt-approach incision
Belt-Fugua hypospadias repair
Belz lacrimal sac rongeur
Belzer apparatus
Belzer machine
Benaron forceps
bench back test
bench knot pusher-tier
bench surgery
bender
bending fracture
Bendixen-Kirschner traction
    bow
Benedict gastroscope
Benedict operating gastroscope
Benedict operation
Benedict-Roth spirometer
benediction hand
Beneventi retractor

Beneventi self-retaining
    retractor
Beneys tonsil compressor
Bengash needle
Bengolea artery forceps
Bengolea forceps
benign adenomatous polyp
benign biliary stricture
benign papillary stenosis
benign prostatic hypertrophy
benign tumor
benign ulcer
benignity
Béniqué catheter guide
Béniqué dilator
Béniqué sound
Benke everter
Bennell bandage
Bennell elevator
Bennell forceps
Bennell fracture
Bennett approach
Bennett bone elevator
Bennett bone retractor
Bennett cilia forceps
Bennett common duct dilator
Bennett dislocation
Bennett elevator
Bennett epilation forceps
Bennett foreign body spud
Bennett fracture
Bennett monitoring spirometer
Bennett operation
Bennett pressure-cycled
    ventilator
Bennett respirator
Bennett retractor
Bennett spud
Bennett tibia retractor
Bennett valve
Bennett ventilator
Benoist scale
benoxinate hydrochloride
    anesthetic agent
Benson pylorus separator
Benson separator
bent blade

bent blade plate
bent fracture
bent hook
bent needle
Bent operation
Bent shoulder excision
Bentall cardiovascular prosthesis
Bentall inclusion technique
Bentall procedure
Bentley button
Bentley filter
Bentley oxygenator
Bentley transducer
Bentson floppy-tip guide wire
Bentson guide wire
Bentson wire
benzocaine anesthetic agent
benzoquinonium chloride anesthetic agent
Beraud valve
Berbecker needle
Berbecker pliers
Berbecker wire cutter
Berbridge scissors
Berci-Shore choledochoscope
Berci-Shore nephroscope
Berci-Ward laryngopharyngoscope
Berens bident electrode
Berens capsule forceps
Berens clamp
Berens compressor
Berens conical eye implant
Berens corneal knife
Berens corneal transplant
Berens corneal transplant forceps
Berens corneal transplant scissors
Berens corneoscleral punch
Berens corneoscleral transplant
Berens dilator
Berens esophageal retractor
Berens everter
Berens expressor

Berens eye implant
Berens eye retractor
Berens eye speculum
Berens forceps
Berens graft
Berens hook
Berens implant
Berens iridocapsulotomy
Berens iridocapsulotomy scissors
Berens keratome
Berens knife
Berens lens expressor
Berens lens loupe
Berens lens scoop
Berens lid elevator
Berens lid everter
Berens loupe
Berens mastectomy retractor
Berens mastectomy skin flap retractor
Berens muscle clamp
Berens muscle forceps
Berens muscle recession forceps
Berens needle holder
Berens operation
Berens orbital compressor
Berens orbital implant
Berens plastic spatula
Berens prosthesis
Berens pterygium transplant
Berens punch
Berens punctum dilator
Berens pyramidal eye implant
Berens retractor
Berens scissors
Berens scleral hook
Berens sclerectomy
Berens sclerotomy knife
Berens scoop
Berens skin flap retractor
Berens spatula
Berens speculum
Berens sphere eye implant
Berens suture forceps
Berens thyroid retractor

Berens-Rosa eye implant
Berens-Rosa scleral implant
Berens-Smith operation
Bereyea transurethral bladder
    suspension
Bergen retractor
Bergenhem implantation of
    ureter into rectum
Bergenhem procedure
Berger crusher
Berger forceps
Berger interscapular amputation
Berger operation
Berger sign
Berger symptom
Bergeron pillar forceps
Bergh cilia forceps
Berghmann-Foerster sponge
    forceps
Bergman bandage scissors
Bergman forceps
Bergman mallet
Bergman plaster scissors
Bergmann hernia
Bergmann hydrocele repair
Bergmann incision
Bergmann layer
Bergmann-Israel incision
Berke cilia forceps
Berke clamp
Berke forceps
Berke operation
Berke ptosis clamp
Berke ptosis correction
Berke ptosis forceps
Berke-Leahy technique
Berkeley cannula
Berkeley clamp
Berkeley forceps
Berkeley retractor
Berkeley suction unit
Berkeley Vacurette machine
Berke-Motais ptosis correction
Berkowitz-Bellis herniorrhaphy
Berlin edema
Berlind-Auvard retractor
Berlind-Auvard speculum

Berman airway
Berman angiographic catheter
Berman aortic clamp
Berman cardiac catheter
Berman catheter
Berman clamp
Berman disposable airway
Berman eye director
Berman intubating pharyngeal
    airway
Berman localizer
Berman locator device
Berman magnet
Berman metal locator
Berman-Gartland technique
Berman-Moorhead locator
Berman-Moorhead metal
    locator
Berman-Werner probe
Berna infant abdominal
    retractor
Berna retractor
Bernard operation
Bernay gauze packer
Bernay hydrocele trocar
Bernay retractor
Bernay tracheal retractor
Bernay uterine packer
Berndt hip ruler
Berne clips hemostat
Berne forceps
Berne nasal forceps
Berne nasal rasp
Berne nasal raspatory
Berne rasp
Bernheimer fibers
Bernstein catheter
Bernstein gastroscope
Bernstein light
Bernstein modification gastro-
    scope
Bernstein retractor
Bernstein test
Berridge gauze scissors
berry aneurysm
Berry circle
Berry clamp

Berry forceps
Berry ligament
Berry operation
Berry raspatory
Berry rib raspatory
Berry rotating sheath
Berry sternal needle holder
Berry uterine-elevating forceps
Berry-Lambert elevator
Bertel x-ray position
Bertin bone
Bertin ligament
Bertrand target
Bertrand tract
Bertrandi sutures
Berwick dye
Best clamp
Best colon clamp
Best common duct stone
    forceps
Best forceps
Best gallstone forceps
Best operation
Best right-angle colon clamp
Best telescope
beta finger-grip catheter
    connector
beta irradiation applicator
beta ray microscope
beta therapy eye applicator
Beta-Cap II closure system
Betacel-Biotronik pacemaker
Betadine
Betadine Helafoam solution
Betadine scrub
Betadine soap
Betadine solution
beta-lactose pack
betatron irradiation
Bethea sheet holder
Bethea sign
Bethke iridectomy
Bethune bone cutter
Bethune clamp
Bethune elevator
Bethune hook
Bethune lobectomy tourniquet

Bethune lung tourniquet
Bethune nerve hook
Bethune periosteal elevator
Bethune phrenic retractor
Bethune retractor
Bethune rib rongeur
Bethune rib shears
Bethune rongeur
Bethune shears
Bethune tourniquet
Bethune-Coryllos rib shears
Bettman empyema tube
Bettman gauze
Bettman-Forash thermopore
Bettman-Forash thoracotome
Bettman-Noyes forceps
Bevan abdominal incision
Bevan forceps
Bevan gallbladder forceps
Bevan hemostatic forceps
Bevan incision
Bevan operation
Bevan vertical elliptical skin
    incision of abdomen
Bevan-Rochet operation
bevel
beveled, bevelled
beveled speculum
beveled vein
Beyea operation
Beyer atticus punch
Beyer bone rongeur
Beyer endaural rongeur
Beyer forceps
Beyer needle
Beyer paracentesis needle
Beyer punch
Beyer rongeur
Beyer rongeur forceps
Beyer-Stille bone rongeur
bezoar
Bezold abscess
Bezold ganglion
Bezold mastoiditis
Bezold perforation
Bezold reflex
Bezold sign

Bezold triad
Bezold-Edelman tuning fork
Bezold-Jarisch reflex
BF large-core bronchoscope
biactive coagulation set cautery
biarticulate
Bias hip prosthesis
Bias porous metal hip
    prosthesis
bias stockinette
Bias total hip system
bias-cut
bias-cut stockinette
bias-cut stockinette dressing
biatrial hypertrophy
biaxial joint
BIB (biliointestinal bypass)
bibasally
bibasilar atelectasis
bibasilar rales
bicap cautery
bicap hemostatic system
bicap probe
bicapsular
bicarotid trunk
bicaval
Bicek retractor
Bicek vaginal retractor
Bi-Centric endoprosthesis
Biceps bipolar coagulator
biceps brachii, musculus
biceps femoris, musculus
biceps jerk
biceps muscle
biceps reflex
biceps tendon sheath
Bicer-val prosthetic valve
bicipital
bicipital groove
bicipital rib
bicipital tendinitis
Bick ectropion repair
Bick procedure
Bickel ring
bicollis uterus
biconcave
biconcave lens

biconvex
biconvex lens
bicornis uterus
bicornuate uterus
bicoudate catheter
bicoudé catheter
bicuspid aortic valve
bicuspid teeth
bicuspid valve
bicuspid valvotomy
bicuspid valvulotomy
bicuspidate
bicuspidization
bicycle dynamometer
bicycle ergometer
bicylindrical lens
bident retractor
bidirectional
bidirectional cavopulmonary
    anastomosis
bidirectional shunt
bidiscoidal placenta
Bielschowsky head tilt test
Bielschowsky operation
Bielschowsky-Jansky disease
Biemer vessel clip
Biemer vessel clip applier
biepicondylar line
Bier amputation
Bier amputation saw
Bier anesthesia
Bier arm block anesthesia
Bier block
Bier block anesthesia unit
Bier combined treatment
Bier local anesthesia
Bier operation
Bier passive hyperemia
Bier treatment
Bierer tenaculum
Bierer vacuum
Bierhoff crutch
Bierman needle
Biesenberger mammaplasty
Biesenberger operation
Biesenberger reduction
    mammaplasty

Biethium ostomy rod
Bietti eye implant
Bietti implant cataract lens
Bietti lens
bifascicular block
bifascicular heart block
biferious pulse
bifid
bifid clitoris
bifid hook
bifid pelvis
bifid pinna
bifid retractor
bifid thumb
bifid tongue
bifid uvula
bifixation
bifocal demand pacemaker
bifocal fixation
bifocal glasses
bifocal lens
bifocal pacer
bifrontal
bifrontal craniotomy
bifurcated aortofemoral
    prosthesis
bifurcated ligament
bifurcated retractor
bifurcated seamless prosthesis
bifurcated vascular graft
bifurcation
bifurcation graft
bifurcation of gallbladder
bifurcation of renal pelvis
bifurcation of trachea
bifurcation of ureter
bifurcation of vessels
bifurcation osteotomy
bifurcation point
bifurcation prosthesis
bifurcational lesion
Bigelow calvarium clamp
Bigelow clamp
Bigelow dislocation
Bigelow evacuator
Bigelow forceps
Bigelow ligament

Bigelow litholapaxy
Bigelow lithotrite
Bigelow operation
Bigelow sutures
bigeminal pregnancy
bigeminal pulse
bigeminal rhythm
bigeminy
Biggs mammaplasty retractor
bike brace
bilabe
bilateral internal mammary
    artery (BIMA)
bilateral lithotomy
bilateral procedures
Bilboa-Dotter nasogastric tube
bile
bile ascites
bile bag
bile canaliculi
bile concretion
bile duct
bile duct adenoma
bile duct lumen
bile duct proliferation
bile duct stone
bile duct stricture
bile lake
bile plug
bile salts
bile stasis
bileaflet heart valve
bileaflet prosthesis
bileaflet tilting-disk prosthetic
    valve
bile-stained fluid
bile-tinged fluid
Bilhaut-Cloquet wedge resec-
    tion
Bili mask
biliary atresia
biliary balloon catheter
biliary balloon probe
biliary calculus
biliary catheter
biliary dilation
biliary duct

biliary duct dilator
biliary duct prosthesis
biliary dyskinesia
biliary endoprosthesis
biliary enteric anastomosis
biliary manometry
biliary obstruction
biliary plexus
biliary procedure
biliary radicle
biliary retractor
biliary sphincter
biliary stent
biliary stone basket
biliary tract
biliary tract stone
biliary tract tray
biliary tree
biliary-cutaneous fistula
biliary-duodenal fistula
biliary-duodenal pressure
    gradient
biliary-enteric fistula
Bili-Dosimeter
Bililite
bilioduodenal prosthesis
bilioenteric fistula
biliointestinal bypass (BIB)
biliopancreatic bypass (BPB)
biliopancreatic shunt
biliopleural fistula
bilious
bilirubin pigment gallstone
bilirubinate stone
Bili-Timer
Bill axis traction handle
Bill traction handle
Billeau curet
Billeau ear curet
Billeau ear knife
Billeau ear loop
Billeau loop
Billeau Teflon-coated loop
billet
Billroth anastomosis
Billroth forceps
Billroth gastrectomy

Billroth gastroduodenoscopy
Billroth gastroenterostomy
Billroth gastrojejunostomy
Billroth gastrostomy
Billroth hypertrophy
Billroth operation
Billroth ovarian trocar
Billroth retractor
Billroth tongue excision
Billroth tube
Billroth tumor forceps
Billroth I anastomosis
Billroth I gastroduodenostomy
Billroth I gastroenterostomy
Billroth I gastrostomy
Billroth I operation
Billroth II anastomosis
Billroth II gastrectomy
Billroth II gastroenterostomy
Billroth II gastrojejunostomy
Billroth II gastrostomy
Billroth II operation
bilobate
bilobate placenta
bilobed
bilobed flap
bilobed gallbladder
bilobed placenta
bilobed skin flap
bilobed skin flap technique
bilocular joint
bilocularis uterus
bilumen mammary implant
BIMA (bilateral internal
    mammary artery)
BIMA reconstruction
bimalleolar fracture
bimanual examination
bimanual pelvic examina-
    tion
bimanual percussion
bimanual version
bimaxillary dentoalveolar
    protrusion
Bi-Metric hip system
Bimler activator
Bimler appliance

binangle
binangled chisel
binary fission
binasal
binasal pharyngeal airway
binaural
binaural stethoscope
binder
Binet scale
Bing sign
Bing-Taussig heart procedure
Binkhorst eye implant
Binkhorst implant
Binkhorst intraocular lens
    implant
Binkhorst lens
Binkhorst lens forceps
Binkhorst lens implant
Binnie operation
binocular
binocular accommodation
binocular bandage
binocular dressing
binocular eye dressing
binocular instrument
binocular loupe
binocular microscope
binocular ophthalmoscope
binocular prism
binocular prism loupe
binocular shield
binocular slit lamp
binocular surgical loupe
binocular tube
Bio Flote
Bio Foam Eggcrate
Bio Gard critical care flotation
    unit
bioacrylic interface
Biobrane adhesive
Biobrane dressing
Biobrane glove
Biobrane skin substitute
bioceramics
Bioclusive drape
Bioclusive dressing
Bioclusive transparent dressing

biocompatible
Biocor heart valve
Biocor prosthetic valve
Biodex machine
Biodex test
Biodrape dressing
biodynamics
BioDyne
bioequivalent
biograft
biograft umbilical prosthesis
Bio-Groove total hip prosthesis
biohazard container
biohazard operating technique
biohazard specimen
bioimplant
bioingrowth
BioKleen
Biolox ceramic femoral head
biomaterial
biomechanical ankle platform
    system (BAPS)
biomechanics
Bio-Med MVP-10 pediatric
    ventilator
Bio-Medicus pump
biomembrane
Biomet bed
Biomet femoral component
Biomet fracture brace
Biomet impactor
Biomet instruments
Biomet plug
Biomet total knee instruments
Biomet Velcro wrist support
biometric profile
biometric prosthesis
biometry probe
biomicroscope
biomicroscopy
Bio-Modular shoulder system
biomort
bion
Bionit II vascular prosthesis
Bionit prosthesis
Bionit vascular graft
Bionit vascular prosthesis

biophotometer
Biophysic Medical laser
biophysical profile (BPP)
BioPolyMeric vascular graft
bioprosthesis
bioprosthetic heart valve
bioprosthetic valve
biopsy
biopsy accessories
biopsy after radiation
biopsy by curettage
biopsy cannula
biopsy curet
biopsy forceps
biopsy instruments
biopsy loop electrode
biopsy needle
biopsy punch
biopsy punch forceps
biopsy set
biopsy specimen forceps
biopsy suction curet
biopsy telescope
biopsy thorascope
biopsy tongs
bioptic aid
bioptic biopsy
bioptic telescope
bioptome
Bio-Pump for bypass surgery
biorbital angle
biorhythm
Biot breathing
Biot sign
BioTac biopsy cannula
biotesting
biotome
Biotronik demand pacemaker
Biotronik pacemaker
Bio-Vascular prosthetic valve
Bi-OX III ear oximeter
biparietal
biparietal craniotomy
biparietal diameter (BPD)
biparietal hump
biparietal suture
bipartite

bipartite patella
bipartite placenta
bipartitus uterus
bipedal
bipedicle digital visor flap
bipedicle flap
bipedicle mucoperiosteal flap
bipennate muscle
bipenniform
biphase external pin fixation
biphase Morris fixation
    apparatus
biplane
biplane angiography
biplane cerebral angiography
biplane cineangiogram
biplane orthogonal angiogram
biplane pelvic arteriogram
biplane projection
biplane quantitative coronary
    arteriogram
biplane sector probe
biplane view
biplaner II control
bipolar catheter
bipolar catheter electrode
bipolar cautery
bipolar coagulating forceps
bipolar coagulation
bipolar coagulation forceps
bipolar coagulation-suction
    forceps
bipolar coagulator
bipolar connecting cord
bipolar cup hip prosthesis
bipolar depth electrode
bipolar electrocoagulation
bipolar electrode
bipolar eye forceps
bipolar forceps
bipolar lead
bipolar limb leads
bipolar Medtronic pacemaker
bipolar microforceps
bipolar needle
bipolar pacemaker
bipolar pacemaker leads

bipolar pacing catheter
bipolar pacing electrode
    catheter
bipolar placement of electrodes
bipolar probe
bipolar prosthesis
bipolar temporary pacemaker
    catheter
bipolar total hip
bipolar transsphenoidal forceps
bipolar version
biprism applanation tonometer
Bipro orthodontic appliance
Birch trocar
Bircher bone-holding clamp
Bircher cartilage clamp
Bircher meniscus knife
Bircher operation
Birch-Hirschfield lamp
Birch-Hirschfield light
Bird pressure-cycled ventilator
Bird respirator
Bird table
bird's beak distal esophagus
birefringence
birefringent
Birkett forceps
Birkett hemostatic forceps
Birkett hernia
Birnberg bow intrauterine
    device
Birnberg traction bow
Birt-A-Switch handle
Birtcher cautery
Birtcher coagulator
Birtcher defibrillator
Birtcher electrode
Birtcher electrosurgery unit
Birtcher electrosurgical instru-
    ments
Birtcher electrosurgical needle
Birtcher hyfrecator
Birtcher hyfrecator cautery
Birtcher Hyfrecutter
Birtcher proctological electrode
    set
Birtcher proctology set

Birtcher proctosigmoid desicca-
    tion set
birth canal
birth injury
birth trauma
birthing room
birthmark
Bischoff corona
Bischoff crown
Bischoff myelotomy
Bischoff operation
bisect
bisected mass
bisection
bisection biopsy
Bishop antrum perforator
Bishop antrum trocar
Bishop bone clamp
Bishop chisel
Bishop gouge
Bishop mastoid gouge
Bishop oscillatory electric bone
    saw
Bishop perforator
Bishop saw
Bishop sphygmoscope
Bishop tendon tucker
Bishop tissue forceps
Bishop-Black tendon tucker
Bishop-Black tucker
Bishop-Coop enterostomy
Bishop-DeWitt tendon tucker
Bishop-DeWitt tucker
Bishop-Harman (B-H)
Bishop-Harman anterior
    chamber cannula
Bishop-Harman anterior
    chamber irrigator
Bishop-Harman cannula
Bishop-Harman dressing
Bishop-Harman dressing
    forceps
Bishop-Harman forceps
Bishop-Harman iris forceps
Bishop-Harman irrigating
    cannula
Bishop-Harman irrigator

Bishop-Harman tip
Bishop-Peter tendon tucker
bisiliac diameter
Bi-Soft contact lens
bispherical lens
bispinous diameter
Bissell operation
bistable imaging
bistoury
    Brophy bistoury
    Brophy bistoury knife
    Converse bistoury
    ear bistoury
    Jackson bistoury
    Jackson tracheotomic
      bistoury
    nasal bistoury
    tracheal bistoury
    tracheotomic bistoury
bistoury blade
bistoury knife
bite biopsy
bite block
bite line
bite splint
bitemporal
bitemporal craniotomy
bitemporal diameter
biterminal electrode
biting forceps
biting punch
Bitoric lens
bivalve, bivalved
bivalved cannula
bivalved ear speculum
bivalved elliptical incision
bivalved incision
bivalved plaster cast
bivalved retractor
bivalved speculum
bivalved tube
biventricular assist device
    (BVAD)
Bivona low-resistance voice
    prosthesis
Bivona tracheostomy tube
Bivona voice prosthesis

Bizzarri-Guiffrida knife
Bizzarri-Guiffrida laryngoscope
Bjerrum scotoma
Bjerrum scotometer
Bjerrum screen
Bjerrum sign
Björk diathermy forceps
Björk drill
Björk operation
Björk-Shiley aortic valve
    prosthesis
Björk-Shiley heart valve
Björk-Shiley mitral valve
    prosthesis
Björk-Shiley prosthesis
Björk-Shiley prosthetic aortic
    valve
Björk-Shiley prosthetic mitral
    valve
Björk-Shiley valve prosthesis
BK amputation (below-knee
    amputation)
BL (buccolingual)
black blood clot
Black bone and skin rasp
black box of upper GI tract
black braided sutures
Black clamp
black faceted stone
black light
Black meatus clamp
black pigment gallstone
Black retractor
black silk sutures
black twisted sutures
Blackburn tractor
Black-Decker needle
black-dot heel
blackened laser instruments
Blackett-Healy position
Blackmon needle
Blackwood meniscal repair
Blackwood suture instrument
Black-Wylie dilator
Black-Wylie obstetric dilator
bladder
bladder biopsy

bladder blade
bladder bubble
bladder calculus
bladder carcinoma classification
bladder catheter
bladder dilator
bladder dome
bladder evacuator
bladder flap
bladder forceps
bladder hernia
bladder irrigating valve
bladder irrigation control clamp
bladder mucosa
bladder neck
bladder neck contracture
bladder neck ridge
bladder neck spreader
bladder pacemaker
bladder pillars
bladder reflection
bladder retractor
bladder specimen forceps
bladder stimulation
bladder suspension
bladder syringe
bladder trocar
bladder tube
bladder wall
bladder-prostate model
blade
    adenotome blade
    Aggressor meniscal blade
    angulated-blade elec-
      trode
    anterior commissure
      laryngoscope blade
    arachnoid-shape Beaver
      blade
    arachnoid-shape blade
    Arthro-Lok system of
      Beaver blades
    ASR blade
    ASSI cranial blades
    AtheroCath spinning
      blade catheter
    autopsy blade

blade *continued*
    autopsy blade handle
    Balfour blade
    Balfour center blade
    Balfour fourth-blade
      extension
    banana (Beaver blade)
    Bard-Parker autopsy
      blade
    Bard-Parker blade
    Bard-Parker surgical
      blade
    Barton blade
    Baxter disposable blade
    Beaver Arthro-Lok blade
    Beaver bent blade
    Beaver blade
    Beaver blade banana
    Beaver blade cataract
      knife
    Beaver blade chuck
      handle
    Beaver blade discission
      knife
    Beaver blade handle
    Beaver blade keratome
    Beaver blade rosette
    Beaver cataract blade
    Beaver cataract knife
      blade
    Beaver DeBakey blade
    Beaver discission blade
    Beaver discission knife
      blade
    Beaver eye surgery blade
    Beaver keratome blade
    Beaver Mini-Blades
    Beaver myringotomy
      blade
    Beaver rhinoplasty blade
    Beaver surgical blade
    Beaver surgical blade
      handle
    Beaver tonsillectomy
      blade
    bent blade
    bent blade plate

blade *continued*
　bistoury blade
　bladder blade
　Blount bent blade
　Blount blade plate
　Blount V-blade
　broad-blade forceps
　cam blade-tipped
　　catheter
　carbolized knife blade
　Castroviejo bladebreaker
　　knife
　Castroviejo razor blade
　　holder
　Castroviejo razor
　　bladebreaker
　cataract blade
　center blade
　cephalic blade forceps
　cervical biopsy blade
　cervical blade
　chondroplastic Beaver
　　blade
　chondroplastic blade
　circular blade
　Cloward blade
　cold blade biopsy
　condylar blade plate
　Converse blade retractor
　Cooley-Pontius blade
　Cooley-Pontius sternal
　　blade
　Cottle single-blade
　　retractor
　crescentic blade
　Crile blade
　Curdy blade
　Deaver blade
　DeBakey Beaver blade
　DeBakey blade
　deep spreader blade
　discission blade
　Dixon blade
　Dixon center blade
　double-angled blade
　double-angled blade
　　plate

blade *continued*
　Dynagrip blade handle
　ear surgery Beaver blade
　ear surgery blade
　Elliot femoral condyle
　　blade plate
　Epstein blade
　Epstein hemilaminec-
　　tomy blade
　expandable blade
　eye blade
　eye knife blade
　eye surgery blade
　fenestrated blade forceps
　flat-blade-tipped catheter
　folding blade
　fourth-blade extension
　Gigli-saw blade
　Gill blade
　Goulian blade
　graft blade plate
　Grieshaber blade
　Guedel blade
　Guedel laryngoscope
　　blade
　Hammond blade
　Hammond winged
　　retractor blade
　Hebra blade
　hemilaminectomy blade
　Hendren blade
　Hendren pediatric
　　retractor blade
　Hendren retractor blade
　Hibbs blade
　Hibbs retractor blade
　Hibbs spinal retractor
　　blade
　Hopp anterior commis-
　　sure laryngoscope
　　blade
　Hopp blade
　Hopp laryngoscope
　　blade
　Horgan blade
　Horgan center blade
　House blade

blade *continued*

House knife blade
keratome blade
Kielland blade
knife blade
LaForce adenotome
blade
laminectomy retractor
blade
laryngoscope blade
laryngoscope folding
blade
LaserSonics EndoBlade
LaserSonics Nd:YAG
LaserBlade scalpel
LaserSonics SurgiBlade
Lemmon blade
Lundsgaard blade
M Beaver blade
M-blade
MacIntosh blade
malleable blade retractor
McPherson-Wheeler
blade
microblade knife
Micro-Sharp blade
microvitreoretinal blade
(MVR)
Morse blade
Mueller tongue blade
Mullins blade
Murphy-Balfour center
blade
MVR blade (microvitreo-
retinal)
Myocure blade
nasal saw blade
ocutome vitreous blade
Oertli razor bladebreaker
knife
Orandi blade
Padgett blade
Park blade
Paufique blade
Personna surgical blade
platinum blade electrode

blade *continued*

razor blade
retractor blade
retrograde Beaver blade
round-blade scissors
scimitar blade
scimitar-blade knife
self-retaining retractor
blade
Sharpoint V-lance blade
shoulder blade
sickle-shaped Beaver
blade
sickle-shaped blade
spinal retractor blade
sternal blade
sternal retractor blade
straight-blade electrode
straight-blade laryngo-
scope
Stryker blade
Superblade
surgical blade
Swann-Morton blade
Swann-Morton surgical
blade
Swiss blade
Swiss blade holder
Swiss bladebreaker
Taylor blade
three-bladed clamp
tongue blade
tongue retractor blade
Tooke blade
trephine blade
tubular blade
Tucker-Luikart blade
two-bladed dilator
V-blade plate
Vascutech circular blade
vectis blade
Weck-blade knife
Weinberg blade
winged retractor blade
wood tongue blade
Zalkind-Balfour blade

blade *continued*
 Ziegler blade
 Zimmer femoral condyle
  blade plate
blade and balloon atrial
 septostomy
blade electrode
blade holder
blade plate
blade plate fixation device
blade retractor
bladebreaker
bladebreaker holder
bladebreaker knife
Blade-Wilde ear forceps
Blair approach
Blair arthrodesis
Blair chisel
Blair cleft palate clamp
Blair cleft palate elevator
Blair cleft palate knife
Blair elevator
Blair Gigli-saw guide
Blair head drape
Blair hook
Blair incision
Blair knife
Blair modification of Gellhorn
 pessary
Blair operation
Blair ptosis correction operation
Blair retractor
Blair saw guide
Blair serrefine
Blair silicone drain
Blair-Brown graft
Blair-Brown implant
Blair-Brown knife
Blair-Brown needle
Blair-Brown needle holder
Blair-Brown operation
Blair-Brown prosthesis
Blair-Brown retractor
Blair-Brown skin graft
Blair-Brown skin graft knife
Blair-Brown vacuum retractor

Blair-Brown-McDowell opera-
 tion
Blair-Byars operation
Blair-Morris technique
Blair-Omer technique
Blair-Wehrbein operation
Blaisdell skin pencil
Blake curet
Blake drain
Blake dressing forceps
Blake ear forceps
Blake esophageal tube
Blake forceps
Blake gallstone forceps
Blake knife
Blake rake
Blake silicone drain
Blakemore esophageal tube
Blakemore tube
Blakemore-Sengstaken
 tube
Blakesley decompressor
Blakesley ethmoid forceps
Blakesley forceps
Blakesley lacrimal trephine
Blakesley retractor
Blakesley septal bone forceps
Blakesley septal compression
 forceps
Blakesley septal forceps
Blakesley tongue depressor
Blakesley trephine
Blakesley uvula retractor
Blakesley-Wilde ear forceps
Blakesley-Wilde ethmoid
 forceps
Blalock anastomosis
Blalock clamp
Blalock forceps
Blalock operation
Blalock procedure
Blalock pulmonary clamp
Blalock pulmonic stenosis
 clamp
Blalock shunt
Blalock sutures

Blalock-Hanlon atrial septectomy
Blalock-Hanlon operation
Blalock-Niedner clamp
Blalock-Niedner pulmonic clamp
Blalock-Niedner pulmonic stenosis clamp
Blalock-Taussig anastomosis
Blalock-Taussig operation
Blalock-Taussig shunt
blanch
Blanchard clamp
Blanchard cryptotome
Blanchard forceps
Blanchard hemorrhoid forceps
Blanchard pile clamp
blanched skin
blanching
blanching of hand
blanching of sclera
blanching of trabecular meshwork
blanching reaction
Blanco retractor
Blanco scissors
Blanco valve spreader
Bland cervical traction forceps
Bland cervical traction vulsellum
Bland perineal retractor
bland thrombosis
Bland vulsellum forceps
Blandy urethroplasty
blanket sutures
Blasius lid operation
Blasius operation
Blaskovics operation
Blaskovics ptosis correction
blast injury
blastic metastasis
blastoma
Blasucci catheter
Blasucci clamp
Blasucci curved-tip ureteral catheter

Blasucci pigtail ureteral catheter
Blasucci tip
Blasucci ureteral catheter
Blatt operation
Blaydes corneal forceps
Blaydes forceps
Blazina patellofemoral repair
Blazina procedure
Blazina prosthesis
BLB mask (Baker-Lima-Baker mask)
BLB mask (Boothby, Lovelace, Bulbulian mask)
bleb
Bleck iliopsoas recession
Bleck technique
bled
Bledsoe brace
Bledsoe cast brace
Bledsoe knee brace
Bledsoe leg brace
Bledsoe passive motion exerciser
bleeder
bleeding
bleeding esophageal varices
bleeding lesion
bleeding point
Bleier clip for tubal sterilization
Blenderm surgical tape dressing
blepharectomy
blepharochalasis
blepharoplasty
blepharoplasty clip
blepharoptosis
blepharorrhaphy
blepharostat
blepharotomy
Blessig cyst
Blessig groove
Blessig-Iwanoff cyst
blighted ovum
blind limb
blind nailing
blind percutaneous liver biopsy
blind Rush nailing
blind stump

blind upper esophageal pouch
blink reflex
blister
blitz bath
Bloch-Paul-Mixter operation
block anesthesia
block anesthesia needle
block dissection
Block entropion repair
Block gastric hemostat
block osteotomy
Block right coronary guiding
    catheter
block technique
blockage
Blockaine anesthetic agent
blocked airway
blocked breathing passage
blocked nasal passage
Blocker operation
Bloedorn applicator
Blohmka hemostat
Blohmka tonsil forceps
Blohmka tonsil hemostat
Blohmka vesicostomy
Blom-Singer post-laryngectomy
    valve
Blom-Singer tracheoesophageal
    fistula
Blom-Singer vocal reconstruc-
    tion
Blom-Singer voice valve
blood blister
blood clot
blood coagulation factor
blood count
blood expander
blood patch injection
blood pressure
blood pressure cuff
blood pump
blood sampling instrument
blood staining
blood supply
blood transfusion
blood vessel bridges
blood vessel supporter

blood vessels
blood warmer cuffs
blood-brain barrier
blood-flow probe
blood-fluid warmer
Bloodgood inguinal hernior-
    rhaphy
Bloodgood operation
bloodless
bloodless amputation
bloodless circumcision clamp
bloodless field
bloodless operation
blood-tinged
blood-tinged ascites
Bloodwell forceps
Bloodwell tissue forceps
Bloodwell vascular tissue
    forceps
Bloodwell-Brown forceps
bloody ascites
bloody peritoneal fluid
bloody stool
bloody tap
Bloominstadt lines
Blot perforator
Blot scissors
blot-and-dot hemorrhage
blotchy
Blotts hemostat
Blount bent blade
Blount blade plate
Blount bone retractor
Blount bone spreader
Blount brace
Blount disease
Blount displacement osteotomy
Blount hip retractor
Blount knee retractor
Blount knee staple
Blount mallet
Blount operation
Blount osteotome
Blount osteotomy
Blount plate
Blount procedure for bone
    growth asymmetry

Blount retractor
Blount scoliosis osteotome
Blount staple
Blount stapling
Blount V-blade
blow-by apparatus
blow-by oxygen
blow-by ventilator
blow-hole ileostomy
blow-in fracture
blowing wound
blown pupil
blow-out fracture
blow-out fracture of orbital
    floor
blow-out lesion
blow-out view projection
blow-up gloves
blue cotton sutures
blue dome cyst
Blue Max triple-lumen catheter
blue nevus
Blue rectal suction tip
blue ring pessary
blue sclera
blue Shepard grommet tube
blue sponge dressing
blue twisted cotton sutures
blue-tip aspirator
Blum arterial scissors
Blum forceps
Blumberg sign
Blumensaal line
Blumenthal bone rongeur
Blumenthal rongeur
Blumer rectal shelf
Blumer shelf
Blundell-Jones operation
Blundell-Jones osteotomy
blunt abdominal trauma
blunt and sharp dissection
blunt dissection
blunt dissection and snare
    technique
blunt dissector
blunt hook
blunt injury

blunt needle
blunt nerve hook
blunt obturator
blunt periosteal elevator
blunt probe
blunt rake retractor
blunt retractor
blunt scissors
blunted costophrenic angle
blunting of calyces
blunting of costophrenic angle
blunting of nerve
blunting of sulcus
blunting of valve
bluntly dissected
board
boardlike retractor
Boari button
Boari flap
Boari operation
Boari-Küss flap
Boari-Ockerblad flap reimplan-
    tation
Boariplasty
Boas point
Boas sign
boat nail
boat-shaped heart
Bobath sling
Bobb cholelithotomy
Bobb operation
bobbin
Bobechko rod
Boberg-Ans implant
Boberg-Ans lens
Bobroff operation
Bocca neck dissection
Bochdalek foramen
Bochdalek hernia
Bochdalek valve
Bock foot
Bock nerve
Bock prosthesis
Bodansky unit
Bodenheimer anoscope
Bodenheimer proctoscope
Bodenheimer rectal speculum

Bodenheimer speculum
Bodian discission knife
Bodian scissors
bodkin
Bodnar knee retractor
body cast
body cavity
body jacket
body of fornix
body of Luys
body scanning technique
body section radiography
Boeck sarcoid disease
Boehler (also Böhler)
Boehler angle of calcaneus
Boehler bone rongeur
Boehler clamp
Boehler fracture frame
Boehler pin
Boehler reducing frame
Boehler splint
Boehler tongs
Boehler traction bow
Boehler tractor
Boehler wire splint
Boehler-Braun frame
Boehler-Braun splint
Boehm anoscope
Boehm cord
Boehm current controller
Boehm proctoscope
Boehm sigmoidoscope
Boerema anterior gastropexy
Boerema-Crile operation
Boerhaave syndrome
Boerhaave tear
Boettcher artery forceps
Boettcher forceps
Boettcher hemostat
Boettcher hook
Boettcher pulmonary artery
    clamp
Boettcher pulmonary artery
    forceps
Boettcher scissors
Boettcher tonsil artery forceps
Boettcher tonsil hook

Boettcher tonsil scissors
Boettcher trocar
Boettcher-Farlow snare
Boettcher-Jennings gag
Boettcher-Schnidt antrum trocar
boggy
boggy prostate
boggy uterus
Bogros space
Bogue operation
Böhler (see *Boehler*)
Bohlet angle
Bohlman pin
Bohlman vertebrectomy
Böhm operation
Bohn nodules
Boies cutting forceps
Boies forceps
Boies nasal elevator
Boies nasal fracture elevator
Boies plastic surgery elevator
Boiler septal trephine
Boiler trephine
Boilo head mirror
Boilo laryngeal mirror
Boilo retinoscope
Bolder hemostat
Boldrey brace
Bolex camera
Bolex cine-camera
Boley gouge
Boley retractor
bolster
        cotton bolster
        cotton bolster dressing
bolster finger
bolster operation
bolster sutures
bolt
        Barr bolt
        Camino ventricular bolt
        cannulated bolt
        DePuy bolt
        Fenton bolt
        hexhead bolt
        Hubbard bolt
        Norman tibial bolt

bolt *continued*
    Nylok bolt
    Richmond bolt
    transfixion bolt
    Webb bolt
    Webb stove bolt
    Wilson bolt
    Zimmer bolt
    Zimmer tibial bolt
Bolt sign
Bolton forceps
Boltzmann distribution
Boltzmann factor
bolus (*pl.* boluses)
bolus dressing
bolus injection
bolus ties over graft
bolused
Bomgart stomal bag
Bonaccolto capsule fragment
    forceps
Bonaccolto eye implant
Bonaccolto forceps
Bonaccolto jeweler's-type
    forceps
Bonaccolto magnet
Bonaccolto scleral ring
Bonaccolto utility forceps
Bonaccolto utility pickup
    forceps
Bonaccolto-Flieringa operation
Bonaccolto-Flieringa scleral ring
Bonchek-Shiley cardiac jacket
Bonchek-Shiley vein distention
    system
Bond forceps
Bond placenta forceps
Bond splint
Bondy mastoidectomy (type I,
    II, III)
Bondy operation
bone
bone age
bone attenuation coefficient
bone bank
bone biopsy instruments
bone block

bone bur
bone calipers
bone callus
bone cement
bone chip
bone chisel
bone clamp
bone crusher
bone curet
bone cutter
bone density
bone dowel
bone drill
bone duction
bone elevator
bone extension clamp
bone file
bone flap
bone gouge
bone graft
bone graft holder
bone graft material
bone graft peg
bone growth stimulation
bone growth stimulator (see
    also *stimulator*)
    AME bone growth
      stimulator
    implantable bone growth
      stimulator
    Orgen SpF spinal bone
      growth stimulator
    OrthoGen bone growth
      stimulator
    OrthoPak bone growth
      stimulator
    OsteoGen bone growth
      stimulator
    Osteo-Stim electrical
      bone growth stimula-
      tor
    Spinal-Stim bone growth
      stimulator
bone hand drill
bone hook
bone hump
bone impactor

bone implant
bone infarct
bone island
bone landmarks
bone lesion
bone lever
bone marrow
bone marrow embolism
bone marrow needle
bone marrow pressure
bone marrow tap
bone marrow transplant
bone morphogenic protein
bone pain
bone plate
bone plug
bone prosthesis
bone rasp
bone remodeling
bone rongeur
bone salts
bone saw
bone scan
bone screw
bone shears
bone skid
bone spur
bone stock
bone wax (see also *wax*)
    casting bone wax
    Horsley bone wax
    Lukens bone wax
      dressing
    Mosetig-Moorhof bone
      wax
    sterile bone wax
bone wax dressing
bone wax hemostatic agent
bone wax sutures
bone whorl
bone windowing
bone-biting rongeur
bone-cutting forceps
bone-cutting rongeur
bone-holding clamp
bone-holding forceps
bone-measuring calipers

bone-splitting forceps
bone-within-a-bone appearance
Bonfiglio bone graft
Bongort ostomy pouch
Bonina-Jacobson tube
Bonn forceps
Bonn hook
Bonn iris forceps
Bonn peripheral iridectomy
    forceps
Bonnano catheter
Bonnano tube
Bonner position
Bonnet enucleation of eyeball
Bonnet operation
Bonnet sign
Bonney blue stress incontinence
    test
Bonney cervical amputation
Bonney cervical dilator
Bonney clamp
Bonney clip
Bonney forceps
Bonney hysterectomy
Bonney inflator
Bonney needle
Bonney operation
Bonney suture needle
Bonney sutures
Bonney tissue forceps
Bonta knife
Bonta mastectomy knife
bony ankylosis
bony deformity
bony forehead
bony heart
bony island
bony labyrinth
bony landmarks
bony orbit of eye
bony overhand
bony palate
bony plate
bony projection
bony prominence
bony protuberance
bony pyramid

bony ridge
bony rongeur
bony spicules
bony spur
bony sutures
bony table
Bonzel iridodialysis
Bonzel operation
Boochai scissors
boomerang bladder needle
boomerang needle holder
Boorman gastric cancer typing
    system (types I-IV)
booster
boot brace
Boothby-Lovelace-Bulbulian
    mask (BLB mask)
bootie cast
boot-shaped heart
boot-top fracture
Boplant graft
Bora procedure
borborygmus
Borchard bone wire guide
Borchard wire threader
Borden-Spencer-Herndon
    osteotomy
border of cardiac dullness
border of ramus
borderline
bore trocar
Boren-Mayo table
Bores forceps
Bores twist fixation ring
Borge bile duct clamp
Borge catheter
Borge clamp
Borggreve operation
borne
Boros esophagoscope
Borsch bandage
Borsch dressing
Borthen operation
Bortz clamp
Bose bar
Bose hook
Bose nail fold removal

Bose operation
Bose retractor
Bose tracheal hook
Bose tracheotomy
Bosher commissurotomy knife
Bosher knife
BosPac cardiopulmonary bypass
    system
boss of bone
Bossalino blepharoplasty
Bossalino operation
bosselated
bosselated surface
bosselated uterus
Bossi dilator
Bost arthrodesis
Bost operation for talipes
    equinovarus
Boston bivalve brace
Boston bivalve cast
Boston brace
Boston Lying-In cervical forceps
Boston Lying-In cervical-
    grasping forceps
Boston model trephine
Bosworth approach
Bosworth coracoclavicular
    screw
Bosworth decompressor
Bosworth drill
Bosworth fusion
Bosworth headband
Bosworth nasal saw
Bosworth nasal snare
Bosworth nasal speculum
Bosworth operation
Bosworth plate
Bosworth procedure
Bosworth retractor
Bosworth saw
Bosworth screw
Bosworth shoulder arthroplasty
Bosworth snare
Bosworth speculum
Bosworth-Shawler incision
Botallo duct
Botallo foramen

Bottini operation
bottle hernia operation
bottle operation
bottle repair
bottlemaker's cataract
bottom out
Botvin forceps
Botvin iris forceps
Botvin-Bradford eye enucleator
Bouchard nodes
Bouchard nodules
Boucheron speculum
Bouchut tube
bougie (see also *searcher,*
   *sound*)
    à-boule bougie
    acorn-tipped bougie
    armed bougie
    Bangs bougie
    bronchoscopic bougie
    Buerger bougie
    Buerger dilating bougie
    bulbous bougie
    caustic bougie
    Celestin dilator bougie
    Chevalier Jackson bougie
    common duct bougie
    conical bougie
    Cooper bougie
    coudé bougie
    cylindrical bougie
    dilatable bougie
    dilating bougie
    Dourmashkin bougie
    Dourmashkin tunneled
     bougie
    ear bougie
    elastic bougie
    elbowed bougie
    eustachian bougie
    exploratory bougie
    filiform bougie
    filiform bougie probe
    filiform Jackson bougie
    Fort bougie
    French bougie
    Friedman-Otis bougie

bougie *continued*
    Friedman-Otis bougie à
     boule
    frontal sinus bougie
    fusiform bougie
    Gabriel Tucker bougie
    Garceau bougie
    Gruber bougie
    Gruber medicated
     bougie
    Guyon bougie
    Guyon exploratory
     bougie
    Harold Hayes eustachian
     bougie
    Hegar bougie
    Hertel bougie
    Hertel bougie-
     urethrotome
    Holinger bougie
    Holinger-Hurst bougie
    Hurst bougie
    Hurst esophageal bougie
    Hurst mercury bougie
    Hurst mercury-filled
     bougie
    infant bougie
    Jackson bougie
    Jackson esophageal
     bougie
    Jackson tracheal bougie
    Klebanoff common duct
     bougie
    large-diameter bougie
    LeFort bougie
    LeFort filiform bougie
    Maloney bougie
    Maloney mercury bougie
    Maloney tapered bougie
    medicated bougie
    mercury-filled bougie
    mercury-filled esopha-
     geal bougie
    mercury-weighted
     bougie
    olive-tipped bougie
    Otis bougie à boule

bougie *continued*
    Otis bougie à boule
      dilator
    Otis urological bougie
    Phillips bougie
    Plummer bougie
    radiopaque bougie
    Ravich bougie
    rectal bougie
    retrograde bougie
    Ritter bougie
    rosary bougie
    Ruschelit bougie
    Ruschelit urethral bougie
    Savary bougie
    soluble bougie
    sounds and bougies
    spiral-tipped bougie
    Storz bougie-
      urethrotome
    tapered bougie
    tapered rubber bougie
    tracheal bougie
    Trousseau bougie
    Tucker bougie
    tunneled bougie
    Urbantschitsch bougie
    urethral bougie
    urethral whip bougie
    Wales bougie
    Wales rectal bougie
    wax bougie
    wax-tipped bougie
    whalebone eustachian
      bougie
    whalebone filiform
      bougie
    whip bougie
    whistle bougie
    woven bougie
    yellow-eyed dilating
      bougie
bougie à boule
bougienage
bougienage biopsy
bougie-urethrotome
Bouillaud sign

Bouilly operation
bounding pulse
bounding pupil
Bourns humidifier
Bourns infant respirator
Bourns infant ventilator
Bourns respirator
Bourns-Bear ventilator
bout of rejection
boutonnière deformity
boutonnière repair
Bovie
    AG Bovie electrosurgical
      unit
    Bantam Bovie coagulator
    Bantam Bovie unit
    clinic Bovie
    coagulating-current
      Bovie
    cutting Bovie knife
    Davis Bovie cautery
    green Bovie
    liquid conductor Bovie
    Ritter Bovie
Bovie accessories
Bovie cautery
Bovie Chuck-It accessories
Bovie chuck-type handle
Bovie coagulating current
Bovie coagulating forceps
Bovie coagulating-current
  hemostat
Bovie coagulation cautery
Bovie coagulation tip
Bovie coagulator
Bovie current
Bovie cutting current
Bovie cutting-current hemostat
Bovie electrocautery
Bovie electrocautery unit
Bovie electrocoagulation unit
Bovie electrode
Bovie electrosurgical unit
Bovie endoscopic connecting
  cord
Bovie knife
Bovie liquid conductor

Bovie needle
Bovie suction device
Bovie unit
bovied
bovine allograft
bovine graft
bovine graft material
bovine heart valve
bovine heterograft
bovine implant
bovine pericardial heart valve
    xenograft
bovine pericardial prosthesis
bovine prosthesis
bow intrauterine device (bow
    IUD)
bow IUD
bowel
bowel axis
bowel bag
bowel contents
bowel dilatation
bowel intussusception
bowel loop
bowel lumen
bowel obstruction
bowel pattern
bowel prep regimen
bowel retractor
bowel sounds
bowel stoma
bowel tones
bowel wall
Bowen AMS rasp
Bowen chisel
Bowen gooseneck chisel
Bowen gouge
Bowen osteotome
Bowen periosteal elevator
Bowen suction loose body
    forceps
Bowen suture drill
Bowen wire cerclage system
Bowen-Grover meniscotome
bowenoid carcinoma of vulva
bowing of fracture
bowing of nail

bowing of vocal cords
bowl
Bowlby splint
bowleg
bowler hat sign
bowler's thumb
Bowles stethoscope
bowling-pin incision
Bowman capsule
Bowman cataract needle
Bowman dilator
Bowman disks
Bowman eye knife
Bowman glands
Bowman iris needle
Bowman iris scissors
Bowman lacrimal dilator
Bowman lacrimal probe
Bowman lamina
Bowman layer
Bowman membrane
Bowman muscle
Bowman needle
Bowman operation
Bowman probe
Bowman scissors
Bowman slitting of canaliculus
Bowman strabismus scissors
Bowman tube
bowstring
bowstring sign
Box adenotome
Box osteotome
boxcarring
Box-DeJager adenotome
boxer's elbow
boxer's fracture
box-joint forceps
Boxwood hammer
Boxwood mallet
Boyce holder
Boyce needle holder
Boyce position
Boyce sign
Boyce tube
Boyd amputation
Boyd approach

Boyd bone graft
Boyd disarticulation
Boyd dissecting scissors
Boyd graft
Boyd implant
Boyd incision
Boyd intraocular implant lens
Boyd lens
Boyd operation
Boyd posterior bone block
    elbow
Boyd posterior incision
Boyd retractor
Boyd scissors
Boyd table
Boyd-Anderson biceps proce-
    dure
Boyden sphincter
Boyd-McLeod tennis elbow
    procedure
Boyd-Sisk shoulder procedure
Boyes clamp
Boyes muscle clamp
Boyes operation
Boyes technique
Boyes-Goodfellow hook
Boyes-Goodfellow hook
    retractor
Boyle-Davis mouth gag
Boyne dental prosthesis
Boynton needle holder
Boys-Allis forceps
Boys-Allis tissue forceps
Boys-Allis tissue-holding
    forceps
Bozeman catheter
Bozeman clamp
Bozeman curet
Bozeman dilator
Bozeman dressing forceps
Bozeman forceps
Bozeman hook
Bozeman needle holder
Bozeman operation
Bozeman position
Bozeman speculum
Bozeman sutures

Bozeman uterine forceps
Bozeman uterine-dressing
    forceps
Bozeman uterine-packing
    forceps
Bozeman-Douglas uterine-
    dressing forceps
Bozeman-Finochietto needle
    holder
Bozeman-Fritsch catheter
Bozeman-Wertheim needle
    holder
Bozzi foramen
BPB (biliopancreatic bypass)
BPD (biparietal diameter)
BPH (benign prostatic hypertro-
    phy)
BPP (biophysical profile)
BPSA (bronchopulmonary
    segmental artery)
Bq (becquerel)
Braasch bladder specimen
    forceps
Braasch bulb
Braasch bulb catheter
Braasch bulb ureteral
    catheter
Braasch catheter
Braasch cystoscope
Braasch direct catheterization
    cystoscope
Braasch direct cystoscope
Braasch forceps
Braasch ureteral catheter
Braasch ureteral dilator
Braasch-Bumpus prostatic
    punch
Braasch-Kaplan direct-vision
    cystoscope
Braastad costal arch retractor
Braastad retractor
brace
    49er knee brace
    AFO brace (ankle-foot
        orthosis brace)
    Aircast air-stirrup leg
        brace

brace *continued*

Aircast brace
Aircast fracture brace
Aircast pneumatic brace
air-stirrup ankle brace
ankle air-stirrup brace
AO brace (ankle orthosis brace)
AOA cervical immobilization brace
Arnold brace
Atlanta hip brace
Atlanta-Scottish Rite brace
back brace
bail-lock brace
bike brace
Biomet fracture brace
Bledsoe brace
Bledsoe cast brace
Bledsoe knee brace
Bledsoe leg brace
Blount brace
Boldrey brace
boot brace
Boston bivalve brace
Boston brace
bracelet test
Buck knee brace
cage-back brace
Callender brace
Camp brace
Can-Am brace
canvas brace
Capener brace
CASH brace
cast brace
cervical brace
cervical collar brace
chair-back brace
Cincinnati ACL brace
clamshell brace
collar brace
Cook walking brace
Count'R-Force arch brace
CTI brace
Cunningham brace

brace *continued*

DePuy fracture brace
derotation brace
Don Joy knee brace
double Becker ankle brace
drop-foot brace
drop-lock knee brace
Duncan shoulder brace
Fisher brace
flexor hinge hand splint brace
Florida brace
Forrester brace
Forrester cervical collar brace
four-point cervical brace
four-poster cervical brace
functional fracture brace
gaiter brace
Galveston metacarpal brace
Gauvain brace
Gillette brace
Goldthwait brace
Guilford brace
hand brace
head brace
high-Knight brace
Hilgenreiner brace
Hudson brace
Hudson brace with bur
Hudson-Jones knee cage brace
hyperextension brace
InCare brace
ischial brace
ischial weightbearing brace
ischial weightbearing leg brace
Jewett brace
Jewett hyperextension brace
Jones brace
King brace
Klenzak brace
Kling cervical brace

brace *continued*

Knight brace
KSO brace
Kuhlman brace
Küntscher-Hudson brace
Kydex brace
LeCocq brace
leg brace
Lenox Hill brace
Lenox Hill knee brace
Lenox Hill Spectralite
    knee brace
Lerman hinge brace
Lofstrand brace
long-leg brace
Lorenz brace
LSU reciprocation-gait
    orthosis brace
Lyman Smith brace
McDavid knee brace
McKee brace
McLight PCL brace
MD brace (Medical
    Design brace)
Medical Design brace
    (MD brace)
Metcalf spring drop
    brace
Miami fracture brace
Milwaukee brace
Milwaukee scoliosis
    brace
Multi-Lock knee brace
Murphy brace
nonweightbearing brace
Omni knee brace
Oppenheim brace
Orthomedics brace
Ortho-Mold spinal brace
Orthoplast fracture brace
Palumbo dynamic
    patellar brace
Palumbo knee brace
Patten Bottom Perthes
    brace
Phelps brace
Power Play knee brace

brace *continued*

PPG-AFO brace (ankle-
    foot orthosis brace)
PPG-TLSO brace
    (thoracolumbar
    standing orthosis
    brace)
PTB brace
Raney flexion jacket
    brace
ratchet-type brace
Rolyan brace
Rolyan tibial fracture
    brace
Sarmiento brace
Schanz brace
Schanz collar brace
scoliosis brace
Scottish Rite brace
seton hip brace
short-leg brace
shoulder brace
shoulder subluxation
    inhibitor brace (SSI
    brace)
Smedberg brace
snap-lock brace
SOMI brace
SSI brace (shoulder
    subluxation inhibitor
    brace)
stirrup brace
Swede-O brace
Taylor back brace
Taylor brace
Teufel brace
Thomas brace
Thomas cervical collar
    brace
Thomas walking brace
thoracolumbar standing
    orthosis brace (TLSO
    brace)
TLSO brace (thoracolum-
    bar standing orthosis
    brace)
toedrop brace

brace *continued*
    Tomasini brace
    Tracker knee brace
    Trinkle brace
    UBC brace (University of British Columbia brace)
    UCLA functional long-leg brace
    University of British Columbia brace (UBC brace)
    Verlow brace
    Von Lackum transection shift jacket brace
    walking brace
    Warm Springs brace
    weightbearing brace
    Wilke boot brace
    Wilke brace
    Williams brace
    Wright Universal brace
brace with burs
bracelet test
brachial
brachial anesthesia
brachial arteriogram
brachial arteriography
brachial artery
brachial bypass
brachial coronary catheter
brachial dance
brachial fascia
brachial muscle
brachial plexus
brachial plexus block
brachial plexus nerve
brachial veins
brachiales, venae
brachialis, arteria
brachialis, musculus
brachialis superficialis, arteria
brachiocarpal articulation
brachiocephalic
brachiocephalic artery
brachiocephalic trunk
brachiocephalic veins
brachiocephalicae (dextra et sinistra), venae
brachiocrural
brachiocubital
brachiocyrtosis
brachiogram
brachioradial ligament
brachioradial muscle
brachioradialis, musculus
brachiotomy
brachioulnar articulation
Bracht-Wachter bodies
Bracht-Wachter lesion
brachybasia
brachycephalic
brachycephaly
brachydactyly
brachymetacarpia
brachymetapody
brachymetatarsia
brachyphalangia
brachystasis
brachytherapy
bracing
Bracken fixation forceps
Bracken forceps
Bracken iris forceps
Bracken irrigating cannula
Bracken scleral fixation forceps
Bracken tissue-grasping forceps
bracketed splint
Brackett dental probe
Brackett hip osteotomy
Brackett operation
Brackett probe
Brackett technique
Brackett-Osgood approach
Brackett-Osgood knee procedure
Brackin incision
Brackin ureterointestinal anastomosis
Brackmann TORP
Braden flushing reservoir
Braden reservoir
Braden-CSF flushing reservoir
Braden-MPF flushing system

Bradford enucleation neu-
    rotome
Bradford forceps
Bradford fracture appliance
Bradford fracture frame
Bradford frame
Bradford thyroid forceps
Bradford thyroid traction
    vulsellum forceps
Bradford-Young Y-V plasty
Bradshaw-O'Neill aorta clamp
Bradshaw-O'Neill clamp
Brady suspension splint
bradyarrhythmia
bradycardia
Brady-Jewett technique
bradykinesia
brady-tachy syndrome
Bragard sign
Bragg-Paul pulsator
Bragg-Paul respirator
Brahms mallet toe procedure
Braid strabismus
braided Ethibond sutures
braided Mersilene sutures
braided Nurolon sutures
braided nylon sutures
braided polyamide sutures
braided silk sutures
braided sutures
braided wire sutures
Brailey operation
Brailey stretching of supratroch-
    lear nerve
brain
brain abscess
brain biopsy cannula
brain biopsy needle
brain cannula
brain clip
brain concussion
brain death
brain depressor
brain electrical activity map/
    mapping (BEAM)
brain elevator
brain forceps

brain hook
brain knife
brain probe
brain retractor
brain scan
brain scissors
brain silicone-coated retractor
brain spatula
brain spatula forceps
brain spatula spoon
brain spatula with insulation
brain speculum
brain spoon
brain stem
brain suction tip
brain suction tube
brain surgery instrument
brain tumor forceps
brain-exploring cannula
brain-exploring trocar
branch
branch vein occlusion
branched calculus
branchial
branchial cleft
branchial cleft sinusectomy
branchial cyst
branchial pouch
branchial sinus
branchiogenous cyst
Brand forceps
Brand opponensplasty
Brand shunt-introducing forceps
Brand tendon forceps
Brand tendon passer
Brand tendon stripper
Brand tendon transfer
Brand tendon-holding forceps
Brand tendon-tunneling forceps
Brandt brassiere
Brandt treatment
Brandt-Andrews maneuver
Branemark osseointegration
    implant
Brannon-Wickstrom technique
Bransford-Lewis dilator
Brant aluminum splint

Brant splint
Brantley-Turner retractor
Brantley-Turner vaginal
    retractor
brash
Brasivol soap
brassiere-type dressing
BRAT system (Baylor rapid
    autologous transfusion
    system)
Brauer cardiolysis
Brauer chisel
Brauer operation
Braun anastomosis
Braun cranioclast
Braun decapitation hook
Braun depressor
Braun episiotomy scissors
Braun forceps
Braun frame
Braun graft
Braun hook
Braun implant
Braun ligature carrier
Braun needle
Braun operation
Braun pinch graft technique
Braun prosthesis
Braun scissors
Braun shoulder procedure
Braun skin graft
Braun technique
Braun tenaculum
Braun uterine tenaculum
Braun uterine tenaculum
    forceps
Braun-Fernwald sign
Braun-Jaboulay gastrectomy
Braun-Jaboulay gastroenteros-
    tomy
Braun-Jaboulay technique
Braun-Jardine-DeLee hook
Braun-Stadler bandage scissors
Braunwald prosthesis
Braunwald valve
Braunwald-Cutter ball-valve
    prosthesis

Braunwald-Cutter caged-ball
    heart valve
Braunwald-Cutter prosthesis
Braunwald-Cutter prosthetic
    valve
Braun-Wangensteen graft
Braun-Wangensteen operation
Braun-Wangensteen prosthesis
Braun-Yasargil right-angle clip
Brawley antrum rasp
Brawley antrum raspatory
Brawley frontal sinus rasp
Brawley nasal suction tip
Brawley rasp
Brawley retractor
Brawley scleral wound retractor
Brawley suction apparatus
Brawley suction tip
Brawley tube
Brawner orbital implant
brawny edema
brawny induration
brawny trachoma
Braxton Hicks contraction
Braxton Hicks sign
Braxton Hicks version
Brazelton neonatal assessment
    scale
bread-and-butter pericardium
bread-knife valvulotome
bread-loaf fashion
breadth
breast architecture
breast augmentation
breast biopsy
breast bone
breast bridge
breast implant
breast plate
breast prosthesis
breast ptosis
breast pump
breast reconstruction after
    mastectomy
breast reduction
breast shadow
breast surgery

breast tenaculum
breast tenaculum forceps
breaststroke injury
breaststroker's knee
breathing tube
Brecht feeder
Breck pin
Breckenmacher tract
breech birth
breech delivery
breech extraction
breech presentation
Breen retractor
bregmatic bone
bregmatic fontanelle
bregmatomastoid suture
bregmocardiac reflex
Breisky pelvimeter
Breisky vaginal speculum
Breisky-Navratil vaginal
    speculum
Breitman adenotome
Bremmer halo
Bremmer halo traction
Bremmer-Breeze splint
Brenner carotid bypass shunt
Brenner forceps
Brenner inguinal herniorrhaphy
Brenner operation
Brent eyebrow reconstruction
Brent pressure earrings for
    keloid surgery
brephoplastic graft
Breschet veins
Brescio-Breisky-Navratil
    speculum
Brescio-Cimino arteriovenous
    fistula
Bresgen cannula
Bresgen catheter
Bresgen probe
Bresgen sinus probe
Breslow microstaging system for
    malignant melanoma
Brett bone graft
Brett operation
Brett osteotomy

Brett technique
Brett-Campbell tibial osteotomy
Breuerton x-ray view
brevicollis
Brevital anesthetic agent
Brewer infarcts
Brewer kidney
Brewer operation
Brewer speculum
Brewer vaginal speculum
Brewser arthrotomy approach
Brewslow melanoma classifica-
    tion
Brewster phrenic retractor
Brewster retractor
Brewster sinus punch
Bricker ileal conduit
Bricker ileoureterostomy
Bricker loop
Bricker operation
Bricker ureteroileostomy
Brickner position
Brickner sign
bridge
Bridge clamp
Bridge deep-surgery forceps
bridge flap
Bridge forceps
bridge of nose
Bridge operation
Bridge prosthesis
Bridge telescope
bridging
bridging osteophytes
bridle stricture
bridle sutures
Briggs laryngoscope
Briggs operation
Briggs retractor
Briggs transilluminator
Brigham brain tumor
Brigham brain tumor forceps
Brigham forceps
Brigham thumb tissue forceps
Brigham total ankle system
Brigham total knee prosthesis
Brightbill cutting block

Brighton balloon
Brighton electrical stimulation
    system
Brighton epistaxis balloon
Bright-Ring keratoscope
brim
brim of pelvis
brimstone liver
Brinkerhoff anoscope
Brinkerhoff proctoscope
Brinkerhoff rectal speculum
Brinkerhoff speculum
Brinton disease
brisement
brisement forcé
brisk
brisk hemorrhage
brisk reflexes
Bristow elevator
Bristow operation
Bristow periosteal elevator
Bristow screw
Bristow zygomatic elevator
Bristow-Latarjet procedure
British test
Britt argon laser
Brittain arthrodesis
Brittain chisel
Brittain fusion
Brittain knee arthrodesis
Brittain operation
Brittain shoulder arthrodesis
Brittain-Dunn arthrodesis
brittle
brittle bone
brittle failure
broach
        barbed broach
        DuaLock broach
        ELP broach
        femoral broach
        femoral prosthetic
          broach
        Fred Thompson broach
        Harris broach
        intramedullary broach
        Mittlemeir broach

broach *continued*
        root-canal broach
        series II femoral broach
        smooth broach
broaching
broad adhesive band
broad band
broad ligament of uterus
broad nasal bridge
broad-based polyp
Broadbent inverted sign
Broadbent operation
Broadbent sign
broadbill hemostat
broad-blade forceps
Broca angle
Broca motor speech area of
    brain
Broca pouch
Broca region
Broca space
Brock auricle clamp
Brock cardiac dilator
Brock cardiac dilator rongeur
Brock clamp
Brock commissurotomy knife
Brock dilator
Brock incision
Brock infundibular punch
Brock infundibulectomy
Brock knife
Brock operation
Brock probe
Brock punch
Brock syndrome
Brock valvotomy
Brock valvulotome
Brockenbrough angiocatheter
Brockenbrough catheter
Brockenbrough commis-
    surotomy
Brockenbrough mapping
    catheter
Brockenbrough modified
    bipolar catheter
Brockenbrough needle
Brockenbrough sign

Brockenbrough transseptal
   catheter
Brockenbrough transseptal
   commissurotomy
Brockman clubfoot procedure
Brockman operation
Brockman technique
Brockman-Nissen arthrodesis
Broders index of tumor
   malignancy
Brodhead uterine gauze
   packing
Brodie abscess
Brodie disease
Brodie finger
Brodie fistula probe
Brodie joint
Brodie knee
Brodie ligament
Brodie probe
Brodney cannula
Brodney catheter
Brodney clamp
Brodney hemostatic bag
Brombach perimeter
Bromley operation
Bromley uterine curet
Brompton cocktail
Brompton Hospital retractor
Brompton mixture
Brompton solution
Bron implant cataract lens
Bron suction tube
bronchi (*sing.* bronchus)
bronchial biopsy
bronchial biopsy forceps
bronchial breath sounds
bronchial brushings
bronchial bud
bronchial catheter
bronchial check-valve
bronchial dilator
bronchial drainage
bronchial forceps
bronchial glands
bronchial lavage
bronchial lumen
bronchial obstruction

bronchial stump
bronchial sutures
bronchial tree
bronchial tube
bronchial veins
bronchial washings
bronchiales, venae
bronchial-grasping forceps
bronchiectasis
bronchiole
bronchoalveolar lavage (BAL)
bronchoalveolar lavage fluid
   (BALF)
Broncho-Cath endotracheal
   tube
bronchocele sound
bronchocentric granulomatosis
bronchocutaneous fistula
bronchodilation
bronchodilator
bronchoesophageal muscle
bronchofiberscope
bronchogenic
bronchogram
bronchography
broncholithiasis
bronchomediastinal
bronchophony
bronchoplasty
bronchoplasty repair
bronchopleural fistula
bronchopneumonia
bronchopulmonary segmental
   artery (BPSA)
bronchopulmonary segments
bronchorrhaphy
bronchoscope
     ACMI bronchoscope
     Albert bronchoscope
     Albert slotted broncho-
       scope
     BF large-core broncho-
       scope
     Broyles bronchoscope
     Bruening broncho-
       scope
     Chevalier Jackson
       bronchoscope

bronchoscope *continued*
- coagulation bronchoscope
- costophrenic bronchoscope
- Davis bronchoscope
- double-channel irrigating bronchoscope
- Dumon bronchoscope
- Dumon-Harrell bronchoscope
- emergency ventilation bronchoscope
- Emerson bronchoscope
- fiberoptic bronchoscope (FOB)
- folding emergency. ventilation bronchoscope
- Foregger bronchoscope
- Fujinon flexible bronchoscope
- Haslinger bronchoscope
- Holinger bronchoscope
- Holinger infant bronchoscope
- Holinger-Jackson bronchoscope
- hook-on bronchoscope
- infant bronchoscope
- irrigating bronchoscope
- Jackson bronchoscope
- Jackson full-lumen standard bronchoscope
- Jesberg bronchoscope
- Jesberg infant bronchoscope
- Kernan-Jackson bronchoscope
- Kernan-Jackson coagulating bronchoscope
- Killian bronchoscope
- Machida bronchoscope
- Michelson bronchoscope
- Michelson infant bronchoscope
- Moersch bronchoscope

bronchoscope *continued*
- Negus bronchoscope
- Negus-Broyles bronchoscope
- Olympus bronchoscope
- Olympus fiberoptic bronchoscope
- Overholt-Jackson bronchoscope
- pediatric bronchoscope
- Pentax bronchoscope
- Pilling bronchoscope
- respiration bronchoscope
- Riecker bronchoscope
- Riecker respiration bronchoscope
- Safar bronchoscope
- Safar ventilation bronchoscope
- slotted bronchoscope
- standard bronchoscope
- Storz bronchoscope
- Storz emergency ventilation bronchoscope
- Storz folding emergency ventilation bronchoscope
- Storz infant bronchoscope
- Storz-Doesel-Huzly bronchoscope tube
- Tucker bronchoscope
- ventilation bronchoscope
- Waterman bronchoscope
- Waterman folding bronchoscope
- Yankauer bronchoscope
bronchoscopic aspirating tube
bronchoscopic aspirator
bronchoscopic battery box
bronchoscopic biopsy forceps
bronchoscopic bougie
bronchoscopic brush
bronchoscopic cleaner
bronchoscopic cleaning tool
bronchoscopic face shield
bronchoscopic forceps

bronchoscopic forceps handle
bronchoscopic guide
bronchoscopic instrument guide
bronchoscopic magnet
bronchoscopic probe
bronchoscopic rotation forceps
bronchoscopic rule
bronchoscopic specimen
    collector
bronchoscopic sponge carrier
bronchoscopic suction tube
bronchoscopic telescope
bronchoscopy
bronchoscopy sponge
bronchoscopy with aspiration
bronchoscopy with biopsy
bronchoscopy with dilatation
bronchoscopy with drainage
bronchoscopy with insertion
bronchoscopy with irrigation
bronchoscopy with removal
bronchospasm
bronchospirometric catheter
bronchospirometry
bronchostomy
bronchotome
bronchotomy
bronchotomy with biopsy
bronchotomy with exploration
bronchotomy with removal
bronchovesicular markings
bronchovesicular respiration
bronchus (*pl.* bronchi)
bronchus clamp
bronchus forceps
bronchus-grasping forceps
Bronson magnet
Bronson operation
Bronson speculum
Bronson-Park speculum
Bronson-Ray curet
Bronson-Turtz iris retractor
bronze mallet
bronze sutures
bronze wire sutures
Brook wire-stitch scissors
Brooke fashion
Brooke ileostomy

Brooker bone classification
    system (grade I, etc.)
Brooker-Wills distal-proximal
    locking system
Brooker-Wills interlocking nail
Brooks adenoid punch
Brooks gallbladder scissors
Brooks punch
Brooks scissors
Brooks-Jenkins fusion
Brooks-Seddon transfer
Broomhead ankle surgery
Broomhead approach
Brophy bistoury
Brophy bistoury knife
Brophy cleft palate knife
Brophy cleft palate operation
Brophy dressing forceps
Brophy elevator
Brophy forceps
Brophy gag
Brophy knife
Brophy mouth gag
Brophy needle
Brophy operation
Brophy periosteal elevator
Brophy periosteotome
Brophy plastic surgery scissors
Brophy plate
Brophy scissors
Brophy tenaculum
Brophy tenaculum retractor
Brophy tissue forceps
Brophy tooth elevator
Brophy-Deschamps needle
Broviac atrial catheter
Broviac catheter
Broviac hyperalimentation
    catheter
brow presentation
brow-down position
Brown applicator
Brown bone elevator
Brown cannula
Brown chisel
Brown clamp
Brown cleft palate knife
Brown cotton applicator

Brown dermatome
Brown ear speculum
Brown electrodermatome
Brown elevator
Brown forceps
Brown hook
Brown knife
Brown mallet
Brown nasal applicator
Brown needle
Brown needle holder
Brown operation
Brown periosteotome
brown pigment gallstone
Brown push-back palato-
    plasty
Brown rasp
Brown raspatory
Brown retractor
Brown saw
Brown scissors
Brown side-grasping forceps
Brown snare
Brown staphylorrhaphy needle
Brown suture hook
Brown technique
Brown tendon sheath syndrome
Brown thoracic forceps
Brown tissue forceps
Brown tissue hook
Brown tonsil snare
Brown tonsillectome
brown tumor
Brown uvula retractor
Brown-Adson forceps
Brown-Adson tissue forceps
Brown-Bahnson forceps
Brown-Blair dermatome
Brown-Blair operation
Brown-Buerger cystoscope
Brown-Buerger dilator
Brown-Buerger forceps
Brown-Buerger hemostat
Brown-Davis gag
Brown-Dodge angiogram
Brown-Dohlman corneal
    implant
Brown-Dohlman eye implant

Brown-Dohlman implant
Browne basket
Browne hypospadias repair
Browne orthosis
Browne retractor set
Browne splint
Browne stone basket
Browne urethral reconstruc-
    tion
Browning vein
Brown-McDowell procedure
Brown-McHardy air-filled
    pneumatic dilator
Brown-McHardy dilator
Brown-McHardy pneumatic
    dilator
Brown-Pusey corneal trephine
Brown-Pusey trephine
Brown-Roberts-Wells headrest
Brown-Roberts-Wells CT
    stereotaxic guide
Brown-Séquard injection
Brown-Séquard lesion
Brown-Séquard paralysis
Brown-Séquard syndrome
Brown-Sharp gauge sutures (BS
    gauge sutures)
brow-up presentation
Broyles anterior commissure
    laryngoscope
Broyles aspirator
Broyles bronchoscope
Broyles dilator
Broyles esophageal dilator
Broyles esophagoscope
Broyles forceps
Broyles laryngoscope
Broyles laryngoscopy
Broyles nasopharyngoscope
Broyles telescope
Broyles tube
Bruce bundle
Bruce protocol
Bruch gland
Bruch mastoid retractor
Bruch membrane
Bruck protocol
Brücke fibers

Brücke lens
Brücke muscle
Bruel-Kjaer transvaginal
    ultrasound probe
Bruel-Kjaer ultrasound scanner
Bruening bronchoscope
Bruening cannula
Bruening chisel
Bruening cutting-tip forceps
Bruening ear snare
Bruening electroscope
Bruening esophagoscope
Bruening ethmoid exenteration
    forceps
Bruening forceps
Bruening nasal snare
Bruening nasal-cutting septum
    forceps
Bruening otoscope
Bruening pneumatic oto-
    scope
Bruening punch
Bruening retractor
Bruening septum forceps
Bruening snare
Bruening speculum
Bruening-Citelli forceps
Bruening-Citelli rongeur
Brughleman needle
Bruhat laser fimbrioplasty
Bruhat maneuver
bruised tissue
bruit
bruit de clapotement
Brun bone curet
Brun bone knife
Brun chisel
Brun curet
Brun ear curet
Brun mastoid curet
Brun plaster shears
Brun plastic shears
Brun plastic surgery scissors
Brun scissors
Bruner vaginal speculum
brunescent
brunescent cataract
Brunetti chisel

Brunn cyst
Brunner adenoma
Brunner chisel
Brunner colon clamp
Brunner dissector
Brunner forceps
Brunner glands
Brunner goiter dissector
Brunner incision
Brunner intestinal clamp
Brunner intestinal forceps
Brunner raspatory
Brunner retractor
Brunner rib shears
Brunner tissue forceps
brunnescent (see *brunescent*)
Brunschwig artery forceps
Brunschwig forceps
Brunschwig operation
Brunschwig pancreatoduo-
    denectomy
Brunschwig retractor
Brunschwig total pelvic
    exenteration
Brunschwig viscera forceps
Brunschwig visceral retractor
Brun-Stadler episiotomy scissors
Brunswick total hip
Brunton otoscope
Bruser approach
Bruser incision
Bruser lateral incision
Bruser skin incision
brush
        Acu-Brush
        Air-Lon tracheal tube
            brush
        Anchor all-nylon hand
            brush
        Anchor brush dispenser
        aortic valve brush
        Ayre brush
        Barraquer brush
        bronchoscopic brush
        bur brush
        cleaning brush
        contour instrument
            cleaning brush

brush *continued*
    Cytobrush
    cytological brush
    denture brush
    Edwards-Carpentier
      aortic valve brush
    endotracheal tube brush
    Gill biopsy brush
    Glassman brush
    Haidinger brush
    hand brush dispenser
    hand nylon scrub brush
    hand scrub brush
    Kurten wire brush
    Mill-Rose cytology brush
    nylon hand scrub brush
    nylon scrub brush
    ophthalmic sable brush
    polishing brush
    protected bronchoscopic
      brush
    sable brush
    stomach brush
    Storz cleaning brush
    tracheal tube brush
    Wagner laryngeal brush
brush biopsy
brush burn
brush cytology
brush dispenser
Brushfield spots
brushings
brusque dilatation of
    esophagus
BRW (Brown-Roberts-Wells)
BRW CT stereotaxic guide
BRW stereotaxic system
Bryan technique
Bryan-Morrey approach
Bryant lumbar colotomy
Bryant nasal forceps
Bryant operation
Bryant sign
Bryant traction
Brymill cryoprobe
BSS (balanced salt solution)
BSU (Bartholin, Skene, and
    urethral glands)

BTM hip system
bubble formation
bubble oxygenator
bubble trap oxygenator
    pump
bubble ventriculography
bubo
bubonocele
buccal artery
buccal crossbite
buccal fat pad
buccal glands
buccal mucosa
buccal nerve
buccal pedicle-flap operation
buccal sulcus
buccal tablet
buccal tube
buccalis, arteria
buccalis, nervus
buccinator muscle
buccinator, musculus
buccolingual (BL)
buccolingual diameter
Buchbinder catheter
Buchholz acetabular cup
Buchholz knee prosthesis
Buchholz prosthesis
Buchholz total hip prosthesis
Buchwalter retractor
Buck applicator
Buck bone curet
Buck curet
Buck dissecting knife
Buck ear applicator
Buck ear curet
Buck ear knife
Buck ear probe
Buck extension
Buck extension bar
Buck extension frame
Buck extension splint
Buck extension traction
Buck fascia
Buck fracture appliance
Buck hook
Buck knee brace
Buck knife

Buck mastoid curet
Buck myringotome
Buck myringotome knife
Buck myringotomy knife
Buck nasal applicator
Buck operation
Buck osteotome
Buck periosteal elevator
Buck probe
Buck restrictor
Buck splint
Buck traction
Buck tractor
bucket
bucket-handle fracture
bucket-handle tear
bucket-handle tear of meniscus
bucket-handle view of facial
    bones
Buck-Gramcko incision
Buck-Gramcko pollicization
buckle fracture of phalanx
buckling
buckling of cortex
buckling of knee
buckling of sclera
buckling operation
Bucknall procedure
Bucknall urethral reconstruction
Buckstein colonic insufflator
Buckstein insufflator
Buckston suture
Bucky diaphragm
Bucky film
Bucky grid
Bucky rays
Bucky studies
Bucky technique
Bucy cordotomy knife
Bucy knife
Bucy laminectomy rongeur
Bucy retractor
Bucy tube
Bucy-Frazier cannula
Bucy-Frazier coagulating-
    suction cannula
Bucy-Frazier suction tube

Bud bur
buddy splint
buddy tape
Budin joint
Budinger blepharoplasty
Budinger operation
Bueleau empyema trocar
Buerger bougie
Buerger dilating bougie
Buerger disease
Buerger exercises
Buerger needle
Buerger snare
Buerger-McCarthy bladder
    forceps
Buerger-McCarthy forceps
Buerger-McCarthy scissors
Buerger-Oliver dilator
Buerhenne catheter
Buerhenne technique
Buettner-Parel cutter
Buettner-Parel vitreous cutter
buffalo hump
buffer
Bugbee electrode
Bugbee fulgurating electrode
Bugg-Boyd procedure
Buie biopsy forceps
Buie cannula
Buie clamp
Buie electrode
Buie fistula probe
Buie forceps
Buie fulguration electrode
Buie hemorrhoidectomy
Buie irrigator
Buie operating scissors
Buie operation
Buie pile clamp
Buie position
Buie probe
Buie rectal irrigator
Buie rectal scissors
Buie rectal suction tip
Buie rectal suction tube
Buie retractor
Buie scissors

Buie sigmoidoscope
Buie specimen forceps
Buie suction tube
Buie technique
Buie tube
Buie-Hirschman anoscope
Buie-Hirschman clamp
Buie-Hirschman pile clamp
Buie-Hirschman proctoscope
Buie-Hirschman speculum
Buie-Smith anal retractor
Buie-Smith retractor
Buie-Smith speculum
build-up eye implant
bulb
bulb catheter
bulb of inferior jugular vein
bulb of occipital horn of lateral
    ventricle
bulb of penis
bulb of vestibule
bulb retractor
bulb suction
bulb suture
bulb syringe
bulb ureteral catheter
bulbar peptic ulcer
bulbi penis, arteria
bulbi penis, vena
bulbi vestibuli vaginae, arteria
bulbi vestibuli, vena
bulbocavernosus, musculus
bulbocavernosus reflex
bulbocavernous glands
bulbocavernous muscle
bulbocavernous reflex
bulbomembranous
bulbomimic reflex
bulboprostatic urethral anasto-
    mosis
bulbosity of nasal tip
bulbospongiosus, musculus
bulbourethral
bulbourethral glands
bulbous bougie
bulbous cervix
bulbous dilatation

bulbous tip of nose
bulbous turbinates
bulbous urethra
bulboventricular fold
bulbus
bulbus urethrae
bulge
bulging disk
bulky compressive dressing
bulky dressing
bulky pressure dressing
bulla (*pl.* bullae)
bulla ethmoidalis
bulldog clamp
bulldog clamp-applier forceps
bulldog clamp-applying forceps
bulldog forceps
bulldog hemostat
bulldog microclamp
bulldog nasal scissors
bulldog scissors
Buller bandage
Buller eye shield
bullet forceps
bullet probe
bullet tenaculum
bullous
bullous pemphigoid
bullous-like edema
bull's eye lamp
bull's eye lesion
Bumgardner dental holder
Bumke pupil
Bumm curet
Bumm placental curet
Bumm uterine curet
bumped up
bumper fracture
bumper-fender fracture
Bumpus forceps
Bumpus resectoscope
Bumpus specimen forceps
bunching sutures
Buncke quartz needle
Buncke technique
bundle branch block
bundle of His

bundle of Kent
Bunge amputation
Bunge exenteration spoon
Bunge meatotome
Bunge scissors
Bunge spoon
Bunim forceps
Bunim urethral forceps
bunion
bunion dissector
bunion operation
bunion osteotomy
bunionectomy
bunionette
Bunke clamp
Bunker forceps
Bunker implant
Bunker intraocular implant lens
Bunker lens
Bunke-Schulz clamp approxi-
    mator
Bunnell active hand splint
Bunnell bipedicle digital visor
    flap
Bunnell dissecting probe
Bunnell dressing
Bunnell drill
Bunnell finger splint
Bunnell flap
Bunnell forwarding probe
Bunnell hand drill
Bunnell knuckle-bender with
    outrigger
Bunnell ligament repair
Bunnell modified safety-pin
    splint
Bunnell needle
Bunnell operation
Bunnell outrigger splint
Bunnell probe
Bunnell procedure
Bunnell pull-out wire
Bunnell splint
Bunnell sutures
Bunnell tendon needle
Bunnell tendon passer
Bunnell tendon repair

Bunnell tendon stripper
Bunnell tendon transfer
Bunnell test
Bunnell-Howard arthrodesis
    clamp
Bunnell-Littler dressing
Bunny boot
Bunt catheter
Bunt forceps holder
Bunt instrument holder
Bunyan bag
bupivacaine anesthesia
bupivacaine hydrochloride
    anesthetic agent
bur
> Acrotorque bur
> Adson bur
> Adson enlarging bur
> Adson perforating bur
> Adson-Rogers cranial bur
> Allport bur
> Allport eustachian bur
> antral bur
> Bailey bur
> Bailey skull bur
> Ballenger bur
> Ballenger mastoid bur
> Ballenger-Lillie bur
> Ballenger-Lillie mastoid
> bur
> bone bur
> brace with burs
> Bud bur
> Burwell bur
> Burwell corneal bur
> Caparosa bur
> Caparosa cutting bur
> carbide bur
> carbide mastoid bur
> cataract bur
> Cavanaugh bur
> Cavanaugh-Israel bur
> choanal bur
> Concept Ophtho-Bur
> Cone bur
> conical bur
> corneal bur

bur *continued*
- cranial bur
- Cross corneal bur
- crosscut bur
- crosscut fissure bur
- curetting bur
- Cushing bur
- Cushing cranial bur
- cutting bur
- Davidson bur
- dental bur
- D'Errico bur
- D'Errico enlarging bur
- D'Errico perforating bur
- diamond bur
- diamond-dust bur
- Doyen bur
- drilled bur hole
- Dyonics bur
- electric bur
- electrically driven bur
- enlarging bur
- eustachian bur
- Farrior bur
- fenestration bur
- Ferris Smith-Halle bur
- Ferris Smith-Halle sinus bur
- fissure bur
- Frey-Freer bur
- Hall bur
- Hall mastoid bur
- Halle bone bur
- Halle bur
- Hannahan bur
- high-speed bur
- high-speed steel bur
- House bur
- Hudson brace with bur
- Hudson bur
- Hudson cranial bur
- Hu-Friedy dental bur
- inverted cone bur
- Jordan bur
- Jordan perforating bur
- Jordan-Day bur
- Jordan-Day cutting bur

bur *continued*
- Jordan-Day fenestration bur
- Jordan-Day polishing bur
- Kopetzky bur
- Kopetzky sinus bur
- Lempert bur
- Light-Veley bur
- Lindeman bur
- M bur (M-1, M-2, etc.)
- Marin bur
- mastoid bone bur
- mastoid bur
- McGhan mini-motor rotary bur machine
- McKenzie bur
- McKenzie enlarging bur
- Mueller bur
- neurosurgical bur
- Patton bur
- pear-shaped bur
- perforating bur
- polishing bur
- round bur
- Sachs bur
- Sachs skull bur
- Scheer-Wullstein cutting bur
- Shea bur
- sinus bur
- skull bur
- slotting bur
- slotting-bur osteotome
- Somerset bur
- sphenoidal bur
- Storz corneal bur
- Surgitome bur
- vulcanite bur
- Wachsberger bur
- Wilkerson bur
- wire pass bur
- Wullstein bur
- Wullstein high-speed bur
- Yazujian bur

bur brush
bur cells
bur drill

bur hole
bur saw
Burch biopsy forceps
Burch bladder suspension
    technique
Burch calipers
Burch evisceration
Burch eye calipers
Burch fixation pick
Burch forceps
Burch operation
Burch ophthalmic pick
Burch pick
Burch procedure
Burch retropubic urethropexy
Burch technique
Burch urethropexy
Burch-Greenwood tendon
    tucker
Burch-Greenwood tucker
Burckhardt operation
Burdach tract
Burdick cautery
Burdick electrosurgical unit
Burdick microtherm diathermy
    unit
Burdick muscle stimulator
    generator
Burdick Zoalite
Burdizzo clamp vasectomy
Burdizzo vasectomy
Buretrol device
Burford clamp
Burford forceps
Burford retractor
Burford rib retractor
Burford rib spreader
Burford spreader
Burford-Finochietto retractor
Burford-Finochietto rib spreader
Burford-Finochietto spreader
Burford-Lebsche knife
Burger technique for scapulo-
    thoracic disarticulation
Burger triangle
Burgess nail
Burgess operation

Burgess table
Burgess technique
bur-hole button
bur-hole cover
bur-hole incision
buried cortex
buried sutures
buried tonsil
Burkhalter procedure
Burkhalter technique
Burkitt lymphoma
Burlar process
Burlar tubercle
Burlisher clamp
Burman technique
Burn amaurosis
burn classification (1st to 4th
    degree)
burn shock
burned out mucosa
Burnett applicator (sizes A, B,
    etc.)
Burnham bandage scissors
Burnham biopsy forceps
Burnham finger bandage
    scissors
Burnham forceps
Burnham scissors
burning pain
burnishing
Burns chisel
Burns forceps
Burns guarded chisel
Burns plate
Burns prism bar
Burns telescope
Burow blepharoplasty
Burow cheiloplasty
Burow flap operation
Burow operation
Burow solution
Burow technique
Burow triangle
Burow vein
Burre hemostat
burred Wright reamer
bursa (*pl.* bursae)

bursal cyst
bursectomy
bursocentesis
bursolith
bursopathy
bursotomy
burst fracture
burst pacemaker
bursting fracture
Burton black light
Burton Fresnel floor light
Burton laryngoscope
Burton line
Burton sign
Buruli lesion
Burwell bur
Burwell corneal bur
burying of appendiceal stump
burying of fimbriae in uterine
    wall
Busacca nodules
Busch scissors
Busch umbilical scissors
Buselmeier shunt
Bush intervertebral curet
Bush stabilized cutting loop
Bush ureteral illuminator
butacaine anesthetic agent
Butcher saw
butethamine hydrochloride
    anesthetic agent
Butler bayonet forceps
Butler dental retractor
Butler retractor
Butler technique
Butler tonsil suction tube
butt
Butte dissector
Butterfield cystoscope
butterfly
butterfly adapter
butterfly clip
butterfly drain
butterfly dressing
butterfly flap
butterfly fracture
butterfly fragment

butterfly heart valve
butterfly IV needle
butterfly needle
butterfly pattern of perihilar
    edema
buttock
button (see also *collar button,
    buttonhook*)
    AEI button for replace-
        ment gastrostomy
    Bentley button
    Boari button
    bur-hole button
    Castelli-Paparella collar-
        button tube
    Chlumsky button
    collar button
    collar-button tube
    collar-button ulceration
    DiaTAP vascular access
        button for dialysis
        patients
    double-button sutures
    Graether buttonhook
    Graether collar button
    Graether collar button-
        hook
    Helsper laryngectomy
        button
    Hughston button for
        meniscal repair
    Husen button for
        meniscal repair
    Jaboulay button
    Joseph button knife
    Joseph button-end
        knife
    Kazanjian button
    Kistner button
    Lardennois button
    Moore button
    Moore tracheostomy
        button
    Murphy button
    Panje voice button
    patellar button
    peritoneal button

button *continued*
    polyethylene collar button
    polypropylene button sutures
    Resnick Button bipolar coagulator
    Reuter button
    Sheehy button
    Sheehy collar-button tube
    Smithwick buttonhook
    Smithwick silk button-hook
    Teflon button
    Todd button
    tracheostomy button
    Villard button
    voice button
button cautery
button drainage
button electrode
button infuser
button knife
button sutures
button technique
button-end knife
buttonhole
buttonhole deformity
buttonhole fracture
buttonhole incision
buttonhole mitral stenosis
buttonhole opening
buttonhole operation
buttonhook (see also *hook*)
    Graether buttonhook
    Graether collar button-hook
    Smithwick buttonhook

buttonhook *continued*
    Smithwick silk button-hook
buttonhook nerve retractor
buttonhook retractor
button-nosed knife
buttress
buttress plate
buttress thread screw
Butyn anesthetic agent
Buxton clamp
Buxton uterine clamp
Buyes air-vent suction tube
Buzzi operation
BV-2 needle
BVAD (biventricular assist device)
by mouth (per os; p.o., po, PO)
Byers flap
Byers prosthesis
Byers repair
Byford retractor
bypass
bypass blockage
bypass graft
bypass machine
bypass occluded segment
bypass prosthesis
bypass surgery
bypass tract
bypass tube
bypass vein graft
bypassable
Byrel pacemaker
Byron intraocular implant lens
Byron lens
Byron Smith correction of ectropion
Byron Smith lazy-T procedure
Byron Smith operation

C&S (culture and sensitivity)
C-area in nose
C-arm fluoroscopy unit
C-arm image intensifier
C-arm portable x-ray unit
C-C (convexo-concave)
C-Casting tape
C-clamp
C-DAK artificial kidney
C-DAK dialyzer
C-fiber
C-graft
C-loop of duodenum
C-P (Chaffin-Pratt)
C-P suction
C-P suction tube
C-section (cesarean section)
C-section delivery
C-splint
C-splint immobilizer
C-sponge
C-washer
C-wire Serter
CA monitor (cardiac-apnea monitor)
CAB (coronary artery bypass)
CABG (coronary artery bypass graft)
CABG'd (slang for coronary artery bypass grafted)
cable
cable graft
cable twister orthosis
cable wire sutures
Cabot leg splint
Cabot ring body
Cabot splint
Cabral coronary reconstruction

CABS (coronary artery bypass surgery)
cacomelia
CAD (computerized assisted design; coronary artery disease)
CAD hip prosthesis
CAD prosthesis
CAD reamer
cadaver
cadaveric donor
cadaveric donor transplantation
cadaveric graft
cadaveric homograft
cadaveric organ
cadaveric organ donation
cadaveric reaction
cadaveric transplant
café au lait spots
Caffey disease
Caffiniere prosthesis
cage-back brace
caged-ball heart valve
caged-ball valve prosthesis
caged-disk heart valve
CAHD (coronary arteriosclerotic/atherosclerotic heart disease)
Cairns clamp
Cairns forceps
Cairns hemostatic forceps
Cairns operation
Cairns retractor
Cairns rongeur
caked breast
caked kidney
Calamary cast boot
Calamary cast shoe
calamus scriptorius

Calandriello open hip reduction
Calandruccio compression
    device
Calandruccio external fixator
Calandruccio frame
Calandruccio nail
calcaneal apophysis occult
    compression injury
calcaneal bone
calcaneal bursa
calcaneal facet
calcaneal region
calcaneal spur
calcaneal sulcus
calcaneal tendon
calcaneal tuberosity
calcaneoapophysitis
calcaneoastragaloid
calcaneoastragaloid articulation
calcaneocavus
calcaneocuboid
calcaneocuboid articulation
calcaneodynia
calcaneofibular
calcaneofibular ligament
calcaneonavicular
calcaneonavicular ligament
calcaneoplantar
calcaneotibial
calcaneovalgocavus
calcaneus
calcar
calcar avis
calcar femorale
calcar pedis
calcareous
calcareous cataract
calcareous deposit
calcareous metastasis
calcarine fissure
calcarine sulcus
calcereous pancreatitis
calcific
calcific change
calcific density
calcific deposit
calcific shadow
calcification

calcified
calcified density
calcified focus
calcified free body
calcified lesion
calcified mass
calcified node
calcified organ
calcified tissue
calcified tissue scissors
calcifying
calcinosis
calcipenia
Calcitite bone graft material
Calcitite hydroxyapatite
calcium alginate applicator
calcium bilirubinate stone
calcium chloride
calcium concretion
calcium pump
calcium sodium alginate wound
    dressing
calciuria
Calculair spirometer
calculated date of confinement
calculated dose
calculi (*sing.* calculus)
calculus (*pl.* calculi)
calculus extraction
Caldani ligament
Caldwell guide
Caldwell operation
Caldwell x-ray view
Caldwell-Coleman technique
Caldwell-Durham procedure
Caldwell-Luc incision
Caldwell-Luc operation
Caldwell-Luc window oper-
    ation
calf (*pl.* calves)
Calgiswab dressing
Calhoun needle
Calhoun-Merz needle
calibrated clubfoot splint
calibrated depth gauge
calibrated guide pin
calibrated position
calibrated V-Lok cuff

calibrated-tip threaded guide
    pin
calibration
calibration gauge
calibration tonometer
calibration well
calibrator
Calibri forceps
caliceal
caliceal cups
caliceal cyst
caliceal dilatation
caliceal diverticulum
caliceal pattern
caliceal stone
caliceal system
calicectasis
calicectomy
calices (*sing.* calix)
caliculus ophthalmicus
caliectasis
caliectomy
calipers
    Albee bone graft calipers
    Austin Moore inside-
        outside calipers
    Austin Moore outside
        calipers
    Austin strut calipers
    Barker calipers
    bone calipers
    bone-measuring calipers
    Burch calipers
    Burch eye calipers
    Castroviejo calipers
    Castroviejo eye calipers
    Cone calipers
    Cottle calipers
    electric calipers
    eye calipers
    Green calipers
    Green eye calipers
    House calipers
    ice-tong calipers
    Jameson calipers
    Jameson eye calipers
    Ladd calipers
    Lange skinfold calipers
    Machemer calipers

calipers *continued*
    ophthalmic calipers
    Paparella calipers
    skinfold calipers
    Stahl calipers
    strut calipers
    Thorpe calipers
    tibial calipers
    tonsillar calipers
    Townley calipers
    Townley femur calipers
    Townley inside-outside
        femur calipers
    Vernier calipers
    V.M. & Co. ruler calipers
calipers strut
calix (*pl.* calices)
Callaghan sutures
Callahan approach
Callahan flange
Callahan forceps
Callahan lens loupe
Callahan operation
Callahan retractor
Callahan scleral fixation forceps
Callahan zonule lens stripper
Callander amputation
Callender brace
Callender clip
Callisen operation
callosomarginal artery
callus
callus formation
Calman carotid clamp
Calman ring clamp
Calnan-Nicole prosthesis
calomel electrode
Calot node
Calot operation
Calot triangle
Caltagirone chisel
Caltagirone knife
Caltagirone skin graft knife
Caluso PEG (percutaneous
    endoscopic gastros-
    tomy)
calvarial
calvarial hook
calvarial lesion

calvarium clamp
Calve cannula
calyceal (see *caliceal*)
calycectasis (see *calicectasis*)
calycectomy (see *calicectomy*)
calyces renales majores
calyces renales minores
calyx (*pl.* calyces) (see *calix*)
cam blade-tipped catheter
Cam tent
cambium
Cambridge defibrillator
Cambridge jelly electrode
Camel tube
camelback sign
Camel-Lindbergh pump
camera
    Anger camera
    anterior bulbi camera
    Beaulieu camera
    Bolex camera
    Bolex cine-camera
    cine-camera
    Circon camera
    Circon video camera
    Docustar fundal camera
    DyoCam arthroscopic
      video camera
    endo-camera
    EndoVideo-Five endo-
      scopic camera
    Fujica gastrocamera
    fundal camera
    fundus-retinal camera
    gamma camera
    gastrocamera
    Keeler camera
    Kowa camera
    Kowa fundus camera
    Kowa hand camera
    Kowa Optimed camera
    Kowa retinal camera
    Medx camera
    Nikon camera
    Olympus gastrocamera
    Olympus operating
      camera

camera *continued*
    ophthalmoscope camera
    Polaroid camera
    Reichert camera
    Schepens binocular
      indirect camera
    scintillation camera
    slit-lamp camera
      attachment
    Storz camera equipment
    Storz endocamera
    Stryker chip camera
    Syn-optics camera
    Topcon camera
    unicameral bone cyst
    Zeiss camera equipment
    Zeiss operating camera
camera attachment
camera equipment
Cameron cautery
Cameron electrosurgical unit
Cameron fracture appliance
Cameron gastroscope
Cameron periosteal elevator
Cameron-Haight elevator
Cameron-Haight periosteal
    elevator
Cameron-Lorenz cautery
Cameron-Miller cautery
Cameron-Miller electrocoagula-
    tion unit
Cameron-Miller electrode
Camey ileocystoplasty
Camey procedure
Camille Bernard lip repair
Camino catheter
Camino ventricular bolt
Camitz opponensplasty
Cammann stethoscope
camouflage
Camp brace
Camp collar
Camp corset
Camp grid cassette
Campbell airplane splint
Campbell applicator
Campbell approach

Campbell arthrodesis
Campbell arthroplasty gouge
Campbell bone block
Campbell catheter
Campbell elevator
Campbell forceps
Campbell gouge
Campbell graft
Campbell infant catheter
Campbell lacrimal sac retractor
Campbell laminectomy rongeur
Campbell ligament
Campbell ligature-carrier
    forceps
Campbell miniature sound
Campbell needle
Campbell nerve root retractor
Campbell operation
Campbell osteotome
Campbell periosteal elevator
Campbell rest strap
Campbell retractor
Campbell rongeur
Campbell self-retaining retractor
Campbell sound
Campbell splint
Campbell suprapubic cannula
Campbell suprapubic retractor
Campbell trocar
Campbell ureteral catheter
Campbell ureteral catheter
    forceps
Campbell urethral catheter
Campbell urethral catheter
    forceps
Campbell urethral sound
Campbell ventricular needle
Campbell-Akbarnia procedure
Campbell-Boyd tourniquet
Campbell-Goldthwait patella
    dislocation operation
Campbell-Molesworth-Campbell
    approach
Campbell-Young incontinence
    repair
Camp-Coventry position
Camp-Lewin collar

Camper chiasm
Camper fascia
campotomy
Camp-Sigraris stockings
camptocormia
camptodactyly
camptospasm
Canadian crutches
canal
canal knife
canal of Cloquet
canal of Corti
canal of Nuck
canal of Petit
canal of Schlemm
canal rays
Canale technique
canalicular scissors
canalicular system
canaliculi (*sing.* canaliculus)
canaliculi cochleae, vena
canaliculitis
canaliculodacryocystostomy
canaliculodacryorhinostomy
canaliculoplasty
canaliculorhinostomy
canaliculus (*pl.* canaliculi)
canaliculus chordae tympani
canaliculus cochleae
canaliculus dilator
canaliculus knife
canaliculus lacrimalis
canaliculus mastoideus
canaliculus of chorda tympani
canaliculus of cochlea
canaliculus probe
canaliculus punch
canaliculus tympanicus
canaliculus vein
canalis adductorius
canalis pterygoidei, nervus
canalis pterygoidei, vena
canalization
canaloplasty
canals and drums
Can-Am brace
cancelled bone

cancelli (*sing.* cancellus)
cancellous bone
cancellous bone graft
cancellous bone screw
cancellous formation
cancellous graft
cancellous screw
cancellous tissue
cancellus (*pl.* cancelli)
cancer
cancer cell collector
cancerous growth
cancerous mass
cancerous region
cancerous tissue
cancrum nasi
cancrum oris
Candela laser lithotriptor
candidiasis
candle vaginal cesium
    implant
Cane bone-holding forceps
Cane forceps
Canfield knife
Canfield operation
Canfield tonsil knife
canine muscle
canine teeth
canine transmissible tumor
canine-to-canine lingual splint
canker sore
Cannon endarterectomy loop
Cannon ring
Cannon stripper
Cannon vein stripper
cannon waves
cannonball metastasis
cannonball pulse
Cannon-Rochester elevator
Cannon-Rochester lamina
    elevator
cannula
        Abelson cannula
        Abelson cricothyrotomy
            cannula
        Abraham cannula
        Abraham laryngeal
            cannula

cannula *continued*
    acorn cannula
    Adson brain-exploring
        cannula
    Adson cannula
    Adson drainage cannula
    Adson exploring can-
        nula
    air cannula
    air injection cannula
    Air-Lon inhalation
        cannula
    alpha-chymotrypsin
        cannula
    anterior chamber
        cannula
    anterior chamber
        irrigating cannula
    antral cannula
    antral sinus cannula
    aortic arch cannula
    aortic cannula
    Aronson-Fletcher antrum
        cannula
    arterial cannula
    aspiration cannula
    aspirator cannula
    atrial cannula
    attic cannula
    B-H irrigating cannula
    Bahnson cannula
    Bailey cannula
    Bard arterial cannula
    Bardic cannula
    Barraquer cannula
    Bechert intraocular lens
        cannula
    Bellocq cannula
    Bellucci cannula
    Berkeley cannula
    biopsy cannula
    BioTac biopsy cannula
    Bishop-Harman anterior
        chamber cannula
    Bishop-Harman cannula
    Bishop-Harman irrigating
        cannula
    bivalve cannula

cannula *continued*
   Bracken irrigating
      cannula
   brain biopsy cannula
   brain cannula
   brain-exploring cannula
   Bresgen cannula
   Brodney cannula
   Brown cannula
   Bruening cannula
   Bucy-Frazier cannula
   Bucy-Frazier coagulating-
      suction cannula
   Buie cannula
   Calve cannula
   Campbell suprapubic
      cannula
   Carabelli cannula
   Casselberry cannula
   Castaneda cannula
   Castroviejo cannula
   cataract-aspirating
      cannula
   caval cannula
   cerebral cannula
   Charlton cannula
   Chilcott cannula
   Chilcott venoclysis
      cannula
   Christmas-tree cannula
   Clagett S-cannula
   Clagett cannula
   clysis cannula
   coagulating-suction
      cannula
   Coakley cannula
   Coakley frontal sinus
      cannula
   Codman cannula
   Cohen cannula
   Cohen intrauterine
      cannula
   Cohen tubal insufflation
      cannula
   Cohen-Eder cannula
   Concorde suction
      cannula
   cone biopsy cannula

cannula *continued*
   Cone cannula
   Cone cerebral cannula
   Cone-Bucy cannula
   Cooper cannula
   Cooper chemopallidec-
      tomy cannula
   Cooper double-lumen
      cannula
   Cope needle introducer
      cannula
   coronary artery cannula
   coronary cannula
   coronary perfusion
      cannula
   cortex-aspirating cannula
   cricothyrotomy cannula
   curved cannula
   cyclodialysis cannula
   dacryocystorhinostomy
      cannula
   Day attic cannula
   Day cannula
   DeWecker cannula
   DeWecker syringe
      cannula
   Digiflex cannula
   DLP aortic root cannula
   Dorsey cannula
   Dorsey ventricular
      cannula
   double-lumen cannula
   Dow Corning cannula
   Drews cannula
   Duke cannula
   Dulaney antral cannula
   Dupuis cannula
   egress cannula
   Elsberg brain-exploring
      cannula
   Elsberg cannula
   Elsberg ventricular
      cannula
   ERCP (endoscopic
      retrograde cholangio-
      pancreatography)
   ERCP cannula
   esophagoscopic cannula

cannula *continued*
exploring cannula
eye and ear cannula
fallopian cannula
Fasanella cannula
Fazio-Montgomery
cannula
Fein cannula
femoral artery cannula
Fisher cannula
Fisher ventricular
cannula
Fletcher-Pierce cannula
Flexicath silicone
subclavian cannula
Ford Hospital ventricular
cannula
Franklin-Silverman
cannula
Frazier brain-exploring
cannula
Frazier cannula
Frazier ventricular
cannula
frontal sinus cannula
Futch cannula
gallbladder cannula
Gans eye cannula
Gass cannula
Gass cataract-aspirating
cannula
Gill sinus cannula
Gills-Welsh irrigating
cannula
Girard irrigating cannula
Goldstein anterior
chamber–irrigating
cannula
Goldstein cannula
Goldstein irrigating
cannula
Goodfellow cannula
Goodfellow frontal sinus
cannula
Gott cannula
Gram cannula
Gregg cannula

cannula *continued*
Hahn cannula
Hasson cannula
Hasson-Eder laparoscope
cannula
Haverfield brain cannula
Haverfield cannula
Havlicek spiral cannula
Haynes cannula
Hepacon cannula
high-flow cannula
Hoen cannula
Hoen ventricular cannula
Holinger cannula
hollow cannula
Holman-Mathieu cannula
Holman-Mathieu
salpingography
cannula
Hudgins cannula
Hudgins salpingography
cannula
Hudson all-clear nasal
cannula
Hulka cannula
Hulka uterine cannula
HUMI cannula
Huse cannula
Hyde "frog" irrigating
cannula
iliac-femoral cannula
Illouz cannula
Illouz suction cannula
infusion cannula
Ingals cannula
Ingals flexible silver
cannula
Ingals rectal injection
cannula
inhalation cannula
injection cannula
inlet cannula
intra-arterial cannula
intracardiac cannula
intraocular cannula
intraocular lens cannula
intrauterine cannula

cannula *continued*

irrigating cannula
Jarcho cannula
Jarcho self-retaining
    uterine cannula
Judd cannula
Kahn cannula
Kahn trigger cannula
Kahn uterine trigger
    cannula
Kanavel brain-exploring
    cannula
Kanavel cannula
Kanavel exploring
    cannula
Kelman cannula
Kesilar cannula
Keyes-Ultzmann-Luer
    cannula
Kidde uterine cannula
Killian antrum cannula
Killian cannula
Killian-Eicken cannula
Kleegman cannula
Knolle cannula
Knolle-Pearce cannula
Kos attic cannula
Kos cannula
Krause cannula
Kreutzmann cannula
lacrimal cannula
Lamb cannula
laparoscopic cannula
laparoscopy cannula
large-bore cannula
laryngeal cannula
lens cannula
Lifemed cannula
Lillie attic cannula
Lillie cannula
Lindeman cannula
Litwak cannula
Look coaxial flexible
    disposable cannula
Luer suction cannula
    adapter
Luer tracheal cannula

cannula *continued*

Lukens cannula
Luongo cannula
Luongo sphenoid
    irrigating cannula
LV apex cannula (left
    ventricular apex
    cannula)
Mandelbaum cannula
maxillary sinus cannula
Mayo cannula
Mayo-Ochsner cannula
Mayo-Ochsner suction
    trocar cannula
McGoon cannula
McIntyre cannula
mediastinal cannula
Medicut cannula
Mercedes tip cannula
metal cannula
metallic-tip cannula
metal-tipped cannula
middle ear suction
    cannula
mirror cannula
Moncrieff cannula
monitoring cannula
Montgomery tracheal
    cannula system
Morris cannula
Myerson-Moncrieff
    cannula
Myles cannula
Myles sinus antral
    cannula
nasal cannula
Neal cannula
Neal fallopian cannula
Neubauer cannula
New York Eye and Ear
    cannula
O'Gawa irrigating
    cannula
Olympus monopolar
    cannula
outlet cannula
pacifico cannula

cannula *continued*

Packo pars plana cannula
Padgett shark-mouth cannula
Padgett-Concorde suction cannula
Paterson cannula
Patton cannula
Pereyra cannula
perfusion cannula
Pierce attic cannula
Pierce cannula
plastic cannula
polyethylene cannula
Polystan perfusion cannula
portal cannula
Portex cannula
Portnoy ventricular cannula
Post washing cannula
Pritchard cannula
Pynchon cannula
Randolph cannula
rectal injection cannula
return-flow cannula
Rigg cannula
Riordan flexible silver cannula
Robb cannula
Rockey cannula
Rockey tracheal cannula
Rolf-Jackson cannula
Roper cannula
Rowsey cannula
Rubin cannula
Rycroft cannula
S-cannula
Sachs brain-exploring cannula
Sachs cannula
Sarns aortic arch cannula
Sarns cannula
Sarns two-stage cannula
Sarns venous drainage cannula

cannula *continued*

Scheie anterior chamber cannula
Scheie cannula
Scott attic cannula
Scott cannula
Scott rubber ventricular cannula
Scott ventricular cannula
Seletz cannula
Seletz ventricular cannula
Semm cannula
Sewall antral cannula
Sewall cannula
Sheets cannula
Shepard cannula
sidewall infusion cannula
Silastic cannula
Silastic coronary artery cannula
silicone cannula
Silver cannula
Sims cannula
sinus antral cannula
sinus cannula
sinus-irrigating cannula
Skillern cannula
Skillern sphenoid cannula
SMI cannula
Soresi cannula
Southey cannula
Spencer cannula
sphenoidal cannula
Spielberg sinus cannula
Storz needle cannula
straight lacrimal cannula
Strauss cannula
stress on cannula
suction cannula
suprapubic cannula
Sylva irrigating cannula
Teflon cannula
Teflon ERCP cannula
Tenner cannula
Tenner eye cannula

cannula *continued*
    Todd-Heyer cannula
      guide
    Topper cannula
    tracheal cannula
    tracheostomy cannula
    tracheotomy cannula
    transseptal cannula
    Trendelenburg cannula
    trigeminus cannula
    trigger cannula
    Troutman alpha-
      chymotrypsin cannula
    Troutman cannula
    tubal insufflation cannula
    Tulevech lacrimal
      cannula
    Turnbull cannula
    two-stage Sarns cannula
    urethral instillation
      cannula
    urethrographic cannula
    USCI cannula
    uterine cannula
    uterine trigger cannula
    uterine vacuum cannula
    Vabra cannula
    vacuum intrauterine
      cannula
    Van Alyea antral cannula
    Van Alyea cannula
    Van Osdel irrigating
      cannula
    Veirs cannula
    vena caval cannula
    Venflon cannula
    venoclysis cannula
    venous cannula
    ventricular cannula
    Veress cannula
    Veress laparoscopic
      cannula
    Visitec anterior chamber
      cannula
    Visitec cannula
    Vitalcor cardioplegia
      infusion cannula

cannula *continued*
    Von Eichen cannula
    Von Eichen antral
      cannula
    washout cannula
    Webb cannula
    Webster infusion cannula
    Weil cannula
    Weil lacrimal cannula
    Weiner cannula
    Wells cannula
    Wells Johnson cannula
    West cannula
    West lacrimal cannula
    wire-wound cannula
    Wolf cannula
    Wolf drainage cannula
    Yankauer middle meatus
      cannula
    Zylik cannula
cannula clamp
cannula scissors
cannula tubing adapter
cannulate
cannulated
cannulated bolt
cannulated bronchoscopic
    forceps
cannulated cortical step drill
cannulated drill
cannulated forceps
cannulated nail
cannulated reamer
cannulated wire threader
cannulation
cannulation catheter
cannulation of aorta
cannulation of femoral artery
    and vein
cannulation of vena cava
cannulization
can-opener capsulotomy
Cantelli sign
cantering rhythm
canthectomy
canthi (*sing.* canthus)
cantholysis

canthomeatal flap
canthomeatal line
canthoplasty
canthorrhaphy
canthotomy
canthus (*pl.* canthi)
cantilever
Cantor intestinal tube
Cantor tube
canvas brace
cap bunionectomy
cap splint
capacitive radiofrequency
Caparosa bur
Caparosa cutting bur
Caparosa wire crimper
CAPD (continuous ambulatory
    peritoneal dialysis)
Cape system
capeline
capeline bandage
Capener brace
Capener technique
Capetown aortic prosthetic
    valve
Capetown prosthesis
capillary
capillary angioma
capillary bed
capillary bronchiectasis
capillary drainage
capillary embolism
capillary fracture
capillary loop
capillary microscope
capillary muscle
capillary points of ooze
capillary pressure
capillary stenosis
capillary wedge pressure
Capiox II oxygenator
capital
capital epiphysis
capital operation
capitate bone
capitate dislocation
capitellum

capitonnage
capitonnage sutures
capitular articulation
capitular process
capitulum
capitulum humerae
capitulum of humerus
capitulum of stapes
Caplan double-action scissors
Caplan nasal scissors
Capner boutonnière splint
Capner gouge
Capner splint
Capp point
capped elbow
capped knee
capping
capsotomy (see *capsulo-
    tomy*)
capsular adhesions
capsular advancement
capsular cataract
capsular decidua
capsular hemiplegia
capsular joint
capsular ligament
capsular occlusion
capsular opacities
capsular reefing
capsule
capsule forceps
capsule fragment forceps
capsule of corpora
capsule of glomerulus
capsule of kidney
capsule of knee
capsule of spleen
capsule of Tenon
capsule tumor
capsulectomy
capsulitis
capsulodesis
capsuloganglionic hemorrhage
capsulolenticular
capsulolenticular cataract
capsuloplasty
capsulorrhaphy

capsulotome
    Darling capsulotome
capsulotomy
capsulotomy scissors
CapSure cardiac pacing lead
capture beats
caput forceps
caput medusae
caput succedaneum
Carabelli aspirator
Carabelli cannula
Carabelli collector
Carabelli irrigator
Carabelli lumen finder
Carabelli tube
CaraGlass fiberglass casting tape
Carapace disposable face shield
Carass ventilator
Carassini spool
carbide bur
carbide mastoid bur
carbide-jaw forceps
carbide-jaw needle holder
carbide-jaw scissors
Carbocaine hydrochloride
    anesthetic agent
carbolize
carbolized knife blade
carbon arc lamp
carbon arc light
carbon dioxide anesthetic agent
carbon dioxide cautery
carbon dioxide insufflation
carbon dioxide laser
carbon dioxide pressure
carbon dioxide therapy
carbon fiber
carbon ion therapy
carbonaceous material
Carborundum disk
Carborundum polisher
carbuncle
Carceau-Brahms ankle
    arthrodesis
carcinectomy
carcinoembryonic antigen
    (CEA)

carcinoid
carcinoid tumor
carcinoma (*pl.* carcinomas,
    carcinomata)
carcinoma in situ (CIS)
carcinomatosis
carcinomatous lesion
CARD (cardiac automatic
    resuscitative device)
Cardarelli sign
cardboard splint
Carden amputation
Carden disarticulation
cardia
cardia of stomach
cardiac aneurysm
cardiac angiogram
cardiac apex
cardiac apnea monitor (C-A
    monitor)
cardiac area
cardiac arrest
cardiac asthma
cardiac automatic resuscitative
    device (CARD)
cardiac balloon pump
cardiac border
cardiac bronchus
cardiac care unit (CCU)
cardiac catheter
cardiac catheter microphone
cardiac catheterization
cardiac chamber
cardiac compensation
cardiac contractility
cardiac decompression
cardiac defect
cardiac defibrillator
cardiac depressant
cardiac dilator
cardiac disease
cardiac Doppler examination
cardiac dullness
cardiac effusion
cardiac failure (CF)
cardiac fibrillation
cardiac fluoroscopy

cardiac function
cardiac ganglion
cardiac glands
cardiac hypertrophy
cardiac impairment
cardiac impulse
cardiac infarction
cardiac instability
cardiac intervention
cardiac irregularity
cardiac massage
cardiac monitor
cardiac monitor strip
cardiac monitoring
cardiac mucosa
cardiac murmur
cardiac muscle
cardiac nerves
cardiac notch
cardiac notch of lung
cardiac orifice
cardiac output
cardiac pacemaker
cardiac pacing
cardiac patch
cardiac perfusion
cardiac plexus
cardiac probe
cardiac profile
cardiac puncture
cardiac rate
cardiac resuscitation
cardiac revascularization
cardiac rhythm
cardiac scissors
cardiac series
cardiac shadow
cardiac shock
cardiac shunt
cardiac shunt detection
cardiac silhouette
cardiac size
cardiac souffle
cardiac sounds
cardiac sphincter
cardiac status
cardiac stimulant

cardiac study
cardiac stump
cardiac syncope
cardiac tamponade
cardiac transplant
cardiac tumor
cardiac tumor plop
cardiac ultrasound
cardiac valve
cardiac valve dilator
cardiac valve leaflets
cardiac veins
cardiac ventriculography
cardiac workup
cardiaci thoracici, nervi
cardiacus cervicalis inferior,
    nervus
cardiacus cervicalis medius,
    nervus
cardiacus cervicalis superior,
    nervus
cardiectomy
Cardillo retractor
cardinal ligaments
cardinal signs of inflammation
cardinal suture
cardinal vein
cardinal vessel
cardioangiogram
cardioangiography
cardiocentesis
Cardio-Cool myocardial
    protection pouch
Cardio-Cuff
cardiodiaphragmatic angle
CardioDiary heart monitor
cardiodilator
cardiodiosis
cardioesophageal
cardioesophageal junction
cardioesophageal sphincter
cardiogenic shock
cardiogram
cardiography
Cardio-Green dye
cardiohepatic angle
cardiohepatic sulcus

cardiohepatic triangle
cardiokymograph
cardiokymographic test
cardiologic magnification
cardiolysis
Cardiomarker catheter
cardiomegaly
Cardiomemo device
cardiometer
cardiometry
cardiomyopathy
cardiomyopexy
cardiomyoplasty
cardiomyotomy
cardio-omentopexy
Cardio-Pace Medical Durapulse
    pacemaker
cardiopathy
cardiopericardiopexy
cardiophrenic angle
cardioplasty
cardioplegia
cardioplegic needle
cardioplegic solution
cardioplegic technique
cardiopneumonopexy
cardiopulmonary arrest
cardiopulmonary bypass
cardiopulmonary circulation
cardiopulmonary murmur
cardiopulmonary resuscitation
cardiopulmonary resuscitator
cardiopuncture
cardiorespiratory arrest
cardiorespiratory failure
cardiorespiratory murmur
cardiorespiratory sign
cardiorrhaphy
cardioschisis
cardioscope
cardiospasm
cardiospasm dilator
cardiosplenopexy
cardiothoracic ratio
cardiothoracic surgery
cardiothymic silhouette
cardiotomy

cardiotomy reservoir chest
    drainage
cardiovalvulotome
cardiovalvulotomy
cardiovascular
cardiovascular anastomotic
    clamp
cardiovascular bulldog clamp
cardiovascular circulation
cardiovascular clamp
cardiovascular collapse
cardiovascular disturbance
cardiovascular forceps
cardiovascular function
cardiovascular implant
cardiovascular physiology
cardiovascular response
cardiovascular scissors
cardiovascular shunt
cardiovascular silhouette
cardiovascular structures
cardiovascular support
cardiovascular surgery
cardiovascular sutures
cardiovascular system
cardiovascular thoracic needle
    holder
cardiovascular tissue forceps
cardiovascular tourniquet
cardioversion
cardioversion paddles
cardioverted
cardioverter-defibrillator
carditis
Cardona corneal prosthesis
    forceps
Cardona corneal prosthesis
    trephine
Cardona eye prosthesis
Cardona forceps
Cardona lens
Carey capsule
Carey-Coombs murmur
Cargile membrane
Cargile sutures
caries
caries of bone

carina
carina fornicis
carina of trachea
carina urethralis vaginae
carious lesion
carious teeth
Carl P. Jones traction splint
Carlens cardioscope
Carlens catheter
Carlens curet
Carlens double-lumen endotra-
    cheal tube
Carlens fiberoptic mediastino-
    scope
Carlens forceps
Carlens mediastinoscope
Carlens needle
Carlens retractor
Carlens tube
Carmack curet
Carmack ear curet
Carmalt artery forceps
Carmalt clamp
Carmalt forceps
Carmalt hemostat
Carmalt hysterectomy forceps
Carmalt splinter forceps
Carmalt tube
Carman rectal tube
Carman tube
Carmel clamp
carmine dye
Carmody aspirator
Carmody drill
Carmody electric aspirator
Carmody forceps
Carmody pump
Carmody thumb tissue forceps
Carmody tissue forceps
Carmody valvulotome
Carmody-Batson operation
Carmody-Brophy forceps
Carnochan operation
carotici externi, nervi
caroticotympanic nerves
caroticotympanici, nervi
caroticus internus, nervus
carotid angiogram

carotid angiography
carotid arterial beds
carotid arteriogram
carotid arteriography
carotid artery
carotid artery block
carotid artery bypass clamp
carotid artery clamp
carotid artery forceps
carotid artery occlusion
carotid artery stenosis
carotid bifurcation
carotid bifurcation endarterec-
    tomy
carotid body
carotid bruit
carotid bypass shunt
carotid canal
carotid cavernous sinus
carotid clamp
carotid compression
carotid endarterectomy (CEA)
carotid endarterectomy shunt
carotid eversion endarterectomy
carotid ganglion
carotid gland
carotid massage
carotid nerve
carotid plexus
carotid pulsation
carotid pulse
carotid pulse tracing
carotid puncture
carotid sheath
carotid shunt
carotid sinus
carotid sinus nerve
carotid sinus reflex
carotid sinus sensitivity
carotid sinus stimulation
carotid sinus syncope
carotid sinus syndrome
carotid steal syndrome
carotid subclavian endarterec-
    tomy
carotid syncope
carotid triangle
carotid vein

carotid vessel
carotid-axillary bypass
carotid-carotid bypass
carotid-subclavian bypass
carotid-subclavian transposition
carotis communis, arteria
carotis externa, arteria
carotis interna, arteria
carpal articulation
carpal bones
carpal boss
carpal canal
carpal fracture
carpal lunate implant
carpal prosthesis
carpal row
carpal scaphoid screw
carpal tunnel
carpal tunnel decompression
carpal tunnel projection
carpal tunnel release
carpal tunnel syndrome
carpals
carpectomy
Carpenter dissector
Carpenter enucleator
Carpenter knife
Carpenter tonsil knife
Carpentier annuloplasty
Carpentier annuloplasty ring
    prosthesis
Carpentier ring
Carpentier stent
Carpentier tricuspid val-
    vuloplasty
Carpentier valve
Carpentier-Edwards aortic valve
    prosthesis
Carpentier-Edwards bio-
    prosthesis
Carpentier-Edwards bio-
    prosthetic valve
Carpentier-Edwards mitral
    annuloplasty valve
Carpentier-Edwards pericardial
    valve
Carpentier-Edwards porcine
    prosthetic valve

Carpentier-Edwards valve
Carpentier-Edwards valve
    prosthesis
Carpentier-Edwards xenograft
Carpentier-Rhone-Poulenc
    mitral rings prosthesis
carpocarpal
carpometacarpal (CMC)
carpometacarpal articulation
carpometacarpal disarticulation
carpometacarpal ligament
carpopedal
carpopedal contraction
carpopedal spasm
carpophalangeal
Carpue operation
Carpue rhinoplasty
Carpule needle
Carpule syringe
carpus
carpus curvus
Carr lobectomy tourniquet
Carr tourniquet
Carrel clamp
Carrel method
Carrel mosquito forceps
Carrel operation
Carrel patch
Carrel sutures
Carrel treatment
Carrel tube
Carrel-Dakin treatment
Carrie traction
carrier (see also *ligature carrier,
    sponge carrier, suture
    carrier, tube carrier*)
    amalgam carrier
    Braun ligature carrier
    bronchoscopic sponge
        carrier
    Campbell ligature-carrier
        forceps
    clamp carrier
    cotton carrier
    DeBakey-Semb ligature-
        carrier clamp
    dermacarrier
    Deschamps carrier

carrier *continued*

    Deschamps ligature carrier
    Favoloro ligature carrier
    fiberoptic light carrier
    Finochietto clamp carrier
    Fitzwater ligature carrier
    foil carrier
    gauze pad carrier
    Jackson sponge carrier
    Kilner suture carrier
    Lahey carrier
    Lahey ligature carrier
    ligature carrier
    light carrier
    London College foil carrier
    Madden ligature carrier
    Mayo carrier
    proctological cotton carrier
    sponge carrier
    Storz cotton carrier
    suture carrier
    Tauber ligature carrier
    tube carrier
    Wangensteen carrier
    Wangensteen ligature carrier
    Young ligature carrier

Carrion penile prosthesis
Carrion-Small penile implant
Carroll aluminum hammer
Carroll arthrodesis
Carroll awl
Carroll bone hook
Carroll bone-holding forceps
Carroll elevator
Carroll forearm tendon stripper
Carroll hook
Carroll hook curet
Carroll needle
Carroll needle holder
Carroll offset hand retractor
Carroll osteotome
Carroll periosteal elevator
Carroll retractor
Carroll rongeur
Carroll technique
Carroll tendon-passing forceps
Carroll-Adson forceps
Carroll-Girard screw
Carroll-Legg osteotome
Carroll-Legg periosteal elevator
Carroll-Smith-Petersen osteotome
Carroll-Taber arthroplasty
carrying angle
Carson catheter
Carson model catheter
Carswell grapes
Carten mitral valve retractor
Carter clamp
Carter curet
Carter elevator
Carter eye elevator
Carter introducer sphere
Carter knife
Carter operation
Carter retractor
Carter speculum
Carter sphere introducer
Carter splenectomy
Carter splint
Carter submucous curet
Carter-Glassman resection clamp
Carter-Rowe view
cartilage
cartilage abrader
cartilage chisel
cartilage clamp
cartilage cutting board
cartilage forceps
cartilage graft
cartilage guide
cartilage implant
cartilage knife
cartilage of nasal septum
cartilage prosthesis
cartilage punch
cartilage ring
cartilage scissors
cartilage stripper

cartilage tear
cartilage-hair hypoplasia
cartilage-holding forceps
cartilaginous
cartilaginous arthroplasty
cartilaginous cup arthroplasty
cartilaginous disk
cartilaginous exostosis
cartilaginous growth
cartilaginous joint
cartilaginous portion
cartilaginous pyramid
cartilaginous ring
cartilaginous septum
cartilaginous tissue
cartilaginous tube
cartilaginous tumor
cartilaginous vault
cartridge base
cartwheel fracture
Cartwright heart prosthesis
Cartwright implant
Cartwright valve prosthesis
Cartwright vascular prosthesis
caruncle
caruncle clamp
caruncle forceps
caruncula (*pl.* carunculae)
caruncula lacrimalis
CAS connector
Casanellas operation
cascade
cascade stomach
Casco heating pad
case
case cart
caseated tissue
caseation
caseocavernous abscess
caseous
caseous cataract
caseous necrosis
caseous pneumonia
Casey operation
Casey pelvic clamp
CASH (cruciform anterior spinal
    hyperextension)

CASH brace
CASH orthosis
Caslick operation
Caspar alligator forceps
Caspar forceps
Caspar ring opacity
Cassel operation
Casselberry cannula
Casselberry position
Casselberry sphenoid washing
    tube
Casselberry tube
Casser fontanelle
Casser muscle
casserian muscle
cassette
cassette cup collecting device
Cassidy-Brophy dressing
    forceps
Cassidy-Brophy forceps
cast
cast book
cast brace
cast cap splint
cast cells
cast cutter
cast lingual splint
cast sock
cast syndrome
CastAlert device
Castallo eyelid retractor
Castallo lid retractor
Castallo retractor
Castallo speculum
Castanares bilateral blepharo-
    plasty
Castanares face-lift scissors
Castanares scissors
Castaneda anastomosis clamp
Castaneda cannula
Castaneda clamp
Castaneda IMM vascular clamp
Castaneda multipurpose clamp
Castaneda suture tag forceps
Castaneda vascular clamp
Castaneda-Mixter clamp
Castellani paint

Castelli tube
Castellino sign
Castelli-Paparella collar-button
    tube
Castelli-Paparella myringotomy
    tube
Castens trocar
Castex rigid dressing
CastGuard
Castillo catheter
casting
casting bone wax
casting tape
Castle laminectomy table
Castle procedure
Castle sterilizer
Castmate plaster bandage
    dressing
castration
Castro-Martinez keratome
Castroviejo adjustable retractor
Castroviejo bladebreaker knife
Castroviejo calipers
Castroviejo cannula
Castroviejo capsule forceps
Castroviejo clamp
Castroviejo compressor
Castroviejo corneal dissector
Castroviejo corneal microscis-
    sors
Castroviejo corneal scissors
Castroviejo corneal trephine
Castroviejo corneoscleral punch
Castroviejo corneoscleral suture
    forceps
Castroviejo cyclodialysis spatula
Castroviejo dermatome
Castroviejo dilator
Castroviejo dissector
Castroviejo double-end dilator
Castroviejo electrode
Castroviejo enucleation snare
Castroviejo erysiphake
Castroviejo eye calipers
Castroviejo eye speculum
Castroviejo forceps
Castroviejo implant

Castroviejo keratome
Castroviejo knife
Castroviejo lacrimal dilator
Castroviejo microneedle holder
Castroviejo microscissors
Castroviejo needle
Castroviejo needle holder
Castroviejo operation
Castroviejo ophthalmic knife
Castroviejo punch
Castroviejo razor
Castroviejo razor blade holder
Castroviejo razor bladebreaker
Castroviejo retractor
Castroviejo scissors
Castroviejo sclerotome
Castroviejo section scissors
Castroviejo snare
Castroviejo spatula
Castroviejo speculum
Castroviejo spoon
Castroviejo suture forceps
Castroviejo transplant forceps
Castroviejo transplant trephine
Castroviejo transplant-grafting
    capsule
Castroviejo trephine
Castroviejo tying forceps
Castroviejo Vital needle holder
Castroviejo-Arruga capsule
    forceps
Castroviejo-Arruga forceps
Castroviejo-Barraquer needle
    holder
Castroviejo-Barraquer speculum
Castroviejo-Colibri corneal
    forceps
Castroviejo-Furniss cornea-
    holding forceps
Castroviejo-Green needle holder
Castroviejo-Kalt needle holder
Castroviejo-Kalt traction handle
Castroviejo-Scheie cyclodia-
    thermy
Castroviejo-Simpson forceps
Castroviejo-Troutman needle
    holder

Castroviejo-Troutman scissors
Castroviejo-Vannas capsulotomy
    scissors
Castroviejo-Wheeler discission
    knife
CAT scan (computerized axial
    tomography scan)
CAT scanner
Catalano tubing
cataract
cataract aspirator
cataract blade
cataract bur
cataract extraction
cataract extractor
cataract flap operation
cataract knife
cataract lamp
cataract lens
cataract mask
cataract needle
cataract operation
cataract probe
cataract scissors
cataract spoon
cataract suction unit
cataract-aspirating cannula
cataract-aspirating needle
catastrophic brain damage
catastrophic brain injury
catgut
catgut ligature
catgut plain ties
catgut sutures (CGS)
cathartic colon
Cathcart endoprosthesis
Cathelin segregator
cathematic catheter
catheter
        3-way catheter
        3-way Foley catheter
        3-way irrigating
            catheter
        5-French angiographic
            catheter
        5-French stiff catheter
        6-eye catheter
        8-lumen catheter

catheter *continued*
    à demeure catheter
    Abramson catheter
    ACMI Alcock catheter
    ACMI catheter
    ACMI Emmett hemostatic
        catheter
    ACMI Owens catheter
    ACMI positive pressure
        catheter
    ACMI ureteral cathe-
        ter
    Acmistat catheter
    acorn-tipped catheter
    Acrad HS catheter (hys-
        terosalpingography
        catheter)
    ACS catheter
    ACS exchange guiding
        catheter
    ACS floppy-tip guiding
        catheter
    ACS JL4 catheter
    ACS Mini catheter
    ACS RX coronary
        dilatation catheter
    adapter catheter
    aero-flo tip catheter
    AgX antimicrobial Foley
        catheter
    Air-Lon inhalation
        catheter
    AL-1 catheter
    Alcock catheter
    Alcock conical catheter
        adapter
    Alcock hemostatic
        catheter
    Alcock return-flow
        hemostatic catheter
    Alcott catheter
    alimentation cathe-
        ter
    Allis catheter
    Alvarez-Rodriguez
        cardiac catheter
    amber latex catheter
    Amcath catheter

catheter *continued*

>Amplatz aortography catheter
>Amplatz cardiac catheter
>Amplatz catheter
>Amplatz coronary catheter
>Amplatz femoral catheter
>Angiocath PRN catheter
>angiocatheter
>angiographic balloon occlusion catheter
>angiographic catheter
>Angio-Kit catheter
>angiopigtail catheter
>angioplasty balloon catheter
>angled balloon catheter
>angulated catheter
>Anthron heparinized catheter
>aortic catheter
>aortogram catheter
>aortographic catheter
>AR-1 catheter
>AR-2 diagnostic catheter
>AR-2 guiding catheter
>Arani catheter
>Arani double-loop guiding catheter
>Argyle catheter
>Argyle Medicut R catheter
>Arrow multilumen catheter
>Arrow pulmonary artery catheter
>Arrow-Berman balloon angioplasty catheter
>Arrow-Berman balloon catheter
>Arrow-Howes multi-lumen catheter
>arterial catheter
>arterial embolectomy catheter
>ASC Monorel catheter

catheter *continued*

>Ash catheter
>ASI uroplasty TCU dilatation catheter
>AtheroCath spinning blade catheter
>Atlantic ileostomy catheter
>Atlas balloon dilatation catheter
>auricular appendage catheter
>automatic catheter
>Axiom DG balloon angioplasty catheter
>bag catheter
>Bailey catheter
>bailout catheter
>Baim catheter
>balloon biliary catheter
>balloon catheter
>balloon dilatation catheter
>balloon dilating catheter
>balloon embolectomy catheter
>balloon flotation catheter
>balloon-tipped angiographic catheter
>Banno catheter
>Bard balloon-directed pacing catheter
>Bard catheter
>Bard guiding catheter
>Bard helical catheter
>Bard x-ray ureteral catheter
>Bardam catheter
>Bardam red rubber catheter
>Bardco catheter
>Bardex catheter
>Bardex Foley catheter
>Bardex Lubricath Foley catheter
>Bardic catheter
>Bardic cutdown catheter

catheter *continued*

Bardic translucent
catheter
Bardic vein catheter
Bartholin gland catheter
Baschui pigtail catheter
bat-wing catheter
Baxter dilatation catheter
Beird eye catheter
Béniqué catheter guide
Berman angiographic
catheter
Berman cardiac catheter
Berman catheter
Bernstein catheter
beta finger-grip catheter
connector
bicoudate catheter
bicoudé catheter
biliary balloon catheter
biliary catheter
bipolar catheter
bipolar pacing catheter
bipolar pacing electrode
catheter
bipolar temporary
pacemaker catheter
bladder catheter
Blasucci catheter
Blasucci curved-tip
ureteral catheter
Blasucci pigtail ureteral
catheter
Blasucci ureteral catheter
Block right coronary
guiding catheter
Blue Max triple-lumen
catheter
Bonnano catheter
Borge catheter
Bozeman catheter
Bozeman-Fritsch catheter
Braasch bulb catheter
Braasch bulb ureteral
catheter

catheter *continued*

Braasch catheter
Braasch ureteral catheter
brachial coronary
catheter
Bresgen catheter
Brockenbrough angio-
catheter
Brockenbrough catheter
Brockenbrough mapping
catheter
Brockenbrough modified
bipolar catheter
Brockenbrough transsep-
tal catheter
Brodney catheter
bronchial catheter
bronchospirometric
catheter
Broviac atrial catheter
Broviac catheter
Broviac hyperalimenta-
tion catheter
Buchbinder catheter
Buerhenne catheter
bulb catheter
bulb ureteral catheter
Bunt catheter
cam blade-tipped
catheter
Camino catheter
Campbell catheter
Campbell infant cathe-
ter
Campbell ureteral
catheter
Campbell urethral
catheter
cannulation catheter
cardiac catheter
cardiac catheter micro-
phone
Cardiomarker catheter
Carlens catheter
Carson catheter
Carson model catheter

catheter *continued*

Castillo catheter
cathematic catheter
Cathlon IV catheter
caval catheter
cecostomy catheter
central catheter
central venous catheter
cephalad catheter
cerebral catheter
Chaffin catheter
Chaffin tube catheter
Chemo-Port catheter
cholangiography catheter
cloverleaf catheter
coaxial catheter
cobra catheter
cobra-shaped catheter
coil-tipped catheter
condom catheter
conductance catheter
conformation of right heart catheter
conical catheter
conical-tip catheter
Constantine catheter
Constantine flexible metal catheter
ConstaVac catheter
continuous irrigation catheter
Cook arterial catheter
Cook catheter
Cook pigtail catheter
Cook TPN catheter
Cooley vena caval catheter clamp
Cordis catheter
Cordis guiding catheter
Cordis Lumelec catheter
Cordis pigtail catheter
Corlon angiocatheter
coronary catheter
coronary dilatation catheter
coronary guiding catheter

catheter *continued*

coronary sinus thermodilution catheter
coudé assist catheter
coudé catheter
coudé urethral catheter
coudé-tip catheter
coudé-tip demeure catheter
Councill catheter
Councill retention catheter
Cournand catheter
Coxeter catheter
Coxeter prostatic catheter
CPV catheter
Critikon balloon thermodilution catheter
Critikon balloon-tipped end-hole catheter
Critikon catheter
cryoablation catheter
Cummings catheter
Cummings four-wing catheter
Cummings-Pezzer catheter
Curl Cath catheter
curved catheter
cutdown catheter
cystocatheter
Dacron catheter
Dakin catheter
Datascope intra-aortic balloon pump catheter
Davol catheter
Davol rubber catheter
de Pezzer catheter
de Pezzer self-retaining catheter
Dearor model catheter
decompressive enteroclysis catheter
DeKock two-way bronchial catheter
DeLee catheter
DeLee infant catheter
DeLee tracheal catheter

catheter *continued*
> Deseret angiocatheter
> Deseret catheter
> Desilets catheter
> Desilets-Hoffman
> catheter introducer
> Devonshire catheter
> DeWeese caval catheter
> Diaflex ureteral dilatation
> catheter
> diagnostic catheter
> dialysis catheter
> dilatation balloon
> catheter
> dilating catheter
> dilating pressure balloon
> catheter
> dilation catheter
> disposable catheter
> DLP cardioplegic
> catheter
> Doppler coronary
> catheter
> Dormia stone basket
> catheter
> Dorros brachial internal
> mammary guiding
> catheter
> Dotter caged-balloon
> catheter
> Dotter coaxial catheter
> double-current catheter
> double-J indwelling
> catheter stent
> double-J silicone internal
> ureteral catheter stent
> double-J stent catheter
> double-lumen Broviac
> catheter
> double-lumen catheter
> double-lumen Hickman
> catheter
> double-lumen Hickman-
> Broviac catheter
> double-lumen Silastic
> catheter
> Dover catheter

catheter *continued*
> Dow Corning catheter
> Dow Corning
> cystocatheter
> Dow Corning ileal pouch
> catheter
> drainage catheter
> Drew-Smythe catheter
> Ducor balloon catheter
> Ducor cardiac catheter
> DVI Simpson AtheroCath
> catheter
> Easy catheter
> Edslab catheter
> Edslab cholangiography
> catheter
> Edwards catheter
> Edwards diagnostic
> catheter
> eight-lumen esophageal
> manometry catheter
> eight-lumen manometry
> catheter
> El Gamal coronary
> bypass catheter
> El Gamal guiding
> catheter
> elbowed catheter
> Elecath catheter
> Elecath thermodilution
> catheter
> electrode catheter
> embolectomy catheter
> en chemise catheter
> end-hole catheter
> endotracheal catheter
> Enhanced Torque 8F
> guiding catheter
> Eppendorfer angio-
> catheter
> Eppendorfer cardiac
> catheter
> Eppendorfer catheter
> ERCP catheter
> Erythroflex catheter
> esophagoscopic catheter
> eustachian catheter

catheter *continued*

Evermed catheter
extrusion balloon catheter
fallopian catheter
FAST balloon catheter (flow-assisted, short-term balloon catheter)
faucial catheter
faucial eustachian catheter
female catheter
female catheter-dilator
femoral guiding catheter
fenestrated catheter
filiform catheter
filiform-tipped catheter
Finesse guiding catheter
Finesse large-lumen guiding catheter
flat-blade-tipped catheter
flexible catheter
flexible metal catheter
Flexitip catheter
floating catheter
flotation catheter
flow-directed balloon-tipped catheter
flow-directed catheter
flow-oximetry catheter
fluid-filled catheter
Fogarty balloon biliary catheter
Fogarty balloon catheter
Fogarty catheter
Fogarty dilation catheter
Fogarty embolus catheter
Fogarty gallstone catheter
Fogarty irrigation catheter
Fogarty occlusion catheter
Fogarty venous thrombectomy catheter
Fogarty-Chin catheter
Fogarty-Chin extrusion balloon catheter

catheter *continued*

Fogarty-Chin peripheral dilatation catheter
Foley acorn-bulb catheter
Foley balloon catheter
Foley catheter
Foley cone-tip catheter
Foley-Alcock bag catheter
Foley-Alcock catheter
Foltz catheter
Foltz-Overton cardiac catheter
four-eye catheter
four-wing catheter
four-wing Malecot retention catheter
Freedom external catheter
French angiographic catheter
French catheter
French curve out-of-plane catheter
French Foley catheter
French in-plane guiding catheter
French MBIH catheter
French mushroom-tipped catheter
French red-rubber Robinson catheter
French Robinson catheter
French Silastic Foley catheter
French tripolar His catheter
Friend catheter
Friend-Hebert catheter
Fritsch catheter
Furniss catheter
Furniss female catheter
Gambro catheter
Ganz-Edwards coronary infusion catheter
Garceau catheter

catheter *continued*

gastroenterostomy catheter
Gauderer-Ponsky catheter
Gensini angiocatheter
Gensini catheter
Gensini Teflon catheter
Gentle-Flo suction catheter
Gibbon catheter
Gibbon urethral catheter
Gilbert balloon catheter
Gilbert catheter
Gilbert pediatric balloon catheter
Gilbert pediatric catheter
Goodale-Lubin catheter
Gore-Tex catheter
Gorlin catheter
Gorlin pacing catheter
Gould PentaCath 5-lumen thermodilution catheter
Gouley catheter
Goutz catheter
graduated catheter
graduated-size catheter
graft-seeker catheter
graft-seeking catheter
Grollman catheter
Grollman pigtail catheter
Groshong catheter
Groshong double-lumen catheter
Gruentzig arterial balloon catheter
Gruentzig balloon catheter
Gruentzig balloon catheter angioplasty
Gruentzig catheter
Gruentzig coronary catheter dilating system
Gruentzig 20-30 dilating catheter

catheter *continued*

Gruentzig D dilating catheter
Gruentzig D-G dilating catheter
Gruentzig Dilaca catheter
Gruentzig G dilating catheter
Gruentzig S dilating catheter
Gruentzig steerable catheter
guide catheter
guiding catheter
Guyon catheter guide
Guyon ureteral catheter
Hagner bag catheter
Hagner catheter
Hakim catheter
Hanafee catheter
Hanafee catheter tip
Harris catheter
Harris uterine injector catheter
Hartmann catheter
Hartmann eustachian catheter
Hartzler catheter
Hartzler dilatation catheter
Hartzler Micro catheter
Hartzler Micro II catheter
Hartzler Micro XT catheter
Hartzler Ultra Lo-Profile catheter
Hatch catheter
headhunter catheter
headhunter visceral angiography catheter
helical catheter
Hemaquet catheter introducer
hemostatic catheter
Hepacon catheter
hexapolar catheter
Hickman catheter

catheter *continued*

Hickman indwelling catheter
Hickman indwelling right atrial catheter
Hickman-Broviac catheter
Hidalgo catheter
Hieshima coaxial catheter
Higgins catheter
high-fidelity catheter
high-flow catheter
His catheter
Hi-Torque floppy guide catheter
Hollister catheter
Hollister self-adhesive catheter
Holt self-retaining catheter
Holter-Hausner catheter
hot-tipped catheter
Hryntschak catheter
HUI catheter (Harris uterine injector catheter)
Hyams catheter
HydraCross TLC PTCA catheter
hydrostatic balloon catheter
hyperalimentation catheter
hysterosalpingography catheter
IAB catheter (intra-aortic balloon catheter)
ICP catheter
Impersol catheter
indwelling catheter
infant catheter
infant female catheter
infant male catheter
inflatable catheter
inflatable Foley bag catheter
infusion catheter

catheter *continued*

Ingram catheter
Inoue balloon catheter
insertion of catheter
Intact catheter
intercostal catheter
internal mammary artery catheter
intra-aortic balloon catheter
intra-arterial chemotherapy catheter
intracardiac catheter
Intracath catheter
intracoronary guiding catheter
intracoronary perfusion catheter
intracranial pressure catheter
intracranial pressure catheter monitor
Intran disposable intrauterine pressure measurement catheter
Intrasil catheter
intrauterine catheter
intrauterine pressure catheter
intravenous catheter
intravenous pacing catheter
introducer catheter
irrigating catheter
irrigation catheter
Itard catheter
IV catheter (intravenous catheter)
J-vac catheter
Jackson-Pratt catheter
Jaeger-Whiteley catheter
Javid catheter
JB catheter
JB-1 catheter
Jelco catheter
Jelm catheter
Jelm two-way catheter

catheter *continued*

JL-4 catheter (Judkins left, 4 cm)
JL-5 catheter (Judkins left, 5 cm)
Josephson catheter
JR-4 catheter (Judkins right, 4 cm)
JR-5 catheter (Judkins right, 5 cm)
Judkins catheter
Judkins coronary catheter
Judkins left coronary catheter
Judkins right coronary catheter
Judkins USCI catheter
Judkins-4 guiding catheter
Karmen catheter
Katon catheter
Kearns bag catheter
Kensey atherectomy catheter
kidney internal splint catheter (KISS)
kidney internal stent catheter (KISS)
Kifa catheter
Kimball catheter
King catheter
King guiding catheter
King multipurpose catheter
King multipurpose coronary graft catheter
kink-resistant catheter
kink-resistant peritoneal catheter
KISS catheter (kidney internal splint/stent catheter)
Lahey catheter
Lane catheter
Lane rectal catheter
Lapides catheter

catheter *continued*

large-bore catheter
large-lumen catheter
laser catheter
latex catheter
LeFort catheter
LeFort male catheter
LeFort urethral catheter
left ventricular clamp catheter
Lehman catheter
Lehman ventriculography catheter
Leroy catheter
LeVeen catheter
Levin tube catheter
Lifecath catheter
Lillehei-Warden catheter
Lloyd catheter
Lloyd esophagoscopic catheter
Lo-Profile balloon catheter
Lo-Profile II balloon catheter
Lo-Profile steerable dilatation catheter
lobster-tail catheter
Longdwel catheter
Longdwel Teflon catheter
LPS catheter
Luer-Lok catheter connection
Lumaguide infusion catheter
lumbar subarachnoid catheter
Lumelec catheter
Mahurkar catheter
Mahurkar dual-lumen catheter
Mahurkar dual-lumen dialysis catheter
Mahurkar dual-lumen femoral catheter
Malecot 2-wing catheter

MCRail

catheter *continued*

Malecot 4-wing catheter
Malecot catheter
Malecot suprapubic cystostomy catheter
Malecot urethral catheter
Mallinckrodt angiographic catheter
Mallinckrodt catheter
Maloney catheter
Mandelbaum catheter
Mani catheter
Mani cerebral catheter
Mansfield balloon catheter
Mansfield dilatation balloon catheter
mastoid catheter
McCarthy catheter
McCaskey catheter
McGoon coronary perfusion catheter
McIntosh double-lumen catheter
McIver catheter
McIver nephrostomy catheter
Med Rad catheter
mediastinal catheter
Medicut catheter
Medina catheter
Medina ileostomy catheter
MediPort-DL double-lumen catheter
Meditech arterial dilatation catheter
Meditech balloon catheter
Meditech catheter
Meditech Mansfield dilating catheter
Meditech steerable catheter
Medtronic balloon catheter
Mercier catheter

catheter *continued*

metal catheter
Metaport catheter
Metras catheter
metro catheter
Micro-Guide catheter
microinvasive catheter
micromanometer-tip catheter
midstream aortogram catheter
Mikro-tip angiocatheter
Millar micromanometer catheter
Millar pigtail angiographic catheter
Miller-Abbott catheter
Mini-Profile dilatation catheter
Mitsubishi angioscopic catheter
Mixtner catheter
Monorail angioplasty catheter
Morris catheter
MPF catheter
Mueller catheter guide
Mullins catheter introducer
Mullins transseptal catheter
multielectrode impedance catheter
multilumen catheter
Multi-Med triple-lumen catheter
Multi-Med triple-lumen infusion catheter
multipolar impedance catheter
multipurpose catheter
Multistim electrode catheter
mushroom catheter
Mylar catheter
nasal catheter
nasobiliary catheter
nasotracheal catheter

Moncrieff Popovich

catheter *continued*

NBIH catheter
Neal catheter
Nélaton catheter
nephrostomy catheter
NIH catheter
NIH left ventriculography catheter
Nutricath catheter
Nycore angiography catheter
Nycore catheter
occlusion catheter
Odman-Ledin catheter
Olbert balloon catheter
Olbert balloon dilatation catheter
olivary catheter
olive-tip catheter
Omni catheter
Omniflex balloon catheter
Optiscope catheter
Owen catheter
oximetric catheter
oximetry catheter
pacemaker catheter
Paceport catheter
pacifico catheter
pacing catheter
Paparella catheter
passage of catheter
Pathfinder catheter
PDT guiding catheter
PE Plus II balloon dilatation catheter
PE Plus II peripheral balloon catheter
pediatric balloon catheter
pediatric catheter
pediatric Foley catheter
peel-away catheter
peel-off catheter
Percor dual-lumen intra-aortic balloon catheter
Percor intra-aortic ballon catheter

catheter *continued*

Percor-DL catheter (dual-lumen catheter)
Percor-Stat-DL catheter (dual-lumen catheter)
percutaneous catheter
percutaneous trans-hepatic biliary drainage catheter
percutaneous trans-hepatic pigtail catheter
perfusion catheter
Peri-Patch peritoneal catheter extension set
peripheral atherectomy catheter
peripheral long-line catheter
peripherally inserted central catheter (PICC)
peritoneal catheter
peritoneal dialysis catheter
Perma-Cath catheter
Per-Stat-DL catheter
pervenous catheter
Pezzer catheter
Pezzer mushroom-tipped catheter
Pezzer suprapubic cystostomy catheter
Pharmaseal catheter
Phillips catheter
Phillips urethral catheter
PIBC catheter (percuta-neous intra-aortic balloon counterpulsa-tion catheter)
PICC (peripherally inserted central catheter)
pigtail catheter
Pilcher bag catheter
Pilcher catheter
Pilotip catheter
plastic catheter
Pleurovac chest catheter

PASport catheter .

catheter *continued*

pneumatic balloon catheter
pneumatic balloon catheter dilation
polyethylene catheter
Polystan catheter
Polystan venous return catheter
polyvinyl catheter
portal catheter
Portnoy catheter
Porto-Vac catheter
Positrol catheter
Positrol USCI catheter
Pousson pigtail catheter
preformed catheter
preformed Cordis catheter
preshaped catheter
Priestly catheter
probe catheter
probing catheter
Profile Plus catheter
Profile Plus dilatation catheter
Proflex dilatation catheter
prostatic catheter
Pruitt irrigation catheter
Pruitt occlusion catheter
PTBD catheter (percutaneous transhepatic biliary drainage catheter)
PTCA catheter
Pudenz-Heyer vascular catheter
pulmonary artery catheter
pulmonary flotation catheter
pulmonary triple-lumen catheter
pusher catheter
quadripolar catheter
Quanticor catheter

catheter *continued*

Quinton biopsy catheter
Quinton catheter
Quinton Mahurkar double-lumen catheter
Quinton Mahurkar dual-lumen peritoneal catheter
Quinton Q-Port catheter
Raaf Cath vascular catheter
Raaf catheter
Raaf double-lumen catheter
Raaf dual-lumen catheter
radial artery catheter
Radiofocus Glidewire angiography catheter
radiopaque catheter
railway catheter
Raimondi catheter
Raimondi spring peritoneal catheter
Raimondi ventricular catheter
Ramirez winged catheter
rapid exchange balloon catheter
Rashkind balloon catheter
Rashkind catheter
Rashkind septostomy balloon catheter
rat-tail catheter
recessed balloon septostomy catheter
rectal catheter
red Robinson catheter
red rubber catheter
RediFurl catheter
Reif catheter
Rentrop catheter
Rentrop infusion catheter
Replogle catheter
retention catheter
retroperfusion catheter
return-flow catheter

catheter *continued*

return-flow hemostatic catheter
Reynolds infusion catheter
RF balloon catheter
right coronary catheter
right-angle chest catheter
Ring biliary drainage catheter
Ring catheter
Ring-McLean catheter
Robinson catheter
Robinson urethral catheter
Rodriguez catheter
Rodriguez-Alvarez catheter
Rolnel catheter
Ross catheter
Rothene catheter
round-tip catheter
Rovenstine catheter-introducing forceps
Royal Flush angiographic flush catheter
rubber catheter
rubber-shod catheter
Rumel catheter
Rusch catheter
Rusch-Foley catheter
Ruschelit catheter
Rutner catheter
Rutner wedge catheter
Saratoga sump catheter
Schneider catheter
Schneider-Shiley catheter
Schneider-Shiley dilatation catheter
Schoonmaker catheter
Schoonmaker femoral catheter
Schoonmaker multipur-pose catheter
Schrotter catheter
Schwarten balloon-dilatation catheter

catheter *continued*

Science-Med balloon catheter
Sci-Med skinny catheter
Scoop transtracheal catheter
Seldinger catheter
Selective-HI catheter
Seletz catheter
self-retaining catheter
Sellheim uterine catheter
semirigid catheter
Semm uterine catheter
sensing catheter
septostomy balloon catheter
Shadow-Stripe catheter
shaver catheter
Sheldon catheter
shellac-covered catheter
Shepherd hook catheter
Shiley catheter
Shiley guiding catheter
Shiley JL-4 guiding catheter
Shiley JR-4 guiding catheter
Shiley MultiPro catheter
Shiley soft-tip guiding catheter
Shiley-Ionescu catheter
SHJR4s catheter (side-hole Judkins right, curve 4, short catheter)
side-hole catheter
side-hole pigtail catheter
sidewinder catheter
Silastic catheter
Silastic mushroom catheter
silicone elastomer catheter
silicone elastomer infusion catheter
silicone rubber Dacron-cuffed catheter
Silicore catheter

catheter *continued*

Silitek catheter
silk-and-wax catheter
Simmons catheter
Simplus catheter
Simplus dilatation catheter
Simpson atherectomy catheter
Simpson AtheroCath catheter
Simpson Ultra Lo-Profile balloon catheter
Simpson-Robert ACS dilatation catheter
Simpson-Robert catheter
single need catheter
single-stage catheter
six-eye catheter
Skene catheter
soft catheter
SOF-T guiding catheter
Softip arteriography catheter
Softip catheter
Softip diagnostic catheter
Softouch guiding catheter
solid-state esophageal manometry catheter
solid-tip catheter
Sones Cardio-Marker catheter
Sones catheter
Sones coronary catheter
Sones Hi-Flow catheter
Sones Positrol catheter
Sones vent catheter
Sorenson catheter for CVP line
Spectraprobe-PLS laser angioplasty catheter
Spetzler catheter
Spetzler subarachnoid catheter
spiral-tip catheter
spiral-tipped catheter

catheter *continued*

split-sheath catheter
Squire catheter
Stack perfusion coronary dilatation catheter
Stamey catheter
Stamey ureteral catheter
standard 6-lumen perfused catheter
Stanford end-hole pigtail catheter
steerable catheter
Stertzer brachial guiding catheter
Stertzer catheter
stimulating catheter
Stitt catheter
Storz bronchial catheter
Storz catheter
Storz-DeKock two-way bronchial catheter
straight catheter
straight flush percutane-ous catheter
Stress Cath catheter
Stretzer bent-tip USCI catheter
styletted catheter
styletted tracheobron-chial catheter
subclavian catheter
subclavian dialysis catheter
suction catheter
Suggs catheter
Sugita catheter
SULP II catheter
sump catheter
sump pump catheter
suprapubic catheter
Sureflow catheter
Surgitek catheter
Surgitek double-J ureteral catheter
Swan-Ganz catheter
Swan-Ganz guide-wire TD catheter

catheter *continued*

Swan-Ganz pulmonary
artery catheter
Swan-Ganz thermodilu-
tion catheter
Switzerland dilatation
catheter
T-tube catheter
TAC atherectomy
catheter
Tauber catheter
Teflon catheter
Teflon-tipped catheter
temporary pacing
catheter
Tenckhoff catheter
Tenckhoff peritoneal
catheter
Tenckhoff renal dialysis
catheter
Tennis Racquet angiogra-
phic catheter
Tennis Racquet catheter
Texas catheter
thermistor catheter
thermodilution balloon
catheter
thermodilution pacing
catheter
thermodilution Swan-
Ganz catheter
Thompson bronchial
catheter
Thompson catheter
three-way catheter
three-way Foley catheter
three-way irrigating
catheter
thrombectomy catheter
Thruflex PTCA balloon
catheter
Tiemann catheter
Tiemann coudé catheter
Tiemann Foley catheter
TLC Baxter balloon
catheter
Tomac catheter
toposcopic catheter

catheter *continued*

Torcon angiographic
catheter
Torcon catheter
TPN catheter
tracheal catheter
transcatheter
transducer-tipped
catheter
transluminal extraction
catheter (TEC)
transseptal catheter
transthoracic catheter
transvenous pacemaker
catheter
Trattner catheter
triple thermistor coronary
sinus catheter
triple-lumen catheter
triple-lumen central
catheter
triple-lumen central
venous catheter
triple-lumen manometric
catheter
tripolar catheter
Tuohy catheter
twist drill catheter
two-way catheter
Tygon catheter
UA catheter (umbilical
artery catheter)
UAC (umbilical artery
catheter)
Ultramer catheter
umbilical artery catheter
(UA catheter, UAC)
umbilical catheter
umbilical vein catheter
ureteral catheter
ureteral catheter obtura-
tor
urethral catheter
urethrographic catheter
urinary catheter
urologic catheter
Uro-San Plus external
catheter
USCI Bard catheter

Turkel

catheter *continued*

USCI catheter
USCI Finesse guiding catheter
USCI guiding catheter
USCI Mini-Profile balloon dilatation catheter
USCI Positrol coronary catheter
Vabra catheter
Vacurette catheter
valvuloplasty balloon catheter
van Sonnenberg catheter
van Sonnenberg sump catheter
Van Tassel angled pigtail catheter
Van Tassel pigtail catheter
Variflex catheter
vascular catheter
venous catheter
venous thrombectomy catheter
venting catheter
ventricular catheter
ventricular catheter introducer
ventriculography catheter
Versaflex steerable catheter
vertebrated catheter
Virden catheter
Vitalcor catheter
Vitalcor venous catheter
Vitalcor venous return catheter
Vitax female catheter
Vivonex jejunostomy catheter
Von Andel catheter
Von Andel dilation catheter
Vygon Nutricath S catheter
Walther catheter

catheter *continued*

Walther female catheter
wash catheter
washing catheter
Watanabe catheter
water-infusion esophageal manometry catheter
wave guide catheter
Weber catheter
Webster coronary sinus catheter
wedge catheter
Wedge Cook catheter
whalebone filiform catheter
whistle-tip catheter
whistle-tip Foley catheter
whistle-tip ureteral catheter
Wholey-Edwards catheter
Wick catheter
Williams L-R guiding catheter
Wilson-Cook catheter
Wilton-Webster coronary sinus catheter
Winer catheter
winged catheter
wire stylet catheter
Wishard catheter
Wishard tip catheter
Wishard ureteral catheter
Witzel enterostomy catheter
Wolf catheter
Wolf nephrostomy bag catheter
Woodruff catheter
Woodruff ureteropyelographic catheter
Word catheter
woven catheter
woven-silk catheter
Wurd catheter
Y-trough catheter
Yankauer catheter

catheter *continued*
    Zavod bronchospirometry catheter
    Zavod catheter
    Zucker cardiac catheter
    Zucker catheter
    Zurich dilatation catheter
catheter ablation of bundle of His
catheter adapter
catheter arteriography
catheter balloon
catheter balloon valvuloplasty (CBV)
catheter care kit
catheter clamp
catheter connector
catheter coudé
catheter deflecting mechanism
catheter dilatation
catheter drainage
catheter fin
catheter forceps
catheter forming wires
catheter gauge
catheter guide
catheter in place
catheter insertion
catheter introducer
catheter mapping
catheter needle
catheter placement
catheter plug
catheter positioned
catheter sepsis
catheter sheath
catheter site
catheter stylet
catheter tip
catheter tray
catheter tubing adapter
catheter was parked
catheter wick
catheter wire stylet
catheter-dilator
catheterization
catheterization of bladder
catheterization of duct
catheterization of eustachian tube
catheterization of heart
catheterization of lacrimonasal duct
catheterize
catheterized specimen
catheter-tip syringe
Cathlon IV catheter
cathode
catlin
catlin amputating knife
catling (see *catlin*)
cat's paw retractor
Cattell tube
Cattell forked-type T-tube
Cattell herniorrhaphy
Cattell operation
Cattell T-tube
Catterall classification of Perthes disease (I–IV)
Catterall prosthesis
cauda equina
caudad
caudal
caudal anesthesia
caudal artery
caudal aspect
caudal block
caudal branch
caudal displacement
caudal elevator
caudal flexure
caudal helix
caudal ligament
caudal needle
caudal pancreaticojejunostomy
caudal pole
caudal sac
caudal septum
caudalward
caudate
caudate lobe
caudate lobe of liver
caudate nucleus
caudate process
caudocephalad

caudocranial hemiaxial view
caudocranial view
cauliflower ear
cauliflower excrescence
Causse-Shea prosthesis
Causse-Shea tube
caustic bougie
caustic pencil
cauterization
cauterization of cervix
cauterization of lesion
cauterization of nose
cauterize
cautery
    Accu-Temp hot wire
      cautery
    actual cautery
    akidogalvanocautery
    Alcon cautery
    Alcon hand cautery
    alkaline battery cautery
    argon laser photocoagu-
      lator cautery
    biactive coagulation set
      cautery
    bicap cautery
    bipolar cautery
    Birtcher cautery
    Birtcher hyfrecator
      cautery
    Bovie cautery
    Bovie coagulation
      cautery
    Bovie electrocautery
    Bovie electrocautery
      unit
    Burdick cautery
    button cautery
    Cameron cautery
    Cameron-Lorenz cautery
    Cameron-Miller cautery
    carbon dioxide cautery
    chemical cautery
    chemicocautery
    chemocautery
    coagulation cautery
    cold cautery

cautery *continued*
    Concept cautery
    Concept eye cautery
    Concept hand-held
      cautery
    Corrigan cautery
    cryocautery
    Currentrol cautery
    cystoscopic electro-
      cautery
    Davis Bovie cautery
    Disposolette cautery
    Downes cautery
    electric cautery
    electrocautery
    electrocautery knife
    electrocautery pattern
    electrocautery snaring
    electrocautery unit
    endoscopic laser cautery
    excision and cautery
    eye cautery
    fine cautery
    galvanic cautery
    galvanocautery
    gas cautery
    Geiger cautery
    Geiger-Downes cautery
    Gonin cautery
    Goodhill cautery
    hand cautery
    Hawkins cervix coniza-
      tion cautery
    heat cautery
    Hildreth cautery
    Hildreth ocular cautery
    I-Stat cautery
    I-Temp cautery
    linear cautery
    looped cautery
    Magielski cautery
    Malis electrocautery
    Mentor cautery
    microcautery unit
    micropoint cautery
    Mills cautery
    Mira cautery

cautery *continued*

  Mira tip eye cautery
  monopolar cautery
  Mueller cautery
  Mueller Currentrol
    cautery
  Muir cautery clamp
  National cautery
  needlepoint electro-
    cautery
  NeoKnife cautery
  Neo-Med cautery
  ocular cautery
  ophthalmic cautery
  Op-Temp cautery
  Oxycel cautery
  Paquelin cautery
  Parker-Heath cautery
  penlight cautery
  Percy cautery
  potential cautery
  Prince cautery
  Prince eye cautery
  retinal puncture cautery
  Rommel cautery
  Rommel-Hildreth cautery
  Scheie cautery
  Scheie electrocautery
  Scheie ophthalmic
    cautery
  silver nitrate cautery
  silver nitrate cautery
    sticks
  Sluder cautery electrode
  snare cautery
  solar cautery
  Souttar cautery
  spot cautery
  Stanton cautery with
    mousetrap clamp
  Statham cautery
  steam cautery
  straight cautery
  sun cautery
  thermocautery
  Todd cautery
  Valley Lab cautery

cautery *continued*

  valvanocautery
  virtual cautery
  von Graefe cautery
  Wadsworth-Todd eye
    cautery
  Walker cautery
  Wappler cautery
  Wappler cold cautery
  wet-field cautery
  wet-field eraser cautery
  Wills Hospital eye
    cautery
  wound cautery
  xenon arc photocoagula-
    tion cautery
  Ziegler cautery
cautery bend
cautery cable
cautery clamp
cautery electrode
cautery for retinal detachment
cautery handle
cautery knife
cautery pencil
cautery snare
cautery transformer
cautery unit
cavagram
caval cannula
caval catheter
caval filter
caval fold
caval nodes
caval occlusion clamp
caval snare
caval tourniquet
caval valve
cavamesenteric shunt
Cavanaugh bur
Cavanaugh-Israel bur
Cavanaugh-Wells tonsil forceps
cavascope
Cave cartilage knife
Cave gouge
Cave incision
Cave knee retractor

Cave knife
Cave operation
Cave retractor
Cave scaphoid gouge
Cave scaphoid spatula
Cave spatula
cavernomatous changes
cavernosae penis, venae
cavernoscope
cavernoscopy
cavernosi clitoridis, nervi
cavernosi penis, nervi
cavernosography
cavernosometry
cavernotomy
cavernous
cavernous nerves of clitoris
cavernous nerves of penis
cavernous portion of urethra
cavernous sinus
cavernous urethra
cavernous veins of penis
Cave-Rowe operation
Cave-Rowe patellar procedure
CAVH (continuous arterio-
    venous hemofiltration)
Cavin osteotome
Cavin shunt
cavitary disease
cavitary lesion
cavitary mass
cavitation of lobe
Cavitron aspirator
Cavitron cataract extraction unit
Cavitron dental unit
Cavitron dissector
Cavitron scalpel
Cavitron ultrasonic aspirator
    (CUSA)
Cavitron-Kelman cataract unit
Cavitron-Kelman phacoemulsifi-
    cation
Cavitron-Kelman surgical unit
cavity
cavogram
cavography
cavopulmonary anastomosis

cavovalgus
cavovarus
CAVU (continuous arterio-
    venous ultrafiltration)
cavum
cavum conchae
cavum epidurale
cavum nasi
cavum septi pellucidi
cavum subarachnoideale
cavum subdurale
cavum trigeminale
cavum tympani
cavum uteri
cavum vergae
Caylor scissors
Cayo saw
CBD (common bile duct)
CBD stone
CBV (catheter balloon val-
    vuloplasty)
CCT (computerized cranial to-
    mography)
CCU (coronary care unit;
    cardiac care unit)
CD (conjugate diameter)
CDH (congenital dislocated hip)
CDH (congenital dysplasia of
    hip)
CDR (cup/disk ratio)
CE angle of Wiberg
CEA (carcinoembryonic
    antigen)
CEA (carotid endarterectomy)
Cebotome drill
cecal
cecal appendage
cecal appendix
cecal block
cecal cystoplasty
cecal fold
cecal hernia
cecal mesocolic lymph nodes
cecal vault
cecal volvulus
cecectomy
Cecil cotton

Cecil dressing
Cecil hypospadias repair
Cecil operation
Cecil transurethral resection of
    prostate
Cecil TURP
Cecil urethral stricture operation
Cecil-Culp hypospadias repair
Cecil-Culp operation
Cecil-Culp urethroplasty
cecocele
cecocolic
cecocolic intussusception
cecocolon
cecocolopexy
cecocoloplicopexy
cecocolostome
cecocolostomy
cecocystoplasty
cecofixation
cecoileostomy
cecopexy
cecoplication
cecoptosis
cecorectal
cecorrhaphy
cecosigmoidostomy
cecostomy
cecostomy catheter
cecostomy retractor
cecostomy trocar
cecotomy
cecum
cecum mobile
CEEA stapler (curved end-to-
    end anastomosis stapler)
cefadroxil
cefamandole
cefazolin sodium
celectome
Celestin dilator bougie
Celestin esophageal tube
Celestin graduated dilator
Celestin graft material
Celestin implant
Celestin latex rubber tube
Celestin prosthesis

Celestin tube
celiac
celiac angiography
celiac arteriography
celiac artery
celiac atresia
celiac axis
celiac clamp
celiac ganglion
celiac glands
celiac lymph nodes
celiac nerves
celiac plexus
celiac trunk
celiacography
celiectomy
celiocentesis
celioenterotomy
celiogastrotomy
celiohysterectomy
celiomyomectomy
celiomyomotomy
celioparacentesis
celiopyosis
celiorrhaphy
celioscope
celioscopy
celiotomy
celiotomy incision
cell and flare
Cell Saver autologous blood
    recovery system
Cell Saver blood
Cell Saver Haemolite
Cellamin bandage
Cellamin resin plaster-of-Paris
    bandage
Cellolite
Cellolite patty
Cellona bandage
Cellona resin plaster-of-Paris
    bandage
cellophane
cellophane dressing
cells
celltrifuge device
cellules

cellulocutaneous
cellulocutaneous flap
celluloid
celluloid graft material
celluloid implant
celluloid linen sutures
celluloid prosthesis
celluloid sutures
celluloid thread
cellulose
cellulose gauze
celoscope
celoscopy
celotomy
celsian amputation
celsian lithotomy
celsian operation
Celsus lithotomy
Celsus operation
cement
cement burn
cement eater
cement eater drill
cement gun
cement mantle
cement restrictor
cemented gingiva
cementless
cementless hip system
cementoma
cementophyte
cementum fracture
cementum hyperplasia
Cenflex central monitoring
    system
Centaur trial cup
center blade
centering collar
centering drill
centering ring
centesis
centigray (cGy)
centimeter (cm)
central amputation
central artery of retina
central callus
central canal

central cataract
central catheter
central cerebral sulcus
central compartment
central iridectomy
central nervous system (CNS)
central nervous system shunt
central sutures incised
central tendon
central tendon of diaphragm
central tendon of perineum
central terminal electrode
central vein of retina
central vein of suprarenal gland
central veins of liver
central vein of retina
central venous catheter
central venous line
central venous pressure (CVP)
central venous pressure line
central vision
centrales hepatis, venae
centralis glandulae suprarenalis,
    vena
centralis retinae, arteria
centralis retinae, vena
centrifuge microscope
centripetal extrusion
centripetal nerve
centripetal venous pulse
centrocecal scotoma
centroparietal regions
Centry bicarbonate dialysis
    control unit
Centry II dialysis machine
cephalad
cephalad aspect
cephalad catheter
cephalagia
cephalgia
cephalic
cephalic blade forceps
cephalic flexure
cephalic presentation
cephalic triangle
cephalic vein
cephalic version

cephalica accessoria, vena
cephalica, vena
cephalocaudad
cephalocaudad diameter
cephalocentesis
cephalogram
cephalography
cephalometric radiography
cephalometric roentgenogram
cephalometry
cephalopelvic disproportion
    (CPD)
cephalotomy
ceraceous
ceramic
ceramic hip prosthesis
ceramic total hip
ceratocricoid muscle
ceratocricoideus, musculus
ceratopharyngeal muscle
ceratopharyngeus, musculus
cerclage
cerclage for retinal detachment
cerclage of cervix
cerclage of fractured bone
cerclage wire
cerebellar artery
cerebellar ataxis
cerebellar attachment
cerebellar cortex
cerebellar degeneration
cerebellar electrodes
cerebellar gliosis
cerebellar hemisphere
cerebellar notch
cerebellar peduncle
cerebellar pontine angle
cerebellar rigidity
cerebellar sclerosis
cerebellar stimulation
cerebellar tonsil
cerebellar veins
cerebelli inferior anterior, arteria
cerebelli inferior posterior,
    arteria
cerebelli inferiores, venae
cerebelli superior, arteria

cerebelli superiores, venae
cerebellomedullary cistern
cerebellopontine angle
cerebellopontine angle cistern
cerebellopontine angle tumor
cerebellum
cerebellum retractor
cerebral air embolism
cerebral anesthesia
cerebral angiogram
cerebral angiography
cerebral angiography needle
cerebral apophysis
cerebral aqueduct
cerebral arteriogram
cerebral arteriography
cerebral artery
cerebral blood flow
cerebral calcification
cerebral cannula
cerebral catheter
cerebral circulation
cerebral compression
cerebral concussion
cerebral contusion
cerebral cortex
cerebral death
cerebral decompression
cerebral edema
cerebral embolism
cerebral epidural space
cerebral fissure
cerebral fornix
cerebral fossa
cerebral function
cerebral hemiplegia
cerebral hemisphere
cerebral hemorrhage
cerebral infarction
cerebral lateralization
cerebral nerve ganglionectomy
cerebral nerves
cerebral origin
cerebral palsy
cerebral paraplegia
cerebral paresis
cerebral paroxysmal activity

cerebral peduncle
cerebral retractor
cerebral seizure
cerebral sinusography
cerebral spasm
cerebral thrombosis
cerebral trauma
cerebral tumor
cerebral vasoconstriction
cerebral vein
cerebral ventricles
cerebral ventriculography
cerebration
cerebri anterior, arteria
cerebri anterior, vena
cerebri inferiores, venae
cerebri internae, venae
cerebri magna, vena
cerebri media, arteria
cerebri media profunda, vena
cerebri media superficialis, vena
cerebri posterior, arteria
cerebri superiores, venae
cerebroangiophotoscintigram
cerebromedullary tube
cerebro-ocular
cerebrospinal
cerebrospinal axis
cerebrospinal endarteritis
cerebrospinal fasciculus
cerebrospinal fluid (CSF)
cerebrospinal fluid otorrhea
cerebrospinal fluid rhinorrhea
cerebrospinal fluid shunt system
cerebrospinal fluid system
cerebrospinal pressure
cerebrostomy
cerebrovascular
cerebrovascular accident (CVA)
cerebrovascular blood circula-
    tion
cerebrovascular insufficiency
cerebrovascular obstructive
    disease
cerebrovascular occlusion
cerebrovascular resistance
cerebrum

cerulean cataract
cerumen
ceruminal impaction
ceruminous gland
ceruminous gland tumor
Cerva Crane halter
cervical abortion
cervical adenopathy
cervical amputation
cervical anesthesia
cervical artery
cervical atypism
cervical biopsy
cervical biopsy blade
cervical biopsy curet
cervical biopsy forceps
cervical biopsy punch forceps
cervical blade
cervical brace
cervical canal
cervical cancer
cervical carcinoma
cervical cauterization
cervical cerclage
cervical cesarean section
cervical chain
cervical collar
cervical collar brace
cervical cone biopsy
cervical conization
cervical conization electrode
cervical cord injury
cervical cordotomy
cervical cordotomy knife
cervical culture
cervical curet
cervical curettage
cervical curvature
cervical curve
cervical dilator
cervical discharge
cervical disk
cervical disk instruments
cervical drill
cervical drill guard
cervical dysplasia
cervical dystocia

cervical ectopy
cervical erosion
cervical esophagus
cervical fascia
cervical flexure
cervical foraminal punch
cervical forceps
cervical fusion
cervical ganglion
cervical glands
cervical heart
cervical hemostatic forceps
cervical incision
cervical incompetence
cervical insertion of radium
cervical intraepithelial neoplasia
    (CIN)
cervical knife
cervical laminectomy punch
cervical lymph node
cervical mallet
cervical mediastinoscopy
cervical mobilization
cervical musculature
cervical needle
cervical neoplasia
cervical nerves
cervical neural canal
cervical node
cervical os
cervical Pap smear
cervical pleura
cervical plexus
cervical plexus nerve block
cervical polyp
cervical pregnancy
cervical punch
cervical punch biopsy
cervical punch forceps
cervical radium insertion
cervical region
cervical retractor
cervical rib
cervical rib syndrome
cervical rongeur
cervical smear
cervical spine

cervical spondylolysis
cervical sprain
cervical stenosis
cervical stump
cervical support
cervical sutures
cervical swab
cervical sympathectomy
cervical sympathetic nerve
cervical tenaculum
cervical traction
cervical traction forceps
cervical traction tongs
cervical vein
cervical vertebrae
cervicales, nervi
cervicalis ascendens, arteria
cervicalis profunda, arteria
cervicalis profunda, vena
cervicectomy
cervicobrachial
cervicobrachialgia
cervicobregmatic diameter
cervicodynia
cervicofacial face lift
cervicoisthmic angle
cervico-occipital
cervicoplasty
cervicothoracic
cervicothoracic ganglion
cervicotrochanteric
cervicouterine ganglion
cervicovaginal adhesions
Cervital partial ossicular
    replacement prosthesis
    (PORP)
Cervital PORP (partial ossicular
    replacement prosthesis)
Cervital TORP (total ossicular
    replacement prosthesis)
Cervital total ossicular replace-
    ment prosthesis (TORP)
cervitome
cervix
cervix forceps
cervix suture needle
cervix uteri

cervix-holding forceps
cesarean birth
cesarean delivery
cesarean forceps
cesarean hysterectomy
cesarean section
cesium applicator
cesium cylinder
cesium insertion
cesium irradiation
cesium mold
cesium radiation
cesium sources
cesium therapy
cesium tube
cesium tube radiation
cessation
Cetacaine anesthetic agent
Cetacaine topical anesthetic
CF (cardiac failure)
CFC pheresis (continuous-flow
    centrifugation pheresis)
CFE Taperloc hip prosthesis
CFLV3UU colonoscope
CFS total hip (contoured
    femoral stem total hip)
CFV (continuous-flow ventila-
    tion)
CGS (catgut suture)
cGy (centigray)
Chadwick scissors
Chaffin catheter
Chaffin suction tube
Chaffin sump tube
Chaffin tube
Chaffin tube catheter
Chaffin-Pratt concept unit
Chaffin-Pratt drain
Chaffin-Pratt percolator hanger
    holder
Chaffin-Pratt suction tube
Chaffin-Pratt suction unit
Chaffin-Pratt tube
chain ligatures
chain saw
chain sutures
chain-of-lakes configuration

chain-of-lakes sign
chair cushion
chair lift
chair pad
chair-back brace
chair-table
Chakirgil technique
chalazion
chalazion clamp
chalazion curet
chalazion excision
chalazion forceps
chalazion knife
chalazion punch
chalazion retractor
chalazion trephine
chalk bones
chalky bones
chamber irrigation
chamber of eye
chamber size
Chamberlain decompressor
Chamberlain incision
Chamberlain line
Chamberlain mediastinoscopy
Chamberlain mediastinotomy
Chamberlain procedure
Chamberlen forceps
Chamberlen obstetrical forceps
Chambers diaphragm
Chambers doughnut pessary
Chambers intrauterine cup
Chambers pessary
Chambers technique
Chamfer cut
Chamfer guide
Chamfer reamer
Chamfer saw
chamfered
Champ elastic bandage
Champetier de Ribes obstetrical
    bag
Champion sutures
Championnière forceps
Champy bone plate
Chan wrist rest
Chance fracture

Chance lumbar spine fracture
Chandler arthrodesis
Chandler bone elevator
Chandler elevator
Chandler forceps
Chandler hammer
Chandler hip fusion
Chandler iridectomy
Chandler iris forceps
Chandler laminectomy retractor
Chandler mallet
Chandler retractor
Chandler spinal perforating
	forceps
Chandler splint
Chandler technique
Chandler V-pacing probe
Chang bone-cutting forceps
channel retractor
channel ulcer
Chaoul tube
Chapchal technique
Chapman-Dintenfass perforator
Chaput forceps
Chaput operation
Charcot arthritis
Charcot arthrosis
Charcot foot
Charcot joint
Charcot operation
Charcot prosthesis
Charcot sign
Charcot triad
Charcot-Bouchard aneurysm
Charcot-Leyden crystals
Charcot-Marie-Tooth atrophy
Chardack Medtronic pacemaker
Chardack pacemaker
Chardack-Greatbatch im-
	plantable cardiac pulse
	generator
Chardack-Greatbatch pace-
	maker
charged particle beam therapy
charged particles
charger
Charles intraocular lens

Charles lens
Charles needle
Charles operation
Charles vacuuming needle
Charlton antrum needle
Charlton cannula
Charlton needle
Charlton trocar
Charnley approach
Charnley arthrodesis
Charnley arthroplasty
Charnley bone clamp
Charnley cemented hip
	prosthesis
Charnley clamp
Charnley compression fusion
Charnley compressor
Charnley cup
Charnley drill
Charnley forceps
Charnley hip prosthesis
Charnley knee prosthesis
Charnley knee retractor
Charnley prosthesis
Charnley reamer
Charnley retractor
Charnley-Barnes hemostat
Charnley-cobra total hip
	prosthesis
Charnley-Ferreira trochanter
	reattachment
Charnley-Moore hip prosthesis
Charnley-Mueller approach
Charnley-Mueller arthroplasty
Charnley-Mueller cemented hip
	prosthesis
Charnley-Mueller rasp
Charretera flap
Charrière bone saw
Charrière saw
Charrière scale
Chassaignac axillary muscle
Chassaignac tubercle
Chassard-Lapiné maneuver
Chassin tube
Chatfield-Girdlestone splint
Chatzidakis implant

Chauffard point
chauffeur's fracture
Chausse view
Chaussier areola
Chaussier tube
Chaves procedure
Chaves scapula surgery
Chaves-Rapp scapula surgery
Chayes handpiece
CHD (congenital heart defect)
CHD (congenital hip disloca-
    tion)
CHD (congestive heart disease)
CHD (coronary heart disease)
Cheatle forceps
Cheatle slit
Cheatle slit for colostomy
    takedown
Cheatle sterilizer forceps
Cheatle-Henry hernia
Cheatle-Henry incision
Cheatle-Henry operation
check ligament
Check-Flo introducer
checkup
check-valve obstruction
check-valve sheath
cheek flap
cheek retractor
cheesy cataract
Cheever tonsillectomy
cheilectomy
cheilognathopalatoschisis
cheilognathoprosoposchisis
cheilognathoschisis
cheilognathouranoschisis
cheiloplasty
cheilorrhaphy
cheiloschisis
cheilostomatoplasty
cheilotomy
cheiromegaly
cheiroplasty
cheiropodalgia
cheirospasm
Chelsea-Eaton anal speculum
Chelsea-Eaton speculum
chemabrasion

chemexfoliation
chemical anesthesia
chemical burn
chemical cardioversion
chemical cautery
chemical decortication
chemical hysterectomy
chemical pallidectomy
chemical peel of skin
chemical shift
chemical sympathectomy
chemicocautery
chemocauterization
chemocautery
chemocoagulation
chemodectomy
chemolysis
chemoneurolysis
chemonucleolysis
chemopallidectomy
chemopallidectomy scissors
chemopallidothalamectomy
chemopeel
Chemo-Port catheter
chemoprophylaxis
chemosis
chemosurgery
chemothalamectomy
chemotherapy
Cherney abdominal incision
Cherney incision
Cherney sutures
Cherney thyroid nodule
Cherney-Winklesnit abdominal
    incision
Chernez incision
Chernov hook
Chernov notched ruler
Chernov tracheostomy hook
Cheron forceps
cherry angioma
Cherry brain probe
Cherry drill
Cherry extractor
Cherry forceps
Cherry laminectomy self-
    retaining retractor
Cherry osteotome

Cherry probe
Cherry retractor
Cherry S-shaped scissors
Cherry S-shaped brain retractor
Cherry scissors
cherry sponge
Cherry tongs
Cherry traction tongs
Cherry-Adson forceps
Cherry-Austin drill
Cherry-Kerrison forceps
Cherry-Kerrison laminectomy
    rongeur
Cherry-Kerrison rongeur for-
    ceps
cherry-picking procedure
chessboard graft
chessboard implant
chessboard prosthesis
chessboard skin graft
chest bellows
chest cardiac massage
chest cavity
chest clear to percussion and
    auscultation
chest compression
chest congestion
chest cuirass
chest diameter
chest drainage
chest dressing
chest film
chest mediastinum
chest muscles
chest nodules
chest pain
chest percussion
chest port
chest position
chest spreader
chest thump
chest tightness
chest tube
chest wall
chest wall defect
chest x-ray
Chester forceps
Chevalier Jackson bougie

Chevalier Jackson broncho-
    scope
Chevalier Jackson esophago-
    scope
Chevalier Jackson forceps
Chevalier Jackson gastroscope
Chevalier Jackson laryngeal
    speculum
Chevalier Jackson laryngectomy
Chevalier Jackson laryngoscope
Chevalier Jackson operation
Chevalier Jackson scissors
Chevalier Jackson speculum
Chevalier Jackson tracheal tube
Chevalier Jackson tube
chevron incision
chevron osteotomy
Cheyne dissector
Cheyne dry dissector
Cheyne operation
Cheyne periosteal elevator
Cheyne retractor
Cheyne-Stokes sign
CHF (congestive heart failure)
Chiari operation for congenital
    hip dislocation
Chiari osteotomy
Chiari-Arnold syndrome
chiasm
chiasm of Camper
chiasm of digitus of hand
chiasm of flexor sublimis
chiasm of musculus flexor
    digitorum
chiasm opticum
chiasma
chiasmatic cistern
Chiazzi operation
Chiba eye needle
Chiba needle
Chiba percutaneous cholangi-
    ogram
Chick fracture table
Chick operating table
Chick sterile dressings
chicken-bill rongeur
chicken-bill rongeur forceps
Chick-Hyde fracture table

Chick-Langren table
Chiene incision
Chiene operation
Chiene test for femoral neck
　　fracture
Chilaiditi syndrome
Chilcott cannula
Chilcott venoclysis cannula
Child classification of liver
　　disease
Child clip-applying forceps
child esophagoscope
Child forceps
Child intestinal forceps
Child operation
Child operative risk grading
　　system (A, B, C)
Child pancreatectomy
Child pancreaticoduodenostomy
Children's Hospital brain
　　spatula
Children's Hospital clip
Children's Hospital forceps
Children's Hospital intestinal
　　forceps
Children's Hospital mallet
Children's Hospital screwdriver
Children's Hospital spatula
Childress operation
Childs Cardio-Cuff
child's rib spreader
child-size eye speculum
Childs-Phillips bowel plication
Childs-Phillips forceps
Childs-Phillips intestinal
　　plication needle
Childs-Phillips needle
Childs-Phillips plication needle
Child-Turcotte classification of
　　liver reserve
chin augmentation
chin implant
chin lift
chin muscle
chin prosthesis
chin protuberance
chin reflex

chin retraction sign
chin strap
Chinese fingerstraps traction
　　device
Chinese twisted silk sutures
chip fracture
chip syringe
chiroplasty
chisel
　　Adson chisel
　　Adson laminectomy
　　　chisel
　　Alexander chisel
　　Alexander mastoid chisel
　　Amico chisel
　　Andrews chisel
　　antral chisel
　　Army pattern chisel
　　Artmann chisel
　　Artmann disarticulation
　　　chisel
　　Austin chisel
　　Austin Moore mortising
　　　chisel
　　Bakelite dental chisel
　　Ballenger chisel
　　Ballenger-Hajek chisel
　　binangled chisel
　　Bishop chisel
　　Blair chisel
　　bone chisel
　　Bowen chisel
　　Bowen gooseneck chisel
　　Brauer chisel
　　Brittain chisel
　　Brown chisel
　　Bruening chisel
　　Brun chisel
　　Brunetti chisel
　　Brunner chisel
　　Burns chisel
　　Burns guarded chisel
　　Caltagirone chisel
　　cartilage chisel
　　Cinelli chisel
　　Cinelli-McIndoe chisel
　　Clawicz chisel

chisel *continued*
    Clevedent-Gardner chi-
      sel
    Clevedent-Wakefield
      chisel
    Cloward chisel
    Cloward puka chisel
    Cloward spinal fusion
      chisel
    Cloward-Harman chisel
    Cobb chisel
    Compere bone chisel
    Compere chisel
    Converse chisel
    Converse guarded chisel
    Converse nasal chisel
    Cooley chisel
    corneal chisel
    costotome chisel
    Cottle antral chisel
    Cottle chisel
    Cottle crossbar chisel
    Cottle crossbar fishtail
      chisel
    Cottle curved chisel
    Cottle fishtail chisel
    Councilman chisel
    Crane bone chisel
    Crane chisel
    crossbar chisel
    crurotomy chisel
    Dautrey chisel
    Derlacki chisel
    Derlacki-Shambaugh
      chisel
    D'Errico chisel
    D'Errico laminectomy
      chisel
    disarticulation chisel
    dissecting chisel
    double-guarded chisel
    Duray-Read chisel
    Duray-Wood chisel
    Eicher chisel
    Eicher tri-fin chisel
    ethmoidal chisel
    Farrior-Derlacki chisel

chisel *continued*
    Farrior-Dworacek canal
      chisel
    Faulkner antrum chisel
    Faulkner chisel
    Faulkner trocar chisel
    Faulkner-Browne chisel
    fishtail chisel
    Fomon chisel
    footplate chisel
    fracture chisel
    Freer bone chisel
    Freer chisel
    Freer lacrimal chisel
    Freer submucous chisel
    French chisel
    frontal sinus chisel
    Gardner bone chisel
    Gardner chisel
    Goldman chisel
    gooseneck chisel
    guarded chisel
    Hajek chisel
    Hajek septal chisel
    Halle chisel
    Heermann chisel
    Henderson chisel
    Hibbs bone chisel
    Hibbs chisel
    hollow chisel
    Holmes chisel
    House chisel
    House footplate chisel
    House-Derlacki chisel
    J.E. Sheehan chisel
    Joseph chisel
    Katsch chisel
    Keyes bone-splitting
      chisel
    Keyes chisel
    Kezerian chisel
    Killian chisel
    Killian frontal sinus
      chisel
    Killian-Claus chisel
    Killian-Reinhard chisel
    Kilner chisel

chisel *continued*
Kreischer bone chisel
Kreischer chisel
lacrimal chisel
Lambotte chisel
Lambotte splitting chisel
laminectomy chisel
Lebsche chisel
Lexer chisel
Lucas chisel
MacAusland chisel
Magielski chisel
mastoid chisel
McIndoe chisel
Metzenbaum chisel
Meyerding chisel
middle ear chisel
Moberg chisel
Moore chisel
Moore hollow chisel
Moore prosthesis
  mortising chisel
mortising chisel
Murphy chisel
nasal chisel
Obwegeser splitting
  chisel
Partsch chisel
Passow chisel
peapod chisel
Peck chisel
pick chisel
puka chisel
Read chisel
Richards chisel
Rish chisel
Roberts chisel
Schuknecht chisel
septal chisel
Sewall chisel
Sewall ethmoidal chisel
Shambaugh-Derlacki
  chisel
Sheehan chisel
Sheehan nasal chisel
Sheehy-House chisel
Silver chisel

chisel *continued*
Simmons chisel
sinus chisel
Skoog nasal chisel
small bone chisel
Smillie chisel
Smillie cartilage chisel
Smith-Petersen chisel
spinal fusion chisel
splitting chisel
Stacke chisel guard
stapes chisel
Stille chisel
Stille pattern bone chisel
submucous chisel
tri-fin chisel
Troutman chisel
Troutman mastoid chisel
twin-pattern chisel
U.S. Army chisel
Virchow chisel
Walsh chisel
West bone chisel
West chisel
White bone chisel
White chisel
Wilmer chisel
Wilmer wedge chisel
Wolf chisel knife
Worth chisel
chisel elevator
chisel fracture
chisel fracture of radius
chisel guard
chisel knife
chisel-osteotome
Chitten-Hill retractor
chloramine
chloramine anesthetic agent
chloramine catgut sutures
chloramphenicol
chloroma
chloromycetin
chloromyeloma
chloroprocaine hydrochloride
  anesthetic agent
Chlumsky button

CHM (hypertrophic cardiomy-
    opathy)
Cho technique
choana (*pl.* choanae)
choana atresia
choana narium
choanal bur
choanal plug
choanal polyp
chocolate cyst
choked disk
cholangiectasis
cholangioadenoma
cholangiocarcinoma
cholangiocholangiostomy
cholangiocholecystocholedoch-
    ectomy
cholangioenterostomy
cholangiogastrostomy
cholangiogram
cholangiography
cholangiography catheter
cholangiography tube
cholangiohepatoma
cholangiojejunostomy
cholangiopancreatogram
cholangiopancreatography
cholangiostomy
cholangiotomy
cholecyst
cholecystalgia
cholecystatony
cholecystectasia
cholecystectomy
cholecystelectrocoagulectomy
cholecystendysis
cholecystenteric
cholecystenteric fistula
cholecystenteroanastomosis
cholecystenterorrhaphy
cholecystenterostomy
cholecystgastrostomy
cholecystic
cholecystitis
cholecystitis with lithiasis
cholecystnephrostomy
cholecystocecostomy

cholecystocholangiogram
cholecystocholangiography
cholecystocholedochal fistula
cholecystocolonic
cholecystocolostomy
cholecystocolotomy
cholecystoduodenal fistula
cholecystoduodenal ligament
cholecystoduodenocolic fistula
cholecystoduodenocolic fold
cholecystoduodenostomy
cholecystoelectrocoagulectomy
cholecystoenterostomy
cholecystogastric
cholecystogastric fistula
cholecystogastrostomy
cholecystogram
cholecystography
cholecystoileostomy
cholecystointestinal fistula
cholecystojejunostomy
cholecystokinetic
cholecystolithiasis
cholecystolithotripsy
cholecystonephrostomy
cholecystopancreatostomy
cholecystopathy
cholecystopexy
cholecystoptosis
cholecystopyelostomy
cholecystorrhaphy
cholecystostomy
cholecystotomy
choledochal
choledochal cyst
choledochal sphincter
choledochal sphincterotomy
choledochectomy
choledochendysis
choledochitis
choledochocholedochorrhaphy
choledochocholedochostomy
choledochocolonic fistula
choledochoduodenal fistula
choledochoduodenal junctional
    stenosis
choledochoduodenostomy

choledochoenterostomy
choledochogastrostomy
choledochogram study
choledochography
choledochohepatostomy
choledochoileostomy
choledochojejunostomy
choledocholith
choledocholithiasis
choledocholithotomy
choledocholithotripsy
choledochopancreatic ductal
    junction
choledochopancreatostomy
choledochoplasty
choledochorrhaphy
choledochoscope
       Berci-Shore choledocho-
         scope
       Fujinon flexible choledo-
         choscope
       Storz choledochoscope
choledochoscope-nephroscope
choledochoscopy
choledochosphincterotomy
choledochostomy
choledochotomy
choledochotomy incision
choledochus
choledochus cyst
choledogram
cholelithiasis
cholelithotomy
cholelithotripsy
cholelithotrity (see *cholelitho-
    tripsy*)
cholemia
cholepathia
choleperitoneum
cholescintigraphy
cholesteatoma
cholesterol calculus
cholesterol gallstone
cholesterol stone
chondral
chondrectomy
chondrification

chondroblastoma
chondrocutaneous flap
chondrodynia
chondroectodermal dysplasia
chondrogenesis
chondroglossus muscle
chondrolysis
chondroma
chondromalacia
chondromatosis
chondrometaplasia
chondromucoid
chondromyxofibroma
chondronecrosis
chondro-osseous
chondro-osteodystrophy
chondropathology
chondropharyngeal muscle
chondroplastic
chondroplastic Beaver blade
chondroplastic blade
chondroplasty
chondrosarcoma
chondroskeleton
chondrosternal
chondrosternal articulation
chondrosternal depression
chondrosternoplasty
chondrotome
        Dyonics chondrotome
        Stryker chondrotome
chondrotomy
chop amputation
Chopart amputation
Chopart ankle dislocation
Chopart cheiloplasty
Chopart dislocation
Chopart fracture
Chopart joint
Chopart operation
choppy sea sign
chorda (*pl.* chordae)
chorda dorsalis
chorda gubernaculum
chorda saliva
chorda spermatica
chorda tendineae cordis

chorda tympani nerve
chorda tympani pusher
chordal tissue
chordate
chordectomy
chordee
chorditis cantorum
chorditis fibrinosa
chorditis nodosa
chorditis tuberosa
chorditis vocalis
chordoma
chordotomy
choreiform movements
chorion
chorion membranes
chorionic
chorionic cyst
chorionic plaque
chorionic tissue
chorionic vesicle
chorionic villi
chorionic villi biopsy (CVB)
chorionic villi sampling
chorioretinal
chorioretinitis
choriovitelline placenta
choroid
choroid artery
choroid atrophy
choroid detachment
choroid plexus
choroid vein
choroidal artery
choroidal atrophy
choroidal cataract
choroidal vessels
choroidea anterior, arteria
choroidea, vena
choroidectomy
Chorus pacemaker
Choyce anterior chamber lens
Choyce eye implant
Choyce implant
Choyce implant cataract lens
Choyce intraocular lens forceps
Choyce lens

Choyce lens forceps
Choyce Mark eye implant
Choyce-Tennant lens
Chrisman-Snook ankle procedure
Christiansen total hip
Christie gallbladder retractor
Christmas-tree cannula
Christmas-tree rasp
Christopher-Williams overtube
Christopher-Williams tube
chromated catgut sutures
chromatography
chromic blue dyed sutures
chromic catgut mattress sutures
chromic catgut sutures
chromic collagen sutures
chromic gut sutures
chromic ligatures
chromic sutures
chromicized catgut sutures
chromocystoscopy
chromohydrotubation
chromopertubation
chromosomal mosaicism
chromotubation
chromoureteroscopy
chronaximeter
chronically infected
chronically inflamed
Chronocor IV external pacemaker
chronology
chronotropic effect
CHS (compression hip screw)
Chubb tonsil forceps
chuck
chuck adapter
chuck cutter
chuck drill
chuck handle
chuck handle holster
chuck key
Chuck-It disposable accessories
Chuinard femoral osteotomy
Chuinard-Petersen arthrodesis
Chun-gun transillumination

Church cardiovascular scissors
Church deep surgery scissors
Church pediatric scissors
Church scissors
Chux incontinent dressing
Chvostek sign
Chvostek-Trousseau sign
Chvostek-Weiss sign
chyle
chyle cyst
chyle fat
chylectasis
chylous
chylous ascites
chylous fluid
Chymodiactin
chymonucleolysis
chymopapain
Cibis electrode
Cibis procedure
Cibis ski needle
cicatrectomy
cicatrices (*sing.* cicatrix)
cicatricial
cicatricial stricture
cicatricotomy
cicatrix (*pl.* cicatrices)
cicatrizant
cicatrization
cicatrize
cicatrizing enteritis
Cicherelli bone rongeur
Cicherelli forceps
Cicherelli rongeur
Cicherelli rongeur forceps
cidal level
Cidex (aqueous glutaraldehyde)
Cidex solution
cigarette drain
Cikloid dressing
Cilastin tube
Cilco extractor
Cilco intraocular lens
Cilco laser
Cilco lens
cilia
cilia base

cilia forceps
ciliares anteriores, arteriae
ciliares breves, nervi
ciliares longi, nervi
ciliares posteriores breves,
    arteriae
ciliares posteriores longae,
    arteriae
ciliares, venae
ciliaris, musculus
ciliarotomy
ciliary arteries
ciliary axis
ciliary body
ciliary disk
ciliary flush
ciliary folds
ciliary ganglion
ciliary glands
ciliary ligament
ciliary margins
ciliary muscle
ciliary nerves
ciliary processes
ciliary reflex
ciliary region
ciliary veins
ciliary vessels
ciliary zonule
ciliectomy
cilioretinal artery
cilioretinal vein
ciliospinal center
cilium pacemaker
Cimino arteriovenous fistula
Cimino arteriovenous shunt
Cimino AV fistula
Cimino fistula
Cimino-Brescia arteriovenous
    fistula
CIN (cervical intraepithelial
    neoplasia)
cinch operation
cinching
cinchocaine anesthetic agent
Cincinnati ACL brace
Cincinnati incision

cinctured
cine CT
cineangiocardiogram
cineangiocardiography
cineangiogram
cineangiography
cinearteriogram
cinebronchogram
cine-camera
cinefluorography
Cinelli chisel
Cinelli elevator
Cinelli guarded osteotome
Cinelli osteotome
Cinelli scissors
Cinelli-Fomon scissors
Cinelli-McIndoe chisel
cinematic amputation
cinematization
cinephonation study
cineplastic amputation
cineplastic procedure
cineplastic surgery
cineplastics
cineplasty
cineradiogram
cineradiographic examination
cineradiography
cines and plain films
cingulate gyrus
cingulate sulcus
cingulectomy
cinguli gyrus
cingulotomy
cingulumotomy
Cintor knee prosthesis
cionectomy
cionorrhaphy
cionotome
cionotomy
circinate
circle absorption anesthesia
circle knife
circle nephrostomy tube
circle of Willis
circling silicone tape
CircOlectric bed

CircOlectric sling
Circon arthroscope
Circon camera
Circon leg holder
Circon video camera
Circon-ACMI electrohydraulic
    lithotriptor probe
circular amputation
circular bandage
circular blade
circular block anesthesia
circular enterorrhaphy
circular fibers
circular flap
circular fold
circular guillotine incision
circular incision
circular lesion
circular muscle
circular myotomy
circular punch
circular rasp
circular saw
circular stapler
circular stapling device
circular sutures
circular tape
circular twin saw
circulating blood volume
circulation
circulator
circulatory
circulatory assist
circulatory collapse
circulatory compromise
circulatory control
circulatory embarrassment
circulatory overload
circulatory system function
circumanal glands
circumareolar incision
circumcaval ureter
circumcise
circumcision
circumcisional clamp
circumcisional incision
circumcisional scissors

circumcisional shield
circumcisional sutures
circumcorneal incision
circumcoronal wire
circumduction
circumferential
circumferential bipolar montage
circumferential fracture
circumferential implantation
circumferential incision
circumferential lesion
circumferential wiring
circumferentially
circumferentiating skin incision
circumflex artery
circumflex artery of scapula
circumflex artery scissors
circumflex coronary artery
circumflex femoral artery
circumflex femoral veins
circumflex humeral artery
circumflex iliac artery
circumflex iliac superficial fascia
circumflex iliac vein
circumflex nerve
circumflex scissors
circumflex vessel
circumflexa femoris lateralis, arteria
circumflexa femoris medialis, arteria
circumflexa humeri anterior, arteria
circumflexa humeri posterior, arteria
circumflexa ilium profunda, arteria
circumflexa ilium profunda, vena
circumflexa ilium superficialis, arteria
circumflexa ilium superficialis, vena
circumflexa scapulae, arteria
circumflexae femoris laterales, venae

circumflexae femoris mediales, venae
circumflexed branch
circumlimbar incision
circummandibular wiring
circumoral incision
circumscribed
circumscribed area
circumscribed lesion
circumscribing incision
circumtractor
circum-umbilical incision
circumvent
cirrhosis
cirrhotic
cirrhotic gastritis
cirrhotic liver
cirsectomy
cirsenchysis
cirsodesis
cirsotome
cirsotome knife
cirsotomy
CIS (carcinoma in situ)
cistern
cisterna
cisterna chyli
cisterna magna
cisternal puncture
cisternal tap
cisternography
Citanest anesthetic agent
Citelli forceps
Citelli laminectomy punch
Citelli punch
Citelli rongeur
Citelli-Bruening ear forceps
Citelli-Meltzer atticus punch
Citelli-Meltzer punch
Civiale forceps
Civiale lithotrity
Civiale operation
Clado anastomosis
Clagett Barrett esophagogastrostomy
Clagett cannula
Clagett closure
Clagett needle

Clagett S-cannula
Clairborne clamp
clamp
    3-bladed clamp
    2-clamp anastomosis
    3-clamp technique
    Abadie clamp
    Abadie enterostomy
      clamp
    Ablaza clamp
    Acland clamp
    Acland clamp approxi-
      mator
    Acland double clamp
      approximator
    Acland microvascular
      clamp
    Acland microvascular
      clamp applier
    Adair breast clamp
    Adair clamp
    Adson-Brown clamp
    agraffe clamp
    Ahlquist-Durham
      embolism clamp
    Alfred M. Large clamp
    Alfred M. Large vena
      cava clamp
    Allen anastomosis clamp
    Allen clamp
    Allen intestinal clamp
    Allen-Kocher clamp
    Allis clamp
    Allison clamp
    Alyea clamp
    Alyea vas clamp
    anastomosis clamp
    aneurysm clamp
    angled clamp
    angled peripheral
      vascular clamp
    Ann Arbor clamp
    Ann Arbor double towel
      clamp
    anterior resection clamp
    AO clamp
    aorta aneurysm clamp

clamp *continued*
    aorta cannulae clamp
    aorta clamp
    aortic aneurysm clamp
    aortic cannula clamp
    aortic clamp
    aortic crossclamp
    aortic crossclamp time
    aortic occlusion clamp
    appendage clamp
    Asch clamp
    Atlee bronchus clamp
    Atlee clamp
    Atra-grip clamp
    atraumatic clamp
    Ault clamp
    Ault intestinal clamp
    Ault intestinal occlusion
      clamp
    auricle clamp
    auricular appendage
      clamp
    auricular artery clamp
    Babcock clamp
    Babcock tissue clamp
    baby pylorus clamp
    Backhaus clamp
    Backhaus towel clamp
    Backhaus-Jones towel
      clamp
    Backhaus-Kocher towel
      clamp
    Bahnson aortic clamp
    Bahnson appendage
      clamp
    Bahnson clamp
    Bailey aortic clamp
    Bailey clamp
    Bailey-Cowley clamp
    Bailey-Morse clamp
    Bainbridge clamp
    Bainbridge intestinal
      clamp
    Bainbridge vessel clamp
    Balfour clamp
    Ballantine clamp
    Bamby clamp

clamp *continued*

  Bard clamp
  Bartley anastomosis
    clamp
  Bartley partial-occlusion
    clamp
  Baumrucker inconti-
    nence clamp
  Baumrucker post-TUR
    irrigation clamp
  Beall bulldog clamp
  Beardsley clamp
  Beardsley intestinal
    clamp
  Beck aortic clamp
  Beck clamp
  Beck miniature aortic
    clamp
  Beck vascular clamp
  Beck-Potts aorta and
    pulmonic clamp
  Beck-Potts clamp
  Beck-Satinsky clamp
  Belcher clamp
  Bell clamp
  Berens clamp'
  Berens muscle clamp
  Berke clamp
  Berke ptosis clamp
  Berkeley clamp
  Berman aortic clamp
  Berman clamp
  Berry clamp
  Best clamp
  Best colon clamp
  Best right-angle colon
    clamp
  Bethune clamp
  Bigelow calvarium clamp
  Bigelow clamp
  Bircher bone-holding
    clamp
  Bircher cartilage clamp
  Bishop bone clamp
  Black clamp
  Black meatus clamp
  bladder irrigation control
    clamp

clamp *continued*

  Blair cleft palate clamp
  Blalock clamp
  Blalock pulmonary
    clamp
  Blalock pulmonic
    stenosis clamp
  Blalock-Niedner clamp
  Blalock-Niedner pul-
    monic clamp
  Blalock-Niedner pul-
    monic stenosis clamp
  Blanchard clamp
  Blanchard pile clamp
  Blasucci clamp
  bloodless circumcision
    clamp
  Boehler clamp
  Boettcher pulmonary
    artery clamp
  bone clamp
  bone extension clamp
  bone-holding clamp
  Bonney clamp
  Borge bile duct clamp
  Borge clamp
  Bortz clamp
  Boyes clamp
  Boyes muscle clamp
  Bozeman clamp
  Bradshaw-O'Neill aorta
    clamp
  Bradshaw-O'Neill clamp
  Bridge clamp
  Brock auricle clamp
  Brock clamp
  Brodney clamp
  bronchus clamp
  Brown clamp
  Brunner colon clamp
  Brunner intestinal clamp
  Buie clamp
  Buie pile clamp
  Buie-Hirschman clamp
  Buie-Hirschman pile
    clamp
  bulldog clamp
  bulldog microclamp

clamp *continued*
Bunnell-Howard
arthrodesis clamp
Bunke clamp
Bunke-Schulz clamp
approximator
Burdizzo clamp vasec-
tomy
Burford clamp
Burlisher clamp
Buxton clamp
Buxton uterine clamp
C-clamp
Cairns clamp
Calman carotid clamp
Calman ring clamp
calvarium clamp
cannula clamp
cardiovascular anasto-
motic clamp
cardiovascular bulldog
clamp
cardiovascular clamp
Carmalt clamp
Carmel clamp
carotid artery bypass
clamp
carotid artery clamp
carotid clamp
Carrel clamp
Carter clamp
Carter-Glassman
resection clamp
cartilage clamp
caruncle clamp
Casey pelvic clamp
Castaneda anastomosis
clamp
Castaneda clamp
Castaneda IMM vascular
clamp
Castaneda multipurpose
clamp
Castaneda vascular
clamp
Castaneda-Mixter clamp
Castroviejo clamp
cautery clamp

clamp *continued*
caval occlusion clamp
celiac clamp
chalazion clamp
Charnley bone clamp
Charnley clamp
circumcisional clamp
Clairborne clamp
cloth-shod clamp
coarctation clamp
Codman cartilage clamp
Codman clamp
Collin clamp
Collin umbilical
clamp
colon clamp
colostomy clamp
columella clamp
Cooley anastomosis
clamp
Cooley aortic aneurysm
clamp
Cooley aortic cannula
clamp
Cooley aortic clamp
Cooley bronchus clamp
Cooley bulldog clamp
Cooley caval occlusion
clamp
Cooley clamp
Cooley coarctation clamp
Cooley graft clamp
Cooley iliac clamp
Cooley multipurpose
clamp
Cooley neonatal vascular
clamp
Cooley partial occlusion
clamp
Cooley patent ductus
clamp
Cooley pediatric clamp
Cooley renal clamp
Cooley vascular clamp
Cooley vena caval
catheter clamp
Cooley vena caval clamp
Cooley-Beck clamp

clamp *continued*

Cooley-Beck vessel clamp
Cooley-Derra anastomosis clamp
Cooley-Derra clamp
Cooley-Satinsky clamp
Cooley-Satinsky multipurpose clamp
Cope clamp
Cope-DeMartel clamp
cordotomy clamp
Cottle clamp
Cottle columella clamp
cotton-roll rubber-dam clamp
Crafoord aortic clamp
Crafoord clamp
Crafoord coarctation clamp
Crawford auricle clamp
Crenshaw caruncle clamp
Crile appendiceal clamp
Crile clamp
Crile crushing clamp
Crile-Crutchfield clamp
Cross clamp
cross-action bulldog clamp
cross-action clamp
crossclamp
Cruickshank clamp
crush clamp
crushing clamp
Crutchfield clamp
Cunningham clamp
Cunningham incontinence clamp
curved clamp
curved Mayo clamp
curved-8 clamp
Cushing clamp
Dacron graft clamp
Daems bronchial clamp
Daems clamp
Dandy clamp

clamp *continued*

Daniel clamp
Daniel colostomy clamp
Davidson clamp
Davidson muscle clamp
Davidson pulmonary vessel clamp
Davidson vessel clamp
Davis aneurysm clamp
Davis aortic aneurysm clamp
Davis clamp
Dean MacDonald clamp
Dean MacDonald gastric resection clamp
Deaver clamp
DeBakey aortic aneurysm clamp
DeBakey aortic clamp
DeBakey arterial clamp
DeBakey bulldog clamp
DeBakey clamp
DeBakey coarctation clamp
DeBakey cross-action bulldog clamp
DeBakey miniature multipurpose clamp
DeBakey multipurpose clamp
DeBakey patent ductus clamp
DeBakey pediatric clamp
DeBakey peripheral vascular clamp
DeBakey right-angled multipurpose clamp
DeBakey ring-handled bulldog clamp
DeBakey tangential clamp
DeBakey tangential occlusion clamp
DeBakey vascular clamp
DeBakey-Bahnson clamp
DeBakey-Bahnson vascular clamp

clamp *continued*
DeBakey-Bainbridge
clamp
DeBakey-Beck clamp
DeBakey-Derra anasto-
mosis clamp
DeBakey-Harken auricle
clamp
DeBakey-Harken clamp
DeBakey-Howard aortic
aneurysmal clamp
DeBakey-Howard clamp
DeBakey-Kay aortic
clamp
DeBakey-Kay clamp
DeBakey-McQuigg-
Mixter bronchial clamp
DeBakey-Satinsky vena
caval clamp
DeBakey-Semb clamp
DeBakey-Semb ligature-
carrier clamp
DeCourcy clamp
DeCourcy goiter clamp
DeMartel clamp
DeMartel vascular clamp
DeMartel-Wolfson
anastomotic clamp
DeMartel-Wolfson clamp
DeMartel-Wolfson colon
clamp
DeMartel-Wolfson
intestinal anastomotic
clamp
DeMartel-Wolfson
intestinal clamp
Demos tibial arterial
clamp
Dennis anastomotic
clamp
Dennis clamp
Derra aortic clamp
Derra clamp
Derra vena cava clamp
Derra vestibular clamp
Desmarres clamp
Desmarres lid clamp

clamp *continued*
DeWeese clamp
DeWeese vena cava
clamp
Dieffenbach clamp
Diethrich clamp
Diethrich shunt clamp
Dingman cartilage clamp
Dingman clamp
disposable muscle
biopsy clamp
dissecting clamp
Dixon-Thomas-Smith
clamp
Dixon-Thomas-Smith
colonic clamp
Dixon-Thomas-Smith
intestinal clamp
Dobbie-Trout clamp
Doctor Collins clamp
Doctor Long clamp
Dogliotti-Guglielmini
clamp
Donald clamp
double towel clamp
Downing clamp
Doyen clamp
Doyen intestinal clamp
dreamer clamp
duckbill clamp
ductus clamp
duodenal clamp
Duval lung clamp
Earle clamp
Earle hemorrhoidal
clamp
Eastman clamp
Eastman intestinal clamp
Edebohls clamp
Edebohls kidney clamp
Edna towel clamp
Edwards clamp
Edwards handleless
clamp
Edwards spring clamp
Efteklar clamp
Eisenstein clamp

clamp *continued*

  enterostomy clamp
  entropion clamp
  Erhardt clamp
  Erhardt lid clamp
  Ewing lid clamp
  exclusion clamp
  extension bone clamp
  extension clamp
  Falk clamp
  Falk vaginal cuff clamp
  Farabeuf-Lambotte bone-holding clamp
  Farabeuf-Lambotte clamp
  Favoloro proximal anastomosis clamp
  Favorite clamp
  feather clamp
  Fehland clamp
  Fehland intestinal clamp
  Fehland right-angled colon clamp
  femoral clamp
  ferrule clamp
  fine-toothed clamp
  Finochietto artery clamp
  Finochietto clamp
  flow-regulator clamp
  Fogarty clamp
  Fogarty-Chin clamp
  Ford clamp
  Forrester clamp
  Foss anterior resection clamp
  Foss clamp
  Foss intestinal clamp
  Frahur clamp
  Frazier-Adson clamp
  Frazier-Adson osteoplastic flap clamp
  Frazier-Sachs clamp
  Freeman clamp
  Friedrich clamp
  Friedrich-Petz clamp
  full-curved clamp
  Furniss anastomotic clamp

clamp *continued*

  Furniss clamp
  Furniss-Clute anastomosis clamp
  Furniss-Clute clamp
  Furniss-Clute duodenal clamp
  Furniss-McClure-Hinton clamp
  Gandy clamp
  Gant clamp
  Garcia aorta clamp
  Gardner skull clamp
  Garland clamp
  Garland hysterectomy clamp
  Gaskell clamp
  gastric clamp
  gastroenterostomy clamp
  gastrointestinal clamp (GI clamp)
  gate clamp
  Gavin-Miller clamp
  Gemini clamp
  Gerbode patent ductus clamp
  GI clamp (gastrointestinal clamp)
  gingival clamp
  Glassman anterior resection clamp
  Glassman clamp
  Glassman gastroenterostomy clamp
  Glassman gastrointestinal clamp
  Glassman intestinal clamp
  Glassman liver-holding clamp
  Glassman-Allis clamp
  Glover auricular-appendage clamp
  Glover bulldog clamp
  Glover clamp
  Glover coarctation clamp
  Glover curved clamp

clamp *continued*

Glover patent ductus
clamp
Glover spoon anasto-
mosis clamp
Glover vascular clamp
Glover-DeBakey clamp
goiter clamp
Goldblatt clamp
Gomco bloodless
circumcision clamp
Gomco circumcision
clamp
Gomco clamp
Gomco umbilical cord
clamp
Gomco-Bell clamp
Goodhill tonsillar
hemostat clamp
Goodwin clamp
graft clamp
Grant abdominal aortic
aneurysmal clamp
Grant aneurysmal clamp
Grant clamp
grasping clamp
Gray clamp
Green clamp
Green lid clamp
Gregory baby profunda
clamp
Gregory bulldog clamp
Gregory carotid bulldog
clamp
Gregory clamp
Gregory external clamp
Gross clamp
Gross coarctation clamp
Gross coarctation
occlusion clamp
Grover clamp
Gusberg hysterectomy
clamp
Gussenbauer clamp
gut clamp
Gutgeman auricular
appendage clamp

clamp *continued*

Gutgeman clamp
Guyon clamp
Guyon kidney clamp
Guyon vessel clamp
Guyon-Péan clamp
Guyon-Péan vessel
clamp
Haberer intestinal clamp
half-curved clamp
Halsted clamp
handleless clamp
Harken auricular clamp
Harken clamp
Harrah lung clamp
Harrington clamp
Harrington hook clamp
Harrington-Carmalt
clamp
Harrington-Mixter clamp
Harvey Stone clamp
Hausmann vascular
clamp
Haverhill clamp
Hayes anterior resection
clamp
Hayes clamp
Hayes colon clamp
Heaney clamp
Heititz clamp
Heitz-Boyer clamp
hemoclip clamp
hemorrhoidal clamp
hemostatic clamp
hemostatic thoracic
clamp
Hendren clamp
Hendren ductus clamp
Hendren megaureter
clamp
Hendren ureteral clamp
Henley subclavian artery
clamp
Henley vascular clamp
Herbert Adams clamp
Herff clamp
Herrick clamp

clamp *continued*

Herrick kidney clamp
Herrick kidney pedicle
clamp
Herrick pedicle clamp
Hesseltine clamp
Heyer-Schulte biopsy
clamp
Heyer-Schulte clamp
Heyer-Schulte muscle
biopsy clamp
Heyer-Schulte Rayport
muscle biopsy clamp
Hibbs clamp
Hirsch mucosal clamp
Hirschman clamp
Hoff towel clamp
Hoffmann clamp
Hohmann clamp
Hollister clamp
Holter pump clamp
Hopkins aortic clamp
Hopkins aortic occlusion
clamp
Hopkins clamp
Hudson clamp
Hufnagel aortic clamp
Hufnagel ascending
aortic clamp
Hufnagel clamp
Hufnagel valve-holding
clamp
Hugh Young pedicle
clamp
Hume clamp
Humphries aortic clamp
Humphries clamp
Humphries reverse-curve
aortic clamp
Hunt clamp
Hunt colostomy clamp
Hurwitz clamp
Hurwitz esophageal
clamp
Hurwitz intestinal clamp
Hyams clamp
Hyams meatus clamp

clamp *continued*

hydraclip clamp
Hydragrip clamp
hysterectomy clamp
iliac clamp
Iliff clamp
incontinence clamp
infant vascular clamp
intestinal anastomosis
clamp
intestinal clamp
intestinal occlusion
clamp
intestinal ring clamp
Jackson bone-extension
clamp
Jackson clamp
Jacob clamp
Jacobson bulldog
clamp
Jacobson clamp
Jacobson microbulldog
clamp
Jacobson modified vessel
clamp
Jacobson vessel clamp
Jacobson-Potts clamp
Jacobson-Potts vessel
clamp
Jahnke anastomosis
clamp
Jahnke-Cook-Seeley
clamp
Jameson muscle clamp
Janko clamp
Jarvis clamp
Jarvis pile clamp
Javid bypass clamp
Javid carotid artery
bypass clamp
Javid carotid artery
clamp
Javid clamp
Jesberg clamp
Johns Hopkins bulldog
clamp
Johns Hopkins clamp

clamp *continued*

Johns Hopkins coarcta-
tion clamp
Johns Hopkins modified
Potts clamp
Johnston clamp
Jones clamp
Jones thoracic clamp
Jones towel clamp
Joseph clamp
Joseph septal clamp
Judd clamp
Judd-Allis clamp
Juevenelle clamp
Julian-Fildes clamp
K-Gar clamp
Kane clamp
Kane umbilical clamp
Kane umbilical cord
clamp
Kantor circumcision
clamp
Kantor clamp
Kantrowitz clamp
Kantrowitz hemostatic
clamp
Kantrowitz thoracic
clamp
Kapp clamp
Kapp microarterial clamp
Kapp-Beck bronchial
clamp
Kapp-Beck clamp
Kapp-Beck coarctation
clamp
Kapp-Beck colon clamp
Kapp-Beck-Thomson
clamp
Karamar-Mailatt tarsor-
rhaphy clamp
Kartchner carotid artery
clamp
Kartchner carotid clamp
Kaufman clamp
Kaufman kidney clamp
Kay aortic clamp
Kay clamp

clamp *continued*

Kay-Lambert clamp
Kelly clamp
Kelsey clamp
Kelsey pile clamp
Kern bone clamp
Kern bone-holding
clamp
Kern clamp
Khodadad clamp
kidney clamp
kidney pedicle clamp
Kiefer clamp
Kindt artery clamp
Kindt carotid artery
clamp
Kindt clamp
Kinsella-Buie clamp
Kinsella-Buie lung clamp
Kitner clamp
Kleinert-Kutz clamp
Kleinschmidt appendec-
tomy clamp
Klute clamp
Kocher clamp
Kocher intestinal clamp
Kolodny clamp
Kutzmann clamp
Ladd clamp
Ladd lid clamp
Lahey clamp
Lahey thoracic clamp
Lambert aortic clamp
Lambert-Kay aorta clamp
Lambert-Kay clamp
Lambert-Kay vascular
clamp
Lambert-Lowman bone
clamp
Lambert-Lowman clamp
Lambotte clamp
Lamis patella clamp
Lane bone-holding
clamp
Lane clamp
Lane gastroenterostomy
clamp

clamp *continued*

Lane intestinal clamp
Lane towel clamp
Large clamp
Large vena caval clamp
    (Alfred M. Large)
laryngectomy clamp
Lee microvascular clamp
Lees clamp
Lees vascular clamp
left ventricular clamp
    catheter
Leland-Jones clamp
Leland-Jones peripheral
    vascular clamp
Leland-Jones vascular
    clamp
Lem-Blay circumcision
    clamp
Lem-Blay clamp
Lewin bone clamp
Lewin bone-holding
    clamp
Lewin clamp
lid clamp
Liddle aorta clamp
Lindner anastomosis
    clamp
Linnartz clamp
Linnartz intestinal clamp
Linnartz stomach clamp
Linton clamp
Linton tourniquet
    clamp
lion-jaw clamp
lip clamp
liver-holding clamp
Lloyd-Davis clamp
Locke bone clamp
locking clamp
Lockwood clamp
Lorna nonperforating
    towel clamp
Lowman bone clamp
Lowman bone-holding
    clamp
Lowman clamp

clamp *continued*

Lowman-Gerster bone
    clamp
Lulu clamp
lung clamp
lung exclusion clamp
MacDonald clamp
Madden clamp
Madden intestinal clamp
Maingot clamp
Malgaigne clamp
Marcuse tube clamp
marginal clamp
Martel clamp
Martin cartilage clamp
Martin clamp
Martin muscle clamp
Mason clamp
Mason vascular clamp
Masters intestinal clamp
Masters-Schwartz
    intestinal clamp
Masters-Schwartz liver
    clamp
Masterson clamp
Mastin clamp
Mastin muscle clamp
Mattox aortic clamp
May kidney clamp
Mayfield skull clamp
Mayo clamp
Mayo kidney clamp
Mayo vessel clamp
Mayo-Guyon clamp
Mayo-Guyon vessel
    clamp
Mayo-Lovelace clamp
Mayo-Robson intestinal
    clamp
McCleery-Miller clamp
McCleery-Miller intestinal
    anastomosis clamp
McCleery-Miller intestinal
    clamp
McDonald clamp
McGuire clamp
McKenzie clamp

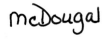

clamp *continued*

McLean clamp
McNealey-Glassman
   clamp
McNealey-Glassman-
   Mixter clamp
McQuigg clamp
meatal clamp
meatus clamp
Meeker gallstone
   clamps
megaureter clamp
meniscal clamp
metal clamp
metallic clamp
Michel aortic clamp
Michel clamp
microarterial clamp
microbulldog clamp
microclamp clip
microvascular clamp
Mikulicz clamp
Mikulicz peritoneal
   clamp
Miles clamp
Miles rectal clamp
Millin clamp
Mini-Ullrich bone clamp
Mitchel aortomy clamp
Mitchel-Adam multipur-
   pose clamp
Mixter clamp
Mixter right-angle clamp
Mogen circumcision
   clamp
Mohr clamp
Moorehead clamp
Moorehead lid clamp
Moreno clamp
Morris aortic clamp
mosquito clamp
mosquito lid clamp
mouse-tooth clamp
Moynihan clamp
Moynihan towel clamp
Mueller clamp
Mueller pediatric clamp

clamp *continued*

Mueller vena caval clamp
Muir cautery clamp
Muir clamp
Muir rectal cautery clamp
multipurpose clamp
muscle biopsy clamp
muscle clamp
mush clamp
Myles clamp
Myles hemorrhoidal
   clamp
myocardial clamp
nephrostomy clamp
Nichol clamp
Nicola clamp
Niedner anastomosis
   clamp
Niedner clamp
Niedner pulmonic clamp
noncrushing bowel
   clamp
noncrushing clamp
noncrushing intestinal
   clamp
noncrushing liver-
   holding clamp
noncrushing vascular
   clamp
nonperforating towel
   clamp
Noon AV fistula clamp
Nunez clamp
Nussbaum clamp
Nussbaum intestinal
   clamp
occluding clamp
occlusion clamp
occlusion multipurpose
   clamp
Ochsner artery clamp
Ochsner clamp
Ochsner thoracic
   clamp
Ockerblad clamp
O'Connor clamp
O'Connor lid clamp

clamp *continued*
- O'Hanlon gastrointestinal clamp
- O'Hanlon intestinal clamp
- Olivecrona aneurysm clamp
- O'Neill cardiac clamp
- O'Neill clamp
- O'Shaughnessy clamp
- osteoplastic flap clamp
- padded clamp
- parametrium clamp
- Parham-Martin bone clamp
- Parham-Martin bone-holding clamp
- Parham-Martin clamp
- Parker clamp
- Parker-Kerr clamp
- partial occlusion clamp
- partially occluding clamp
- Partipilo clamp
- patellar clamp
- patent ductus clamp
- Payr clamp
- Payr gastrointestinal clamp
- Payr pylorus clamp
- Payr resection clamp
- Péan clamp
- Péan hemostatic clamp
- Péan hysterectomy clamp
- pediatric bulldog clamp
- pediatric vascular clamp
- pedicle clamp
- Peers towel clamp
- pelvic clamp
- Pemberton clamp
- Pemberton sigmoid anastomosis clamp
- Pemberton sigmoid clamp
- Pemberton spur-crushing clamp
- penile clamp
- penis clamp

clamp *continued*
- Pennington clamp
- Percy clamp
- pericortical clamp
- peripheral vascular clamp
- peritoneal clamp
- Petz clamp
- Phaneuf clamp
- phantom clamp
- Phillips clamp
- Phillips rectal clamp
- pile clamp
- Pilling clamp
- pinchcock clamp
- placenta clamp
- placing of clamps
- Plastibell clamp
- Pomeranz aortic clamp
- Poppen clamp
- Poppen-Blalock carotid artery clamp
- Poppen-Blalock clamp
- Poppen-Blalock-Salibi clamp
- post-TUR clamp
- post-TUR irrigation clamp
- post-TUR irrigation control clamp
- Potts aortic clamp
- Potts cardiovascular clamp
- Potts clamp
- Potts coarctation clamp
- Potts divisional clamp
- Potts ductus clamp
- Potts patent ductus clamp
- Potts-Niedner aorta clamp
- Potts-Niedner clamp
- Potts-Satinsky clamp
- Potts-Smith aortic clamp
- Potts-Smith aortic occlusion clamp
- Poutasse clamp

clamp *continued*

Presbyterian Hospital clamp
Presbyterian Hospital occluding clamp
Presbyterian Hospital T-clamp
Preshaw clamp
Price muscle biopsy clamp
Price-Thomas bronchial clamp
Price-Thomas clamp
Prince clamp
Pringle clamp
Providence Hospital clamp
ptosis clamp
Pudenz-Heyer clamp
pulmonary artery clamp
pulmonary clamp
pulmonary embolism clamp
pulmonary vessel clamp
pulmonic clamp
pulmonic stenosis clamp
pylorus clamp
Ralks clamp
Ramstedt clamp
Rankin clamp
Rankin intestinal clamp
Ranzewski clamp
Ravich clamp
Rayport muscle clamp
Redo intestinal clamp
Reich-Nechtow clamp
renal artery clamp
renal clamp
renal pedicle clamp
resection clamp
reverse-curve clamp
Reynolds clamp
Reynolds resection clamp
Reynolds vascular clamp
Rhinelander clamp
Richards bone clamp

clamp *continued*

Richards clamp
Rienhoff arterial clamp
Rienhoff clamp
right-angle clamp
Rochester clamp
Rochester-Péan clamp
Rockey clamp
Roe aortic clamp
Roeder clamp
Roeder towel clamp
Roosevelt clamp
Roosevelt gastroenteros-tomy clamp
Roosevelt gastrointestinal clamp
rubber-dam clamp
rubber-shod clamp
Rubin bronchus clamp
Rubin clamp
Rubovits clamp
Ruel aorta clamp
Rumel clamp
Rumel myocardial clamp
Rumel rubber clamp
Rumel thoracic clamp
Rush bone clamp
Rush clamp
Salibi carotid artery clamp
Salibi carotid clamp
Salibi clamp
Santulli clamp
Sarnoff aortic clamp
Sarnoff clamp
Sarot artery clamp
Sarot bronchial clamp
Sarot clamp
Satinsky aortic clamp
Satinsky clamp
Satinsky vascular clamp
Satinsky vena cava clamp
Schlein clamp
Schlesinger clamp
Schnidt clamp

clamp *continued*

Schumacher aorta
clamp
Schutz clamp
Schwartz arterial
aneurysm clamp
Schwartz bulldog clamp
Schwartz clamp
Schwartz intracranial
clamp
Scoville-Lewis clamp
Scudder clamp
Scudder intestinal clamp
Scudder stomach clamp
Sehrt clamp
Seidel bone-holding
clamp
Sellor clamp
Selman clamp
Selverstone carotid artery
clamp
Selverstone carotid
clamp
Selverstone clamp
Senning bulldog clamp
Senning clamp
Senning-Stille clamp
septal clamp
serrefine clamp
Sheehy ossicle-holding
clamp
Shoemaker intestinal
clamp
shutoff clamp
side-biting clamp
Siegler-Hellman clamp
sigmoid clamp
Singley clamp
Singley intestinal
clamp
skull clamp
Slocum meniscal
clamp
Smith bone clamp
Smith clamp
Smith cordotomy clamp
Smith marginal clamp

clamp *continued*

Smithwick anastomotic
clamp
Smithwick clamp
Softjaw clamp
Softjaw handleless clamp
Somers clamp
Somers uterine clamp
Southwick clamp
speed lock clamp
sponge clamp
spoon anastomosis
clamp
spoon clamp
spur-crushing clamp
St. Mark clamp
St. Vincent tube clamp
stainless steel clamp
Stanton cautery clamp
Stanton clamp
stenosis clamp
Stepita clamp
Stepita meatus clamp
Stetten intestinal clamp
Stevenson clamp
Stille clamp
Stille kidney clamp
Stille vessel clamp
Stille-Crawford clamp
Stille-Crawford coarcta-
tion clamp
Stockman clamp
Stockman penis
clamp
stomach clamp
Stone clamp
Stone-Holcombe
anastomosis clamp
Stone-Holcombe clamp
Stone-Holcombe
intestinal clamp
Stony splenorenal shunt
clamp
Storz meatus clamp
straight clamp
straight Crile clamp
Stratte clamp

clamp *continued*

Strauss clamp
Strauss meatus clamp
Strelinger colon clamp
Strelinger right-angle
    colon clamp
Subramanian aortic
    clamp
Subramanian clamp
Subramanian miniature
    aortic clamp
Sugarbaker retrocolic
    clamp
Sumner clamp
Surgi-Med clamp
Swan aortic clamp
Swan clamp
swan-neck clamp
Swiss bulldog clamp
Sztehlo clamp
Sztehlo umbilical clamp
Tamai clamp approxima-
    tor
tangential clamp
tangential occlusion
    clamp
Tatum clamp
Tehl clamp
Textor vasectomy clamp
Thoma clamp
Thompson carotid artery
    clamp
Thompson clamp
Thompson carotid
    vascular clamp
thoracic clamp
three-bladed clamp
three-clamp technique
tissue occlusion clamp
tonsillar clamp
towel clamp
Trendelenburg-Crafoord
    clamp
Trendelenburg-Crafoord
    coarctation clamp
trochanter-holding clamp
truncus clamp

clamp *continued*

Trusler clamp
tube-occluding clamp
tubing clamp
tubing clamp forceps
Tucker appendix clamp
turkey-claw clamp
two-clamp anastomosis
Tydings tonsil clamp
Tyrrell clamp
Ullrich tubing clamp
umbilical clamp
umbilical cord clamp
umbiliclamp
ureteral clamp
urethrographic cannula
    clamp
urethrographic clamp
urinary incontinence
    clamp
vaginal cuff clamp
Valdoni clamp
Vanderbilt clamp
Vanderbilt University
    vessel clamp
Vanderbilt vessel clamp
Varco dissecting clamp
vas clamp
Vasconcelos-Barretto
    clamp
vascular clamp
vascular graft clamp
vasovasotomy clamp
Veidenheimer clamp
vena caval clamp
Verbrugge bone clamp
Verbrugge clamp
vessel clamp
vessel peripheral clamp
vessel-occluding clamp
vestibular clamp
voltage clamp
von Petz clamp
von Petz intestinal clamp
von Petz stomach clamp
Vorse occluding clamp
Vorse-Webster clamp

clamp *continued*
  Vorse-Webster tube-
    occluding clamp
  Wadsworth lid clamp
  Walther clamp
  Walther kidney pedicle
    clamp
  Walther pedicle clamp
  Walther-Crenshaw clamp
  Walther-Crenshaw
    meatus clamp
  Walton clamp
  Walton meniscus clamp
  Wangensteen anasto-
    mosis clamp
  Wangensteen clamp
  Wangensteen gastric-
    crushing anastomotic
    clamp
  Warthen clamp
  Warthen spur-crushing
    clamp
  Watts clamp
  Watts locking clamp
  Weaver chalazion
    clamp
  Weaver clamp
  Weber aortic clamp
  Weck clamp
  wedge resection clamp
  Wells clamp
  Wells pedicle clamp
  Wertheim clamp
  Wertheim-Cullen clamp
  Wertheim-Cullen pedicle
    clamp
  Wertheim-Reverdin
    clamp
  Wertheim-Reverdin
    pedicle clamp
  Wester clamp
  Whitver clamp
  Willett clamp
  Williams clamp
  Wilman clamp
  Wilson clamp
  wire-tightening clamp

clamp *continued*
  Wirthlin splenorenal
    clamp
  Wirthlin splenorenal
    shunt clamp
  Wister clamp
  Wolfson clamp
  Wood bulldog clamp
  Wylie carotid artery
    clamp
  Wylie clamp
  Wylie hypogastric clamp
  X-clamp
  Yasargil carotid clamp
  Yasargil clamp
  Yellen clamp
  Young clamp
  Young renal pedicle
    clamp
  Zachary-Cope clamp
  Zachary-Cope-DeMartel
    clamp
  Zachary-Cope-DeMartel
    colon clamp
  Zachary-Cope-DeMartel
    triple-colon clamp
  Ziegler-Furniss clamp
  Zimmer cartilage clamp
  Zimmer clamp
  Zipser clamp
  Zipser penis clamp
  Zutt clamp
clamp carrier
clamp clip
clamp forceps
clamp-carrier forceps
clamped, cut, and ligated
clamped, cut, and tied
clamping and tying
clamp-on telescope
clamshell brace
Clancy whipstitch
Clancy-Zoellner procedure
Clar-73 headlight
Clark applicator
Clark capsule fragment for-
  ceps

Clark classification of malignant
    melanomas (levels I-IV)
Clark common duct dilator
Clark dilator
Clark eye speculum
Clark forceps
Clark level melanoma (levels I-IV)
Clark operation
Clark perineorrhaphy
Clark speculum
Clark technique
Clark vein stripper
Clark-Axer technique
Clark-Guyton forceps
Clark-McGovern classification of
    malignant melanoma
Clark-Verhoeff capsule forceps
Clark-Verhoeff forceps
clasp bar
clasp-knife reflex
clasp-knife rigidity
clasp-knife spasticity
Classen-Demling papillotome
classic, classical
classical approach
classical cesarean section
classical incision
classical sign of rejection
classical technique
Classix pacemaker
Classon deep surgery scissors
Classon pediatric scissors
Classon scissors
Claude hyperkinesis sign
claudicant
claudication
claustrum
clavate clove-hitch sutures
clavate sutures
clavicle
clavicle bone
clavicle splint
clavicle strap sling
clavicopectoral
clavicotomy
clavicular

clavicular cross splint
clavicular fracture fragment
clavicular incisure of sternum
clavicular notch
clavicular notch of sternum
clavicular region
clavipectoral
clavipectoral fascia
clavipectoral triangle
clavus (pl. clavi)
clavus durum
clavus mollum
claw retractor
claw toe
clawfoot
clawhand
Clawicz chisel
claw-toe position
Clayman forceps
Clayman intraocular implant
    lens
Clayman lens
Clayman lens forceps
Clayman lens implant
Clayman-Kelman intraocular
    lens forceps
Clayman-Kelman lens
Clayman-Knolle lens loop
clay-shoveler's fracture
Clayton laminectomy shears
Clayton operation
Clayton osteotome
Clayton shears
Clayton splint
CLBBB (complete left bundle
    branch block)
clean acrylic template splint
clean and dry incision
clean case
clean cervix
clean closure
clean wound
clean-contaminated case
cleaning brush
cleaning pistol
cleaning tool

cleanse
cleanser
cleansing blood
cleansing emulsion
cleansing enema
cleanup
clear airways
clear lung fields
clear to auscultation
clear to percussion
clear urine
Cleasby iridectomy
Cleasby iris spatula
cleavage
cleavage fracture
cleavage line
cleavage plane
Cleaves position
Cleeman sign
cleft
cleft foot
cleft hand
cleft jaw
cleft lip
cleft lip repair
cleft mitral valve
cleft nose
cleft palate
cleft palate elevator
cleft palate forceps
cleft palate impression
cleft palate instruments
cleft palate knife
cleft palate needle
cleft palate operation
cleft palate prosthesis
cleft palate repair
cleft palate tenaculum
cleft tongue
cleidocranial
cleidotomy
cleidotripsy
Cleland cutaneous ligament
Cleland ligaments
Clemons Tube-Tainer
clenched fist sign
Clerf aspirating tip

Clerf aspirator
Clerf cancer cell collector
Clerf dilator
Clerf forceps
Clerf laryngeal saw
Clerf laryngoscope
Clerf saw
Clerf tube
Clerf-Arrowsmith pin closer
Clerf-Arrowsmith safety pin
    closure
Clevedan positive pressure
    respirator
Clevedent crossbar elevator
Clevedent forceps
Clevedent retractor
Clevedent-Gardner chisel
Clevedent-Lucas curet
Clevedent-Miller elevator
Clevedent-Wakefield chisel
Cleveland bone rongeur
Cleveland bone-cutting forceps
Cleveland-Bosworth-Thompson
    operation
Clevis dressing
clicking rales
clicking sensation
clicking sound
click-murmur syndrome
clinch
clincher nail
clinic Bovie
clinical sign
clinical signs and symptoms
clinical surgery
Clinidine
Clinitron air-fluidized bed
clip (see also *clip applier*)
        Acland clip
        Adams orthodontic clip
        Adams-DeWeese vena
            caval clip
        Adams-DeWeese vena
            caval serrated clip
        Adson brain clip
        Adson clip
        Adson scalp clip

clip *continued*

Adson scalp hemostasis clip
Ahlquist-Durham clip
Ahlquist-Durham vena cava clip
aneurysm clip
aneurysm clip case
Austin clip
Autoclip
Auto-Suture Surgiclip
Avalox skin clip
Backhaus clip
Berne clip hemostat
Biemer vessel clip
Bleier clip for tubal sterilization
blepharoplasty clip
Bonney clip
brain clip
Braun-Yasargil right-angle clip
butterfly clip
Callender clip
Children's Hospital clip
clamp clip
Codman clip
cranial aneurysm clip
Cushing clip
Cushing-McKenzie clip
Dandy clip
Dermaclip
DeWeese-Hunter clip
Drake aneurysm clip
Drake clip
Drew clip
Duane U-clip
Edwards clip
Edwards parallel jaw spring clip
Elgiloy-Heifitz aneurysm clip
Ethicon clip
Feldstein blepharoplasty clip
fenestrated Drake clip
Filshie clip

clip *continued*

Friedman clip
gate clip
Heath clip
Hegenbarth clip
Hegenbarth-Adams clip
Heifitz aneurysm clip
Heifitz clip
hemoclip
hemostasis clip
hemostasis scalp clip
hemostasis silver clip
hemostatic clip
Hesseltine umbiliclip
Hoxworth clip
hydraclip
Ingraham-Fowler tantalum clip
Kapp clip
Keer aneurysm clip
Kerr clip
Khodadad clip
Kifa clip
Koln clip
LDS clip
LeRoy clip
LeRoy disposable scalp clip
Liga surgical clip
Ligaclip
Mayfield aneurysmal clip
Mayfield clip
McDermott clip
McFadden aneurysm clip
McFadden clip
McKenzie clip
McKenzie silver brain clip
metal clip
Michel clip
Michel scalp clip
Michel suture clip
Michel wound clip
microanastomosis clip
microclamp clip
microclip

clip *continued*
   Miles clip
   Miles skin clip
   Miles Teflon clip
   Miles vena cava clip
   Moren-Moretz vena caval
      clip
   Moretz clip
   Moynihan clip
   Multiclip
   Multiclip disposable
      ligating clip device
   Olivecrona aneurysm
      clip
   Olivecrona clip
   Olivecrona silver clip
   parallel-jaw spring clip
   Paterson long-shank
      brain clip
   Penfield clip
   Penfield silver clip
   Petz clip
   Phynox clip
   Phynox cobalt alloy clip
   Platina clip implant
      cataract lens
   Platina clip lens
   Pool Pfeiffer self-locking
      clip
   Raney clip
   Raney scalp clip
   Raney stainless steel
      scalp clip
   scalp clip
   scalp hemostasis clip
   Schaedel clip
   Schepens clip
   Schutz clip
   Schwartz clip
   Scoville clip
   Scoville-Lewis clip
   Secu clip
   Selman clip
   Seraphim clip
   Serature clip
   Serature spur clip
   silver clip

clip *continued*
   Silverstein malleus clip
      wire
   skin clip
   Smith aneurysmal clip
   Smith clip
   Smithwick clip
   Smithwick silver clip
   spring clip
   Sugar aneurysm clip
   Sugar clip
   Sugita aneurysm clip
   Sugita clip
   Sundt clip
   Sundt encircling clip
   Sundt-Kees aneurysm
      clip
   Sundt-Kees clip
   Surgiclip
   Surgidev iris clip
   suture clip
   tantalum clip
   tantalum hemostasis
      clip
   temporary clip
   temporary vascular clip
   temporary vessel clip
   Tomac clip
   Tonnis clip
   Totco Autoclip
   Totco clip
   towel clip
   Tru-Clip
   U-clip
   umbilical clip
   umbiliclip
   V-clip
   vascular clip
   vena caval clip
   vessel clip
   Vitallium clip
   von Petz clip
   Wachtenfeldt clip
   Wachtenfeldt butterfly
      clip
   Wachtenfeldt wound clip
   Weck clip

clip *continued*
    Weck hemoclip
    wing clip
    wound clip
    Yasargil aneurysmal clip
    Yasargil clip
    Yasargil microclip
clip applier (see also *clip*)
    aneurysm clip applier
    Autoclip applier
    Auto-Suture Clip-A-Matic clip applier
    Biemer vessel clip applier
    cranial aneurysm clip applier
    Heifitz clip applier
    hemoclip applier
    pivot aneurysm clip applier
    pivot microanastomosis clip applier
    microclip applier
    Scoville clip applier
    suture clip applier
    vari-angle clip applier
clip approximator
clip forceps
clip remover
clip-applying forceps
clip-introducing forceps
clip-on attachment
clip-on light bundles
clitoral incision
clitoridectomy
clitoridotomy
clitoris
clitorotomy
clivogram
clivography
clivus
cloaca (*pl.* cloacae)
clockwise rotation of heart
clogged artery
clonic contraction
clonic convulsion
clonic seizure

clonic spasm
clonk
clonus
Cloquet canal
Cloquet fascia
Cloquet ganglion
Cloquet hernia
Cloquet needle
Cloquet node
closed amputation
closed anesthesia
closed chest cardiac massage
closed chest drainage
closed circle system
closed commissurotomy
closed drain
closed drainage
closed drainage tube
closed flap amputation
closed fracture
closed heart surgery
closed in a routine manner
closed in anatomic layers
closed in layers
closed injury
closed iris forceps
closed loop
closed mitral commissurotomy
closed pneumothorax
closed reduction
closed reduction and internal fixation
closed reduction of dislocation
closed reduction of fracture
closed reduction of fracture-dislocation
closed skull fracture
closed subcondylar osteotomy
closed suction drain
closed suction drainage tube
closed suction tube
closed technique
closed thoracic drainage system
closed thoracostomy
closed tube drainage
closed valvotomy
closed vitrectomy

closed water-seal drainage
closed water-seal suction tube
closed water-seal thoracic
    drainage system
closed wedge osteotomy
closed-angle glaucoma
closed-box suction
closed-end ostomy pouch
closed-loop intestinal obstruc-
    tion
closed-plaster method
closely spaced electrodes
closer forceps
closer water-seal drainage
closer wire
closing ABD wedge bunionec-
    tomy
closing forceps
closing pressure
Clostridium perfringens
Clostridium tetani
closure (see also *sutures*)
closure of colostomy
closure of defect
closure of fistula
closure of ostomy
closure of wound
clot evacuator
clot stripper
cloth disk
cloth scissors
clothesline drain
clothespin graft
cloth-shod clamp
cloudy ascites
cloudy fluid
cloudy iris
cloudy urine
Cloutier knee prosthesis
Cloutier operation
clove hitch
clove-hitch knot
clove-hitch sutures
cloverleaf catheter
cloverleaf counterbore
cloverleaf deformity
cloverleaf excision

cloverleaf nail
cloverleaf pin
cloverleaf pin extractor
cloverleaf plate
cloverleaf rod
cloverleaf skull
cloverleaf-type deformity
Cloward back fusion
Cloward blade
Cloward chisel
Cloward curet
Cloward drill
Cloward dural hook
Cloward elevator
Cloward guide
Cloward hammer
Cloward hook
Cloward intervertebral punch
Cloward laminectomy instru-
    ment
Cloward operation
Cloward osteotome
Cloward periosteal elevator
Cloward procedure
Cloward puka chisel
Cloward puka operation
Cloward punch
Cloward retractor
Cloward rongeur
Cloward self-retaining retractor
Cloward spinal fusion chisel
Cloward spinal fusion osteo-
    tome
Cloward stitch suture
Cloward trephine
Cloward vertebral spreader
Cloward-Cone ring curet
Cloward-Cushing vein retractor
Cloward-Dowel cutter
Cloward-Dowel punch
Cloward-English laminectomy
    rongeur
Cloward-English punch
Cloward-Harman chisel
Cloward-Harper laminectomy
    rongeur
Cloward-Harper punch

Cloward-Hoen laminectomy
    retractor
Cloward-Hoen retractor
CLS cementless hip system
CLS total hip
clubbed finger
clubbed penis
clubbing
clubbing of distal phalanges
clubbing of extremities
clubbing of fingers
clubfoot
clubfoot splint
clubhand
clump kidney
clunial nerves
clunium inferiores, nervi
clunium medii, nervi
clunium superiores, nervi
Clute incision
Clutton joint
Clyburn Colles fixator
Clyburn dynamic Colles
    fixator
Clyman endometrial curet
clysis
clysis cannula
clyster
clysterize
cm (centimeter)
CMC (carpometacarpal)
CMG (cystometrogram)
CMV (continuous mandatory
    ventilation)
CMW bone cement
CNS (central nervous sys-
    tem)
CO1 cartridge
CO2 cartridge
CO2 laser
CO2 muscle prosthesis
co-abrasion
coagulate
coagulated bleeders
coagulated bleeding
    points
coagulating current
coagulating current Bovie

coagulating electrode
coagulating forceps
coagulating knife
coagulating-suction cannula
coagulating-suction forceps
coagulation
coagulation bronchoscope
coagulation cautery
coagulation electrode
coagulation factor
coagulation forceps
coagulation-aspiration tube
coagulator (see also *photoco-
    agulator*)
    American Optical
        photocoagulator
    argon laser photocoagu-
        lator
    Ball coagulator
    Ballantine-Drew coagula-
        tor
    Bantam Bovie coagulator
    Bantam coagulator
    Biceps bipolar coagula-
        tor
    bipolar coagulator
    Birtcher coagulator
    Bovie coagulator
    Codman-Mentor wet-
        field coagulator
    Coherent argon laser
        photocoagulator
    Concept bipolar coagula-
        tor
    electrocoagulator
    endocoagulator
    Fabry coagulator
    hyfrecator coagulator
    Magielski electroco-
        agulator
    Malis coagulator
    Mentor wet-field
        coagulator
    Mentor wet-field cordless
        coagulator
    Mira photocoagulator
    National coagulator
    photocoagulator

coagulator *continued*
    Polar-Mate bipolar
       microcoagulator
    Poppen coagulator
    Resnick Button bipolar
       coagulator
    Ritter coagulator
    suction-electrocoagulator
    wet-field coagulator
    xenon arc photocoagula-
       tor
    xenon photocoagulator
    Zeiss photocoagulator
coagulopathy
coagulum
coagulum pyelolithotomy
Coakley antrum curet
Coakley cannula
Coakley curet
Coakley forceps
Coakley frontal sinus cannula
Coakley hemostat
Coakley nasal curet
Coakley nasal probe
Coakley nasal speculum
Coakley probe
Coakley sinus curet
Coakley sinus operation
Coakley speculum
Coakley sutures
Coakley tonsil hemostat
Coakley trocar
Coakley tube
Coakley-Allis forceps
coalescence
coalition
coapt
coaptation
coaptation plate
coaptation splint
coaptation sutures
coarctate retina
coarctation
coarctation clamp
coarctation forceps
coarctation hook
coarctation of aorta

coarctation of pulmonary
    arteries
coarctation of thoracic aorta
coarctectomy
coarctotomy
coarse
coarse crepitation
coarse folds
coarse nodular cirrhosis
coarse rales
coarse trabeculation
coarse tremor
coarsened mucosal fold
    pattern
coarsening
coat-sleeve amputation
coated carbon fiber
coated polyester sutures
coated sutures
coated Vicryl sutures
Coats ring
Co-Axa Lite light
coaxial cable
coaxial catheter
coaxial headlight
cobalt
cobalt-60 irradiation
cobalt-60 therapy
cobalt-chrome
cobalt-chromium alloy
Coban bandage
Coban dressing
Coban elastic dressing
Coban wrap
Coban wrapping
Cobb chisel
Cobb curet
Cobb elevator
Cobb gouge
Cobb method
Cobb osteotome
Cobb periosteal elevator
Cobb retractor
Cobb spinal elevator
Cobb technique
Cobbett knife
cobbler's sutures
cobblestone degeneration

cobblestone lesion
cobblestone mucosa
cobblestoning
cobblestoning of mucosa
cobblestoning sign
Cobb-Ragde bladder neck
    suspension
Cobb-Ragde needle
Cobe dialyzer
Cobe double blood pump
Cobe staple gun
Cobe stapler
Cobelli glands
cobra catheter
cobra plate
cobra retractor
cobra-head anastomosis
cobra-head plate
cobra-hood technique for
    transecting graft
cobra-shaped catheter
Coburg-Connell airway
Coburn anterior chamber
    intraocular lens implant
Coburn intraocular lens
Coburn lens
Coburn Mark IX eye
    implant
cocaine anesthetic agent
cocaine atomizer
cocaine hydrochloride
cocaine hydrochloride anes-
    thetic agent
cocainization
cocainize
coccydynia
coccygeal artery
coccygeal bone
coccygeal ganglion
coccygeal glands
coccygeal muscle
coccygeal nerve
coccygeal plexus
coccygeal vertebrae
coccygectomy
coccygeopubic diameter
coccygeus, musculus
coccygeus, nervus

coccygodynia
coccygotomy
coccyx
coccyx bone
cochlea (*pl.* cochleae)
cochlear branch
cochlear canal
cochlear cells
cochlear degeneration
cochlear duct
cochlear electrical stimulation
cochlear implant
cochlear joint
cochlear nerve
cochlear nucleus
cochlear prosthesis
cochlear recess of vestibule
cochleariform process
cochleate uterus
cochleo-orbicular reflex
cochleopalpebral reflex
cochleopapillary reflex
cochleostapedial reflex
Cock urethrotomy
cock-up arm splint
cock-up hand splint
cocoon dressing
cocoon thread sutures
cod liver oil-soaked strips
    dressing
codfish appearance of vertebrae
Codivilla bone graft
Codivilla extension
Codivilla graft
Codivilla operation
Codivilla operation for pseu-
    darthrosis
Codman angle
Codman approach
Codman cannula
Codman cartilage clamp
Codman clamp
Codman clip
Codman drill
Codman exercises
Codman incision
Codman patty
Codman shunt

Codman sign
Codman sponge
Codman triangle
Codman vein stripper
Codman x-ray angle
Codman-Kerrison laminectomy
    rongeur
Codman-Leksell laminectomy
    rongeur
Codman-Mentor erasure
Codman-Mentor microscope
Codman-Mentor wet-field
    coagulator
Codman-Schlesinger cervical
    rongeur
Codman-Shurtleff cranial drill
Cody magnetic probe
Cody sacculotomy tack
Cody tack
Cody tack inserter
Cody tack procedure
Coe Comfort tissue-conditioning
    liner
coefficient of joint friction
Coe-pak cement
cofferdam
Coffey incision
Coffey operation
Coffey technique (I, II, III)
Coffey ureterointestinal
    anastomosis
Coffey uterine suspension
Cogan-Boberg-Ans lens implant
Cogsell tip aspirator
cog-tooth of malleus
cogwheel
cogwheel motion
cogwheel respiration
cogwheel rigidity
cogwheel sign
Cohan corneal utility forceps
Cohan microscope
Cohan needle holder
Cohan-Barraquer microscope
Cohan-Vannas scissors
Cohan-Westcott scissors
Cohen cannula

Cohen elevator
Cohen intrauterine cannula
Cohen nasal-dressing forceps
Cohen operation
Cohen rasp
Cohen reimplantation
Cohen retractor
Cohen sinus raspatory
Cohen tubal insufflation
    cannula
Cohen urethroplasty
Cohen uterine incision
Cohen-Eder cannula
Cohen-Eder tongs
Coherent argon laser photoco-
    agulator
Coherent radiation argon laser
Coherent system of CO2
    surgical laser
cohesive dressing
coil
coil dialyzer
coil hemodialyzer
coil intrauterine device (coil
    IUD)
Coil magnifier
coil vascular stent
coiled bony structure
coiled cochlea
coiled position
coiled upon itself
coiled-spring appearance
coil-tipped catheter
coin lesion
Colclough rongeur
cold biopsy
cold blade biopsy
cold bone scan
cold cardioplegic solution
cold cautery
cold conization
cold conization of cervix
cold cup biopsy forceps
cold cup forceps
cold defect
cold infusion
cold knife

cold light fountain
cold nodule
cold pack
cold pressor test
cold snare
cold to the opposite, warm to the same (COWS)
cold-cone knife
cold-knife conization
Coldlite speculum
Coldlite transilluminator
Coldlite vaginal speculum
Coldlite-Graves vaginal speculum
coldness of extremity
cold-punch resectoscope
Cole duodenal retractor
Cole fracture frame
Cole operation
Cole osteotomy
Cole pediatric tube
Cole polyethylene vein stripper
Cole procedure
Cole pull-out wire
Cole retractor
Cole sign
Cole tube
Cole vein stripper
colectomy
Coleman operation for talipes valgus
Coleman retractor
Coleman-Noonan technique
Coleman-Stelling-Jarrett technique
Colibri corneal forceps
Colibri corneal utility forceps
Colibri eye forceps
Colibri forceps
Colibri microforceps
Colibri speculum
Colibri-Pierce forceps
Colibri-Storz forceps
colic
colic artery
colic flexure
colic omentum

colic patch
colic surface of spleen
colic valve
colic vein
colica dextra, arteria
colica dextra, vena
colica media, arteria
colica media, vena
colica sinistra, arteria
colica sinistra, vena
coliplication
colipuncture
collagen
collagen graft
collagen implant
collagen prosthesis
collagen sutures
collagen tape prosthesis
collagenase
collagenous
collagenous colitis
collagenous fibers
collapse
collapse of lung
collapsed jugular vein
collapsed lung
collar bone
collar brace
collar button (see also *button*)
    Castelli-Paparella collar-button tube
    Graether collar button
    Graether collar buttonhook
    polyethylene collar button
    Sheehy collar-button tube
collar button-like ulcer
collar dressing
collar incision
collar-button abscess
collar-button tube
collar-button ulceration
collateral
collateral artery
collateral circulation

collateral eminence
collateral ligaments
collateral vessels
collateralis media, arteria
collateralis radialis, arteria
collateralis ulnaris inferior,
     arteria
collateralis ulnaris superior,
     arteria
collateralization
collecting structures
collecting system
collecting tube
collecting tubule
collection tube
collector
     cancer cell collector
     Carabelli collector
     Clerf cancer cell collector
     Davidson collector
     Lukens collector
Coller artery forceps
Coller forceps
Coller hemostatic forceps
Colles fascia
Colles fracture
Colles operation
Colles sling
Colles space
Colles splint
collet
colliculus
Collier eye needle holder
Collier forceps
Collier hemostatic forceps
Collier needle holder
Collier-Crile hemostatic forceps
Collier-DeBakey hemostatic
     forceps
Collier-Martin hook
collimation
collimator helmet
Collin abdominal retractor
Collin amputating knife
Collin clamp
Collin dissector

Collin forceps
Collin intestinal forceps
Collin lung-grasping forceps
Collin mucous forceps
Collin osteoclast
Collin pelvimeter
Collin pleural dissector
Collin rib shears
Collin sound
Collin speculum
Collin sternal self-retaining
     retractor
Collin tissue forceps
Collin tongue forceps
Collin tube
Collin umbilical clamp
Collin vaginal speculum
Collin-Beard procedure
Collin-Duvall intestinal forceps
Collings electrode
Collings fulguration electrode
Collings knife
Collins dynamometer
Collins solution
Collins-Mayo mastoid retractor
Collis antireflux operation
Collis Eagle I spirometry unit
Collis forceps
Collis gastroplasty
Collis microutility forceps
Collis mouth gag
Collis repair
Collis scissors
Collis spirometer
Collis technique
Collis-Belsey repair
Collis-Maumenee corneal
     forceps
Collis-Nissen fundoplication
Collis-Nissen operation
Collison body drill
Collison cannulated hand drill
Collison drill
Collison plate
Collison screw
Collison screwdriver

Collison tap drill
collodion
collodion dressing
collodion gauze
collodion solution
collodion strip
colloid
colloid adenocarcinoma
colloid bodies
colloid cyst
colloid goiter
colloid milium
Collostat hemostatic sponge
Collostat sponge
collum
Collyer pelvimeter
coloanal anastomosis
coloboma
colocecostomy
colocentesis
colocholecystostomy
coloclyster
colocolic anastomosis
colocolic intussusception
colocolostomy
colocutaneous
colocutaneous fistula
colocystoplasty
colofixation
cologastrostomy
colohepatopexy
coloileal
coloileotomy
cololysis
colon
colon ascendens
colon clamp
colon cut-off sign
colon descendens
colon resection
colon resection and anasto-
    mosis
colon sigmoideum
colon transversum
Colonial retractor
colonic adenoma
colonic anesthesia

colonic distention
colonic diverticulum
colonic inertia
colonic insufflator
colonic lavage
colonic loop
colonic myenteric plexus
colonic obstruction
colonic patch
colonic pit
colonic polyp
colonic varices
colonic volvulus
Colonlite bowel prep
Colonna arthroplasty
Colonna operation
Colonna reconstruction
Colonna-Ralston approach
Colonna-Ralston operation
colonofiberoptic scope
colonorrhagia
colonorrhea
colonoscope
    CFLV3UU colonoscope
    fibercolonoscope
    Fujinon colonoscope
    OES colonoscope
    Olympus colonoscope
    short bundle colono-
        scope
    video image colono-
        scope
colonoscope syringe
colonoscopic evaluation
colonoscopic polypectomy
colonoscopy
colopexia
colopexostomy
colopexotomy
colopexy
Coloplast bag
Coloplast colostomy bag
Coloplast colostomy pouch
Coloplast dressing
Coloplast flange
Coloplast flange pouch
Coloplast pouch

coloplication
coloproctectomy
coloproctostomy
coloptosis
colopuncture
color contrast microscope
Colorcode instrument identification
color-coded Doppler system
color-coding tape
colorectal cancer
colorectal mucosa
colorectal polyp
colorectosigmoidostomy
colorectostomy
colored tape
color-flow Doppler echocardiogram
color-flow Doppler system
colorrhaphy
coloscope
coloscopy
Coloset ostomy pouch
colosigmoidostomy
colostomy
colostomy bag
colostomy bridge
colostomy clamp
colostomy loop
colostomy pouch
colostomy rod
colostomy site
colostomy tube
colostrum
colotomy
colovesical fistula
Colpacs
colpectomy
Colp-Hofmeister operation
colpocele
colpoceliocentesis
colpoceliotomy
colpocentesis
colpocleisis
colpocystotomy
colpocystoureterocystotomy
colpocystourethropexy

colpohysterectomy
colpohysterotomy
colpomyomectomy
colpoperineoplasty
colpoperineorrhaphy
colpopexy
colpoplasty
colpopoiesis
colporectopexy
colporrhaphy
colposcope
colposcopic examination
colposcopic-directed punch biopsy
colposcopy
Colpostar-V6 colpostat
colpostat
Colpostats applicator
colpotomy
colpoureterocystotomy
colpoureterotomy
Colson vaporizer
Coltart arthrodesis
Coltart talus fracture operation
Colton empyema tube
Columbia staging system for breast carcinoma
columella
columella clamp
columella implant
columellar type II tympanoplasty
columnar cells
columnar mucosa
columnar-lined esophagus
Colver dissector
Colver examining retractor hook
Colver forceps
Colver hook
Colver knife
Colver needle
Colver retractor
Colver tonsil forceps
Colver tonsil hemostat
Colver tonsil needle
Colver tonsil retractor

Colver tonsil-seizing forceps
Colver-Coakley forceps
Colver-Coakley tonsil forceps
Colver-Dawson decompressor
comatose
Comberg contact lens
Comberg operation
combination forceps/needle
    holder
combination mallet
combination sleeve bridge
combination stethoscope
combined femoral-inguinal
    herniorrhaphy
combined frontal-ethmoid-
    sphenoid sinusotomy
combined hemorrhoids
combined internal and external
    version
combined needle holder and
    scissors
combined penetrating and
    lamellar corneal graft
combined sacral and caudal
    block anesthesia
combined version
comblike redness sign
Comby sign
comedo (*pl.* comedones)
comedo extractor
comedocarcinoma
comedomastitis
comedones (*sing.* comedo)
Comfeel Ulcus occlusive
    dressing
comitans nervi hypoglossi,
    vena
comitans nervi ischiadici, arteria
Command PS pacemaker
Commando glossectomy
Commando resection
comma-shaped vertebral out-
    growth
comminuted fracture
comminution
commissural bundle
commissural myelotomy

commissural pulmonary valve
commissure
commissure laryngoscope
commissure of fornix
commissure of Gudden
commissurorrhaphy
commissurotomy
commissurotomy knife
committed mode pacemaker
common anterior facial vein
common atrium
common bile duct (CBD)
common bile duct dilator
common bile duct obstruction
common bile duct stone
common carotid artery
common component
common digital vein of foot
common duct
common duct bougie
common duct cholangiogram
common duct dilator
common duct exploration
common duct obstruction
common duct probe
common duct scoop
common duct sound
common duct stone
common duct tumor
common duct-holding forceps
common extensor muscle of
    digits
common extensors
common facial vein
common fibular nerve
common hepatic duct
common iliac artery
common iliac lymph nodes
common iliac vein
common interosseous artery
common McPherson forceps
common palmar digital arteries
common palmar digital nerves
common peroneal nerve
common plantar digital arteries
common plantar digital nerves
common tendinous ring

common tendon
common wart
communicans anterior cerebri, arteria
communicans posterior cerebri, arteria
communicating artery
communis tendon
compact bone
compact tissue
comparison film
comparison microscope
comparison views
compartment of knee
compartment syndrome
compartmental total knee prosthesis
compatible findings
compensated
compensated cardiac status
compensatory
compensatory atrophy
compensatory circulation
compensatory curvature of spine
compensatory curve
compensatory hypertrophy
Compere bone chisel
Compere chisel
Compere femoral lengthening procedure
Compere fixation wire
Compere gouge
Compere operation
Compere osteotome
Compere pin
Compere threaded pin
competent ileocecal valve
competent valve
complement
complemental air
complementary hypertrophy
complementary induction
complete abortion
complete closure
complete dislocation
complete emptying of bladder
complete excision
complete filling
complete fracture
complete heart block
complete left bundle branch block (CLBBB)
complete obstruction
complete procedure
complete remission
complete weightbearing
complex simple fracture
compliance
complicated
complicated birth
complicated cataract
complicated delivery
complicated dislocation
complicated fracture
complicated labor
complicated postoperative course
complicated recovery
component
component pusher
component ribs
composite flap
composite fracture
composite graft
composite joint
composite materials
composite odontoma
composite operation
composite resection
composite valve graft
composition
compound comminuted fracture
compound cyst
compound dislocation
compound dressing
compound flap
compound fracture
compound ganglion
compound joint
compound microscope
compound nevus
compound presentation
compound scanner

compound skin flap
compound skull fracture
compound sutures
compress
compressed nerves
compression
compression anesthesia
compression arthrodesis
compression bandage
compression boot
compression bra
compression deformity
compression device
compression dressing
compression forceps
compression fracture
compression hip screw (CHS)
compression hook
compression instruments for
    bone plating
compression of brain
compression of carotid artery
compression of spinal cord
compression paddle
compression plate
compression reflex
compression rod
compression screw
compression screw plate
compression splint
compression stockings
compression syndrome
compression tape
compression wrench
compression-type deformity
compressor (see also *decom-*
    *pressor*)
    Adair screw compressor
    air compressor
    Anthony compressor
    Anthony enucleation
      compressor
    Anthony orbital enuclea-
      tion compressor
    Barnes compressor
    Beneys tonsil compres-
      sor

compressor *continued*
    Berens compressor
    Berens orbital compres-
      sor
    Castroviejo compressor
    Charnley compressor
    continuous air compres-
      sor
    Deschamps compressor
    DeVilbiss air compressor
    DeVilbiss compressor
    enucleation compressor
    orbital enucleation
      compressor
    screw compressor
    Sehrt compressor
    shot compressor
    tonsillar compressor
    tubing compressor
compressor muscle of naris
Comprol dressing
compromise
compromised
computed axial tomography
    (CAT)
computed tomography (CT)
computer dose calculation
computer tomography
computer-assisted operation
computerized assisted design
    (CAD)
computerized assisted design
    prosthesis
computerized axial tomography
    (CAT)
computerized cranial tomogra-
    phy (CCT)
computerized muscle-joint
    evaluation
computerized tomography (CT)
concave
concave anterior surface
concave gouge
concave lens
concave posterior surface
concave sheath and obturator
concavity

concavity and depression
concavity of spine
concavoconcave
concavoconcave lens
concavoconvex
concavoconvex lens
concealed hemorrhage
concealed hernia
concentric atrophy
concentric constriction
concentric hypertrophy
concentric needle electrode
concentric pantomography
concentric swabbing
concentric-needle electrode
Concept bipolar coagulator
Concept cautery
Concept dermatome
Concept eye cautery
Concept hand-held cautery
Concept Intra-Arc drive
Concept Multi-Liner lining
    needle
Concept nerve stimulator
Concept Ophtho-Bur
Concept screw
concha (*pl.* conchae)
concha auriculae
concha bullosa
concha nasalis
concha nasoturbinal
concha of auricle
concha of Santorini
concha sphenoidalis
conchal cartilage
conchal flap
conchal fossa
conchal mastoid angle
conchectomy
conchotome
conchotomy
Conco tractor
concomitant
Concorde suction cannula
concrete burn
concretion
concurrent findings

concussion
condenser
condom catheter
condom catheter attachment
Condon antibiotic prep
conductance catheter
conducting cord
conduction
conduction anesthesia
conduction defect
conduction disturbance
conduction nerve study
conduction system
conduction system of heart
conduction time
conduction velocity
conductive base
conductive device
conductive V-Lok cuff
conductivity
conductor
    Adson conductor
    Adson saw conductor
    Bailey conductor
    Bailey saw conductor
    Bovie liquid conductor
    Davis conductor
    Davis saw conductor
    esophageal conductor
    flexible esophageal
        conductor
    Gigli-saw conductor
    Kanavel conductor
    liquid conductor Bovie
    nonconductor
    saw conductor
    Storz conductor
    Storz esophageal
        conductor
    Storz flexible esophageal
        conductor
    Xomed Audiant bone
        conductor
conduit
conduitogram
conduitography
condylar

condylar articulation
condylar blade plate
condylar canal
condylar emissary vein
condylar fossa
condylar fracture
condylar guide inclination
condylar implant arthroplasty
condylar prosthesis
condyle
condyle bone
condyle of mandible
condylectomy
condylocephalic nail
condyloid fossa
condyloid joint
condyloid process
condyloma (*pl.* condylomata,
    condylomas)
condyloma acuminatum
condylomata (*sing.* condyloma)
condylotomy
cone arthrodesis
cone biopsy
cone biopsy cannula
cone biopsy knife
cone biopsy needle
Cone bone punch
Cone bur
Cone calipers
Cone cannula
cone cells
Cone cerebral cannula
Cone curet
Cone forceps
Cone guide
Cone knife
Cone nasal curet
Cone needle
cone projection
Cone punch
Cone retractor
Cone ring curet
Cone scalp retractor
Cone self-retaining retractor
Cone skull punch
cone specimen

Cone suction biopsy curet
Cone suction tube
Cone tube
Cone ventricular needle
Cone wire twister
Cone wire-twisting forceps
Cone-Bucy cannula
coned AP projection
coned-down view
coned-down x-ray view
cone-down projection
cone-down view
cone-shaped amputation stump
configuration and size
confinement
confirmatory incision
confluence
confluence of sinuses
confluent
confluent rash
confluent shadows
conformation of right heart
    catheter
conformer
    acrylic conformer
    acrylic conformer eye
        implant
    eye conformer
    eye implant conformer
    Fox conformer
    Fox eye conformer
    implant conformer
    plastic conformer
    Universal conformer
conformer for eye
confrontation fields
confrontation of visual fields
congenerous muscles
congenital abnormality
congenital absence of (organ,
    organ part, tissue)
congenital amputation
congenital anomaly
congenital birth defect
congenital condition
congenital defect
congenital deformity

congenital disease
congenital dislocated hip (CDH)
congenital dislocation
congenital disorder
congenital dysplasia of hip
    (CDH)
congenital failure
congenital fracture
congenital heart defect (CHD)
congenital hernia
congenital hip dislocation
    (CHD)
congenital lesion
congenital malformation
congenital mass
congenital megacolon
congested kidney
congested vascular structures
congestion
congestive cardiac failure
congestive failure
congestive glaucoma
congestive heart disease (CHD)
congestive heart failure (CHF)
congestive splenomegaly
conglobate gland
conglutinant
conglutination
Congo red dye
conic, conical
conical bougie
conical bur
conical catheter
conical cornea
conical eye implant
conical implant
conical stump
conical trocar
conical-tip catheter
conical-tip electrode
coniotomy
conization biopsy
conization electrode
conization instrument
conization knife
conization of cervix
conization of uterine cervix

conization technique
conjoined nerve root
conjoined organs
conjoined tendon
conjugate deviation
conjugate diameter (CD)
conjugate eye movement
conjugate gaze
conjugate measurements
conjugate movement
conjugate paralysis
conjunctiva (pl. conjunctivae)
conjunctival abscess
conjunctival adhesions
conjunctival arteries
conjunctival cul-de-sac
conjunctival flap
conjunctival fold
conjunctival forceps
conjunctival fornix
conjunctival incision
conjunctival injection
conjunctival lipoma
conjunctival tumor
conjunctival veins
conjunctivales anteriores,
    arteriae
conjunctivales posteriores,
    arteriae
conjunctivales, venae
conjunctivocystorhinostomy
conjunctivodacryocystorhinos-
    tomy
conjunctivodacryocystostomy
conjunctivoplasty
conjunctivorhinostomy
conjunctivotarsal area
conjunctivotarsal surface
Conley incision
Conley neck incision
Conley pin
Conley prosthesis
Conley radical neck incision
Conn operation
Conn technique
Conn tourniquet
connate teeth

connecting cord
connecting neurons
connecting nipple
connection cord
connective tissue
connective tissue cells
connective tissue disorder
connective tissue sheath
connective tissue stalk
connector
  ACS angioplasty Y-
    connector
  beta finger-grip catheter
    connector
  CAS connector
  catheter connector
  CSF shunt connector
    forceps
  Hemmer connector
    flusher
  major connector bar
  mediastinal sump
    connector
  metal connector
  metal suction connector
  minor connector bar
  neurosurgical connector
  Storz catheter connector
  straight connector
  suction connector
  swivel connector tubing
  T-vent connector
  U-connector
  Y-connector
connector bar
connector forceps
connector tubing
Connell airway
Connell breathing tube
Connell cystoscope
Connell ether vapor tube
Connell gastrectomy
Connell incision
Connell inverting suture
Connell operation
Connell sutures
conoid lens

conoid ligament
conoid process
Conrad operation
Conrad-Crosby biopsy needle
Conrad-Crosby needle
consanguineous donor
conscious
consciousness
consecutive amputation
consecutive dislocation
consensual reflex
conservative
conservative approach
conservative surgery
conservative treatment
consistency
consistent findings
consolidant
consolidation
consolidation of lungs
consonating rales
conspicuous
constant
Constantine catheter
Constantine flexible metal
  catheter
ConstaVac catheter
constipation
constrained hinged knee
  prosthesis
constrained knee prosthesis
constrained nonhinged knee
  prosthesis
constrained total knee prosthesis
constricted
constricted blood vessels
constricting esophageal
  lesion
constricting pain
constriction
constriction of pupil
constrictive edema
constrictive hyperemia
constrictive ring
constrictor muscle
constrictor muscle of pharynx

constrictor pharyngis inferior, musculus
constrictor pharyngis medius, musculus
constrictor pharyngis superior, musculus
construction
consultation
consumption
contact
contact burn
contact lens
contact metastasis
contact ring
contact shell implant
contact splint
contaminant
contaminated case
contaminated field
contaminated wound
contamination
contiguous
contiguous loop
contiguous rib
contiguous ventricular septal defect
continence
continent ileal pouch
continent ileal reservoir
continent ileostomy
Continent operation
continuity
continuous air compressor
continuous ambulatory peritoneal dialysis (CAPD)
continuous arteriovenous hemofiltration (CAVH)
continuous arteriovenous ultrafiltration (CAVU)
continuous blanket
continuous catgut sutures
continuous caudal anesthesia
continuous circular inverting sutures
continuous cuticular sutures
continuous epidural anesthesia
continuous hemostatic sutures

continuous Holter monitor
continuous interlocking sutures
continuous inverting sutures
continuous irrigation
continuous irrigation catheter
continuous irrigation-suction resectoscope
continuous key pattern sutures
continuous Lembert sutures
continuous locked sutures
continuous loop wire
continuous loop wiring
continuous mandatory ventilation (CMV)
continuous mattress sutures
continuous nasogastric suction
continuous over-and-over sutures
continuous passive motion device
continuous pericardial lavage
continuous peridural anesthesia
continuous positive airway pressure (CPAP)
continuous pull-through technique
continuous running locked sutures
continuous running sutures
continuous silk sutures
continuous spinal anesthesia
continuous suction
continuous suction drainage
continuous suction pump
continuous suction thoracic drainage system
continuous suction tube
continuous sutures
continuous tension
continuous U-shaped sutures
continuous wave
continuous-flow nebulizer
continuous-flow resectoscope
continuous-flow ventilation (CFV)
continuous-locking manner

continuously perfused probe
continuous-wave Doppler
    imaging
continuous-wave ultrasound
contour defect
contour instrument cleaning
    brush
contour line
contour of heart
contour of nasal bones
contour retractor
contour scalp retractor
contoured Dow Corning Silastic
    prosthesis
contra-angle
contra-aperture
contracted abdomen
contracted heart
contracted heel cord
contracted kidney
contracted pelvis
contracted shoulder
contracted toe
contracted urinary bladder
contracted uterus
contractile stricture
contractility
contracting and relaxing of
    muscles
contraction
contraction of muscles
contraction of pupil
contraction of uterus
contraction on ventriculo-
    gram
contraction pattern
contraction reflex
contraction time
contraction-relaxation cycle
contractor (see also *rib contrac-
    tor*)
    Adams rib contractor
    baby rib contractor
    Bailey baby rib contrac-
      tor
    Bailey contractor
    Bailey rib contractor

contractor *continued*
    Bailey-Gibbon contrac-
      tor
    Bailey-Gibbon rib
      contractor
    Cooley rib contractor
    Effenberger contractor
    Graham rib contractor
    Lemmon contractor
    Medicon contractor
    Rienhoff-Finochietto rib
      contractor
    rib contractor
    Sellor contractor
    Sellor rib contractor
    Waterman rib contractor
contracture
contracture of hip
contracture of knee
contracture of ligament
contraincision
contraindication
contraindication to surgery
contralateral
contralateral aspect
contralateral breast
contralateral ear
contralateral movement
contralateral organ
contralateral radiation
contralateral sign
contrast agent
contrast angiogram
contrast aortogram
contrast CT scan
contrast echocardiography
contrast enema
contrast enhancement
contrast examination
contrast material
contrast medium
contrast selective cholangi-
    ogram
contrast-enhanced scan
Contraves microscope
contrecoup contusion
contrecoup fracture

contrecoup injury
contributing factor
control belt
control cable
control syringe
controlled drain
controlled procedure
controlled respiration
controller
Control-Release needle
Contura cast
Contura medicated dressing
contused
contused wound
contusion
contusion cataract
contusions and abrasions
conus branch
conus elasticus
conus elasticus laryngis
conus medullaris
convalescence
convalescent
convalescing patient
ConvaTec ostomy products
Conveen drip collector
conventional concentric
    electromyography
conventional method
conventional reform eye
    implant
conventional reform implant
conventional shell-type eye
    implant
conventional shunt
conventional surgery
conventional treatment
convergence
convergence of eyes
convergent
convergent ray
convergent squint
convergent strabismus
converging lens
Converse alar elevator
Converse alar retractor
Converse bistoury

Converse blade retractor
Converse chisel
Converse curet
Converse double-ended
    retractor
Converse guarded chisel
Converse guarded osteotome
Converse hinged skin hook
Converse hook
Converse knife
Converse method
Converse nasal chisel
Converse nasal retractor
Converse nasal rongeur
Converse nasal root rongeur
Converse nasal saw
Converse nasal speculum
Converse nasal tip scissors
Converse needle holder
Converse operation
Converse osteotome
Converse periosteal elevator
Converse plastic surgery
    scissors
Converse rasp
Converse raspatory
Converse retractor
Converse rongeur
Converse saw
Converse scissors
Converse skin hook
converse skin lines
Converse speculum
Converse splint
Converse-Gillies needle holder
Converse-MacKenty elevator
conversion
conversion of position
conversion table
converted rhythm
converter
convertible cystoscope
convertible telescope and fin
Convertors surgical drapes
convex
convex lens
convex sheath and obturator

convexes of brain
convexity
convexity of lens
convexity of spine
convexoconcave disk prosthetic
    valve
convexoconcave lens
convexoconcave valve pros-
    thesis
conveyor
convoluted seminiferous
    tubules
convolution
convolutional artery
convolutional markings
convolutions of cerebrum
convolutions of Gratiolet
convulsion
convulsive disorder
Conway eye retractor
Conway lid retractor
Conway operation
Conzett goniometer
Cook arterial catheter
Cook catheter
Cook County aspirator
Cook County Hospital aspirator
Cook County suction tube
Cook County tracheal suction
    tube
Cook eye speculum
Cook helical stone dislodger
Cook introducer
Cook pacemaker
Cook pigtail catheter
Cook rectal retractor
Cook rectal speculum
Cook retractor
Cook shingle
Cook speculum
Cook TPN catheter
Cook transseptal sheath
Cook ureteral stent
Cook Urosoft stent
Cook walking brace
Cook-Amplatz dilator
cookie cutter

cookie cutter areolar marker
Cooley anastomosis
Cooley anastomosis clamp
Cooley anastomosis forceps
Cooley aorta retractor
Cooley aortic aneurysm clamp
Cooley aortic cannula clamp
Cooley aortic clamp
Cooley aortic forceps
Cooley aortic vent needle
Cooley arterial occlusion
    forceps
Cooley arteriotomy scissors
Cooley atrial retractor
Cooley auricular appendage
    forceps
Cooley bronchus clamp
Cooley bulldog clamp
Cooley cardiac tucker
Cooley cardiovascular forceps
Cooley cardiovascular scissors
Cooley cardiovascular suction
    tube
Cooley caval occlusion clamp
Cooley chisel
Cooley clamp
Cooley coarctation clamp
Cooley coarctation forceps
Cooley coronary dilator
Cooley CSR forceps
Cooley curved forceps
Cooley dilator
Cooley double-angled jaw
    forceps
Cooley first-rib shears
Cooley forceps
Cooley graft clamp
Cooley graft forceps
Cooley iliac clamp
Cooley iliac forceps
Cooley intrapericardial anasto-
    mosis
Cooley microvascular needle
    holder
Cooley modification of Water-
    ston anastomosis
Cooley multipurpose clamp

Cooley multipurpose forceps
Cooley needle holder
Cooley neonatal instruments
Cooley neonatal retractor
Cooley neonatal vascular clamp
Cooley operation
Cooley partial occlusion clamp
Cooley patent ductus clamp
Cooley patent ductus forceps
Cooley pediatric aortic forceps
Cooley pediatric clamp
Cooley pediatric dilator
Cooley peripheral vascular
    forceps
Cooley probe-point scissors
Cooley renal clamp
Cooley retractor
Cooley reverse-cut scissors
Cooley rib contractor
Cooley rib retractor
Cooley scissors
Cooley sternotomy retractor
Cooley suction tube
Cooley sump tube
Cooley tangential pediatric
    forceps
Cooley tissue forceps
Cooley U-sutures
Cooley valve dilator
Cooley vascular clamp
Cooley vascular forceps
Cooley vascular tissue forceps
Cooley vena caval catheter
    clamp
Cooley vena caval clamp
Cooley Vital microvascular
    needle holder
Cooley-Baumgarten aortic
    forceps
Cooley-Beck clamp
Cooley-Beck vessel clamp
Cooley-Bloodwell low profile
    valve
Cooley-Bloodwell mitral valve
    prosthesis
Cooley-Bloodwell-Cutter
    prosthesis
Cooley-Bloodwell-Cutter valve
Cooley-Cutter disk prosthetic
    valve
Cooley-Cutter prosthesis
Cooley-Derra anastomosis
    clamp
Cooley-Derra clamp
Cooley-Merz sternum retractor
Cooley-Pontius blade
Cooley-Pontius shears
Cooley-Pontius sternal blade
Cooley-Pontius sternum shears
Cooley-Satinsky clamp
Cooley-Satinsky multipurpose
    clamp
Coolidge tube
Cool-Vapor vaporizer
Coombs cord
Coonrad prosthesis
Coonrad total elbow
Coonrad wrist prosthesis
Cooper argon laser
Cooper basal ganglia guide
Cooper bougie
Cooper cannula
Cooper chemopallidectomy
    cannula
Cooper chemopallidectomy
    needle
Cooper cryoprobe
Cooper cryostat
Cooper director
Cooper double-lumen cannula
Cooper elevator
Cooper gouge
Cooper guide
Cooper hernia
Cooper lens
Cooper ligament
Cooper ligament repair
Cooper mallet
Cooper nasal ganglia guide
Cooper needle
Cooper operation
Cooper scissors
Cooper spinal fusion elevator
Coopernail sign

CooperVision argon laser
CooperVision Fragmatome
CooperVision J-loop intraocular
    lens
CooperVision laser
CooperVision ocutome
CooperVision system VI
Cooper-Xenotec system
coordinate convulsion
coordinate muscle movement
coordinated reflexes
coordinates
coordination
Cope biopsy needle
Cope bronchography
Cope clamp
Cope double-ended retractor
Cope lung forceps
Cope needle
Cope needle introducer cannula
Cope nephrostomy tube
Cope pleural biopsy needle
Cope thoracentesis needle
Cope-DeMartel clamp
Copeland intraocular lens
    implant
Copeland lens
Copeland lens implant
Copeland radial pan-chamber
    intraocular lens
Copeland retinoscope
copious
copious bleeding
copious drainage
copious irrigation
copious lavage
copper sulphate cone
copper wire appearance
copper wire arteries
copper wire effect
copper wiring
Copper-7 IUD
copper-clad steel needle
Coppridge forceps
Coppridge grasping forceps
Coppridge urethral forceps
coquille plano lens

cor biloculare
cor pacemaker
cor pulmonale
cor triatriatum
cor triloculare biatriatum
coracoacromial
coracoacromial ligament
coracobrachial muscle
coracobrachialis, musculus
coracoclavicular ligament
coracoclavicular screw
coracohumeral ligament
coracoid notch
coracoid process
coral calculus
coralliform cataract
coralliformis cataract
Coratomic pacemaker
Coratomic prosthetic valve
Coratomic R-wave inhibited
    pacemaker
Coratomic R-wave inhibited
    pulse generator
Corb biopsy trocar
Corbett bone-cutting forceps
Corbett bone-cutting rongeur
Corbett forceps
Corbett foreign body spud
Corbett spud
Corbin technique
Corbin-Farnsworth defibril-
    lator
Corboy hemostat
Corboy needle holder
cord
cord bladder
cord block
cord blood
cord handle
cord injury
cord length
cord lengthening
cord stripping
cord tumor
cordate
cordectomy
Cordes forceps

Cordes punch
Cordes punch forceps tip
Cordes sphenoid punch
Cordes-New elevator
Cordes-New forceps
Cordes-New laryngeal punch
Cordes-New laryngeal punch
    elevator
Cordes-New laryngeal punch
    forceps
Cordes-New punch
cordiform tendon of diaphragm
cordiformis uterus
Cordis Ancar pacing lead
cordis anteriores, venae
Cordis Atricor pacemaker
Cordis catheter
Cordis Chronocor pacemaker
Cordis Ectocor pacemaker
Cordis fixed-rate pacemaker
Cordis Gemini pacemaker
Cordis guiding catheter
Cordis Hakim pump
Cordis Hakim shunt
Cordis Lumelec catheter
cordis magna, vena
cordis media, vena
cordis minimae, venae
Cordis Multicor pacemaker
Cordis Omni Stanicor Theta
    transvenous pacemaker
Cordis Omnicor Stanicor
    pacemaker
Cordis pacemaker
cordis parva, vena
Cordis pigtail catheter
Cordis Sequicor pacemaker
Cordis sheath
Cordis Ventricor pacemaker
cordless dermatome
cordoma
Cordonnier ureteroileal loop
cordopexy
cordotomy
cordotomy clamp
cordotomy hook
cordotomy knife

Cordran tape
cordy pulse
core cooling
core mold stent
core wire guide
corectomy
corelysis
coreometrics
coreoplasty
coretomy
Core-Vent implant
Corey forceps
Corey ovum forceps
Corey tenaculum
Cor-Flex guide
Cor-Flex wire guide
Corgill punch
Corit canal
corkscrew
corkscrew arteries
corkscrew dural hook
corkscrew esophagus
corkscrew femoral head
    remover
Corlon angiocatheter
Cormed infusion pump
cornea
cornea farinata
cornea globosa
cornea guttata
cornea opaca
cornea plana
cornea scissors
cornea-holding forceps
corneal abrader
corneal abrasion
corneal abscess
corneal abscission
corneal applicator
corneal astigmatism
corneal bur
corneal burn
corneal chisel
corneal contusion
corneal curet
corneal debrider
corneal degeneration

corneal deposits
corneal dissector
corneal ectasia
corneal edema
corneal erosion
corneal eye implant
corneal fistula
corneal flap
corneal forceps
corneal graft
corneal hook
corneal implant
corneal incision
corneal infiltrate
corneal keloid
corneal knife
corneal knife dissector
corneal loupe
corneal luster
corneal margin
corneal microscope
corneal needle
corneal opacity
corneal rasp
corneal reflex
corneal rust ring remover
corneal scarring
corneal scissors
corneal section
corneal section scissors
corneal space
corneal staining
corneal suture needle
corneal sutures
corneal swelling
corneal thickness measuring
    equipment
corneal transplant
corneal transplant forceps
corneal transplant scissors
corneal transplantation
corneal trephination
corneal trephine
corneal tube
corneal ulcer
corneal utility forceps
corneal wound

cornea-suturing forceps
corneoconjunctivoplasty
corneomandibular reflex
corneomental reflex
corneopterygoid reflex
corneoscleral forceps
corneoscleral incision
corneoscleral junction
corneoscleral punch
corneoscleral scissors
corneoscleral sutures
corneoscleral trephination
corneoscleral wound
corneoscleroconjunctival
    sutures
Corner plug
corner retractor
Corner tampon
Cornet forceps
corniculate cartilage
corniculate tubercle
Corning anesthesia
Corning implant
Corning puncture
Corning silicone
Cornish wool dressing
Cornman dissecting knife
cornu (*pl.* cornua)
cornual implantation
cornual portion of uterus
cornual pregnancy
cornual resection of fallopian
    tube
cornuradicular zone
corollary incision
corona (*pl.* coronae)
corona ciliaris
corona dentis
corona glandis
corona radiata
corona vascularis
coronal arc technique
coronal bipolar montage
coronal incision
coronal orientation
coronal plane
coronal sulcus

coronal suture
coronal suture lines
coronaria dextra, arteria
coronaria sinistra, arteria
coronary angiogram
coronary angiography
coronary angioplasty
coronary arteries
coronary arteriogram
coronary arteriography
coronary arteriosclerotic heart
   disease (CAHD)
coronary artery aneurysm
coronary artery angioplasty
coronary artery bypass (CAB)
coronary artery bypass graft
   (CABG)
coronary artery bypass grafted
   (CABG'd) (slang)
coronary artery bypass surgery
   (CABS)
coronary artery cannula
coronary artery disease (CAD)
coronary artery endarterectomy
coronary artery perfusion
coronary artery scissors
coronary atherosclerotic heart
   disease (CAHD)
coronary blood flow
coronary bypass
coronary bypass surgery
coronary cannula
coronary care unit (CCU)
coronary cataract
coronary cataract of Vogt
coronary catheter
coronary catheterization
coronary cineangiogram
coronary cineangiography
coronary circulation
coronary cusps
coronary dilatation catheter
coronary dilator
coronary embolism
coronary endarterectomy
coronary fistula
coronary guiding catheter
coronary heart disease (CHD)

coronary insufficiency
coronary ligaments
coronary occlusion
coronary opacification
coronary perfusion
coronary perfusion cannula
coronary perfusion components
coronary perfusion tip
coronary reflex
coronary scissors
coronary sinus
coronary sinus suction tube
coronary sinus thermodilution
   catheter
coronary steal phenomenon
coronary sulcus
coronary tendon
coronary thrombosis
coronary vasodilator
coronary veins
coronary wire
Coronet magnet
coronoid
coronoid flap
coronoid fossa
coronoid process
coronoidectomy
Corpak feeding tube
corpora (*sing.* corpus)
corpora albicantia
corpora cavernosa penis
corpora quadrigemina
corporeal cesarean section
corporis callosi
corpus (*pl.* corpora)
corpus adiposum orbitae
corpus albicans
corpus callosum
corpus cavernosum clitoridis
corpus cavernosum penis
corpus cavernosum urethrae
corpus cerebelli
corpus ciliaris
corpus clitoridis
corpus luteal cyst
corpus luteum
corpus of uterus
corpus spongiosum penis

corpus spongiosum urethrae
    muliebris
corpus uteri
corpus vitreum
corpuscle
corpuscular volume
corrected condition
correction
corrective cast
corrective operation
corrective procedure
corrective therapy
correlation
Corrigan cautery
Corrigan sign
corroborate
corrugator muscle
corrugator supercilii, musculus
corset
Cortac monitoring electrode
Cortel insertion of steel rods
Cortel technique
cortex (*pl.* cortices)
cortex avulsion
cortex lentis
cortex of kidney
cortex reflex
cortex retractor
cortex screw
cortex-aspirating cannula
Corti ganglion
Corti rods
cortical
cortical adhesions
cortical area
cortical atrophy
cortical bone
cortical bone graft
cortical buckling
cortical cataract
cortical cyst
cortical desmoid
cortical destruction
cortical electrode
cortical electroencephalogram
cortical evoked responses
cortical fracture
cortical fragment

cortical function
cortical graft
cortical incision
cortical lesion
cortical lobules of kidney
cortical medullary junction
cortical opacification
cortical peel
cortical process
cortical scarring of kidney
cortical screw
cortical spoking
cortical step drill
cortical surface
cortical thickening
cortical thickness
cortical thumb
corticectomy
cortices (*sing.* cortex)
corticoadrenal tumor
corticobulbar tract
corticocancellous graft
corticospinal
corticospinal lesion
corticospinal tract
corticospinal tract lesion
corticosteroids
corticostriatal
corticotomy
Corwin forceps
Corwin hemostat
Corwin tonsillar forceps
Corwin tonsillar hemostat
Corwin tonsillar hemostatic
    forceps
Coryllos periosteal elevator
Coryllos rasp
Coryllos raspatory
Coryllos retractor
Coryllos rib raspatory
Coryllos rib shears
Coryllos thoracoscope
Coryllos-Bethune rib shears
Coryllos-Doyen periosteal
    elevator
Coryllos-Moure rib shears
Coryllos-Shoemaker rib shears
Cosman ICM Tele-Sensor

Cosman ICP Tele-Sensor
Cosman monitor
Cosman telemonitoring
cosmesis
Cosmet lens
cosmetic
cosmetic appearance
cosmetic operation
cosmetic reconstruction
cosmetic surgery
Cosmos pacemaker
Cosmos pulse-generator
    pacemaker
costa (*pl.* costae)
costal angle
costal arch
costal arch retractor
costal bone
costal cartilage
costal elevator
costal excursion
costal incisures of sternum
costal margin
costal notch of sternum
costal periosteal elevator
costal periosteotome
costal pleura
costatectomy
costectomy
Costen rongeur
Costen tube
Costen-Kerrison rongeur
costicartilage
costicervical
costispinal
costoaxillary vein
costocentral articulation
costocervical trunk
costochondral joint
costochondral margin
costochondrectomy
costoclavicular
costoclavicular ligament
costoclavicular maneuver
costocolic fold
costodiaphragmatic recess
costoinferior

costomediastinal
costomediastinal recess
Coston eye decompressor
Coston iris needle
costophrenic
costophrenic angle
costophrenic bronchoscope
costophrenic sinus
costophrenic sulcus
costoprostatectomy
costosternal
costosternal angle
costosternal articulation
costosternoplasty
costotome
        Tudor-Edwards costo-
        tome
costotome chisel
costotomy
costotransverse articulation
costotransverse ligament
costotransversectomy
costoversion thoracoplasty
costovertebral
costovertebral angle
costovertebral articulation
Cotrel body cast
Cotrel cast technique
Cotrel casting
Cotrel traction
Cotrel-Dubousset rod
Cotrel-Dubousset spinal
    instrumentation
Cotrel-Dubousset spinal rod
    fixation
Cotte neurectomy
Cotte operation
Cotting operation
Cottle alar protector
Cottle alar retractor
Cottle alar elevator
Cottle angular scissors
Cottle antral chisel
Cottle biting forceps
Cottle bone crusher
Cottle bone guide
Cottle bone lever

Cottle bulldog scissors
Cottle calipers
Cottle cartilage guide
Cottle chisel
Cottle chisel osteotome
Cottle clamp
Cottle columella clamp
Cottle crossbar chisel
Cottle crossbar fishtail chisel
Cottle curved chisel
Cottle dorsal scissors
Cottle double hook
Cottle double-edged knife
Cottle dressing scissors
Cottle elevator
Cottle elevator-feeler
Cottle fishtail chisel
Cottle forceps
Cottle four-prong retractor
Cottle graduated elevator
Cottle guide
Cottle heavy septum scissors
Cottle hook
Cottle incision
Cottle insertion forceps
Cottle instrument tray and
    spring holder
Cottle knife
Cottle knife guide
Cottle knife handle
Cottle lower lateral forceps
Cottle mallet
Cottle modified knife handle
Cottle nasal knife
Cottle nasal saw
Cottle nasal scissors
Cottle nasal speculum
Cottle nasal-biting rongeur
Cottle needle holder
Cottle operation
Cottle osteotome
Cottle periosteal comb
Cottle periosteal elevator
Cottle pillar retractor
Cottle profilometer
Cottle pronged retractor
Cottle protected knife handle

Cottle rasp
Cottle raspatory
Cottle retractor
Cottle saw
Cottle scissors
Cottle septum elevator
Cottle septum speculum
Cottle sharp prong retractor
Cottle sharp tenaculum
Cottle single-blade retractor
Cottle skin elevator
Cottle soft palate retractor
Cottle speculum
Cottle spicule sweeper
Cottle spring scissors
Cottle stent scissors
Cottle suction tube
Cottle sweeper
Cottle tenaculum
Cottle tenaculum hook
Cottle tissue forceps
Cottle Universal nasal saw
Cottle upper lateral retractor
Cottle Vital dorsal angled
    scissors
Cottle weighted retractor
Cottle-Arruga forceps
Cottle-Jansen bone rongeur
Cottle-Jansen forceps
Cottle-Jansen rongeur
Cottle-Jansen rongeur forceps
Cottle-Joseph hook
Cottle-Joseph retractor
Cottle-Joseph saw
Cottle-Kazanjian bone rongeur
Cottle-Kazanjian forceps
Cottle-Kazanjian nasal forceps
Cottle-Kazanjian nasal-cutting
    forceps
Cottle-MacKenty elevator
Cottle-MacKenty elevator rasp
Cottle-MacKenty septal elevator
Cottle-Medicon osteotome
Cottle-Neivert retractor
Cottle-Walsham forceps
Cottle-Walsham septal straight-
    ener

Cottle-Walsham septum-
    straightening forceps
Cottle-Walsham straightener
Cotton ankle fracture
cotton applicator
cotton balls
cotton bolster
cotton bolster dressing
cotton carrier
Cotton cartilage graft to
    cricolaryngeal area
cotton Deknatel sutures
cotton ear applicator
cotton elastic bandage
cotton elastic dressing
Cotton fracture
cotton gauze
cotton nasal applicator
Cotton osteotomy
cotton pledgets
cotton pledgets dressing
cotton plug
cotton receptacle
cotton screw
cotton sutures
cotton wadding
cotton wool
cotton-ball dressing
cotton-ball hemorrhage of eye
Cottonoid dissector
Cottonoid patty
Cottonoid strips
cotton-roll gingivitis
cotton-roll rubber-dam clamp
cotton-tipped applicator
cotton-wadding dressing
cotton-wool bandage
cotton-wool exudate
cotton-wool patch
cotyledon
cotyloid cavity
cotyloid ligament
cotyloid notch
Couch-DeRosa-Throop hip
    procedure
couching needle
coudé assist catheter

coudé bag
coudé bougie
coudé catheter
coudé electrode
coudé hemostatic bag
coudé urethral catheter
coudé-tip catheter
coudé-tip demeure catheter
cough fracture
Coulevaire uterus
Coulter counter
Coumadin
Councill basket
Councill catheter
Councill dilator
Councill retention catheter
Councill stone basket
Councill stone dislodger
Councill stone extractor
Councill stone scoop
Councilman chisel
Counsellor vaginal mold
Counsellor-Davis artificial-
    vagina operation
count
counterbalance
counterbore
    cloverleaf counterbore
    Curry hip nail counter-
        bore
    Curry hip nail counter-
        bore with Lloyd
        adapter
    round counterbore
counterextension
counterincision
counteropening
counterpressure
counterpulsation
counterpulsation balloon
counterpuncture
counterrotating saw
countershock
countersink
countertraction
countertraction splint
Count'R-Force arch brace

coup de sabre deformity
coup-contrecoup
Coupland elevator
Coupland nasal suction tube
Coupland suction tube
coupled pulse
coupled rhythm
coupling interval
coupling microscope
Cournand arterial needle
Cournand catheter
Cournand needle
Cournand-Grino angiography
    needle
Cournand-Grino needle
course of dialysis
course of radiation
coursing
Courvoisier gallbladder
Courvoisier gastroenterostomy
Courvoisier incision
Coventry arthroplasty
Coventry nail
Coventry osteotomy
Coventry staple
Coventry total hip replacement
Coventry wiring
Coventry-Johnson classification
Coverlet adhesive dressing
Cover-Pad dressing
Cover-Roll adhesive gauze
Cover-Roll dressing
Cover-Roll stretch bandage
Cover-Strip wound closure
    strips
coving
cowhorn tooth-extracting
    forceps
Cowper glands
Cowper ligament
COWS (cold to the opposite,
    warm to the same)
Cox skin lines
Cox technique
coxa adducta
coxa flexa
coxa magna

coxa plana
coxa valga
coxa vara
coxa vara luxans
coxarthrosis
Coxeter catheter
Coxeter prostatic catheter
Cox-Uphoff double-lumen
    breast prosthesis
Cox-Uphoff implant
Cox-Uphoff International tissue
    expander (CUI tissue
    expander)
Cox-Uphoff prosthesis
Cox-Uphoff skin expander
Cozen approach
Cozen-Brockway operation
Cozen-Brockway Z-plasty
CPAP (continuous positive
    airway pressure)
CPD (cephalopelvic dispropor-
    tion)
CPI Astra pacemaker
CPI Maxilith pacemaker
CPI Microthin pacemaker
CPI Minilith pacemaker
CPI pacemaker
CPI Ultra II pacemaker
CPM (continuous passive
    motion)
CPM device
CPV catheter
Crabtree dissector
Cracchiolo forefoot arthro-
    plasty
crack fracture
crack growth
crack lung
cracked heel
cracked pot note
cracked-pot resonance
cracked-pot sound
cradle arm sling
cradling instrument
cradling system
Crafon-Oretorp arthroscopy
    pump

Crafoord aortic clamp
Crafoord bronchial forceps
Crafoord clamp
Crafoord coarctation clamp
Crafoord coarctation forceps
Crafoord forceps
Crafoord hemostat
Crafoord lobectomy scissors
Crafoord operation
Crafoord pulmonary forceps
Crafoord retractor
Crafoord scissors
Crafoord thoracic scissors
Crafoord-Cooley tucker
Crafoord-Cooley tunneler
Crafoord-Sellors hemostatic
    forceps
Craig abduction splint
Craig angular scissors
Craig forceps
Craig headrest
Craig headrest holder
Craig needle
Craig pin
Craig scissors
Craig septum-cutting forceps
Craig splint
Craig tonsil-seizing forceps
Craig vertebral body biopsy set
Craig-Sheehan retractor
Cramer cleft palate elevator
Cramer splint
Cramer wire splint
cramping abdominal pain
Crampton muscle
Crane bone chisel
Crane chisel
Crane flap
Crane gouge
Crane hammer
Crane mallet
Crane osteotome
Crane pick
cranial aneurysm clip
cranial aneurysm clip applier
cranial arteritis
cranial bone rongeur

cranial bur
cranial cavity
cranial defect
cranial diameter
cranial drill
cranial forceps
cranial fossa
cranial halo
cranial insufflation
cranial nerve I (olfactory)
cranial nerve II (optic)
cranial nerve III (oculomotor)
cranial nerve IV (trochlear)
cranial nerve V (trigeminal)
cranial nerve VI (abducens)
cranial nerve VII (facial)
cranial nerve VIII (vestibulo-
    cochlear)
cranial nerve IX (glossopharyn-
    geal)
cranial nerve X (vagus)
cranial nerve XI (accessory)
cranial nerve XII (hypoglossal)
cranial nerve sign
cranial nerves (I-XII, also 1-12)
cranial neurectomy
cranial operating instruments
cranial perforator
cranial puncture
cranial reflex
cranial retractor
cranial rongeur
cranial rongeur forceps
cranial segment
cranial sinus
cranial sutures
cranial synostosis
cranial trauma
cranial trephine
cranial twist drill perforator
cranial vault
craniales, nervi
craniamphitomy
craniectomy
craniocaudad position
craniocaudad views
craniocaudal views

craniocerebral injury
craniocerebral topography
cranioclasis
cranioclast
    Auvard cranioclast
    Braun cranioclast
    DeLee-Zweifel cranio-
       clast
    Zweifel-DeLee cranio-
       clast
craniodiaphyseal dysplasia
craniofacial
craniofacial anomaly
craniofacial appliance
craniofacial cleft
craniofacial disjunction
craniofacial dysostosis
craniofacial fracture appliance
craniofacial suspension wiring
craniometric diameter
cranioplastic kit
cranioplastic material dressing
cranioplasty
craniopuncture
craniosacral
craniosacral division
craniospinal irradiation
craniostenosis
craniostosis
craniosynosectomy
craniosynostosis
craniotome
    B-1 craniotome attach-
       ment (also B-2, etc.)
    B-craniotome
    Hall craniotome
    Hall in-and-out cranio-
       tome
    Hall neurosurgical
       craniotome
    Muehr craniotome
    turbo-bit craniotome
    Verbrugge-Souttar
       craniotome
    Williams craniotome
craniotomy
craniotomy flap

craniotomy instrument set
craniotomy scissors
craniotrypesis
craniovac drain
cranium
Cranley-Graff phleborrheogram
Crapeau nasal snare
Crapeau snare
crash cart
crash cesarean section
crater
craterization
cravat
cravat bandage
Crawford aortic retractor
Crawford auricle clamp
Crawford canaliculus hook
Crawford canaliculus probe
Crawford crutches
Crawford dural elevator
Crawford fascial forceps
Crawford fascial needle
Crawford fascial stripper
Crawford fracture frame
Crawford low-lithotomy
    crutches
Crawford needle
Crawford operation
Crawford retractor
Crawford suture ring
Crawford-Adams acetabular cup
Crawford-Adams arthroplasty
Crawford-Adams cup
Crawford-Adams cup arthro-
    plasty
Crawford-Adams hip arthro-
    plasty
crease
crease incision
crease line
Credé maneuver
Credé method
Credé prophylaxis
Credo operation
Creech aorto-iliac graft
Creech manner
Creed dissector

Creench insertion of vascular
    prosthesis
creeping thrombosis
Creevy biopsy forceps
Creevy bladder evacuator
Creevy calyx dislodger
Creevy dilator
Creevy evacuator
Creevy irrigator
Creevy operation
Creevy stone dislodger
Creevy-Bumpus hemostat
Crego bow traction
Crego closed reduction
Crego elevator
Crego Gigli-saw
Crego operation
Crego osteotomy
Crego periosteal elevator
Crego retractor
Crego traction
Crego wire traction
cremaster fascia
cremaster muscle
cremaster, musculus
cremasteric artery
cremasteric fascia
cremasteric layer
cremasteric muscle
cremasteric reflex
cremasterica, arteria
cremnocele
Crenshaw carbuncle forceps
Crenshaw caruncle clamp
Crenshaw caruncle forceps
Crenshaw forceps
crepe bandage
crepitant rales
crepitation
crepitus
crepitus at fracture site
crescendo
crescendo angina
crescendo murmur
crescendo pattern
crescendo TIAs (crescendo
    transient ischemic attacks)

crescendo-decrescendo murmur
crescent
crescent choroid
Crescent graft
crescent incision
crescent of cardia
crescent operation
Crescent plaster knife
crescentic blade
crescentic bunionectomy
crescentic glomerulonephritis
crescentic lobule
crescent-shaped incision
crest
crevice
Crib-O-Gram
cribriform compress
cribriform fascia
cribriform hymen
cribriform plate
cribriform process
cribriform sinus
cribriform tissue
Cricket stapling device
cricoarytenoid joint ankylosis
cricoarytenoid ligament
cricoarytenoid muscle
cricoarytenoideus lateralis,
    musculus
cricoarytenoideus, musculus
cricoarytenoideus posterior,
    musculus
cricoesophageal tendon
cricoid cartilage
cricoidectomy
cricopharyngeal diverticulum
cricopharyngeal muscle
cricopharyngeal sphincter
cricopharyngeus, musculus
cricothyroarytenoid ligament
cricothyroid
cricothyroid ligament
cricothyroid membrane
cricothyroid muscle
cricothyroid needle puncture
cricothyroid trocar
cricothyroidectomy

cricothyroideus, musculus
cricothyroidotomy
cricothyroidotomy and trache-
    ostomy
cricothyrostomy
cricothyrotomy
cricothyrotomy cannula
cricothyrotomy trocar
cricotomy
cricotracheal ligament
cricotracheotomy
Crigler evaluator
Crikelair otoplasty
Crile appendiceal clamp
Crile arterial forceps
Crile blade
Crile clamp
Crile cleft palate knife
Crile crushing clamp
Crile dissector
Crile forceps
Crile gall duct forceps
Crile gall duct hemostat
Crile head traction
Crile hemostat
Crile hook
Crile incision
Crile knife
Crile Micro-Line artery forceps
Crile needle holder
Crile nerve hook
Crile retractor
Crile single hook
Crile spatula
Crile stripper
Crile thyroid double-ended
    retractor
Crile vagotomy stripper
Crile-Barnes hemostatic forceps
Crile-Crutchfield clamp
Crile-Duval lung-grasping
    forceps
Crile-Murray needle holder
Crile-Wood needle holder
Crile-Wood Vital needle holder
crimped Dacron prosthesis
crimped wire

crimped woven prosthesis
crimper (see also *wire crimper*)
    Caparosa wire crimper
    Francis-Gray wire
        crimper
    Gruppe wire crimper
    House crimper forceps
    Juers crimper
    McGee crimper
    McGee-Caparosa wire
        crimper
    Schuknecht crimper
    Schuknecht Teflon
        crimper
    Schuknecht wire crimper
    Shiffrin wire crimper
    wire crimper
    wire-crimper forceps
crimper closer forceps
crimper forceps
crimper wire
crinkle
crinkle line
Crinotene dressing
Cripps obturator
Cripps operation
crisis
Crisp aneurysm
crisscross
crisscross fashion
crisscross heart
Critchett excision of anterior
    eyeball
Critchett operation
criterion (*pl.* criteria)
critical level
critical mass
Critikon balloon thermodilution
    catheter
Critikon balloon-tipped end-
    hole catheter
Critikon catheter
Critikon pressure infuser
Crobin technique
crochet hook
crocodile forceps
crocodile tongue

Cröhnlein procedure
Crombie tongue
Cronin cheiloplasty
Cronin cleft palate elevator
Cronin implant
Cronin mammary implant
Cronin method
Cronin operation
Cronin palate elevator
Cronin palate knife
Cronin Silastic mammary
    prosthesis
Cronin-Matthews eave flap
crook measuring prosthesis
Crookes lens
Crookes tube
CROS hearing aid prosthesis
Crosby capsule
Crosby knife
Crosby-Cooney operation for
    ascites
Crosby-Kugler capsule
cross circulation
Cross clamp
cross contamination
Cross corneal bur
cross femoral-femoral bypass
Cross needle trocar
Cross osteotome
Cross scleral trephine
cross section (noun; see also
    *cross-section*)
cross union
cross-action bulldog clamp
cross-action clamp
cross-action forceps
cross-arm flap
crossbar (see also *bar*)
    Clevedent crossbar
      elevator
    Cottle crossbar chisel
    Cottle crossbar fishtail
      chisel
crossbar chisel
crossbar chisel-osteotome
crossbar elevator
crossbite

crossclamp
crossclamp time
crossclamped aorta
crossclamping
crosscut
crosscut bur
crosscut fissure bur
crosscut saw
crossed coil
crossed reflex
crossed renal ectopia
crossed sword fashion
Crossen puncturing tenaculum
cross-finger flap
cross-friction massage
crosshatch
crosshatch incision
crossing over
Cross-Jones disk valve prosthe-
    sis
Cross-Jones mitral valve
Cross-Jones valve prosthesis
cross-leg bypass graft
cross-leg flap
cross-leg graft
cross-leg skin flap
crossmatch
crossover
crossover bypass
crossover graft
crossover vasectomy
crosspiece
cross-pin teeth
cross-reactivity
cross-section (verb; see also
    *cross section*)
cross-sectional
cross-sectional echocardiogra-
    phy
cross-sectional image
cross-sectional plane
cross-sectional view
cross-shaped incision
cross-slot screwdriver
cross-sword technique of Park
cross-table lateral position
cross-talk pacemaker

Crotti retractor
Crotti thyroid retractor
Croupette
Crouzon disease
Crouzon facial deformity
Crowe-Davis mouth gag
Crowel-Beard ptosis procedure
Crowe-tip pin
crown and bridge scissors
crown debridement
crown drill
crown drill screw
crown saw
crown stitch
crown sutures
crown-collar scissors
crown-crimping pliers
crowning of infant's head
crown-of-thorns head holder
crown-rump length
crown-to-heel
crown-to-rump
crow's feet
Crozat appliance
crucial anastomosis
crucial bandage
crucial incision
cruciate head screw
cruciate incision
cruciate ligament guide
cruciate ligament tear
cruciate ligaments
cruciate pulley
cruciate screw
cruciform anterior spinal
    hyperextension (CASH)
cruciform head-bone screw
cruciform screw
cruciform screwdriver
Cruickshank clamp
Crump dilator
Crump vessel dilator
Crump-Himmelstein dilator
crunching sound
crura (*sing.* crus)
crura anthelicis

crura cerebelli
crura cerebri
crura hook
crura of clitoris
crural area
crural canal
crural fascia
crural hernia
crural ligament
crural nipper
crural nipper forceps
crural region
crural repair
Cruricast dressing
crurotomy
crurotomy chisel
crurotomy nipper
crurotomy saw
crus (*pl.* crura)
crus anterius stapedis
crus anthelicis
crus breve incudis
crus cerebri
crus clitoridis
crus fornicis
crus glandis clitoridis
crus guide fork
crus helicis
crus laterale
crus mediale
crus of clitoris
crus of diaphragm
crus of fornix
crus of helix
crus of incus
crus of stapes
crus penis
crus posterius stapedis
crush clamp
crush injury
crush kidney
crush vasectomy technique
crushed chest injury
crushed muscle
crusher (see also *spur crusher*)
crushing

crushing and removal of calculi
crushing chest discomfort
crushing clamp
crushing fracture
crushing injury
crushing of calculus
crushing of nerve
crushing of vas deferens
crushing sensation in chest
crust
crusting
Crutchfield clamp
Crutchfield drill
Crutchfield hand drill
Crutchfield operation
Crutchfield reduction technique
Crutchfield skeletal traction
Crutchfield skull tongs
Crutchfield skull-tip pin
Crutchfield tongs
Crutchfield tongs prosthesis
Crutchfield tongs traction
Crutchfield traction
Crutchfield traction bow
Crutchfield traction tongs
Crutchfield-Raney drill
Crutchfield-Raney drill point
Crutchfield-Raney tongs
Crutchfield-Raney traction
     tongs
Cruveilhier atrophy
Cruveilhier joint
Cruveilhier nodules
Cruveilhier sign
Cruveilhier tumor
Cruveilhier ulcer
crux of heart
Cryer elevator
Cryer Universal forceps
cryoablation catheter
cryoanalgesia
cryocardioplegia
cryocataract extraction
cryocautery
cryoconization
cryodestruction
cryoextraction of cataract

cryoextractor (see also *extractor*)
    Alcon cryoextractor
    Amoils cryoextractor
    Beaver cryoextractor
    Bellows cryoextractor
    disposable cryoextractor
    Frigitronics cryoextractor
    Krwawicz cryoextractor
    Thomas cryoextractor
cryofrigitronics
cryogenic cataract extraction
cryogenic eye surgery
cryogenic probe
cryogenic surgery
cryoglue
cryohypophysectomy
cryoleucotomy
Cryolife valvular graft
cryomagnet
cryo-ophthalmic unit
cryopencil
cryopexy
cryophake
    Alcon cryophake
    Frigitronics cryophake
    Keeler cryophake
    Keeler cryophake unit
cryoprecipitate
cryopreservation
cryopreserved allograft
cryoprobe (see also *probe*)
    Amoils cryoprobe
    Brymill cryoprobe
    Cooper cryoprobe
    Frigitronics cryoprobe
    Kry-Med 300 cryoprobe
    Rubinstein cryoprobe
cryopter
    Thomas cryopter
cryoretinopexy
cryostat
    Cooper cryostat
cryostylet
    disposable cryostylet
    Frigitronics cryostylet
    Kelman cryostylet
cryosurgery

cryosurgical apparatus
cryosurgical interruption of AV
    node
cryosurgical technique
cryothalamectomy
cryothalmotomy
cryotherapy
cryounit
crypt
crypt hook
crypt knife
cryptectomy
cryptic tonsil
cryptitis
cryptorchidectomy
cryptorchidism
cryptorchidopexy
cryptotomy
crypts of Lieberkühn
crypts of Luschka
crypts of palatine tonsil
crypts of pharyngeal tonsil
crypts of tonsils
crystal
crystalline
crystalline lens
crystallization
crystallized trypsin
crystalloid
Csapo abortion
Csapody operation
CSF (cerebrospinal fluid)
CSF flushing reservoir
CSF flushing valve
CSF shunt connector forceps
CSF shunt instruments
CSF shunt system
CSF shunt-introducing forceps
CT (computed tomography,
    computerized tomography)
CT gantry
CT scan
CT scanner
CT-guided needle aspiration
    biopsy
CTI brace
CTT scanner

CTX needle
Cu-7 intrauterine device
CU-8 needle
Cubbins approach
Cubbins incision
Cubbins screw
Cubbins screwdriver
Cubbins shoulder arthroplasty
Cubbins-Callahan-Scuderi
    approach
Cube urinary drainage system
cubital fossa
cubital lymph nodes
cubital nerve
cubital region
cubital tunnel
cubital tunnel syndrome
cubital vein
cubitocarpal
cubitoradial
cubitus valgus
cubitus varus
cuboid bone
cueing
cuff
    aortic cuff
    Astropulse cuff
    atrial cuff
    blood pressure cuff
    blood warmer cuff
    calibrated V-Lok cuff
    Cardio-Cuff
    Childs Cardio-Cuff
    conductive V-Lok cuff
    elephant cuff
    Falk vaginal cuff clamp
    Honan cuff
    inflatable cuff
    inflatable tourniquet
        cuff
    inflatable tracheal tube
        cuff
    Kidde tourniquet cuff
    mucosal cuff
    musculotendinous cuff
    nerve cuff
    pneumatic cuff

cuff *continued*
- pressure cuff
- rectal muscle cuff
- reefed vaginal cuff
- right atrial cuff
- rotator cuff
- sphygmomanometer cuff
- suprahepatic caval cuff
- tourniquet cuff
- tracheal tube cuff
- uterine cuff
- vaginal cuff
- Vitacuff
- Wolfe uterine cuff forceps

cuff abscess
cuff electrode
cuff pressure
cuff resection
cuff salpingostomy
cuff sign
cuffed endotracheal tube
cuffed sheet
cuffed tube
cuffless tube
cuff-type inactive electrode
CUI tissue expander (Cox-Uphoff International tissue expander)
cuirass
cuirass jacket
cuirass respirator
Cukier nasal forceps
Culbertson canal knife
Culcher-Sussman pelvic inlet measurement
cul-de-sac
cul-de-sac of Douglas
cul-de-sac of vagina
culdocentesis
culdoplasty
culdoscope
- Decker culdoscope
- fiberoptic culdoscope
- photoculdoscope

culdoscopy
culdotomy

culdotomy incision
Cullen abduction splint
Cullen obstetrical forceps
Cullen sign
Culler eye forceps
Culler fixation forceps
Culler iris spatula
Culler lens spoon
Culler rectus muscle hook
Culler spatula
Culley splint
Cullom septal forceps
Cullom-Mueller adenotome
culmen
Culp biopsy needle
Culp pyeloplasty
Culp ureteropelvioplasty
Culp-Calhoon operation
Culp-Scardino operation
culture
culture and sensitivity (C&S)
culture tubes
Cummings catheter
Cummings four-wing catheter
Cummings tube
Cummings-Pezzer catheter
cumulative dose
cumulative radiation effect
cumulative toxicity index
cuneiform
cuneiform bone
cuneiform cartilage
cuneiform joint
cuneiform ligament
cuneiform osteotomy
cuneiform tubercle
cuneiforms 1, 2, 3
cuneocuboid
cuneonavicular
cuneonavicular ligament
cuneoscaphoid
Cunningham brace
Cunningham clamp
Cunningham incontinence clamp
cup
- Accu-Path acetabular cup system

cup *continued*
    acetabular cup
    Alivium prosthesis cup
    Aufranc cup
    Buchholz acetabular cup
    caliceal cups
    Centaur trial cup
    Chambers intrauterine
        cup
    Charnley cup
    Crawford-Adams
        acetabular cup
    Crawford-Adams cup
    dry cup
    ear cup
    Harris-Galante cup
    iodine cup
    Laing concentric hip cup
    large physiological cup
    magnetic cups
    McBride cup
    McGoey-Evans acetabu-
        lar cup
    McGoey-Evans cup
    McKee-Farrar acetabular
        cup
    McKee-Farrar cup
    medicine cup
    nasal suction cup
    Natural-Loc RM acetabu-
        lar cups
    New England Baptist
        acetabular cup
    O'Connor finger cup
    ocular cup
    O'Harris-Petruso cup
    ophthalmic cup
    optic cup
    porous coat cup for
        Richards hip prosthesis
    Rickham cup
    Rotalok cup
    Silastic obstetrical
        vacuum cup
    Smith-Petersen cup
    Spectron metal-backed
        cup for Richards hip
        prosthesis

cup *continued*
    stainless steel cup
    suction cup
    Titan hip cup
    trial acetabular cup
    trial cup
    Vitallium cup
    wet cup
cup arthroplasty
cup biopsy forceps
cup forceps
cup hip prosthesis
cup impactor
cup pessary
cup positioner
cup-and-ball osteotomy
cup-and-spill stomach
cup-biting forceps
cup-biting punch
cup/disk ratio (CDR)
cupid's bow
cupped disk
cupped forceps
cupping
cupping glass
cupping of disk
cupping of nerve
Cupraphane dialyzer reaction
cup-shaped ear forceps
cup-shaped electrode
cup-shaped forceps
cup-shaped inner ear forceps
cup-shaped middle ear forceps
cupula (*pl.* cupulae)
cupula cristae ampullaris
cupula of cochlea
cupula of pleura
cupula technique
cupular cecum of cochlear duct
cupuliform cataract
Curad plastic bandage
Curad plastic dressing
curare anesthetic agent
curative
curative dose
curative result
curative surgery
curb tenotomy

Curdy blade
Curdy knife
Curdy sclerotome
Curdy sclerotome knife
cure
curet

adenoid curet
Alvis curet
Alvis foreign body curet
Anderson curet
Angell curet
angled curet
antral curet
aortic curet
aspirating curet
Auto-Suture curet
B-12 dental curet
Ballantine uterine curet
Ballenger curet
Ballenger ethmoid
    curet
banjo curet
Bardic curet
Barnhill adenoid curet
Barnhill curet
Barnhill-Jones curet
Barth curet
Barth mastoid curet
Beaver curet
Berkeley Vacurette
    machine
Billeau curet
Billeau ear curet
biopsy curet
biopsy suction curet
Blake curet
bone curet
Bozeman curet
Bromley uterine curet
Bronson-Ray curet
Brun bone curet
Brun curet
Brun ear curet
Brun mastoid curet
Buck bone curet
Buck curet
Buck ear curet

curet *continued*

Buck mastoid curet
Bumm curet
Bumm placental curet
Bumm uterine curet
Bush intervertebral curet
Carlens curet
Carmack curet
Carmack ear curet
Carroll hook curet
Carter curet
Carter submucous curet
cervical biopsy curet
cervical curet
chalazion curet
Clevedent-Lucas curet
Cloward curet
Cloward-Cone ring curet
Clyman endometrial
    curet
Coakley antrum curet
Coakley curet
Coakley nasal curet
Coakley sinus curet
Cobb curet
Cone curet
Cone nasal curet
Cone ring curet
Cone suction biopsy
    curet
Converse curet
corneal curet
Daubenspeck bone curet
DeLee curet
Dench ear curet
Dench uterine curet
DePuy bone curet
DePuy curet
Derlacki curet
Derlacki ear curet
dermal curet
diagnostic curet
disk curet
disposable vacuum curet
double-ended bone curet
double-ended curet
double-lumen curet

curet *continued*
- down-biting curet
- Duncan curet
- Duncan endometrial biopsy curet
- Duncan endometrial curet
- ear curet
- elevator-curet
- embolectomy curet
- endaural curet
- endocervical biopsy curet
- endocervical curet
- endometrial biopsy curet
- endometrial curet
- endotracheal curet
- Epstein curet
- ethmoidal curet
- Faulkner antrum curet
- Faulkner curet
- Faulkner ethmoid curet
- Faulkner nasal curet
- fenestration curet
- Ferguson bone curet
- Ferguson curet
- fine curet
- fine-angled curet
- Fink chalazion curet
- Fink curet
- foreign-body curet
- Fox curet
- Fox dermal curet
- Franklin-Silverman curet
- Franseen rectal curet
- Freimuth curet
- Freimuth ear curet
- frontal sinus curet
- Garcia-Rock endometrial suction curet
- Gifford corneal curet
- Gifford curet
- Goldman curet
- Goldstein curet
- Govons curet
- Gracey curet
- Green corneal curet

curet *continued*
- Green curet
- Greene uterine curet
- Greene endocervical curet
- Greene placental curet
- Gross curet
- Gross ear curet
- Gusberg cervical biopsy curet
- Gusberg cervical cone curet
- Gusberg curet
- Gusberg endocervical biopsy curet
- Gusberg endocervical curet
- Halle curet
- Halle ethmoidal curet
- Halle sinus curet
- Hannon curet
- Hannon endometrial biopsy curet
- Hannon endometrial curet
- Hardy microcuret
- Harrison curet
- Harrison scarifying curet
- Harrison-Shea curet
- Hartmann adenoidal curet
- Hartmann curet
- Hatfield bone curet
- Hayden curet
- Hayden tonsil curet
- Heaney curet
- Heaney uterine curet
- Heath chalazion curet
- Heath curet
- Hebra chalazion curet
- Hebra corneal curet
- Hibbs bone curet
- Hibbs curet
- Hibbs-Spratt curet
- Hibbs-Spratt spinal fusion curet

curet *continued*

Hofmeister endometrial
biopsy curet
Holden curet
Holden uterine curet
Holtz curet
Holtz ear curet
Holtz endometrial curet
hook-type dermal curet
horizontal ring curet
Hotz curet
Hotz ear curet
House curet
House stapes curet
House-Paparella curet
House-Paparella stapes
curet
Howard spinal curet
Hunter curet
Hunter large uterine
curet
Hunter uterine curet
Ingersoll adenoid curet
Ingersoll curet
Innomed bone curet
Innomed curet
intervertebral curet
irrigating curet
irrigating uterine curet
Jansen bone curet
Jansen curet
Jones adenoid curet
Jones curet
Jordan-Rosen curet
Juers ear curet
K-curette
Kelly curet
Kelly-Gray curet
Kelly-Gray uterine curet
Kevorkian curet
Kevorkian endocervical
curet
Kevorkian-Younge
biopsy curet
Kevorkian-Younge curet
Kevorkian-Younge
endocervical biopsy
curet

curet *continued*

Kezerian curet
Kirkland curet
Kushner-Tandatnick
curet
Kushner-Tandatnick
endometrial biopsy
curet
labyrinth curet
large bowel curet
laryngeal curet forceps
Laufe aspirating curet
Laufe-Novak diagnostic
curet
Laufe-Randall curet
Lempert curet
long-handle curet
Lounsbury curet
Lounsbury placenta curet
Lucas curet
Luer bone curet
Luer curet
Luongo curet
Lynch curet
Magielski curet
Malis microcuret
Maroon lip curet
Martin dermal curet
mastoid curet
Mayfield curet
Mayfield spinal curet
McCaskey antral curet
McCaskey curet
McElroy curet
Meigs curet
Meigs endometrial curet
Meyerding curet
Meyerding saw-toothed
curet
Meyhoeffer chalazion
curet
Meyhoeffer curet
microbone curet
microcuret
middle ear curet
middle ear ring curet
Middleton adenoid curet
Middleton curet

curet *continued*

Milan uterine curet
Miles antral curet
Miller curet
Molt curet
Mosher curet
Mosher ethmoid curet
Moult curet
Mueller curet
Munchen endometrial
  biopsy curet
Myles antral curet
Myles curet
nasal curet
Noland-Budd cervical
  curet
Noland-Budd curet
Novak biopsy curet
Novak curet
Novak uterine-suction
  curet
Novak-Schoeckaert
  endometrial biopsy
  curet
O'Connor double-edge
  curet
Orban curet
oval-window curet
Paparella curet
Piffard curet
Piffard dermal curet
Piffard placental curet
Pipelle endometrial
  suction curet
pituitary curet
placenta curet
plastic curet
polyvinyl curet
Pratt antrum curet
Pratt curet
Pratt ethmoid curet
Pratt nasal curet
Randall biopsy curet
Randall curet
Randall endometrial
  biopsy curet
Raney curet
Raney spinal fusion curet

curet *continued*

Ray curet
Ray pituitary curet
Read facial curet
Read oral curet
Récamier curet
rectal curet
Reich curet
Reich-Nechtow cervical
  biopsy curet
Reich-Nechtow curet
Reiner curet
resectoscope curet
reverse-angle skid curet
Rheinstaedter curet
Rheinstaedter uterine
  curet
Richards bone curet
Richards curet
Richards mastoid curet
Richards mastoid
  ethmoid curet
Ridpath curet
Ridpath ethmoid curet
right-angle curet
ring curet
Rock endometrial suction
  curet
Rosen curet
Rosenmueller curet
ruptured disk curet
salpingeal curet
saw-toothed curet
scarifying curet
Schaeffer curet
Schaeffer ethmoid curet
Schaeffer mastoid curet
Schede curet
Schroeder curet
Schroeder uterine curet
Schwartz curet
Schwartz endocervical
  curet
Scoville curet
Scoville ruptured disk
  curet
Seemes spinal fusion
  curet

curet *continued*
serrated curet
Shapleigh curet
Shapleigh ear curet
sharp curet
Sharp derma curet
Shea curet
Simon bone curet
Simon spinal curet
Simpson antral curet
Simpson curet
Sims curet
Sims uterine curet
sinus curet
Skeele chalazion curet
Skeele corneal curet
Skeele curet
Skeele eye curet
Skene uterine curet
Skene uterine spoon
    curet
Skillern curet
Skillern sinus curet
Smith-Petersen curet
soft rubber curet
sonic curet
spinal curet
spinal fusion curet
Spratt bone curet
Spratt curet
Spratt ear curet
Spratt mastoid curet
St. Clair-Thompson
    adenoid curet
St. Clair-Thompson curet
stapes curet
stirrup-loop curet
Storz resectoscope curet
Strully curet
Strully ruptured disk
    curet
Stubbs adenoid curet
Stubbs curet
submucous curet
suction curet
suction tip curet
Synthes facial curet

curet *continued*
Tabb curet
Taylor curet
Temens curet
Thomas curet
Thomas uterine curet
Thompson curet
Thorpe curet
toxemia curet
uterine curet
uterine irrigating curet
uterine suction curet
Vacurette
Vacurette suction curet
vacuum curet
vertical ring curet
V.M. & Co. mastoid curet
Vogel adenoid curet
Vogel curet
Vogel infant adenoid
    curet
Volkmann bone curet
Volkmann curet
Volkmann oval curet
Voller curet
Walker curet
Walker ruptured disk
    curet
Wallich curet
Walsh curet
Walsh dermal curet
Walsh hook-type dermal
    curet
Walton curet
Weaver chalazion curet
Weisman curet
Weisman ear curet
Weisman infant ear curet
West-Beck spoon curet
Williger bone curet
Wolff dermal curet
Wullstein curet
Wullstein ring curet
Yankauer curet
Yankauer ear curet
Yankauer salpingeal
    curet

curet *continued*
    Yasargil curet
    Younge uterine biopsy
       curet
    Younge uterine curet
curet forceps
curettage
curettage and irrigation
curette (see *curet*)
curetted
curetted bone
curettement
curetting bur
curettings
Curity dressing
Curl Cath catheter
curl-back shell eye implant
curled enamel
Curlex cranioplasty
Curling stress ulcer
Curling ulcer
curly toes
Curon dressing
Curran eye knife
currant jelly clot
currant jelly thrombus
current
current controller
current transformer
Currentrol cautery
Curry hip nail
Curry hip nail counterbore
Curry hip nail counterbore with
    Lloyd adapter
Curry needle
Curry splint
Curry walking splint
Curschmann trocar
Curtin operation
Curtin technique
Curtis arthroplasty
Curtis forceps
Curtis operation
Curtis technique
Curtis tissue forceps
curvature
curvature site

curve of Spee
curved awl
curved cannula
curved catheter
curved clamp
curved end-to-end anastomosis
    stapler (CEEA stapler)
curved forceps
curved gouge
curved hemostat
curved hook
curved incision
curved knife
curved Mayo clamp
curved Mayo scissors
curved needle
curved needle eye spud
curved needle holder
curved needle spud
curved nerve hook
curved periosteal elevator
curved periscapular incision
curved scissors
curved suture needle
curved toenails
curved tractor
curved tying forceps
curved valvulotome
curved zonule separator
curved-8 clamp
curved-downward incision
curved-on-flat scissors
curvilinear
curvilinear calcification
curvilinear flattening
curvilinear incision
curvilinear skin incision
curving incision
CUSA (Cavitron ultrasonic
    aspirator)
CUSA aspirator
CUSA dissector
Cusco speculum
Cusco vaginal speculum
Cushing aluminum retractor
Cushing angled retractor
Cushing bipolar forceps

Cushing bone rongeur
Cushing brain depressor
Cushing brain forceps
Cushing brain instruments
Cushing brain retractor
Cushing brain spatula
Cushing brain spatula spoon
Cushing bur
Cushing clamp
Cushing clip
Cushing cranial bur
Cushing cranial drill
Cushing cranial perforator
Cushing cranial rongeur forceps
Cushing decompression forceps
Cushing decompression
    retractor
Cushing disease
Cushing dressing forceps
Cushing drill
Cushing dural hook
Cushing dural hook knife
Cushing dural knife
Cushing elevator
Cushing forceps
Cushing Gigli-saw guide
Cushing hook
Cushing knife
Cushing needle
Cushing nerve retractor
Cushing operation
Cushing perforator
Cushing perforator drill
Cushing periosteal elevator
Cushing pituitary spoon
Cushing reflex
Cushing retractor
Cushing rongeur
Cushing S-retractor
Cushing S-shaped brain spatula
Cushing self-retaining retractor
Cushing spatula
Cushing spatula spoon
Cushing spoon
Cushing staphylorrhaphy
    elevator
Cushing straight retractor

Cushing stress ulcer
Cushing sutures
Cushing thumb forceps
Cushing tissue forceps
Cushing tumor
Cushing ulcer
Cushing vein retractor
Cushing Vital tissue forceps
Cushing-Brown tissue forceps
Cushing-Hopkins periosteal
    elevator
Cushing-Kocher retractor
Cushing-Landolt trans-
    sphenoidal speculum
Cushing-McKenzie clip
Cushing-Taylor carbide-jaw
    forceps
cushion defects
cushioned heel shoe
cushioning sutures
Cushman drain
Cusick eye knife
Cusick operation
cusp
cusp height
cuspid
cuspid teeth
custocolic fold
Custodis implant
Custodis operation
Custodis scleral buckle opera-
    tion
Custodis sponge
Custodis sutures
custom pectus excavatum per
    moulange prosthesis
custom-contoured implant
cut and ligated
cut edge
cut end of bone
cut section
cut snare wire
cut surface
cut, clamped, and ligated
cut-and-sew technique
cutanea tarda, vena
cutanea, vena

cutaneous abscess
cutaneous amputation
cutaneous edges approximated
cutaneous ileostomy
cutaneous ligaments of
    phalanges
cutaneous muscle
cutaneous nerve
cutaneous punch
cutaneous reaction
cutaneous stimulators
cutaneous striae
cutaneous suture of palate
cutaneous sutures
cutaneous tag
cutaneous ureterostomy
cutaneous vasostomy
cutaneous vein
cutaneous vesicostomy
cutaneus antebrachii lateralis,
    nervus
cutaneus antebrachii medialis,
    nervus
cutaneus antebrachii posterior,
    nervus
cutaneus brachii lateralis
    inferior, nervus
cutaneus brachii lateralis
    superior, nervus
cutaneus brachii medialis,
    nervus
cutaneus brachii posterior,
    nervus
cutaneus dorsalis intermedius,
    nervus
cutaneus dorsalis lateralis,
    nervus
cutaneus dorsalis medialis,
    nervus
cutaneus femoris lateralis,
    nervus
cutaneus femoris posterior,
    nervus
cutaneus, musculus
cutaneus surae lateralis, nervus
cutaneus surae medialis, nervus
cutdown

cutdown catheter
cutdown incision
cutdown instruments
cuticle
cuticle nipper
cuticle scissors
cuticular fold
cuticular sutures
cutin
Cutinova dressing
cutis elastica
cutis graft
Cutler eye implant
Cutler flap
Cutler forceps
Cutler implant
Cutler operation
Cutler repair
Cutler-Beard bridge flap
Cutler-Beard operation
Cutler-Beard reconstruction
Cutler-Beard technique
cutoffs
cutter (see also *wire cutter*)
        atherectomy cutter
        Beaver cutter
        Berbecker wire cutter
        Bethune bone cutter
        Birtcher Hyfrecutter
        bone cutter
        Buettner-Parel cutter
        Buettner-Parel vitreous
            cutter
        cast cutter
        chuck cutter
        Cloward-Dowel cutter
        cookie cutter
        cookie cutter areolar
            marker
        diamond-pin cutter
        double-action bone
            cutter
        Douvas cutter
        Douvas vitreous cutter
        dowel cutter
        Dyonics cutter
        Dyonics meniscal cutter

cutter *continued*
    electric cutter
    Expand-O-Graft dispos-
        able cutter
    finger ring cutter
    Freeman cookie-cutter
        areolar marker
    Hyfrecutter
    Intra-Articular Surgical
        System cutter
    Kloti cutter
    Kloti vitreous cutter
    Kuhlman cast cutter
    Leather valve cutter
    Lempert malleus cutter
    Machemer cutter
    Machemer VISC (vitreous
        infusion suction cutter)
    Machemer vitreous
        cutter
    Maguire-Harvey cutter
    Maguire-Harvey vitreous
        cutter
    malleus cutter
    Martin wire cutter
    Martini bone cutter
    nail cutter
    nasal stent cutter
    O'Malley-Heintz cutter
    Parel-Crock cutter
    Parel-Crock vitreous
        cutter
    pin cutter
    plaster cast cutter
    rectal cutter
    rib cutter
    right-angled bone cutter
    Roos rib cutter
    SCDK-Cutter valve
    Schuknecht cutter
    Sklar bone pin cutter
    Sklar cutter
    Stengstrom nerve
        cutter
    Stryker cast cutter
    suction cutter
    Tolentino cutter
    Tolentino vitreous cutter

cutter *continued*
    VISC (vitreous infusion
        suction cutter)
    vitreous infusion suction
        cutter (VISC)
    wire cutter
    Wister wire-and-pin
        cutter
    Woelfe-Boehler cutter
Cutter aortic valve prosthesis
Cutter cast
Cutter cast for disk lesion
Cutter cast tape
cutter gamma
Cutter mitral valve
Cutter SCDK prosthesis
Cutter-Smeloff aortic valve
    prosthesis
Cutter-Smeloff cardiac valve
    prosthesis
Cutter-Smeloff disk valve
Cutter-Smeloff heart valve
Cutter-Smeloff mitral valve
cutting block
cutting board
cutting Bovie knife
cutting bur
cutting current
cutting device
cutting disk
cutting edge
cutting forceps
cutting loop
cutting loop electrode
cutting needle
cuttlefish disk
Cuvier ducts
CVA (cerebrovascular acci-
    dent)
CVB (chorionic villi biopsy)
CVIS imaging device
CVOD (cerebrovascular
    obstructive disease)
CVP (central venous pressure)
C.W. Mayo instruments (see
    *Mayo*)
cyanoacrylate adhesive
cyanoacrylate embolization

cyanosis
cyanotic
Cyberlith demand pacemaker
Cyberlith pacemaker
CyberTach pacemaker
Cybex evaluation
Cybex machine
Cyclaine anesthetic agent
cycle
cyclectomy
cyclic irregularity
cyclic loading
cyclic therapy
cyclic treatment
cyclicotomy
cycloanemization
cyclocryotherapy
cyclodialysis
cyclodialysis cannula
cyclodialysis spatula
cyclodiathermy
cyclodiathermy needle
cycloelectrolysis
cycloergometer
cyclographic tomogram
cyclolithopexy
cyclomethycaine sulfate
    anesthetic agent
cyclopentane anesthetic agent
cyclophotocoagulation
cycloplegia
cyclopropane anesthetic
    agent
cyclotomy
cyesis
cylinder aneurysm
cylinder axis
cylinder cast
cylinder process
cylindrical
cylindrical bougie
cylindrical lens
cylindrical reamer
cylindrical zonule separator
cylindrical-object forceps
Cymed Micro skin pouch
Cyriax technique
cyst

cyst wall
cystadenocarcinoma
cystadenoma
cystauchenotomy
cystduodenostomy
cystectasia
cystectasy
cystectomy
cystgastrostomy
cystic
cystic artery
cystic breast
cystic carcinoma
cystic cataract
cystic change
cystic dilatation
cystic disease
cystic duct
cystic duct cholangiogram
cystic duct forceps
cystic duct lumen
cystic duct scoop
cystic enlargement
cystic goiter
cystic hernia
cystic lesion
cystic mass
cystic mastitis
cystic membrane
cystic plexus
cystic structure
cystic tumor
cystic vein
cystica, arteria
cystica, vena
cystic-choledochal junction
cysticolithectomy
cysticolithotripsy
cysticorrhaphy
cysticotomy
cystidoceliotomy
cystidolaparotomy
cystidotrachelotomy
cystine urinary tract stones
cystis
cystis fellea
cystitome (see also *cystotome*)
    Azar cystitome

cystitome *continued*
    eye cystitome
    Graefe cystitome
    Knolle cystitome
    Knolle-Kelman
      cystitome
    Lieppman cystitome
    McIntyre cystitome
    Nevyas cystitome
    Worth cystitome
Cystocath
cystocatheter
cystocele
cystocele repair
cystochromoscopy
cystocolostomy
cystodiaphanoscopy
cystodrain
cystoduodenostomy
cystoelytroplasty
cystoenterocele
cystoepiplocele
cystogastrostomy
cystogenic aneurysm
cystogram
cystography
cystohepatic triangle
cystohydrodistention
cystojejunostomy
cystolithectomy
cystolitholapaxy
cystolithotomy
cystometer
    Lewis cystometer
    recording cystometer
    water cystometer
cystometer chart
cystometric study
cystometrogram (CMG)
cystometrography
cystometry
cystopanendoscope
cystopericystectomy
cystopexy
cystophotography
cystoplasty
cystoplasty augmentation
cystoproctostomy
cystopyelogram

cystopyelography
cystoradium insertion
cystorectostomy
cystoreductive surgery
cystorrhaphy
cystosarcoma
cystosarcoma phylloides
cystoscope
    ACMI cystoscope
    Albarran cystoscope
    Albarran cystoscope
      attachment
    Bard cystoscope tip
    Beard cystoscope
    Braasch cystoscope
    Braasch direct catheteri-
      zation cystoscope
    Braasch direct
      cystoscope
    Braasch-Kaplan direct-
      vision cystoscope
    Brown-Buerger
      cystoscope
    Butterfield cystoscope
    electrocystoscope
    female cystoscope
    fiberoptic cystoscope
    Foroblique cystoscope
    French Brown-Buerger
      cystoscope
    French-Wappler
      cystoscope
    Graefe cystoscope
    Holth cystoscope
    infant cystoscope
    Judd female urethro-
      cystoscope
    Kelly cystoscope
    Kirwin cystoscope
    Laidley cystoscope
    Leiter cystoscope
    Lowsley-Peterson
      cystoscope
    McCarthy cystoscope
    McCarthy-Campbell
      cystoscope
    McCarthy-Peterson
      cystoscope
    McCrea cystoscope

cystoscope *continued*
- National cystoscope
- National general-purpose cystoscope
- Nesbit cystoscope
- obturator cystoscope
- Olympus cystoscope
- Otis bulb cystoscope
- Otis-Brown cystoscope
- Ravich convertible cystoscope
- Ravich cystoscope
- sheath cystoscope
- Storz cystoscope
- Storz cystoscope-urethroscope
- Storz direct-vision cystoscope
- Storz suprapubic cystoscope
- suprapubic cystoscope
- telescope of cystoscope
- Universal cystoscope
- ureterocystoscope
- Wappler cystoscope
- Wheeler cystoscope
- Wilder cystoscope
- Young cystoscope

cystoscope cord
cystoscope obturator
cystoscope sheath
cystoscope tip
cystoscope-urethroscope
cystoscope-urethroscope adapter
cystoscopic biopsy
cystoscopic connecting nipple
cystoscopic cord
cystoscopic electrocautery
cystoscopic electrode
cystoscopic examination
cystoscopic findings
cystoscopic forceps
cystoscopic fulgurating electrode
cystoscopic fulguration
cystoscopic rongeur
cystoscopic scissors
cystoscopic snare
cystoscopic ulcer
cystoscopic urography
cystoscopy
cystoscopy and dilatation
cystostomy
cystostomy tube
cystotome (see also *cystitome*)
- Beard cystotome
- Graefe cystotome
- Graefe flexible cystotome
- Holth cystotome
- Kelman cystotome
- Knapp cystotome
- Mendez ultrasonic cystotome
- Visitec cystotome
- Wheeler cystotome
- Wilder cystotome

cystotomy
cystotrachelotomy
cystotrocar
cystoureterogram
cystoureterolithotomy
cystourethral suspension
cystourethrogram
cystourethrography
cystourethropexy
cystourethroplasty
cystourethroscope
- ACMI cystourethroscope
- ACMI microlens cystourethroscope
- Foroblique cystourethroscope

cystourethroscope bridge
cystourethroscope parts
cystourethroscopy
Cytobrush
cytocidal
cytologic, cytological
cytological biopsy
cytological brush
cytology

Cytoxan
Czermak eye knife
Czermak keratome
Czermak operation
Czermak spaces
Czerny herniorrhaphy

Czerny incision
Czerny operation
Czerny rectal speculum
Czerny sutures
Czerny-Lembert sutures

D&C (dilation and curettage;
    dilatation and curettage)
D&E (dilation and evacuation)
D&G sutures
D&N (distant and near)
D/3 (distal third)
D3 dialyzer
D-Tach needle
Dacomed Omni Phase penile
    prosthesis
Dacomed Rigidscan
Dacomed Snap-Gauge
Dacron arterial prosthesis
Dacron bifurcation prosthesis
Dacron bolstered sutures
Dacron catheter
Dacron graft
Dacron graft clamp
Dacron implant
Dacron knitted graft
Dacron mesh
Dacron onlay patch graft
Dacron patch
Dacron patch graft
Dacron preclotted graft
Dacron prosthesis
Dacron Sauvage patch
Dacron shield
Dacron stent
Dacron sutures
Dacron tape
Dacron tightly woven graft
Dacron traction sutures
Dacron tubular graft
Dacron valve prosthesis
Dacron vascular prosthesis
Dacron velour graft
Dacron vessel prosthesis
Dacron Weave Knit graft
dacryoadenectomy

dacryoadenotomy
dacryocystectomy
dacryocystogram
dacryocystography
dacryocystorhinostomy
dacryocystorhinostomy cannula
dacryocystorhinostomy needle
dacryocystorhinostomy retractor
dacryocystorhinostomy trephine
dacryocystostomy
dacryocystosyringotomy
dacryocystotomy
dacryolith
dacryostomy
dacryotrephine
dactylocostal rhinoplasty
dactylolysis
Daems bronchial clamp
Daems clamp
Dagnini reflex
Dahlgren rongeur
Dahlgren scissors
Dahlgren-Hudson forceps
Daig atrial screw-in lead
Daig pacemaker
Daig screw-in lead
Daily cataract needle
Daily cataract operation
Daily eye knife
Daily fixation hook
Daily keratome
Daily sutures
Daisy vitrectomy machine
Dakin catheter
Dakin dressing
Dakin fluid
Dakin solution
Dakin tube
Dakin tubing
Dakin-Carrel method

Dale abdominal binder
Dale abdominal support
Dale ankle support
Dale femoral-popliteal anasto-
    mosis forceps
Dale first rib rongeur
Dale forceps
Dale knee support
Dale pelvic support
Dale rib support
Dale tennis elbow support
Dale traction
Dale wrist support
Dalen-Fuchs nodules
Dalgleish operation
Dallas operation
Dallas retractor
D'Allesandro serial suture-
    holding forceps
Dalrymple sign
dam
dam drain
D'Amato sign
Dammann-Muller operation
Damon Scan Mate
damped waveform
Damshek needle
Damshek sternal trephine
Damshek trephine
Dan chalazion forceps
Dana operation
Dana rhizotomy
DANA shoulder system
Danberg forceps
Danberg iris forceps
Dandy clamp
Dandy clip
Dandy forceps
Dandy hemostat
Dandy hemostatic forceps
Dandy hook
Dandy needle
Dandy nerve hook
Dandy neurosurgical scissors
Dandy operation
Dandy rhizotomy
Dandy scalp forceps

Dandy scalp hemostat
Dandy scissors
Dandy suction tube
Dandy trigeminal scissors
Dandy ventricular needle
Dandy ventriculostomy
Dandy-Cairns brain needle
Dandy-Cairns ventricular needle
Dandy-Walker deformity
Dandy-Walker syndrome
Danforth method
Danforth operation
Dan-Gradle cilial forceps
Daniel clamp
Daniel colostomy clamp
Daniel operation
Daniels hemostatic tonsillec-
    tome
Daniels operation
Daniels tonometer
Daniels tonsillectome
Danis retractor
Danis-Weber ankle fracture
    classification (types A, B,
    C)
Danker-Wohlk contact lens
Dann respirator
Dannheim eye implant
Dann-Jennings mouth gag
Dansac ileal pouch
Dansac karaya seal pouch
Dansac ostomy pouch
Dap II biopsy needle guide
Dappen jar
Darby surgical shoe
Darco medical-surgical shoe
    and toe alignment splint
Darco shoe
Darco toe alignment splint
Dardik biograft
Dardik graft
Dardik human graft
Dardik umbilical graft
Dardik umbilical prosthesis
Dardik vein substitute
Darin intraocular implant lens
Darin lens

darkening of nipples
darkfield microscope
Darling capsulotome
Darling popliteal retractor
Darmstruck lymphoma
Darrach elevator
Darrach procedure
Darrach resection
Darrach retractor
Darrach technique
Darrach ulnar resection
Darrach wrist arthroplasty
Darrach-McLaughlin approach
Dartigues uterine-elevating
    forceps
dartoid tissue
dartos fascia
dartos pouch
Darwin tubercle
Das Gupta scapula procedure
dashboard fracture
dashboard perineum
D'Assumpcao rhytidoplasty
    marker
Datascope balloon
Datascope intra-aortic balloon
    pump
Datascope intra-aortic balloon
    pump catheter
Daubenspeck bone curet
Daubenton plane
d'Aubigne operator
d'Aubigne prosthesis
daughter cyst
Dautrey chisel
Dautrey osteotome
Dautrey osteotomy
Dautrey retractor
Dautrey-Munro osteotome
Davat operation for varicocele
David drainage
David rectal speculum
David technique
Davidoff cordotomy knife
Davidoff knife
Davidoff retractor
Davidson bur

Davidson clamp
Davidson collector
Davidson forceps
Davidson muscle clamp
Davidson periosteal elevator
Davidson pneumothorax
    apparatus
Davidson pulmonary vessel
    clamp
Davidson pulmonary vessel
    forceps
Davidson retractor
Davidson scapular retractor
Davidson syringe
Davidson thoracic trocar
Davidson trocar
Davidson vessel clamp
Davidson-Mathieu elevator
Davidson-Mathieu raspatory
Davidson-Mathieu-Alexander
    elevator
Davidson-Mathieu-Alexander
    elevator rasp
Davidson-Sauerbruch elevator
Davidson-Sauerbruch rasp
Davidson-Sauerbruch rib
    raspatory
Davidson-Sauerbruch-Doyen
    elevator
Davidson-Sauerbruch-Doyen
    periosteal elevator
Daviel cataract extraction
Daviel chalazion knife
Daviel knife
Daviel lens loupe
Daviel lens spoon
Daviel loupe
Daviel operation
Daviel scoop
Daviel spoon
Davies-Colley operation
Davis aneurysm clamp
Davis aortic aneurysm clamp
Davis bone skid
Davis Bovie cautery
Davis brain retractor
Davis brain spatula

Davis bronchoscope
Davis capsule forceps
Davis clamp
Davis coagulating forceps
Davis coagulation electrode
Davis conductor
Davis double-ended retractor
Davis electrode
Davis forceps
Davis foreign body spud
Davis graft
Davis hemostat
Davis hip arthrodesis
Davis hook
Davis hysteropexy
Davis implant
Davis knife
Davis knife needle
Davis loop stone dislodger
Davis metacarpal splint
Davis monopolar bayonet
    forceps
Davis mouth gag
Davis needle
Davis needle holder
Davis nerve separator
Davis operation
Davis periosteal elevator
Davis pillar retractor
Davis pin
Davis prosthesis
Davis raspatory
Davis retractor
Davis rib spreader
Davis saw conductor
Davis saw guide
Davis scissors
Davis self-retaining scalp
    retractor
Davis separator
Davis skid
Davis sound
Davis spatula
Davis splint
Davis spud
Davis stone dislodger
Davis thoracic tissue forceps
Davis tonsillar hemostat

Davis tonsillar knife
Davis tonsillar needle
Davis tooth plate
Davis uterine suspension
Davis-Crowe mouth gag
Davis-Geck eye sutures
Davis-Geck incision
Davis-Geck surgical stapler
Davis-Geck sutures
Davis-Kitlowski otoplasty
Davis-Rockey incision
Davol bag
Davol catheter
Davol colon tube
Davol dermatome
Davol drain
Davol forceps
Davol pillows
Davol punch
Davol rongeur
Davol rongeur forceps
Davol rubber catheter
Davol suction drain
Davol suction tube
Davol sump drain
Davol tourniquet
Davol tube
Davol-Simon dermatome
Davy speculum
DAW (dispense as written)
Dawson-Yuhl spinal instru-
    ments
Day attic cannula
Day cannula
Day ear hook
Day hook
Day knife
Day tonsillar knife
db (decibel)
DC plate
DCFAO plate
DCP (dynamic compression
    plate)
DCS (dynamic condylar
    screw)
DCS implant (dorsal column
    stimulator/stimulation
    implant)

DDD (degenerative disk disease)
DDD pacemaker (dual-sensing, -pacing, -mode)
DDI mode pacemaker
De Alvarez forceps
de Andrade-MacNab technique
de Grandmont operation
de la Caffiniere trapeziometacarpal prosthesis
de la Camp sign
de Musset sign
De Paco implant
De Paco prosthesis
de Pezzer (see also *Pezzer*)
de Pezzer catheter
de Pezzer self-retaining catheter
de Quervain (also *Quervain*)
de Quervain fracture
de Quervain incision
de Quervain release
de Quervain tenolysis
de Signeux dilator
de Vincentiis operation
dead bowel
dead space
deafferentation
de-aired graft
Dean antral rasp
Dean antral trocar
Dean applicator
Dean bone rongeur
Dean cotton applicator
Dean curved eye knife
Dean ear snare
Dean forceps
Dean hemostat
Dean iris knife
Dean iris knife needle
Dean knife
Dean MacDonald clamp
Dean MacDonald gastric resection clamp
Dean mastoid rongeur
Dean needle
Dean needle knife
Dean periosteotome
Dean rasp

Dean raspatory
Dean rongeur
Dean scissors
Dean tonsillar forceps
Dean tonsillar hemostat
Dean tonsillar hemostatic forceps
Dean tonsillar knife
Dean tonsillar scissors
Dean trocar
Deane tube
Dean-Senturia needle
Dean-Shallcross tonsil-seizing forceps
Dean-Trusler scissors
Dearor model catheter
dearterialization
Deaver blade
Deaver clamp
Deaver hemostat
Deaver incision
Deaver operating scissors
Deaver retractor
Deaver scissors
Deaver skin incision
Deaver T-drain
Deaver T-tube
DeBakey aortic aneurysm clamp
DeBakey aortic clamp
DeBakey arterial clamp
DeBakey arterial forceps
DeBakey Autraugrip forceps
DeBakey ball-valve prosthesis
DeBakey Beaver blade
DeBakey blade
DeBakey bulldog clamp
DeBakey cardiovascular needle holder
DeBakey chest retractor
DeBakey clamp
DeBakey coarctation clamp
DeBakey cross-action bulldog clamp
DeBakey dissecting forceps
DeBakey endarterectomy scissors
DeBakey forceps

DeBakey graft
DeBakey heart pump oxygena-
tor
DeBakey heart valve
DeBakey implant
DeBakey intraluminal stripper
DeBakey miniature multipur-
pose clamp
DeBakey multipurpose clamp
DeBakey needle
DeBakey needle holder
DeBakey patent ductus clamp
DeBakey pediatric clamp
DeBakey peripheral vascular
clamp
DeBakey prosthesis
DeBakey retractor
DeBakey rib spreader
DeBakey right-angled multipur-
pose clamp
DeBakey ring-handled bulldog
clamp
DeBakey scissors
DeBakey stitch scissors
DeBakey stripper
DeBakey suction tube
DeBakey tangential clamp
DeBakey tangential occlusion
clamp
DeBakey thoracic forceps
DeBakey tissue forceps
DeBakey tucker
DeBakey tunneler
DeBakey valve hook
DeBakey valve prosthesis
DeBakey valve scissors
DeBakey vascular clamp
DeBakey vascular dilator
DeBakey vascular forceps
DeBakey vascular prosthesis
DeBakey vascular scissors
DeBakey vascular tissue forceps
DeBakey Vasculour-II vascular
prosthesis
DeBakey Vital needle holder
DeBakey-Bahnson clamp
DeBakey-Bahnson forceps
DeBakey-Bahnson vascular
clamp

DeBakey-Bainbridge clamp
DeBakey-Bainbridge forceps
DeBakey-Balfour retractor
DeBakey-Beck clamp
DeBakey-Colovira-Rumel
thoracic forceps
DeBakey-Cooley anastomosis
forceps
DeBakey-Cooley cardiovascular
forceps
DeBakey-Cooley dilator
DeBakey-Cooley forceps
DeBakey-Cooley retractor
DeBakey-Cooley-Deaver
retractor
DeBakey-Creech aneurysm
repair
DeBakey-Creech manner
DeBakey-Creech procedure
DeBakey-Derra anastomosis
clamp
DeBakey-Diethrich vascular
forceps
DeBakey-Harken auricle
clamp
DeBakey-Harken clamp
DeBakey-Howard aortic
aneurysmal clamp
DeBakey-Howard clamp
DeBakey-Kay aortic clamp
DeBakey-Kay clamp
DeBakey-Kelly hemostatic
forceps
DeBakey-McQuigg-Mixter
bronchial clamp
DeBakey-Metzenbaum dissect-
ing scissors
DeBakey-Metzenbaum
scissors
DeBakey-Mixter thoracic
forceps
DeBakey-Péan cardiovascular
forceps
DeBakey-Potts scissors
DeBakey-Rankin hemostatic
forceps
DeBakey-Reynolds anastomosis
DeBakey-Reynolds anastomosis
forceps

DeBakey-Rumel thoracic
    forceps
DeBakey-Satinsky vena caval
    clamp
DeBakey-Semb clamp
DeBakey-Semb forceps
DeBakey-Semb ligature-carrier
    clamp
DeBakey-Surgitool prosthetic
    valve
Debeyre rotator cuff operation
Debeyre-Patte-Elmelik tech-
    nique
Deboisans drain
Debove membrane
Debove tube
debride
debrided bone surface
debrided necrotic tissue
debridement
debridement and irrigation
debridement and revision
debridement needle
debridement of bruised tissue
debridement of compound skull
    fracture
debridement of necrotic tissue
debridement of wound
debridement technique
debrider
        corneal debrider
        Nordson debrider
        Sauer debrider
debris
Debrisan
Debrisan dressing
debulking
debulking of tumor
debulking operation
decalcification
decalcify
decamethonium bromide
    anesthetic agent
decamethonium iodide anes-
    thetic agent
decannulation of aorta
decannulation of femoral artery
    and vein

decannulation of vena cava
decannulation of ventricle
decannulation plug
decapitation
decapitation hook
decapitation scissors
decapsulation
decapsulation of kidney
Decasone
decay
decayed teeth
decelerated breathing
deceleration
deceleration injury
deceleration of heart rate
decentered lens
decentration of lenses
decerebrate
decerebrate posturing
decerebrate rigidity
dechondrified
decibel (db)
decidua
decidua basalis
decidua capsularis
decidua menstrualis
decidua parietalis
decidua reflexa
decidua serotina
decidua vera
decidual endometritis
decidual fragment
decidual tissue
deciduous cuspid
deciduous placenta
deciduous teeth
deciduous tissue
deciliter
Decker culdoscope
Decker culdoscopy
Decker microforceps
Decker microrongeur
Decker operation
Decker pituitary rongeur
Decker retractor
Decker scissors
declination angle
declinator

declive
declotting
decompensation
decompression
decompression of abdomen
decompression of heart
decompression of imperforate
    anus
decompression of orbit
decompression of pericardium
decompression of rectum
decompression of spinal cord
decompression operation
decompressive
decompressive colostomy
decompressive craniotomy
decompressive enteroclysis
    catheter
decompressive laminectomy
decompressive retractor
decompressive trocar
decompressive tube
decompressor (see also
    *compressor*)
    Andrews decompressor
    Andrews-Pynchon
        decompressor
    Balmer decompressor
    Beatty decompressor
    Blakesley decompressor
    Bosworth decompressor
    Chamberlain decompres-
        sor
    Colver-Dawson decom-
        pressor
    Coston eye decompres-
        sor
    Dorsey decompressor
    Dunn decompressor
    Farlow decompressor
    Fraser decompressor
    Granberry decompressor
    Hamilton decompressor
    Israel decompressor
    Jobson-Pynchon
        decompressor
    Kellogg decompressor

decompressor *continued*
    Layman decompressor
    Lewis decompressor
    Mullins decompressor
    Pirquet decompressor
    Proetz decompressor
    Pynchon decompressor
    Savage intestinal
        decompressor
    Schepens eye decom-
        pressor
    Sims vaginal decompres-
        sor
    Titus decompressor
    Wieder decompressor
decontamination
decortical position
decorticate posturing
decorticate rigidity
decortication
decortication of heart
decortication of kidney
decortication of lung
DeCourcy clamp
DeCourcy goiter clamp
decreased peristalsis
decrescendo early systolic
    murmur
decrescendo murmur
decrescent arteriosclerosis
Decubi-Care pad dressing
decubital necrosis
decubitus
decubitus cushion
decubitus film
decubitus position
decubitus ulcer
decussation
Deddish-Potts intestinal forceps
Dedo laryngoscope
Dedo machine
Dedo-Jako microlaryngoscope
dedolation
Dedo-Pilling laryngoscope
Dee elbow prosthesis
deep abdominal reflexes
deep abdominal tenderness

deep and regular respirations
deep artery of clitoris
deep artery of penis
deep auricular artery
deep brachial artery
deep brain stimulation
deep cervical artery
deep cervical fascia
deep cervical vein
deep cervical jugulodigastric
    nodes
deep circumflex iliac artery
deep circumflex iliac vein
deep closure
deep coma
deep dissection
deep dorsal vein
deep epigastric vessels
deep external pudendal artery
deep facial vein
deep fascia
deep femoral artery
deep femoral vein
deep flexor muscle
deep inguinal ring
deep interloop abscess
deep keratitis
deep knife
deep layer
deep lingual artery
deep lingual vein
deep middle cerebral artery
deep muscle
deep nerve
deep palmar arch
deep palpation
deep penetrating wound
deep perineal fascia
deep perineal space
deep peroneal nerve
deep petrosal nerve
deep rake retractor
deep retractor
deep spreader blade
deep temporal artery
deep temporal nerve
deep temporal vein

deep tendon reflexes (DTRs)
deep transverse fibers
deep transverse ligament
deep transverse muscle of
    perineum
deep tumor
deep ulceration
deep vein
deep veins of clitoris
deep veins of penis
deep venous thrombosis (DVT)
deep volar arch
deepened incision
deepening reamer
de-epicardialization
de-epithelialized
deeply anesthetized patient
deep-seated lesion
deep-surgery forceps
deep-surgery scissors
Dees holder
Dees needle
Dees operation
Dees suture needle
Dees-Young procedure
defatted
defatted skin graft
defatting of skin
defecation
defecogram
defecography
defect
defect closed with sutures
defective
Defer method
deferent duct
deferentectomy
deferential
deferential artery
deferentialis, arteria
deferred fracture
deferred shock
defervesce
defervescence
defibrillated heart
defibrillating patient
defibrillation

defibrillation and electrical
    cardioversion
defibrillation paddle
defibrillation technique
defibrillator
defibrillator implant
defibrillator paddle
deficiency
deficient
deficit
definite
definite mass
definition
definitive callus
definitive diagnosis
definitive irradiation
definitive surgery
definitive therapy
definitive treatment
deflated tourniquet
deflation
deflected skin flap
deflecting obturator
deflection
defocused beam
deformation
deformed
deformity
Defourmental bone rongeur
Defourmental forceps
Defourmental rongeur
Defourmental rongeur forceps
defunctionalized
degenerated tissue
degenerating decidual tissue
degeneration
degeneration of adrenal gland
degenerative bone changes
degenerative cataract
degenerative change
degenerative disease
degenerative disk disease
    (DDD)
degenerative disorder
degenerative heart disease
degenerative joint disease (DJD)
degenerative spurring

degenerative status
degloving
degloving injury
degloving technique
deglutition
deglutition mechanism
deglutitory cough
deglycerated
Degnon sutures
degree
dehiscence
dehiscence of iris
dehiscence of uterus
dehiscence of wound
dehydrated
dehydration
deionized water
Deiter operation
Deiter terminal frame
DeJager elevator
Dejerine sign
Dejerine-Davis percussion
    hammer
Dejerine-Landouzy dystrophy
Dejerine-Sottas atrophy
dekalon sutures
DeKlair operation
Deklene sutures
Deknatel K-needle
Deknatel needle
Deknatel silk sutures
Deknatel sutures
Deknatel tape
DeKock two-way bronchial
    catheter
Del Toro operation
Delaborde dilator
Delaborde tracheal dilator
DeLaginiere abdominal retractor
Delaney phrenic retractor
Delaney retractor
delayed closure of wound
delayed conduction
delayed emptying
delayed flap
delayed graft
delayed healing

delayed operative cholangiography
delayed primary closure
delayed reaction
delayed reflex
delayed skin flap
delayed skin flap technique
delayed sutures
delayed transfer flap
delayed union
Delbet hip classification
Delbet splint
Delbet splint for heel fracture
Delclos applicator
Delclos dilator
Delclos ovoid
Delclos vaginal cylinder
DeLee catheter
DeLee cervix-holding forceps
DeLee corner retractor
DeLee curet
DeLee dressing forceps
DeLee forceps
DeLee infant catheter
DeLee knife
DeLee maneuver
DeLee obstetrical forceps
DeLee operation
DeLee ovum forceps
DeLee pelvimeter
DeLee retractor
DeLee speculum
DeLee spoon tissue forceps
DeLee suction
DeLee tenaculum
DeLee tracheal catheter
DeLee tracheal trap
DeLee trap aspirator
DeLee trap meconium aspirator
DeLee tube
DeLee Universal retractor
DeLee uterine forceps
DeLee uterine packing forceps
DeLee vaginal retractor
DeLee vesical retractor
DeLee-Breisky pelvimeter

DeLee-Hillis obstetrical head stethoscope
DeLee-Hillis obstetrical stethoscope
DeLee-Hillis stethoscope
DeLee-Perce perforator
DeLee-Simpson forceps
DeLee-Zweifel cranioclast
Delgado electrode
delicate balance
delicate scissors
delicate skin hook
delicate structure
delimiting keratotomy
delineate
Delitala T-nail
Delitala T-pins
delivered
delivery
Dellon generator
Delmege sign
Delore method
Delorme operation
Delorme rectal prolapse operation
Delorme-Fowler operation
Delphian lymph node
Delphian node
Delrin frame of valve prosthesis
Delrin heart valve
delta activity
Delta pacemaker
delta phalanx
Delta-FormCast reinforcing resin
Delta-lite casting tape
Delta-lite S-casting tape
Delta-Net stockinette
deltoid fascia
deltoid ligament
deltoid muscle
deltoid region
deltoid-splitting approach
deltoideus, musculus
deltopectoral groove
deltopectoral incision
demand pacemaker
demarcated border

demarcated lesion
demarcated margin
demarcation
Demarest forceps
Demarest septal forceps
Demarquay sign
DeMartel appendix forceps
DeMartel clamp
DeMartel forceps
DeMartel neurosurgical scissors
DeMartel retractor
DeMartel scalp forceps
DeMartel scissors
DeMartel sutures
DeMartel vascular clamp
DeMartel vascular scissors
DeMartel-Wolfson anastomotic
    clamp
DeMartel-Wolfson clamp
DeMartel-Wolfson colon clamp
DeMartel-Wolfson forceps
DeMartel-Wolfson intestinal
    anastomotic clamp
DeMartel-Wolfson intestinal
    clamp
Demel forceps
Demel wire-tightening forceps
Demel wire-twisting forceps
Demel-Ruttin operation
Demerol anesthetic agent
demifacet
demigauntlet
demigauntlet bandage
demigauntlet dressing
demineralization
demineralization of bone
demineralized bone matrix
demineralized bony structure
Deming nephropexy
Demling-Classen
    sphincterotome
Demme method
demonstrable evidence
Demos tibial arterial clamp
demucosation
demyelinate
demyelinating

demyelinating disease
demyelination
demyelinization
Denans operation
Dench atomizer
Dench ear
Dench ear curet
Dench forceps
Dench insufflator
Dench knife
Dench nebulizer
Dench rongeur
Dench uterine curet
Dench vaporizer
dendrite
dendrites and axons
dendritic calculus
dendritic lesion
dendritic ulcer
Denecke headlight
denervate
denervated bladder
denervated heart
denervated muscle atrophy
denervation
Denham pin
Denham skeletal fixation
Denhardt mouth gag
Denhardt-Dingman mouth gag
Denholtz appliance
Denis Browne adult retractor
    set
Denis Browne bucket
Denis Browne forceps
Denis Browne needle
Denis Browne operation
Denis Browne pediatric
    retractor set
Denis Browne procedure
Denis Browne ring retractor
Denis Browne splint
Denis Browne talipes hobble
    splint
Denis Browne tray
Denis Browne Universal
    retractor set
Denker operation

Denker trocar
Denker tube
Denman spontaneous version
Dennie lines
Dennie-Morgan infraorbital
  folds
Dennis anastomosis
Dennis anastomotic clamp
Dennis clamp
Dennis forceps
Dennis intestinal forceps
Dennis intestinal tube
Dennis operation
Dennis tube
Dennis-Brooke ileostomy
Dennis-Brown abdominal
  retractor
Dennis-Brown pouch
Denniston dilator
Dennis-Varco pancreaticoduo-
  denostomy
Dennyson-Fulford arthrodesis
Denonvilliers aponeurosis
Denonvilliers blepharoplasty
Denonvilliers fascia
Denonvilliers operation
Denonvilliers space
Dens view of cervical spine
dense
dense adhesions
dense bony structure
densitometry
density
Dent sleeve
dental alveoli
dental amalgam
dental anatomy
dental anesthesia
dental appliance
dental arch
dental arch bar
dental arch bar frame
dental artery
dental bridge
dental bur
dental caries
dental cavity

dental crown
dental debridement
dental disease
dental drill
dental elevator
dental excavator
dental exostosis
dental extraction
dental fistula
dental flange
dental forceps
dental handpiece
dental impaction
dental implant
dental impression
dental knife
dental mold
dental nerve
dental operculum
dental plaque
dental plate
dental pliers
dental procedure
dental prosthesis
dental pulp
dental repair
dental restorative surgery
dental retractor
dental shelf
dental splint
dental syringe
dental tool
dental tophus
dentate fascia
dentate fissure
dentate fracture
dentate gyrus
dentate ligament
dentate line
dentate nucleus
dentate sutures
denticular hymen
denticulate ligament
dentinocemental junction
dentinogenesis imperfecta
dentinoma
dentitio difficilis

dentition
dentitional odontectomy
dentoalveolar abscess
dentofacial surgery
dentosurgical
dentulous
denture adhesive
denture brush
denture impression
denture splint
dentures
denudation
denudation of cornea
denude
denuded
Denuse operation
Denver hydrocephalus shunt
Denver nasal splint
Denver peritoneal-venous
    shunt
Denver splint
Denver-Krupin valve
deorsumduction of eye
deossification
deoxygenated blood
Depage position
Depage-Janeway gastrostomy
DePalma hip prosthesis
DePalma knife
Depaul tube
dependency
dependency skin lines
dependent
dependent drainage
depilation
depilatory dermal forceps
depolarizing electrode
deposit
deposition
depot intramuscular injection
depressed
depressed chest wall
depressed fracture
depressed skull fracture
depressed systolic pressure

depression
depressor (see also *tongue
    depressor*)
    Andrews tongue
        depressor
    Andrews-Pynchon
        tongue depressor
    Balmer depressor
    Blakesley tongue
        depressor
    brain depressor
    Braun depressor
    Cushing brain depressor
    Dorsey tongue depressor
    Dunn tongue depressor
    Farlow tongue depressor
    Fraser depressor
    Hamilton tongue
        depressor
    Israel depressor
    Lewis tongue depressor
    O'Connor depressor
    oral screw tongue
        depressor
    Proetz tongue depressor
    Pynchon tongue
        depressor
    Pynchon-Lillie tongue
        depressor
    Schepens depressor
    Schocket depressor
    scleral depressor
    Titus tongue depressor
    tongue depressor
    Weder tongue depressor
    Wilder scleral depressor
depressor anguli oris, musculus
depressor labii inferioris,
    musculus
depressor muscle
depressor nerve
depressor reflex
depressor septi nasi, musculus
depressor supercilii, musculus
deprivation

depth electrode
depth gauge
Depthalon monitoring electrode
depth-gain compensation
DePuy arthroplasty
DePuy awl
DePuy bolt
DePuy bone curet
DePuy bone mill
DePuy curet
DePuy drill
Depuy dual-lock hip prosthesis
DePuy extractor
DePuy fracture brace
DePuy fracture frame
DePuy fracture-reducing frame
DePuy head halter
DePuy nail
DePuy nerve hook
DePuy open-thimble splint
DePuy orthopedic implant
DePuy pin
DePuy plate
DePuy Porocoat hemiarthro-
    plasty
DePuy prosthesis
DePuy reamer
DePuy retractor
DePuy rocking-leg splint
DePuy rongeur
DePuy screwdriver
DePuy splint
DePuy-Potts splint
derangement of joint
derangement of knee
derangement of vasomotor
    nerves
Derby operation
Derch vaporizer
Dercum disease
Derf ear knife
Derf forceps
Derf holder
Derf needle holder
Derf Vital needle holder
derivation

derivative circulation
Derlacki capsule knife
Derlacki chisel
Derlacki curet
Derlacki ear curet
Derlacki elevator
Derlacki gouge
Derlacki knife
Derlacki mobilizer
Derlacki operation
Derlacki ossicle holder
Derlacki punch
Derlacki-Hough mobilizer
Derlacki-Juers head holder
Derlacki-Shambaugh chisel
Derlacki-Shambaugh micro-
    scope
Derma Care dressing
Dermablend
dermabrader (see also *abrader*)
    diamond dermabrader
    Iverson dermabrader
    lid dermabrader
    sandpaper dermabrader
    Stryker dermabrader
dermabrasion
dermacarrier
Dermaclip
dermagraft
dermal bone
dermal curet
dermal cyst
dermal elevator
dermal graft
dermal instrument
dermal pedicle
dermal punch
dermal sinus
dermal sutures
dermal tension nonabsorbing
    sutures
dermal tissue
Dermalene sutures
Dermalon cuticular sutures
Dermalon sutures
Dermamesh graft expander

Dermascrub
Dermatape
Dermatex compound
dermatoautoplasty
dermatofibrosarcoma protuber-
    ans
dermatoheteroplasty
dermatome
    air dermatome
    Bard-Parker dermatome
    Brown dermatome
    Brown electrodermatome
    Brown-Blair dermatome
    Castroviejo dermatome
    Concept dermatome
    cordless dermatome
    Davol dermatome
    Davol-Simon dermatome
    DeSilva dermatome
    Down hand dermatome
    Duval dermatome
    Duval disposable
        dermatome
    electric dermatome
    electrodermatome
    Hall dermatome
    Hood dermatome
    manual dermatome
    Meek-Wall dermatome
    Meek-Wall microder-
        matome
    microdermatome
    Padgett dermatome
    Padgett-Hood der-
        matome
    Padgett-Hood electroder-
        matome
    Pitkin dermatome
    Reese dermatome
    Simon dermatome
    single-use dermatome
    Stryker dermatome
    Stryker Rolo-dermatome
    Tanner-Vandeput mesh
        dermatome
    Weck dermatome
dermatomic

dermatoplastic
dermatoplasty
Dermex wrap
dermic graft
Dermicel dressing
Dermicel tape
Dermiclear tape
Dermilite tape
dermis
dermodesis
dermoepidermal junction
dermoid cancer
dermoid cyst
dermoid tumor
Dermo-Jet injector
Dermoplast spray
dermoplasty
Dermostat implant
Dermostat orbital implant
Dermot-Pierse ball-tipped knife
DeRoaldes nasal speculum
derotation brace
derotation osteotomy
Derra aortic clamp
Derra cardiac valve dilator
Derra clamp
Derra commissurotomy knife
Derra dilator
Derra forceps
Derra guillotine
Derra knife
Derra urethral forceps
Derra valve dilator
Derra valvulotome
Derra vena cava clamp
Derra vestibular clamp
D'Errico bur
D'Errico chisel
D'Errico dressing forceps
D'Errico drill
D'Errico enlarging bur
D'Errico forceps
D'Errico hypophyseal forceps
D'Errico knife
D'Errico laminectomy chisel
D'Errico nerve elevator
D'Errico nerve retractor

D'Errico perforating bur
D'Errico perforating drill
D'Errico perforator
D'Errico periosteal elevator
D'Errico retractor
D'Errico skull trephine
D'Errico spatula
D'Errico tissue forceps
D'Errico trephine
D'Errico-Adson retractor
Desault apparatus
Desault bandage
Desault dislocation
Desault dressing
Desault fracture
Desault hip sign
Desault ligation
Desault sign
Desault wrist dislocation
Descemet membrane
Descemet operation
descemetocele
descended diaphragm
descended testicle
descending aorta
descending brain stem
descending colon
descending duodenum
descending genicular artery
descending loop colostomy
descending palatine artery
descending thoracic aorta to
    pulmonary artery shunt
descending urogram
descending urography
descensus
descensus uteri
descensus ventriculi
Deschamps carrier
Deschamps compressor
Deschamps ligature carrier
Deschamps ligature needle
Deschamps needle
Deschamps-Navratil ligature
    needle
Deschamps-Navratil needle
desensitization

desensitize
Deseret angiocatheter
Deseret catheter
Deseret sump drain
desiccate
desiccated lesion
desiccated thyroid
desiccation
desiccation needle
desiccation-fulguration needle
designated donor
designated recipient
Desilets catheter
Desilets-Hoffman catheter
    introducer
Desilets-Hoffman introducer
Desilets-Hoffman micropunc-
    ture introducer
Desilets-Hoffman pacemaker
    introducer
DeSilva dermatome
Desjardins forceps
Desjardins gall duct scoop
Desjardins gallbladder scoop
Desjardins gallstone forceps
Desjardins gallstone probe
Desjardins gallstone scoop
Desjardins point
Desjardins probe
Desjardins scoop
Desmarres chalazion forceps
Desmarres clamp
Desmarres corneal dissector
Desmarres dissector
Desmarres elevator
Desmarres eye dissector
Desmarres forceps
Desmarres knife
Desmarres lid clamp
Desmarres lid elevator
Desmarres lid forceps
Desmarres lid retractor
Desmarres needle
Desmarres operation
Desmarres paracentesis knife
Desmarres paracentesis needle
Desmarres retractor

Desmarres scarifier
desmoid
desmoid lesion
desmology
desmotomy
desquamated cells
desquamating debris
desquamation
desquamative gingivitis
desquamative nephritis
desquamative pneumonia
destruction of lesion
destruction of lesion by
    cauterization
destruction of lesion by
    curettage
destruction of lesion by
    fulguration
destructive injury
destructive process
desultory labor
desultory pain
detached loose body
detached retina
detachment
detachment of ligament
detachment of retina
DeTakats-McKenzie brain clip-
    applying forceps
DeTakats-McKenzie clip-
    applying forceps
DeTakats-McKenzie forceps
detector
Detergicide
Detergiclene
deteriorated condition
deteriorating neurological
    disorder
deteriorating patient
deterioration
determinant
detorsed
detorsion
detrusor function
detrusor pattern
detrusor response
detrusor sphincter dyssynergia

detrusor urinae
detubation
Deucher abdominal retractor
deutan axis
Deutschman cataract knife
Deutschman knife
devascularization
devascularize
DeVega annuloplasty
DeVega prosthesis
DeVega tricuspid valve
    annuloplasty
developed flap
developmental cataract
Deventer diameter
Deventer pelvis
deviated nasal septum
deviation
device (see also *intrauterine
    device*)
    abdominal aortic
        counterpulsation
        device
    abdominal left ventricu-
        lar assist device
    Abiomed BVAD 5000
        (biventricular assist
        device)
    ACMI ulcer-measuring
        device
    Agee 4-pin fixation
        device
    AICD device
    ALVAD (abdominal left
        ventricular assist
        device)
    anti-siphon device
    application of traction
        device
    Aqua-Purator suction
        device
    Arrow-Clarke thoracen-
        tesis device
    atherectomy device
    automatic stapling device
    automatic suction device
    Berman locator device

device *continued*

biventricular assist device (BVAD)
blade plate fixation device
Bovie suction device
Buretrol device
BVAD (biventricular assist device)
Calandruccio compression device
CARD (cardiac automatic resuscitative device)
cardiac automatic resuscitative device (CARD)
Cardiomemo device
cassette cup collecting device
CastAlert device
celltrifuge device
Chinese fingerstraps traction device
circular stapling device
compression device
conductive device
continuous passive motion device
CPM device
Cricket stapling device
Cu-7 intrauterine device
cutting device
CVIS imaging device
Dinamap automated blood pressure device
Doppler device
Doppler sound device
double-headed P190 stapling device
EEA stapling device
EID (emergency infusion device)
emergency infusion device (EID)
Erlangen magnetic colostomy device
exterior pelvic device

device *continued*

external vascular compression device
Finn chamber patch test device
fixation device
Fox internal fixation device
G-suit device
GIA stapling device
Grass pressure-recording device
Hare splint device
Hare traction device
Hershey left ventricular assist device
Hoffmann external fixation device
Hoffmann traction device
Hollister circumcision device
HUI device for tubal lavage
HUMI device for tubal lavage
ILA stapling device
IMED infusion device
infusion device
input device
insertion of fixation device
insertion of traction device
Inspiron device
insufflation device
internal fixating device
internal fixation device
intra-aortic balloon assist device
intramedullary device
intramedullary fixation device
intrauterine contraceptive device (IUCD)
intrauterine device (IUD)
IUD (intrauterine device)

Dubin

device *continued*

KED (Kendrick extrication device)

Kendrick extrication device (KED)

Kennedy ligament augmentation device (LAD)

kinetic continuous passive motion device

kinetic CPM device

LAD (ligament augmentation device)

left ventricular assist device (LVAD)

leg-holding device

Lewis intramedullary device

Lewis suspension device

ligament augmentation device (LAD)

linear stapling device

Loewi suspension device

LVAD (left ventricular assist device)

manipulation of prosthetic device

McAtee compression screw device

McAtee olecranon device

mechanical device

MediPort implanted vascular device

metallic fixation device

Mouradian humeral fixation device system

Multiclip disposable ligating clip device

Nimbus Hemopump cardiac assist device

Novacor left ventricular assist device

Orthofix external fixation device

Ortholav irrigation and suction device

orthotic device

device *continued*

output device

ParaGard intrauterine device

Pierce-Donachy ventricular assist device

Pisces device

Plastizote orthotic device

PPT orthotic device

Progestasert intrauterine device

prosthetic device

pulsatile assist device

Response external suction device for impotence

retaining device

Richards compression device

Richards external fixation device for fractures

right ventricular assist device

Roger Anderson external skeletal fixation device

rotational atherectomy device

Sanders jet ventilation device respirator

Sengstaken-Blakemore device

SGIA stapling device

Shug device for male contraception

Simpson PET balloon atherectomy device

SMI Surgi-Med CPM devices

Soluset device

Sorbothane orthotic device

Spenco orthotic device

Spetzler MacroVac surgical suction device

Spitz-Holter flushing device

stapling device

device *continued*
   stereotaxic device
   stone locking device
   suction device
   Symbion pneumatic
     assist device
   Tenderfoot incision-
     making device
   Tessier disimpaction
     device forceps
   Thoratec biventricular
     assist device
   Thoratec right ventricular
     assist device
   Thoratec ventricular
     assist device
   Travenol infusor device
   Ultroid device for
     hemorrhoid treatment
   Universal joint device
   vacuum tumescence-
     constrictor device
   VAD (ventricular assist
     device; vascular/
     venous access device)
   VED (vacuum erection
     device)
   Venodyne pneumatic
     inflation device
   ventricular assist device
   Vidal device
   Vidal-Ardrey modified
     Hoffman device
   Wagner leg-lengthening
     device
   Wallach freezer cryosur-
     gical device
   Wallach pencil cryosurgi-
     cal device
   Wallach surgical device
   Wizard disposable
     inflation device
   Wolvek fixation device
   Wright Care-TENS device
   Zilkie device
Devices, Ltd., pacemaker
DeVilbiss air compressor

DeVilbiss atomizer
DeVilbiss bottle
DeVilbiss compressor
DeVilbiss cranial forceps
DeVilbiss cranial rongeur
DeVilbiss cranial trephine
DeVilbiss cutoffs
DeVilbiss eye irrigator
DeVilbiss forceps
DeVilbiss irrigating syringe
DeVilbiss irrigator
DeVilbiss nebulizer
DeVilbiss powder blower
DeVilbiss rack
DeVilbiss rongeur
DeVilbiss rongeur forceps
DeVilbiss skull trephine
DeVilbiss speculum
DeVilbiss spirometer
DeVilbiss suction tube
DeVilbiss trephine
DeVilbiss Vacu-Aide aspirator
DeVilbiss vaginal speculum
DeVilbiss vaporizer
DeVilbiss-Stacey speculum
Devine colostomy
Devine hypospadias repair
Devine operation
Devine pyloroplasty
Devine tube
Devine-Millard-Aufricht retractor
Devine-Millard-Frazier suction
   tube
devisceration
devitalization
devitalize
devitalized tissue
Devonshire catheter
Devonshire knife
Devonshire needle
Devonshire operation for talipes
   valgus
Devonshire roller
Dewald halo spinal appliance
DeWall bubbler-type pump
Dewar elevator
Dewar flask

Dewar procedure
Dewar-Barrington procedure
Dewar-Harris operation
dewebbing
DeWecker anterior sclerotomy
DeWecker cannula
DeWecker eye implant
DeWecker eye scissors
DeWecker forceps
DeWecker iridectomy scissors
DeWecker iris scissors
DeWecker iris spatula
DeWecker operation
DeWecker scissors
DeWecker sclerotomy
DeWecker syringe cannula
DeWecker-Pritikin scissors
DeWeerd ureteropelvioplasty
DeWeese axis traction forceps
DeWeese caval catheter
DeWeese clamp
DeWeese vena cava clamp
DeWeese-Hunter clip
Dewey forceps
Dewey obstetrical forceps
Dexon
Dexon mesh
Dexon Plus sutures
Dexon subcuticular sutures
Dexon sutures
Dextra surgical table
dextran
dextranomer
dextrocardia
dextroduction of eye
dextroposition
dextropositioned aorta
dextrorotatory
dextrorotatory scoliosis
dextrorotoscoliosis
dextroscoliotic curvature
dextroversion
Deyerle apparatus
Deyerle drill
Deyerle hip fracture reduction
Deyerle nail
Deyerle pin
Deyerle plate

Deyerle procedure
Deyerle punch
Deyerle screw
DG Softgut sutures
Dia pump
Dia pump aspirator
Dia suction
diabetes mellitus
diabetic cataract
diabetic puncture
Diabeticorum dressing
diaclasis
diaclastic amputation
diacondylar fracture
Diacyte fine-needle aspiration
    biopsy system
diafiltrate
diafiltration
Diaflex dilator
Diaflex nephrostomy
Diaflex ureteral dilatation
    catheter
diagnostic catheter
diagnostic curet
diagnostic curettage
diagnostic D&C
diagnostic dilatation and
    curettage
diagnostic ear tube
diagnostic laparoscopy
Diagnostic Medical Instruments
    (DMI)
diagnostic mirror
diagnostic otoscope
diagnostic procedure
diagnostic set
diagnostic spinal tap
diagnostic study
diagnostic surgery
diagnostic therapy
diagnostic tube
diagnostic ultrasound
diagnostic x-ray
dial lock
dial osteotomy
dial-type ophthalmodyna-
    mometer
Dialyflex dialysis fluid

dialysate bag
dialysis
dialysis catheter
dialysis fluid
dialysis procedure
dialysis shunt
dialysis therapy
dialysis unit
dialysis-related ascites
dialyzation unit
dialyzed patient
dialyzer
diamagnetic
diameter
diamond bur
diamond dermabrader
diamond disk
diamond drill
diamond fraise
diamond green marker
diamond inlay bone graft
diamond knife
diamond nail
diamond nasal rasp
diamond needle holder
diamond rasp
Diamond tube
diamond-dust bur
diamond-dusted tip
diamond-edge scissors
Diamond-Gould technique
diamond-pin cutter
diamond-point suture needle
diamond-shaped murmur
Diamox (acetazolamide)
Dianoux trichiasis operation
diaphanography
diaphanoscope
diaphanoscopy
diaphanous
diaphragm
diaphragm pacing system
diaphragm pessary
diaphragm stethoscope
diaphragma
diaphragmatic
diaphragmatic artery
diaphragmatic excursions

diaphragmatic hernia
diaphragmatic hernia repair
diaphragmatic herniorrhaphy
diaphragmatic hiatus
diaphragmatic injury
diaphragmatic muscle
diaphragmatic nerve
diaphragmatic pleura
diaphragmatic pulmonary
    infarct
diaphragmatic silhouette
diaphragmatic surface of heart
diaphragmatocele
diaphyseal
diaphyseal-epiphyseal fusion
diaphysectomy
diaphysis
diarthrodial joint
diascopic examination
diascopy
Dias-Gingerich technique
Diasonics transducer
diastalsis
diastasis
diastasis cordis
diastasis of cranial bone
diastasis of muscle
diastasis recti
diastasis recti abdominis
diastatic fracture
diastatic skull fracture
diastole
diastolic blood pressure
diastolic murmur
diastolic pressure
diastolic rumble
DiaTAP vascular access button
    for dialysis patients
diathermia knife
diathermic electrode
diathermic eye electrode
diathermic forceps
diathermic loop
diathermic loop biopsy
diathermic needle
diathermic retinal electrode
diathermic scissors
diathermy

diathermy and massage
diathesis
diatrizoate meglumine
diazepam
DIB (duodenoileal bypass)
Dibbell cleft lip-nasal revision
dibucaine hydrochloride
    anesthetic agent
DIC (diffuse intravascular
    coagulopathy)
DIC (disseminated intravascular
    coagulation)
diced cartilage graft
dichorionic placenta
dichromography
Dick cardiac valve dilator
Dick combination container
Dick dilator
Dick operation
Dick treatment stand
Dick valve dilator
Dickerson intraocular implant
    lens
Dickerson lens
Dickey operation
Dickey ptosis repair
Dickey-Fox operation
Dickson operation
Dickson osteotomy
Dickson shelf operation
Dickson technique
Dickson-Diveley operation
Dickson-Willien technique
Dickson-Wright orbit decom-
    pression
dicrotic notch
dicrotic pulse
didactylism
didelphic uterus
Diederich empyema trocar
Dieffenbach amputation
Dieffenbach clamp
Dieffenbach forceps
Dieffenbach knife
Dieffenbach operation
Dieffenbach otoplasty
Dieffenbach plastic closure
Dieffenbach serrefine

Dieffenbach-Duplay operatio
Dieffenbach-Szymanowski-
    Kuhnt operation
Dieffenbach-Warren operatio
Dieffenbach-Webster operati
Diener forceps
dieresis
Diertz shears
Dieter forceps
Dieter nipper
Dieter-House nipper
Diethrich apparatus
Diethrich clamp
Diethrich coronary artery set
Diethrich coronary scissors
Diethrich right-angled
    hemostatic forceps
Diethrich scissors
Diethrich shunt clamp
Diethrich valve scissors
diethyl oxide anesthetic agen
Dieulafoy aspirator
Dieulafoy erosion
Dieulafoy triad
Dieulafoy ulcer
differential
differential diagnosis
differential spinal anesthesia
differentiated
differentiated carcinoma
differentiation
difficult vaginal delivery
diffraction pattern
diffuse
diffuse atrophy
diffuse condition
diffuse enlargement
diffuse idiopathic sclerosing
    hyperostosis (DISH)
diffuse swelling
digastric fossa
digastric muscle
digastric nerve
digastric triangle
digastricus, musculus
digestive tract
digestive tube
Digiflex cannula

Digilab pneumatonographer
Digilab pneumatonometer
Digit Span
digital
digital artery
digital biometric rule
digital block
digital block anesthesia
digital compression
digital examination
digital image score
digital nerve
digital nerve block
digital readout
digital runoff
digital subtraction angiogram
digital subtraction angiography
    (DSA)
digital subtraction supra-
    valvular aortogram
digital tonometry
digital vein
digital venous arch
digitalate pulse
digitales dorsales hallucis
    lateralis et digiti secundi
    medialis, nervi
digitales dorsales manus,
    arteriae
digitales dorsales nervi radialis,
    nervi
digitales dorsales nervi ulnaris,
    nervi
digitales dorsales pedis, arteriae
digitales dorsales pedis, nervi
digitales dorsales pedis, venae
digitales palmares communes,
    arteriae
digitales palmares communes
    nervi mediani, nervi
digitales palmares communes
    nervi ulnaris, nervi
digitales palmares propriae,
    arteriae
digitales palmares proprii nervi
    mediani, nervi
digitales palmares proprii nervi
    ulnaris, nervi

digitales palmares, venae
digitales plantares communes,
    arteriae
digitales plantares communes
    nervi plantaris lateralis,
    nervi
digitales plantares communes
    nervi plantaris medialis,
    nervi
digitales plantares propriae,
    arteriae
digitales plantares proprii nervi
    plantaris lateralis, nervi
digitales plantares proprii nervi
    plantaris medialis, nervi
digitales plantares, venae
digitalis
digitalization of heart
digitalize
digital-to-analog converter
Digitate microsurgical instru-
    ment
digitation
digitized subtraction angiogra-
    phy
digitoxin
Dilamezinsert dilator
Dilamezinsert penile prosthesis
Dilantin
Dilaprobe
Dilaprobe dilator
dilatable bougie
dilatation
dilatation and aspiration
    (D&A)
dilatation and curettage
    (D&C)
dilatation balloon catheter
dilatation of cervix
dilatation of colon
dilatation of common bile duct
dilatation of esophagus
dilatation of organ
dilatation of urethra
dilate
dilated gallbladder
dilated organ
dilated pupil

dilated stricture
dilated vessel
dilating bougie
dilating catheter
dilating forceps
dilating pressure balloon
   catheter
dilating probe
dilation
dilation and curettage (D&C)
dilation and evacuation (D&E)
dilation catheter
dilation instrument
dilation of cervix
dilation with metal sound
dilator
   Ambler dilator
   American Dilation
     System dilator
   American endoscopy
     dilator
   American endoscopy
     esophageal dilator
   Amplatz dilator
   anal dilator
   aortic dilator
   Arnott dilator
   Atlee dilator
   Atlee uterine dilator
   Backhaus dilator
   Bailey dilator
   Bakes bile duct dilator
   Bakes common duct
     dilator
   Bakes dilator
   Bakes-Pearce dilator
   Bard dilator
   Bard urethral dilator
   Barnes dilator
   Beardsley aortic dilator
   Beardsley dilator
   Béniqué dilator
   Bennett common duct
     dilator
   Berens dilator
   Berens punctum dilator
   biliary duct dilator

dilator *continued*
   Black-Wylie dilator
   Black-Wylie obstetric
     dilator
   bladder dilator
   Bonney cervical dilator
   Bossi dilator
   Bowman dilator
   Bowman lacrimal dilator
   Bozeman dilator
   Braasch ureteral dilator
   Bransford-Lewis dilator
   Brock cardiac dilator
   Brock cardiac dilator
     rongeur
   Brock dilator
   bronchial dilator
   bronchodilator
   Brown-Buerger dilator
   Brown-McHardy air-filled
     pneumatic dilator
   Brown-McHardy dilator
   Brown-McHardy
     pneumatic dilator
   Broyles dilator
   Broyles esophageal
     dilator
   canaliculus dilator
   cardiac dilator
   cardiac valve dilator
   cardiodilator
   cardiospasm dilator
   Castroviejo dilator
   Castroviejo double-end
     dilator
   Castroviejo lacrimal
     dilator
   catheter-dilator
   Celestin dilator bougie
   Celestin graduated
     dilator
   cervical dilator
   Clark common duct
     dilator
   Clark dilator
   Clerf dilator
   common bile duct dilator

dilator *continued*
    common duct dilator
    Cook-Amplatz dilator
    Cooley coronary dilator
    Cooley dilator
    Cooley pediatric dilator
    Cooley valve dilator
    coronary dilator
    coronary vasodilator
    Councill dilator
    Creevy dilator
    Crump dilator
    Crump vessel dilator
    Crump-Himmelstein dilator
    de Signeux dilator
    DeBakey vascular dilator
    DeBakey-Cooley dilator
    Delaborde dilator
    Delaborde tracheal dilator
    Delclos dilator
    Denniston dilator
    Derra cardiac valve dilator
    Derra dilator
    Derra valve dilator
    Diaflex dilator
    Dick cardiac valve dilator
    Dick dilator
    Dick valve dilator
    Dilamezinsert dilator
    Dilaprobe dilator
    Dotter dilator
    Dourmashkin dilator
    Eder-Puestow dilator
    Einhorn dilator
    Einhorn esophageal dilator
    esophageal dilator
    esophagospasm dilator
    expansile dilator
    Falope-ring dilator
    Feldbausch dilator
    female catheter-dilator
    Fenton dilator
    Ferris biliary duct dilator

dilator *continued*
    Ferris dilator
    Ferris filiform dilator
    French dilator
    French-McRea dilator
    Frommer dilator
    frontal sinus dilator
    Galezowski dilator
    Galezowski lacrimal dilator
    gall duct dilator
    Garrett dilator
    Garrett vascular dilator
    Gerbode dilator
    Gerbode mitral dilator
    Gerbode mitral valvulotomy dilator
    Gerbode valve dilator
    Glover dilator
    Godelo dilator
    Gohrbrand cardiac dilator
    Gohrbrand dilator
    Goodell dilator
    Goodell uterine dilator
    Gouley dilator
    grooved director dilator
    Gruentzig balloon dilator
    Guyon dilator
    Hank uterine dilator
    Hank-Bradley uterine dilator
    Hayman dilator
    Hearst dilator
    Heath dilator
    Heath punctum dilator
    Hegar dilator
    Hegar rectal dilator
    Hegar uterine dilator
    Hegar-Goodell dilator
    Heinkel-Semm dilator instruments
    Henley dilator
    Henning dilator
    Hertel rigid dilator stone forceps
    Hiebert vascular dilator

dilator *continued*
Hohn vessel dilator
Hopkins dilator
Hosford dilator
Hosford eye dilator
Hosford lacrimal dilator
Hurst bullet-tip dilator
Hurst dilator
Hurst esophageal dilator
Hurst esophagus dilator
Hurst mercury dilator
Hurst mercury-filled dilator
Hurst-Maloney dilator
Hurst-Tucker pneumatic dilator
Hurtig dilator
hydrostatic dilator
Iglesias dilator
infant dilator
Ivinsco cervical dilator
Jackson dilator
Jackson-Mosher dilator
Jackson-Plummer dilator
Jackson-Trousseau dilator
Johnston dilator
Jolly dilator
Jolly uterine dilator
Jones canaliculus dilator
Jones dilator
Jones lacrimal canaliculus dilator
Jordan dilator
Jordan wire loop dilator
K-Pratt dilator
Kahn dilator
Kahn uterine dilator
Kearns bladder dilator
Kearns dilator
Kelly dilator
Kelly orifice dilator
Kelly uterine dilator
Kleegman dilator
Kohlman dilator
Kohlman urethral dilator
Kron bile duct dilator

dilator *continued*
Kron dilator
Kron gall duct dilator
Laborde dilator
Laborde tracheal dilator
lacrimal dilator
laminaria seaweed obstetrical dilator
Landau dilator
laryngeal dilator
Laufe cervical dilator
Leader-Kohlman dilator
LeFort dilator
Lucchese mitral valve dilator
Mahoney dilator
Maloney dilator
Maloney esophageal dilator
Maloney mercury-filled dilator
Maloney mercury-filled esophageal dilator
Maloney tapered-tip dilator
mandrin dilator
Mantz dilator
Mantz rectal dilator
Marax bronchodilator
McCrae dilator
meatal dilator
mercury-filled dilator
mercury-weighted dilator
Miller dilator
mitral dilator
mitral valve dilator
Mixter dilator
Moersch cardiospasm dilator
Mosher cardiospasm dilator
Muldoon dilator
Muldoon lacrimal dilator
Murphy common duct dilator
Murphy dilator
myocardial dilator

dilator *continued*

nasal dilator
Nettleship dilator
Nettleship-Wilder dilator
Nettleship-Wilder
  lacrimal dilator
olivary dilator
olive dilator
Otis bougie à boule
  dilator
Ottenheimer common
  duct dilator
Ottenheimer dilator
Outerbridge uterine
  dilator
Palmer dilator
Palmer uterine dilator
Parsonnet dilator
Patton dilator
Phillips dilator
Plummer dilator
Plummer esophageal
  dilator
Plummer water-filled
  pneumatic esophageal
  dilator
Plummer-Vinson dilator
pneumatic balloon
  dilator
pneumatic dilator
Potts dilator
Potts expansile dilator
Potts-Riker dilator
Pratt dilator
Pratt rectal dilator
Pratt uterine dilator
probe dilator
Puestow dilator
punctum dilator
pyloric stenosis dilator
pylorodilator
Ramstedt dilator
Ramstedt pyloric stenosis
  dilator
Ravich dilator
Ravich ureteral dilator
rectal dilator

dilator *continued*

Reich-Nechtow dilator
Richards-Moeller pneu-
  matic air-filled dilator
Rider-Moeller pneumatic
  dilator
Rigiflex balloon dilator
Rigiflex dilator
Ritter dilator
Ritter meatal dilator
Roland dilator
Rolf dilator
Rolf punctum dilator
Royal Hospital dilator
Russell dilator
Savary dilator
Savary esophageal dilator
Savary tapered thermo-
  plastic dilator
Savary-Gilliard dilator
Savary-Gilliard esophag-
  eal dilator
sheath-dilator
Simpson lacrimal dilator
Simpson uterine dilator
Sims dilator
Sims uterine dilator
Sinexon dilator
sinus dilator
Sippy dilator
Sippy esophageal dilator
Smedberg dilator
sphincter dilator
Spielberg dilator
stapes dilator
Starck cardiodilator
Starck dilator
Starlinger dilator
Starlinger uterine dilator
Steele bronchial dilator
Steele dilator
Stille uterine dilator
Stucker bile duct dilator
Theobald lacrimal dilator
through-the-scope dilator
  (TTS)
tracheal dilator

dilator *continued*

    transventricular dilator
    Trousseau dilator
    Trousseau-Jackson dilator
    Trousseau-Jackson esophageal dilator
    Trousseau-Jackson tracheal dilator
    TTS dilator (through-the-scope dilator)
    Tubbs dilator
    Tubbs mitral valve dilator
    Tucker dilator
    Turner dilator
    two-bladed dilator
    ureteral dilator
    urethral dilator
    urethral meatus dilator
    uterine dilator
    vaginal dilator
    valve dilator
    van Buren dilator
    Vantec dilator
    vascular dilator
    vasodilator
    vein dilator
    Vibrodilator
    Wales dilator
    Walther dilator
    Walther urethral dilator
    Wilder dilator
    Williams dilator
    Williams lacrimal dilator
    wire loop dilator
    wire loop stapes dilator
    Wise dilator
    Wylie dilator
    Wylie uterine dilator
    Young dilator
    Young rectal dilator
    Ziegler dilator
dilator muscle of nose
dilator muscle of pupil
dilator naris, musculus
dilator probe

dilator pupillae, musculus
dilator-sheath
Dilaudid anesthetic agent
Dileant osteotome
Dillwyn Evans procedure
diluting fluid
dimethylpolysiloxane
diminished bowel sounds
diminished breath sounds
diminished function
diminished reflexes
diminution
Dimitry dacryocystorhinostomy trephine
Dimitry erysiphake
Dimitry trephine
Dimitry-Bell erysiphake
Dimitry-Thomas erysiphake
dimness
dimpling
dimpling of breast skin
dimpling of eyeball
dimpling of skin
Dinamap automated blood pressure device
Dinamap blood pressure monitor
Dinamap monitor
Dingman abrader
Dingman bone-holding forceps
Dingman breast dissector
Dingman cartilage clamp
Dingman clamp
Dingman elevator
Dingman flexible retractor
Dingman Flexsteel retractor
Dingman forceps
Dingman mouth gag
Dingman needle
Dingman ostectomy
Dingman osteotome
Dingman passing needle
Dingman periosteal elevator
Dingman retractor
Dingman wire passer
Dingman zygoma elevator
Dingman zygoma hook

Dingman-Denhardt mouth gag
Dingman-Senn retractor
dinner fork deformity
Dintenfass ear knife
Dintenfass-Chapman knife
Diomet plug
diopter
diopter prism
dip and plateau at cardiac
    catheterization
dip coating autoradiography
diphasic wave
diploic vein
diploica frontalis, vena
diploica occipitalis, vena
diploica temporalis anterior,
    vena
diploica temporalis posterior,
    vena
diplopia
Diplos pacemaker
dipstick
dipyridamole-thallium imaging
    (DTI)
direct catheterizing cystocope
direct component
direct current
direct cystoscope
direct drainage
direct fecal contamination
direct field
direct forward-vision telescope
direct fracture
direct hernia
direct inguinal hernia
direct inspection
direct laryngeal operating
    instruments
direct laryngoscope
direct metastasis
direct microlaryngoscopy
direct ophthalmoscope
direct ophthalmoscopy
direct radial sutures
direct transfer flap
direct transverse traction (DTT)
direct visualization

direct-focus headlight
directed biopsy
director
    angled director
    Berman eye director
    Cooper director
    Durnin angled director
    gorget director
    grooved director
    Larry director
    Larry grooved director
    Larry rectal director
    Leksell director
    Pratt director
    Pratt rectal director
    Putti-Platt director
    Quickert grooved
        director and tongue tie
    rectal director
    Teale director
    Wylie uterine director
direct-vision adenotome
direct-vision cystoscope
direct-vision internal ure-
    throtomy (DVIU)
direct-vision liver biopsy
direct-vision telescope
dirty wound
dirty-lung appearance
disarticulated
disarticulation
disarticulation chisel
disc (see *disk*)
discharge
discharge tube
discission
discission blade
discission knife
discission needle
discission of cataract
discission of cervix
discission of cervix uteri
discission of lens
discission of pleura
discogenic
discogenic disease
discoid valve prosthesis

discoidectomy
discoloration
discolored
discomfort
disconjugate gaze (also
    dysconjugate)
discopathy
discrepancy
discrete aneurysm
discrete lesion
discrete mass
discrete nodule
discrimination
discriminator
diseased condition
diseased organ
diseased tissue
disembowelment
DISH (diffuse idiopathic
    sclerosing hyperostosis)
dishpan fracture
DISI (dorsal intercalated
    segmental instability)
DISIDA scan
disimpaction
disimpaction forceps
disinfectant
disinfecting fluid
disinfection
disintegrating stones
disintegration
disjoint
disjunction
disjunctive nystagmus
disk
disk cupping
disk curet
disk diameter
disk disease
disk electrode
disk elevation
disk endoscope
disk explorer
disk forceps
disk grabber
disk herniation
disk oxygenator

disk oxygenator pump
disk poppet
disk protrusion
disk space
disk valve
disk valve prosthesis
diskectomy
diskectomy with Cloward fusion
diskiform process
diskogram
diskographic needle
diskography
dislocated joint
dislocation
dislocation fracture
dislocation of bone
dislocation of cartilage
dislocation of joint
dislocation procedure
dislodged
dislodger (see also *stone
    dislodger*)
    Cook helical stone
        dislodger
    Councill stone dislodger
    Creevy calyx dislodger
    Creevy stone dislodger
    Davis loop stone
        dislodger
    Davis stone dislodger
    Dormia dislodger
    Dormia stone dislodger
    Dormia ureteral stone
        dislodger
    Ellik loop stone dis-
        lodger
    filiform stone dislodger
    Howard spiral dislodger
    Howard stone dislodger
    Howard-Flaherty spiral
        dislodger
    Johnson stone dislodger
    Levant dislodger
    Levant stone dislodger
    Morton dislodger
    Morton stone dislodger
    Ortved dislodger

dislodger *continued*
    Porges stone dislodger
    Robinson dislodger
    Robinson stone dislodger
    spiral stone dislodger
    stone dislodger
    Storz stone dislodger
    Tessier dislodger
    ureteral basket stone
      dislodger
    ureteral stone dislodger
    woven-loop dislodger
    woven-loop stone
      dislodger
    Wullen dislodger
    Wullen stone dislodger
    Zeiss stone dislodger
dismemberment
disorganized globe
dispense as written (DAW)
dispensing tablet
dispersing electrode
dispersing lens
displaced fracture
displacement
displacement of fracture
displacement osteotomy
displacement syringe
display technique
disposable airway
disposable catheter
disposable cord
disposable cryoextractor
disposable cryostylet
disposable ear tip
disposable electrode
disposable electrode pad
disposable electrosurgical cord
disposable electrosurgical
    electrode
disposable electrosurgical pencil
disposable endoscopic conduct-
    ing cord
disposable endoscopic electro-
    surgical cord
disposable forceps
disposable ground plate

disposable instrument
disposable iris retractor
disposable laryngoscope
disposable muscle biopsy clamp
disposable otoscopic ear tips
disposable probe
disposable retractor
disposable scalpel
disposable sigmoidoscope
disposable specimen trap
disposable speculum
disposable sterile scalpel
disposable stone basket
disposable stripper
disposable surgical electrode
disposable syringe
disposable TUR drape
disposable vacuum curets
disposable vaginal speculum
Disposolette cautery
disproportion
disrupted operative wound
disruption of operative wound
Disse space
dissected
dissecting aneurysm
dissecting chisel
dissecting clamp
dissecting forceps
dissecting hook
dissecting probe
dissecting scissors
dissecting tonsillar scissors
dissecting vital scissors
dissection
dissection and snare
dissection and stripping
dissection bench
dissection forceps
dissection hook
dissection probe
dissector
    Adson dissector
    Allerdyce dissector
    Allis dissector
    Allis dry dissector
    Angell-James dissector

dissector *continued*

Aspiradeps lipodissector
aspirating dissector
attic dissector
Aufranc dissector
Austin dissector
Ball dissector
Barraquer corneal
    dissector
Beaver dissector
blunt dissector
Brunner dissector
Brunner goiter dissector
bunion dissector
Butte dissector
Carpenter dissector
Castroviejo corneal
    dissector
Castroviejo dissector
Cavitron dissector
Cheyne dissector
Cheyne dry dissector
Collin dissector
Collin pleural dissector
Colver dissector
corneal dissector
corneal knife dissector
Cottonoid dissector
Crabtree dissector
Creed dissector
Crile dissector
CUSA dissector
Desmarres corneal
    dissector
Desmarres dissector
Desmarres eye dissector
Dingman breast dissector
double-ended dissector
Doyen rib dissector
ear dissector
Effler-Groves dissector
elevator-dissector
endarterectomy dissector
facial nerve dissector
Fager pituitary dissector
Falcao dissector
Falcao suction dissector
Fisher tonsil dissector

dissector *continued*

Freer dissector
Freer elevator-dissector
Gannetta dissector
goiter dissector
Green corneal dissector
Green dissector
Green eye dissector
Hajek-Ballenger dissector
Hajek-Ballenger septal
    dissector
Hamrick suction
    dissector
Hardy dissector
Hardy pituitary dissector
Harris dissector
Hartmann tonsillar
    dissector
Heath dissector
Heath trephine flap
    dissector
Henke tonsillar dissector
Herczel dissector
Holinger dissector
Holinger endarterectomy
    dissector
Holinger laryngeal
    dissector
Hood dissector
House dissector
House-Urban dissector
House-Urban rotary
    dissector
Hunt dissector
Hurd dissector
Hurd tonsil dissector
Hurd-Weder tonsil
    dissector
hydrostatic dissector
Israel dissector
Israel tonsillar dissector
Jackson-Pratt dissector
Jannetta aneurysm neck
    dissector
Jannetta dissector
Jazbi dissector
Jazbi suction tonsillar
    dissector

dissector *continued*

Jazbi tonsil dissector
joker dissector
Judet dissector
Kennerdell-Maroon
dissector
King-Hurd dissector
King-Hurd tonsil
dissector
Kistner dissector
Kitner dissector
Kleinert-Kutz dissector
Kocher dissector
Kocher goiter dissector
Kocher periosteal
elevator and dissector
Kurze dissector
Kurze microdissector
lamina dissector
Lane dissector
Lang dissector
laryngeal dissector
Lemmon intimal dissec-
tor
Lewin bunion dissector
Lewin dissector
Lewin sesamoidectomy
dissector
lipodissector
Logan dissector
Lothrop dissector
Lynch dissector
Lynch laryngeal dissec-
tor
Lynch tonsillar dissector
MacAusland dissector
MacDonald dissector
Madden dissector
Malis microdissector
Manhattan Eye and Ear
corneal dissector
Maroon-Jannetta neuro-
dissector
Martinez knife-dissector
McCabe dissector knife
McCabe facial nerve
dissector
McCabe flap knife
dissector

dissector *continued*

McWhinnie dissector
microdissector
microsurgery dissector
Miller tonsillar dissector
Milligan double-ended
dissector
Molt dissector
Moorehead dissector
Morrison-Hurd dissec-
tor
Morrison-Hurd tonsillar
dissector
Mulligan dissector
nasal dissector
nerve root laminectomy
dissector
neurosurgical dissector
Oldberg dissector
Olivecrona dissector
Olivecrona double-
ended dissector
Olivecrona-Stille
dissector
Paton corneal dissector
peanut dissector
Penfield dissector
Penfield neurodissector
Pierce dissector
Pierce submucous
dissector
pleural dissector
Potts dissector
prostatic dissector
Raney dissector
Rayport dural dissector
Rhode Island dissector
Rhoton neurodissector
Rienhoff dissector
Rochester dissector
Rochester laminar
dissector
Roger dissector
Roger submucous
dissector
Rosen dissector
rotary dissector
Ruddy dissector
Sachs-Freer dissector

dissector *continued*
Schmieden-Taylor
neurodissector
Sens dissector
sesamoidectomy
dissector
Sheldon-Pudenz
dissector
Sloan dissector
Sloan goiter flap
dissector
Smith dissector
Smith tonsillar dissector
Smithwick dissector
sponge dissector
spud dissector
square-tipped artery
dissector
Stallard  dissector
Stolte dissector
submucous dissector
suction dissector
suction tonsillar dissector
Tonnis-Adson neurodis-
sector
tonsil dissector
tonsil-suction dissector
Troutman corneal
dissector
Troutman eye dissector
ultrasonic dissector
vascular dissector
Walker dissector
Walker tonsil dissector
Walker tonsil-suction
dissector
Wangensteen dissector
Watson-Cheyne dissector
Watson-Cheyne dry
dissector
West hand dissector
West plastic dissector
Wieder dissector
Woodson double-ended
dissector
Wynne-Evans tonsil
dissector

dissector *continued*
Yasargil dissector
Yoshida dissector
Yoshida tonsil dissector
Young dissector
Young urological
dissector
dissector and pillar
dissector hook
disseminate
disseminated carcinoma
disseminated disease
disseminated intravascular
coagulation (DIC)
dissemination
dissemination of disease
dissipate
dissolution of stone
dissolvable
dissolving blood clot
dissolving gallstone
dissolving kidney stone
distal antrum
distal arteriotomy
distal aspect
distal bile duct
distal colon
distal duodenum
distal endarterectomy
distal esophageal ring
distal esophagectomy
distal esophagus
distal femoral resector
distal femoral tensor
distal fibula
distal flap
distal gastrectomy
distal hypospadias
distal ileitis
distal ileum
distal interphalangeal joint
distal ischemia
distal occlusion
distal pancreatectomy
distal pancreaticojejunostomy
distal portion of organ

distal procedure
distal Roux-en-Y gastric
    operation
distal runoff
distal splenorenal shunt
distal tunnel technique
distal ulna
distant flap
distant metastasis
distant metastatic disease
distant skin flap
distend
distention
distortion
distraction hook
distraction rod
distress
distribution of hair
disturbance
disuse atrophy
Dittel operation
Dittel sound
Dittrich plug
diuresed patient
diuresis
diuretic
divergent
divergent dislocation
divergent outlet forceps
divergent strabismus
diversion
diversion of blood flow
diversionary ileostomy
diverticula (*sing.* diverticulum)
diverticular disease
diverticular hernia
diverticulectomy
diverticulitis
diverticulogram
diverticulography
diverticulopexy
diverticulosis
diverticulum (*pl.* diverticula)
diverting colostomy
diverting loop ileostomy
diverting stoma
divided and separated

divided and tied
divided colostomy
divided respiration
divided tendon
divided-stoma colostomy
divinyl ether
divinyl ether anesthetic agent
division
division line
division of adhesions
division skin lines
divulse
divulsion
divulsor
Dix foreign body spud
Dix gouge
Dix needle
Dix spud
Dix spud probe
Dix-Hallpike maneuver
Dix-Hallpike test
Dixon blade
Dixon center blade
Dixon-Lovelace hemostatic
    forceps
Dixon-Thomas-Smith clamp
Dixon-Thomas-Smith colonic
    clamp
Dixon-Thomas-Smith intestinal
    clamp
Dixon-Thorpe vitreous foreign
    body forceps
DLP aortic root cannula
DLP cardioplegic catheter
DLP cardioplegic needle
DMI (Diagnostic Medical
    Instruments)
DMI ambulatory surgery table
DNR (do not resuscitate)
do not resuscitate (DNR)
Doane knee retractor
Dobbhoff feeding tube
Dobbie-Trout clamp
Dobie globule
Dobutrex support
dock wire
docking needle

docking wire
Docktor forceps
Docktor needle
Docktor suture
Docktor tissue forceps
Doc's ear plugs
Doctor Collins clamp
Doctor Long clamp
documentation sheath
Docustar fundal camera
Doderlein operation
Doderlein-Kronig operation
Doesel-Huzly bronchoscopic
    tube
dog ears
dog-ear sign
dog-earing
dog-legged filiforms
Dogliotti valvulotome
Dogliotti-Guglielmini clamp
Doherty eye implant
Doherty eye sphere
Doherty graft
Doherty implant
Doherty prosthesis
Doherty sphere eye implant
Doherty sphere implant
Dohlman endoscope
Dohlman hook
Dohlman incus hook
Dohlman operation
Dohlman plug
Dohn-Carton brain retractor
Dolan extractor
Doléris operation
Doléris uterine suspension
Dolfin extensor tenotomy
dolichocephaly
dolichopellic pelvis
Doll method
doll's eye maneuver
doll's eye reflex
doll's eye sign
dome fracture
dome of bladder
dome of diaphragm
Dome paste boot

domed angle-tipped electrode
dominant hemisphere
dominant pattern
dominant skin lines
doming of mitral valve leaflet
doming of valve
Dominici tube
domino reflex
Don Joy knee brace
Donald clamp
Donald operation
Donald vulsellum
Donald-Fothergill operation
Donaldson eustachian tube
Donaldson eye patch
Donaldson myringotomy tube
Donaldson Silastic ear tube
Donaldson Teflon tube
Donaldson tube
donated body
donated organ
Donberg iris forceps
Donnati sutures
Donnheim implant
Donoghue knee procedure
donor
donor bank
donor cadaver
donor island harvesting
donor organs and tissues
donor recipient
donor screening
donor transfusion
donor transplant
donor typing
donor-specific transfusion (DST)
Dooley nail
dopamine
Doplette monitor
Doppler analysis
Doppler apparatus
Doppler blood flow detector
Doppler coronary catheter
Doppler device
Doppler echocardiogram
Doppler echocardiography
Doppler effect

Doppler flow detector
Doppler flow probe
Doppler flowmeter
Doppler monitor
Doppler operation
Doppler probe
Doppler sound device
Doppler stethoscope
Doppler ultrasonic flowmeter
Doppler ultrasonography
Doppler ultrasound
Doppler-Cavin monitor
dopplergram
dopplergraphy
Doptone
Doptone fetal stethoscope
Doptone monitor
Doptone monitoring
Dorello canal
Dorendorf sign
Dorian rib stripper
Dormia basket
Dormia biliary stone basket
Dormia dislodger
Dormia stone basket
Dormia stone basket catheter
Dormia stone dislodger
Dormia ureteral basket
Dormia ureteral stone dislodger
Dornier extracorporeal shock-
    wave lithotripsy system
Dornier gallstone lithotriptor
Dornier lithotriptor
Dornier waterbath lithotriptor
Dorno rays
Dorrance operation
Dorrance palatal pushback
Dorros brachial internal
    mammary guiding catheter
dorsal aponeurotic fascia
dorsal artery
dorsal artery of clitoris
dorsal artery of foot
dorsal artery of nose
dorsal artery of penis
dorsal aspect
dorsal branch of nerve

dorsal bunion
dorsal calcaneocuboid ligament
dorsal carpal ligament
dorsal columella implant
dorsal column
dorsal column stimulation
dorsal column stimulator
    implant (DCS implant)
dorsal cornu
dorsal decubitus position
dorsal digital arteries
dorsal digital nerves
dorsal digital veins
dorsal elevated position
dorsal fascia
dorsal flap
dorsal flexure
dorsal hood
dorsal hump
dorsal inertia position
dorsal intercalated segmental
    instability (DISI)
dorsal intercarpal ligament
dorsal interosseous fascia
dorsal interosseous muscles
dorsal ligament
dorsal lingual veins
dorsal lithotomy position
dorsal metacarpal arteries
dorsal metacarpal veins
dorsal metatarsal arteries
dorsal metatarsal veins
dorsal muscle
dorsal nasal branch of ophthal-
    mic artery
dorsal nerve
dorsal nerve of clitoris
dorsal nerve of penis
dorsal nerve root
dorsal penile nerve block
    (DPNB)
dorsal plaster spine
dorsal plate
dorsal point
dorsal position
dorsal radiocarpal ligament
dorsal recumbent position

dorsal reflex
dorsal region
dorsal retinaculum
dorsal rhizotomy
dorsal rigid position
dorsal root entry zone lesion
    (DREZ lesion)
dorsal sacrococcygeal muscle
dorsal scapular nerve
dorsal scissors
dorsal sclerosis
dorsal sensory branch of ulnar
    nerve
dorsal slit of prepuce
dorsal spine
dorsal strut
dorsal supine incision
dorsal surface
dorsal talonavicular ligament
dorsal vein
dorsal veins of clitoris
dorsal veins of penis
dorsal veins of tongue
dorsal venous arch of foot
dorsal vertebra
dorsal vertebrae
dorsal view
dorsal-angled scissors
dorsales clitoridis superficiales,
    venae
dorsales linguae, venae
dorsales penis superficiales,
    venae
dorsalis clitoridis, arteria
dorsalis clitoridis, nervus
dorsalis clitoridis profunda,
    vena
dorsalis nasi, arteria
dorsalis pedis, arteria
dorsalis pedis pulse
dorsalis penis profunda, vena
dorsalis scapulae, nervus
Dorsey bayonet forceps
Dorsey cannula
Dorsey cervical foraminal
    punch
Dorsey decompressor

Dorsey dural separator
Dorsey forceps
Dorsey leukotome
Dorsey needle
Dorsey punch
Dorsey retractor
Dorsey screwdriver
Dorsey separator
Dorsey spatula
Dorsey tongue depressor
Dorsey transorbital leukotome
Dorsey ventricular cannula
dorsiflexion
dorsiflexion sign
dorsiflexor
dorsiflexor wedge osteotomy
dorsispinal vein
dorsoanterior
dorsocuboidal reflex
dorsodecubitus position
dorsolateral
dorsolateral incision
dorsolateral surface
dorsomedial thalamotomy
dorsomedian
dorsoplantar projection
dorsoposterior
dorsoradial
dorsorecumbent position
dorsorostral
dorsosacral position
dorsoscapular
dorsosupine position
dorsoventral
dorsum
dorsum nasi
dorsum rotundum
dorsum sella
Dos Santos aortography needle
Dos Santos lumbar aortography
    needle
Dos Santos needle for aortogra-
    phy
dosage adjustment
dosage boost
dosage of medication
dosage range

dose
dose and beams
dose calculation
dose fractionation
dose of chemotherapy
dose of medication
dose of radiation
dose profile
dose response
dosimeter
dosimetry
dot hemorrhage
Dott mouth gag
Dott operation
Dott retractor
dotted line
Dotter caged-balloon catheter
Dotter coaxial catheter
Dotter dilator
Dotter operation
Dotter-Judkins percutaneous
    transluminal angioplasty
Dotter-Judkins technique
Dott-Kilner mouth gag
Doubilet sphincterotome
Doubilet sphincterotomy
double aortic arch
double armboard
double Becker ankle brace
double bladder
double concave
double contrast technique
double convex
double decidual sac sign
double elevator
double fracture
double harelip
double hip spica
double hook
double injection
double J-shaped reservoir
double kidney
double knot
double lip
double pedicle flap
double pyloroplasty
Double Seal Tubegauze

double simultaneous stimulation
    (DSS)
double spatula
double stockinette
double towel clamp
double ureter
double urethra
double uterus
double vagina
double-action ankle joint
double-action bone cutter
double-action bone-cutting
    forceps
double-action hump forceps
double-action rongeur
double-action rongeur forceps
double-angled blade
double-angled blade plate
double-angled retractor
double-angled valve
double-armed mattress sutures
double-armed retention sutures
double-armed sutures
double-articulated broncho-
    scopic forceps
double-articulated laryngeal
    forceps tip
double-ball separator
double-balloon valvotomy
double-balloon valvuloplasty
double-barreled colostomy
double-barreled ileostomy
double-barreled loop colostomy
double-barreled needle
double-barreled reservoir
double-biting rongeur
double-blind procedure
double-bubble flushing
    reservoir
double-bubble sign
double-button sutures
double-camelback sign
double-cataract mask
double-catheterizing cysto-
    scope
double-catheterizing telescope
double-channel endoscope

double-channel irrigating
bronchoscope
double-compartment knee
replacement
double-concave forceps
double-concave rat-tooth
forceps
double-concave rotating saw
double-contrast barium meal
double-contrast study
double-crank retractor
double-crush syndrome
double-cuffed tube
double-cupped forceps
double-current catheter
doubled black silk sutures
doubled chromic catgut sutures
doubled pursestring sutures
doubled sutures
double-edged knife
double-end, double-ended
double-ended bone curet
double-ended curet
double-ended dissector
double-ended elevator
double-ended flap
double-ended flap knife
double-ended graft
double-ended needle forceps
double-ended periosteal
elevator
double-ended probe
double-ended retractor
double-ended spatula
double-ended suture forceps
double-ended tissue forceps
double-fixation hook
double-flanged valve-sewing
ring
double-flap amputation
double-flap operation
double-footling delivery
double-guarded chisel
double-headed P190 stapler
double-headed P190 stapling
device
double-hook skin tenaculum

double-J indwelling catheter
stent
double-J silicone internal
ureteral catheter stent
double-J silicone splint
double-J stent catheter
double-J ureteral stent
double-lumen breast implant
double-lumen breast implant
material
double-lumen Broviac catheter
double-lumen cannula
double-lumen catheter
double-lumen curet
double-lumen endobronchial
tube
double-lumen endoprosthesis
double-lumen Hickman catheter
double-lumen Hickman-Broviac
catheter
double-lumen Silastic catheter
double-lumen tube
double-needle cataract operation
double-occlusal splint
double-outlet right ventricle
double-pedicle skin flap
double-pigtail endoprosthesis
double-pigtail stent
double-pronged hook
double-puncture laparoscopy
double-reverse alpha sigmoid
loop
double-rod penile prosthesis
double-spoon forceps
double-stop sutures
double-threaded Herbert screw
double-tooth tenaculum
double-velour graft
double-velour knitted graft
double-woven wire
double-Y incision
doubling time for tumor
doubly armed sutures
doubly clamped
doubly clamped and divided
doubly clamped and ligated

doubly ligated
doubly ligated suture
Dougherty eye irrigator
Dougherty irrigator
doughnut headrest
doughnut kidney
doughnut lesion
doughnut pessary
doughnut sign
Douglas antral trocar
Douglas bag
Douglas cilia forceps
Douglas cul-de-sac
Douglas eye forceps
Douglas fold
Douglas forceps
Douglas graft
Douglas knife
Douglas line
Douglas mesh skin graft
Douglas method
Douglas mucosal snare
Douglas mucosal speculum
Douglas nasal scissors
Douglas operation
Douglas pelvimeter
Douglas pouch
Douglas rectal snare
Douglas skin graft
Douglas snare
Douglas speculum
Douglas suture needle
Douglas sutures
Douglas trocar
douglascele
Douglas-Roberts snare
Dourmashkin bougie
Dourmashkin cystoscope
Dourmashkin dilator
Dourmashkin operation
Dourmashkin tunneled bougie
Douvas cutter
Douvas roto-extractor
Douvas vitreous cutter
Douvas-Barraquer speculum
Dover catheter
dovetail

Dow Corning antifoam agent
    dressing
Dow Corning cannula
Dow Corning catheter
Dow Corning contoured Silastic
    prosthesis
Dow Corning cystocatheter
Dow Corning ileal pouch
    catheter
Dow Corning implant
Dow Corning mammary
    prosthesis
Dow Corning shunt
Dow Corning Silastic prosthesis
Dow Corning Silastic prosthetic
    sizer
Dow Corning silicone
Dow Cystocath
Dow hollow-fiber artificial
    kidney dialyzer
Dow hollow-fiber dialyzer
Dow hollow-fiber hemodialyzer
dowager hump
dowel
dowel cutter
Dowell hernia repair
Dowell operation
Dower bone plugger
Down epiphyseal knife
Down flow generator
Down hand dermatome
down-biting curet
Downes cautery
down-fracture
downgoing
downgoing Babinski bilaterally
downgoing toes
downhill course
downhill esophageal varices
Downing cartilage knife
Downing clamp
Downing hot air bath
Downing knife
Downing retractor
Downs arthroscope
downward compression
downward curvature

downward displacement
downward movement
downward tilting
Doyen abdominal retractor
Doyen abdominal scissors
Doyen bur
Doyen clamp
Doyen costal elevator
Doyen electrode
Doyen elevator
Doyen forceps
Doyen gallbladder forceps
Doyen hysterectomy
Doyen intestinal clamp
Doyen intestinal forceps
Doyen mouth gag
Doyen needle
Doyen needle holder
Doyen operation
Doyen periosteal elevator
Doyen raspatory
Doyen retractor
Doyen rib dissector
Doyen rib elevator
Doyen rib hook
Doyen rib rasp
Doyen rib raspatory
Doyen rib shears
Doyen scissors
Doyen screw
Doyen speculum
Doyen trocar
Doyen tumor screw
Doyen uterine forceps
Doyen vaginal retractor
Doyen vulsellum forceps
Doyen-Jansen mouth gag
Doyle nasal splint
Doyle nasal tampon
Doyle operation
Doyle vein stripper
DPA (dual photoabsorptiometry)
DPNB (dorsal penile nerve block)
Dr. Light-Veley (see *Light-Veley*)
Dr. Twiss duodenal tube

Draeger high-vacuum erysiphake
Draeger tonometer
Drager Volumeter
Dragstedt feeding gastrostomy
Dragstedt gastrostomy
Dragstedt graft
Dragstedt implant
Dragstedt operation
Dragstedt prosthesis
Dragstedt skin graft
Dragstedt vagotomy and gastrojejunostomy
Dragstedt-Tanner operation
drain
Abramson sump drain
accordion drain
ACMI Pezzer drain
Adson drainage cannula
angle drain
Angle-Pezzer drain
antral drain
Atraum with Clotstop drain
Axiom drain
Bardex drain
Bellini drain
Blair silicone drain
Blake drain
Blake drain and J-Vac suction reservoir
Blake silicone drain
butterfly drain
Chaffin-Pratt drain
cigarette drain
closed drain
closed suction drain
clothesline drain
controlled drain
craniovac drain
Cushman drain
cystodrain
dam drain
Davol drain
Davol suction drain
Davol sump drain
Deaver T-drain

drain *continued*

Deboisans drain
Deseret sump drain
dual-sump silicone drain
DuoDerm drain
flute-ended right-angle
    drain
fluted J-Vac drain
four-wing drain
four-wing Malecot drain
Freyer drain
Freyer suprapubic drain
Gomco drain
grommet drain tube
Hemovac drain
Hendrickson drain
Hendrickson suprapubic
    drain
Heyer-Schulte suction
    drain system
high-capacity drain
high-capacity silicone
    drain
Hysterovac drain
Hysto-vac drain
intercostal drain
J-vac drain
Jackson-Pratt drain
Jackson-Pratt suction
    drain
Keith drain
Lahey drain
latex drain
Leydig drain
Malecot 2-wing drain
Malecot 4-wing drain
Malecot drain
Mantisol drain
Marion drain
mediastinal drain
mesonephric drain
Mikulicz drain
Miller-vac drain
Monaldi drain
Morris drain
Mosher drain
myringotomy drain tube

drain *continued*

Nélaton rubber tube
    drain
papilla drain
Penrose drain
Perma-Cath drain
Pezzer drain
Pharmaseal drain
pigtail nephrostomy
    drain
polyethylene drain
polyvinyl drain
Quad-Lumen drain
quarantine drain
Ragnell drain
Redivac drain
Redon drain
Reliavac drain
removal of drain
Reuter bobbin stainless
    steel drain tube
Ritter drain
Ritter suprapubic suction
    drain
Robertson suprapubic
    drain
rubber drain
rubber-dam drain
Sacks biliary drain
Salem sump drain
seton drain
Silastic drain
Silastic thyroid drain
silicone drain
silicone sump drain
silicone thoracic drain
Snyder Hemovac drain
Snyder mini-Hemovac
    drain
soft rubber drain
Sof-Wick drain
Sovally suprapubic
    suction cup drain
spaghetti drain
stab drain
stab-wound drain
Sterivac drain

drain *continued*
suction drain
sump drain
sump Penrose drain
suprapubic drain
suprapubic suction drain
Surgilav drain
T-drain
T-tube drain
Teflon nasobiliary drain
thoracic drain
thyroid drain
tissue drain
TLS drain
TLS suction drain
transnasal drain
transpapillary drain
triple-lumen sump drain
two-wing drain
two-wing Malecot drain
umbilical tape drain
Vacutainer drain
vacuum drain
van Sonnenberg sump
     drain
Vigilon drain
Wangensteen drain
Waterman sump drain
water-seal drain
whistle-tip drain
Wolf drainage cannula
Wolff drain
wolffian drain
wound drain
Wylie drain
Y-drain
drain site
drain tube
drainable ostomy pouch
drainage bag
drainage catheter
drainage from wound
drainage gastroscopy
drainage of abscess
drainage of ascites
drainage of bone
drainage of chest

drainage of cyst
drainage of gland
drainage of muscle
drainage of organ
drainage of sinus
drainage of tissues
drainage of wound
drainage pump
drainage system
drainage to gravity
drainage tube
drainage with myringotomy
drained abscess
draining abscess
draining incisional site
draining lesion
draining wound
Drake aneurysm clip
Drake clip
Drake machine
Drake uroflometer
Drake-Willock automatic
     delivery system
Drake-Willock dialyzer
Drapanas mesocaval shunt
Drapanas shunt
drape
3M drape
3M Vi-Drape
adhesive drape
adhesive plastic drape
Auto-Band Steri-drape
Bioclusive drape
Biodrape dressing
Blair head drape
Convertors surgical
     drape
disposable TUR drape
eye drape
Eye-Pak drape
fenestrated drape
fenestrated sterile drape
head drape
incise drape
Ioban antimicrobial
     incise drape
Ioban drape

drape *continued*
   Ioban Steri-drape
   iodophor Steri-drape
   J&J Band-Aid sterile
     drape
   MMM drape (3M drape)
   MMM Vi-Drape (3M Vi-
     Drape)
   Nevyas drape retractor
   operation drape
   operation microscope
     drape   *1010*
   Opraflex drape
   Opraflex incise drape
   paper drape
   plastic drape
   procedure drape
   sewn-in waterproof
     drape
   split drape
   Steri-Drape
   sterile drape
   surgical drape
   Thompson drape
   Transelast surgical
     drape
   transparent drape
   transparent drape
   Vi-Drape
draped area
draped free
draped in a routine fashion
draped in a routine manner
draped operative field
draped out of the field
Drapier needle
draping of field
draping of surgical patient
Drato bunionectomy
drawn ankle clonus
drawn back
dreamer clamp
Dreiling tube
Dreisse meatotome
dressed tube
dressed wound

dressing (see also *bandage*)
   3M dressing
   ABD dressing
   absorbable dressing
   Ace adherent dressing
   Ace elastic dressing
   Ace longitudinal strips
     dressing
   Ace rubber elastic
     dressing
   Ace-Hesive dressing
   acrylic resin dressing
   Acu-derm wound
     dressing
   Adaptic dressing
   Adaptic gauze dressing
   AD-Hese-Away dress-
     ing
   adhesive absorbent
     dressing
   adhesive dressing
   Aeroplast dressing
   air pressure dressing
   aloe tape dressing
   anorectal dressing
   antiseptic dressing
   Aquaflo dressing
   Aquamatic dressing
   Aquaphor gauze dressing
   Aureomycin gauze
     dressing
   B-D butterfly swab
     dressing
   bacitracin dressing
   Band-Aid dressing
   Barnes-Hind ophthalmic
     dressing
   barrel dressing
   Barton dressing
   Baynton dressing
   bias cut stockinette
     dressing
   binocular dressing
   binocular eye dressing
   Biobrane dressing
   Bioclusive dressing

dressing *continued*

Bioclusive transparent dressing
Biodrape dressing
Bishop-Harman dressing
Blenderm surgical tape dressing
blue sponge dressing
bolus dressing
bone wax dressing
Borsch dressing
brassiere-type dressing
bulky compressive dressing
bulky dressing
bulky pressure dressing
Bunnell dressing
Bunnell-Littler dressing
butterfly dressing
calcium sodium alginate wound dressing
Calgiswab dressing
Castex rigid dressing
Castmate plaster bandage dressing
Cecil dressing
cellophane dressing
chest dressing
Chick sterile dressing
Chux incontinent dressing
Cikloid dressing
Clevis dressing
Coban dressing
Coban elastic dressing
cocoon dressing
cod liver oil-soaked strips dressing
cohesive dressing
collar dressing
collodion dressing
Coloplast dressing
Comfeel Ulcus occlusive dressing
compound dressing
compression dressing
Comprol dressing

dressing *continued*

Contura medicated dressing
Cornish wool dressing
cotton bolster dressing
cotton elastic dressing
cotton pledgets dressing
cotton-ball dressing
cotton-wadding dressing
Coverlet adhesive dressing
Cover-Pad dressing
Cover-Roll dressing
cranioplastic material dressing
Crinotene dressing
Cruricast dressing
Curad plastic dressing
Curity dressing
Curon dressing
Cutinova dressing
Dakin dressing
Debrisan dressing
Decubi-Care pad dressing
demigauntlet dressing
Derma Care dressing
Dermicel dressing
Desault dressing
Diabeticorum dressing
Dow Corning antifoam agent dressing
Dri-Site dressing
dry dressing
dry pressure dressing
dry sterile dressing (DSD)
dry-and-occlusive dressing
DSD (dry sterile dressing)
DuoDerm dressing
DuoDerm porous dressing
Dyna-Flex dressing
elastic foam pressure dressing

dressing *continued*
    Elastikon dressing
    Elastikon wristlet
        dressing
    Elasto dressing
    Elastomull dressing
    Elastoplast dressing
    Elastoplast pressure
        dressing
    Elastopore dressing
    Epigard dressing
    Epilock dressing
    Esmarch roll dressing
    ethylene oxide dressing
    Expo eye dressing
    Exudry dressing
    eye dressing
    EZ-Derm dressing
    Fastrak traction strip
        dressing
    felt dressing
    figure-eight dressing
    figure-of-eight dressing
    filiform dressing
    fine-mesh dressing
    finger-cot dressing
    fixed dressing
    flats of dressing
    Flex foam dressing
    Flex-Aid knuckle
        dressing
    Flexinet dressing
    fluff dressing
    fluffed gauze dressing
    fluffy compression
        dressing
    foam rubber dressing
    Foille dressing
    four-tailed dressing
    Fowler dressing
    Fricke dressing
    Fricke scrotal dressing
    Fuller rectal dressing
    Fuller shield dressing
    Fuller shield rectal
        dressing
    Furacin dressing

dressing *continued*
    Furacin gauze dressing
    Galen dressing
    Garretson dressing
    gauze dressing
    gauze stent dressing
    Gauztex dressing
    Gelfilm dressing
    Gelfoam dressing
    Gelocast dressing
    Gibney dressing
    Gibson dressing
    Gio-occlusive dressing
    Glasscock dressing
    Glasscock ear dressing
    Griffin bandage lens
        dressing
    GU irrigant dressing
    Gypsona plaster dressing
    hammock dressing
    Harrison interlocked
        mesh dressing
    Hexcel cast dressing
    hip spica dressing
    Hueter perineal dressing
    immobilizing dressing
    impermeable dressing
    impregnated dressing
    InteguDerm dressing
    IPOP cast dressing
        (immediate postopera-
        tive prosthesis cast
        dressing)
    Ivalon dressing
    J&J dressing
    jacket-type chest
        dressing
    jelly dressing
    Jobst dressing
    Jobst mammary support
        dressing
    Jones dressing
    Kaltostat wound dressing
    karaya dressing
    Kerlix conforming
        bandage dressing
    Kerlix dressing

dressing *continued*

Kling adhesive dressing
Kling conform dressing
Kling dressing
Kling gauze dressing
Koagamin dressing
Koch-Mason dressing
Koylon foam rubber dressing
Larrey dressing
Lister dressing
Lubafax dressing
Lukens bone wax dressing
LYOFOAM dressing
LYOFOAM wound dressing
mammary support dressing
Manchu cotton dressing
many-tailed dressing
Martin rubber dressing
mastoid dressing
mechanic's waste dressing
Medici aerosol adhesive tape remover dressing
Mersilene dressing
Mersilene mesh dressing
Merthiolate dressing
Metaline dressing
Microdon dressing
Microfoam dressing
Micropore surgical tape dressing
Minnesota Mining Company (3M) dressing
MMM dressing (3M dressing)
moist dressing
moleskin traction hitch dressing
monocular dressing
monocular eye dressing
Montgomery strap dressing
muslin dressing

dressing *continued*

mustache dressing
N-terface graft dressing
neoprene dressing
nonadhering dressing
nonadhesive dressing
Nu-Gauze dressing
Nu-wrap rolls dressing
occlusive dressing
O'Donoghue dressing
oiled silk dressing
Op-Site dressing
Op-Site occlusive dressing
Orthoflex dressing
Orthoplast dressing
Ostic plaster dressing
Owen cloth dressing
Owen gauze dressing
Oxycel dressing
oxyquinoline dressing
Paracine dressing
paraffin dressing
patch dressing
peacock dressing
PEG self-adhesive elastic dressing
Peries medicated hygienic wipe dressing
petrolatum dressing
petrolatum gauze dressing
Piedmont all-cotton elastic dressing
plaster dressing
plaster pants dressing
plaster-of-Paris dressing
plastic dressing
pledget dressing
PolyFlex traction dressing
Pope halo dressing
postnasal dressing
Preptic dressing
Presso-Elastic dressing
Pressoplast compression dressing
Presso-Superior dressing

dressing *continued*

pressure dressing
Priessnitz dressing
Primaderm dressing
propylene dressing
protective dressing
pulped muscle dressing
Quadro dressing
Queen Anne dressing
Qwik-Clean dressing
Ray-Tec dressing
Red Cross adhesive
    dressing
Reston dressing
Reston foam dressing
Rezifilm dressing
Reziplast spray-on
    dressing
Ribble dressing
Richet dressing
Robert Jones compres-
    sive dressing
Robert Jones dressing
Rochester dressing
roller dressing
Rondic sponge dressing
Rose bed dressing
rubber Scan spray
    dressing
saline dressing
Sayre dressing
Scan spray dressing
scarlet red gauze
    dressing
scrotal dressing
scultetus binder dress-
    ing
scultetus dressing
Selofix dressing
Selopor dressing
semicompressive
    dressing
semipermeable mem-
    brane dressing
semipressure dressing
Septisol soap dressing
Shantz dressing
sheepskin dressing

dressing *continued*

sheer spot Band-Aid
    dressing
sheet-wadding dressing
Silastic dressing
silicone dressing
Silverstein dressing
sling dressing
Sof-Rol dressing
Sof-Wick dressing
Sommers compression
    dressing
Sorbsan dressing
spica dressing
Spray Band dressing
squares of dressing
Sta-Tite gauze dressing
stent dressing
Steri-pads dressing
sterile compression
    dressing
sterile dressing
stockinette dressing
Styrofoam dressing
subclavian Tegaderm
    dressing
Superflex elastic dressing
Super-Trac adhesive
    traction dressing
Surfasoft dressing
surgical dressing
Surgicel dressing
Surgicel gauze dressing
Surgifix dressing
Surgi-Pad combined
    dressing
Surgitube dressing
suspensory dressing
Synthaderm dressing
T-bandage dressing
T-binder pressure
    dressing
Tegaderm dressing
Tegaderm occlusive
    dressing
Tegaderm transparent
    dressing
Telfa dressing

*Profore compression dressing*

dressing *continued*

Telfa gauze dressing
Telfa plastic film dressing
Tensoplast elastic
adhesive dressing
Tensor elastic dressing
Tes Tape dressing
Thillaye dressing
tie-over dressing
Tomac foam rubber
traction dressing
Tomac knitted rubber
elastic dressing
transparent dressing
Transpore surgical tape
dressing
triangular dressing
tube dressing
tubular dressing
tulle gras dressing
twill dressing
Uniflex dressing
upper body dressing
Usher Marlex mesh
dressing
Varick elastic dressing
Vaseline dressing
Vaseline gauze dressing
Vaseline petrolatum
gauze dressing
Vaseline wick dressing
Velcro dressing
Velcro fastener dressing
Velpeau dressing
Velpeau sling-dressing
Velpeau stockinette
dressing
Velroc dressing
Ventfoam traction
dressing
Victorian collar dressing
Victorian collar-type
dressing
Vi-Drape dressing
Vigilon dressing
Vioform dressing
Vioform gauze dressing

dressing *continued*

Wangensteen dressing
water dressing
Watson-Jones dressing
Webril dressing
Weck-cel dressing
wet dressing
wet-to-dry dressing
whisk-packets dressing
wick dressing
wool roll dressing
wound dressing
wraparound dressing
Xeroflo dressing
Xeroform dressing
Y-bandage dressing
Zephyr rubber elastic
dressing
Zim-Flux dressing
Zimocel dressing
Zobec sponge dressing
Zonas porous adhesive
tape dressing
Zoroc resin plaster
dressing
dressing forceps
dressing jar
Drew clip
Drews cannula
Drews cilia forceps
Drews forceps
Drews hook
Drews intraocular implant lens
Drews intraocular lens forceps
Drews iris retractor
Drews lavage needle
Drews lens
Drews pick
Drews polisher
Drews suture
Drews suture pickup spatula
Drew-Smythe catheter
Drews-Rosenbaum retractor
DREZ (dorsal route entry zone)
DREZ lesion
drill

ACL drill

drill *continued*
    Adson drill
    Adson spiral drill
    Adson twist drill
    Adson-Rogers perforating
      drill
    agility drill
    air drill
    Amico drill
    Archimedean drill
    ASIF twist drills
    ASSI wire pass drill
    automatic cranial drill
    autotome drill
    Bailey drill
    Björk drill
    bone drill
    bone hand drill
    Bosworth drill
    Bowen suture drill
    Bunnell drill
    Bunnell hand drill
    bur drill
    cannulated cortical step
      drill
    cannulated drill
    Carmody drill
    Cebotome drill
    cement eater drill
    centering drill
    cervical drill
    Charnley drill
    Cherry drill
    Cherry-Austin drill
    chuck drill
    Cloward drill
    Codman drill
    Codman-Shurtleff cranial
      drill
    Collison body drill
    Collison cannulated hand
      drill
    Collison drill
    Collison tap drill
    cortical step drill
    cranial drill
    crown drill

drill *continued*
    Crutchfield drill
    Crutchfield hand drill
    Crutchfield-Raney drill
    Cushing cranial drill
    Cushing drill
    Cushing perforator drill
    dental drill
    DePuy drill
    D'Errico drill
    D'Errico perforating drill
    Deyerle drill
    diamond drill
    eye drill in arthrotomy
    fingernail drill
    Fisch drill
    flat drill
    Galt drill
    Gray drill
    Hall air drill
    Hall drill
    Hall power drill
    Hall-Osteon drill system
    hand drill
    Harold Crowe drill
    Harris-Smith anterior
      interbody drill
    Hewson drill
    high-speed drill
    Hudson cerebellar
      attachment drill
    Hudson drill
    intramedullary drill
    Jacobs chuck drill
    Jordan-Day drill
    Kerr drill
    Kerr hand drill
    Kirschner bone drill
    Kirschner wire drill
    Lentulo drill
    Lentulo spiral drill
    Light-Veley automatic
      cranial drill
    Light-Veley cranial drill
    Light-Veley drill
    Luck bone drill
    Luck drill

drill *continued*
Lusskin drill
Macewen drill
Magnuson twist drill
Mathews drill
McKenzie drill
McKenzie perforating twist drill
McKenzie perforator drill
Micro-Aire drill
Microtek drill system
Midas Rex drill
Mini Stryker power drill
Minos air drill
Mira drill
Moore drill
Neurain drill
Neurairtome drill
Orthairtome II drill
orthopedic drill
Osteone air drill
ototome drill
Pease bone drill
penetrating drill
Penn drill
perforating drill
perforating twist drill
pilot drill
Ralks bone drill
Ralks drill
Ralks fingernail drill
Raney bone drill
Raney cranial drill
Raney drill
rib drill
Richter bone drill
Shea drill
Shea ear drill
Sherman-Stille drill
skull traction drill
Smedberg drill
Smith drill
spiral drill
Spirec drill
step-down drill
Stille cranial drill
Stille drill

drill *continued*
Stille pattern bone drill
Stryker drill
suture hole drill
Synthes facial drill
tap drill
Thornwald antral drill
Thornwald drill
Treace drill
Treace microdrill
Treace stapes drill
trephine drill
Trinkle power drill
twist drill
Universal drill
Universal hand drill with chuck key
Universal two-speed hand drill
Vitallium drill
Warren-Mack drill
Wolferman drill
Wullstein drill
Zimalate drill
Zimalate twist drill
Zimmer drill
Zimmer hand drill
Zimmer Universal drill
Zimmer-Kirschner hand drill
drill guard
drill guide
drill hole
drill point
drill reamer
drilled bur hole
Drinker respirator
drip chamber
drip infusion
drip phleboclysis
drip pyelogram
drip pyelography
Dri-Site dressing
driver (see also *screwdriver*)
Allen-headed screwdriver
automatic screwdriver
Becker screwdriver

driver *continued*

Children's Hospital
screwdriver
Collison screwdriver
cross-slot screwdriver
cruciform screwdriver
Cubbins screwdriver
DePuy screwdriver
Dorsey screwdriver
Flatt driver
Hall driver
Hansen-Street driver-
extractor
Harrington hook driver
heavy cross-slot screw-
driver
hexhead screwdriver
Jewett driver
Johnson screwdriver
Ken driver
Ken driver-extractor
Küntscher driver
Küntscher nail driver
Lane screwdriver
lever-type screwdriver
light cross-slot screw-
driver
Lok-it screwdriver
Lok-screw double-slot
screwdriver
Lok-screw screwdriver
Massie driver
Massie screwdriver
Master screwdriver
Maxi-Driver
McNutt driver
McReynolds driver
McReynolds driver-
extractor
medium screwdriver
mini-driver instruments
Moore driver
Moore-Blount driver
Moore-Blount screw-
driver
Neufeld driver
Phillips screwdriver

driver *continued*

plain screwdriver
prostatic driver
Pugh driver
Richards Phillips
screwdriver
Richter screwdriver
Rush driver
Rush driver-bender-
extractor
Rush pin driver-bender-
extractor
Schneider driver-
extractor
Schneider nail driver
screwdriver
Shallcross screwdriver
Sherman screwdriver
Sherman-Pierce screw-
driver
single cross-slot screw-
driver
Stryker screwdriver
tibial driver
Trenkle screwdriver
White screwdriver
Williams screwdriver
Woodruff screwdriver
Zimmer driver
Zimmer driver-extractor
Zimmer Orthair ream
driver
Zimmer screwdriver
driver-bender extractor
driver-extractor
dromedary hump
drooping
drop anesthesia
drop finger
drop foot
drop hand
drop metastasis
drop shoulder
drop-back procedure
Droperidol anesthesia
drop-foot brace
drop-foot procedure

drop-foot splint
drop-lock knee brace
drop-lock ring
dropped beat
dropper
dropper bottle
Drualt bundle
Druck-Schrauben screw
drug allergy
drug dosage
drug interaction
drug intolerance
drug intoxication
drug reaction
drug regimen
drug release capsule
drug sensitivity
drug therapy
drug use
drug withdrawal
drug-induced abortion
drug-induced condition
drug-induced hypothermia
drug-infusion pump
drug-resistant
drum elevator
drum elevator knife
drum membrane
drum probe
drum scraper
drumhead
drumhead elevator
Drummond wire technique
Drummond-Morison operation
drums of skin graft
drumstick finger
dry adhesions
dry amputation
dry colostomy
dry compress
dry cup
dry dressing
dry field
dry gangrene
dry hernia
dry incision
dry labor

dry lithotripsy
dry needle holder
dry pack
dry packing
dry packs
dry pressure dressing
dry socket
dry sterile dressing (DSD)
dry sterilizer thermometer door
dry swallows
dry-and-occlusive dressing
Dryden-Quickert tube
dryness
DSA (digital subtraction angiography)
DSD (dry sterile dressing)
DSS (double-simultaneous stimulation)
DST (donor-specific transfusion)
DTAF-F bypass (descending thoracic aortofemoral-femoral bypass)
DTI (dipyridamole-thallium imaging)
DTRs (deep tendon reflexes)
DTT (direct transverse traction)
dual adapter
dual distal-lighted laryngoscope
dual photoabsorptiometry (DPA)
dual-beam fiberoptic light source
dual-chamber AV sequential pacemaker
dual-chamber pacemaker
dual-contrast study
dual-inlay bone graft
dual-lead electrode
dual-lock Depuy hip prosthesis
dual-lock hip prosthesis
dual-lock prosthesis
dual-lock total hip replacement system
DuaLock broach
DuaLock total hip
dual-onlay bone graft
dual-onlay graft

Dualoupe
dual-pass pacemaker
dual-sump silicone drain
Duane U-clip
DUB (dysfunctional uterine bleeding)
Duberstein intraluminal tube wick
Dubinet prosthesis
Dubois decapitation scissors
Dubois method
Dubois scissors
Dubois shears
Dubowitz syndrome
Duchenne disease
Duchenne trocar
Duchenne-Erb paralysis
Duchenne-Landouzy dystrophy
duckbill clamp
duckbill elevator
duckbill forceps
duckbill rongeur
duckbill speculum
Duckett procedure for hypospadias repair
Duckworth-Smith technique
Ducor balloon catheter
Ducor cardiac catheter
duct
duct cancer
duct carcinoma
duct cell carcinoma
duct ectasia
duct exploration
duct fistula
duct lumen
duct of Cuvier
duct of Santorini
duct of epididymis
duct of Wirsung
duct stone
duct tumor
ductal
ductal cannulation
ductal carcinoma
ductal cyst
ductal dilatation

ductal dilation
ductal sinus
ductile
ductile failure
ductility
duction
ductions and versions
ductless glands
ductogram
ductography
duct-to-duct anastomosis
ductus
ductus arteriosus
ductus choledochus
ductus clamp
ductus deferens
ductus deferentis, arteria
ductus lacrimalis
ductus perilymphatici
ductus spreader
Duddell membrane
Dudley hook
Dudley operation
Dudley rectal tenaculum hook
Dudley tenaculum
Dudley tenaculum hook
Dudley-Smith rectal speculum
Dudley-Smith speculum
Duecollement hemicolectomy
Duecollement maneuver
Duehr-Allen eye implant
Duffield cardiovascular scissors
Duffield scissors
Duhamel colon operation
Duhamel operation
Duhamel pull-through procedure of colon
Dührssen incision
Dührssen operation
Dührssen tampon
Dührssen vaginofixation
Duke bleeding time
Duke cannula
Duke pistol-grip cane
Duke trocar
Duke tube
Duke-Elder lamp

Dubin device (sent to path in a .....)

Duke-Elder operation
Duke-Elder ultraviolet light
Dukes carcinoma (A, B, C, or D)
Dulaney antral cannula
Dulaney intraocular implant lens
Dulaney lens
Dulcolax bowel prep
dull aching pain
dull curettage
dull retractor
dulled sense of pain
dullness to percussion
dull-pointed forceps
dull-pronged retractor
Dulox sutures
dumbbell incision
dummy seeds
dummy sources in cesium implant
Dumon bronchoscope
Dumon-Gilliard prosthesis pushing tube
Dumon-Harrell bronchoscope
Dumon-Harrell tracheal tube
Dumont angular scissors
Dumont dissecting forceps
Dumont forceps
Dumont retractor
Dumont scissors
Dumont Swiss dissecting forceps
Dumont thoracic scissors
Dumont tweezers
dumping of barium meal
dumping stomach
dumping syndrome
Duncan curet
Duncan endometrial biopsy curet
Duncan endometrial curet
Duncan fold
Duncan position
Duncan shoulder brace
Dundas Grant tube
Dunhill forceps

Dunhill hemostat
Dunlop elbow traction
Dunlop sleeve
Dunlop stripper
Dunlop thrombus stripper
Dunlop traction
Dunn anterior spinal system
Dunn decompressor
Dunn operation
Dunn tongue depressor
Dunn-Brittain foot arthrodesis
Dunn-Brittain operation
Dunn-Brittain triple arthro-desis
Dunn-Dautrey condylar head elevator
Dunn-Hess femoral component
Dunn-Hess osteotomy
Dunning elevator
Dunning periosteal elevator
Dunnington operation
Duo adhesive cement
duobiotic
Duocondylar knee prosthesis
duodenal artery
duodenal atresia
duodenal bulb
duodenal bulb deformity
duodenal clamp
duodenal constriction
duodenal deformity
duodenal erosion
duodenal fistula
duodenal fold
duodenal fossa
duodenal gland
duodenal loop
duodenal lumen
duodenal mucosa
duodenal obstruction
duodenal opening
duodenal perforation
duodenal pin
duodenal polyp
duodenal recess
duodenal retractor
duodenal spasm

duodenal stasis
duodenal stump
duodenal sweep
duodenal tube
duodenal ulcer
duodenal ulceration
duodenal vein
duodenal villi
duodenal wall hamartoma
duodenal web
duodenectomy
duodenitis
duodenobiliary pressure
    gradient
duodenocholedochostomy
duodenocholedochotomy
duodenocolic
duodenocolic fistula
duodenocolic ligament
duodenocystostomy
duodenoduodenostomy
duodenoenterostomy
duodenogram
duodenography
duodenoileal bypass (DIB)
duodenoileostomy
duodenojejunal
duodenojejunal flexure
duodenojejunal fold
duodenojejunal hernia
duodenojejunal junction
duodenojejunal obstruction
duodenojejunostomy
duodenolysis
duodenomesocolic fold
duodenopancreatectomy
duodenopyloric
duodenopyloric constriction
duodenorrhaphy
duodenoscope
    ACMI duodenoscope
    fiberduodenoscope
    Machida FDS (fiberduo-
        denoscope)
    Machida fiberduodeno-
        scope (FDS)
    Olympus duodenoscope

duodenoscopy
duodenostomy
duodenotomy
duodenum
DuoDerm drain
DuoDerm dressing
DuoDerm porous dressing
Duo-Drive cortical bone screw
Duo-Lock hip prosthesis
Duo-Patella knee prosthesis
Duo-Sonic stehoscope
Duplay bursitis
Duplay hook
Duplay hypospadias repair
Duplay nasal speculum
Duplay operation
Duplay tenaculum
Duplay tenaculum forceps
Duplay tube
Duplay uterine tenaculum
Duplay uterine tenaculum
    forceps
Duplay-Lynch nasal speculum
Duplay-Lynch speculum
duplex placenta
duplex scanner
duplex scanning
duplex ultrasound
duplication
duplication cyst
duplication of organ
Dupuis cannula
Dupuy-Dutemps blepharoplasty
Dupuy-Dutemps needle
Dupuy-Dutemps operation
Dupuytren amputation
Dupuytren contracture
Dupuytren enterotome
Dupuytren fracture
Dupuytren hydrocele
Dupuytren knife
Dupuytren operation
Dupuytren sign
Dupuytren splint
Dupuytren sutures
Dupuytren tourniquet
Dupuy-Weiss needle

dura
dura mater
Durafilm
Duraglit instrument polish
dural confluence of sinuses
dural covering
dural defect
dural elevator
dural film sheeting
dural forceps
dural hook
dural hook knife
dural implant
dural incision
dural knife
dural plate
dural protector
dural protector drill guide
dural retractor
dural sac
dural scissors
dural separator
dural sinus
dural tenting suture
Duran annuloplasty ring
Duranest anesthetic agent
Duran-Houser wire splint
Durapatite
DuraPhase semirigid penile
    prosthesis
duraplasty
Durapore hypoallergenic tape
DuraPrep
Durapulse pacemaker
Durasoft lens
Dura-T contact lens
Duray-Read chisel
Duray-Read gouge
Duray-Read osteotome
Duray-Ward osteotome
Duray-Wood chisel
Dürck node
Duret hemorrhage
Durham needle
Durham operation
Durham plasty for flatfoot
Durham tracheostomy tube
Durham tracheotomy trocar

Durham trocar
Durham tube
Durham-Caldwell operation
Durman operation
Durnin angled director
durotomy
Duroziez sign
Durr operation
Duryea retractor
duskiness
dusky
dusky stoma
Dutch pessary
duToit procedure
duToit rotator cuff procedure
duToit staple
duToit-Roux capsulorrhaphy
duToit-Roux shoulder proce-
    dure
Duval bag
Duval dermatome
Duval disposable dermatome
Duval forceps
Duval irrigating syringe
Duval lung clamp
Duval lung forceps
Duval lung-grasping forceps
DuVal pancreatic drainage
DuVal pancreaticojejunos-
    tomy
Duval Vital intestinal forceps
Duval-Allis forceps
Duval-Coryllos rib shears
Duval-Crile forceps
Duval-Crile intestinal forceps
Duval-Crile lung forceps
Duval-Crile tissue forceps
DuVal-Puestow pancreaticoje-
    junostomy
Duvergier sutures
Duverney fracture
Duverney fracture of ilium
Duverney plantar condylec-
    tomy
DuVries condylectomy
DuVries hammer toe repair
DuVries lateral ankle recon-
    struction

Dura-Kold wrap

DuVries needle
DuVries osteotomy
DuVries procedure
DVI pacemaker
DVI Simpson AtheroCath
    catheter
DVIU (direct vision internal
    urethrotomy)
DVT (deep venous thrombosis)
Dwyer cable
Dwyer cancellous screw
Dwyer clubfoot procedure
Dwyer collar
Dwyer gouge
Dwyer instrumentation
Dwyer instrumentation and
    fusion
Dwyer operation for talipes
    equinovarus
Dwyer osteotomy
Dwyer rod
Dwyer scoliosis procedure
Dwyer screw
Dwyer staple
Dwyer-Wickham electrical
    stimulation system
Dycen pad
Dyclone anesthetic agent
dyclonine hydrochloride
    anesthetic agent
dye allergy
dye dilution technique
dye laser
Dyna-Flex dressing
Dynagrip blade handle
Dynagrip handle
dynamic aorta
dynamic block
dynamic compression plate
    (DCP)
dynamic computed tomography
dynamic condylar screw (DCS)
dynamic facial skin lines
dynamic ileus
dynamic image
dynamic line
dynamic penile prosthesis

dynamic splint
dynamic splinting
dynamization
dynamometer
    Collins dynamometer
    dial-type ophthalmody-
        namometer
    Dynoptor ophthalmody-
        namometer
    squeeze dynamometer
    suction ophthalmodyna-
        mometer
    Reichert ophthalmodyna-
        mometer
    electronic ophthalmody-
        namometer
    hand dynamometer
    Jamar dynamometer
    Preston dynamometer
    Bailliart ophthalmodyna-
        mometer
    suction ophthalmodyna-
        mometer
dynamoscope
dynamoscopy
Dynaplex knee
Dynoptor ophthalmodyna-
    mometer
DyoCam arthroscopic video
    camera
Dyonics arthroscope
Dyonics arthroscopic instru-
    ment
Dyonics bur
Dyonics chondrotome
Dyonics cutter
Dyonics meniscal cutter
Dyonics meniscal trimmer
Dyonics meniscotome
Dyonics microsurgical instru-
    ment
Dyonics motorized meniscal
    shaver
Dyonics needle scope arthro-
    scope
Dyonics Pace Setter 3500
    arthroscopic system

Dyonics shaver
DyoVac suction punch
dysarthrosis
dyschondroplasia
dysconjugate gaze (also
    disconjugate)
dyscrasic fracture
dysesthesia
dysfunction
dysfunctional
dysfunctional uterine bleeding
dyskinesia
dyskinetic and dystonic
    reactions
dyskinetic labor
dyskinetic reaction
dysmenorrhea

dysmotility
dysplasia
dysplastic type
dysplastic valve
dyspnea
dyspneic
dysrhythmia
dysrhythmic activity
dyssynchrony
dyssynergia
dyssynergic bladder
dystocia
dystonic movement
dystonic reactions
dystopic calcification
dystrophy
dysuria

8-channel cross-sectional anal
    sphincter probe
8-lumen catheter
E&J restrictor
E-C junction
E-CABG (endarterectomy and
    coronary artery bypass
    graft)
E-cotton bandage
E-point septal separation (EPSS)
E-rosette
E-rosette cell marker
E-rosette receptor
E-rosetting
E-sign
E-Z-EM Cut biopsy needle
E-Z-ON surgical bra
EAB (elective abortion)
Eagle arthroscope
Eagle spirometer
Eagle styloid process
    syndrome
Eagle-Barrett syndrome
Eagleton operation
ear
ear applicator
ear basin
ear bistoury
ear block
ear bone
ear bougie
ear canal
ear cartilage
ear cavity
ear cup
ear curet
ear cut snare wire
ear dissector
ear elevator
ear forceps

ear hook
ear instrument
ear instrument rack
ear knife
ear loop
ear loupe
ear marker
ear mobilizer
ear operating instrument
ear oximeter
ear oximetry
ear pinna
ear pinna prosthesis
ear piston prosthesis
ear probe
ear punch
ear punch forceps
ear reconstruction
ear rongeur
ear scissors
ear setback
ear snare
ear speculum
ear speculum holder
ear spoon
ear spoon and hook
ear suction adapter
ear suction tube
ear surgery Beaver blade
ear surgery blade
ear syringe
ear-dressing forceps
eardrum
eardrum elevator
ear-grasping forceps
Earle clamp
Earle hemorrhoidal clamp
Earle probe
Earle rectal probe
earlobe

earlobe crease
early detection
early opening of valve
ears, nose, and throat (ENT)
easily reducible hernia
EAST (Emory angioplasty vs. surgery trial)
Eastman clamp
Eastman cystic duct forceps
Eastman forceps
Eastman intestinal clamp
Eastman retractor
Eastman tube
Eastman vaginal retractor
Easton cock-up splint
East-West retractor
Easy catheter
easy-out retractor
Eatol plate arthroplasty
Eaton agent
Eaton nasal speculum
Eaton prosthesis
Eaton speculum
Eaton upper limb prosthesis
Eaton-Littler technique
Eber forceps
Eber holder
Eber needle holder
Eberbusch ptosis correction procedure
Eberle release
EBI bone stimulator
EBI bone-healing system
EBI unit
EBL (estimated blood loss)
Ebner gland
ebonation
ébranlement
Ebstein angle
Ebstein anomaly
Ebstein cardiac anomaly
eburnated bone
eburnation
eburnized bone end
écarteur
ECC (endocervical curettings)
ECCE (extracapsular cataract extraction)

eccentric amputation
eccentric atrophy
eccentric hypertrophy
eccentric implantation
Eccentric locked rib shears
eccentric monocuspid tilting-disk prosthetic valve
eccentric occlusion
Eccentric syringe
ecchondrotome
ecchymosis (*pl.* ecchymoses)
ecchymotic area
ecchymotic discoloration
eccrine duct
eccrine gland
ECG (electrocardiogram)
ECG triggering unit
ECG-synchronized digital subtraction angiogram
echelon sutures
echinococcosis
echinococcotomy
Echinococcus
echinococcus cyst
echinococcus liver cyst
Echlin bone rongeur
Echlin duckbill rongeur
Echlin rongeur forceps
Echlin-Luer rongeur
echo Doppler
echo intensity
echo pattern
echo scan
echo scanner
echo time
echocardiogram
echocardiographic probe
echocardiographic study
echocardiography
echo-dense valve
echoencephalogram
echoencephalography
echo-free space
echogenic area
echogenic liver
echogenic mass
echogenic pattern
echogenic sludge

echogenicity
echo-guided ultrasound
Echols retractor
echoplanar imaging
echo-signal shape
echo-spared area
ECIC bypass (extracranial-intracranial bypass)
Eck fistula
Eck fistula in reverse
Eckhout gastroplasty
Eckhout vertical gastroplasty
eclampsia
eclamptic toxemia
ECMO (extracorporeal membrane oxygenation)
economy line instrument
écouvillon
écrasement
écraseur
ECRB (extensor carpi radialis brevis)
ECRL (extensor carpi radialis longus)
ECT (emission computerized tomography)
ECT (European compression technique)
ECT internal fracture fixation and bone screw
ectasia
ectasia of abdominal aorta
ectasia of aorta
ectasia of cornea
ectasia of sclera
ectasia of thoracic aorta
ectatic aneurysm
ectatic aortic valve
ectocolostomy
Ectocor pacemaker
ectocuneiform bone
ectoderm
ectodermal
ectokelostomy
ectopia
ectopia lentis
ectopia of lens
ectopia vesicae

ectopic
ectopic activity
ectopic anus
ectopic atrial pacemaker
ectopic beat
ectopic bladder
ectopic kidney
ectopic ossification
ectopic pacemaker
ectopic pregnancy
ectopic testis
ectopic tissue
ectopy
ectropion
ectropion of eyelid
ectropion repair
ectropion senilis
ECU (extensor carpi ulnaris)
ECU tenodesis
EDB (extensor digitorum brevis)
EDC (expected date of confinement)
eddy current
Edebohls clamp
Edebohls incision
Edebohls kidney clamp
Edebohls operation
Edebohls position
Edelmann-Galton whistle
edema
edematous
edematous change
Eden technique
Eden-Hybbinette operation for shoulder dislocation
Eden-Hybbinette shoulder arthroplasty
Eden-Lange procedure
Eden-Lawson operation
Eder esophagoscope
Eder forceps
Eder gastroscope
Eder laparoscope
Eder photostrobe unit
Eder sigmoidoscope
Eder tongs
Eder Totalap system
Eder-Chamberlin gastroscope

Eder-Cohn endoscope
Eder-Hufford esophagoscope
Eder-Hufford gastroscope
Eder-Palmer gastroscope
Eder-Palmer semiflexible
    fiberoptic endoscope
Eder-Puestow dilation
Eder-Puestow dilator
Eder-Puestow wire
EDF cast
edge effect
edge trimmed
edge undermined
edge-to-edge occlusion
edge-to-edge sutures
Edinburgh retractor
Edinburgh sutures
Edinger-Westphal nucleus
EDL (extensor digitorum
    longus)
Edlich gastric lavage tube
Edlich lavage tube
Edlich tube lavage
Edmark mitral valve
Edmondson grading system
Edna towel clamp
EDQ (extensor digiti quinti)
edrophonium chloride anes-
    thetic agent
Edslab applicator
Edslab catheter
Edslab cholangiography
    catheter
Edwards catheter
Edwards clamp
Edwards clip
Edwards diagnostic catheter
Edwards graft
Edwards handleless clamp
Edwards heart valve
Edwards hook
Edwards implant
Edwards parallel-jaw spring clip
Edwards patch
Edwards prosthesis
Edwards raspatory
Edwards rectal hook

Edwards seamless prosthesis
Edwards septectomy
Edwards spring clamp
Edwards Teflon intracardiac
    implant
Edwards Teflon intracardiac
    patch graft
Edwards Teflon intracardiac
    patch prosthesis
Edwards Teflon intracardiac
    prosthesis
Edwards Ventrac pulse genera-
    tor
Edwards-Carpentier aortic valve
    brush
Edwards-Duromedics bileaflet
    valve heart valve
Edwards-Duromedics prosthetic
    valve
Edwards-Duromedics valve
Edwards-Tapp arterial graft
EEA (end-to-end anastomosis)
EEA Auto-Suture stapler
EEA circular stapler
EEA stapler
EEA stapling device
EEG (electroencephalogram)
EEG activity
EEG channel
EEG feedback
EEG record
EEG recording
EEG tracing
EEG wave
EENT (eyes, ears, nose, and
    throat)
EF (ejection fraction)
EF slope
effaced cervix
effacement
effacement and dilatation
effacement of calyx
effacement of cervix
effacement of mucosa
effective
effectiveness
Effenberger contractor

Effenberger retractor
efferent
efferent artery
efferent duct
efferent glomerular arteriole
efferent limb
efferent loop
efferent nerve
efferent neuron
efferent vessel
effervescent
efficacious
efficacy
Effler operation
Effler tack
Effler-Groves cardiovascular
    forceps
Effler-Groves dissector
Effler-Groves forceps
Effler-Groves operation
effleurage
effleurage of uterus
effluent gas
effluxed clear urine
effused fluid
effusion
effusion of joint
EFM (electronic fetal monitor-
    ing)
Efteklar clamp
Efteklar technique
Efteklar-Charnley hip prosthesis
Egawa classification
EGD (esophagogastroduode-
    noscopy)
eggcrate mattress
Eggers bone plate
Eggers contact splint
Eggers operation
Eggers plate
Eggers screw
Eggers splint
Eggers tendon transfer
eggshell calcification
eggshell nail
egress cannula
egress needle

EHL (extensor hallucis longus)
Ehmke ear prosthesis
Ehmke platinum Teflon implant
Ehmke platinum Teflon
    prosthesis
Ehrhardt forceps
Ehrhardt lid forceps
Ehrlich-Türck line
EHT electrode (electrohydro-
    thermoelectrode)
Eicher chisel
Eicher femoral prosthetic head
Eicher hip prosthesis
Eicher prosthesis
Eicher rasp
Eicher raspatory
Eicher tri-fin chisel
EIC-negative breast tumor
EID (emergency infusion
    device)
Eidemiller tunneler
Eifrig intraocular implant lens
Eifrig lens
eight-ball hemorrhage
eight-ball hyphema
eighth cranial nerve (VIII)
eight-lumen esophageal
    manometry catheter
eight-lumen manometry
    catheter
eikonometer
Einhorn chemotherapy regimen
Einhorn dilator
Einhorn esophageal dilator
Einhorn string test
Einhorn tube
Einthoven triangle
EIP (extensor indicis proprius)
Eiselberg uterine scissors
Eiselberg-Mathieu needle holder
Eisenmenger complex
Eisenstein clamp
Eisenstein forceps
Eissner prostatic cooler
Eitner operation
ejaculation center
ejaculatory duct

ejection click
ejection fraction (EF)
ejection murmur
ejection rate
ejection time
Ekehorn operation
EKG (electrocardiogram)
EKG monitor strip
EKG silence
El Gamal coronary bypass
    catheter
El Gamal guiding catheter
Ela pacemaker
Elasta-Wrap elastic gauze
elastic
elastic adhesive bandage
elastic band
elastic band ligation
elastic bandage
elastic bougie
elastic compression stockings
elastic fibers
elastic foam bandage
elastic foam pressure dressing
elastic gauze
elastic hose
elastic ligature
elastic line
elastic membrane
elastic modulus
elastic orthosis
elastic pulse
elastic rubber band
elastic skin lines
elastic sutures
elastic tissue
elastic traction
elasticity
elasticity of skin
elastic-thread ligature
Elastikon bandage
Elastikon dressing
Elastikon elastic tape
Elastikon wristlet dressing
elastin
Elasto dressing
elastomer
Elastomull bandage

Elastomull dressing
Elastomull elastic gauze
    bandage
Elastoplast bandage
Elastoplast dressing
Elastoplast pressure dressing
Elastopore dressing
elbow jerk
elbow joint
elbow prosthesis
elbow reflex
elbow structure
elbowed bougie
elbowed catheter
Eldridge-Green color vision
    light
Eldridge-Green lamp
Elecath catheter
Elecath pacemaker
Elecath thermodilution catheter
elective abortion (EAB)
elective correction
elective repair
elective surgery
elective therapy
electively fibrillated
electric, electrical
electric activity
electric anesthesia
electric aspirator
electric bed
electric bur
electric burn
electric calipers
electric capacity
electric cardiac pacemaker
electric cardioversion
electric cautery
electric charge
electric current
electric cutter
electric defibrillation
electric dermatome
electric evacuator
electric field
electric hair clippers
electric head lamp
electric impedance

electric implant
electric knife
electric laryngofissure saw
electric meatotome
electric nerve stimulation
electric potential
electric probe
electric retinoscope
electric saw
electric shock
electric stimulation
electric stimulus
electric surgical clippers
electric therapy
electric trephine
electrically driven bur
electricator
electricity-induced anesthesia
electroacoustic locator
electroacupuncture
electroanalgesia
electroanesthesia
electrocardiogram (ECG, EKG)
electrocardiographic leads
electrocardiographic monitor
electrocardiography
electrocardioscope
electrocauterization
electrocauterize
electrocautery
electrocautery knife
electrocautery pattern
electrocautery snaring
electrocautery unit
electrocholecystectomy
electrocholecystocausis
electrocoagulated bleeders
electrocoagulating biopsy
    forceps
electrocoagulation
electrocoagulator
electrocochleogram
electrocochleography
electroconductive cream
electroconization
electroconization of cervix
electrocorticogram study
electrocorticography

electrocystoscope
electrode
    10–20 electrode system
    ACMI biopsy loop
        electrode
    ACMI monopolar
        electrode
    ACMI retrograde
        electrode
    air-spaced electrode
    angled ball-end electrode
    angle-tip electrode
    angular-tip electrode
    angulated-blade elec-
        trode
    Arrowsmith electrode
    Arruga surface electrode
    Arzco electrode
    atrial electrode
    ball electrode
    Ball reusable electrode
    Ballenger electrode
    Ballenger follicle
        electrode
    Bard electrode
    bayonet-tip electrode
    Beaver electrode
    Berens bident electrode
    biopsy loop electrode
    bipolar catheter elec-
        trode
    bipolar depth electrode
    bipolar electrode
    Birtcher electrode
    Birtcher proctological
        electrode set
    biterminal electrode
    blade electrode
    Bovie electrode
    Bugbee electrode
    Bugbee fulgurating
        electrode
    Buie electrode
    Buie fulguration elec-
        trode
    button electrode
    calomel electrode
    Cambridge jelly electrode

electrode *continued*

Cameron-Miller electrode
Castroviejo electrode
cautery electrode
central terminal electrode
cerebellar electrodes
cervical conization
  electrode
Cibis electrode
closely spaced electrodes
coagulation electrode
Collings electrode
Collings fulguration
  electrode
concentric needle
  electrode
conical-tip electrode
conization electrode
Cortac monitoring
  electrode
cortical electrode
coudé electrode
cuff electrode
cuff-type inactive
  electrode
cup-shaped electrode
cutting loop electrode
cystoscopic electrode
cystoscopic fulgurating
  electrode
Davis coagulation
  electrode
Davis electrode
Delgado electrode
depolarizing electrode
depth electrode
Depthalon monitoring
  electrode
diathermic electrode
diathermic eye electrode
diathermic retinal
  electrode
disk electrode
dispersing electrode
disposable electrode
disposable electrosurgi-
  cal electrode

electrode *continued*

disposable surgical
  electrode
domed angle-tipped
  electrode
Doyen electrode
dual-lead electrode
EHT electrode (electro-
  hydrothermoelectrode)
electrohydrothermoelec-
  trode (EHT electrode)
EMG electrode
ENT electrode
epicardial electrode
epidural electrode
equipotential electrode
exploring electrode
external electrode
eye diathermy electrode
fine-needle electrode
fine-wire electrode
flat-tip electrode
flat-wire eye electrode
flexible radiothermal
  electrode
follicle electrode
fulgurating electrode
fulguration electrode
Galloway electrode
glass pH electrode
Gradle electrode
Gradle needle electrode
Grantham electrode
Guyton electrode
Hamm electrode
Hamm fulgurating
  electrode
Hamm resectoscope
  electrode
Hubbard electrode
Hurd bipolar diathermy
  electrode
Hurd electrode
Hyams-Timberlake wire
  loop for electrode
Iglesias electrode
impedance electrode

electrode *continued*

- implanted electrode
- impregnated electrode
- inactive electrode
- indifferent electrode
- interelectrode distance
- intracerebral electrode
- Jewett electrode
- karaya electrode
- knife electrode
- Kronfeld electrode
- LaCarrere electrode
- Lane ureteral meatotomy electrode
- large-loop electrode
- Levin electrode
- lobotomy electrode
- localizing electrode
- loop electrode
- Lynch electrode
- McCarthy coagulation electrode
- McCarthy electrode
- McCarthy fulguration electrode
- McWhinnie electrode
- meatotomy electrode
- Medtronic corkscrew electrode pacemaker
- metal electrode
- microelectrode
- midoccipital electrode
- Moersch electrode
- multielectrode impedance catheter
- multilead electrode
- multiple-point electrode
- multipurpose ball electrode
- Multistim electrode catheter
- Myerson electrode
- myocardial electrode
- Nashold electrode
- National cautery electrode
- needle electrode

electrode *continued*

- Neil-Moore electrode
- neutral electrode
- New electrode
- New York Hospital electrode
- ophthalmic cautery electrode
- pacemaker electrode
- pacing electrode
- pacing wire electrode
- pad electrode
- panendoscope electrode
- parallel loop electrode
- patient electrode
- Pischel electrode
- platinum blade electrode
- point electrode
- pointed-tip electrode
- proctological ball electrode
- proctoscopic fulguration electrode
- proximal electrode
- punctate electrode
- pyramidal electrode
- Ray rhizotomy electrode
- reference electrode
- reimplanted electrode
- retinal diathermy electrode
- retrograde electrode
- Riba electrourethrotome electrode
- rod electrode
- roller electrode
- round-loop electrode
- round-wire electrode
- scalp electrode
- Schepens electrode
- semi-flat tip electrode
- Shealy facet rhizotomy electrode
- single-fiber EMG electrode
- single-wire electrode
- Sluder cautery electrode
- Sluder-Mehta electrode

electrode *continued*
   small-loop electrode
   Smith electrode
   Stern-McCarthy electrode
   stick-on electrode
   Storz cystoscopic
      electrode
   Storz resectoscope
      electrode
   straight-blade electrode
   straight-point electrode
   straight-tipped electrode
   surface electrode
   surgical electrode
   sutureless pacemaker
      electrode
   temporal electrode
   TENS (terminal electrode
      nerve stimulator)
   terminal adapter
      electrode
   terminal electrode
   Timberlake electrode
   tongue plate electrode
   tonsillar electrode
   transvenous electrode
   turbinate electrode
   Turner cystoscopic
      fulguration electrode
   ultrasonic electrode
   underwater electrode
   unipolar electrode
   USCI pacing electrode
   ventroposterolateral
      thalamic electrode
      (VPL electrode)
   VPL thalamic electrode
      (ventroposterolateral
      thalamic electrode)
   Walker electrode
   Walker ureteral mea-
      totomy electrode
   Wappler electrode
   Williams tonsil electrode
   Wyler electrode
   Wyler subdural strip
      electrode

electrode *continued*
   Ziegler cautery electrode
   Zuker bipolar pacing
      electrode
electrode catheter ablation
electrode cream
electrode fixation
electrode gel
electrode introducer
electrode pad
electrodermal response
electrodermatome
electrodesiccate
electrodesiccation
electrodesiccation and curet-
      tage
electrodesiccation of wart
electrodiagnostic testing
electrodialyzer
electrodiaphake
electrodiaphane
electrodiaphanoscope
electrodiaphanoscopy
Electrodyne cardiac monitor
Electrodyne defibrillator
Electrodyne pacemaker
electrodynogram
electroencephalic response
electroencephalogram (EEG)
electroencephalographic
electroencephalography
electroenterostomy
electroexcision
electrofulguration
electrofulguration hemostasis
electrogalvanic stimulation
electrogastroenterostomy
electrogastrogram
electrogastrography
electrogoniometer
electrohemostasis
electrohydraulic cystolithola-
      paxy
electrohydraulic lithotripsy
electrohydraulic lithotriptor
      probe
electrohydraulic shock waves

electrohydrothermoelectrode
    (EHT electrode)
electrokeratotomy
electrokymogram
electrokymography
electrolithotripsy
electrolithotrity
electrolysis
electrolyte
electromagnet
electromagnetic
electromagnetic flow probe
electromicrokeratome
electromotive force
electromuscular sensibility
electromyogram (EMG)
electromyograph
electromyography
electron beam
electron beam therapy
electron microscope
electron volt
electronarcosis agent
electroneurolysis
electroneuronography (ENOG)
electronic
electronic component
electronic diaphragm pacing
electronic endoscope
electronic fetal monitoring
    (EFM)
electronic flash generator
electronic larynx
electronic mass
electronic nerve stimulator
electronic neurostimulation
electronic ophthalmodyna-
    mometer
electronic stethoscope
electronic stimulation
electronic stimulation of bone
    growth
electronic stimulator
electronic thermometer
electronic tonographer
electronic tonometer
electronic ureteral stimulator

electronically provoked
    response
electronystagmograph (ENG)
electronystagmography
electro-oculogram (EOG)
electro-oculogram apparatus
electroparacentesis
electrophoresis
electrophoretic
electrophysiologic study
electrophysiologic testing
electroresection
electroretinogram (ERG)
electroretinography
electroscission
electroscope
    Bruening electroscope
    Haslinger electroscope
electrosection
electroshock
electrospinal orthosis (ESO)
electrostatic
electrostatic generator
electrostatic unit
electrostimulation
electrosurgery
electrosurgical
electrosurgical biopsy forceps
electrosurgical cauterization
electrosurgical cord
electrosurgical cutting knife
electrosurgical dispersive pad
electrosurgical equipment
electrosurgical knife
electrosurgical pencil
electrosurgical resectoscope tip
electrosurgical snare
electrosurgical snare polypec-
    tomy
electrosurgical unit
    AG Bovie electrosurgical
        unit
    Bovie electrosurgical unit
    Burdick electrosurgical
        unit
    Cameron electrosurgical
        unit

electrosurgical unit *continued*
    Ellman Surgitron
      electrosurgical unit
    ultrasonic diathermy
      electrosurgical unit
    Viamonte-Hobbs
      electrosurgical unit
    Viamonte-Jutzy electro-
      surgical unit
electrotherapy
electrotherm
electrotome
    infant electrotome
    McCarthy electrotome
    McCarthy miniature
      electrotome
    miniature electrotome
    Nesbit electrotome
    punctate electrotome
    Stern-McCarthy elec-
      trotome
electrotomy
electrotorque motor
electrourethrotome
Elema pacemaker
Elema-Schonander pacemaker
element
elephant cuff
elephant-ear clavicle splint
elephantiasis operation
elevated diaphragm
elevated lesion
elevated position
elevated pressure
elevated scapula
Elevath pacemaker
elevating forceps
elevating lens
elevation
elevation of diaphragm
elevation of skull fracture
elevator (see also *periosteal*
    *elevator*)
    Abbott elevator
    Abbott table elevator
    Abraham elevator
    Adson elevator

elevator *continued*
    Adson periosteal elevator
    Alexander elevator
    Allerdyce elevator
    Allis periosteal elevator
    Amerson bone elevator
    angular elevator
    Anthony elevator
    Antole-Condale elevator
    Artmann elevator
    Ashley elevator
    Aufranc periosteal
      elevator
    Aufricht elevator
    Aufricht nasal elevator
    Austin duckbill elevator
    Austin elevator
    Bailey rib elevator
    ball-end elevator
    Ballenger elevator
    Ballenger septal elevator
    Ballenger-Hajek elevator
    Baron elevator
    Baron palate elevator
    Barsky elevator
    Batson-Carmody elevator
    beat-up periosteal
      elevator
    Behrend periosteal
      elevator
    Bellucci elevator
    Bennell elevator
    Bennett bone elevator
    Bennett elevator
    Berens lid elevator
    Berry-Lambert elevator
    Bethune elevator
    Bethune periosteal
      elevator
    Blair cleft palate elevator
    Blair elevator
    blunt periosteal elevator
    Boies nasal elevator
    Boies nasal fracture
      elevator
    Boies plastic surgery
      elevator

elevator *continued*

bone elevator
Bowen periosteal elevator
brain elevator
Bristow elevator
Bristow periosteal elevator
Bristow zygomatic elevator
Brophy periosteal elevator
Brophy tooth elevator
Brown bone elevator
Brown elevator
Buck periosteal elevator
Cameron periosteal elevator
Cameron-Haight elevator
Cameron-Haight periosteal elevator
Campbell elevator
Campbell periosteal elevator
Cannon-Rochester elevator
Cannon-Rochester lamina elevator
Carroll elevator
Carroll periosteal elevator
Carroll-Legg periosteal elevator
Carter elevator
Carter eye elevator
caudal elevator
Chandler bone elevator
Chandler elevator
Cheyne periosteal elevator
chisel elevator
Cinelli elevator
cleft palate elevator
Clevedent crossbar elevator
Clevedent-Miller elevator

elevator *continued*

Cloward elevator
Cloward periosteal elevator
Cobb elevator
Cobb periosteal elevator
Cobb spinal elevator
Cohen elevator
Converse alar elevator
Converse periosteal elevator
Converse-MacKenty elevator
Cooper elevator
Cooper spinal fusion elevator
Cordes-New elevator
Cordes-New laryngeal punch elevator
Coryllos periosteal elevator
Coryllos-Doyen periosteal elevator
costal elevator
costal periosteal elevator
Cottle alar elevator
Cottle elevator
Cottle elevator-feeler
Cottle graduated elevator
Cottle periosteal elevator
Cottle septum elevator
Cottle skin elevator
Cottle-MacKenty elevator
Cottle-MacKenty septal elevator
Coupland elevator
Cramer cleft palate elevator
Crawford dural elevator
Crego elevator
Crego periosteal elevator
Cronin cleft palate elevator
Cronin palate elevator
crossbar elevator
Cryer elevator

elevator *continued*
- curved periosteal elevator
- Cushing elevator
- Cushing periosteal elevator
- Cushing staphylorrhaphy elevator
- Cushing-Hopkins periosteal elevator
- Darrach elevator
- Davidson periosteal elevator
- Davidson-Mathieu elevator
- Davidson-Mathieu-Alexander elevator
- Davidson-Sauerbruch elevator
- Davidson-Sauerbruch-Doyen elevator
- Davidson-Sauerbruch-Doyen periosteal elevator
- Davis periosteal elevator
- DeJager elevator
- dental elevator
- Derlacki  elevator
- dermal elevator
- D'Errico nerve elevator
- D'Errico periosteal elevator
- Desmarres elevator
- Desmarres lid elevator
- Dewar elevator
- Dingman elevator
- Dingman periosteal elevator
- Dingman zygoma elevator
- double elevator
- double-ended elevator
- double-ended periosteal elevator
- Doyen costal elevator
- Doyen elevator
- Doyen periosteal elevator

elevator *continued*
- Doyen rib elevator
- drum elevator
- drumhead elevator
- duckbill elevator
- Dunn-Dautrey condylar head elevator
- Dunning elevator
- Dunning periosteal elevator
- dural elevator
- ear elevator
- eardrum elevator
- ethmoidal elevator
- Farabeuf elevator
- Farabeuf periosteal elevator
- Farrior-Shambaugh elevator
- Farris elevator
- Fay suction elevator
- Federspiel periosteal elevator
- fenestration elevator
- Ferris Smith elevator
- file elevator
- Fiske periosteal elevator
- flap elevator
- Fomon elevator
- Fomon nostril elevator
- Fomon periosteal elevator
- Frazier dural elevator
- Frazier elevator
- Frazier suction elevator
- Freer double elevator
- Freer double-ended elevator
- Freer double-ended septum elevator
- Freer elevator
- Freer elevator-dissector
- Freer nasoseptal elevator
- Freer periosteal elevator
- Freer septal elevator
- Freer single-ended elevator
- Friedman elevator

elevator *continued*
    Friedrich rib elevator
    Gill cleft palate elevator
    Gillies elevator
    Gillies zygomatic
      elevator
    Gimmick elevator
    Goldman elevator
    Goodwillie periosteal
      elevator
    Graham elevator
    Haight periosteal
      elevator
    Hajek-Ballenger elevator
    Hajek-Ballenger septal
      elevator
    Halle elevator
    Halle nasal elevator
    Halle septal elevator
    Hamrick elevator
    hand and plastic surgery
      elevator
    hand surgery elevator
    Harper periosteal
      elevator
    Harrington spinal
      elevator
    Hatt golf-stick elevator
    hawk's beak elevator
    Hayden elevator
    Hayden palate elevator
    Hayes phalangeal
      elevator
    heavy elevator
    Hedblom costal elevator
    Hedblom elevator
    Henner elevator
    Herczel elevator
    Herczel periosteal
      elevator
    Herczel raspatory
      elevator
    Herczel rib elevator
    Hibbs chisel elevator
    Hibbs costal elevator
    Hibbs elevator
    Hibbs periosteal elevator

elevator *continued*
    Hibbs spinal fusion
      chisel elevator
    hockey-stick elevator
    Hoen elevator
    Hoen periosteal elevator
    Holly elevator
    Hopkins elevator
    Horsley elevator
    Hough elevator
    Hough spatula elevator
    House drum elevator
    House elevator
    House endaural elevator
    House flap elevator
    House Gimmick drum
      elevator
    House Gimmick stapes
      elevator
    House stapes elevator
    Howorth elevator
    Hudson double-ended
      elevator
    Hudson elevator
    Hurd elevator
    Hurd septal elevator
    Hurd tonsil elevator
    inclined-plane elevator
    Iowa periosteal elevator
    Iowa University elevator
    Iowa University perios-
      teal elevator
    Jackson elevator
    Jacobson elevator
    Jannetta elevator
    joker elevator
    Jordan elevator
    Joseph elevator
    Joseph periosteal
      elevator
    Joseph periosteotome
      elevator
    Joseph-Killian elevator
    Key periosteal elevator
    Killian double-ended
      elevator
    Killian elevator
    Killian septal elevator

elevator *continued*
  Kilner elevator
  Kinsella elevator
  Kinsella periosteal
    elevator
  Kirmisson elevator
  Kirmisson periosteal
    elevator
  Kleesattel elevator
  Kleinert-Kutz elevator
  Kocher elevator
  Kocher periosteal
    elevator
  Koenig elevator
  L-shaped elevator
  Ladd elevator
  Lambotte elevator
  lamina elevator
  Lamont elevator
  Lane elevator
  Lane periosteal elevator
  Langenbeck elevator
  Langenbeck periosteal
    elevator
  Lee-Cohen elevator
  Lemmon sternal elevator
  lemon squeezer obstetri-
    cal elevator
  Lempert elevator
  Lewis periosteal elevator
  lid elevator
  Logan elevator
  long periosteal elevator
  Love-Adson elevator
  Love-Adson periosteal
    elevator
  Lowis periosteal elevator
  Luongo elevator
  MacDonald periosteal
    elevator
  MacKenty elevator
  MacKenty periosteal
    elevator
  MacKenty septal elevator
  Magielski elevator
  malar elevator
  Malis elevator

elevator *continued*
  Matson elevator
  Matson periosteal
    elevator
  Matson rib elevator
  Matson-Alexander
    elevator
  Matson-Alexander rib
    elevator
  McCabe elevator
  McClamary elevator
  McIndoe elevator
  MGH elevator
  MGH periosteal elevator
  middle ear elevator
  Miller-Apexo elevator
  Molt elevator
  Molt periosteal elevator
  Moore elevator
  Moorehead elevator
  mucoperiosteal elevator
  mucosa elevator
  narrow elevator
  nasal elevator
  Neurological Institute
    elevator
  Neurological Institute
    periosteal elevator
  neurosurgical elevator
  nostril elevator
  Obwegeser periosteal
    elevator
  osteophyte elevator
  Overholt double-ended
    elevator
  Overholt elevator
  Overholt periosteal
    elevator
  Pace periosteal elevator
  palate elevator
  Paparella elevator
  Paparella otologic
    surgery elevator
  Penfield elevator
  Pennington elevator
  Pennington septum
    elevator

elevator *continued*
    perichondrial elevator
    periosteal elevator
    periosteum elevator
    Perkins elevator
    Phemister elevator
    Pierce double-ended
      elevator
    Pierce elevator
    Pischel elevator
    pituitary elevator
    plastic surgery elevator
    Poppen elevator
    Poppen periosteal
      elevator
    Potts elevator
    Presbyterian Hospital
      elevator
    pressure elevator
    Proctor elevator
    Proctor mucosal elevator
    Quervain elevator
    Ralks elevator
    Raney periosteal elevator
    Ray-Parsons-Sunday
      elevator
    Ray-Parsons-Sunday
      staphylorrhaphy
      elevator
    Read periosteal elevator
    rib elevator
    rib elevator and raspatory
    rib elevator and stripper
    Roberts-Gill periosteal
      elevator
    Rochester elevator
    Rochester laminar
      elevator
    Roger septal elevator
    root elevator
    Rosen elevator
    Rowe elevator
    Sachs elevator
    Sauerbruch elevator for
      first rib

elevator *continued*
    Sauerbruch-Frey rib
      elevator
    Sayre double-ended
      elevator
    Sayre elevator
    Sayre periosteal elevator
    scalene elevator
    Scheer elevator
    Schuknecht elevator
    Scott-McCracken elevator
    Scott-McCracken
      periosteal elevator
    screw elevator
    Sebileau elevator
    Sédillot elevator
    Sédillot elevator-
      raspatory
    Sédillot periosteal
      elevator
    septal elevator
    Sewall elevator
    Sewall ethmoidal
      elevator
    Sewall mucoperiosteal
      elevator
    Shambaugh elevator
    Shambaugh endaural
      elevator
    Shambaugh-Derlacki
      elevator
    Shambaugh-Derlacki
      endaural elevator
    sharp elevator
    Shea elevator
    Sisson fracture-reducing
      elevator
    skin elevator
    Slocum elevator
    Smith-Petersen elevator
    soft tissue elevator
    Sokolec elevator
    Somers uterine elevator
    Soonawalla uterine
      elevator
    spinal elevator
    spinal fusion elevator

elevator *continued*

- spiral elevator
- Spurling periosteal elevator
- stapes elevator
- staphylorrhaphy elevator
- Steele periosteal elevator
- Stevens elevator
- Stille periosteal elevator
- Stille-Langenbeck elevator
- straight elevator
- stripper and elevator
- submucous elevator
- suction elevator
- Sumner elevator
- Sunday elevator
- Sunday staphylorrhaphy elevator
- T-bar elevator
- T-handled elevator
- Tabb ear elevator
- Tabb elevator
- Takahashi elevator
- Tarlov nerve elevator
- Tenzel elevator
- Tenzel periosteal elevator
- Tessier disimpaction elevator
- Tessier elevator
- Tobolsky elevator
- tonsillar elevator
- tooth elevator
- Tronzo elevator
- Turner elevator
- Turner periosteal elevator
- uterine elevator
- Veau elevator
- von Langenbeck periosteal elevator
- Walker elevator
- Ward elevator
- Watson-Jones elevator
- wedge elevator
- West blunt elevator

elevator *continued*

- Willauer-Gibbon periosteal elevator
- Williger elevator
- Winter elevator
- Woodson elevator
- Yankauer periosteal elevator
- zygoma elevator

elevator and dissector
elevator and raspatory
elevator and stripper
elevator-curet
elevator-dissector
elevator-raspatory
elevator-stripper
eleventh cranial nerve
Elgiloy frame of prosthetic valve
Elgiloy lead-tip pacemaker
Elgiloy pacemaker
Elgiloy-Heifitz aneurysm clip
Elgin table
elicited
elimination
Ellik bladder evacuator
Ellik evacuator
Ellik kidney stone basket
Ellik loop stone dislodger
Ellik meatotome
Ellik sound
Ellik stone basket
ellik'd (slang for removal of bladder chips with Ellik evacuator)
Ellik-Shaw obturator
Ellingson intraocular implant lens
Ellingson lens
Elliot corneal trephine
Elliot eye trephine
Elliot femoral condyle blade plate
Elliot femoral condyle plate
Elliot operation
Elliot plate
Elliot position
Elliot treatment

Elliot trephination
Elliot trephine
Elliott gallbladder forceps
Elliott hemostatic forceps
Elliott obstetrical forceps
ellipse
ellipsoid joint
ellipsoid of spleen
ellipsoidal articulation
elliptic, elliptical
elliptical amputation
elliptical excision
elliptical incision
elliptical sagittal incision
Ellis eye needle holder
Ellis foreign body spud
Ellis holder
Ellis operation
Ellis plate
Ellis probe
Ellis sign
Ellis spud
Ellis technique
Ellis Vital needle holder
Ellis-Jones operation
Ellis-Jones peroneal tendon
   procedure
Ellison fixation staple system
Ellison knee procedure
Ellison procedure
Ellman Surgitron electrosurgical
   unit
Ellsner gastroscope
Elmed coagulation
Elmed hysteroscope
Elmslie ankle reconstruction
Elmslie ligament repair
Elmslie modification of ankle
   reconstruction
Elmslie procedure
Elmslie-Cholmeley operation
Elmslie-Trillat patellar tendon
   transplant
Elmslie-Trillat technique
Eloesser flap
Eloesser operation
elongated aorta

elongated gland
elongated S-incision
elongated uvula
elongation
elongation and torsion
elongation of thoracic aorta
ELP broach
ELP femoral prosthesis
ELP stem for hip arthroplasty
Elsberg brain-exploring cannula
Elsberg cannula
Elsberg incision
Elsberg ventricular cannula
Elschnig blepharorrhaphy
Elschnig bodies
Elschnig canthorrhaphy
Elschnig capsular forceps
Elschnig cataract knife
Elschnig cyclodialysis forceps
Elschnig cyclodialysis spatula
Elschnig eye spoon
Elschnig fixation forceps
Elschnig forceps
Elschnig iridectomy
Elschnig keratoplasty
Elschnig knife
Elschnig lens scoop
Elschnig lens spoon
Elschnig lid retractor
Elschnig needle holder
Elschnig operation
Elschnig pearl
Elschnig pterygium knife
Elschnig retractor
Elschnig scoop
Elschnig secondary membrane
   forceps
Elschnig spatula
Elschnig spoon
Elschnig tissue-grasping forceps
Elschnig-O'Brien fixation
   forceps
Elschnig-O'Brien forceps
Elschnig-O'Brien tissue-grasping
   forceps
Elschnig-O'Connor fixation
   forceps

Elschnig-O'Connor forceps
Ely operation
emanation
EMB (endomyocardial biopsy)
embarrassed respiration
embarrassment
embedded
embedded tissue
embole
embolectomy
embolectomy catheter
embolectomy curet
emboli (*sing.* embolus)
embolia
embolic aneurysm
embolic occlusion
embolic pneumonia
embolic thrombosis
embolism
embolization
embolization treatment
embolized atheroma
embolomycotic aneurysm
embolus (*pl.* emboli)
embouchment
embrace reflex
embrasure
embryo
embryoma
embryonal carcinoma
embryonal cyst
embryonal tumor
embryonic
embryotomy
embryotomy knife
emedullate
emergency infusion device
    (EID)
emergency laparotomy
emergency operation
emergency room
emergency surgery
emergency tracheostomy set
emergency ventilation broncho-
    scope
emergent operation
Emerson bronchoscope

Emerson cuirass respirator
Emerson pump
Emerson respirator
Emerson restrictor
Emerson stripper
Emerson suction
Emerson suction tube
Emerson vein stripper
emery disk
Emesco 9NS handpiece
Emesco handpiece
emesis
emesis basin
emesis pan
emetic
EMG (electromyogram)
EMG electrode
EMI scan
EMI scanner
eminectomy
eminence
eminence of face
eminent
eminoplasty
emissaria condylaris, vena
emissaria mastoidea, vena
emissaria occipitalis, vena
emissaria parietalis, vena
emissary vein
emission
emission computerized to-
    mography (ECT)
Emko foam
Emmert-Gellhorn pessary
Emmet forceps
Emmet hemostatic bag
Emmet needle
Emmet operation
Emmet ovarian trocar
Emmet probe
Emmet retractor
Emmet scissors
Emmet sutures
Emmet tenaculum
Emmet tenaculum hook
Emmet trocar
Emmet uterine probe

Emmet uterine scissors
Emmet uterine tenaculum
Emmet uterine tenaculum hook
Emmet-Murphy needle
emmetropia
Emmet-Studdiford perineor-
    rhaphy
Emory angioplasty vs. surgery
    trial (EAST)
emphysematous
emplastrum
empty sella syndrome
emptying
emptying time
empyema
empyema trocar
empyema tube
empyematic scoliosis
emulgent vein
emulsion
EMV grading of Glasgow coma
    scale
en bissac
en bloc
en bloc dissection
en bloc distal pancreatectomy
en bloc removal
en bloc resection
en bloc vulvectomy
en chemise catheter
en coin fracture
en cuirasse
en cull
en face
en face irradiation field
en face visualization
en masse
en rave fracture
enamel
enamel rod
enamel rod sheath
enarthrodial joint
encapsulated
encapsulated empyema
encapsulated pleural fluid
encapsulated tumor
encased heart

encased in plaster
encatarrhaphy
encephalic angioma
encephalic region
encephaloarteriogram
encephalocentesis
encephalogram
encephalography
encephalomalacia
encephalomyelitis
encephalomyelopathy
encephalon
encephalopathy
encephalopuncture
encephalorrhagia
encephaloscope
encephaloscopy
Encerin soap
encircling band
encircling endocardial ventricu-
    lotomy
encircling operation for scleral
    buckle
encircling procedure for retinal
    detachment
encircling silicone tube
encircling tape ligature
encircling tube
Encor lead
Encor pacemaker
encountered
encroach
encroachment
encrustation
encrusted pyelitis
encrusted tongue
encysted
encysted calculus
encysted hernia
encysted hydrocele
encysted pleurisy
end artery
end colostomy
end ileostomy
end point
end tube
endaortitis

endarterectomized
endarterectomy
endarterectomy and coronary artery bypass graft (E-CABG)
endarterectomy and embolectomy
endarterectomy dissector
endarterectomy loop
endarterectomy scissors
endarterectomy spatula
endarterectomy stripper
endaural
endaural approach
endaural curet
endaural incision
endaural nystagmus
endaural retractor
endaural rongeur
endaural speculum
end-diastolic murmur
end-diastolic pressure
end-diastolic volume
endemic goiter
Ender intramedullary nail
Ender nail
Ender nailing
Ender pin
endermic injection
end-hole catheter
end-loop colostomy
end-loop ileocolostomy
end-loop ileostomy
endoaneurysmorrhaphy
endobronchial anesthesia
endobronchial tree
endobronchial tube
endocamera
endocardial bipolar pacemaker
endocardial cushion defect
endocardial murmur
endocardial pacemaker
endocardial pressure
endocardial sclerosis
endocardial tumor
endocardial-to-epicardial resection
endocarditis

endocardium
endocavitary radiation therapy
endocervical biopsy
endocervical biopsy curet
endocervical biopsy punch
endocervical canal
endocervical culture
endocervical curet
endocervical curettage
endocervical curettings (ECC)
endocervical glands
endocervical lesion
endocervical mucosa
endocervical os
endocervical polyp
endocervical polypectomy
endocervical probe
endocervical smear
endocervix
endocholedochal
endochondral bone
endochondral bone deposit
endochondroma
endocoagulator
endocrine
endocrine disorder
endocrine fracture
endocrine glands
endocrine neoplasia
endocrine system
endodermal cyst
endodermal sinus
endodontia
endodontitis
EndoDynamics suction polyp trap
endoesophageal prosthesis
endogenous anastomosis
endoherniorrhaphy
endoilluminator
endolaryngeal brachytherapy mold
endolaryngeal lesion
endoluminal stent
endolymphatic duct
endolymphatic fluid
endolymphatic sac

endolymphatic sac enlargement
    instrument
endolymphatic shunt tube
endolymphatic shunt tube
    introducer
endolymphatic subarachnoid
    shunt
endolymphatic tube
endomagnifier
endometrectomy
endometrial biopsy
endometrial biopsy curet
endometrial carcinoma
endometrial cavity
endometrial curet
endometrial forceps
endometrial glands
endometrial hyperplasia
endometrial implant
endometrial lesion
endometrial polyp
endometrial polyp forceps
endometrial tissue
endometriosis
endometriotic implant
endometritis
endometrium
endomyocardial
endomyocardial biopsy (EMB)
endomyocardial disease
endomyocardial fibrosis
end-on mattress sutures
endoneurolysis
end-organ damage
endo-osseous dental
    implant
endo-osseous implant
endoplasmic reticulum
endoplastic amputation
endoprosthesis
endoprosthetic arthroplasty
endoprosthetic femoral head
    replacement
endopyelotomy
endorectal ileal pull-through
    operation
endorectal pull-through
    procedure
endorectal ultrasound (ERU)

endoscope
    ACMI endoscope
    cystopanendoscope
    disk endoscope
    Dohlman endoscope
    double-channel endo-
        scope
    Eder-Cohn endoscope
    Eder-Palmer semiflexible
        fiberoptic endoscope
    electronic endoscope
    end-viewing endoscope
    fiberoptic endoscope
    fiberoptic panendoscope
    flexible endoscope
    Foroblique panendo-
        scope
    forward-viewing
        endoscope
    French-McCarthy
        panendoscope
    Fujinon endoscope
    Fujinon EVE video
        endoscope
    Fujinon EVG-F upper GI
        video endoscope
    Fujinon flexible endo-
        scope
    Fujinon flexible lower GI
        endoscope
    Fujinon UGI-FP endo-
        scope
    GIF-HM endoscope
    GIF-XQ endoscope
    JFB III endoscope
    Kelly endoscope
    Kelly panendoscope
    Lowsley-Peterson
        endoscope
    McCarthy panendoscope
    mother-daughter
        endoscope
    Olympus endoscope
    Olympus panendoscope
    oral panendoscope
    panendoscope
    pediatric endoscope
    Pentax side-viewing
        endoscope

endoscope *continued*
    rigid endoscope
    Rockey endoscope
    semiflexible endoscope
    semirigid endoscope
    side-viewing endoscope
    TJF endoscope
    Toshiba video endo-
      scope
    video endoscope
    Wolf panendoscope
endoscopic
endoscopic bicap probe
endoscopic biopsy
endoscopic biopsy forceps
endoscopic bladder litholapaxy
endoscopic cholangiogram
endoscopic connecting cord
endoscopic decompression
endoscopic dilation
endoscopic Doppler ultra-
    sonography
endoscopic electrosurgical cord
endoscopic examination
endoscopic grasping forceps
endoscopic heat probe
endoscopic instrumentation
endoscopic laser cautery
endoscopic magnet
endoscopic manipulation
endoscopic papillotomy
endoscopic polypectomy
endoscopic procedure
endoscopic retrograde
    cholangiogram (ERC)
endoscopic retrograde
    cholangiopancreatography
    (ERCP)
endoscopic retrograde
    sphincterotomy (ERS)
endoscopic snare
endoscopic sphincterotomy (ES)
endoscopic sterilizing case
endoscopic study
endoscopic suture-cutting
    forceps
endoscopic technique

endoscopic telescope
endoscopic trolley
endoscopic tube
endoscopic visualization
endoscopist
endoscopy
endoskeletal prosthesis
endoskeleton
endospeculum
endospeculum forceps
endosteal
endosteum
Endotek urodynamic monitor
endothelial cancer
endothelial dystrophy
endothelial lining
endothelial tissue
endothelialization
endothelialization of vascular
    graft
endotheliochorial placenta
endothelioma
endothelium
endotherm knife
endothermy
endothoracic fascia
endothyropexy
Endotome intra-articular tissue
    resection system
endotoxic shock
endotracheal
endotracheal anesthesia
endotracheal catheter
endotracheal curet
endotracheal general anesthesia
endotracheal insufflation
    anesthesia
endotracheal intubation
endotracheal stripper
endotracheal suctioning
endotracheal tube
endotracheal tube brush
endotracheal tube forceps
endotracheal tumor
Endotrol endotracheal tube
Endotrol tracheal tube
endourologic treatment

end-over-end running sutures
EndoVideo-Five endoscopic
    camera
endplate
endplate of vertebrae
end-sigmoid colostomy
end-stage disease
end-stage failure
end-systolic murmur
end-systolic pressure
end-systolic volume
end-to-back bowel anastomosis
end-to-end anastomosis (EEA)
end-to-end ileocolostomy
end-to-end jejunoileal bypass
end-to-end occlusion
end-to-side anastomosis
end-to-side choledochojejunos-
    tomy
end-to-side colostomy
end-to-side ileotransverse
    colostomy
end-to-side jejunoileal bypass
end-to-side portacaval shunt
end-to-side vein bypass
end-viewing endoscope
Enertrax pacemaker
enflurane
ENG (electronystagmograph)
Engel saw
Engel-Lysholm maneuver
Engelmann disease
Engelmann disk
Engelmann splint
Engel-May nail
Engh porous metal hip
    prosthesis
engine reamer
Engle plaster saw
Englehardt femoral prosthesis
English cane
English forceps
English position
English rhinoplasty
English tissue forceps
English-McNab shoulder
    prosthesis

English-pattern tissue forceps
engorged vasculature
engorgement
engraftment
Engstrom respirator
enhanced scan
Enhanced Torque 8F guiding
    catheter
enhancement surgery
enhancing lesion
Enker brain retractor
Enker self-retaining brain
    retractor
enlarged adenoids
enlarged incision
enlarged mass
enlarged organ
enlarged uterus
enlargement
enlargement of organ
enlarging bur
Enneking staging
Ennis forceps
ENOG (electroneuronography)
ensheathing callus
ensiform
ensiform appendix
ensiform cartilage
ensiform process
ENT (ears, nose, and throat)
ENT chair
ENT electrode
ENT procedure instrument set
ENT treatment unit
enterauxe
enterectasis
enterectomy
enteric
enteric anastomosis
enteric cyst
enteric isolation
enteric precautions
enteroanastomosis
enterobiliary operation
enterocele
enterocele sac
enterocelectomy

enterocentesis
enterocholecystostomy
enterocholecystotomy
enterocleisis
enteroclysis
enterocolectomy
enterocolitis
enterocolostomy
enterocutaneous fistula
enterocystocele
enteroenteric fistula
enteroenterostomy
enteroepiplocele
enterogastric reflex
enterogenous cyst
enterohepatic circulation
enterohepatopexy
enteroinsular atresia
enterolith
enterolithiasis
enterolithotomy
enterolysis
enteromerocele
enteromesenteric
enteromesenteric occlusion
enteropancreatostomy
enteropathogenic Escherichia
enteropathy
enteroperitoneal abscess
enteropexy
enteroplasty
enteroptosis
enteroptychia
enteroptychy
enterorrhaphy
enteroscope
enterostomal
enterostomal therapy
enterostomy
enterostomy clamp
enterotome
    Abraham enterotome
    Dupuytren enterotome
    laryngeal enterotome
    Lukens enterotome
enterotomy
enterotomy incision

enterotomy scissors
enterourethral fistula
enterovesical fistula
enthesis
enthetic
enthetobiosis
entirety
entity
entocuneiform bone
entoptic pulse
entrapment
entrapment syndrome
EntriFlex small-bowel feeding
    tube
entropion
entropion clamp
entropion forceps
entropion operation
entropion repair
entropium
enucleated
enucleation
enucleation compressor
enucleation neurotome
enucleation of cyst
enucleation of eye
enucleation of eyeball
enucleation scissors
enucleation scoop
enucleation snare
enucleation spoon
enucleator
    Carpenter enucleator
    Hardy enucleator
    Meding tonsil enucleator
    prostatic enucleator
    tonsil enucleator
    tonsillar enucleator
    Van Osdel tonsillar
      enucleator
    Young prostatic enuclea-
      tor
enuresis
enuretic
envelope flap
envelope of tissue
environmental contamination

environmental decontamination
enzymatic debridement
enzymatic decortication
EOG (electro-oculogram)
EOM (extraocular motion)
EOM (extraocular movement)
EOM (extraocular muscles)
epactal bones
epallobiosis
eparterial bronchus
epaulet shoulder pad
epauxesiectomy
EPB (extensor pollicis brevis)
ependyma
ependymoma
epi (slang for epinephrine)
epibulbar carcinoma
epic microscope
epicanthal repair
epicanthic fold
epicanthus
epicardial coronary artery
epicardial Doppler flow
    transducer
epicardial electrode
epicardial implantation of
    pacemaker electrode
epicardial pacemaker
epicardial pacing wire
epicardial retractor
epicardial space
epicardial surface
epicardiectomy
epicardiolysis
epicardium
epicondyle
epicranius muscle
epicritic sensorium
epicystotomy
epidermal cancer
epidermal cyst
epidermal inclusion cyst
epidermatoplasty
epidermic graft
epidermis
epidermization
epidermoid

epidermoid cancer
epidermoid carcinoma
epidermoid carcinoma in situ
epidermoid cyst
epidermoid tumor
epididymectomy
epididymis (*pl.* epididymides)
epididymodeferentectomy
epididymogram
epididymography
epididymoplasty
epididymorrhaphy
epididymotomy
epididymovasostomy
epidural abscess
epidural anesthesia
epidural block
epidural blood patch
epidural cavity
epidural electrode
epidural hematoma
epidural hemorrhage
epidural metastasis
epidural space
epiesophageal cancer
epifascial injection
Epigard dressing
epigastric
epigastric angle
epigastric artery
epigastric discomfort
epigastric fold
epigastric fossa
epigastric hernia
epigastric herniorrhaphy
epigastric incision
epigastric inferior vein
epigastric pain
epigastric puncture
epigastric reflex
epigastric region
epigastric tenderness
epigastric vein
epigastrica inferior, arteria
epigastrica superficialis, arteria
epigastrica superficialis, vena
epigastrica superior, arteria

epigastricae superiores, venae
epigastrium
epigastrocele
epigastrorrhaphy
epiglottectomy
epiglottic cartilage
epiglottidectomy
epiglottis retractor
epikeratophakia
epilating forceps
epilation
epilation forceps
epilation needle
Epilock dressing
epimeric muscle
epimicroscope
epinephrine
epipharynx
epiphrenic diverticulum
epiphyseal
epiphyseal arrest
epiphyseal dysplasia
epiphyseal fracture
epiphyseal line
epiphyseal osteochondroma
epiphyseal plate
epiphyseal stapling
epiphyseal-diaphyseal fusion
epiphysiodesis
epiphysiolysis
epiphysis (*pl.* epiphyses)
epiplocele
epiploectomy
epiploenterocele
epiploic
epiploic appendages
epiploic foramen
epiploic foramen of Winslow
epiploitis
epiplomerocele
epiplomphalocele
epiploon
epiplopexy
epiploplasty
epiplorrhaphy
epiplosarcomphalocele
epiploscheocele

episclera
episcleral artery
episcleral bleeder
episcleral forceps
episcleral lamina
episcleral tissue
episcleral vein
episclerales, arteriae
episclerales, venae
episioperineoplasty
episioperineorrhaphy
episioplasty
episioproctotomy
episiorrhaphy
episiotomy
episiotomy scissors
episodic pain
epispadias
episquamous cells
epistasis
epistatic
epistaxis
epistaxis balloon
epistropheus
epithelial cancer
epithelial carcinoma
epithelial cast
epithelial cells
epithelial cyst
epithelial dysplasia
epithelial inlay operation
epithelial lining
epithelial onlay operation
epithelial outlay operation
epithelial sloughing
epithelial tissue
epithelialization
epithelialize
epithelialized
epithelioid sarcoma
epithelioma
epithelium
epithelization
epithesis
Epitrain active elbow support
Epitrain-N elbow support
epitrochlea

epitrochleoanconaeus, musculus
epitrochleoanconeus muscle
epitympanic
epitympanic recess
epitympanum
epivaginal connective tissue
epizootic abortion
EPL (extensor pollicis longus)
EPL (extracorporeal piezoelectric lithotriptor)
épluchage
eponychial fold
eponychium
Eppendorfer angiocatheter
Eppendorfer biopsy punch
Eppendorfer biopsy punch forceps
Eppendorfer cardiac catheter
Eppendorfer catheter
Eppendorfer cervical biopsy forceps
Eppendorfer punch
Eppendorfer uterine biopsy forceps
Epping epoxy
Eppright osteotomy
epsilon tip
epsilon wave
EPSS (E-point septal separation)
Epstein anomaly
Epstein blade
Epstein bone rasp
Epstein curet
Epstein hammer
Epstein hemilaminectomy blade
Epstein lens implant
Epstein needle
Epstein nephrosis
Epstein osteotome
Epstein rasp
EPTFE vascular suture (expanded polytetrafluoroethylene vascular sutures)
epulosis
epulotic
equal and active bilaterally

equal and brisk reflexes
equal and symmetrical extremities
equal bilaterally
equal pulses bilaterally
equal reflexes bilaterally
equalization
equator
equator of eye
Equen magnet
Equen stomach magnet
Equen-Neuffer knife
Equen-Neuffer laryngeal knife
equilateral hemianopia
equilibrating
equilibrating operation
equilibration
equilibratory ataxia
equilibratory coordination
equilibrium
equilibrium radionuclide angiogram
equinocavovarus
equinocavus
equinovalgus
equinovarus
equinus
equinus deformity
equipotential electrode
equipotential line
Equisetene sutures
equivalent
equivalent fraction
equivocal diagnosis
equivocal response
eradication
erasing of joint
erasing of vein
erasion
Erb point
Erb sign
Erbakan operation
Erben reflex
Erbium-YAG laser
Erbotom F2 electrocoagulation unit
ERC (endoscopic retrograde cholangiogram)

ERCP (endoscopic retrograde cholangiopancreatography)
ERCP cannula
ERCP catheter
ERCP manometry
ERCP-guided biopsy
Erdheim-Chester disease
ErecAid system for impotence
erect position
erect spine
erectile elements of the penis
erectile tissue
erection
erector muscle
erector spinae, musculus
erector spinae retractor
ERG (electroretinogram)
Erhardt clamp
Erhardt ear speculum
Erhardt eyelid forceps
Erhardt forceps
Erhardt lid clamp
Erhardt lid forceps
Erhardt speculum
Eric Lloyd extractor
Eric Lloyd introducer
Erich arch bar
Erich arch bar application and intermaxillary fixation
Erich arch malleable bar
Erich biopsy forceps
Erich facial fracture appliance
Erich facial fracture frame
Erich forceps
Erich laryngeal biopsy forceps
Erich maxillary splint
Erich nasal splint
Erich operation
Erich splint
Erichsen ligature
Erichsen sign
Erich-Winter arch bar
Erickson-Leider-Brown technique
Erie oxygen system
Eriksson cruciate reconstruction
Eriksson knee procedure

Eriksson ligament technique
Eriksson-Paparella holder
erisiphake (see *erysiphake*)
Erlangen endoscopic sphincterotome
Erlangen magnetic colostomy device
Erlangen papillotome
Ermold needle holder
Ernst applicator
Ernst radium application
Ernst radium applicator
Ernst radium capsule
Ernst radium tandem
erosion
erosion of cervix
erosive anastomosis
erratic heart rhythm
ERS (endoscopic retrograde sphincterotomy)
ERU (endorectal ultrasound)
erupted incisor
erupted teeth
eruption
erysiphake
> Barraquer erysiphake
> Bell erysiphake
> Castroviejo erysiphake
> Dimitry erysiphake
> Dimitry-Bell erysiphake
> Dimitry-Thomas erysiphake
> Draeger high-vacuum erysiphake
> Falcao erysiphake
> Flayol-Grant erysiphake
> Harken erysiphake
> Harrington erysiphake
> Johnson erysiphake
> Johnson-Bell erysiphake
> Kara erysiphake
> L'Esperance erysiphake
> Maumenee erysiphake
> Maumenee-Park erysiphake
> Nugent erysiphake
> Nugent-Green-Dimitry erysiphake

erysiphake *continued*
    Post-Harrington erysiphake
    right-angled erysiphake
    Sakler erysiphake
    Searcy erysiphake
    Storz-Bell erysiphake
    Viers erysiphake
    Welsh erysiphake
erythema
erythematosus
erythematous
erythematous changes
Erythroflex catheter
erythromycin
ES (endoscopic sphincterotomy)
escape beats
escape interval
escape of air
escape of gastroduodenal contents
escape pacemaker
escape rhythm
escaped ventricular contraction
Escapini operation
eschar
escharectomy
escharotomy
ESI battery cord
ESI bile block
ESI laryngoscope
ESI sigmoidoscope
ESKA Jonas Silicon-Silver semirigid penile prosthesis
Esmarch bandage
Esmarch operation
Esmarch plaster scissors
Esmarch plaster shears
Esmarch probe
Esmarch roll dressing
Esmarch scissors
Esmarch shears
Esmarch tin bullet probe
Esmarch tourniquet
Esmarch tube
ESO (electrospinal orthosis)
esodic nerve
esophageae, venae

esophageal
esophageal A-ring
esophageal abscess
esophageal airway
esophageal anastomosis
esophageal artery
esophageal atresia
esophageal B-ring
esophageal balloon
esophageal biopsy
esophageal bougie
esophageal bougienage
esophageal cardiogram
esophageal conductor
esophageal contractile ring
esophageal dilatation
esophageal dilation
esophageal dilator
esophageal diverticulectomy
esophageal diverticulum
esophageal dysmotility
esophageal fistula
esophageal fistula closure
esophageal forceps
esophageal groove
esophageal hernia
esophageal hiatus
esophageal inlet
esophageal introitus
esophageal lesion
esophageal lumen
esophageal manometry
esophageal motility
esophageal motility disorder
esophageal mucosa
esophageal mucosal ring
esophageal muscular ring
esophageal myotomy
esophageal obstruction
esophageal perforation
esophageal plexus
esophageal prosthesis
esophageal prosthetic placement
esophageal repair
esophageal resection
esophageal retractor
esophageal scissors

esophageal shears
esophageal shunt
esophageal sound
esophageal spasm
esophageal speculum
esophageal sphincter
esophageal stenosis
esophageal stent
esophageal stethoscope
esophageal stricture
esophageal tamponade
esophageal tear
esophageal tube
esophageal ulcer
esophageal ulceration
esophageal variceal bleed
esophageal varices
esophageal varix (*pl.* varices)
esophageal vein
esophageal web
esophagectomy
esophagobronchial fistula
esophagocardiomyotomy
esophagocologastrostomy
esophagocoloplasty
esophagocolostomy
esophagoduodenostomy
esophagoenterostomy
esophagoesophagostomy
esophagofundopexy
esophagogastrectomy
esophagogastric
esophagogastric anastomosis
esophagogastric flap valve
esophagogastric intubation
esophagogastric junction
esophagogastric mucosal
    junction
esophagogastric tamponade
esophagogastric varix
esophagogastroanastomosis
esophagogastroduodenoscopy
    (EGD)
esophagogastromyotomy
esophagogastropexy
esophagogastroplasty
esophagogastroscopy

esophagogastrostomy
esophagogram
esophagography
esophagoileostomy
esophagojejunal anastomosis
esophagojejunogastrostomosis
esophagojejunogastrostomy
esophagojejunoplasty
esophagojejunostomy
esophagolaryngectomy
esophagomyotomy
esophagonasogastric tube
esophagopharynx
esophagoplasty
esophagoplication
esophagorrhaphy
esophagosalivary reflex
esophagoscope
    ACMI esophagoscope
    ACMI fiberoptic esoph-
        agoscope
    ballooning esophago-
        scope
    Boros esophagoscope
    Broyles esophagoscope
    Bruening esophagoscope
    Chevalier Jackson
        esophagoscope
    child esophagoscope
    Eder esophagoscope
    Eder-Hufford esophago-
        scope
    fiberoptic esophago-
        scope
    Foregger rigid esophago-
        scope
    Foroblique esophago-
        scope
    full-lumen esophago-
        scope
    Haslinger esophago-
        scope
    Haslinger tracheobron-
        choesophagoscope
    Holinger child esophago-
        scope
    Holinger esophagoscope

esophagoscope *continued*
   Holinger infant esophagoscope
   Hufford esophagoscope
   infant esophagoscope
   Jackson esophagoscope
   Jackson full-lumen esophagoscope
   Jackson standard full-lumen esophagoscope
   Jasbee esophagoscope
   Jesberg esophagoscope
   Jesberg upper esophagoscope
   Lell esophagoscope
   Moersch esophagoscope
   Mosher esophagoscope
   Moure esophagoscope
   Olympus esophagoscope
   operating esophagoscope
   optical esophagoscope
   oval esophagoscope
   pediatric esophagoscope
   Roberts esophagoscope
   Sam Roberts esophagoscope
   Schindler esophagoscope
   Storz esophagoscope
   Storz operating esophagoscope
   Storz optical esophagoscope
   Storz pediatric esophagoscope
   Tesberg esophagoscope
   Universal esophagoscope
   upper esophagoscope
   Yankauer esophagoscope
esophagoscopic cannula
esophagoscopic catheter
esophagoscopic forceps
esophagoscopic tube
esophagoscopy
esophagospasm

esophagospasm dilator
esophagostoma
esophagostomy
esophagotome
esophagotomy
esophagram
esophagus
esotropia
Esser eyelid operation
Esser graft
Esser implant
Esser inlay graft
Esser inlay operation
Esser operation
Esser prosthesis
Esser skin graft
Essex-Lopresti classification
Essex-Lopresti fracture
Essex-Lopresti fracture reduction
Essex-Lopresti maneuver
Essex-Lopresti method
Essex-Lopresti reduction technique
Essig wire acrylic splint
Essig wiring
Essrig dissecting scissors
Essrig forceps
Essrig scissors
Essrig tissue forceps
Estecar prosthesis
Estes operation
estimated blood loss (EBL)
Estlander cheiloplasty
Estlander flap
Estlander flap cheiloplasty
Estlander operation
Estridge ventricular needle
estrogen assay
ESW-C1
ESWL (extracorporeal shock wave lithotripsy)
Etch-Master instrument marker
ethacrynic acid
ether anesthesia
ether anesthetic agent
ether bed

Etheron augmentation mam-
mography
Ethibond polyester sutures
Ethibond sutures
Ethicon clip
Ethicon paste
Ethicon silk sutures
Ethicon slip
Ethicon staple
Ethicon sutures
Ethicon-Atraloc sutures
Ethiflex retention sutures
Ethiflex sutures
Ethilon nylon sutures
Ethilon sutures
Ethi-pack sutures
ethmoid
ethmoid cornu
ethmoidal artery
ethmoidal bone
ethmoidal bulla
ethmoidal cells
ethmoidal chisel
ethmoidal curet
ethmoidal elevator
ethmoidal exenteration forceps
ethmoidal fissure
ethmoidal forceps
ethmoidal fossa
ethmoidal infundibulum
ethmoidal lamina cribrosa
ethmoidal nerve
ethmoidal process
ethmoidal punch
ethmoidal sinus
ethmoidal veins
ethmoidales, venae
ethmoidalis anterior, arteria
ethmoidalis anterior, nervus
ethmoidalis posterior, arteria
ethmoidalis posterior, nervus
ethmoid-cutting forceps
ethmoidectomy
ethmoidomaxillary suture
ethmoidotomy
ethocaine anesthetic agent
Ethox lavage tube

Ethrane anesthetic agent
Ethridge forceps
Ethridge hysterectomy forceps
Ethrone graft
Ethrone implant
Ethrone prosthesis
ethyl chloride anesthetic agent
ethyl ether anesthetic agent
ethyl oxide anesthetic agent
ethyl vinyl ether anesthetic
agent
ethylene anesthetic agent
ethylene oxide
ethylene oxide dressing
etidocaine hydrochloride
anesthetic agent
etiological conclusion
etiology
EUA (examination under
anesthesia)
Euchidia technique
eugenic sterilization
eunuchism
eunuchoid gigantism
euplastic
eustachian applicator
eustachian attachment
eustachian bougie
eustachian bur
eustachian canal
eustachian cartilage
eustachian catheter
eustachian muscle
eustachian probe
eustachian sound
eustachian tonsil
eustachian tube
eustachian valve
euthyroid
evacuate
evacuation
evacuation of barium
evacuation of blood clots
evacuation of bowel
evacuation of clots
evacuation of subdural
hematoma

evacuator
    Bigelow evacuator
    bladder evacuator
    clot evacuator
    Creevy bladder evacuator
    Creevy evacuator
    electric evacuator
    Ellik bladder evacuator
    Ellik evacuator
    Ewald evacuator
    Hutch evacuator
    ice clot evacuator
    Iglesias evacuator
    Kennedy-Cornwell bladder evacuator
    Lempert evacuator
    McCarthy bladder evacuator
    McCarthy evacuator
    McKenna Tide-Ur-Ator evacuator
    Sklar evacuator
    Snyder Hemovac evacuator
    Storz bladder evacuator
    Storz evacuator
    Storz-Ellik evacuator
    suction evacuator
    Thompson evacuator
    Timberlake evacuator
    Toomey bladder evacuator
    Toomey evacuator
evagination
Eva-Hewes reconstruction
evaluate
evaluation
evaluative staging
evanescent
Evans ankle ligament repair
Evans blue dye
Evans foot procedure
Evans forceps
Evans fusion
Evans operation
Evans procedure

Evans staging of neuroblastoma
Evans Vital tissue forceps
evaporation
event
eventration
Everclear laryngeal mirror
Everett forceps
Everett-TeLinde operation
Evermed catheter
Eversbusch operation
Eversbusch ptosis operation
eversion
eversion of organ
eversion position
eversion stress test
eversion tape strapping
everted
everted lid
everted nipple
everter (see also *lid everter*)
    Benke everter
    Berens everter
    Berens lid everter
    Keizer everter
    lid everter
    Struble everter
    Vail everter
    Walker everter
    Walker lid everter
everting interrupted sutures
everting sutures
Eves snare
Eves tonsillar knife
Eves tonsillar snare
Eves-Neivert tonsillar snare
évidement
evidence
évideur
Evipal anesthetic agent
evisceration
evisceration knife
evisceration of eyeball
evisceration of orbital contents
evisceration spoon
evoked action potential
evoked potential
evoked response

evolving
evulsion
Ewald elbow arthroplasty
Ewald elbow prosthesis
Ewald evacuator
Ewald forceps
Ewald gastroscope
Ewald lavage
Ewald prosthesis
Ewald scoring system
Ewald stomach tube
Ewald total elbow
Ewald total elbow replacement
Ewald tube
Ewald-Hudson brain forceps
Ewald-Hudson dressing forceps
Ewald-Walker knee implant
Ewart sign
Ewing capsule forceps
Ewing eye implant
Ewing forceps
Ewing lid clamp
Ewing operation
Ewing sarcoma
Ewing sign
Ewing tumor
ex vivo
exacerbation
exacerbation of pain
exacerbation of symptoms
exact nature unknown
exam
examination
examination insert tube
examination retractor
examination under anesthesia
    (EUA)
examine
examining arthroscope
examining gastroscope
examining hook
examining hysteroscope
examining light
examining stool
examining telescope
exarticulation
excavated tumor

excavation
excavation of tumor
excavator
    Austin excavator
    dental excavator
    Farrior excavator
    Farrior oval-window
        excavator
    Farrior oval-window
        piston gauge excavator
    fenestration excavator
    Hough excavator
    Hough oval-window
        excavator
    Hough whirlybird
        excavator
    House excavator
    Lempert excavator
    Merlis obstetrical
        excavator
    middle ear excavator
    oval-window excavator
    Schuknecht excavator
    sinus tympani excavator
    stapes excavator
    whirlybird excavator
    whirlybird stapes
        excavator
excavator hoe
excess
excessive callus formation
excessive fluid retention
exchange transfusion
ExciMed 200 ultraviolet laser
    surgery
excimer cool laser
excimer laser
excised adenoids
excision
excision and biopsy
excision and cautery
excision and fulguration
excision and wedge biopsy
excision of cyst
excision of duct
excision of fissure
excision of joint

excision of lesion
excision of organ
excision of sinus
excision of tissue
excision of tumor
excisional biopsy
excisional conization
excisional scar
excisional thoracoscopy
exclusion
exclusion clamp
excochleation
excoriated
excoriation
excrement
excresence
excretion
excretion and secretion
excretion cystogram
excretion cystography
excretion of dye
excretion of protein
excretion pyelogram
excretion pyelography
excretion rate
excretion urogram
excretion urography
excretory
excretory cystogram
excretory duct
excretory function
excretory pyelogram
excretory system
excretory urethrogram
excretory urogram
excretory urography
excruciating pain
exenterated
exenteration
exenteration forceps
exenteration of eye
exenteration of orbital contents
exenteration of pelvic organs
exenteration of sinus
exenteration spoon
exenterative
exeresis

Exeter total hip system
exfoliation
exfoliative
Exner plexus
Exner rib shears
exocardial murmur
exoccipital bone
exocervix
exocrine gland
exodontia
exogenous aneurysm
exolever forceps
exomphalos
exophoria
exophthalmic
exophthalmic goiter
exophthalmometer
    Hertel exophthalmome-
        ter
    Luedde exophthalmome-
        ter
exophthalmometry
exophthalmos
exophytic
exophytic adenocarcinoma
exophytic carcinoma
exophytic lesion
exophytic mass
exoskeleton
exostectomy
exostosectomy
exostosis (*pl.* exostoses)
exostosis bursata
exostosis cartilaginea
exostosis formation
exotropia
expandable blade
expandable breast implant
expandable olive
expanded lung
expanded polytetrafluoroeth-
    ylene vascular sutures
    (EPTFE)
expander
expanding reamer
Expand-O-Graft disposable
    cutter

expansile
expansile abdominal mass
expansile dilator
expansile knife
expansile pulsation
expansile valvulotome
expansion
expansion and excursion
expansion of chest
expansion of lung
expected date of confinement
    (EDC)
expelled afterbirth
expelled fetus
expelled flatus
expelled placenta
experimental surgery
experimental therapy
experimental treatment
expiration and inspiration
expiration-inspiration ratio
expiratory curve
expiratory flow
expiratory flow rate
expiratory pressure
expiratory rhonchi
expiratory sounds
expiratory wheezes
exploration
exploration and repair
exploratory
exploratory biopsy
exploratory bougie
exploratory incision
exploratory laparotomy
exploratory meatoantrotomy
exploratory operation
exploratory pneumonotomy
exploratory procedure
exploratory puncture
exploratory suction tip
exploratory surgery
exploratory thoracotomy
exploratory trephine
explorer
        disk explorer
        Hoen explorer
exploring cannula

exploring electrode
exploring needle
explosive decompression
Expo eye dressing
exposed bone
exposed capsule
exposed organ
exposed tissue
exposing peritoneum
exposure
express lens
expressed skull fracture
expression
expressive
expressor (see also *lens
        expressor*)
        Arruga expressor
        Arruga lens expressor
        Bagley-Wilmer expressor
        Berens expressor
        Berens lens expressor
        follicle expressor
        follicle lid expressor
        Goldmann expressor
        Heath expressor
        Heath lid expressor
        Hess expressor
        Hess tonsil expressor
        intracapsular lens
            expressor
        Kirby expressor
        Kirby hook expressor
        Kirby intracapsular
            expressor with curved
            zonal separator
        Kirby intracapsular lens
            expressor
        Kirby lens expressor
        lens expressor
        lid expressor
        Medallion lens expressor
        Rizzuti eye expressor
        Rizzuti iris expressor
        Smith expressor
        Smith lens expressor
        Smith lid expressor
        tonsillar expressor
        Verhoeff expressor

expressor *continued*
    Wilmer-Bagley expressor
expressor lens
expulsion contraction
expulsive hemorrhage
expulsive pain
exquisite
exquisite pain
exquisite tenderness
exquisitely
EXS femoropopliteal bypass
    graft
EXS vascular graft
exsanguinate
exsanguinating hemorrhage
exsanguination
exsanguination transfusion
exsanguinotransfusion
exsect
exsection
exsector
exstrophy of bladder
extended position
extended radical mastectomy
Extendex tubing
extensile
extension
extension bone clamp
extension bridge
extension clamp
extension splint
extension traction
extension tractor
extensive
extensive debridement
extensive resection
extensor carpi radialis brevis,
    musculus (ECRB)
extensor carpi radialis longus,
    musculus (ECRL)
extensor carpi ulnaris, musculus
    (ECU)
extensor digiti minimi, muscu-
    lus
extensor digiti quinti, musculus
    (EDQ)
extensor digiti quinti proprius,
    musculus

extensor digitorum brevis,
    musculus (EDB)
extensor digitorum communis,
    musculus
extensor digitorum longus,
    musculus (EDL)
extensor digitorum, musculus
extensor hallucis brevis,
    musculus
extensor hallucis longus,
    musculus (EHL)
extensor indicis, musculus
extensor indicis proprius,
    musculus (EIP)
extensor muscle
extensor pollicis brevis,
    musculus (EPB)
extensor pollicis longus,
    musculus (EPL)
extensor retinaculum
extensor retinaculum of ankle
extensor retinaculum of wrist
extensor tendon
extensor wad of three
exterior pelvic device
exteriorization
exteriorization colostomy
exteriorization of rectum
exteriorize
external
external acoustic meatus
external anal sphincter muscle
external angle
external asynchronous pace-
    maker
external biliary fistula
external calcaneoastragaloid
    ligament
external canal
external canthotomy
external capsule
external cardiac massage
external carotid artery
external carotid nerve
external carotid vein
external chest compression
external compression
external cruciate ligament

external demand pacemaker
external ear canal
external electrode
external ethmoidectomy
external fixator
external frontal sinusotomy
external genitalia
external hemorrhage
external hemorrhoid
external hemorrhoidectomy
external hernia
external iliac artery
external iliac lymph node
external iliac vein
external iliac vessel
external inguinal ring
external intercostal muscles
external jugular vein
external landmark
external lateral ligament
external levator resection to
    repair blepharoptosis
external levator resection for
    ptosis
external ligament
external ligament of malleus
external mammary vein
external mastoid process
external meatus
external musculature
external nasal nerve
external nasal splint
external nasal veins
external oblique fascia
external oblique muscle
external obturator muscle
external occipital protuberance
external orifice
external os
external osteotomy
external pacemaker
external palatine vein
external perineal fascia
external photography
external pillar
external pin fixation
external popliteal nerve

external proctotomy
external prosthesis
external pterygoid muscle
external pterygoid nerve
external pterygoid vein
external pudendal artery
external pudendal vein
external pudic vessel
external radial vein
external radiation therapy
external rectal sphincter
external rectus muscle
external rectus sheath
external ring
external rotation
external rotator
external secretion
external semilunar cartilage
external sinusotomy
external skin tag
external spermatic artery
external spermatic fascia
external spermatic nerve
external sphenoid sinusotomy
external sphincter
external splint
external stripper
external table
external traction
external transthoracic pace-
    maker
external urethral orifice
external urethral sphincter
external urethrotomy
external vascular compression
    device
external vein stripper
external version
external-internal pacemaker
externalize
externally controlled noninva-
    sive programmed stimula-
    tion pacemaker
externally rotated
externofrontal retractor
extirpation
extra digit

extra-alveolar crown
extra-articular
extra-articular arthrodesis
extra-axial brain tumor
extracanthic diameter
extracapsular
extracapsular ankylosis
extracapsular cataract extraction
    (ECCE)
extracapsular extraction of
    cataract
extracapsular eye forceps
extracapsular fracture
extracapsular lens extraction
extracardiac graft
extracardiac shunt
extracellular
extracerebral factors
extrachromic sutures
extracorporeal
extracorporeal bypass
extracorporeal circulation
extracorporeal exchange
    hypothermia
extracorporeal heart
extracorporeal irradiation of
    blood, lymph
extracorporeal membrane
    oxygenation (ECMO)
extracorporeal perfusion
extracorporeal piezoelectric
    lithotriptor (EPL)
extracorporeal pump
extracorporeal shock wave
    lithotripsy (ESWL)
extracostal bundle
extracostal muscle
extracranial-intracranial bypass
    (ECIC bypass)
extracting forceps
extraction
extraction of calculus
extraction of cataract
extraction of kidney stone
extraction of lens
extraction of teeth
extraction of tooth

extraction of ureteral stone
extraction test
extractor (see also *cryoextrac-
    tor*)
    Alcon cryoextractor
    Amico extractor
    Amoils cryoextractor
    Andrews comedo
        extractor
    Austin Moore extractor
    Beaver cryoextractor
    Bellows cryoextractor
    cataract extractor
    Cherry extractor
    Cilco extractor
    cloverleaf pin extractor
    comedo extractor
    Councill stone extractor
    cryoextractor
    DePuy extractor
    disposable cryoextractor
    Dolan extractor
    Douvas roto-extractor
    driver-bender extractor
    driver-extractor
    Eric Lloyd extractor
    femoral head extractor
    fetal head extractor
    Frigitronics cryoextractor
    Gills-Welsh cortex
        extractor
    Grieshaber extractor
    Hansen-Street driver-
        extractor
    hatchet extractor
    head extractor
    hoe extractor
    hooked extractor
    impactor-extractor
    Jewett bone extractor
    Kelman extractor
    Ken driver-extractor
    Krwawicz cataract
        extractor
    Krwawicz cryoextractor
    Lempert extractor
    Massie extractor

extractor *continued*
    McDermott extractor
    McLaughlin extractor
    McNutt extractor
    McReynolds driver-
      extractor
    McReynolds extractor
    Moore extractor
    Moore prosthesis
      extractor
    Moore-Blount extractor
    Murless fetal head
      extractor
    Murless head extractor
    Murless vector head
      extractor
    phacoemulsifier-extractor
    prosthesis extractor with
      hand grip
    Rush driver-bender
      extractor
    Rush extractor
    Rush pin driver-bender
      extractor
    Rush pin lead-filled head
      mallet with extractor
    Rush pin prosthesis
      extractor with hand
      grip
    Saalfeld comedo
      extractor
    Schamberg extractor
    Schneider driver-
      extractor
    Schneider nail extractor
    Smith-Petersen extractor
    Smith-Petersen nail
      extractor
    Southwick screw
      extractor
    stone extractor
    Thomas cryoextractor
    Thompson root extractor
    Troutman cataract
      extractor
    Unna comedo extractor
    Unna extractor

extractor *continued*
    ureteral stone extractor
    Walton extractor
    Zimmer driver-extractor
    Zimmer extractor
extractor hook
extradural
extradural anesthesia
extradural block
extradural compression
extradural cord compression
extradural defect
extradural hematoma
extradural hemorrhage
extradural metastatic disease
extraesophageal reflux
extrafascial apicolysis
Extrafil breast implant
extrahepatic
extrahepatic bile duct
extrahepatic biliary atresia
extrahepatic biliary cystic
    dilation
extrahepatic biliary obstruction
extrahepatic obstruction
extrahepatic venous obstruction
extraluminal
extraluminal stripper
extramammary disease
extramedullary
extraneous
extraneous electrode potential
extranodal extension
extraocular motion (EOM)
extraocular movement (EOM)
extraocular muscles (EOM)
extraocular tension
extraoral appliance
extraoral incision
extraoral open reduction of
    mandible
extraosseous
extrapelvic disease
extraperiosteal plombage
extraperiosteal pneumonolysis
extraperitoneal
extraperitoneal approach

extraperitoneal cesarean section
extraperitoneal tissue
extrapetrosal drainage
extrapleural apicolysis
extrapleural fascia
extrapleural pneumonolysis
extrapleural pneumothorax
extrapleural resection of rib
extrapolar region
extrapyramidal
extrapyramidal signs
extrasaccular
extrasaccular hernia
extrasphincteric anal fistula
extrastimulus technique
extrasystole
extrathoracic carotid subclavian
    bypass graft
extrathoracic spread of cancer
extrauterine pelvic mass
extrauterine pregnancy
extravasated contrast medium
extravasation
extravasation of blood
extravasation of contrast
    medium
extravasation of urine
extreme pain
extreme Trendelenburg posi-
    tion
extremity perfusion
extremity strength
extrinsic
extrinsic colon deformity
extrinsic compression
extrinsic defect
extrinsic mass
extrinsic muscle
extrinsic obstruction
extrinsic pressure
extruded disk
extrusion
extrusion balloon catheter
extrusion needle
extubate
extubated
extubation

exuberant
exuberant granulation
exudate
exudation
exudative
exudative ascites
exudative tonsillitis
Exudry dressing
exumbilication
eye and ear cannula
eye bandage
eye blade
eye bottle rack
eye bubble
eye calipers
eye cautery
eye conformer
eye cystitome
eye diathermy electrode
eye drape
eye dressing
eye drill in arthrotomy
eye dropper bottle
eye drops
eye enucleation snare
eye evisceration spoon
eye fixation forceps
eye fixation hook
eye forceps
eye heating pad
eye hook
eye implant (see also *implant*)
    acrylic ball eye implant
    acrylic conformer eye
        implant
    acrylic eye implant
    Allen eye implant
    Appolionio eye implant
    Arruga eye implant
    Arruga movable eye
        implant
    Azar Tripod eye implant
    Berens conical eye
        implant
    Berens eye implant
    Berens pyramidal eye
        implant

eye implant *continued*
- Berens sphere eye implant
- Berens-Rosa eye implant
- Bietti eye implant
- Binkhorst eye implant
- Bonaccolto eye implant
- Brown-Dohlman eye implant
- build-up eye implant
- Choyce eye implant
- Choyce Mark eye implant
- Coburn Mark IX eye implant
- conical eye implant
- conventional reform eye implant
- conventional shell-type eye implant
- corneal eye implant
- curl-back shell eye implant
- Cutler eye implant
- Dannheim eye implant
- DeWecker eye implant
- Doherty sphere eye implant
- Doherty eye implant
- Duehr-Allen eye implant
- Ewing eye implant
- Federov eye implant
- Fox eye implant
- Frey eye implant
- front build-up eye implant
- Garcia-Novito eye implant
- glass sphere eye implant
- gold eye implant
- gold sphere eye implant
- Guist eye implant
- Guist sphere eye implant
- hemisphere eye implant
- Hoffmann eye implant
- hollow sphere eye implant

eye implant *continued*
- hook-type eye implant
- hordeolum eye implant
- Hughes eye implant
- Ivalon eye implant
- Jordan eye implant
- Lemoine eye implant
- Levitt eye implant
- Lincoff eye implant
- lucite eye implant
- magnetic eye implant
- McGhan eye implant
- Medical Optics eye implant
- Mules eye implant
- Mules sphere eye implant
- Nocito eye implant
- peanut eye implant
- plastic ball eye implant
- plastic sphere eye implant
- Plexiglas eye implant
- polyethylene eye implant
- Precision eye implant
- pyramidal eye implant
- Rayner-Choyce eye implant
- reform eye implant
- reverse-shape eye implant
- Ruedemann eye implant
- scleral buckle eye implant
- scleral eye implant
- semishell eye implant
- shell-type eye implant
- shell eye implant
- Silastic eye implant
- silicone eye implant
- Simcoe eye implant
- Simcoe-Amo eye implant
- Snellen eye implant
- sphere eye implant
- spherical eye implant
- Stone eye implant
- surface eye implant

eye implant *continued*
    tantalum eye implant
    tire eye implant
    Troutman eye implant
    tunneled eye implant
    Vitallium eye implant
    Wheeler eye implant
    Wheeler sphere eye
      implant
    wire mesh eye implant
eye implant conformer
eye infection
eye irrigator
eye knife
eye knife blade
eye knife box
eye knife plastic box
eye lesion
eye loupe
eye magnet
eye motion
eye movement
eye movement artifact
eye needle
eye needle holder
eye needle holder forceps
eye occluder
eye pad
eye patch
eye response
eye retractor
eye scissors
eye shield (see also *shield*)
    aluminum eye shield
    Barraquer eye shield
    Buller eye shield
    Fox aluminum eye shield
    Fox eye shield
    protective eye shield
    Universal eye shield
eye speculum
eye sphere implant
eye sphere introducer

eye spoon
eye spud
eye surgery blade
eye suture forceps
eye sutures
eyeball
eyeball movement
eyeball under tension
eyebrow
eyed needle
eyed obturator
eyed probe
eyed suture needle
eye-dressing forceps
eyeglasses
eye-irrigating tip
eyelash loss
eyelashes
eyeless atraumatic suture needle
eyeless needle
eyeless suture needle
eyelet clasp
eyelet lag screw
eyelid
eyelid forceps
eyelid ptosis operation
eyelid resection
eyelid retractor
eyelid speculum
eyelid swelling
Eye-Pak drape
eyepiece
eyepiece attachment
eyes, ears, nose, and throat
    (EENT)
Eyler elbow procedure
Eyler operation
Eyler procedure
EZ-Derm dressing
EZ-Derm temporary skin
    substitute
Ezvue violet haptic one-piece
    lenses

1st-degree burn
4 x 4 gauze
4 x 4 sponge
4 x 4s
4-A Magovern heart valve
4-A Magovern prosthesis
4-A Magovern valve prosthesis
4-prong rake retractor
40-day chromic catgut suture
49er knee brace
5-French angiographic catheter
5-French stiff catheter
F&R (force and rhythm)
F.R. Thompson hip prosthesis
F.R. Thompson rasp
FAB staging of carcinoma
    (French, American, British
    staging)
fabella (*pl.* fabellae)
fabellofibular ligament
fabere (flexion, abduction,
    external rotation, exten-
    sion)
fabere abduction test
fabere extension test
fabere external rotation test
fabere fixation test
fabere sign
fabere-Patrick test
Fabry coagulator
face presentation
face shield
face-down position
face-lift
face-lift operation
face-lift scissors
face-shield headband
facet
facet cartilage
facet eroder
facet joints

facet of cornea
facet rasp
facet raspatory
facet rhizotomy
facet subluxation
facetectomy
faceted (also facetted)
faceted gallstone
faceted stone
facial abrasions
facial artery
facial asymmetry
facial bones
facial canal
facial deformity
facial fracture
facial nerve (cranial nerve
    VII)
facial nerve dissector
facial nerve knife
facial nerve monitor
facial nerve sign
facial nerve stimulator
facial neuralgia
facial palsy
facial prosthetic
facial triangle
facial vein
facial weakness
facialis, arteria
facialis, nervus
facialis, vena
faciei profunda, vena
facies
facile reflex
facilitation
facilitative
facility
faciobrachial hemiplegia
faciolingual hemiplegia
facioplasty

facioscapulohumeral artery
Facit uterine polyp forceps
factor
Faden procedure
Faden retropexy
Faden strabismus operation
Faden sutures
fadir (flexion, abduction, internal rotation) sign
Fager pituitary dissector
Fahey approach
Fahey hip pin
Fahey operation
Fahey pin
Fahey-Compere pin
Fahey-O'Brien procedure
Fahrenheit scale
failed forceps delivery
failed nipple valve
failure
faint diastolic murmur
faint opacification
Fairbanks operation
Fairbanks-Sever shoulder procedure
Fairline instruments
fait accompli
Fajersztajn sign
Falcao dissector
Falcao erysiphake
Falcao fixation forceps
Falcao suction dissector
falces (*sing.* falx)
falcial
falciform
falciform cartilage
falciform fold of fascia lata
falciform hymen
falciform ligament
falciform lobule
falciform process
falcine region
Falconer maneuver
Falk appendectomy spoon
Falk clamp
Falk forceps
Falk operation

Falk retractor
Falk spoon
Falk vaginal cuff clamp
Falk vaginal retractor
Falk-Shukuris operation
falling palate
fallopian
fallopian aqueduct
fallopian artery
fallopian cannula
fallopian catheter
fallopian pregnancy
fallopian tube repair prosthesis
fallopian tubes
Fallot pentalogy
Fallot tetralogy
Fallot trilogy
Falope ring
Falope tubal sterilization ring
Falope-ring applicator
Falope-ring dilator
Falope-ring dual-incision instruments
Falope-ring guide kit
Falope-ring mini-laparotomy instruments
Falope-ring single-incision instruments
Falope-ring tubal sterilization
false aneurysm
false ankylosis
false bruit
false colonic obstruction
false cords
false diverticulum
false Dupuytren contracture
false joint
false labor
false ligament
false membrane
false pregnancy
false ribs
false stricture
false sutures
false teeth
false vocal cord
false-negative

false-positive
Falta triad
falx (*pl.* falces)
falx cerebelli
falx cerebri
falx inguinalis
falx ligamentosa
falx of maxillary antrum
familial
familial defect
familial disease
familial disorder
familial predisposition
familial tendency
fanning of toes
Fansler anoscope
Fansler proctoscope
Fansler rectal speculum
Fansler speculum
Fansler-Frykman operation
Fanta eye speculum
Fanta operation
fantascope
far field
far sight
far sutures
Farabeuf amputation
Farabeuf bone-holding forceps
Farabeuf double-ended retractor
Farabeuf elevator
Farabeuf forceps
Farabeuf operation
Farabeuf periosteal elevator
Farabeuf rasp
Farabeuf raspatory
Farabeuf retractor
Farabeuf saw
Farabeuf-Collen rasp
Farabeuf-Lambotte bone-
    holding clamp
Farabeuf-Lambotte bone-
    holding forceps
Farabeuf-Lambotte clamp
Farabeuf-Lambotte forceps
Faraci punch
Faraci-Skillern punch
Faraday shield

faradic current
faradic electrostimulation
faradic stimulation
far-and-near sutures
Farill operation
Farkas urethral speculum
Farlow decompressor
Farlow snare
Farlow tongue depressor
Farlow tonsil snare
Farlow-Boettcher snare
Farlow-Boettcher tonsil snare
Farmer hallux valgus operation
Farmer operation
Farmer technique
far-near sutures
Farnham forceps
Farnham nasal-cutting forceps
Farr retractor
Farr self-retaining retractor
Farr spring retractor
Farre line
Farre tubercles
Farrell applicator
Farrell nasal applicator
Farrington forceps
Farrington nasal polyp forceps
Farrington septum forceps
Farrior anterior footplate pick
Farrior applicator
Farrior blunt palpator
Farrior bur
Farrior chuck handle
Farrior ear speculum
Farrior excavator
Farrior flap exposure instru-
    ments
Farrior footplate pick
Farrior forceps
Farrior knife
Farrior oval ear speculum
Farrior oval speculum
Farrior oval-window excavator
Farrior oval-window pick
Farrior oval-window piston
    gauge excavator
Farrior posterior footplate pick

Farrior raspatory
Farrior speculum
Farrior wire-crimping forceps
Farrior-Derlacki chisel
Farrior-Dworacek canal chisel
Farrior-Joseph nasal saw
Farrior-McHugh knife
Farrior-Shambaugh elevator
Farris elevator
Farris tissue forceps
Fasanella cannula
Fasanella iris retractor
Fasanella operation
Fasanella retractor
Fasanella-Servat operation
Fasanella-Servat ptosis correc-
    tion procedure
Fasano test during rhizotomy
fascia (*pl.* fasciae)
fascia bulbi
fascia graft
fascia lata
fascia lata femoris
fascia lata graft
fascia lata implant
fascia lata prosthesis
fascia lata sling operation
fascia needle
fascia stripper
fascia transversalis
fasciae (*sing.* fascia)
fascial
fascial arthroplasty
fascial cleft
fascial defect
fascial flap
fascial graft
fascial layer
fascial planes
fascial sheath
fascial sling for facial
    paralysis
fascial stranding
fasciaplasty
fascicle
fascicular graft

fascicular heart block
fasciculated bladder
fasciculation
fasciculation potential
fasciculi (*sing.* fasciculus)
fasciculoventricular bypass tract
fasciculoventricular connection
fasciculus (*pl.* fasciculi)
fasciculus aberrans of Monakow
fasciculus cuneatus
fasciculus gracilis
fasciculus lenticularis
fasciculus of Gowers
fasciculus of Rolando
fasciectomy
fasciitis
fasciodesis
fasciogram
fascioplasty
fasciorrhaphy
fascioscapulohumeral
fasciotome
        Luck fasciotome
fasciotomy
fashion
FAST balloon catheter (flow-
    assisted, short-term balloon
    catheter)
fast twitch muscle
Fast-Fit vascular stocking
Fast-Pass endocardial lead
Fast-Pass lead pacemaker
Fastrak scanner
Fastrak traction material
Fastrak traction strip dressing
fat deposits
fat embolism
fat embolization
fat embolus
fat graft
fat hernia
fat marrow
fat necrosis
fat pad
fat towels
fat transplant

fatal complications
fatal heart attack
fatal seizure
fatality rate
fatigability
fatigue
fatigue fracture
fatigued
fat-pad retractor
fat-pad sign
fatty ascites
fatty atrophy
fatty capsule of kidney
fatty cardiopathy
fatty deposits
fatty liver
fatty material
fatty tissue
fatty tumor
faucet aspirator
Faucher stomach tube
faucial and lingual tonsillec-
    tomy
faucial arch
faucial area
faucial catheter
faucial eustachian catheter
faucial reflex
faucial tonsil
faucial tonsillectomy
Faught sphygmomanometer
Faulkner antrum chisel
Faulkner antrum curet
Faulkner antrum gouge
Faulkner chisel
Faulkner curet
Faulkner ethmoid curet
Faulkner nasal curet
Faulkner trocar
Faulkner trocar chisel
Faulkner-Browne chisel
faulty valve action
Faure forceps
Faure uterine biopsy forceps
Fauvel forceps
Fauvel laryngeal forceps
Favoloro atrial retractor
Favoloro ligature carrier

Favoloro proximal anastomosis
    clamp
Favoloro retractor
Favoloro scissors
Favoloro self-retaining sternal
    retractor set
Favoloro sternal retractor
Favoloro tunneler
Favoloro-Morse sternal spreader
Favorite clamp
Fay suction elevator
Fay suction tube
Fazio-Montgomery cannula
Fazio-Montgomery tube
FB (fingerbreadths)
FB (foreign body)
FCR (flexor carpi radialis)
FCU (flexor carpi ulnaris)
FDB (flexor digitorum brevis)
FDL (flexor digitorum longus)
FDM (flexor digiti minimi)
FDP (flexor digitorum profun-
    dus)
FDQ (flexor digiti quinti)
FDS (flexor digitorum
    sublimis)
FDS (flexor digitorum superfi-
    cialis)
feather clamp
febrile convulsion
febrile reaction
febrile state
fecal
fecal contents
fecal excretion
fecal fistula
fecal impaction
fecal incontinence
fecal material
fecal obstruction
fecal reservoir
fecal residue
fecalith
fecalith obstruction
fecal-oral route
feces
feces and gas
Fechner intraocular implant lens

Fechner lens
fecopurulent
Federici sign
Federov eye implant
Federov implant
Federov lens implant
Federov operation
Federov splenectomy
Federov type I lens implant
Federov type II lens implant
Federspiel cheek retractor
Federspiel needle
Federspiel periosteal elevator
Federspiel scissors
feeble pulse
feedback
feeding gastrostomy
feeding gastrostomy tube
feeding tube
Fegerstra wire
Fehland clamp
Fehland intestinal clamp
Fehland right-angled colon
    clamp
Feilchenfeld forceps
Feilchenfeld splinter forceps
Fein antrum trocar
Fein cannula
Fein needle
Fein trocar
Feist-Mankin position
Feldbausch dilator
Feldenkrais method
Feldman lip retractor
Feldman retractor
Feldstein blepharoplasty clip
Feleky instrument
Felig insulin pump
Fell sucker tip
Fell-O'Dwyer apparatus
felon
Felson silhouette sign
felt dressing
felt pads
felt patch
felt strip
felt-collar splint
felt-foam padding

felt-gauze pad
female catheter
female catheter-dilator
female cystoscope
female reproductive organs
female urethroscope
fem-fem bypass (femoral-
    femoral bypass)
femoral
femoral AP-sizing guide
femoral arteriogram
femoral arteriography
femoral arteriotomy
femoral artery
femoral artery cannula
femoral artery decannulation
femoral artery sheath
femoral bone
femoral broach
femoral bypass
femoral canal
femoral clamp
femoral component
femoral component pusher
femoral condyle
femoral condyle plate
femoral cortex
femoral crossover bypass
femoral dislocation
femoral displacement
femoral embolectomy
femoral epiphysis
femoral fracture
femoral graft
femoral guiding catheter
femoral head
femoral head extractor
femoral head prosthesis
femoral head reamer
femoral head saw
femoral hernia
femoral hernia repair
femoral herniorrhaphy
femoral intermuscular septum
femoral length
femoral ligament
femoral muscle
femoral neck

femoral neck fracture
femoral neck reamer
femoral neck retractor
femoral nerve
femoral nerve traction test
femoral nodes
femoral plate
femoral prosthesis
femoral prosthetic broach
femoral prosthetic head
femoral prosthetic pusher
femoral pulse
femoral pusher
femoral reflex
femoral resector
femoral septum
femoral shaft
femoral shaft rasp
femoral sheath
femoral shortening osteotomy
femoral sizer
femoral splint
femoral tensor
femoral torque
femoral trials
femoral triangle
femoral vein
femoral vein cannulation
femoral vein decannulation
femoral vein-femoral artery
    bypass
femoral-femoral bypass (fem-
    fem bypass)
femoral-inguinal herniorrhaphy
femoralis, arteria
femoralis, nervus
femoralis, vena
femoral-peroneal in situ vein
    bypass graft
femoral-popliteal bypass (fem-
    pop bypass)
femoral-popliteal bypass graft
    (FPB graft)
femoral-popliteal occlusive
    disease
femoral-tibial bypass (fem-tib
    bypass)

femoral-tibial-peroneal bypass
femoroaxillary bypass
femorocele
femorodistal bypass
femorodistal vein graft
femorofemoral bypass
femorofemoral crossover bypass
femorofemoral crossover
    prosthesis
femoroiliac
femoropopliteal bypass
femoropopliteal bypass graft
femoropopliteal saphenous vein
    bypass
femoropopliteal vein
femorotibial
femorotibial bypass
fem-pop bypass (femoral-
    popliteal bypass)
fem-tib bypass (femoral-tibial
    bypass)
femtoliter (fL, fl)
femtomole
femur
fence splint
fenestra (*pl.* fenestrae)
fenestra bone graft
fenestra choledocha
fenestra cochleae
fenestra implant
fenestra ovalis
fenestra prosthesis
fenestra rotunda
fenestra vestibuli
fenestrae (*sing.* fenestra)
fenestrated blade forceps
fenestrated catheter
fenestrated compress
fenestrated cup biopsy forceps
fenestrated Drake clip
fenestrated drape
fenestrated forceps
fenestrated hymen
fenestrated lens scoop
fenestrated membrane
fenestrated septum
fenestrated sheet

fenestrated sterile drape
fenestrated tracheostomy tube
fenestrated tube
fenestrated valve
fenestrating
fenestration
fenestration bur
fenestration cavity
fenestration curet
fenestration elevator
fenestration excavator
fenestration hook
fenestration instruments
fenestration of semicircular
    canal
fenestration operation
fenestration saw
fenestrator
        Rosen fenestrator
fenestrometer
        Paparella fenestrometer
Fenger forceps
Fenger gall duct probe
Fenger gallbladder probe
Fenger gallstone probe
Fenger probe
Fenger spiral gallstone probe
fentanyl anesthesia
fentanyl citrate
Fenton bolt
Fenton bulldog vulsellum
Fenton dilator
Fenton nail
Fenton operation
Fenzel hook
FEP-ringed Gore-Tex vascular
    graft
Ferciot splint
Ferciot technique
Ferciot wire guide
Feree-Rand perimeter
Fergus operation
Fergus percutaneous introducer
    kit
Ferguson abdominal scissors
Ferguson angiotribe
Ferguson angiotribe forceps

Ferguson basket
Ferguson bone curet
Ferguson bone-holding forceps
Ferguson brain suction tube
Ferguson curet
Ferguson forceps
Ferguson gallstone scoop
Ferguson implant
Ferguson inguinal hernior-
    rhaphy
Ferguson mouth gag
Ferguson needle
Ferguson probang
Ferguson probe
Ferguson retractor
Ferguson scissors
Ferguson scoop
Ferguson stone basket
Ferguson suture needle
Ferguson technique
Ferguson tenaculum
Ferguson-Ackland mouth gag
Ferguson-Brophy mouth gag
Ferguson-Coley operation
Ferguson-Frazier suction tube
Ferguson-Gwathmey mouth gag
Ferguson-Metzenbaum scissors
Ferguson-Moon rectal retractor
Ferguson-Moon retractor
Ferguson-Thompson-King
    osteotomy
Fergusson bone knife
Fergusson excision of maxilla
Fergusson incision
Fergusson operation
Fergusson speculum
Fergusson tubular vaginal
    speculum
Ferkel technique
fermentation tube
fern test
Fernandez osteotomy
Ferrein canal
Ferris biliary duct dilator
Ferris colporrhaphy forceps
Ferris common duct scoop
Ferris dilator

Ferris filiform dilator
Ferris forceps
Ferris scoop
Ferris Smith bone-biting forceps
Ferris Smith cup rongeur
    forceps
Ferris Smith elevator
Ferris Smith forceps
Ferris Smith fragment forceps
Ferris Smith intervertebral disk
    rongeur
Ferris Smith knife
Ferris Smith needle holder
Ferris Smith operation
Ferris Smith pituitary rongeur
Ferris Smith punch
Ferris Smith retractor
Ferris Smith rongeur
Ferris Smith tissue forceps
Ferris Smith-Gruenwald punch
Ferris Smith-Gruenwald rongeur
Ferris Smith-Gruenwald
    sphenoid punch
Ferris Smith-Halle bur
Ferris Smith-Halle sinus bur
Ferris Smith-Kerrison neurosur-
    gical ronguer
Ferris Smith-Kerrison rongeur
Ferris Smith-Kerrison rongeur
    forceps
Ferris Smith-Lyman periosteo-
    tome
Ferris Smith-Sewall orbital
    retractor
Ferris Smith-Sewall retractor
Ferris Smith-Spurling rongeur
Ferris Smith-Takahashi forceps
Ferris Smith-Takahashi rongeur
Ferris tissue forceps
Ferris-Robb knife
Ferris-Robb tonsil knife
ferromagnetic
ferromagnetic silicone
ferromagnetic tamponade
ferrule
ferrule clamp
fetal abnormality

fetal age
fetal basiotripsy
fetal blood-sampling instrument
fetal cardiac activity
fetal circulation
fetal cleidotomy
fetal cord
fetal cord clamp
fetal cranial diameters
fetal cranioclasis
fetal craniotomy
fetal death
fetal decelerations
fetal distress
fetal giantism
fetal growth parameters
fetal growth retardation
fetal head
fetal head extractor
fetal heart
fetal heart sounds (FHS)
fetal heart tones (FHT)
fetal hydrops
fetal ischiopubiotomy
fetal lie
fetal lung maturity
fetal macrosomia
fetal malrotation
fetal membranes
fetal monitor
fetal movement
fetal pelvic disproportion
fetal placenta
fetal pole
fetal position
fetal respiration
fetal rhythm
fetal small parts
fetal somatic activity
fetal stethoscope
fetal substantia nigra implants
fetal tissue
fetal viability
fetal wastage
fetogram
fetography
fetomaternal hemorrhage

fetopelvic disproportion
fetoscope
fetoscopy
fetus
fetus expulsion
Feuerstein ear tube
Feuerstein myringotomy drain
    tube
fever
FHB (flexor hallucis brevis)
FHS (fetal heart sounds)
FHT (fetal heart tones)
FIA (fluorescent immunoassay)
fiber
fiber cell
fiber of Remak
fibercolonoscope
fiberduodenoscope
fibergastroscope
fiberglass
fiberglass casting tape
fiberglass graft
fiberglass sleeve trocar
fiberhead hammer
fiber-illuminated
fibermallet
fiberoptic
fiberoptic anoscope
fiberoptic bronchoscope
fiberoptic bronchoscopy (FOB)
fiberoptic cable
fiberoptic cable adapter
fiberoptic cold light source
fiberoptic culdoscope
fiberoptic cystoscope
fiberoptic endoscope
fiberoptic esophagoscope
fiberoptic gastroscope
fiberoptic headlight
fiberoptic hysteroscope
fiberoptic instrument
fiberoptic laryngoscope
fiberoptic lens
fiberoptic light
fiberoptic light bundle
fiberoptic light cable
fiberoptic light carrier

fiberoptic light cord
fiberoptic light source
fiberoptic lighted suction tube
fiberoptic Lite-Piper cable
fiberoptic otoscope
fiberoptic panendoscope
fiberoptic photographic sheath
fiberoptic probe
fiberoptic proctosigmoidoscope
fiberoptic right-angle telescope
fiberoptic sheath
fiberoptic sigmoidoscope
fiberoptic system
fiberoptic telescope
fiberoptic tube
fiberoptics
fibers
fiberscope
    bronchofiberscope
    gastroduodenal fiber-
        scope
    gastrofiberscope
    Hirschowitz fiberscope
    Olympus choledocho-
        fiberscope
    Olympus duodenofiber-
        scope
    Olympus esophagofiber-
        scope
    Olympus fiberscope
    Olympus ureteroreno-
        fiberscope
    Pentax colonofiberscope
    SC-5A fiberscope
    side-viewing fiberscope
fiberscopic transduodenal duct
    injection
Fibrel gelatin matrix implant
fibrillar mass of Flemming
fibrillar twitching
fibrillary contractions
fibrillary glia
fibrillary tremor
fibrillary waves
fibrillate
fibrillating action potentials
fibrillating waves

fibrillation
fibrillation potential
fibrillator subclavian-subclavian
    bypass
fibrillatory tremors
fibrils
fibrin
fibrin bodies
fibrin calculus
fibrin deposit
fibrin film
fibrin foam
fibrin glue
fibrin peel
fibrin plug
fibrin sponge
Fibrindex test
fibrinolytic hemorrhage
fibrinopurulent
fibrinous
fibrinous bronchitis
fibrinous material
fibrinous pericarditis
fibrinous tissue
fibroadenoma
fibroadenomatous hyperplasia
    of prostate
fibroadenosis
fibroadipose tissue
fibroblastoma
fibrocalcareous disease
fibrocalcareous scarring
fibrocalcific
fibrocartilage
fibrocartilaginous
fibrocartilaginous disk
fibrocartilaginous joint
fibrocartilaginous material
fibrocaseous
fibrocystic
fibrocystic disease
fibrocystic nodules
fibroelastosis
fibroepithelial polyp
fibroepithelial polypoid
    anorectal lesion
fibrofatty tissue

fibrohyaline nodule
fibrohyaline tissue
fibroid
fibroid cataract
fibroid heart
fibroid hook
fibroid induration
fibroid of uterus
fibroid tumor of uterus
fibroid uterus
fibroidectomy
fibrolipomatous tissue
fibroma (*pl.* fibromas, fibro-
    mata)
fibromatosis
fibromatosis gingivae
fibromectomy
fibrometer
fibromuscular
fibromuscular hyperplasia
fibromuscular junction
fibromuscular stoma
fibromuscular walls
fibromyelinic plaques
fibromyoma (*pl.* fibromyomas,
    fibromyomata)
fibromyomata uteri
fibromyomectomy
fibromyotomy
fibroplasia
fibroplastic endocarditis
fibrosarcoma
fibrosing myopathy
fibrosis
fibrotic
fibrotic changes
fibrotic infiltration
fibrotic markings
fibrotic mitral valve
fibrotic scarring
fibrotic strands
fibrous
fibrous anal tags
fibrous ankylosis
fibrous appendix hepatis
fibrous capsule
fibrous connective tissue

fibrous dysplasia
fibrous goiter
fibrous joint
fibrous membrane
fibrous nodule
fibrous organ
fibrous process
fibrous renal capsule
fibrous sac
fibrous sheath
fibrous tissue
fibrous union
fibrovascular polyp
fibrovascular stroma
fibula
fibular
fibular artery
fibular bone
fibular collateral ankle sprain
fibular collateral ligament
fibular facet
fibular head
fibular muscle
fibular neck
fibular nerve
fibular notch
fibular shaft
fibular veins
fibulares, venae
fibularis, nervus
fibulocalcaneal
fibulotalar joint
Ficat staging for avascular
    necrosis (I–IV)
Fick halo
Fick measurement of cardiac
    output
Fick operation
Fick perforation of footplate
Fick position
Fick technique
fiddle-string adhesions
field
field block
field block anesthesia
field gradient
field lock

field of vision (FOV)
field size
Fielding classification
fifth cranial nerve (V)
fifth intercostal space
FIGO (International Federation
    of Gynecology and
    Obstetrics)
FIGO staging of carcinoma of
    reproductive system
figure-eight cast
figure-eight dressing
figure-four position
figure-four test
figure-of-eight bandage
figure-of-eight dressing
figure-of-eight sutures
fil d'Arion tube
filament
filament sutures
filamented form
filamentous adhesion
filamentous appendage
filamentous component
filamentous form
filariasis
Filatov keratoplasty
Filatov operation
Filatov-Marzinkowsky operation
file
        bone file
file elevator
filiform
filiform bougie
filiform bougie probe
filiform catheter
filiform dressing
filiform follower
filiform guide
filiform implantation
filiform Jackson bougie
filiform papillae
filiform pulse
filiform stone dislodger
filiforms and followers
filiform-tipped catheter
filipuncture

Fillauer bar
Fillauer night splint
Fillauer splint
filler graft
fillet
filleting
filling defect
filling factor
filling of bladder
filling of pulp canal
filling of right atrium
film
    absorbable film
    absorbable gelatin film
    Bucky film
    chest film
    cines and plain films
    comparison film
    decubitus film
    Durafilm
    dural film sheeting
    fibrin film
    gallbladder film
    gelatin film
    gelatinous film
    glycocalyx-enclosed
      biofilm
    Heyer-Schulte dural film
      sheeting
    lateral film
    localization films
    oblique film
    PA film (posteroanterior
      film)
    Panorex film
    plain film
    plain film of abdomen
    Polaroid film
    portable film
    posteroanterior film (PA
      film)
    postevacuation film
    postreduction film
    postvoiding film
    pre-evacuation film
    preliminary film
    prereduction film

film *continued*
    recumbent film
    scout film
    semiupright film
    serial films
    skull film
    spot film
    strain film
    subtraction films
    sulfa film
    supine film
    surgical film
    Telfa plastic film
    translateral film
    upright film
    Vi-Drape surgical film
film dosimetry
film oxygenator
film packs
filmy adhesions
filmy tongue
filopressure
Filshie clip
filter
    Amicon diafilter
    Bentley filter
    caval filter
    Gianturco-Roehm bird's
      nest vena caval filter
    Greenfield filter
    Greenfield inferior vena
      caval filter
    Greenfield vena caval
      filter
    Kimray-Greenfield anti-
      embolus filter
    Kimray-Greenfield filter
    Kimray-Greenfield vena
      caval filter
    mediastinal sump filter
    Millipore filter
    Mobin-Uddin filter
    Mobin-Uddin umbrella
      filter
    Mobin-Uddin vena caval
      filter
    platinum filter

filter *continued*
    umbrella filter
    vena caval umbrella
      filter
    Wrattan eye filter
filtered
filtered-back projection
filtering cicatrix
filtering operation
filtration
filtration rate
Filtzer corkscrew
Filtzer interbody rasp
filum terminale
fimbria (*pl.* fimbriae)
fimbria ovarica
fimbrial repair kit
fimbriated
fimbriated end
fimbriated fold
fimbriated oviduct
fimbriectomy
fimbrioplasty
fin
final closure
final diagnosis
final impression
final pathological diagnosis
final stage of labor
findings
Findley folding pessary
fine artery forceps
fine cautery
fine chromic sutures
fine crepitant rales
fine curet
fine forceps
fine moist rales
fine needle
fine plain catgut
fine rales
Fine scissors
fine silk sutures
Fine suture-tying forceps
fine sutures
fine tremor
fine-angled curet

Fine-Castroviejo suturing
    forceps
fine-dissecting forceps
fine-dissecting scissors
Fine-Gill corneal knife
fine-mesh dressing
fine-mesh gauze
fine-needle aspiration (FNA)
fine-needle aspiration biopsy
    (FNAB)
fine-needle aspiration cytology
    (FNAC)
fine-needle biopsy
fine-needle electrode
fine-needle percutaneous
    cholangiogram
fine-needle transhepatic
    cholangiogram
fine-pointed hemostat
Finesse aspiration system
Finesse guiding catheter
Finesse large-lumen guiding
    catheter
fine-stitch scissors
fine-suture scissors
fine-tissue forceps
fine-toothed clamp
fine-toothed forceps
fine-wire electrode
finger agnosia
finger cot
finger dissection
finger drop
finger flap
finger flexion reflex
finger fracture
finger fracture dissection
finger fracture technique
finger goniometer
finger jerk
finger joint implant
finger motion
finger plate
finger prick test
finger prosthesis
finger pursuit drift
finger rake retractor

finger retractor
finger ring cutter
finger ring saw
finger splint
finger tamponade
finger vision
fingerbreadth (*pl.* finger-
    breadths) (FB)
finger-cot dressing
finger-cot pack
finger-cot splint
finger-like villi
fingernail
fingernail drill
finger-thumb reflex
fingertip
fingertip amputation
fingertip fracture
fingertip lesion
finishing ball reamer
finishing cup reamer
Fink cataract operation
Fink chalazion curet
Fink curet
Fink fixation forceps
Fink forceps
Fink hook
Fink irrigator
Fink lacrimal retractor
Fink laryngoscope
Fink muscle hook
Fink retractor
Fink tendon tucker
Fink tucker
Finkelstein sign for synovitis
Fink-Jameson forceps
Fink-Jameson oblique muscle
    forceps
Fink-Rowland keratome
Finn chamber patch test device
finned pacemaker lead
Finney gastroduodenostomy
Finney gastroenterostomy
Finney operation
Finney penile implant
Finney penile prosthesis
Finney prosthesis

Finney pyloroplasty
Finney-flexirod penile prosthe-
    sis
Finnoff laryngoscope
Finnoff transilluminator
Finochietto artery clamp
Finochietto clamp
Finochietto clamp carrier
Finochietto forceps
Finochietto laminectomy
    retractor
Finochietto lobectomy forceps
Finochietto needle
Finochietto needle holder
Finochietto operation
Finochietto retractor
Finochietto rib retractor
Finochietto rib spreader
Finochietto scissors
Finochietto spreader
FInochietto stirrup
Finochietto thoracic forceps
Finochietto thoracic scissors
Finochietto Vital needle
    holder
Finochietto-Billroth I gastrec-
    tomy
Finochietto-Geissendorfer rib
    retractor
Finsen carbon arc light
Finsen retractor
Finsen-Reya light
Finsterer operation
Finsterer suction tube
Finsterer sutures
Finsterer-Hofmeister operation
Finzi-Harmer operation
Firland nebulizer
Firlene eye magnet
firm cell mass
firm tissue
firm uterus
first impression
FIRST instrumentation with
    Synatomic Total Knee
    System
first stage of labor

first trimester of pregnancy
first-degree burn (1st-degree
   burn)
first-degree sprain
first-pass nuclide rest and
   exercise angiogram
first-pass radionuclide angio-
   gram
first-pass scintigraphy
first-pass technique
first-stage draining of liver
   abscess
first-stage procedure
first-toe Jones repair
Fisch drill
Fisch dural hook
Fischer arthrodesis
Fischer needle
Fischer pneumothoracic needle
Fischer shunt
Fischer sign
Fischer syringe
Fischl forceps
Fischl skin hook
Fischmann angiotribe forceps
Fischmann urethroplasty
Fish antral probe
Fish forceps
Fish grasping forceps
Fish nasal forceps
Fish sinus probe
fish vertebrae
Fisher advancement forceps
Fisher bed
Fisher brace
Fisher cannula
Fisher capsular forceps
Fisher eye needle
Fisher forceps
Fisher guide
Fisher knife
Fisher needle
Fisher operation
Fisher quartz "cold" generator
Fisher rasp
Fisher retractor
Fisher spoon

Fisher spud
Fisher tape board
Fisher technique
Fisher tonsil dissector
Fisher tonsil knife
Fisher tonsil retractor
Fisher ventricular cannula
Fisher-Arlt forceps
Fisher-Arlt iris forceps
fisherman's pliers
Fisher-Nugent retractor
Fisher-Smith spatula
fish-flesh consistency
fishhook
fishhook needle
fish-mouth amputation
fish-mouth cervix
fish-mouth incision
fish-mouth mitral stenosis
fish-mouth suture
fishnet pattern
fish-scale gallbladder
fishtail chisel
fishtail raspatory
fishtail spatula
Fiske periosteal elevator
fissula
fissure
fissure bur
fissure forceps
fissure fracture
fissure in ano
fissurectomy
fissured fracture
fissuring
fist percussion
fistula (*pl.* fistulas, fistulae)
fistular closure
fistular hook
fistular knife
fistular needle
fistular probe
fistulation
fistulatome
fistulectomy
fistulization
fistuloenterostomy

fistulogram
fistulography
fistulotome
fistulotome knife
fistulotomy
fistulous
fistulous tract
Fitzgerald aortic aneurysm
    forceps
Fitzgerald forceps
Fitzpatrick suction tube
Fitzwater forceps
Fitzwater ligature carrier
Fitzwater peanut sponge-
    holding forceps
five-in-one repair
fixation
fixation anchor
fixation apparatus
fixation bandage
fixation device
fixation forceps
fixation graft
fixation hook
fixation in vivo
fixation pin
fixation point
fixation ring
fixation sutures
fixation test
fixation with osteogenesis
fixative
fixative solution
fixator
fixator muscle of base of stapes
fixator muscles
fixed appliance
fixed arch bar
fixed bridge
fixed dressing
fixed perfusion defect
fixed-rate asynchronous atrial
    pacemaker
fixed-rate asynchronous
    ventricular pacemaker
fixed-rate pacemaker
fixing screw

fixing time
fL, fl (femtoliter)
FL pheresis (filtration
    leukapheresis)
FL4 guide
flaccid
flaccidity
Flack node
Flagg laryngoscope
flail
flail chest
flail extremity
flail joint
flail mitral valve
Flajani operation
flaking
flaking skin
Flanagan gouge
Flanagan spinal fusion gouge
Flanagan-Burem graft
flange
    Callahan flange
    Coloplast flange
    dental flange
    hip flange
    labial flange
    lingual flange
    Scuderi-Callahan flange
    Syed template flange
flange of Syed template
flank
flank area
flank bone
flank incision
flank pain
flank stripe
flank tenderness
flank wound
flank-strip sign on supine
    abdominal film
Flannery ear speculum
Flannery speculum
flap
    Abbé flap
    Abbé lip flap
    Abbé-Estlander flap
    abdominothoracic flap

flap *continued*

Abrams-Lucas flap heart valve
advancement flap
advancement of rectal flap
artery island flap
avulsion flap injury
Bakamjian flap
Bakamjian pedicle flap
Bakamjian tubed flap
Beer cataract flap operation
Berens mastectomy skin flap retractor
Berens skin flap retractor
bilobed flap
bilobed skin flap
bipedicle digital visor flap
bipedicle flap
bipedicle mucoperiosteal flap
bladder flap
Boari flap
Boari-Küss flap
Boari-Ockerblad flap reimplantation
bone flap
bridge flap
buccal pedicle-flap operation
Bunnell bipedicle digital visor flap
Bunnell flap
Burow flap
butterfly flap
Byers flap
canthomeatal flap
cellulocutaneous flap
Charretera flap
cheek flap
chondrocutaneous flap
circular flap
closed flap
composite flap
compound flap

flap *continued*

compound skin flap
conchal flap
conjunctival flap
corneal flap
coronoid flap
Crane flap
craniotomy flap
Cronin-Matthews eave flap
cross-arm flap
cross-finger flap
cross-leg flap
cross-leg skin flap
Cutler flap
Cutler-Beard bridge flap
deflected skin flap
delayed flap
delayed skin flap
delayed transfer flap
developed flap
direct transfer flap
distal flap
distant flap
distant skin flap
dorsal flap
double-end flap
double-ended flap
double-pedicle flap
double-pedicle skin flap
Eloesser flap
envelope flap
esophagogastric flap valve
Estlander flap
fascial flap
finger flap
fleur-de-lis flap
fleur-de-lis forehead flap
forehead flap
fornix-based conjunctival flap
free flap
French flap
French sliding flap
gauntlet flap
Gillies flap

flap *continued*

Gillies up-and-down flap
Gunderson conjunctival flap
Gunter Von Noorden flap
H-flap
horseshoe flap
horseshoe-shaped skin flap
HUMI cervical forceps skate flap
immediate transfer flap
Imre flap operation
Indian flap
Indian rotation flap
Indian skin flap operation
interpolated flap
inverted horseshoe flap
island flap
island leg flap
island pedicle flaps
Italian distant flap
Italian flap
jump flap
jump skin flap
Juri skin flap
Kapetansky flap
Karadanzic flap
Knapp flap operation
Koerner flap
Kutler V-Y flaps
Langenbeck flap
Langenbeck pedicle mucoperiosteal flap
leg flap
LeMesurier rectangular flap
Limberg flap
lingual tongue flap
Linton flap
lip flap
liver flap
local flap
localized advancement flap

flap *continued*

long rectangular flap
MacFee neck flap
marsupial flap
marsupial skin flap
McGregor forehead flap
McHugh flap knife
medial flap
Millard forehead flap
Millard island flap
Monks-Esser flap
Monks-Esser island flap
Morrison toe flap
mucoperiosteal flap
mucoperiosteal pedicle flap
muscle flap
musculocutaneous flap
myocutaneous flap
Nahai tensor fascia lata flap
Nahigian butterfly flap
Nassif parascapular flap
osteoplastic flap
over-and-out cheek flap
parrot-beak flap
pedicle flap
pedicle mucoperiosteal flap
pharyngeal flap
posterolateral flap
raised skin flaps
RAM flap (rectus abdominis myocutaneous flap)
rectangular flap
rectus abdominis myocutaneous flap (RAM flap)
reflected skin flap
rollflap
rope flap
rotation advancement flap
rotation flap
rotation skin flap
rotational flap graft

flap *continued*
    S-flap incision
    sandwich flap
    scleral flap
    Sewell-Boyden flap
    short rectangular flap
    skate flap
    skin flap
    sliding flap
    spiral flap
    Stein-Abbé lip flap
    Stein-Kazanjian flap
    Stenstrom foot flap
    surgical flap
    switch flap
    synovial flap
    Tagliacozzi flap
    Tait flap
    Tenzel semicircular flap
    Tham flap
    thenar flap
    Thom flap
    Truc flap
    tube flap
    tubed pedicle flap
    tumble flap
    tumbler flap
    tumbler skin flap
    tunnel flap
    tympanomeatal flap
    tympanotomy flap
    up-and-down flap
    V-Y advancement flap
    V-Y flap
    Van Lint conjunctival flap
    Vasconez tensor fascia
       lata flap
    volar flap
    von Langenbeck
       bipedicle mucoperios-
       teal flap
    von Langenbeck flap
    Von Noorden flap
    waltzed skin flap
    Washio skin flap
    Weir pattern skin flap
       technique

flap *continued*
    winged-V flap
    Wookey neck flap
    Z-flap
    Zimany bilobed flap
    Zimany flap
flap advancement procedure
flap amputation
flap elevator
flap knife
flap of conjunctiva
flap of periosteum
flap operation
flap otoplasty
flap rotation
flap scissors
flap technique
flap valve after hiatal hernia
    repair
flapless amputation
flapping of conjunctiva
flapping sound
flapping tremor
flapping tremor sign
flap-type laceration
flap-valve mechanism
flare
flare-up
flaring
flaring of nostrils
flaring tool
flash burn
flash generator
flash ophthalmia
flash pan
flash stimulation
flash tube
flashlight
flask
flask-shaped heart
flat abdomen
flat chest
flat curve
flat drill
flat electrocardiogram
flat encephalogram
flat eye bandage

flat eye spud
flat feet
flat hand
flat lip
flat pelvis
flat plate
flat plate of abdomen
flat spatula
flat spatula needle
flat sutures
flat zonule separator
flat-blade-tipped catheter
flatfoot
flats of dressing
Flatt driver
Flatt prosthesis
Flatt thumb prosthesis
flattened
flattened duodenal fold
flattened nose
flattening
flattening of T-wave
flat-tip electrode
flatulent
flatus
flat-wire eye electrode
flaval ligament
flavectomy
Flaxedil sutures
Flayol-Grant erysiphake
fleck of barium
Fleck preparation
Fleet bowel prep
Fleet enema
fleeting chest pain
Fleischer corneal ring
Fleischer ring
Fleischner lines
Fleming conization instrument
Fleming conization of cervix
Fleming operation
flesh
flesh trabeculae of heart
Fletcher afterloading colpostat
Fletcher afterloading tandem
Fletcher AL tandem (afterload-
    ing tandem)

Fletcher dressing forceps
Fletcher forceps
Fletcher knife
Fletcher loading applicator
Fletcher tandem
Fletcher tonsil knife
Fletcher-Pierce cannula
Fletcher-Suit afterloading
    applicator
Fletcher-Suit afterloading
    tandem
Fletcher-Suit application
Fletcher-Suit applicator
Fletcher-Suit polyp forceps
Fletcher-Van Doren forceps
Fletcher-Van Doren sponge-
    holding forceps
Fletcher-Van Doren uterine
    forceps
Fletcher-Van Doren uterine
    polyp forceps
Fletcher-Van Doren uterine
    polyp sponge-holding
    forceps
fleur-de-lis flap
fleur-de-lis forehead flap
fleurette
Flex foam dressing
Flex guide wire
Flex-Aid knuckle dressing
flexed incision
Flexguide intubation
Flexguide intubation guide
flexibility
flexible biopsy instrument
flexible bronchoscopic biopsy
    instrument
flexible catheter
flexible dental suction
flexible Dualens implant
flexible endoscope
flexible erection
flexible esophageal conductor
flexible fiberoptic sigmoido-
    scopy
flexible fiberoptic system
flexible foreign body forceps

flexible gastroscope
flexible guide wire
flexible injection needle
flexible laparoscopic instruments
flexible metal catheter
flexible penile prosthesis
flexible pes planus
flexible probe
flexible radiothermal electrode
flexible retractor
flexible rod penile implant
flexible round silicone rod
flexible rubber endoscopic tube
flexible rubber tube
flexible shaft retractor
flexible sigmoidoscope
flexible steerable wire
flexible suction tube
flexible tourniquet
flexible tubing
flexible-J guide wire
Flexicair low-air-loss bed
Flexicath silicone subclavian cannula
Flexicon elastic gauze
Flexicon gauze bandage
Flexi-Flate II penile implant
Flexi-Flate inflatable penile prosthesis
Flexi-Flate penile implant
Flexilite conforming elastic bandage
Flexilite gauze bandage
Flexinet dressing
flexing
flexion
flexion, abduction, external rotation, extension (fabere)
flexion, abduction, internal rotation (fadir)
flexion contracture
flexion crease
flexion position
flexion reflex
flexion skin lines
flexion-extension projection

Flexi-rod II penile implant
Flexi-rod penile prosthesis
Flexi-rod semirigid penile prosthesis
Flexiscope arthroscope
Flexisplint flexed-arm board
Flexitip catheter
Flex-i-Tip
Flexitone sutures
Flexlens
Flex-Lok pegs
Flexon steel sutures
Flexon sutures
flexor carpi radialis, musculus (FCR)
flexor carpi ulnaris, musculus (FCU)
flexor digiti minimi brevis manus, musculus
flexor digiti minimi brevis pedis, musculus
flexor digiti minimi, musculus (FDM)
flexor digiti quinti, musculus (FDQ)
flexor digitorum brevis, musculus (FDB)
flexor digitorum brevis pedis, musculus
flexor digitorum longus, musculus (FDL)
flexor digitorum longus pedis, musculus
flexor digitorum profundus, musculus (FDP)
flexor digitorum sublimis, musculus (FDS)
flexor digitorum superficialis, musculus (FDS)
flexor hallucis brevis, musculus (FHB)
flexor hallucis longus, musculus (FHL)
flexor hinge hand splint brace
flexor muscle
flexor origin
flexor origin syndrome

flexor pollicis brevis, musculus (FPB)
flexor pollicis longus, musculus (FPL)
flexor retinaculum
flexor tendon
flexor tone
flexor wad of five
flexor zone
flexorplasty
Flexsteel retractor
Flexsteel ribbon retractor
flexure
flexure line
flexure of colon
flexure of duodenum
flexure of rectum
flexure skin lines
Flieringa fixation ring
Flieringa scleral ring
flip angle
floaters
floating cartilage
floating catheter
floating disk heart valve
floating gallbladder
floating gallstone
floating kidney
floating knee
floating patella
floating ribs
floating spleen
floating thumb
floor cells
floor of mouth
floor of orbit
floor of orifice
floppy mitral valve
floppy disk
floppy guide wire
floppy valve syndrome
floppy-tipped guide
floppy-tipped guide wire
floppy-type of Nissen fundoplication
Florentine iris
Florester vascular occluder

florid duct lesion
Florida brace
floridic pain
floriform cataract
flotation catheter
flow capacity
flow cytometry of DNA
flow mapping technique
flow of blood
flow of urinary stream
flow probe
flow rate
flow tract
flow volume
flow-cytometry analysis
flow-directed balloon-tipped catheter
flow-directed catheter
flowmeter
    Doppler flowmeter
    Doppler ultrasonic flowmeter
    Gould electromagnetic flowmeter
    Statham flowmeter
flowmetry
flow-oximetry catheter
flow-regulator clamp
Floyd needle
Floyd-Barraquer speculum
flucrylate
fluctuant
fluctuate
fluctuating
fluctuation
fluff dressing
fluffed gauze
fluffed gauze dressing
fluffs
fluffy compression dressing
fluffy excrescences
fluffy periostitis
Fluhrer rectal probe
fluid aspiration
fluid formation
fluid intake
fluid output

fluid pressure
fluid reservoir
fluid retention
fluid volume
fluid wave
fluid-filled
fluid-filled catheter
fluid-filled sac
fluorescein
fluorescein angiogram
fluorescein angiography
fluorescein angioscopy
fluorescein dye
fluorescein strip
fluorescein uptake
fluorescence
fluorescence microscope
fluorescent antibody
fluorescent imaging
fluorescent immunoassay (FIA)
fluorescent microscope
fluorescent ray
fluorescent scan
fluorography
fluorometric technique
fluoroscope
fluoroscopic control
fluoroscopic foreign body
    forceps
fluoroscopic monitor
fluoroscopic study
fluoroscopy
Fluosol artificial blood
Fluotec vaporizer
Fluothane anesthetic agent
flush
flush aortogram
flush heparin lock
flush out kidneys
flush tube
flush with saline
flush with skin stoma
flushing of artery
flushing reservoir
flushing valve
Flute needle
fluted J-Vac drain

flute-ended right-angle drain
flutter
flux
flying "T" pelvic area
Flynn technique
Flynn-Richards-Saltzman
    technique
Flynt needle
FNA (fine-needle aspiration)
FNAB (fine-needle aspiration
    biopsy)
FNAC (fine-needle aspiration
    cytology)
foam embolus
foam rubber
foam rubber dressing
foam rubber graft
foam rubber stent
foam rubber vaginal stent
FoaMTrac traction bandage
FOB (fiberoptic bronchoscopy)
focal abnormality
focal accumulation
focal and lateralizing neurologic
    signs
focal area of hemorrhage
focal atrophy
focal colonic mucosal ulcer
focal defect
focal disease
focal edema
focal finding
focal infarction
focal lesion
focal motor sign
focal point
focal tenderness
focal tumor
focalizing signs
foci (sing. focus)
foci of infection
focus (pl. foci)
focus of atelectasis
focus of infection
focused beam
focused grid
Foerger airway

Foerster (also Förster)
Foerster abdominal retractor
Foerster abdominal ring
    retractor
Foerster eye forceps
Foerster forceps
Foerster iris forceps
Foerster operation
Foerster photometer
Foerster snare
Foerster sponge forceps
Foerster tissue forceps
Foerster uterine forceps
Foerster uveitis
Foerster-Bauer sponge-holding
    forceps
Foerster-Fuchs black spot
Foerster-Mueller forceps
Foerster-Penfield operation
Foerster-Van Doren sponge-
    holding forceps
Fog maneuver
Fogarty arterial embolectomy
Fogarty balloon
Fogarty balloon biliary catheter
Fogarty balloon catheter
Fogarty biliary balloon probe
Fogarty biliary probe
Fogarty bulldog clamp-applying
    forceps
Fogarty catheter
Fogarty clamp
Fogarty dilation catheter
Fogarty embolus catheter
Fogarty forceps
Fogarty gallstone catheter
Fogarty irrigation catheter
Fogarty occlusion catheter
Fogarty probe
Fogarty vascular clamp
Fogarty venous thrombectomy
    catheter
Fogarty-Chin catheter
Fogarty-Chin clamp
Fogarty-Chin extrusion balloon
    catheter
Fogarty-Chin peripheral
    dilatation catheter

foil carrier
Foille dressing
Foimson biceps tendon repair
fold
fold line
fold of colon
fold of cystic duct
fold of duodenum
fold of ear
fold of large intestine
fold of peritoneum
fold of rectum
fold of skin
fold of stomach
fold of tympanic membrane
fold of uterine tube
fold pattern
folding blade
folding emergency ventilation
    bronchoscope
folding esophagoscope
folding laryngoscope
Foley acorn-bulb catheter
Foley bag
Foley balloon catheter
Foley catheter
Foley cone-tip catheter
Foley forceps
Foley hemostatic bag
Foley operation
Foley plate
Foley pyeloplasty
Foley three-way catheter
Foley ureteropelvioplasty
Foley vas isolation forceps
Foley Y-plasty
Foley Y-type ureteropel-
    vioplasty
Foley Y-V pyeloplasty
Foley-Alcock bag
Foley-Alcock bag catheter
Foley-Alcock catheter
Foley-Alcock hemostatic bag
Foley-Temp
folium
Folius muscle
follicle
follicle electrode

follicle expressor
follicle lid expressor
follicle stimulating hormone
     (FSH)
follicular
follicular adenoma
follicular cyst
follicular membranes
follicular ulcer
folliculi (*sing.* folliculus)
folliculi lymphatici aggregati
folliculi lymphatici aggregati
     appendicis vermiformis
folliculi lymphatici gastrici
folliculi lymphatici lienales
folliculi lymphatici recti
folliculi lymphatici solitarii
     intestini crassi
folliculi lymphatici solitarii
     intestini tenuis
folliculus (*pl.* folliculi)
Follmann balanitis
follow through (verb; see also
     *follow-through*)
follow up (verb; see also
     *followup*)
followers
follow-through (adj, noun; see
     also *follow through*)
followup (adj, noun; see also
     *follow up*)
followup care
followup procedure
followup studies
Foltz catheter
Foltz CSF-flushing reservoir
Foltz flushing reservoir
Foltz needle
Foltz reservoir
Foltz shunt
Foltz to-and-fro flusher
Foltz valve
Foltz-Overton cardiac catheter
Foltz-Overton shunt
fomite
Fomon angular scissors
Fomon chisel
Fomon chisel guard

Fomon dorsal scissors
Fomon double-edged knife
Fomon elevator
Fomon knife
Fomon lower lateral scissors
Fomon nasal rasp
Fomon nostril elevator
Fomon nostril retractor
Fomon operation
Fomon osteotome
Fomon periosteal elevator
Fomon periosteotome
Fomon rasp
Fomon raspatory
Fomon retractor
Fomon scissors
Fomon upper lateral scissors
Fomon Vital dorsal scissors
Fontan atriopulmonary anasto-
     mosis
Fontan modification of Nor-
     wood procedure
Fontan operation
Fontan tricuspid atresia
fontanel (fontanelle preferred)
fontanelle (also fontanel)
fontanelle flat
fontanelle open
Fontan-Kreutzer repair
food bolus obstruction
foot bones
foot holder
foot pods of alar cartilage
football knee
footboard
footboard extension
footdrop
footling breech
footling breech presentation
footling delivery
footling presentation
footpiece
footplate
footplate auger
footplate chisel
footplate fragments
footplate hook
footplate pick

footprint
footprinted in delivery room
footstool
forage
foramen (*pl.* foramina)
foramen of Bochdalek
foramen of Bochdalek hernia
foramen of Luschka
foramen of Monro
foramen of Morgagni
foramen of sclera
foramen of Winslow
foramen magnum
foramen ovale
foramen ovale basis cranii
foramen ovale ossis sphe-
    noidalis
foramen sphenopalatinum
foramen spinosum
foramen stylomastoideum
foramen transversarium
foramen venae cavae
foramen-plugging forceps
foramina (*sing.* foramen)
foramina of Scarpa
foraminal
foraminal hernia
foraminal punch
foraminotomy
Forane anesthetic agent
Forane general anesthetic
Forbes amputation
Forbes graft technique
Forbes procedure for tibial
    fracture nonunion
Forbes speculum
Forbes uterine-dressing forceps
force and rhythm (F&R)
force fluids
force line
forced beat
forced duction
forced duction of eye
forced duction test
forced exhalation
forced expiration

forced expiratory flow
forced expiratory spirogram
forced expiratory time
forced expiratory volume
forced extension
forced flexion
forced movement
forced respiration
forced ventilation
forceful extension
forceful flexion
forceps (see also *vulsellum*)
    Abbott-Mayfield forceps
    abscess forceps
    ACMI forceps
    ACMI Martin endoscopy
        forceps
    ACMI Martin forceps
    Acufex curved basket
        forceps
    Acufex rotary basket
        forceps
    Acufex straight basket
        forceps
    Acufex straight forceps
    Adair breast tenaculum
        forceps
    Adair forceps
    Adair tenaculum forceps
    Adair tissue-holding
        forceps
    Adair uterine forceps
    Adair uterine tenaculum
        forceps
    Adair-Allis forceps
    Adair-Allis tissue forceps
    adenoid forceps
    Adler bone forceps
    Adler forceps
    Adler punch forceps
    Adson artery forceps
    Adson bayonet dressing
        forceps
    Adson brain forceps
    Adson clip-applying
        forceps

forceps *continued*

Adson clip-introducing forceps
Adson cranial rongeur forceps
Adson dressing forceps
Adson forceps
Adson hemostatic forceps
Adson hypophyseal forceps
Adson microbipolar forceps
Adson microdressing forceps
Adson microtissue forceps
Adson scalp clip-applying forceps
Adson thumb forceps
Adson tissue forceps
Adson Vital tissue forceps
Adson-Brown forceps
Adson-Brown tissue forceps
Adson-Mixter forceps
Adson-Mixter neurosurgical forceps
advancement forceps
Aesculap forceps
Alabama University forceps
Alabama University utility forceps
Alderkreutz forceps
Alexander dressing forceps
Allen forceps
Allen intestinal forceps
Allen uterine forceps
alligator crimper forceps
alligator ear forceps
alligator forceps
alligator grasping forceps
alligator nasal forceps

forceps *continued*

alligator-type grasping forceps
Allis forceps
Allis intestinal forceps
Allis Micro-Line pediatric forceps
Allis thoracic forceps
Allis tissue forceps
Allis tissue-holding forceps
Allis-Abramson breast biopsy forceps
Allis-Adair forceps
Allis-Adair tissue forceps
Allis-Coakley forceps
Allis-Coakley tonsil forceps
Allis-Coakley tonsil-seizing forceps
Allis-Duval forceps
Allis-Ochsner forceps
Allis-Ochsner tonsil forceps
Allis-Willauer forceps
Allis-Willauer tissue forceps
Alvis fixation forceps
Alvis forceps
Ambrose eye forceps
Amenabar capsule forceps
anastomosis forceps
Andrews forceps
Andrews tonsil forceps
Andrews tonsil-seizing forceps
Andrews-Hartmann forceps
aneurysm forceps
Angell-James hypophysectomy forceps
angiotribe forceps
angled stone forceps
angular forceps
angulated forceps
Anis corneal forceps

forceps *continued*

Anis corneoscleral
forceps
Anis forceps
Anis microsurgical tying
forceps
Anis tying forceps
anterior capsule forceps
anterior forceps
anterior segment forceps
Anthony-Fisher forceps
antral forceps
aorta aneurysm forceps
aorta forceps
aortic forceps
aortic aneurysm forceps
aortic occlusion forceps
application of obstetric
forceps
applicator forceps
approximation forceps
Archer forceps
Archer splinter forceps
Arrowsmith-Clerf pin-
closing forceps
Arruga capsule forceps
Arruga tip forceps
Arruga-Gill forceps
Arruga-McCool capsule
forceps
Arruga-McCool forceps
arterial forceps
artery forceps
Asch forceps
Asch nasal-straightening
forceps
Asch septal forceps
Asch septal-straightening
forceps
Ash dental forceps
Ashby fluoroscopic
foreign body forceps
Ashby forceps
ASSI bipolar coagulating
forceps
ASSI forceps
Athens forceps

forceps *continued*

Atra-grip forceps
atraumatic forceps
atraumatic tissue forceps
aural forceps
auricular appendage
forceps
Auto–Suture forceps
Autraugrip forceps
Autraugrip tissue for-
ceps
Auvard-Zweifel forceps
axis-traction forceps
Ayers chalazion forceps
Ayers forceps
Azar forceps
Azar tying forceps
Azar utility forceps
B-H forceps
Babcock forceps
Babcock intestinal
forceps
Babcock thoracic tissue-
holding forceps
Babcock tissue forceps
Babcock Vital intestinal
forceps
Babcock Vital tissue
forceps
baby dressing forceps
baby hemostatic forceps
baby intestinal tissue
forceps
baby Lane bone-holding
forceps
baby tissue forceps
backbiting forceps
Backhaus forceps
Backhaus towel forceps
Bacon cranial forceps
Bacon cranial rongeur
forceps
Bacon forceps
Baer bone-cutting
forceps
Baer forceps
Bahnson-Brown forceps

forceps *continued*

Bahnson-Brown tissue
forceps
Bailey aortic valve-
cutting forceps
Bailey chalazion forceps
Bailey forceps
Bailey-Williamson
forceps
Bailey-Williamson
obstetrical forceps
Bainbridge forceps
Bainbridge hemostatic
forceps
Bainbridge intestinal
forceps
Bainbridge resection
forceps
Baird chalazion forceps
Baird forceps
Baker forceps
Baker tissue forceps
Ballantine forceps
Ballantine hysterectomy
forceps
Ballantine-Peterson
forceps
Ballantine-Peterson
hysterectomy forceps
Ballenger forceps
Ballenger sponge forceps
Ballenger sponge-
holding forceps
Ballenger tonsil forceps
Ballenger tonsil-seizing
forceps
Ballenger-Foerster
forceps
Bane forceps
Bane rongeur forceps
Bangerter forceps
Bangerter muscle forceps
Bardeleben bone-holding
forceps
Bard-Parker forceps
Bard-Parker transfer
forceps

forceps *continued*

Barkan forceps
Barkan iris forceps
Barlow forceps
Barnes-Crile forceps
Barnes-Simpson forceps
Barnes-Simpson obstetri-
cal forceps
Baron forceps
Barraquer cilia forceps
Barraquer conjunctiva
forceps
Barraquer fixation
forceps
Barraquer forceps
Barraquer mosquito
forceps
Barraquer suture for-
ceps
Barraquer-Troutman
forceps
Barraquer-von Mandach
clot forceps
Barraya forceps
Barraya tissue forceps
Barrett forceps
Barrett intestinal forceps
Barrett placenta forceps
Barrett tenaculum
forceps
Barrett uterine tenaculum
forceps
Barrett-Allen forceps
Barrett-Allen placenta
forceps
Barrett-Allen uterine-
elevating forceps
Barrett-Murphy forceps
Barrett-Murphy intestinal
forceps
Barrie-Jones forceps
Barsky forceps
Barton forceps
Barton obstetrical
forceps
basket forceps
basket-cutting forceps

forceps *continued*

basket-type crushing
forceps
Bauer dissecting forceps
Bauer forceps
Bauer sponge forceps
Baum-Hecht forceps
Baum-Hecht tarsor-
rhaphy forceps
Baumgartner forceps
bayonet bipolar electro-
surgical forceps
bayonet forceps
bayonet molar forceps
bayonet-type forceps
Bead ethmoid forceps
beaked cowhorn forceps
bean forceps
Beardsley forceps
Beasley-Babcock forceps
Beaupre cilia forceps
Beaupre epilation
forceps
Beaupre forceps
Bechert forceps
Beck forceps
Beebe forceps
Beebe hemostatic
forceps
Beebe wire-cutting
forceps
Beer cilia forceps
Beer forceps
Behrend cystic duct
forceps
Bellucci forceps
Benaron forceps
Bengolea artery forceps
Bengolea forceps
Bennell forceps
Bennett cilia forceps
Bennett epilation forceps
Berens capsule forceps
Berens corneal transplant
forceps
Berens forceps
Berens muscle forceps

forceps *continued*

Berens muscle recession
forceps
Berens suture forceps
Berger forceps
Bergeron pillar forceps
Bergh cilia forceps
Berghmann-Foerster
sponge forceps
Bergman forceps
Berke cilia forceps
Berke forceps
Berke ptosis forceps
Berkeley forceps
Berne forceps
Berne nasal forceps
Berry forceps
Berry uterine-elevating
forceps
Best common duct stone
forceps
Best forceps
Best gallstone forceps
Bettman-Noyes forceps
Bevan forceps
Bevan gallbladder
forceps
Bevan hemostatic
forceps
Beyer forceps
Beyer ronguer forceps
Bigelow forceps
Billroth forceps
Billroth tumor forceps
Binkhorst lens forceps
biopsy forceps
biopsy punch forceps
biopsy specimen forceps
bipolar coagulating
forceps
bipolar coagulation-
suction forceps
bipolar eye forceps
bipolar forceps
bipolar microforceps
bipolar transsphenoidal
forceps

forceps *continued*
   Birkett forceps
   Birkett hemostatic
    forceps
   Bishop tissue forceps
   Bishop-Harman dressing
    forceps
   Bishop-Harman forceps
   Bishop-Harman iris
    forceps
   biting forceps
   Björk diathermy forceps
   bladder forceps
   bladder specimen
    forceps
   Blade-Wilde ear forceps
   Blake dressing forceps
   Blake ear forceps
   Blake forceps
   Blake gallstone forceps
   Blakesley ethmoid
    forceps
   Blakesley forceps
   Blakesley septal bone
    forceps
   Blakesley septal com-
    pression forceps
   Blakesley septal forceps
   Blakesley-Wilde ear
    forceps
   Blakesley-Wilde ethmoid
    forceps
   Blalock forceps
   Blanchard forceps
   Blanchard hemorrhoid
    forceps
   Bland cervical traction
    forceps
   Bland vulsellum for-
    ceps
   Blaydes corneal forceps
   Blaydes forceps
   Blohmka tonsil forceps
   Bloodwell forceps
   Bloodwell tissue forceps
   Bloodwell vascular tissue
    forceps

forceps *continued*
   Bloodwell-Brown
    forceps
   Blum forceps
   Boettcher artery forceps
   Boettcher forceps
   Boettcher pulmonary
    artery forceps
   Boettcher tonsil artery
    forceps
   Boies cutting forceps
   Boies forceps
   Bolton forceps
   Bonaccolto capsule
    fragment forceps
   Bonaccolto forceps
   Bonaccolto jeweler's-
    type forceps
   Bonaccolto utility
    forceps
   Bonaccolto utility pickup
    forceps
   Bond forceps
   Bond placenta forceps
   bone-cutting forceps
   bone-holding forceps
   bone-splitting forceps
   Bonn forceps
   Bonn iris forceps
   Bonn peripheral
    iridectomy forceps
   Bonney forceps
   Bonney tissue forceps
   Bores forceps
   Boston Lying-In cervical
    forceps
   Boston Lying-In cervical-
    grasping forceps
   Botvin forceps
   Botvin iris forceps
   Bovie coagulating
    forceps
   Bowen suction loose
    body forceps
   box-joint forceps
   Boys-Allis forceps
   Boys-Allis tissue forceps

forceps *continued*

Boys-Allis tissue-holding forceps
Bozeman dressing forceps
Bozeman forceps
Bozeman uterine forceps
Bozeman uterine-dressing forceps
Bozeman uterine-packing forceps
Bozeman-Douglas uterine-dressing forceps
Braasch bladder specimen forceps
Braasch forceps
Bracken fixation forceps
Bracken forceps
Bracken iris forceps
Bracken scleral fixation forceps
Bracken tissue-grasping forceps
Bradford forceps
Bradford thyroid forceps
Bradford thyroid traction vulsellum forceps
brain forceps
brain spatula forceps
brain tumor forceps
Brand forceps
Brand shunt-introducing forceps
Brand tendon forceps
Brand tendon-holding forceps
Brand tendon-tunneling forceps
Braun forceps
Braun uterine tenaculum forceps
breast tenaculum forceps
Brenner forceps
Bridge deep-surgery forceps
Bridge forceps

forceps *continued*

Brigham brain tumor forceps
Brigham forceps
Brigham thumb tissue forceps
broad-blade forceps
bronchial biopsy forceps
bronchial forceps
bronchial-grasping forceps
bronchoscopic biopsy forceps
bronchoscopic forceps
bronchoscopic forceps handle
bronchoscopic rotation forceps
bronchus forceps
bronchus-grasping forceps
Brophy dressing forceps
Brophy forceps
Brophy tissue forceps
Brown forceps
Brown side-grasping forceps
Brown thoracic forceps
Brown tissue forceps
Brown-Adson forceps
Brown-Adson tissue forceps
Brown-Bahnson forceps
Brown-Buerger forceps
Broyles forceps
Bruening cutting-tip forceps
Bruening ethmoid exenteration forceps
Bruening forceps
Bruening nasal-cutting septum forceps
Bruening septum forceps
Bruening-Citelli forceps
Brunner forceps
Brunner intestinal forceps

forceps *continued*
Brunner tissue forceps
Brunschwig artery
forceps
Brunschwig forceps
Brunschwig viscera
forceps
Bryant nasal forceps
Buerger-McCarthy
bladder forceps
Buerger-McCarthy
forceps
Buie biopsy forceps
Buie forceps
Buie specimen forceps
bulldog clamp-applier
forceps
bulldog clamp-applying
forceps
bulldog forceps
bullet forceps
Bumpus forceps
Bumpus specimen
forceps
Bunim forceps
Bunim urethral forceps
Bunker forceps
Bunt forceps holder
Burch biopsy forceps
Burch forceps
Burford forceps
Burnham biopsy forceps
Burnham forceps
Burns forceps
Butler bayonet forceps
Cairns forceps
Cairns hemostatic
forceps
Calibri forceps
Callahan forceps
Callahan scleral fixation
forceps
Campbell forceps
Campbell ligature-carrier
forceps
Campbell urethral
catheter forceps

forceps *continued*
Cane bone-holding
forceps
Cane forceps
cannulated broncho-
scopic forceps
cannulated forceps
capsule forceps
capsule fragment forceps
caput forceps
carbide-jaw forceps
cardiovascular forceps
cardiovascular tissue
forceps
Cardona corneal
prosthesis forceps
Cardona forceps
Carlens forceps
Carmalt artery forceps
Carmalt forceps
Carmalt hysterectomy
forceps
Carmalt splinter forceps
Carmody forceps
Carmody thumb tissue
forceps
Carmody tissue forceps
Carmody-Brophy forceps
carotid artery forceps
Carrel mosquito forceps
Carroll bone-holding
forceps
Carroll tendon-passing
forceps
Carroll-Adson  forceps
cartilage forceps
cartilage-holding forceps
caruncle forceps
Caspar alligator forceps
Caspar forceps
Cassidy-Brophy dressing
forceps
Cassidy-Brophy forceps
Castaneda suture tag
forceps
Castroviejo capsule
forceps

forceps *continued*

Castroviejo corneoscleral suture forceps
Castroviejo forceps
Castroviejo suture forceps
Castroviejo transplant forceps
Castroviejo tying forceps
Castroviejo-Arruga capsule forceps
Castroviejo-Arruga forceps
Castroviejo-Colibri corneal forceps
Castroviejo-Furniss corneal-holding forceps
Castroviejo-Simpson forceps
Cavanaugh-Wells tonsil forceps
cephalic blade forceps
cervic hemostatic forceps
cervical biopsy forceps
cervical biopsy punch forceps
cervical forceps
cervical punch forceps
cervical traction forceps
cervix forceps
cervix-holding forceps
cesarean forceps
chalazion forceps
Chamberlen forceps
Chamberlen obstetrical forceps
Championnière forceps
Chandler forceps
Chandler iris forceps
Chandler spinal perforat-ing forceps
Chang bone-cutting forceps
Chaput forceps
Charnley forceps
Cheatle forceps

forceps *continued*

Cheatle sterilizer forceps
Cheron forceps
Cherry forceps
Cherry-Adson forceps
Cherry-Kerrison forceps
Cherry-Kerrison rongeur forceps
Chester forceps
Chevalier Jackson forceps
chicken-bill rongeur forceps
Child clip-applying forceps
Child forceps
Child intestinal forceps
Children's Hospital forceps
Children's Hospital intestinal forceps
Childs-Phillips forceps
Choyce intraocular lens forceps
Choyce lens forceps
Chubb tonsil forceps
Cicherelli forceps
Cicherelli rongeur forceps
cilia forceps
Citelli forceps
Citelli-Bruening ear forceps
Civiale forceps
clamp forceps
Clark capsule fragment forceps
Clark forceps
Clark-Guyton forceps
Clark-Verhoeff capsule forceps
Clark-Verhoeff forceps
Clayman forceps
Clayman lens forceps
Clayman-Kelman intraocular lens forceps

forceps *continued*
    cleft palate forceps
    Clerf forceps
    Clevedent forceps
    Cleveland bone-cutting
      forceps
    clip forceps
    clip-applying forceps
    clip-introducing forceps
    closed iris forceps
    closer forceps
    closing forceps
    coagulating forceps
    coagulating-suction
      forceps
    coagulation forceps
    Coakley forceps
    Coakley-Allis forceps
    coarctation forceps
    Cohan corneal utility
      forceps
    Cohen nasal-dressing
      forceps
    cold cup biopsy forceps
    cold cup forceps
    Colibri corneal forceps
    Colibri corneal utility
      forceps
    Colibri eye forceps
    Colibri forceps
    Colibri microforceps
    Colibri-Pierce forceps
    Colibri-Storz forceps
    Coller artery forceps
    Coller forceps
    Coller hemostatic forceps
    Collier forceps
    Collier hemostatic
      forceps
    Collier-Crile hemostatic
      forceps
    Collier-DeBakey
      hemostatic forceps
    Collin forceps
    Collin intestinal forceps
    Collin lung-grasping
      forceps

forceps *continued*
    Collin mucous forceps
    Collin tissue forceps
    Collin tongue forceps
    Collin-Duvall intestinal
      forceps
    Collis forceps
    Collis microutility forceps
    Collis-Maumenee corneal
      forceps
    Colver forceps
    Colver tonsil forceps
    Colver tonsil-seizing
      forceps
    Colver-Coakley forceps
    Colver-Coakley tonsil
      forceps
    combination forceps/
      needle holder
    common duct-holding
      forceps
    common McPherson
      forceps
    compression forceps
    Cone forceps
    Cone wire-twisting
      forceps
    conjunctival forceps
    connector forceps
    Cooley anastomosis
      forceps
    Cooley aortic forceps
    Cooley arterial occlusion
      forceps
    Cooley auricular
      appendage forceps
    Cooley cardiovascular
      forceps
    Cooley coarctation
      forceps
    Cooley CSR forceps
    Cooley curved forceps
    Cooley double-angled
      jaw forceps
    Cooley forceps
    Cooley graft forceps
    Cooley iliac forceps

forceps *continued*

Cooley multipurpose forceps
Cooley patent ductus forceps
Cooley pediatric aortic forceps
Cooley peripheral vascular forceps
Cooley tangential pediatric forceps
Cooley tissue forceps
Cooley vascular forceps
Cooley vascular tissue forceps
Cooley-Baumgarten aortic forceps
Cope lung forceps
Coppridge forceps
Coppridge grasping forceps
Coppridge urethral forceps
Corbett bone-cutting forceps
Corbett forceps
Cordes forceps
Cordes punch forceps tip
Cordes-New forceps
Cordes-New laryngeal punch forceps
Corey forceps
Corey ovum forceps
cornea-holding forceps
corneal forceps
corneal transplant forceps
corneal utility forceps
cornea-suturing forceps
corneoscleral forceps
Cornet forceps
Corwin forceps
Corwin tonsillar forceps
Corwin tonsillar hemo-static forceps
Cottle biting forceps
Cottle forceps

forceps *continued*

Cottle insertion forceps
Cottle lower lateral forceps
Cottle tissue forceps
Cottle-Arruga forceps
Cottle-Jansen forceps
Cottle-Jansen rongeur forceps
Cottle-Kazanjian forceps
Cottle-Kazanjian nasal forceps
Cottle-Kazanjian nasal-cutting forceps
Cottle-Walsham forceps
Cottle-Walsham septum-straightening forceps
cowhorn tooth-extracting forceps
Craafoord bronchial forceps
Craafoord coarctation forceps
Craafoord forceps
Craafoord pulmonary forceps
Craafoord-Sellors hemostatic forceps
Craig forceps
Craig septum-cutting forceps
Craig tonsil-seizing forceps
cranial forceps
cranial rongeur forceps
Crawford fascial forceps
Creevy biopsy forceps
Crenshaw carbuncle forceps
Crenshaw caruncle forceps
Crenshaw forceps
Crile arterial forceps
Crile forceps
Crile gall duct forceps
Crile Micro-Line artery forceps

forceps *continued*

Crile-Barnes hemostatic forceps
Crile-Duval lung-grasping forceps
crimper closer forceps
crimper forceps
crocodile forceps
cross-action forceps
crural nipper forceps
Cryer Universal forceps
CSF shunt connector forceps
CSF shunt-introducing forceps
Cukier nasal forceps
Culler eye forceps
Culler fixation forceps
Cullom septal forceps
cup biopsy forceps
cup forceps
cup-biting forceps
cupped forceps
cup-shaped ear forceps
cup-shaped forceps
cup-shaped inner ear forceps
cup-shaped middle ear forceps
curet forceps
Curtis forceps
Curtis tissue forceps
curved forceps
curved tying forceps
Cushing bipolar forceps
Cushing brain and tissue forceps
Cushing brain forceps
Cushing cranial rongeur forceps
Cushing decompression forceps
Cushing dressing forceps
Cushing forceps
Cushing thumb forceps
Cushing tissue forceps

forceps *continued*

Cushing Vital tissue forceps
Cushing-Brown tissue forceps
Cushing-Taylor carbide-jaw forceps
Cutler forceps
cutting forceps
cylindrical-object forceps
cystic duct forceps
cystoscopic forceps
D'Allesandro serial suture-holding forceps
Dahlgren-Hudson forceps
Dale femoral-popliteal anastomosis forceps
Dale forceps
Dan chalazion forceps
Danberg forceps
Danberg iris forceps
Dandy forceps
Dandy hemostatic forceps
Dandy scalp forceps
Dan-Gradle cilial forceps
Dartigues uterine-elevating forceps
Davidson forceps
Davidson pulmonary vessel forceps
Davis capsule forceps
Davis coagulating forceps
Davis forceps
Davis monopolar bayonet forceps
Davis thoracic tissue forceps
Davol forceps
Davol rongeur forceps
De Alvarez forceps
Dean forceps
Dean tonsillar forceps
Dean tonsillar hemostatic forceps

forceps *continued*

Dean-Shallcross tonsil-seizing forceps
DeBakey arterial forceps
DeBakey Autraugrip forceps
DeBakey dissecting forceps
DeBakey forceps
DeBakey thoracic forceps
DeBakey tissue forceps
DeBakey vascular forceps
DeBakey vascular tissue forceps
DeBakey-Bahnson forceps
DeBakey-Bainbridge forceps
DeBakey-Colovira-Rumel thoracic forceps
DeBakey-Cooley anastomosis forceps
DeBakey-Cooley cardiovascular forceps
DeBakey-Cooley forceps
DeBakey-Diethrich vascular forceps
DeBakey-Kelly hemostatic forceps
DeBakey-Mixter thoracic forceps
DeBakey-Péan cardiovascular forceps
DeBakey-Rankin hemostatic forceps
DeBakey-Reynolds anastomosis forceps
DeBakey-Rumel thoracic forceps
DeBakey-Semb forceps
Decker microforceps
Deddish-Potts intestinal forceps
deep-surgery forceps

forceps *continued*

D'Errico dressing forceps
D'Errico forceps
D'Errico hypophyseal forceps
D'Errico tissue forceps
Defourmental forceps
Defourmental rongeur forceps
DeLee cervix-holding forceps
DeLee dressing forceps
DeLee forceps
DeLee obstetrical forceps
DeLee ovum forceps
DeLee spoon tissue forceps
DeLee uterine forceps
DeLee uterine-packing forceps
DeLee-Simpson forceps
Demarest forceps
Demarest septal forceps
DeMartel appendix forceps
DeMartel forceps
DeMartel scalp forceps
DeMartel-Wolfson forceps
Demel forceps
Demel wire-tightening forceps
Demel wire-twisting forceps
Dench forceps
Denis Browne forceps
Dennis forceps
Dennis intestinal forceps
dental forceps
depilatory dermal forceps
Derf forceps
Derra forceps
Derra urethral forceps
Desjardins forceps
Desjardins gallstone forceps

forceps *continued*

Desmarres chalazion forceps
Desmarres forceps
Desmarres lid forceps
DeTakats-McKenzie brain clip-applying forceps
DeTakats-McKenzie clip-applying forceps
DeTakats-McKenzie forceps
DeVilbiss cranial forceps
DeVilbiss forceps
DeVilbiss rongeur forceps
DeWecker forceps
DeWeese axis traction forceps
Dewey forceps
Dewey obstetrical forceps
diathermic forceps
Dieffenbach forceps
Diener forceps
Dieter forceps
Diethrich right-angled hemostatic forceps
dilating forceps
Dingman bone-holding forceps
Dingman forceps
disimpaction forceps
disk forceps
disposable forceps
dissecting forceps
dissection forceps
divergent outlet forceps
Dixon-Lovelace hemostatic forceps
Dixon-Thorpe vitreous foreign body forceps
Docktor forceps
Docktor tissue forceps
Donberg iris forceps
Dorsey bayonet forceps
Dorsey forceps

forceps *continued*

double-action bone-cutting forceps
double-action hump forceps
double-action rongeur forceps
double-articulated bronchoscopic forceps
double-articulated laryngeal forceps tip
double-concave forceps
double-concave rat-tooth forceps
double-cupped forceps
double-ended needle forceps
double-ended suture forceps
double-ended tissue forceps
double-spoon forceps
Douglas cilia forceps
Douglas eye forceps
Douglas forceps
Doyen forceps
Doyen gallbladder forceps
Doyen intestinal forceps
Doyen uterine forceps
Doyen vulsellum forceps
dressing forceps
Drews cilia forceps
Drews forceps
Drews intraocular lens forceps
duckbill forceps
dull-pointed forceps
Dumont dissecting forceps
Dumont forceps
Dumont Swiss dissecting forceps
Dunhill forceps
Duplay tenaculum forceps

forceps *continued*

Duplay uterine tenaculum forceps
dural forceps
Duval forceps
Duval lung forceps
Duval lung-grasping forceps
Duval Vital intestinal forceps
Duval-Allis forceps
Duval-Crile forceps
Duval-Crile intestinal forceps
Duval-Crile lung forceps
Duval-Crile tissue forceps
ear forceps
ear punch forceps
ear-dressing forceps
ear-grasping forceps
Eastman cystic duct forceps
Eastman forceps
Eber forceps
Echlin rongeur forceps
Eder forceps
Effler-Groves cardiovascular forceps
Effler-Groves forceps
Ehrhardt forceps
Ehrhardt lid forceps
Eisenstein forceps
electrocoagulating biopsy forceps
electrosurgical biopsy forceps
elevating forceps
Elliott forceps
Elliott gallbladder forceps
Elliott hemostatic forceps
Elliott obstetrical forceps
Elschnig capsular forceps
Elschnig cyclodialysis forceps
Elschnig fixation forceps

forceps *continued*

Elschnig forceps
Elschnig secondary membrane forceps
Elschnig tissue-grasping forceps
Elschnig-O'Brien fixation forceps
Elschnig-O'Brien forceps
Elschnig-O'Brien tissue-grasping forceps
Elschnig-O'Connor fixation forceps
Elschnig-O'Connor forceps
Emmet forceps
endometrial forceps
endometrial polyp forceps
endoscopic biopsy forceps
endoscopic grasping forceps
endoscopic suture-cutting forceps
endospeculum forceps
endotracheal tube forceps
English forceps
English tissue forceps
English-pattern tissue forceps
Ennis forceps
entropion forceps
epilating forceps
epilation forceps
episcleral forceps
Eppendorfer biopsy punch forceps
Eppendorfer cervical biopsy forceps
Erhardt eyelid forceps
Erhardt forceps
Erhardt lid forceps
Erich biopsy forceps
Erich forceps

forceps *continued*

Erich laryngeal biopsy
forceps
esophageal forceps
esophagoscopic forceps
Essrig forceps
Essrig tissue forceps
ethmoidal exenteration
forceps
ethmoidal forceps
ethmoid-cutting forceps
Ethridge forceps
Ethridge hysterectomy
forceps
Evans forceps
Evans Vital tissue forceps
Everett forceps
Ewald forceps
Ewald-Hudson brain
forceps
Ewald-Hudson dressing
forceps
Ewing capsule forceps
Ewing forceps
exenteration forceps
exolever forceps
extracapsular eye forceps
extracting forceps
eye fixation forceps
eye forceps
eye needle holder
forceps
eye suture forceps
eye-dressing forceps
eyelid forceps
Facit uterine polyp
forceps
failed forceps delivery
Falcao fixation forceps
Falk forceps
Farabeuf bone-holding
forceps
Farabeuf forceps
Farabeuf-Lambotte bone-
holding forceps
Farabeuf-Lambotte
forceps

forceps *continued*

Farnham forceps
Farnham nasal-cutting
forceps
Farrington forceps
Farrington nasal polyp
forceps
Farrington septum
forceps
Farrior forceps
Farrior wire-crimping
forceps
Farris tissue forceps
Faure forceps
Faure uterine biopsy
forceps
Fauvel forceps
Fauvel laryngeal forceps
Feilchenfeld forceps
Feilchenfeld splinter
forceps
fenestrated blade forceps
fenestrated cup biopsy
forceps
fenestrated forceps
Fenger forceps
Ferguson angiotribe
forceps
Ferguson bone-holding
forceps
Ferguson forceps
Ferris colporrhaphy
forceps
Ferris forceps
Ferris Smith bone-biting
forceps
Ferris Smith cup rongeur
forceps
Ferris Smith forceps
Ferris Smith fragment
forceps
Ferris Smith tissue
forceps
Ferris Smith-Kerrison
rongeur forceps
Ferris Smith-Takahashi
forceps

forceps *continued*
- fine artery forceps
- fine forceps
- Fine suture-tying forceps
- Fine-Castroviejo suturing forceps
- fine-dissecting forceps
- fine-tissue forceps
- fine-toothed forceps
- Fink fixation forceps
- Fink forceps
- Fink-Jameson forceps
- Fink-Jameson oblique muscle forceps
- Finochietto forceps
- Finochietto lobectomy forceps
- Finochietto thoracic forceps
- Fischl forceps
- Fischmann angiotribe forceps
- Fish forceps
- Fish grasping forceps
- Fish nasal forceps
- Fisher advancement forceps
- Fisher capsular forceps
- Fisher forceps
- Fisher-Arlt forceps
- Fisher-Arlt iris forceps
- fissure forceps
- Fitzgerald aortic aneurysm forceps
- Fitzgerald forceps
- Fitzwater forceps
- Fitzwater peanut sponge-holding forceps
- fixation forceps
- Fletcher dressing forceps
- Fletcher forceps
- Fletcher-Suit polyp forceps
- Fletcher-Van Doren forceps
- Fletcher-Van Doren sponge-holding forceps

forceps *continued*
- Fletcher-Van Doren uterine forceps
- Fletcher-Van Doren uterine polyp forceps
- Fletcher-Van Doren uterine polyp sponge-holding forceps
- flexible foreign body forceps
- fluoroscopic foreign body forceps
- Foerster eye forceps
- Foerster forceps
- Foerster iris forceps
- Foerster sponge forceps
- Foerster tissue forceps
- Foerster uterine forceps
- Foerster-Bauer sponge-holding forceps
- Foerster-Mueller forceps
- Foerster-Van Doren sponge-holding forceps
- Fogarty bulldog clamp-applying forceps
- Fogarty forceps
- Foley forceps
- Foley vas isolation forceps
- foramen-plugging forceps
- Forbes uterine-dressing forceps
- foreign body cystoscopy forceps
- foreign body eye forceps
- foreign body forceps
- Förster (see *Foerster*)
- forward-grasping forceps
- Foss cardiovascular forceps
- Foss forceps
- Foss intestinal clamp forceps
- Fox bipolar forceps
- Fox tissue forceps

forceps *continued*
- F.R. Thompson hip prosthesis forceps
- F.R. Thompson rasp forceps
- Fraenkel (also Fränkel)
- Fraenkel forceps
- Fraenkel cutting-tip forceps
- Fraenkel double-articulated-tip forceps
- Fraenkel forceps
- fragment forceps
- Francis chalazion forceps
- Francis forceps
- Frangenheim biopsy punch forceps
- Frangenheim forceps
- Frangenheim hook-punch forceps
- Fränkel (see *Fraenkel*)
- Frankfeldt forceps
- Frankfeldt grasping forceps
- Fraser forceps
- Freer septal forceps
- Freer-Gruenwald forceps
- Freer-Gruenwald punch forceps
- French-pattern forceps
- Friedman rongeur forceps
- Fry nasal forceps
- Fuchs capsule forceps
- Fuchs capsulotomy forceps
- Fuchs forceps
- Fujinon biopsy forceps
- Fujinon forceps
- Fulpit forceps
- Fulpit tissue forceps
- Furniss cornea-holding forceps
- Furniss forceps
- Furniss polyp forceps
- Furniss-Castroviejo forceps

forceps *continued*
- Furniss-Clute forceps
- Furniss-Rizzuti forceps
- Gabriel Tucker forceps
- galea forceps
- gall duct forceps
- gallbladder forceps
- gallstone forceps
- Gardner hysterectomy forceps
- Garland forceps
- Garland hysterectomy forceps
- Garrigue forceps
- Garrigue uterine-dressing forceps
- Garrison forceps
- gastrointestinal forceps
- Gavin-Miller colon forceps
- Gavin-Miller intestinal forceps
- Gavin-Miller tissue forceps
- Gaylor forceps
- Gaylor uterine biopsy forceps
- Gaylor uterine specimen forceps
- Geissendorfer forceps
- Gelfoam forceps
- Gelfoam pressure forceps
- Gellhorn forceps
- Gellhorn uterine biopsy forceps
- Gelpi forceps
- Gelpi hysterectomy forceps
- Gelpi-Lowrie forceps
- Gelpi-Lowrie hysterectomy forceps
- Gemini forceps
- Gemini gall duct forceps
- Gemini Mixter forceps
- Gemini thoracic forceps
- general wire forceps
- Gerald bipolar forceps

forceps *continued*

Gerald dressing forceps
Gerald forceps
Gerald tissue forceps
Gerbode cardiovascular tissue forceps
Gerbode forceps
GI forceps
Gifford fixation forceps
Gifford forceps
Gifford iris forceps
Gilbert cystic duct forceps
Gilbert forceps
Gill forceps
Gill iris forceps
Gill-Chandler iris forceps
Gillespie obstetrical forceps
Gill-Fuchs forceps
Gill-Hess forceps
Gill-Hess iris forceps
Gillies forceps
Gillies tissue forceps
Gill-Safar forceps
Ginsberg forceps
Ginsberg tissue forceps
Girard forceps
Glassman forceps
Glassman noncrushing pickup forceps
Glassman pickup forceps
Glassman-Allis common duct-holding forceps
Glassman-Allis forceps
Glassman-Allis intestinal forceps
Glassman-Allis miniature intestinal forceps
Glassman-Allis noncrushing tissue-holding forceps
Glenn diverticulum forceps
Glenner forceps
Glenner hysterectomy forceps

forceps *continued*

Glenner vaginal hysterectomy forceps
globular object forceps
Glover curved forceps
Glover forceps
Glover infundibular rongeur forceps
Glover rongeur forceps
Glover spoon-shaped forceps
goiter forceps
goiter vulsellum forceps
Gold forceps
Gold hemostatic forceps
Goldman-Kazanjian forceps
Goldman-Kazanjian nasal forceps
Gomco forceps
Good forceps
Good obstetrical forceps
Goodhill forceps
Goodhill tonsillar forceps
Goodhill tonsillar hemostatic forceps
Goodyear-Gruenwald forceps
Gordon cilia forceps
Gordon forceps
Gordon uterine forceps
Gordon uterine vulsellum forceps
Gradle cilia forceps
Gradle forceps
Graefe (also von Graefe)
Graefe fixation forceps
Graefe forceps
Graefe iris forceps
Graefe nonmagnetic fixation forceps
Graefe tissue-grasping forceps
grasping and cutting forceps
grasping biopsy forceps
grasping forceps

forceps *continued*

Gray cystic duct forceps
Gray forceps
Grayton corneal forceps
Grayton forceps
Green chalazion forceps
Green fixation forceps
Green forceps
Green tissue-grasping forceps
Green-Armytage forceps
Greene tube-holding forceps
Greenwood bipolar coagulation-suction forceps
Greenwood forceps
Gregory forceps
Grey Turner forceps
Grieshaber forceps
Grieshaber iris forceps
Gross forceps
Grotting forceps
Gruenwald dissecting forceps
Gruenwald dressing forceps
Gruenwald ear forceps
Gruenwald forceps
Gruenwald nasal forceps
Gruenwald nasal-cutting forceps
Gruenwald nasal-dressing forceps
Gruenwald tissue forceps
Gruenwald-Bryant forceps
Gruenwald-Bryant nasal forceps
Gruenwald-Bryant nasal-cutting forceps
Gruenwald-Jansen forceps
Gruenwald-Love forceps
Gruppe forceps
Gruppe wire prosthesis-crimping forceps

forceps *continued*

Gruppe wire-crimping forceps
Guggenheim adenoid forceps
guide forceps
Guist fixation forceps
Guist forceps
Gunderson muscle forceps
Gunderson recession forceps
Gunnar-Hey roller forceps
Gusberg uterine forceps
Gutglass cervix hemostatic forceps
Gutglass forceps
Gutierrez-Najar grasping forceps
Guyton forceps
Guyton-Clark capsule fragment forceps
Guyton-Noyes fixation forceps
Guyton-Noyes forceps
Haberer gastrointestinal forceps
Haberer intestinal forceps
Haig Ferguson obstetrical forceps
Hajek antral punch forceps
Hajek forceps
Hajek sphenoid punch forceps
Hajek-Koffler forceps
Hajek-Koffler punch forceps
Hajek-Koffler sphenoidal punch forceps
Halberg forceps
Hale forceps
Hale obstetrical forceps
hallux forceps
Halsey forceps

forceps *continued*

Halsted curved mosquito forceps
Halsted forceps
Halsted hemostatic forceps
Halsted Micro-Line artery forceps
Halsted mosquito forceps
Halsted-Swanson tendon-passing forceps
Hamby forceps
Hamilton forceps
hammer forceps
Hank-Dennen obstetrical forceps
Hannahan forceps
Hardy microbipolar forceps
harelip forceps
Harken cardiovascular forceps
Harken forceps
Harken-Cooley forceps
Harman forceps
Harms forceps
Harms microtying forceps
Harms tying forceps
Harms-Tubingen forceps
Harms-Tubingen tying forceps
Harrington clamp forceps
Harrington forceps
Harrington thoracic forceps
Harrington-Mayo forceps
Harrington-Mayo tissue forceps
Harrington-Mixter clamp forceps
Harrington-Mixter forceps
Harrington-Mixter thoracic forceps
Harris forceps

forceps *continued*

Harris suture-carrying forceps
Hartmann alligator forceps
Hartmann ear forceps
Hartmann ear-dressing forceps
Hartmann forceps
Hartmann hemostatic forceps
Hartmann mosquito forceps
Hartmann nasal-dressing forceps
Hartmann-Citelli alligator forceps
Hartmann-Citelli ear punch forceps
Hartmann-Citelli forceps
Hartmann-Gruenwald forceps
Hartmann-Gruenwald nasal-cutting forceps
Hartmann-Herzfeld ear forceps
Hartmann-Herzfeld forceps
Hartmann-Noyes nasal-dressing forceps
Hartmann-Proctor ear forceps
Hawkins forceps
Hawks-Dennen forceps
Hawks-Dennen obstetrical forceps
Hayes anterior resection forceps
Hayes Martin forceps
Hayes-Olivecrona forceps
Hayton-Williams forceps
Healy forceps
Healy gastrointestinal forceps
Healy intestinal forceps

forceps *continued*

Healy suture-removing
forceps
Heaney forceps
Heaney hysterectomy
forceps
Heaney-Ballantine
forceps
Heaney-Ballantine
hysterectomy
forceps
Heaney-Kantor forceps
Heaney-Kantor hysterec-
tomy forceps
Heaney-Rezek forceps
Heaney-Rezek hysterec-
tomy forceps
Heaney-Simon forceps
Heaney-Simon hysterec-
tomy forceps
Heaney-Stumf forceps
Heath chalazion forceps
Heath forceps
Heermann alligator ear
forceps
Heermann alligator
forceps
Heermann ear forceps
Heermann forceps
Hegenbarth clip forceps
Hegenbarth clip-applying
forceps
Hegenbarth clip-
removing forceps
Hegenbarth forceps
Hegenbarth-Michel clip-
applying forceps
Heidelberg fixation
forceps
Heiss arterial forceps
Heiss forceps
hemoclip-applying
forceps
hemorrhoid forceps
hemorrhoidal forceps
hemostasis clip-applying
forceps

forceps *continued*

hemostasis forceps
hemostatic cervix forceps
hemostatic forceps
hemostatic neurosurgical
forceps
hemostatic tissue forceps
hemostatic tonsillar
forceps
hemostatic tracheal
forceps
Hendren cardiovascular
forceps
Hendren forceps
Hendren pediatric
forceps
Henke forceps
Henke forceps tip
Henke punch forceps tip
Henrotin forceps
Henrotin uterine
vulsellum forceps
Henrotin vulsellum
forceps
Henry cilia forceps
Herff membrane-
puncturing forceps
Herget biopsy forceps
Herman forceps
Herrick forceps
Hertel forceps
Hertel kidney stone
forceps
Hertel rigid dilator stone
forceps
Hertel rigid kidney stone
forceps
Hertel stone forceps
Herzfeld ear forceps
Herzfeld forceps
Hess capsule forceps
Hess capsule iris forceps
Hess forceps
Hess iris forceps
Hess-Barraquer forceps
Hess-Barraquer iris
forceps

forceps *continued*

Hess-Gill eye forceps
Hess-Gill forceps
Hess-Gill iris forceps
Hess-Horwitz forceps
Hess-Horwitz iris forceps
Hevesy polyp forceps
Heyman forceps
Heyman nasal forceps
Heywood-Smith dressing forceps
Heywood-Smith sponge-holding forceps
Hibbs biting forceps
Hibbs forceps
high forceps
Hildebrandt uterine hemostatic forceps
Hildyard forceps
Hinderer cartilage forceps
Hinderer cartilage-holding forceps
Hirschman forceps
Hirschman hemorrhoidal forceps
Hirschman jeweler's forceps
Hirschman lens forceps
Hirst forceps
Hirst-Emmet obstetrical forceps
Hirst-Emmet placental forceps
Hodge forceps
Hodge obstetrical forceps
Hoen forceps
Hoen scalp forceps
Hoffmann ear forceps
Hoffmann ear punch forceps
Hoffmann forceps
Holinger forceps
hollow-object forceps
Holmes fixation forceps
Holmes forceps

forceps *continued*

Holth forceps
Holth punch forceps
Holzbach hysterectomy forceps
Hook basket forceps
hook forceps
Hopkins aortic forceps
Hopkins forceps
Horsley bone-cutting forceps
Horsley forceps
Horsley-Stille bone-cutting forceps
Hosemann choledochus forceps
Hosemann forceps
Hosford-Hicks forceps
Hosford-Hicks transfer forceps
hot biopsy forceps
hot flexible forceps
Hough alligator forceps
Hough forceps
House alligator crimper forceps
House alligator forceps
House alligator grasping forceps
House alligator-strut forceps
House crimper forceps
House cup forceps
House forceps
House Gelfoam pressure forceps
House grasping forceps
House pressure forceps
House strut forceps
House-Dieter eye forceps
Housepian clip-applying forceps
House-Wullstein cup forceps
House-Wullstein ear forceps
House-Wullstein forceps

forceps *continued*

House-Wullstein oval
cup forceps
Howard closing forceps
Howard forceps
Howard tonsil forceps
Howard tonsil-ligating
forceps
Hoxworth forceps
Hoyt forceps
Hoyt hemostatic forceps
Hoytenberger tissue
forceps
Hubbard corneoscleral
forceps
Hubbard forceps
Hudson brain forceps
Hudson cranial rongeur
forceps
Hudson dressing for-
ceps
Hudson forceps
Hudson rongeur forceps
Hudson tissue-dressing
forceps
Hufnagel forceps
Hufnagel mitral valve-
holding forceps
Hulka-Kenwick forceps
Hulka-Kenwick uterine-
manipulating forceps
HUMI cervical forceps
skate flap
hump forceps
Hunt chalazion forceps
Hunt forceps
Hunter splinter forceps
Hunt-Yasargil pituitary
forceps
Hurd bone forceps
Hurd forceps
Hurd septal forceps
Hurd septum-cutting
forceps
Hurdner tissue forceps
Hyde corneal forceps
hyoid-cutting forceps

forceps *continued*

hypogastric artery
forceps
hypophyseal forceps
hypophysectomy forceps
hysterectomy forceps
iliac forceps
Iliff blepharochalasis
forceps
Imperatori forceps
Imperatori laryngeal
forceps
implant forceps
infant biopsy forceps
infundibular forceps
infundibular rongeur
forceps
Ingraham-Fowler clip-
applying forceps
inlet forceps
insertion forceps
instrument-grasping
forceps
instrument-handling
forceps
insulated bayonet
forceps
insulated forceps
insulated monopolar
forceps
insulated tissue forceps
interchangeable forceps
tip
interchangeable laryn-
geal forceps tip
intervertebral disk
forceps
intervertebral disk
rongeur forceps
intestinal forceps
intestinal tissue-holding
forceps
intraocular forceps
intraocular irrigating
forceps
intraocular lens forceps
Iowa forceps

forceps *continued*

Iowa membrane-puncturing forceps
Iowa State fixation forceps
Iowa State forceps
Iowa trumpet forceps guide
iris forceps
iris microforceps
isolation forceps
IV disk forceps
Jackson alligator forceps
Jackson biopsy forceps
Jackson bronchoscopic forceps handle
Jackson forceps
Jackson hemostatic forceps
Jackson infant biopsy forceps
Jackson infant forceps
Jackson laryngeal applicator forceps
Jackson laryngeal forceps
Jackson laryngeal punch forceps
Jackson laryngeal rotation forceps
Jackson laryngofissure forceps
Jackson punch forceps
Jackson ring-rotation forceps
Jackson rotation forceps
Jackson tracheal forceps
Jackson tracheal hemostatic forceps
Jacob forceps
Jacob uterine vulsellum forceps
Jacob vulsellum forceps
Jacobson dressing forceps
Jacobson forceps
Jacobson hemostatic forceps

forceps *continued*

Jacobson microdressing forceps
Jacobson mosquito forceps
Jako laryngeal micro-forceps
James wound approximation forceps
Jameson forceps
Jameson muscle forceps
Jameson recession forceps
Jameson tracheal muscle recession forceps
Jannetta bayonet forceps
Jannetta forceps
Jannetta microbayonet forceps
Jansen bayonet forceps
Jansen bayonet nasal forceps
Jansen ear forceps
Jansen forceps
Jansen nasal-dressing forceps
Jansen thumb forceps
Jansen-Gruenwald forceps
Jansen-Middleton forceps
Jansen-Middleton nasal-cutting forceps
Jansen-Middleton septal forceps
Jansen-Middleton septotomy forceps
Jansen-Middleton septum-cutting forceps
Jansen-Mueller forceps
Jansen-Struyken forceps
Jansen-Struyken septal forceps
Jarcho forceps
Jarcho tenaculum forceps
Jarcho uterine tenaculum forceps
Jarit-Allis tissue forceps

forceps *continued*

Jarit-Crafoord forceps
Jarit-Liston bone-cutting forceps
Jarvis forceps
Jarvis hemorrhoid forceps
Javerts placental forceps
Javerts polyp forceps
Jayles forceps
Jensen forceps
Jensen intraocular lens forceps
Jensen lens forceps
Jervey forceps
Jesberg forceps
Jesberg grasping forceps
jeweler's bipolar forceps
jeweler's forceps
jeweler's microforceps
jeweler's pickup forceps
Johns Hopkins forceps
Johns Hopkins gallbladder forceps
Johns Hopkins occluding forceps
Johnson brain tumor forceps
Johnson forceps
Johnson thoracic forceps
Jones forceps
Jones hemostatic forceps
Jones IMA forceps
Jones towel forceps
Joplin forceps
Judd forceps
Judd strabismus forceps
Judd suture forceps
Judd-Allis forceps
Judd-Allis intestinal forceps
Judd-Allis tissue forceps
Judd-DeMartel forceps
Judd-DeMartel gallbladder forceps
Juers forceps
Juers-Lempert forceps

forceps *continued*

Juers-Lempert rongeur forceps
jugum forceps
Julian forceps
Julian splenorenal forceps
Julian thoracic forceps
Julian thoracic hemostatic forceps
jumbo biopsy forceps
Jurasz forceps
Jurasz laryngeal forceps
Kahler biopsy forceps
Kahler bronchial biopsy forceps
Kahler bronchial forceps
Kahler bronchoscopic forceps
Kahler bronchus-grasping forceps
Kahler forceps
Kahler laryngeal biopsy forceps
Kahler laryngeal forceps
Kahler polyp forceps
Kahn forceps
Kalman forceps
Kalman occluding forceps
Kalt capsule forceps
Kalt forceps
Kantor forceps
Kantrowitz dressing forceps
Kantrowitz forceps
Kantrowitz thoracic forceps
Kantrowitz tissue forceps
Kapp applying forceps
Kapp-Beck forceps
Karp aortic punch forceps
Katzin-Barraquer Colibri forceps
Katzin-Barraquer forceps

forceps *continued*
Kaufman forceps
Kaufman insulated
forceps
Kazanjian cutting forceps
Kazanjian forceps
Kazanjian nasal forceps
Kazanjian nasal hump
forceps
Kazanjian nasal hump-
cutting forceps
Kazanjian nasal-cutting
forceps
Kazanjian-Cottle forceps
Kelly artery forceps
Kelly dressing forceps
Kelly forceps
Kelly placenta forceps
Kelly tissue forceps
Kelly urethral forceps
Kelly-Gray uterine
forceps
Kelly-Murphy forceps
Kelly-Murphy hemostatic
forceps
Kelly-Murphy hemostatic
uterine vulsellum
forceps
Kelly-Rankin forceps
Kelman forceps
Kelman irrigator forceps
Kelman-McPherson
forceps
Kelman-McPherson
microtying forceps
Kelman-McPherson
tissue forceps
Kennedy forceps
Kennedy uterine
vulsellum forceps
Kent forceps
keratotomy forceps
Kern bone-holding
forceps
Kern forceps
Kern-Lane bone-holding
forceps

forceps *continued*
Kerrison forceps
Kevorkian forceps
Kevorkian-Younge
biopsy forceps
Kevorkian-Younge
cervical biopsy forceps
Kevorkian-Younge
forceps
Kevorkian-Younge
uterine biopsy forceps
Khodadad microclip
forceps
kidney stone forceps
kidney-elevating forceps
Kielland (also Kjelland)
Kielland forceps
Kielland obstetrical
forceps
Kielland-Luikart forceps
Kielland-Luikart obstetri-
cal forceps
Killian cutting forceps
tip
Killian double-articulated
forceps tip
Killian forceps
Killian septal compres-
sion forceps
Killian septal forceps
Killian-Jameson forceps
King tissue forceps
King-Prince forceps
King-Prince recession
forceps
Kingsley forceps
Kirby corneoscleral
forceps
Kirby fixation forceps
Kirby forceps
Kirby intracapsular lens
forceps
Kirby iris forceps
Kirby lens forceps
Kirby tissue forceps
Kirby-Arthus fixation
forceps

forceps *continued*
- Kirby-Bracken iris forceps
- Kirkpatrick forceps
- Kirkpatrick tonsil forceps
- Kitner forceps
- Kitner thyroid-packing forceps
- Kjelland (see *Kielland*)
- KleenSpec forceps
- Kleinert-Kutz bone-cutting forceps
- Kleinert-Kutz tendon retriever forceps
- KLI bipolar forceps
- KLI forceps
- KLI monopolar forceps
- Knapp forceps
- Knapp trachoma forceps
- Knight forceps
- Knight nasal forceps
- Knight nasal septum-cutting forceps
- Knight polyp forceps
- Knight septum-cutting forceps
- Knight turbinate forceps
- Knight-Sluder forceps
- knot-holding forceps
- Kocher artery forceps
- Kocher forceps
- Kocher intestinal forceps
- Kocher kidney-elevating forceps
- Kocher Micro-Line intestinal forceps
- Kocher-Ochsner hemostatic forceps
- Koeberlé forceps
- Koenig vascular forceps
- Koerte gallstone forceps
- Koffler forceps
- Koffler septum bone forceps
- Koffler septum forceps
- Koffler-Lillie forceps

forceps *continued*
- Koffler-Lillie septum forceps
- Kogan endospeculum forceps
- Kolb bronchus forceps
- Kolb forceps
- Kolodny forceps
- Kramer forceps
- Krause biopsy forceps
- Krause forceps
- Krause Universal forceps
- Kronfeld forceps
- Kronfeld micropin forceps
- Kronfeld suture forceps
- Krönlein hemostatic forceps
- K/S-Allis forceps
- Kuhnt capsule forceps
- Kuhnt fixation forceps
- Kuhnt forceps
- Kulvin-Kalt forceps
- Kulvin-Kalt iris forceps
- Kurze forceps
- Kurze microbiopsy forceps
- Kurze micrograsping forceps
- Kurze pickup forceps
- Küstner uterine tenaculum forceps
- Laborde forceps
- Lahey forceps
- Lahey gall duct forceps
- Lahey hemostatic forceps
- Lahey thoracic forceps
- Lahey thyroid traction forceps
- Lahey thyroid traction vulsellum forceps
- Lahey-Babcock forceps
- Lahey-Péan forceps
- Lahey-Sweet dissecting forceps
- Lambert chalazion forceps

forceps *continued*
- Lambert forceps
- Lambotte bone-holding forceps
- Lambotte forceps
- Lancaster-O'Connor forceps
- lancet-shaped biopsy forceps
- Lane bone-holding forceps
- Lane forceps
- Lane intestinal forceps
- Lange approximation forceps
- Langenbeck bone-holding forceps
- Langenbeck forceps
- laparoscopic forceps
- Laplace forceps
- Larsen tendon forceps
- laryngeal biopsy forceps
- laryngeal curet forceps
- laryngeal forceps
- laryngeal punch forceps
- laryngeal rotation forceps
- laryngeal sponging forceps
- laryngofissure forceps
- Lauer forceps
- Laufe forceps
- Laufe obstetrical forceps
- Laufe uterine polyp forceps
- Laufe-Barton-Kielland obstetrical forceps
- Laufe-Barton-Kielland-Piper obstetrical forceps
- Laufe-Piper forceps
- Laufe-Piper obstetrical forceps
- Laufe-Piper uterine polyp forceps
- Lawrence deep forceps
- Lawrence forceps
- Lawton forceps

forceps *continued*
- Lawton-Schubert biopsy forceps
- Lawton-Wittner cervical biopsy forceps
- Leader forceps
- Leader vas isolation forceps
- Leahey marginal chalazion forceps
- Lebsche forceps
- Ledhey forceps
- Lee delicate hemostatic forceps
- Lees arterial forceps
- Lees nontraumatic forceps
- Lefferts forceps
- Leigh capsule forceps
- Leigh forceps
- Lejeune forceps
- Lejeune thoracic forceps
- Leksell forceps
- Leland-Jones forceps
- Lemmon-Russian forceps
- Lemoine forceps
- Lempert forceps
- Lempert rongeur forceps
- lens forceps
- lens implant forceps
- Leo Schwartz sponge-holding forceps
- Leonard deep forceps
- Leonard forceps
- Leriche forceps
- Leriche hemostatic forceps
- Leriche tissue forceps
- LeRoy scalp clip-applying forceps
- Lester fixation forceps
- Lester forceps
- Levenson tissue forceps
- Levora fixation forceps
- Levret forceps
- Lewin bone-holding forceps

forceps *continued*

Lewin forceps
Lewis forceps
Lewis septal forceps
Lewis tonsillar hemo-
   static forceps
Lewkowitz forceps
Lewkowitz lithotomy
   forceps
Lexer tissue forceps
Leyro-Diaz forceps
lid forceps
Lieberman forceps
Lieberman suturing
   forceps
Lieberman tying forceps
Lieb-Guerry forceps
ligamenta flava forceps
ligamentum-grasping
   forceps
ligature forceps
ligature-carrying aneu-
   rysm forceps
ligature-carrying forceps
Lillehei forceps
Lillehei valve forceps
Lillehei valve-grasping
   forceps
Lillie forceps
Lillie intestinal forceps
Lillie tissue-holding
   forceps
Lillie-Killian forceps
Lillie-Killian septal bone
   forceps
lingual forceps
Linn-Graefe iris forceps
Linnartz forceps
lion-jaw bone-holding
   forceps
lion-jaw forceps
Lister conjunctival
   forceps
Lister forceps
Liston bone-cutting
   forceps
Liston forceps

forceps *continued*

Liston-Littauer bone-
   cutting forceps
Liston-Stille forceps
lithotomy forceps
Litt forceps
Littauer cilia forceps
Littauer ear-dressing
   forceps
Littauer forceps
Littauer nasal-dressing
   forceps
Littauer-Liston bone-
   cutting forceps
Littauer-Liston forceps
Littauer-West cutting
   forceps
Livingston forceps
Llobera fixation forceps
Llobera forceps
lobectomy forceps
lobe-grasping forceps
lobe-holding forceps
Lobell splinter forceps
Lobenstein-Tarnier
   forceps
Lockwood forceps
Lockwood intestinal
   forceps
Lockwood-Allis forceps
Lockwood-Allis intestinal
   forceps
Lombard-Beyer forceps
Lombard-Beyer rongeur
   forceps
London forceps
London tissue forceps
Long forceps
Long hysterectomy
   forceps
Long Island College
   Hospital placenta
   forceps
Long Island forceps
loop-type snare forceps
loop-type stone-crushing
   forceps

forceps *continued*

- loose body forceps
- Lordan chalazion forceps
- Lordan forceps
- Lore forceps
- Lore suction tip-holding forceps
- Lore suction tube-holding forceps
- Lothrop forceps
- Lothrop ligature forceps
- Love-Gruenwald forceps
- Love-Kerrison forceps
- Lovelace bladder forceps
- Lovelace forceps
- Lovelace hemostatic forceps
- Lovelace thyroid traction vulsellum forceps
- low forceps
- Löw-Beer forceps
- Löwenberg forceps
- Lower forceps
- Lower gall duct forceps
- Lower lateral forceps
- low-forceps delivery
- low-forceps operation
- Lowis IV disk rongeur forceps
- Lowman forceps
- Lowsley forceps
- Lowsley grasping forceps
- Lowsley prostatic lobe-holding forceps
- Lowsley-Luc forceps
- Luc ethmoid forceps
- Luc forceps
- Luc septum forceps
- Luc septum-cutting forceps
- Lucae dressing forceps
- Lucae forceps
- Luer forceps
- Luer hemorrhoidal forceps
- Luer-Whiting forceps
- Luikart forceps

forceps *continued*

- Luikart obstetrical forceps
- Luikart-Kielland forceps
- Luikart-McLean forceps
- Luikart-Simpson forceps
- lung forceps
- lung-grasping forceps
- Lutz forceps
- Lutz septal forceps
- Lutz septal ridge forceps
- Lutz septal ridge-cutting forceps
- Lynch forceps
- Lyon forceps
- MacGregor conjunctival forceps
- MacGregor forceps
- MacKenty forceps
- MacKenty tissue forceps
- Madden forceps
- Madden-Potts forceps
- Magielski forceps
- Magielski tonsil forceps
- Magielski-Heermann forceps
- Magill catheter-introducing forceps
- Magill forceps
- Maier dressing forceps
- Maier forceps
- Maier uterine-dressing forceps
- Mailler colon forceps
- Mailler cut-off forceps
- Mailler intestinal forceps
- Mailler rectal forceps
- Maingot hysterectomy forceps
- Malis angled-up bipolar forceps
- Malis forceps
- Malis titanium micro-surgical forceps
- malleus forceps
- Manhattan Eye & Ear suture forceps

forceps *continued*

Mann forceps
Manning forceps
Mansfield forceps
March-Barton forceps
Marcuse forceps
marginal chalazion forceps
Markwalder forceps
Marshik forceps
Marshik tonsillar forceps
Marshik tonsil-seizing forceps
Martin forceps
Martin nasopharyngeal biopsy forceps
Martin thumb forceps
Martin tissue forceps
Martin uterine tenaculum forceps
Maryan biopsy punch forceps
Maryan forceps
Masterson hysterectomy forceps
mastoid rongeur forceps
Mathieu forceps
Mathieu tongue-seizing forceps
Mathieu urethral forceps
Mathews forceps
Maumenee corneal forceps
Maumenee cross-action capsule forceps
Maumenee forceps
Maumenee straight-action capsule forceps
Maumenee tissue forceps
Maumenee-Colibri forceps
Max Fine forceps
Max Fine tying forceps
Max forceps
Mayfield aneurysmal forceps

forceps *continued*

Mayfield applying forceps
Mayfield forceps
May-Harrington forceps
Mayo bone-cutting forceps
Mayo forceps
Mayo tissue forceps
Mayo ureter isolation forceps
Mayo-Blake forceps
Mayo-Blake gallstone forceps
Mayo-Harrington forceps
Mayo-Ochsner forceps
Mayo-Péan forceps
Mayo-Robson forceps
Mayo-Robson gastro-intestinal forceps
Mayo-Robson intestinal forceps
Mayo-Russian forceps
Mayo-Russian gastro-intestinal forceps
McCarthy forceps
McCarthy visual he-mostatic forceps
McCarthy-Alcock for-ceps
McCarthy-Alcock hemostatic forceps
McClintock placenta forceps
McCoy forceps
McCoy septal forceps
McCoy septum-cutting forceps
McCullough forceps
McCullough suture forceps
McCullough suture-tying forceps
McCullough utility forceps
McGannon forceps
McGannon lens forceps

forceps *continued*

McGee wire-closure forceps
McGee wire-crimper forceps
McGee-Paparella wire-crimping forceps
McGee-Priest forceps
McGee-Priest wire-crimping forceps
McGee-Priest-Paparella closure forceps
McGee-Priest-Paparella crimper-forceps
McGill forceps
McGivney hemorrhoidal forceps
McGravey forceps
McGravey tissue forceps
McGregor forceps
McGuire forceps
McHenry forceps
McHenry tonsillar artery forceps
McIndoe dressing forceps
McIndoe forceps
McIntosh forceps
McIntosh suture-holding forceps
McKay ear forceps
McKay forceps
McKenzie brain clip-applying forceps
McKenzie forceps
McKenzie grasping forceps
McLean forceps
McLean-Tucker obstetrical forceps
McLean-Tucker-Kielland obstetrical forceps
McLean-Tucker-Luikart obstetrical forceps
McLean capsule forceps
McLean ophthalmological forceps

forceps *continued*

McNealey-Glassman-Babcock forceps
McNealey-Glassman-Babcock viscera-holding forceps
McNealey-Glassman-Babcock visceral forceps
McNealey-Glassman-Mixter forceps
McNealey-Glassman-Mixter ligature-carrying aneurysm forceps
McPherson angled forceps
McPherson cornea forceps
McPherson forceps
McPherson lens forceps
McPherson suturing forceps
McPherson tying forceps
McPherson-Pierse forceps
McQuigg forceps
McQuigg-Mixter bronchial forceps
McQuigg-Mixter forceps
McWhorter tonsillar forceps
meat forceps
meat-grasping forceps
mechanical finger forceps
mechanical forceps
Medicon forceps
Medicon wire-twister forceps
Medicon-Jackson forceps
Medicon-Jackson rectal forceps
Medicon-Packer mosquito forceps
medium forceps
Meeker forceps

forceps *continued*

Meeker gallbladder
forceps
Meeker hemostatic
forceps
meibomian expressor
forceps
meibomian forceps
Meltzer adenoid punch
forceps
membrane-puncturing
forceps
Mendel ligature
forceps
Mengert membrane-
puncturing forceps
Merlin stone forceps
Merz hysterectomy
forceps
Metzenbaum forceps
Metzenbaum tonsillar
forceps
Metzenbaum-Tydings
forceps
Meyhoeffer chalazion
forceps
MGH forceps
MGH vulsellum forceps
Michel clip-applying
forceps
Michel forceps
Michel tissue forceps
Michigan forceps
Michigan intestinal
forceps
Micrins forceps
microbayonet forceps
microbiopsy forceps
microbipolar forceps
microbronchoscopic
tissue forceps
microclamp forceps
microclip forceps
microdressing forceps
microextractor forceps
microforceps
Micro-Line artery for-
ceps

forceps *continued*

microneedle holder
forceps
microneurosurgery
forceps
micropin forceps
microsurgery biopsy
forceps
microsuture forceps
microsuture-tying for-
ceps
microtip bipolar forceps
microtissue forceps
microtying eye forceps
microtying forceps
microutility forceps
microvascular forceps
middle ear forceps
middle ear strut forceps
midforceps
Mikulicz forceps
Mikulicz peritoneal
forceps
Mikulicz tonsillar forceps
Milex forceps
Miller bayonet forceps
Miller forceps
Miller rectal forceps
Millin capsule forceps
Millin capsule-grasping
forceps
Millin forceps
Millin lobe-grasping
forceps
Millin T-shaped angled
forceps
Millin T-shaped forceps
Mill-Rose biopsy forceps
Mills forceps
Mills tissue forceps
miniature forceps
miniature intestinal
forceps
mini-micro forceps
Mitchell-Diamond biopsy
forceps
Mitchell-Diamond
forceps

forceps *continued*

mitral forceps
mitral valve-holding
forceps
Mixter forceps
Mixter full-curve forceps
Mixter gall duct forceps
Mixter gallbladder
forceps
Mixter gallstone forceps
Mixter-McQuigg forceps
Mixter-O'Shaugnessy
dissecting and ligature
forceps
Mixter-Paul hemostatic
forceps
Moberg forceps
Moehle corneal forceps
Moehle forceps
Moersch bronchoscopic
specimen forceps
Moersch forceps
Molt forceps
monopolar coagulating
forceps
monopolar forceps
monopolar insulated
forceps
Montenovesi cranial
rongeur forceps
Moody forceps
Moore forceps
Morgenstein blunt
forceps
Moritz-Schmidt forceps
Moritz-Schmidt laryngeal
forceps
Morson forceps
Mosher ethmoid punch
forceps
Mosher forceps
mosquito forceps
mosquito hemostatic
forceps
Mount forceps
Mount intervertebral disk
rongeur forceps
Mount-Mayfield forceps

forceps *continued*

Mount-Olivecrona
forceps
mouse-tooth forceps
Moynihan forceps
Moynihan gall duct
forceps
Moynihan-Navratil
forceps
Muck forceps
Muck tonsillar forceps
mucus forceps
Mueller forceps
Mueller-Markham patent
ductus forceps
Muir hemorrhoidal
forceps
Muldoon meibomian
forceps
multipurpose forceps
Mundie forceps
Mundie placenta
forceps
Murless head extractor
forceps
Murphy forceps
Murphy tonsillar forceps
Murphy-Péan hemostatic
forceps
Murray forceps
muscle forceps
Museux forceps
Museux uterine vulsel-
lum forceps
Museux-Collins uterine
vulsellum forceps
Museholdt forceps
Musial tissue forceps
Myerson forceps
Myerson miniature
laryngeal biopsy
forceps
Myles forceps
Myles hemorrhoidal
forceps
Myles nasal-cutting
forceps
nail-extracting forceps

forceps *continued*
    nasal alligator forceps
    nasal bone forceps
    nasal cartilage-holding
      forceps
    nasal forceps
    nasal hump-cutting
      forceps
    nasal insertion forceps
    nasal lower lateral
      forceps
    nasal needle holder
      forceps
    nasal polyp forceps
    nasal polypus forceps
    nasal septal forceps
    nasal-cutting forceps
    nasal-dressing forceps
    nasal-grasping forceps
    nasal-packing forceps
    nasopharyngeal biopsy
      forceps
    needle forceps
    needle holder forceps
    Negus forceps
    Negus-Green forceps
    Nelson forceps
    Nelson lung-dissecting
      forceps
    Nelson tissue forceps
    Nelson-Martin forceps
    nephrolithotomy forceps
    Neubauer forceps
    Neubauer vitreous
      microextractor for-
      ceps
    neurosurgical dressing
      forceps
    neurosurgical forceps
    neurosurgical ligature
      forceps
    neurosurgical tissue
      forceps
    Nevins forceps
    Nevins tissue forceps
    New biopsy forceps
    New forceps

forceps *continued*
    New Orleans Eye and
      Ear forceps
    New Orleans forceps
    New tissue forceps
    New York Eye and Ear
      fixation forceps
    New York Eye and Ear
      forceps
    Newman forceps
    Newman tenaculum
      forceps
    Newman uterine
      tenaculum forceps
    Nicola microforceps
    Niedner dissecting
      forceps
    Niedner forceps
    NIH mitral valve forceps
    NIH mitral valve-
      grasping forceps
    Niro wire-twister for-
      ceps
    Nisbet fixation forceps
    Nissen cystic forceps
    Nissen forceps
    Nissen gall duct forceps
    Noble forceps
    Noble iris forceps
    noncrushing forceps
    noncrushing pickup
      forceps
    noncrushing tissue-
      holding forceps
    nonfenestrated forceps
    nonmagnetic dressing
      forceps
    nonmagnetic forceps
    nonmagnetic tissue
      forceps
    nonslipping forceps
    nontoothed forceps
    nontraumatizing forceps
    nontraumatizing viscera
      forceps
    Norwood forceps
    Noto dressing forceps

forceps *continued*

Noto sponge-holding forceps
Novak fixation forceps
Noyes forceps
Noyes nasal-dressing forceps
Nugent forceps
Nugent utility forceps
Nugowski forceps
Nussbaum intestinal forceps
Oberhill obstetrical forceps
O'Brien forceps
O'Brien-Elschnig forceps
obstetrical forceps
occluding forceps
occlusion forceps
Ochsner artery forceps
Ochsner forceps
Ockerblad forceps
O'Connor biopsy forceps
O'Connor eye forceps
O'Connor forceps
O'Connor grasping forceps
O'Connor-Elschnig fixation forceps
O'Gawa-Castroviejo forceps
Ogura cartilage forceps
Ogura forceps
Ogura tissue forceps
O'Hanlon forceps
O'Hara forceps
Oldberg forceps
Olivecrona aneurysm forceps
Olivecrona clip-applying forceps
Olivecrona forceps
Olivecrona-Toennis clip-applying forceps
Olympus alligator-jaw endoscopic forceps

forceps *continued*

Olympus basket-type endoscopic forceps
Olympus biopsy forceps
Olympus endoscopic biopsy forceps
Olympus FBK 13 endoscopic biopsy
Olympus hot biopsy forceps
Olympus magnetic extractor forceps
Olympus minisnare forceps
Olympus pelican-type endoscopic forceps
Olympus rat-tooth endoscopic forceps
Olympus rubber-tip endoscopic forceps
Olympus shark-tooth endoscopic forceps
Olympus tripod-type endoscopic forceps
Olympus W-shaped endoscopic forceps
Ombrédanne forceps
optical biopsy forceps
oral forceps
oral rongeur forceps
Orr forceps
Orr gall duct forceps
O'Shaughnessy forceps
ossicle-holding forceps
Ostrom antrum punch-tip forceps
Ostrom forceps
Ostrom punch forceps
Otto forceps
outlet forceps
oval cup forceps
Overholt forceps
Overholt thoracic forceps
Overholt-Geissendoerfer dissecting forceps
Overholt-Mixter dissecting forceps

forceps *continued*

Overstreet endometrial polyp forceps
Overstreet forceps
Overstreet polyp forceps
ovum forceps
Pace-Potts forceps
Packer mosquito forceps
Page forceps
Page tonsillar forceps
Palmer biopsy drill forceps
Palmer biopsy forceps
Pang forceps
papilloma forceps
parametrium forceps
Parker fixation forceps
Parker-Kerr forceps
partial occlusion forceps
patent ductus forceps
Paterson forceps
Paterson laryngeal forceps
Paton corneal forceps
Paton corneal transplant forceps
Paton forceps
Patterson forceps
Paufique forceps
Paufique suture forceps
Pauwels fracture forceps
Payne-Ochsner arterial forceps
Payne-Ochsner forceps
Payne-Péan arterial forceps
Payne-Péan forceps
Payne-Rankin arterial forceps
Payne-Rankin forceps
Payr forceps
Payr pylorus forceps
Péan forceps
Péan GI forceps
Péan hemostatic forceps
Péan hysterectomy forceps

forceps *continued*

Péan sponge forceps
peanut forceps
peanut sponge-holding forceps
peanut-fenestrated forceps
peanut-grasping forceps
peapod intervertebral disk forceps
pediatric forceps
Peet forceps
Peet mosquito forceps
Peet splinter forceps
Pelkmann sponge forceps
Pelkmann uterine forceps
Pelkmann uterine-dressing forceps
Pemberton forceps
Penfield forceps
Penfield suture forceps
Pennington forceps
Pennington hemostatic forceps
Pennington tissue-grasping forceps
Percy forceps
Percy intestinal forceps
Percy tissue forceps
Percy-Wolfson gallbladder forceps
Perdue tonsillar hemostat forceps
perforating forceps
peripheral blood vessel forceps
peripheral iridectomy forceps
peripheral vascular forceps
Perritt fixation forceps
Perritt forceps
Perry forceps
Peter-Bishop forceps
Peters tissue forceps

forceps *continued*

Peyman vitreous-
grasping forceps
Peyman-Green vitreous
forceps
Pfau forceps
Pfister-Schwartz basket
forceps
phalangeal forceps
Phaneuf artery forceps
Phaneuf forceps
Phaneuf uterine artery
forceps
Phaneuf vaginal forceps
Phillips fixation forceps
Phillips forceps
phimosis forceps
Phipps forceps
phrenicectomy forceps
physician's pickup
forceps
physician's splinter
forceps
pickup forceps
pickup noncrushing
forceps
Pierse corneal forceps
Pierse forceps
Pierse Colibri forceps
Pierse-Hoskins forceps
pile forceps
pillar forceps
pillar-grasping forceps
Pilling forceps
Pilling-Liston bone utility
forceps
pin-bending forceps
pinch forceps
Piper forceps
Piper obstetrical forceps
Pischel forceps
Pitanguy forceps
Pitha forceps
Pitha urethral forceps
pituitary forceps
pituitary rongeur forceps
placenta forceps

forceps *continued*

placenta previa forceps
placental forceps
plain forceps
plain thumb forceps
plain tissue forceps
platform forceps
pleurectomy forceps
Pley capsule forceps
Pley forceps
Plondke uterine-
elevating forceps
point forceps
Polk sponge forceps
Pollock double corneal
forceps
Pollock forceps
polyp forceps
polypus forceps
Poppen forceps
Porter duodenal forceps
Porter forceps
Post forceps
posterior forceps
postnasal sponge forceps
Potter sponge forceps
Potter tonsillar forceps
Potts bronchial forceps
Potts bulldog forceps
Potts coarctation forceps
Potts fixation forceps
Potts forceps
Potts patent ductus
forceps
Potts thumb forceps
Potts-Smith forceps
Potts-Smith tissue forceps
Poutasse forceps
Poutasse renal artery
forceps
Pozzi tenaculum forceps
Pratt forceps
Pratt T-shaped hemo-
static forceps
Pratt-Smith forceps
Pratt-Smith tissue-
grasping forceps

forceps *continued*
    prepuce forceps
    Presbyterian Hospital
      forceps
    pressure forceps
    Preston ligamentum
      flavum forceps
    Price-Thomas bronchial
      forceps
    Price-Thomas forceps
    Primbs suturing forceps
    Prince advancement
      forceps
    Prince forceps
    Prince muscle forceps
    Prince trachoma forceps
    proctological biopsy
      forceps
    proctological forceps
    proctological grasping
      forceps
    proctological polyp
      forceps
    Proctor phrenectomy
      forceps
    Proctor phrenicectomy
      forceps
    prostatic forceps
    prostatic lobe forceps
    prostatic lobe-holding
      forceps
    Providence Hospital
      artery forceps
    Providence Hospital
      classic forceps
    Providence Hospital
      forceps
    Providence Hospital
      hemostatic forceps
    ptosis forceps
    pulmonary artery forceps
    pulmonary vessel for-
      ceps
    punch forceps
    Puntenney forceps
    Puntenney tying forceps
    Quervain cranial forceps

forceps *continued*
    Quervain cranial rongeur
      forceps
    Quervain forceps
    Quevedo forceps
    Quire finger forceps
    Quire forceps
    Quire mechanical finger
      forceps
    Raaf forceps
    Raaf-Oldberg interverte-
      bral disk forceps
    Raimondi forceps
    Raimondi scalp hemo-
      static forceps
    Ralks ear forceps
    Ralks forceps
    Ralks splinter forceps
    Ralks wire-cutting
      forceps
    Rampley forceps
    Rand forceps
    Randall forceps
    Randall kidney stone
      forceps
    Randall stone forceps
    Raney clip forceps
    Raney forceps
    Raney scalp clip-
      applying forceps
    Rankin forceps
    Rankin hemostatic
      forceps
    Rankin-Crile forceps
    Rankin-Crile hemostatic
      forceps
    Rankin-Kelly hemostatic
      forceps
    Rapp forceps
    Ratliff-Blake forceps
    Ratliff-Blake gallstone
      forceps
    Ratliff-Mayo forceps
    Ratliff-Mayo gallstone
      forceps
    rat-tooth forceps
    Ray forceps

forceps *continued*

reach-and-pin forceps
Read forceps
recession forceps
rectal biopsy forceps
rectal forceps
Reese advancement
    forceps
Reese forceps
Reese muscle forceps
Reich-Nechtow forceps
Reich-Nechtow hysterec-
    tomy forceps
Reiner-Knight ethmoid-
    cutting forceps
Reisinger forceps
Reisinger lens-extracting
    forceps
renal artery forceps
Rezek forceps
Rhoton forceps
Rhoton ring tumor
    forceps
rib rongeur forceps
Richards forceps
Richards tonsil-grasping
    forceps
Richards tonsil-seizing
    forceps
Richmond forceps
Richter forceps
Richter suture clip-
    removing forceps
Richter-Heath clip-
    removing forceps
Richter-Heath forceps
ridge forceps
Ridley forceps
Rienhoff arterial forceps
Rienhoff forceps
right-angle forceps
rigid biopsy forceps
rigid kidney stone
    forceps
ring forceps
ring-rotation forceps
Ripstein arterial forceps

forceps *continued*

Ripstein forceps
Ripstein tissue forceps
Ritter forceps
Rizzutti forceps
Rizzuti-Furness cornea-
    holding forceps
Rizzuti-Verhoeff forceps
Robb forceps
Robb tonsillar forceps
Robb tonsillar sponge
    forceps
Roberts bronchial
    forceps
Roberts forceps
Robertson forceps
Robertson tonsil-seizing
    forceps
Robertson tonsillar
    forceps
Robson intestinal forceps
Rochester forceps
Rochester gallstone
    forceps
Rochester-Carmalt
    forceps
Rochester-Carmalt
    hemostatic forceps
Rochester-Davis forceps
Rochester-Ewald tissue
    forceps
Rochester-Harrington
    forceps
Rochester-Mixter artery
    forceps
Rochester-Mixter forceps
Rochester-Ochsner
    forceps
Rochester-Ochsner
    hemostat forceps
Rochester-Péan forceps
Rochester-Rankin forceps
Rochester-Rankin
    hemostatic forceps
Rochester-Russian
    forceps
Rockey forceps

forceps *continued*
- Roeder forceps
- Roeder towel forceps
- Roger forceps
- Roger vascular-toothed hysterectomy forceps
- Rogge sterilizing forceps
- Rolf forceps
- Rolf jeweler's forceps
- roller forceps
- rongeur forceps
- Ronis cutting forceps
- Rose disimpaction forceps
- rotating forceps
- rotation forceps
- round punch forceps
- Rovenstine catheter-introducing forceps
- Rowe disimpaction forceps
- Rowe forceps
- Rowe-Killey forceps
- Rowland double-action hump forceps
- Rowland forceps
- Rowland nasal hump forceps
- Royce forceps
- rubber-dam clamp forceps
- rubber-shod forceps
- Rudd Clinic forceps
- Rudd Clinic hemorrhoidal forceps
- Ruel forceps
- Rugby deep-surgery forceps
- Rugby forceps
- Rumel forceps
- Rumel lobectomy forceps
- Rumel rubber forceps
- Rumel thoracic forceps
- Rumel thoracic-dissecting forceps
- Rumel thoracic forceps

forceps *continued*
- Ruskin bone-cutting forceps
- Ruskin bone-splitting forceps
- Ruskin forceps
- Ruskin-Liston forceps
- Ruskin-Rowland forceps
- Russell forceps
- Russell hysterectomy forceps
- Russell-Davis forceps
- Russian forceps
- Russian thumb forceps
- Russian tissue forceps
- Russian-Péan forceps
- Sachs forceps
- Sachs tissue forceps
- Saenger ovum forceps
- Sajou laryngeal forceps
- Sam Roberts bronchial biopsy forceps
- Sam Roberts forceps
- Samuels forceps
- Samuels hemoclip-applying forceps
- Sanders forceps
- Sanders vasectomy forceps
- Sanders-Castroviejo forceps
- Sandt utility forceps
- Santy dissecting forceps
- Santy forceps
- Sarot artery forceps
- Sarot forceps
- Sarot pleurectomy forceps
- Satinsky forceps
- Satterlee advancement forceps
- Satterlee muscle forceps
- Sauer forceps
- Sauerbruch forceps
- Sauerbruch pickup forceps
- Sawtell forceps

forceps *continued*

Sawtell gallbladder forceps
Sawtell hemostatic forceps
Sawtell tonsillar forceps
Sawtell-Davis forceps
Sawtell-Davis tonsillar hemostat forceps
scalp clip forceps
scalp clip-applying forceps
scalp forceps
Scanzoni forceps
Schaaf foreign body forceps
Schaedel towel forceps
Schanzioni craniotomy forceps
Scheer crimper forceps
Scheie-Graefe fixation forceps
Scheinmann forceps
Scheinmann laryngeal forceps
Schepens forceps
Schick forceps
Schindler peritoneal forceps
Schlesinger forceps
Schlesinger intervertebral disk forceps
Schnidt forceps
Schnidt gall duct forceps
Schnidt thoracic forceps
Schnidt tonsillar forceps
Schnidt tonsillar hemostatic forceps
Schnidt-Rumpler forceps
Schoenberg forceps
Schoenberg intestinal forceps
Schoenberg uterine forceps
Schoenberg uterine-elevating forceps
Schroeder forceps

forceps *continued*

Schroeder tenaculum forceps
Schroeder uterine tenaculum forceps
Schroeder vulsellum forceps
Schroeder-Braun forceps
Schroeder-Braun uterine tenaculum forceps
Schroeder-Van Doren tenaculum forceps
Schubert forceps
Schubert uterine biopsy forceps
Schubert uterine biopsy punch forceps
Schubert uterine tenaculum forceps
Schumacher biopsy forceps
Schutz forceps
Schwartz clip-applying forceps
Schwartz forceps
Schwartz obstetrical forceps
Schweigger capsular forceps
Schweigger extracapsular forceps
Schweigger forceps
Schweizer cervix-holding forceps
Schweizer forceps
scissors forceps
sclerectomy punch forceps
Scobee-Allis forceps
Scoville brain forceps
Scoville brain spatula forceps
Scoville forceps
Scoville-Greenwood forceps
Scudder forceps

forceps *continued*
  Scudder intestinal
    forceps
  Scuderi forceps
  Searcy capsule forceps
  Searcy forceps
  Segond forceps
  Segond tumor forceps
  Segond-Landau hysterec-
    tomy forceps
  Seiffert forceps
  Seletz foramen-plugging
    forceps
  Seletz forceps
  Selman forceps
  Selman nonslip tissue
    forceps
  Selman peripheral blood
    vessel forceps
  Selman tissue forceps
  Selman vessel forceps
  Selverstone forceps
  Semb bone-cutting
    forceps
  Semb dissecting forceps
  Semb forceps
  Semb ligature forceps
  Semb-Ghazi dissecting
    forceps
  Semken forceps
  Semken infant forceps
  Semken tissue forceps
  Semmes dural forceps
  Senn forceps
  Senning forceps
  Senturia forceps
  septal bone forceps
  septal compression
    forceps
  septal forceps
  septal ridge forceps
  septum-cutting forceps
  septum-straightening
    forceps
  sequestrum forceps
  serrated forceps
  serrefine forceps

forceps *continued*
  Sewall brain clip-
    applying forceps
  Sewall forceps
  Seyfert forceps
  Shaaf eye forceps
  Shaaf forceps
  Shaaf foreign body
    forceps
  Shallcross forceps
  Shallcross gallbladder
    forceps
  Shallcross hemostatic
    forceps
  Shallcross nasal forceps
  Shallcross nasal-packing
    forceps
  sharp-pointed forceps
  Shearer chicken-bill
    forceps
  Shearer forceps
  sheathed flexible gastric
    forceps
  sheathed flexible
    gastroscopic forceps
  Sheehy forceps
  Sheehy ossicle-holding
    forceps
  Sheets lens forceps
  Sheinmann laryngeal
    forceps
  Shepard forceps
  Shepard intraocular lens
    forceps
  Shepard intraocular lens-
    inserting forceps
  Shepard lens forceps
  Shepard-Reinstein
    intraocular lens
    forceps
  short-tooth forceps
  Shuppe biting forceps
  Shuster forceps
  Shuster suture forceps
  Shuster tonsillar forceps
  Shutt forceps
  Shutt grasping forceps

forceps *continued*
    shuttle forceps
    side-curved forceps
    side-grasping forceps
    sigmoidoscope biopsy
        forceps
    Silver forceps
    Simons stone-removing
        forceps
    Simpson forceps
    Simpson obstetrical
        forceps
    Simpson-Luikart forceps
    Simpson-Luikart obstetri-
        cal forceps
    Sims-Maier sponge and
        dressing forceps
    Singley forceps
    Singley intestinal forceps
    Singley intestinal tissue
        forceps
    Singley tissue forceps
    Singley-Tuttle dressing
        forceps
    Singley-Tuttle tissue
        forceps
    Sinskey forceps
    Sinskey intraocular lens
        forceps
    Sinskey-McPherson
        forceps
    Sinskey-Wilson forceps
    Sinskey-Wilson foreign
        body forceps
    sinus biopsy forceps
    Sisson forceps
    Skene forceps
    Skene uterine forceps
    Skene vulsellum forceps
    Skillern forceps
    Skillern phimosis for-
        ceps
    Skillman forceps
    Skillman hemostatic
        forceps
    Skillman prepuce forceps
    skin forceps

forceps *continued*
    sleeve-spreading dilating
        forceps
    sliding capsule forceps
    small bone-cutting
        forceps
    Smart chalazion forceps
    Smart forceps
    Smart nonslipping
        chalazion forceps
    Smellie obstetrical
        forceps
    Smith forceps
    Smith grasping forceps
    Smith-Petersen forceps
    Smithwick clip-applying
        forceps
    Smithwick forceps
    Smithwick-Hartmann
        forceps
    smooth tissue forceps
    smooth-tooth forceps
    Snellen entropion
        forceps
    Snellen forceps
    Snowden-Pencer forceps
    Snyder deep surgery
        forceps
    Snyder forceps
    Somers forceps
    Somers uterine forceps
    Somers uterine-elevating
        forceps
    Soonawalla vasectomy
        forceps
    Sparta micro iris forceps
    specimen forceps
    speculum forceps
    Spence forceps
    Spence-Adson clip-
        introducing forceps
    Spence-Adson forceps
    Spencer chalazion
        forceps
    Spencer forceps
    Spencer-Wells chalazion
        forceps

forceps *continued*

Spencer-Wells forceps
Spencer-Wells hemostatic forceps
Spero forceps
Spero meibomian expressor forceps
Spero meibomian forceps
sphenoidal punch forceps
spicule forceps
spinal perforating forceps
spinal rongeur forceps
spiral forceps
splinter forceps
splitting forceps
sponge forceps
sponge-and-dressing forceps
sponge-holding forceps
sponging forceps
spoon-shaped forceps
spring-handled forceps
Spurling forceps
Spurling IV disk forceps
Spurling tissue forceps
Spurling-Kerrison forceps
square specimen forceps
squeeze-handle forceps
SSW forceps
St. Clair forceps
St. Clair-Thompson abscess forceps
St. Clair-Thompson forceps
St. Clair-Thompson peritonsillar abscess forceps
St. Martin eye forceps
St. Martin forceps
St. Martin suturing forceps
St. Vincent forceps
St. Vincent tube-clamping forceps

forceps *continued*

standard artery forceps
stapedectomy forceps
stapes forceps
staple forceps
Starr fixation forceps
Starr forceps
Staude forceps
Staude tenaculum forceps
Staude uterine tenaculum forceps
Staude-Jackson tenaculum forceps
Staude-Moore forceps
Staude-Moore uterine tenaculum forceps
Steinmann intestinal forceps
Steinmann intestinal grasping forceps
sterilizer forceps
Stern-Castroviejo forceps
Stevens fixation forceps
Stevens forceps
Stevens iris forceps
Stevenson forceps
Stevenson grasping forceps
Stieglitz splinter forceps
Stille forceps
Stille gallstone forceps
Stille tissue forceps
Stille-Adson forceps
Stille-Barraya intestinal forceps
Stille-Barraya intestinal-grasping forceps
Stille-Björk forceps
Stille-Crile forceps
Stille-Halsted forceps
Stille-Horsley bone-cutting forceps
Stille-Horsley forceps
Stille-Liston bone forceps
Stille-Liston bone-cutting forceps

forceps *continued*

Stille-Liston forceps
Stille-Liston rib-cutting forceps
Stille-Luer forceps
Stille-Russian forceps
Stone forceps
Stone tissue forceps
stone-crushing forceps
stone-extraction forceps
stone-grasping forceps
Stoneman forceps
Storey forceps
Storey gall duct forceps
Storey-Hillar dissecting forceps
Storz biopsy forceps
Storz bronchoscopic forceps
Storz cystoscopic forceps
Storz esophagoscopic forceps
Storz forceps
Storz grasping biopsy forceps
Storz kidney stone forceps
Storz miniature forceps
Storz nasopharyngeal biopsy forceps
Storz optical biopsy forceps
Storz sinus biopsy forceps
Storz stone-crushing forceps
Storz stone-extraction forceps
Storz-Bonn forceps
Storz-Bonn suturing forceps
strabismus forceps
straight forceps
straight single tenaculum forceps
straight-end cup forceps

forceps *continued*

Strassmann uterine-elevating forceps
Stratte forceps
Strelinger catheter-introducing forceps
Stringer catheter-introducing forceps
Stringer forceps
Stringer newborn throat forceps
Struempel ear alligator forceps
Struempel ear punch forceps
Struempel forceps
Struempel-Voss ethmoidal forceps
Strully dressing forceps
Strully tissue forceps
strut forceps
Struyken forceps
Struyken nasal forceps
Struyken nasal-cutting forceps
Struyken turbinate forceps
subglottic forceps
suction forceps
Suker iris forceps
superior rectus forceps
suture and tying forceps
suture forceps
suture-carrying forceps
suture-holding forceps
suture-pulling forceps
suture-tying forceps
suture-tying platform forceps
suturing forceps
Sweet clip-applying forceps
Sweet dissecting forceps
Sweet forceps
Sweet ligature forceps
Syark vulsellum forceps
synovium biopsy forceps

forceps *continued*
Szuler forceps
T-shaped forceps
tack-and-pin forceps
Takahashi cutting
forceps
Takahashi ethmoid
forceps
Takahashi forceps
Takahashi nasal forceps
Takahashi neurological
forceps
tangential forceps
Tarnier forceps
Tarnier obstetrical
forceps
Taylor dissecting forceps
Taylor forceps
Taylor tissue forceps
Teale forceps
Teale uterine vulsellum
forceps
Teale vulsellum forceps
tenaculum forceps
tendon forceps
tendon-holding forceps
tendon-tunneling forceps
Tennant forceps
Tennant intraocular lens
forceps
Tennant-Maumenee
forceps
Terson capsule forceps
Terson forceps
Tessier disimpaction
device forceps
Theurig sterilizer forceps
Thomas Allis forceps
Thomas Allis tissue
forceps
Thomas shot compres-
sion forceps
Thomas uterine tissue-
grasping forceps
Thoms forceps
Thoms tissue-grasping
forceps

forceps *continued*
Thoms-Allis forceps
Thoms-Allis tissue
forceps
Thoms-Gaylor biopsy
forceps
Thoms-Gaylor forceps
Thoms-Gaylor uterine
forceps
thoracic artery forceps
thoracic forceps
thoracic hemostatic
forceps
thoracic tissue forceps
Thorek gallbladder
forceps
Thorek-Mixter forceps
Thorek-Mixter gall duct
forceps
Thorek-Mixter gallblad-
der forceps
Thorpe corneal forceps
Thorpe fixation forceps
Thorpe forceps
three-armed basket
forceps
three-pronged forceps
three-pronged grasping
forceps
throat forceps
through-cutting forceps
tip
thumb forceps
thumb tissue forceps
thumb-dressing forceps
Thurston-Holland
fragment forceps
thyroid forceps
thyroid traction forceps
Tickner forceps
Tiemann bullet forceps
Tilley dressing forceps
Tischler cervical biopsy
forceps
Tischler cervical forceps
Tischler forceps
tissue forceps

forceps *continued*

    tissue forceps with teeth

    tissue forceps without teeth

    tissue-dressing forceps

    tissue-grasping forceps

    tissue-holding forceps

    Tivnen forceps

    Tivnen tonsil-seizing forceps

    Tobey forceps

    Tobold forceps

    Tobold laryngeal forceps

    Tobold-Fauvel forceps

    Tobold-Fauvel grasping forceps

    Toennis tumor-grasping forceps

    Toennis-Adson forceps

    Tomac forceps

    tongue forceps

    tongue-seizing forceps

    tonsil-holding forceps

    tonsillar abscess forceps

    tonsillar artery forceps

    tonsillar forceps

    tonsillar hemostatic forceps

    tonsillar needle holder forceps

    tonsil-ligating forceps

    tonsil-seizing forceps

    tonsil-suturing forceps

    Tooke corneal forceps

    Toomey forceps

    toothed forceps

    toothed thumb forceps

    toothed tissue forceps

    tooth-extracting forceps

    torsion forceps

    towel clip forceps

    towel forceps

    Tower forceps

    Tower muscle forceps

    Townley forceps

    Townley tissue forceps

    tracheal forceps

forceps *continued*

    tracheal hemostatic forceps

    trachoma forceps

    traction forceps

    transfer forceps

    transplant-grafting forceps

    transsphenoidal forceps

    triangular punch forceps

    Troeltsch ear forceps

    Troeltsch forceps

    Trotter forceps

    Trousseau forceps

    Troutman corneal forceps

    Troutman forceps

    Troutman rectal forceps

    Troutman-Barraquer Colibri forceps

    Troutman-Barraquer iris forceps

    Troutman-Llobera fixation forceps

    Troutman-Llobera Flieringa forceps

    tubing clamp forceps

    tubular forceps

    Tucker forceps

    Tucker-McLean obstetrical forceps

    Tuffier forceps

    tumor forceps

    turbinate forceps

    Turnbull forceps

    Turner-Babcock tissue forceps

    Turner-Warwick stone forceps

    Turner-Warwick-Adson forceps

    Turrell biopsy forceps

    Turrell forceps

    Turrell specimen forceps

    Turrell-Wittner rectal biopsy forceps

forceps *continued*

Turrell-Wittner rectal forceps
Tuttle forceps
Tuttle tissue forceps
Twisk forceps
two-toothed forceps
Tydings forceps
Tydings tonsil forceps
Tydings-Lakeside forceps
Tydings-Lakeside tonsil-seizing forceps
Tyrrell foreign body forceps
U-shaped forceps
Ullrich forceps
Universal forceps
University forceps
University of Kansas forceps
University of Michigan Mixter thoracic forceps
upbiting biopsy forceps
upbiting cup forceps
upbiting forceps
Uppsala gall duct forceps
Urbantschitsch forceps
ureteral catheter forceps
ureteral isolation forceps
ureteral stone forceps
urethral forceps
uterine artery forceps
uterine biopsy forceps
uterine forceps
uterine polyp forceps
uterine specimen forceps
uterine tenaculum forceps
uterine vulsellum forceps
uterine-dressing forceps
uterine-elevating forceps
uterine-holding forceps
uterine-manipulating forceps
uterine-packing forceps
utility forceps

forceps *continued*

Utrata capsulorrhexis forceps
vaginal hysterectomy forceps
van Buren forceps
van Buren sequestrum forceps
Van Doren forceps
Van Doren uterine biopsy punch forceps
Van Doren uterine forceps
Van Mandach capsule fragment and clot forceps
Van Struyken forceps
Van Struyken nasal forceps
Vander Pool sterilizer forceps
Vanderbilt deep vessel forceps
Vanderbilt forceps
Vanderbilt University hemostatic forceps
Vannas fixation forceps
Vantage tube-occluding forceps
Varco forceps
Varco gallbladder forceps
Varco thoracic forceps
vas isolation forceps
vascular forceps
vascular tissue forceps
vasectomy forceps
Vaughn sterilizer forceps
vectis cesarean section forceps
vectis forceps
vena caval forceps
Verbrugge bone-holding forceps
Verbrugge forceps
Verhoeff capsule forceps
Verhoeff cataract forceps

forceps *continued*

Verhoeff forceps
vessel clip-applying
forceps
vessel forceps
vessel pediatric forceps
vessel peripheral forceps
Vick-Blanchard forceps
Vick-Blanchard hemor-
rhoidal forceps
Vigger-5 eye forceps
Virtus forceps
Virtus splinter forceps
viscera-holding forceps
visceral forceps
vise forceps
visual hemostatic forceps
Vital forceps
Vital intestinal forceps
Vital lung-grasping
forceps
Vital needle holder
forceps
Vital tissue forceps
vitreous-grasping forceps
Vogt forceps
vomer forceps
vomer septal forceps
von Graefe (see *Graefe* )
von Mondak forceps
von Petz forceps
Voris-Oldberg IV disk
ronguer forceps
Voris-Wester forceps
vulsella forceps
vulsellum forceps
Wachtenfeldt clip-
applying forceps
Wachtenfeldt clip-
removing forceps
Wachtenfeldt forceps
Wadsworth lid forceps
Waldeau fixation
forceps
Waldeau forceps
Waldeyer forceps
Walker forceps

forceps *continued*

Wallace cesarean forceps
Walsh forceps
Walsham forceps
Walsham nasal forceps
Walsham septal forceps
Walsham septum-
straightening forceps
Walter forceps
Walter splinter forceps
Walther forceps
Walther tissue forceps
Walton forceps
Walton-Allis tissue
forceps
Walton-Schubert forceps
Walton-Schubert uterine
biopsy forceps
Walzl hysterectomy
forceps
Wangensteen forceps
Wangensteen tissue
forceps
Warthen forceps
Watson forceps
Watson tonsil-seizing
forceps
Watson-Williams
ethmoid-biting forceps
Watson-Williams forceps
Watson-Williams nasal
forceps
Watson-Williams polyp
forceps
Waugh dissection
forceps
Waugh tissue forceps
Weaver chalazion
forceps
Weaver forceps
Weck forceps
Weck towel forceps
Weck–Harms forceps
Weeks eye forceps
Weiger-Zollner forceps
Weil ear forceps
Weil ethmoidal forceps

forceps *continued*

Weil forceps
Weingartner ear forceps
Weingartner forceps
Weisenbach forceps
Weisman forceps
Weisman uterine
tenaculum forceps
Welch Allyn anal biopsy
forceps
Welch Allyn forceps
Weller cartilage forceps
Wells forceps
Welsh ophthalmological
forceps
Welsh pupil spreader-
retractor forceps
Wertheim forceps
Wertheim hysterectomy
forceps
Wertheim vaginal
forceps
Wertheim-Cullen forceps
Wertheim-Cullen pedicle
forceps
West nasal-dressing
forceps
Westmacott dressing
forceps
Westmacott forceps
Westphal forceps
Westphal gall duct
forceps
Wheeler vessel forceps
White forceps
White tonsil forceps
White tonsil hemostat
forceps
White tonsil-seizing
forceps
White-Lillie forceps
White-Lillie tonsil forceps
White-Oslay forceps
White-Oslay prostatic
lobe-holding forceps
White-Smith forceps

forceps *continued*

Wickman uterine forceps
Wiener hysterectomy
forceps
Wies chalazion forceps
Wies forceps
Wikstroem artery forceps
Wilde ear forceps
Wilde ethmoidal
exenteration forceps
Wilde ethmoidal forceps
Wilde forceps
Wilde laminectomy
forceps
Wilde septal forceps
Wilde-Blakesley
ethmoidal forceps
Wilde-Troeltsch forceps
Wilder dilating forceps
Willauer-Allis forceps
Willauer-Allis thoracic
forceps
Willauer-Allis thoracic
tissue forceps
Willauer-Allis tissue
forceps
Willett forceps
Willett placental forceps
Williams forceps
Williams gastrointestinal
forceps
Williams intestinal
forceps
Williams uterine forceps
Williams vessel-holding
forceps
Wills Hospital forceps
Wills Hospital ophthal-
mology forceps
Wills Hospital utility
forceps
Wilmer iris forceps
Wilson vitreous foreign
body forceps
Wilson-Cook biopsy
forceps

forceps *continued*

wire-closure forceps
wire-crimper forceps
wire-pulling forceps
wire-twisting forceps
Wittner forceps
Wittner uterine biopsy
forceps
Wolf biopsy forceps
Wolf biting basket
forceps
Wolf curved basket
forceps
Wolfe eye forceps
Wolfe uterine cuff
forceps
Wolfson forceps
Woodward forceps
Woodward hemostatic
forceps
Woodward thoracic
hemostatic forceps
Worth advancement
forceps
Worth forceps
Worth muscle forceps
Worth strabismus forceps
wound forceps
wound-clip forceps
Wrigley forceps
Wullstein ear forceps
Wullstein forceps
Wullstein tympanoplasty
forceps
Wullstein-House cup-
shaped forceps
Wullstein-House forceps
Wullstein-Paparella
forceps
Wylie forceps
Wylie uterine forceps
Wylie uterine tenaculum
forceps
Yankauer ethmoid
forceps
Yankauer ethmoid-
cutting forceps

forceps *continued*

Yankauer forceps
Yankauer-Little forceps
Yankauer-Little tube
forceps
Yasargil artery forceps
Yasargil forceps
Yeoman forceps
Yeoman rectal biopsy
forceps
Yeoman uterine forceps
Yeoman-Wittner rectal
biopsy forceps
Yeoman-Wittner rectal
forceps
Young intestinal forceps
Young tongue forceps
Young tongue-seizing
forceps
Younge uterine biopsy
forceps
Younge uterine forceps
Zenker dissecting and
ligature forceps
Ziegler cilia forceps
Ziegler forceps
Zimmer-Hoen forceps
Zimmer-Schlesinger
forceps
Zollinger multipurpose
tissue forceps
Zweifel angiotribe
forceps
forceps delivery
forceps handle
forceps jar
forceps operation
forceps point
forceps tip
forcible feeding
forcipressure
Ford clamp
Ford Hospital ventricular
cannula
Ford stethoscope
Ford-Deaver retractor
fore-and-aft splint

forearm
forearm aluminum shelf crutch
forearm and metacarpal splint
forearm flow
forearm fracture
forearm splint
forebrain
forebrain bundle
Foredom-Oster vibrator
forefoot
forefoot amputation
forefoot equinus
forefoot valgus
forefoot varus
Foregger bronchoscope
Foregger laryngoscope
Foregger rigid esophagoscope
Foregger tube
forehead
forehead flap
forehead prominence
forehead-plasty
foreign body (FB)
foreign body contamination
foreign body curet
foreign body cystoscopy
    forceps
foreign body extraction
foreign body eye forceps
foreign body eye spud
foreign body forceps
foreign body impaction
foreign body in organ
foreign body loop
foreign body obstruction
foreign body passed
foreign body probe
foreign body removed
foreign body retained
foreign body screw
foreign body seen on x-ray
foreign body spud
foreign body trauma
foreign substance
Forel commissure
Forel decussation
Forel field

Forel space
forequadrant incision
forequarter amputation
foreskin
Forestier disease
fork
    aluminum alloy fork
    Bezold-Edelman tuning
        fork
    Cattell forked-type T-
        tube
    crus guide fork
    Gardiner-Brown tuning
        fork
    Hardy implant fork
    Hartmann tuning fork
    implant fork
    Leasure tuning forks
    magnesium tuning forks
    Penn tuning fork
    Ralks tuning fork
    silver-fork deformity
    silver-fork fracture
    tuning fork
forked T-tube
forklike stump
Formad kidney
formal protocol
formaldehyde
formaldehyde catgut
formalin-fixed specimen
formation
formation of fistula
FormFlex intraocular lens
FormFlex lens
forming wires
formocresol
formocresol pulpotomy
forniceal invasion
fornix (pl. fornices)
fornix cerebri
fornix longus of Forel
fornix of superior conjunctiva
fornix-based conjunctival flap
Foroblique cystoscope
Foroblique cystourethroscope
Foroblique esophagoscope

Foroblique lens
Foroblique panendoscope
Foroblique resectoscope
Foroblique telescope
Forrester brace
Forrester cervical collar brace
Forrester clamp
Forrester collar
Forrester head halter
Forrester splint
Forrester-Brown head halter
Förster (see *Foerster*)
Fort bougie
forward bending
forward displacement
forward flexion
forward movement
forward subluxation
forward-bending maneuver
forward-grasping forceps
forwarding probe
forward-viewing endoscope
forward-viewing scope
Fosler splint
Foss anterior resection clamp
Foss bifid gallbladder retractor
Foss bifid retractor
Foss biliary retractor
Foss cardiovascular forceps
Foss clamp
Foss forceps
Foss gallbladder retractor
Foss intestinal clamp
Foss intestinal clamp forceps
Foss retractor
fossa (*pl.* fossae)
fossa of Rosenmüller
Foster bed
Foster defibrillator
Foster fracture frame
Foster frame
Foster needle holder
Foster scissors
Foster snare
Foster turning frame
Foster-Ballenger nasal speculum
Foster-Ballenger speculum

Foster-Gillies needle holder
Fothergill operation
Fothergill sutures
Fothergill-Donald operation
Fothergill-Hunter operation
Fothergill-Shaw operation
Fould operation
foul-smelling
foul-smelling amniotic fluid
fountain decussation of Meynert
fountain syringe
four by fours (4 x 4s)
four-chamber view of heart
fourchette
four-eye catheter
four-flanged nails
four-flap cleft palate repair
four-flap palatoplasty
four-flap procedure
four-flap Z-plasty
Fourier transform
four-lumen tube
Fournier teeth
Fournier test
four-point biopsy
four-point cervical brace
four-point gait
four-portal technique
four-poster cervical brace
four-prong retractor
four-pronged polyp grasper
four-quadrant biopsy
four-quadrant cervical punch
    biopsy
four-tailed bandage
four-tailed dressing
fourth blade extension
fourth cranial nerve
fourth ventricle
four-vessel angiogram
four-vessel arteriogram
four-view chest x-ray
four-wing catheter
four-wing drain
four-wing Malecot drain
four-wing Malecot retention
    catheter

FOV (field of vision)
fovea (*pl.* foveae)
foveal ligament
foveal vision
foveolar gastric mucosa
foveolar reflex
Foville tract
Fowler angular incision
Fowler dressing
Fowler incision
Fowler maneuver
Fowler operation
Fowler position
Fowler procedure for bouton-
    nière deformity
Fowler self-retaining retractor
Fowler sound
Fowler technique
Fowler thoracoplasty
Fowler urethral sound
Fowler-Murphy treatment
Fowler-Stephens orchiopexy
Fowler-Weir incision
Fowles technique
Fox aluminum eye shield
Fox balloon
Fox bipolar forceps
Fox blepharoplasty
Fox cartilage forceps
Fox clavicle splint
Fox conformer
Fox curet
Fox dermal curet
Fox entropion operation
Fox eye conformer
Fox eye implant
Fox eye shield
Fox eye speculum
Fox eyelid implant
Fox graft
Fox implant
Fox internal fixation device
Fox irrigator
Fox operation
Fox prosthesis
Fox scissors
Fox speculum

Fox sphere implant
Fox splint
Fox tissue forceps
Fox wrench
Fox-Blazina knee procedure
Fox-Blazina prosthesis
FPB (femoral-popliteal bypass)
FPB (flexor pollicis brevis)
FPL (flexor pollicis longus)
fps (frames per second)
Frackelton needle
Frackelton wire threader
fraction
fractional anesthesia
fractional biopsy
fractional culture
fractional curettage
fractional D&C (fractional
    dilatation and curettage)
fractional epidural anesthesia
fractional spinal anesthesia
fractional sterilization
fractionated high-dose rate
fractionated radiotherapy
fractionation rate
fractionation with chemother-
    apy
fractionation without chemo-
    therapy
Fractomed splint
Fractura Flex bandage
Fractura Flex elastic bandage
fracture
fracture alignment
fracture appliance (see also
    *appliance*)
        arch bars facial fracture
            appliance
        Bradford fracture
            appliance
        Buck fracture appliance
        Cameron fracture
            appliance
        craniofacial fracture
            appliance
        Erich facial fracture
            appliance

fracture appliance *continued*
   facial fracture appliance
   Gerster fracture appliance
   Goldthwait fracture appliance
   Hibbs fracture appliance
   Janes fracture appliance
   Jewett fracture appliance
   Joseph septal fracture appliance
   Roger Anderson facial fracture appliance
   Vasocillator fracture appliance
   Whitman fracture appliance
   Wilson fracture appliance
fracture band
fracture bar
fracture bed
fracture blister
fracture bowing
fracture by contrecoup
fracture chip
fracture chisel
fracture dislocation
fracture en coin
fracture en rave
fracture fragments
fracture frame (see also *frame*)
   Alexian Brothers overhead fracture frame
   Balkan fracture frame
   Böhler fracture frame
   Bradford fracture frame
   Erich facial fracture frame
   Foster fracture frame
   fracture frame
   Goldthwait fracture frame
   head fracture frame
   Hibbs fracture frame
   hyperextension fracture frame

fracture frame *continued*
   occluding fracture frame
   overhead fracture frame
   Rainbow fracture frame
   reducing fracture frame
   Stryker CircOlectric fracture frame
   Stryker fracture frame
   Thomas fracture frame
   Thompson fracture frame
   trial fracture frame
   turning fracture frame
   Whitman fracture frame
fracture fusion
fracture healing
fracture line
fracture nail
fracture of bone
fracture of cartilage
fracture position
fracture reduced
fracture reduction
fracture site
fracture splint
fracture table
fracture union
fracture with cross union
fracture with delayed union
fracture with malunion
fracture with nonunion
fracture-banding apparatus
fractured bone
fracture-dislocation
fracturing the stricture
Fraenkel (also Fränkel)
Fraenkel appliance
Fraenkel cutting-tip forceps
Fraenkel double-articulated-tip forceps
Fraenkel exercises
Fraenkel forceps
Fraenkel headband
Fraenkel line
Fraenkel quadriplegia grading system
Fraenkel sign
Fraenkel sinus probe
Fraenkel speculum

Fragen anterior commissure
    microlaryngoscope
Fragen scope
fragility
fragmatic buttress
Fragmatome
Fragmatome tip with ultrasound
    spatula
fragment
fragment forceps
fragment of bone
fragment of placenta
fragment pared with motor saw
fragment splintered to pieces
fragment wound
fragmentary filling
fragmentation
fragmentation probe
fragmentation process
Frahur clamp
Frahur scissors
fraise
frame (see also *fracture frame*)
    A-frame orthosis
    Ace-Fischer frame
    Alexian Brothers
        overhead fracture
        frame
    Andrews frame
    arch bars frame
    Balkan fracture frame
    Balkan frame
    Böhler fracture frame
    Böhler reducing frame
    Böhler-Braun frame
    Bradford fracture frame
    Bradford frame
    Braun frame
    Buck extension frame
    Elgiloy frame of pros-
        thetic valve
    Erich facial fracture
        frame
    Foster fracture frame
    Foster frame
    Foster turning frame

frame *continued*
    Goldthwait fracture
        frame
    Goligher retractor frame
    head fracture frame
    Heffington lumbar seat
        spinal surgery frame
    Herzmark hyperexten-
        sion frame
    Hibbs fracture frame
    Hibbs frame
    hyperextension fracture
        frame
    Jewett frame
    Joseph septal frame
    laminectomy frame
    Leksell frame
    Leksell stereotaxic
        frame
    Lex-Ton lumbar laminec-
        tomy frame
    occluding fracture frame
    overhead fracture frame
    Pittsburgh triangular
        frame
    Putti frame
    quadriplegic standing
        frame
    Rainbow fracture frame
    reducing fracture frame
    Relton-Hall frame
    Russell frame
    Slatis frame
    standing frame orthosis
    Stryker CircOlectric
        fracture frame
    Stryker fracture frame
    Stryker frame
    Stryker turning frame
    Thomas fracture frame
    Thomas hyperextension
        frame
    Thompson fracture frame
    trial fracture frame
    trial frame
    turning fracture frame

frame *continued*
    Vidal-Hoffman fixator
      frame
    Whitman fracture frame
    Whitman frame
    Wilson frame
    Wilson spinal frame
    Wingfield frame
    Zimcode traction frames
      tractor
    Zimmer frame
frames per second (fps)
framework
Franceschetti keratoplasty
Franceschetti operation
Franceschetti trephine
Francis chalazion forceps
Francis forceps
Francis knife spud
Francis spud
Francis-Gray forceps
Francis-Gray wire crimper
Francke needle
Franco operation
Frangenheim biopsy punch
    forceps
Frangenheim forceps
Frangenheim hook-punch
    forceps
Frangenheim laparoscope
Frangenheim-Goebell-Stoeckel
    fascia lata suspension
frank
frank breech
frank breech presentation
frank fronds
Frank gastrostomy
frank lead system
Frank operation
frank prolapse
Franke tabes operation
Franke technique
Fränkel (see *Fraenkel*)
Frankfeldt forceps
Frankfeldt grasping forceps
Frankfeldt hemorrhoidal needle
Frankfeldt needle

Frankfeldt rectal snare
Frankfeldt sigmoidoscope
Frankfeldt snare
Frankfeldt snare accessories
Frankfort horizontal plane
Franklin malleable retractor
Franklin retractor
Franklin-Silverman biopsy
    needle
Franklin-Silverman cannula
Franklin-Silverman curet
Franklin-Silverman needle
Frank-Starling curve
Franseen rectal curet
Franz abdominal retractor
Franz retractor
frappage
Fraser decompressor
Fraser depressor
Fraser forceps
Frater intracardiac retractor
Frater retractor
Fraunhofer lines
Frazier brain suction tube
Frazier brain-exploring cannula
Frazier brain-exploring trocar
Frazier cannula
Frazier cordotomy knife
Frazier dural elevator
Frazier dural hook
Frazier dural scissors
Frazier dural separator
Frazier elevator
Frazier hook
Frazier insulated suction tube
Frazier knife
Frazier laminectomy retractor
Frazier modified suction tube
Frazier nasal suction tip
Frazier nasal suction tube
Frazier needle
Frazier operation
Frazier osteotome
Frazier retractor
Frazier scissors
Frazier separator
Frazier straight suction tube

Frazier suction elevator
Frazier suction tip
Frazier suction tube
Frazier trocar
Frazier tube
Frazier ventricular cannula
Frazier ventricular needle
Frazier-Adson clamp
Frazier-Adson osteoplastic flap
    clamp
Frazier-Fay retractor
Frazier-Paparella mastoid tube
Frazier-Paparella suction tube
Frazier-Paparella tube
Frazier-Sachs clamp
Frazier-Spiller operation
freckled
Freckner operation
Fred Thompson broach
Frederick needle
Frederick pneumothorax needle
Fredet-Ramstedt operation
Fredet-Ramstedt pyloromyot-
    omy
Fredricks mammary prosthesis
Fredricks mammary support
free abdominal air
free air
free band of colon
free body
free flap
free flow
free fluid
free graft
free implant
free induction decay
free induction signal
free jejunal graft
free ligature
free ligature suture
free margin of eyelid
free of disease
free of obstruction
free peritoneal air
free prosthesis
free sponge
free tenotomy

free tie
free-body analysis
free-body spinal fusion
freed by blunt dissection
freed by sharp dissection
freed up
Freedom external catheter
free-hand allograft valve
freeing of adhesions
freeing up of adhesions
Free-Lock hip fixation system
freely mobile
freely mobile uterus
freely movable
freely movable mass
freely movable uterus
Freeman clamp
Freeman cookie-cutter areolar
    marker
Freeman face-lift retractor
Freeman leukotome
Freeman operation
Freeman polisher
Freeman resurfacing technique
Freeman retractor
Freeman rhytidectomy scissors
Freeman scissors
Freeman total hip replacement
Freeman transorbital leukotome
Freeman-Samuelson knee
    prosthesis
Freeman-Swanson knee
    prosthesis
Freemont spinal sphygmoma-
    nometer
Freenseen liver biopsy needle
Freer bone chisel
Freer chisel
Freer dissector
Freer double elevator
Freer double-ended elevator
Freer double-ended septum
    elevator
Freer double-pronged hook
Freer elevator
Freer elevator-dissector
Freer gouge

Freer hook
Freer knife
Freer lacrimal chisel
Freer mucosa knife
Freer nasal gouge
Freer nasoseptal elevator
Freer periosteal elevator
Freer periosteotome
Freer retractor
Freer septal elevator
Freer septal forceps
Freer septal knife
Freer single-ended elevator
Freer skin hook
Freer spatula
Freer submucous chisel
Freer submucous instrument
Freer submucous retractor
free-revascularized autograft
Freer-Gruenwald forceps
Freer-Gruenwald punch forceps
Freer-Ingal septal knife
Freer-Ingal submucous knife
free-skin patch graft
free-tie sutures
free-toe transfer
Freeway speculum
Freeway-Graves speculum
freeze-dried bone
freeze-dried bone graft
freeze-dried graft
freeze-drying
freezing
Freiberg cartilage knife
Freiberg disease
Freiberg hip retractor
Freiberg knife
Freiberg retractor
Freiberg traction
Freiberg tractor
Freiburg Injecttimer
Freidenwald-Guyton sling
Freimuth curet
Freimuth ear curet
Frejka hip pillow
Frejka orthosis
Frejka pillow

Frejka pillow splint
Frejka splint
fremitus
frena (*sing.* frenum)
French, American, British
    staging of carcinoma (FAB)
French angiographic catheter
French bougie
French brain retractor
French Brown-Buerger
    cystoscope
French catheter
French catheter scale
French chest tube
French chisel
French curve out-of-plane
    catheter
French dilator
French elbow osteotomy
French flap
French Foley catheter
French in-plane guiding
    catheter
French MBIH catheter
French mushroom-tipped
    catheter
French needle
French operation
French red-rubber Robinson
    catheter
French retractor
French Robinson catheter
French S-shaped brain retractor
French S-shaped retractor
French scale for sizing tubular
    instruments
French Silastic Foley catheter
French skin flap operation
French sliding flap
French sound
French stent
French sutures
French tripolar His catheter
French-Daid introducer
French-eye needle
French-eye needle holder
French-eye Vital needle holder

French-following metal sound
French-Iglesias resectoscope
French-McCarthy panendoscope
French-McRea dilator
French-pattern eye spatula
French-pattern forceps
French-pattern lacrimal probe
French-pattern osteotome
French-pattern raspatory
French-pattern spatula
French-Stern-McCarthy retractor
French-Wappler cystoscope
frenectomy
frenoplasty
frenotomy
frenula (*sing.* frenulum)
frenuloplasty
frenulum (*pl.* frenula)
frenulum of clitoris
frenulum of penis
frenum (*pl.* frena)
Frenzel ear operating head
Frenzel lenses
frequency
frequent
Fresgen frontal sinus probe
fresh bleeding
fresh blood clot
fresh frozen plasma
Fresnel floor light
Fresnel lens
Freund hysterectomy
Freund operation
Frey eye implant
Freyer  operation
Freyer drain
Freyer operation
Freyer suprapubic drain
Frey-Freer bur
Frey-Sauerbruch rib shears
friability
friable
friable cervix
friable mucosa
friable tissue
fricative sounds
Fricke bandage

Fricke dressing
Fricke eyelid operation
Fricke operation
Fricke scrotal dressing
Frickman I operation
Frickman II operation
friction
friction burn        *Fryokman*
friction fremitus    *hand fracture*
friction knot
friction rub
friction sound
Fried clubfoot technique
Friedenwald operation
Friedenwald ophthalmoscope
Friedenwald ptosis operation
Friedenwald-Guyton operation
Fried-Green foot procedure
Fried-Hendel technique
Friedman bone rongeur
Friedman clip
Friedman elevator
Friedman perineal retractor
Friedman retractor
Friedman rongeur forceps
Friedman vein stripper
Friedmann sutures
Friedman-Otis bougie
Friedman-Otis bougie à
    boule
Friedreich ataxia
Friedreich foot operation
Friedreich sign
Friedreich tabes
Friedrich clamp
Friedrich operation
Friedrich raspatory
Friedrich rib elevator
Friedrich-Ferguson retractor
Friedrich-Petz clamp
Friend aspirating tube
Friend catheter
Friend-Hebert catheter
Friesner ear knife
Friesner ear perforator
Friesner knife
Frigitronics cryoextractor

Frigitronics cryophake
Frigitronics cryoprobe
Frigitronics cryostylet
Frigitronics nitrous oxide
    cryosurgery apparatus
Frigitronics probe
Frigitronics retinal probe unit
fringe joint
Fritsch catheter
Fritsch operation
Fritsch retractor
Fritsch uterine douche
Fritz aspirator
Fritz automatic drainage
    treatment unit
frog splint
frog-leg projection
frog-leg splint
frog-leg view
frog-legged position
froglike position
Fröhlich syndrome
Frohm mouth gag
Frohse arcade
Froimson biceps procedure
Frommel operation
Frommer dilator
frondlike filling defect
fronds
front build-up eye implant
frontal
frontal antrotomy
frontal antrum
frontal artery
frontal bone
frontal diploic vein
frontal fontanelle
frontal gyrectomy
frontal gyrus
frontal leads
frontal lobe
frontal lobotomy
frontal nerve
frontal notch
frontal paranasal sinus
frontal plane
frontal process

frontal process of maxilla
frontal projection
frontal region
frontal release sign
frontal segment
frontal sinus
frontal sinus bougie
frontal sinus cannula
frontal sinus chisel
frontal sinus curet
frontal sinus dilator
frontal sinus operation
frontal sinus probe
frontal sinus rasp
frontal sinus wash tube
frontal sinusotomy
frontal suture
frontal vein
frontal zygomatic suture line
frontalis, musculus
frontalis, nervus
frontalis sling
frontoanterior position
frontocentral region
frontodextra posterior
frontodextra transversa
frontoethmoidal sphenoidec-
    tomy
frontoethmoidal suture
frontolacrimal suture
frontomalar suture
frontomaxillary suture
frontomental diameter
frontonasal process
frontonasal suture
fronto-occipital
fronto-occipital diameter
frontoparietal
frontoparietal area
frontoparietal suture
frontoposterior position
frontosphenoid suture
frontotemporal
frontotemporal craniotomy
    incision
frontotransverse position
frontozygomatic suture

front-tap reflex
front-viewing scope
Frosh procedure for ingrown
    nail
frost anesthesia
Frost operation
Frost sutures
Frost-Lang operation
frostbite
frozen section
frozen section diagnosis
frozen shoulder
frozen tissue
Fruehevald splint
Fry nasal forceps
Frye portable aspirator
Frykholm bone rongeur
Frykholm goniometer
Frykholm rongeur
Frykman classification of hand
    fractures
Frykman fracture
FSH (follicle stimulating
    hormone)
FTSG (full-thickness skin graft)
Fuchs capsule forceps
Fuchs capsulotomy forceps
Fuchs crypt
Fuchs forceps
Fuchs keratome
Fuchs operation
Fuchs position
Fuchs two-way eye syringe
Fujica gastrocamera
Fujinon biopsy forceps
Fujinon colonoscope
Fujinon disposable injector
Fujinon endoscope
Fujinon EVE video endo-
    scope
Fujinon EVG-F upper GI video
    endoscope
Fujinon flexible bronchoscope
Fujinon flexible choledocho-
    scope
Fujinon flexible endoscope
Fujinon flexible ENT scope

Fujinon flexible lower GI
    endoscope
Fujinon flexible sigmoidoscope
Fujinon flexible upper GI
    endoscope
Fujinon forceps
Fujinon UGI-FP endoscope
Fujinon variceal injector
Fukala operation
fulcrum
fulgurate
fulgurating electrode
fulgurating unit
fulguration
fulguration electrode
fulguration of bleeding points
full and equal bilaterally
full breech presentation
full extension
full flexion
full function
full occlusal splint
full pack
full range of motion
full weightbearing (FWB)
full-blown infection
full-column barium enema
full-curve sound
full-curved clamp
Fuller bivalve trach tube
Fuller operation
Fuller rectal dressing
Fuller shield
Fuller shield dressing
Fuller shield rectal dressing
Fuller tube
full-lumen esophagoscope
fullness
full-radius synovial resector
full-term delivery
full-term fetus
full-term infant
full-thickness
full-thickness graft
full-thickness implant
full-thickness prosthesis
full-thickness skin graft (FTSG)

full-view lumen finder
full-weightbearing exercises
fully automatic pacemaker
fully automatic, atrioventricular
    universal dual-channel
    pacemaker
fully roused
fulminant
fulminate
fulminating
fulminating appendicitis
fulminating disease
fulmination
Fulpit forceps
Fulpit tissue forceps
Fulton deep-surgery scissors
Fulton laminectomy rongeur
Fulton mouth gag
Fulton retractor
Fulton rongeur
Fulton scissors
Ful-Vue ophthalmoscope
Ful-Vue spot retinoscope
Ful-Vue streak retinoscope
function
function of joint
function study
functional
functional activity
functional cardiac murmur
functional change
functional condition
functional congestion
functional cystic duct obstruc-
    tion
functional death
functional disorder
functional fracture brace
functional illness
functional neurosurgery
functional position
functional range of motion
functional splint
functional stricture
functioning
fundal angioscopy
fundal camera

fundal glands
fundal height
fundal placenta
fundal plication
fundal portion of uterus
fundal to cervical end
fundal varices
fundamental cause
fundectomy
fundi (*sing.* fundus)
fundi intact
fundic gland
fundic mucosa
fundic-antral junction
fundoplication
fundus (*pl.* fundi)
fundus photography
funduscope
funduscopic examination
funduscopy
fundusectomy
fundus-retinal camera
fungating
fungating excrescence
fungating lesion
fungating mass
fungating tumor
fungating wound
fungous excrescence
fungus
fungus ball
funicular
funicular artery
funicular hernia
funicular hydrocele
funicular inguinal hernia
funicular repair
funicular suture
funiculopexy
funiculus (*pl.* funiculi)
funiculus spermaticus
funnel
funnel chest
funnel deformity
funnel-shaped pelvis
Funsten supination splint
Furacin dressing

Furacin gauze
Furacin gauze dressing
Furacin gauze holder
Furadantin
furcate placenta
Furlow cylinder inserter
Furlow inserter
Furlow introducer
Furlow needle holder
Furman type II electrogram
Furniss anastomosis
Furniss anastomotic clamp
Furniss catheter
Furniss clamp
Furniss cornea-holding forceps
Furniss female catheter
Furniss forceps
Furniss incision
Furniss otoplasty
Furniss polyp forceps
Furniss sutures
Furniss ureterointestinal
    anastomosis
Furniss-Castroviejo forceps
Furniss-Clute anastomosis
    clamp
Furniss-Clute clamp
Furniss-Clute duodenal clamp
Furniss-Clute forceps
Furniss-Clute pin
Furniss-McClure-Hinton clamp
Furniss-Rizzuti forceps
Furosemide
furrier's sutures
furrow
furrowed tongue
furuncle

furuncular
furuncular otitis
furunculosis
fused commissures
fused hips
fused kidney
fused teeth
fused vertebrae
fused vulva
fuser pump
fusiform
fusiform aneurysm
fusiform bougie
fusiform cataract
fusiform deformity
fusiform dilatation
fusiform fossa
fusiform gyrus
fusiform lobule
fusiform muscle
fusiform skin revision
fusiform widening of abdominal
    aorta
fusiform widening of duct
fusimotor
fusion
fusion defect
fusion instruments
fusion of bone
fusion of joint
fusion operation
fusion procedure
fusion reflex
fusion tube
Futch cannula
Futura splint
FWB (full weightbearing)

G-banding technique
G-suit device
Gabarro graft
Gabarro operation
Gabarro retractor
Gabbay-Frater suture guide
Gabriel proctoscope
Gabriel syringe
Gabriel Tucker bougie
Gabriel Tucker forceps
Gabriel Tucker tube
Gaenslen incision
Gaenslen procedure
Gaenslen sign
Gaenslen test
Gaffee speculum
gag (see also *mouth gag*)
    Boettcher-Jennings gag
    Boyle Davis mouth gag
    Brophy mouth gag
    Brown-Davis gag
    Collis mouth gag
    Crowe-Davis mouth gag
    Dann-Jennings mouth
      gag
    Davis mouth gag
    Davis-Crowe mouth gag
    Denhardt mouth gag
    Denhardt-Dingman
      mouth gag
    Dingman mouth gag
    Dingman-Denhardt
      mouth gag
    Dott mouth gag
    Dott-Kilner mouth gag
    Doyen mouth gag
    Doyen-Jansen mouth gag
    Ferguson mouth gag

gag *continued*
    Ferguson-Ackland mouth
      gag
    Ferguson-Brophy mouth
      gag
    Ferguson-Gwathmey
      mouth gag
    Frohm mouth gag
    Fulton mouth gag
    Green mouth gag
    Green-Sewall mouth gag
    Hayton-Williams mouth
      gag
    Heister mouth gag
    Hibbs mouth gag
    Jansen mouth gag
    Jennings Loktite mouth
      gag
    Jennings mouth gag
    Jennings-Skillern mouth
      gag
    Kilner mouth gag
    Kilner-Dott mouth gag
    Kilner-Doughty mouth
      gag
    Lane mouth gag
    Lange mouth gag
    Lewis mouth gag
    Maunder oral screw gag
    McDowell mouth gag
    McIvor mouth gag
    McKesson mouth gag
    Molt mouth gag
    Negus mouth gag
    Newkirk mouth gag
    oral screw mouth gag
    oral speculum mouth
      gag

gag *continued*
- Proetz mouth gag
- Proetz-Jansen mouth gag
- Pynchon mouth gag
- Ralks-Davis mouth gag
- Roser mouth gag
- side mouth gag
- Sluder mouth gag
- Sluder-Ferguson mouth gag
- Sluder-Jansen mouth gag
- Sydenham mouth gag
- Wesson mouth gag
- Whitehead mouth gag
- Wolf Loktite gag
- Wolf mouth gag

gag reflex
Gage sign
Gaillard operation
Gaillard-Arlt sutures
Gaillard-Thomas excision
gait plate
gaiter brace
galactocele
Galant abdominal reflex
Galant abdominal response
Galante hip guide
Galante hip prosthesis
Galaxy pacemaker
Galbiati bilateral fetal ischio-pubiotomy
galea
galea forceps
galeaplasty
Galeati gland
Galeazzi fracture
Galeazzi fracture of radius
Galeazzi procedure
Galeazzi sign
Galen anastomosis
Galen bandage
Galen dressing
Galen foramen
Galen vein
Galen ventricle

Galezowski dilator
Galezowski lacrimal dilator
Galin intraocular lens implant
Galin lens
gall duct
gall duct dilator
gall duct forceps
gall duct obstruction
gall duct probe
gall duct scoop
gall duct spoon
Gallagher antral frontal raspatory
Gallagher rasp
Gallagher trocar
gallamine anesthetic agent
gallbladder (GB)
gallbladder aspirator
gallbladder bed
gallbladder calculus
gallbladder cannula
gallbladder colic
gallbladder contraction
gallbladder distention
gallbladder films
gallbladder forceps
gallbladder function
gallbladder fundus
gallbladder ileus
gallbladder inflammation
gallbladder operation
gallbladder retractor
gallbladder scan
gallbladder scissors
gallbladder scoop
gallbladder series
gallbladder shadow
gallbladder spoon
gallbladder stone
gallbladder trocar
gallbladder tube
gallbladder wall
gallbladder wall abscess
Gallie fascia needle
Gallie herniorrhaphy
Gallie needle

Gallie operation
Gallie technique
Gallie tendon passer
Gallie transplant
Gallie-LeMesurier operation
gallop
gallop rhythm
Galloway electrode
gallows-type retractor
gallstone
gallstone colic
gallstone disease
gallstone forceps
gallstone ileus
gallstone migration
gallstone obstruction
gallstone probe
gallstone scoop
Gallvardin systolic click
GALT (gut-associated lymphoid tissue)
Galt drill
Galt saw
Galt skull trephine
Galt trephine
Galton ear whistle
Galton whistle
galvanic cautery
galvanic current
galvanic eye current controller
galvanic probe
galvanic response
galvanic stimulation
galvanocaustic
galvanocaustic amputation
galvanocaustic snare
galvanocautery
galvanoionization
galvanometer
galvanosurgery
galvanotonic contractions
Galveston metacarpal brace
Galveston splint
Galveston technique
Gambee anastomosis
Gambee stitch
Gambee sutures

Gambro catheter
Gambro dialyzer
Gambro Lundia Minor hemo-dialyzer
gamekeeper's thumb
gamekeeper's thumb fracture
gamete intrafallopian transfer (GIFT)
Gamgee tissue
gamma camera
gamma globulin
Gamma knife
Gamma knife machine
Gamma locking nail for hip
gamma ray
Gamma transverse colon loop
Gamna nodules
Gamna-Gandy nodule
Gamon eye knife
Gamophen suture
Gandhi knife
Gandy clamp
Gandy-Gamna nodule
ganglia (*sing.* ganglion)
gangliated nerve
gangliectomy
gangliolysis
ganglion (*pl.* ganglia, ganglions)
ganglion block
ganglion hook
ganglion injection needle
ganglion knife
ganglion of nerve
ganglion of vagus
ganglionated chain
ganglionectomy
ganglioneuroma
ganglionic blocking agent
ganglionic center
ganglionostomy
ganglioside
gangliosympathectomy
gangrene
gangrenosum
gangrenous
gangrenous organ
Gannetta dissector

Gans cyclodialysis
Gans eye cannula
Ganser diverticulum
Ganser ganglion
Gant arthrodesis
Gant clamp
Gant gallbladder retractor
Gant hemostat
Gant hip osteotomy
Gant line
Gant operation
Gant osteotomy
Gant probe
Gantrisin
gantry
gantry angle
gantry stretcher
Gantzer muscle
Ganz-Edwards coronary
    infusion catheter
Ganzfeld stimulator
gap
gape
gaping
gaping wound
gaping wound edges
Garceau approach
Garceau bougie
Garceau catheter
Garceau clubfoot procedure
Garceau-Brahms clubfoot
    procedure
Garcia aorta clamp
Garcia-Novito eye implant
Garcia-Rock endometrial
    suction curet
Garden femoral neck fracture
    classification system (I–IV)
Garden procedure
garden variety
Gardiner-Brown tuning fork
Gardner bone chisel
Gardner chair
Gardner chisel
Gardner headrest
Gardner hysterectomy forceps
Gardner needle

Gardner needle holder
Gardner operation
Gardner shoulder approach
Gardner skull clamp
Gardner suture needle
Gardner tongs
Gardner-Pearson growth grid
    scale
Gardner-Wells headrest
Gardner-Wells skull tongs
Gardner-Wells tongs
Gardner-Wells traction tongs
Garfield-Holinger laryngoscope
gargoylism
Gariel pessary
Garland clamp
Garland forceps
Garland hysterectomy clamp
Garland hysterectomy forceps
Garlock spur crusher
Garner balloon shunt
Garré osteomyelitis
Garren gastric bubble
Garren-Edwards balloon
Garren-Edwards gastric bubble
Garretson bandage
Garretson dressing
Garrett dilator
Garrett retractor
Garrett vascular dilator
Garrigue forceps
Garrigue speculum
Garrigue uterine-dressing
    forceps
Garrigue vaginal retractor
Garrigue vaginal speculum
Garrison forceps
Garrison knife
Garrison rongeur
Garron spatula
garrote tourniquet
Gartner cyst
Gartner duct
Gärtner tonometer
gartnerian cyst
gas analyzer
gas cautery

gas chromatography
gas density line
gas gangrene
gas laser
gas machine
gas pack
gas pattern
gas sterilization
gas tube
gas volume
gaseous
gaseous agent
gaseous cholecystitis
gaseous dilatation
gaseous distention
gaseous injection
gases
gasiness and cramping
Gaskell clamp
gas-liquid chromatography
Gass cannula
Gass cataract-aspirating cannula
Gass cervical punch
Gass corneoscleral punch
Gass endarterectomy spatula
Gass hook
Gass muscle hook
Gass punch
Gass scleral marker
Gass scleral punch
gasserectomy
gasserian ganglion
gasserian ganglion hook
gasserian ganglionectomy
gas-solid chromatography
gastralgia
gastrectomy
gastric acidity
gastric air bubble
gastric analysis
gastric antral erosion
gastric arteries
gastric aspiration tube
gastric atony
gastric atrophy
gastric balloon
gastric bubble

gastric bypass (GBP)
gastric bypass operation
gastric calculus
gastric cardia
gastric clamp
gastric contents
gastric cytology
gastric decompression
gastric dilatation
gastric distention
gastric duplication cyst
gastric emptying
gastric emptying scan
gastric erosion
gastric fistula
gastric folds
gastric freezing
gastric fundal wrap
gastric fundus
gastric gavage
gastric glands
gastric hypersecretion
gastric lavage
gastric lavage tube
gastric loop-type bypass
gastric motility disorder
gastric neurectomy
gastric notch
gastric omentum
gastric outlet
gastric outlet obstruction
gastric partitioning
gastric pit
gastric plexus
gastric pouch
gastric pressure
gastric procedure
gastric pylorus
gastric resection
gastric resection retractor
gastric rugae
gastric rugal fold
gastric sclerosis
gastric secretion
gastric sling muscle
gastric stapling procedure
gastric stoma

gastric stump
gastric suction
gastric surface of spleen
gastric tear
gastric tube
gastric tumor
gastric ulcer
gastric ulceration
gastric varices
gastric veins
gastric vena caval shunt
gastric volvulus
gastric washings
gastrica dextra, arteria
gastrica dextra, vena
gastrica sinistra, arteria
gastrica sinistra, vena
gastricae breves, arteriae
gastricae breves, venae
gastrinoma
gastrin-secreting non-beta islet
    cell tumor
gastritis
gastrocamera
gastrocardiac syndrome
Gastroccult
gastrocele
gastrocnemius
gastrocnemius equinus
gastrocnemius muscle
gastrocnemius, musculus
gastrocnemius reflex
gastrocolic
gastrocolic fistula
gastrocolic ligament
gastrocolic omentum
gastrocolic reflex
gastrocolitis
gastrocolostomy
gastrocolotomy
gastrocolpotomy
gastrocs (slang for gastroc-
    nemius muscles)
gastrodiaphane
gastrodiaphanoscopy
gastrodiaphany
gastroduodenal

gastroduodenal anastomosis
gastroduodenal artery
gastroduodenal contents
gastroduodenal fiberscope
gastroduodenal lumen
gastroduodenal mucosa
gastroduodenal tube
gastroduodenal ulcer
gastroduodenalis, arteria
gastroduodenectomy
gastroduodenitis
gastroduodenopancreatectomy
gastroduodenoscopy
gastroduodenostomy
gastroenteric
gastroenteroanastomosis
gastroenterocolostomy
gastroenterogenous cyst
gastroenteroplasty
gastroenterostomy
gastroenterostomy catheter
gastroenterostomy clamp
gastroenterostomy stoma
gastroenterostomy tube
gastroenterotomy
gastroepiploic
gastroepiploic artery
gastroepiploic branch
gastroepiploic lymph node
gastroepiploic vein
gastroepiploic vessels
gastroepiploica dextra, arteria
gastroepiploica dextra, vena
gastroepiploica sinistra, arteria
gastroepiploica sinistra, vena
gastroesophageal
gastroesophageal hernia
gastroesophageal incompetence
gastroesophageal junction
gastroesophageal reflux
gastroesophageal reflux disease
    (GERD)
gastroesophageal sphincter
gastroesophageal variceal
    plexus
gastroesophagostomy
gastrofiberscope

gastrogalvanization
gastrogastrostomy
gastrogavage
gastrogram
gastrography
gastrohepatic
gastrohepatic ligament
gastrohepatic omentum
gastroileal anastomosis
gastroileal reflex
gastroileitis
gastroileostomy
gastrointestinal (GI)
gastrointestinal biopsy
gastrointestinal bleed
gastrointestinal bleeding
gastrointestinal clamp
gastrointestinal continuity
gastrointestinal disease
gastrointestinal forceps
gastrointestinal instrument
gastrointestinal intubation
gastrointestinal malignancy
gastrointestinal mucosa
gastrointestinal needle
gastrointestinal perforation
gastrointestinal series
gastrointestinal spasm
gastrointestinal stoma
gastrointestinal surgery
gastrointestinal surgical gut
    sutures
gastrointestinal surgical linen
    sutures
gastrointestinal surgical silk
    sutures
gastrointestinal symptomatology
gastrointestinal system
gastrointestinal tract
gastrointestinal tube
gastrointestinal ulcer
gastrojejunal
gastrojejunal anastomosis
gastrojejunal ulcer
gastrojejunocolic
gastrojejunocolic fistula
gastrojejunostomy

gastrolienal ligament
gastrolysis
gastromegaly
gastromotor insufficiency
gastromyotomy
gastronesteostomy
gastropancreatic fold
gastropancreatic ligament
gastropancreatic reflex
gastroparesis
gastropexy
gastrophotography
gastrophrenic
gastrophrenic ligament
gastroplasty
gastroplication
GastroPort enteral feeding
gastroptosis
gastropylorectomy
gastropyloric
gastrorrhaphy
gastrorrhea
gastrorrhexis
gastroscope
    ACMI examining
        gastroscope
    ACMI gastroscope
    Benedict gastroscope
    Benedict operating
        gastroscope
    Bernstein gastroscope
    Bernstein modification
        gastroscope
    Cameron gastroscope
    Chevalier Jackson
        gastroscope
    Eder gastroscope
    Eder-Chamberlin
        gastroscope
    Eder-Hufford gastro-
        scope
    Eder-Palmer gastroscope
    Ellsner gastroscope
    Ewald gastroscope
    examining gastroscope
    fibergastroscope
    fiberoptic gastroscope

gastroscope *continued*
    flexible gastroscope
    GFC gastroscope
    GTF-A gastroscope
    Herman-Taylor gastro-
      scope
    Hirschowitz fiberscope
      gastroscope
    Hirschowitz gastroscope
    Housset-Debray gastro-
      scope
    Janeway gastroscope
    Kelling gastroscope
    Krentz photogastroscope
    Olympus gastroscope
    operating gastroscope
    Pentax gastroscope
    peroral gastroscope
    photogastroscope
    Schindler gastroscope
    Universal gastroscope
    Wolf-Schindler gastro-
      scope
gastroscopic
gastroscopy
gastrosoleus muscle
gastrosphincteric pressure
    gradient
gastrosplenic
gastrosplenic ligament
gastrosplenic omentum
gastrostogavage
gastrostolavage
gastrostoma
gastrostomy
gastrostomy plug
gastrostomy pump
gastrostomy scoop
gastrostomy tube
gastrosuccorrhea
gastrotome
gastrotomy
Gatch bed
gate clamp
gate clip
gate control
gated blood pool angiogram

gated blood pool scan
gated nuclear angiogram
gated pool scan
gated pool test
gated radionuclide angiogram
gated technique
gated test
Gatellier incision
Gatellier operation
Gau gastric balloon
Gaucher splenomegaly
Gauderer-Ponsky catheter
Gauderer-Ponsky PEG (Gaud-
    erer-Ponsky percutaneous
    endoscopic gastrostomy
    procedure)
gauge
    abdominal strain gauge
    acetabular cup gauge
    Austin gauge
    B&S gauge sutures
      (Brown-Sharp gauge
      sutures)
    Brown-Sharp gauge
      sutures (B&S gauge
      sutures)
    calibrated depth gauge
    calibration gauge
    catheter gauge
    Dacomed Snap-Gauge
    depth gauge
    Farrior oval-window
      piston gauge excavator
    heavy gauge suture
    Intermedics intraocular
      radius gauge
    mercury-in-Silastic strain
      gauge
    pressure gauge
    Preston pinch gauge
    Reichert radius gauge
    snap gauge band
    Statham strain gauge
    strain gauge
Gault cochleopalpebral reflex
gauntlet anesthesia
gauntlet bandage

gauntlet flap
gauntlet flap procedure
gauntlet graft
gauntlet splint
Gauss sign
Gauthier retractor
Gauvain brace
gauze (see also *bandage,*
    *dressing, gauze bandage,*
    *gauze dressing, gauze*
    *packer, gauze packing*)
    absorbable gauze
    absorbent gauze
    Adaptic gauze
    adhesive gauze
    Aureomycin gauze
    Bettman gauze
    cellulose gauze
    collodion gauze
    cotton gauze
    Cover-Roll adhesive
        gauze
    Double Seal Tubegauze
    Elasta-Wrap elastic gauze
    elastic gauze
    Elastomull elastic gauze
        bandage
    4 x 4 gauze
    felt-gauze pad
    fine-mesh gauze
    Flexicon elastic gauze
    fluffed gauze
    Furacin gauze
    Gelfoam gauze
    impregnated gauze
    iodoform gauze
    Kerlix gauze
    Kling elastic gauze
    Kling gauze
    Nuform gauze
    Nu-Gauze
        Mersilene gauze
    Owen rayon gauze
    Oxycel gauze
    packed with gauze
    petrolatum gauze
    petrolatum-impregnated
        gauze

gauze *continued*
    plain gauze
    rayon gauze
    Ray-Tec gauze
    sterile absorbent gauze
    strip of gauze
    surgical gauze
    Surgicel gauze
    Teletrast gauze
    Telfa gauze
    trailer gauze
    tube gauze
    Vaseline gauze
    Vaseline petrolatum
        gauze
    Vioform gauze
    Xeroform gauze
    zinc gelatin-impregnated
        gauze
gauze bandage (see also *gauze;*
    *gauze dressing*)
    Elastomull elastic gauze
        bandage
    Flexicon gauze bandage
    Flexilite gauze bandage
    Gauztec bandage
gauze dressing (see also *gauze,*
    *gauze bandage*)
    Adaptic gauze dressing
    Aquaphor gauze dressing
    Aureomycin gauze
        dressing
    fluffed gauze dressing
    Furacin gauze dressing
    Gauztec dressing
    Kling gauze dressing
    Nu-Gauze dressing
    Owen gauze dressing
    petrolatum gauze
        dressing
    scarlet red gauze
        dressing
    Sta-Tite gauze dressing
    Surgicel gauze dressing
    Telfa gauze dressing
    Vaseline gauze dressing
    Vaseline petrolatum
        gauze dressing

gauze dressing *continued*
    Vioform gauze dressing
gauze packer (see also *packer*)
    Allport gauze packer
    Bernay gauze packer
    iodoform gauze packer
    Kitchen postpartum
        gauze packer
gauze packing (see also
    *packing*)
    Adaptic gauze packing
    Brodhead uterine gauze
        packing
    iodoform gauze packing
    Nu-Gauze packing
gauze pad
gauze pad carrier
gauze scissors
gauze sponge
gauze stent dressing
gauze strip
gauze tissue bag
gauze wick
Gauztex bandage
Gauztex dressing
gavage
gavage feeding
gavage tube
Gavard muscle
Gavello operation
Gavin-Miller clamp
Gavin-Miller colon forceps
Gavin-Miller intestinal forceps
Gavin-Miller tissue forceps
gavinofixation
Gay glands
Gayet operation
Gaylor forceps
Gaylor punch
Gaylor tenaculum
Gaylor uterine biopsy forceps
Gaylor uterine specimen
    forceps
Gaylor-Alexander punch
Gaylord pneumatic tourniquet
Gaynor-Hart position
Gaza operation
GB (gallbladder)

GBP (gastric bypass)
GC (general closure)
GC needle
GE pacemaker
GEE oculoplethysmography
GEE-OPG (GEE oculopleth-
    ysmography)
Gehrung pessary
Geiger cautery
Geiger-Downes cautery
Geiger-Mueller counter
Geissendorfer forceps
Geissendorfer rib retractor
Geissler tube
Geissler-Pluecker tube
gel barrier
gel cast
Gel Clean
gel electrophoresis
gelatin
gelatiniform carcinoma
gelatinous
gelatinous capsule
gelatinous carcinoma
gelatinous compression boot
gelatinous disk
gelatinous film
gelatinous marrow
gelatinous material
gelatinous sponge
gelatinous tissue
Gelcast
Geldmacher tendon-passing
    probe
gel-filled implant
gel-filled prosthesis
Gelfilm cap
Gelfilm dressing
Gelfilm plate
Gelfilm retinal orbital implant
Gelfoam
Gelfoam cookie
Gelfoam dressing
Gelfoam forceps
Gelfoam gauze
Gelfoam pack
Gelfoam packing
Gelfoam powder

Gelfoam pressure forceps
Gelfoam sponge
Gelfoam strip
Gelfoam-soaked pledget
Gellhorn forceps
Gellhorn pessary
Gellhorn punch
Gellhorn uterine biopsy forceps
Gellhorn uterine biopsy punch
Gelocast
Gelocast dressing
gelotripsy
Gelpi forceps
Gelpi hysterectomy forceps
Gelpi perineal retractor
Gelpi retractor
Gelpi self-retaining retractor
Gelpi-Lowrie forceps
Gelpi-Lowrie hysterectomy
Gelpi-Lowrie hysterectomy
    forceps
gel-saline mammary implant
gel-saline Surgitek prosthesis
Gély sutures
gemellary pregnancy
gemellus inferior, musculus
gemellus muscle
gemellus superior, musculus
geminate teeth
Gemini clamp
Gemini forceps
Gemini gall duct forceps
Gemini Mixter forceps
Gemini pacemaker
Gemini thoracic forceps
genal glands
Gendelach sphenoid punch
gene mapping
general anatomy
general anesthesia
general cataract
general closure (GC)
general closure needle
general closure sutures
General Electric pacemaker
general endotracheal anesthesia
    (GET)
general eye surgery sutures
general inhalation anesthesia
general insufflation anesthesia
general operating scissors
general surgery
general surgery instrument
    set
general wire forceps
generalized
generalized fatigue
generalized malignancy
generalized metastasis
generalized pain
generalized tenderness
generalized weakness
generator
generous in size
genetic abnormality
genetic amniocentesis
genetic defect
genetic disease
genetic factor
genetic markers
genetic pattern
genetic risk
genetic structures
genetic therapy
genetically at risk
Geneva lens clock
Genga bandage
genial apophysis
genicular artery
genicular branch
genicular veins
geniculate bodies
geniculate ganglion
geniculocalcarine tract
geniculum
geniocheiloplasty
genioglossus muscle
geniohyoid muscle
geniohyoideus, musculus
genioplasty
Genisis dual-chamber pace-
    maker
Genisis pacemaker
genital area

genital fold
genital neoplasia
genital swelling
genitalia
genitofemoral
genitofemoral nerve
genitofemoralis, nervus
genitoplasty
genitospinal center
genitourinary
genitourinary cancer
genitourinary region
genitourinary system
genitourinary tract
Gensini angiocatheter
Gensini catheter
Gensini Teflon catheter
gentian violet
gentle active flexion
gentle exercise
gentle rocking motion
gentle traction
Gentle-Flo suction catheter
gently brought into view
genu corporis callosi
genu impressum
genu nervi facialis
genu recurvatum
genu valgum
genu valgus
genu varum
Genucom total knee analysis
    system
genucubital position
genufacial position
Genupak tampon
genupectoral position
genus descendens, arteria
genus inferior lateralis, arteria
genus inferior medialis, arteria
genus media, arteria
genus superior lateralis, arteria
genus superior medialis, arteria
genus, vena
Genutrain knee support
genyplasty
geographic landmarks
geographic tongue

Geo-Matt foam system
Geomedic arthroplasty
Geomedic femoral condyle
    prosthesis
Geomedic femoral pusher
Geomedic jig
Geomedic knee prosthesis
Geomedic prosthesis
Geomedic total knee prosthesis
Geometric knee prosthesis
geopatellar-type knee replace-
    ment
Georgariou operation
George Lewis technique
George Winter elevation torque
    technique
Georgiade breast prosthesis
Georgiade intraoral traction
Georgiade visor halo fixation
    apparatus
Gerad resurfacing procedure
Gerald bipolar forceps
Gerald dressing forceps
Gerald forceps
Gerald tissue forceps
Gerbode anuloplasty
Gerbode cardiovascular tissue
    forceps
Gerbode dilator
Gerbode forceps
Gerbode mitral dilator
Gerbode mitral valvulotome
Gerbode mitral valvulotomy
    dilator
Gerbode patent ductus clamp
Gerbode rib spreader
Gerbode sternal retractor
Gerbode valve dilator
GERD (gastroesophageal reflux
    disease)
Gerdy fontanelle
Gerdy interauricular loop
Gerdy knee tubercle
Gerdy tubercle
Gerhardt triangle
Gerlach tonsil
germ
Germafect

German A-O hip compression screw
germ-free environment
germinal infection
germinal layer
germinal matrix
germinal rod
germ-laden air
Gerota capsule
Gerota fascia
Gerow Small-Carrion penile implant
Gerster fracture appliance
Gerster traction bar
Gersuny operation
Gerzog ear knife
Gerzog hammer
Gerzog knife
Gerzog mallet
Gerzog mastoid mallet
Gerzog nasal speculum
Gerzog speculum
Gerzog-Ralks ear knife
Gerzog-Ralks knife
Gesco aspirator
gestation
gestational age
gestational diabetes
gestational period
gestational sac
gestational size
gestational weeks
gesticulatory tic
GET anesthesia (general endotracheal anesthesia)
Getty technique for spinal stenosis
Geuder corneal needle
Geuder keratoplasty needle
GFC gastroscope
Ghajar guide
Ghazi rib retractor
Ghon complex
Ghon focus
Ghon lesion
Ghon primary lesion
Ghon tubercle
Ghormley operation
ghost ophthalmoscope
ghost vessels
ghoul hand
GI (gastrointestinal)
GI bleed
GI clamp
GI forceps
GI pop-off silk suture
GI silk suture
GIA (gastrointestinal anastomosis)
GIA circular stapler
GIA instrument
GIA staple
GIA stapler
GIA stapling device
Giannestras metatarsal procedure
Giannestras procedure
Giannestras turnbuckle
Giannini needle holder
giant cell adenocarcinoma
giant cell carcinoma
giant cell tumor
giant swelling
Gianturco coil
Gianturco stent
Gianturco sutures
Gianturco wool-tufted wire coil
Gianturco-Roehm bird's nest vena caval filter
Gibbon catheter
Gibbon hydrocele
Gibbon indwelling ureteral stent
Gibbon stent
Gibbon ureteral stent
Gibbon urethral catheter
gibbous deformity
gibbus
Gibney bandage
Gibney boot
Gibney dressing
Gibney perispondylitis
Gibney strapping
Gibson approach
Gibson dressing

Gibson eye irrigator
Gibson incision
Gibson irrigator
Gibson murmur
Gibson operation
Gibson splint
Gibson sutures
Gibson vestibule
Gibson-Balfour abdominal
    retractor
Gibson-Balfour retractor
Gibson-Foley incision
Gibson-Gibson posterior
    muscle-cutting incision
Giertz rib guillotine
Giertz rib shears
Giertz rongeur
Giertz-Shoemaker rib shears
Giertz-Shoemaker shears
Giesy ureteral dilatation
    balloon
GIF-HM endoscope
Gifford applicator
Gifford corneal applicator
Gifford corneal curet
Gifford curet
Gifford fixation forceps
Gifford forceps
Gifford holder
Gifford iris forceps
Gifford keratotomy
Gifford maneuver
Gifford mastoid retractor
Gifford needle holder
Gifford operation
Gifford reflex
Gifford retractor
Gifford scalp retractor
Gifford sign
Gifford-Galassie reflex
Gifford-Jansen mastoid
    retractor
GIFT (gamete intrafallopian
    transfer)
GIF-XQ endoscope
GIF-XQ fiberoptic instrument
gigahertz
gigantism

Gigli operation
Gigli pubiotomy
Gigli saw
Gigli-saw blade
Gigli-saw conductor
Gigli-saw guide
Gigli-saw handle
Gigli-saw wire
Gilbert balloon catheter
Gilbert catheter
Gilbert cystic duct forceps
Gilbert forceps
Gilbert pediatric balloon
    catheter
Gilbert pediatric catheter
Gilbert prosthesis
Gilbert sign
Gilbert-Graves speculum
Giliberty cup hip prosthesis
Giliberty prosthesis
Giliberty total hip prosthesis
Gill biopsy brush
Gill blade
Gill cleft palate elevator
Gill corneal knife
Gill dropfoot procedure
Gill forceps
Gill iris forceps
Gill knife
Gill laminectomy
Gill needle
Gill needle holder
Gill operation
Gill procedure
Gill respirator
Gill scissors
Gill shoulder arthrodesis
Gill sinus cannula
Gill-Chandler iris forceps
Gillespie obstetrical forceps
Gillespie operation
Gillespie wrist excision
Gillette brace
Gill-Fuchs forceps
Gill-Hess forceps
Gill-Hess iris forceps
Gilliam operation
Gilliam suspension of uterus

Gilliam uterine suspension
Gilliam-Doléris operation
Gillies approach
Gillies construction of replacement thumb
Gillies ectropion graft
Gillies elevation procedure
Gillies elevator
Gillies fashion
Gillies flap
Gillies forceps
Gillies graft
Gillies hook
Gillies horizontal dermal suture
Gillies implant
Gillies incision
Gillies needle holder
Gillies operation
Gillies prosthesis
Gillies scissors
Gillies skin hook
Gillies suture scissors
Gillies tissue forceps
Gillies up-and-down flap
Gillies zygomatic elevator
Gillies zygomatic hook
Gillies-Dingman tenaculum hook
Gillies-Fry operation
Gillies-Kilner operation
Gillies-Millard technique
Gillies-Sheehan needle holder
Gill-Jonas procedure
Gill-Manning decompression laminectomy
Gill-Manning-White fusion
Gillmore needle
Gillquist approach
Gills intraocular implant lens
Gills lens
Gills technique
Gill-Safar forceps
Gill-Stein arthrodesis of wrist
Gill-Stein operation
Gill-Stein radiocarpal arthrodesis
Gills-Welsh cortex extractor
Gills-Welsh irrigating cannula

Gilman-Abrams gastric tube
Gilman-Abrams tube
Gilmer intermaxillary fixation
Gilmer splint
Gilmer tooth splint
Gilmer wiring
Gilmore intraocular implant lens
Gilmore lens
Gilmore probe
Gilquest approach
Gilquist arthroscopy
Gilquist incision
Gilquist procedure
Gil-Vernet dissection
Gil-Vernet lumbotomy retractor
Gil-Vernet operation
Gil-Vernet pyelolithotomy
Gil-Vernet renal sinus retractor
Gil-Vernet retractor
Gimbernat ligament
Gimmick elevator
gingiva (*pl.* gingivae)
gingival cartilage
gingival clamp
gingival crevice
gingival incision
gingival lancet
gingival line
gingival margin
gingival sulcus
gingival trough
gingivectomy
gingivitis
gingivobuccal
gingivolabial incision
gingivolabial sulci
gingivoplasty
gingivostomatitis
Ginsberg forceps
Ginsberg tissue forceps
Gio-occlusive dressing
Giordano operation
Giordano sphincter
Giralde operation
Girard forceps
Girard Fragmatome

Girard irrigating cannula
Girard irrigating tip
Girard keratoprosthesis
Girard needle
Girard operation
Girard phakofragmatome
Girard probe
Girard-Swan knife-needle
girdle
Girdlestone excision of femoral
   head and neck
Girdlestone hip resection
Girdlestone joint resection
Girdlestone operation
Girdlestone-Taylor operation for
   claw toes
Girdner probe
girth
Gissane angle
Gissane spike
Gissane spike nail
Givner eye retractor
glabellar rasp
glabelloalveolar line
gladiolus
gladiolus bone
gland
glandular
glandular cancer
glandular carcinoma
glandular tissue
glans
glans clitoridis
glans of penis
glans penis
Glaser laminectomy retractor
Glaser retractor
glaserian fissure
Glasgow coma scale
Glasgow sign
Glass abdominal retractor
glass bottle
glass hand
glass hand operation
glass jar
glass nasal suction tip
glass nasal tip
glass pH electrode

Glass retractor
glass rod
glass sphere eye implant
glass suction tip
glass vaginal plug
glassblower's cataract
Glasscock dressing
Glasscock ear dressing
Glasscock-House knife
Glasser gastrostomy tube
glasses
Glassman anterior resection
   clamp
Glassman basket
Glassman brush
Glassman clamp
Glassman forceps
Glassman gastroenterostomy
   clamp
Glassman gastrointestinal clamp
Glassman gastrostomy
Glassman intestinal clamp
Glassman liver-holding clamp
Glassman noncrushing instru-
   ments
Glassman noncrushing pickup
   forceps
Glassman pickup forceps
Glassman scissors
Glassman-Allis clamp
Glassman-Allis common duct-
   holding forceps
Glassman-Allis forceps
Glassman-Allis intestinal forceps
Glassman-Allis miniature
   intestinal forceps
Glassman-Allis noncrushing
   tissue-holding forceps
glassy cell carcinoma
glassy swelling
Glattelast elastic knee support
glaucoma
glaucoma knife
glaucomatous cataract
glaucomatous halo
Gleason headband
Gleason prostatic carcinoma
   score

Gleason rasp
Gleason raspatory
Gleason score of prostatic
    carcinoma
Gleason speculum
Gleason staging of prostate
    cancer
Glen Anderson ureteroneo-
    cystostomy
Glenn anastomosis
Glenn diverticulum forceps
Glenn operation
Glenn shunt
Glenner forceps
Glenner hysterectomy forceps
Glenner retractor
Glenner vaginal hysterectomy
    forceps
Glenner vaginal retractor
glenohumeral ligaments
glenoid cavity
glenoid fossa
glenoid labrum
glenoid ligaments
glenoid process
glenoid punch
glenoplasty
glial membrane
glial sheath
gliding joint
gliding motion
gliding prosthesis
glioma
gliosis
Glisson capsule
Glisson sling
Glisson sling splint
glistening fragments
glistening transparent meninges
globe
globe of eye
globe prolapsus pessary
globular
globular object forceps
globule
globulin
globus

globus abdominalis
globus hystericus
globus major epididymidis
globus minor epididymidis
globus of heel
globus pallidus
Glolite infrared light
glomectomy
glomerular arteriole
glomerular basement membrane
glomerular capsule
glomerular filtration
glomerular infiltration
glomerular nephritis
glomerulocapsular nephritis
glomerulonephritis
glomerulus (pl. glomeruli)
glomus jugulare tumor
glomus tumor
Glori post-keloid surgery
    pressure earrings
glossectomy
glossitis
glossoepiglottic fold
glossopalatine gland
glossopalatine muscle
glossopexy
glossopharyngeal muscle
glossopharyngeal nerve (cranial
    nerve IX)
glossopharyngeal nerve sign
glossopharyngeal neurotomy
glossopharyngeus, nervus
glossoplasty
glossorrhaphy
glossosteresis
glossotomy
glottic carcinoma
glottic extension
glottis
glove anesthesia
gloved-fist technique
Glover auricular-appendage
    clamp
Glover bulldog clamp
Glover clamp
Glover coarctation clamp

Glidewire guide wire

Glover curved clamp
Glover curved forceps
Glover dilator
Glover drainage system
Glover forceps
Glover infundibular rongeur
    forceps
Glover patent ductus clamp
Glover rongeur
Glover rongeur forceps
Glover spoon anastomosis
    clamp
Glover spoon-shaped forceps
Glover suction tube
Glover vascular clamp
Glover-DeBakey clamp
glover's sutures
gloving technique
GLR (gravity lumbar reduction)
glucagonoma
Gluck rib shears
Gluck shears
glue
glue-in sutures
glueophytes (slang)
glutaraldehyde
glutaraldehyde-tanned bovine
    carotid artery graft
glutaraldehyde-tanned bovine
    collagen tube
glutaraldehyde-tanned bovine
    heart valve
glutaraldehyde-tanned porcine
    heart valve
glutea inferior, arteria
glutea superior, arteria
gluteae inferiores, venae
gluteae superiores, venae
gluteal artery
gluteal bonnet
gluteal cleft
gluteal fascia
gluteal fold
gluteal hernia
gluteal line
gluteal muscle
gluteal nerve

gluteal reflex
gluteal veins
gluteal vessels
gluten
gluteofemoral
gluteus
gluteus inferior, nervus
gluteus maximus, musculus
gluteus medius, musculus
gluteus minimus, musculus
gluteus superior, nervus
glycerin
glyceryl guaiacolate
glyceryl methacrylate
glyceryl trinitrate
glycine
glycocalyx-enclosed biofilm
glycogen
glycosuria
gnarled enamel
gnathalgia
gnathodynia
gnathological splint
gnathoplasty
gnawing pain
gnawing sensation
Godart expirograph
Godelo dilator
Goebel-Frangenheim-Stoeckel
    operation
Goebel-Stoeckel operation
Goebel-Stoeckel sling
Goeckerman light therapy
Goelet double-ended retractor
Goelet retractor
Goethe sutures
Goffe colporrhaphy
Goffe operation
goggles
Gohrbrand cardiac dilator
Gohrbrand dilator
Gohrbrand valvulotome
goiter
goiter clamp
goiter dissector
goiter forceps
goiter retractor

goiter scissors
goiter tenaculum
goiter vulsellum forceps
Golaski graft
Golay coil
gold crown
gold ear marker
gold eye implant
Gold forceps
Gold hemostatic forceps
gold implant
gold sphere
gold sphere eye implant
gold strip
Goldbacher anoscope
Goldbacher anoscope speculum
Goldbacher needle
Goldbacher proctoscope
Goldbacher speculum
Goldblatt clamp
Goldblatt hypertension
Goldblatt kidney
Golden sign
Goldenhar syndrome
Goldman bar
Goldman cartilage punch
Goldman chisel
Goldman curet
Goldman elevator
Goldman guillotine nerve knife
Goldman hook
Goldman knife
Goldman nerve
Goldman punch
Goldman saw
Goldman scissors
Goldman score of cardiovascular risk
Goldman serrated knife
Goldman Universal nerve hook
Goldman-Fox knife
Goldman-Kazanjian forceps
Goldman-Kazanjian nasal forceps
Goldman-McNeill blepharostat
Goldmann applanation tonometer
Goldmann expressor

Goldmann goniolens
Goldmann lens
Goldmann multi-mirrored lens implant
Goldmann perimeter
Goldmann perimetry
Goldmann tonometer
Goldmann-Favre syndrome
Goldnamer ear basin
Goldner anterior fusion
Goldner-Clippinger technique
gold-plated bandage scissors
Goldstein anterior chamber–irrigating cannula
Goldstein cannula
Goldstein curet
Goldstein eye syringe
Goldstein irrigating cannula
Goldstein irrigator
Goldstein lacrimal sac retractor
Goldstein mucosa speculum
Goldstein retractor
Goldstein speculum
Goldstein spine fusion
Goldstein syringe
Goldthwait bar
Goldthwait brace
Goldthwait fracture appliance
Goldthwait fracture frame
Goldthwait operation
Goldthwait procedure
Goldthwait sign
golf tee-shaped polyvinyl prosthesis
golf-club eye spud
golf-club spud
Golgi apparatus
Golgi cells
Golgi complex
Goligher extraperitoneal ileostomy
Goligher ileostomy
Goligher retractor
Goligher retractor frame
Goligher speculum
Goll tract
Golub lead on EKG
GoLytely bowel prep

gomangioma of ear
Gomco aspirator
Gomco bell
Gomco bloodless circumcision
   clamp
Gomco circumcision clamp
Gomco clamp
Gomco drain
Gomco ENT treatment unit
Gomco forceps
Gomco hemostat
Gomco portable suction
   aspirator
Gomco pump
Gomco suction
Gomco suction aspirator
Gomco suction tube
Gomco thermotic pump
Gomco thoracic drainage pump
Gomco umbilical cord clamp
Gomco uterine aspirator
Gomco-Bell clamp
gomectomy
Gomez fundoplasty
Gomez gastroplasty
Gomez horizontal gastroplasty
Gomez retractor
Gomez-Marquez operation
gonad shield
gonadal agenesis
gonadal aplasia
gonadal dysgenesis
gonadal veins
gonadectomy
gonadotropin
gonads
gonarthrotomy
Gonda reflex
gonial angle
Gonin cautery
Gonin operation
Gonin-Amsler scleral marker
Gonin-Amsler scleral marker
   scissors
goniolens
goniometer
   Conzett goniometer
   electrogoniometer

goniometer *continued*
   finger goniometer
   Frykholm goniometer
   international standard
      goniometer
   Polk goniometer
   Tomac goniometer
goniophotography
gonioprism
goniopuncture
goniopuncture operation
gonioscope
   Allen-Thorpe gonio-
      scope
   Barkan gonioscope
   Koeppe gonioscope
   Richards-Schaefer
      gonioscope
   Troncoso gonioscope
   Zeiss Formair gonio-
      scope
gonioscopy
gonioscopy lens
goniotomy
goniotomy knife
Gooch mastoid retractor
Gooch retractor
Good forceps
Good frontal raspatory
Good obstetrical forceps
Good rasp
Good retractor
Good scissors
Good speculum
Good tonsillar scissors
Goodale-Lubin catheter
Goodall-Power operation
Goode knife
Goode nasal splint
Goode T-tube
Goode tube
Goodell dilator
Goodell sign
Goodell uterine dilator
Goodell-Power operation
Goode-Magne nasal airway
   splint
Goodfellow cannula

Goodfellow frontal sinus
    cannula
Goodhill cautery
Goodhill forceps
Goodhill hook
Goodhill knife
Goodhill prosthesis
Goodhill retractor
Goodhill tonsillar forceps
Goodhill tonsillar hemostatic
    clamp
Goodhill tonsillar hemostatic
    forceps
Goodhill-Down knife
Goodhill-Pynchon tube
Goodley cervical traction
Good-Lite headband
Good-Lite super headlight
Good-Reiner scissors
Good-Reiner tonsil scissors
Goodwillie periosteal elevator
Goodwin clamp
Goodyear knife
Goodyear retractor
Goodyear tonsillar knife
Goodyear tonsillar retractor
Goodyear uvula retractor
Goodyear-Gruenwald for-
    ceps
Goosen vascular punch
gooseneck chisel
gooseneck light
gooseneck rongeur
gooseneck sign
Gordh needle
Gordon arm splint
Gordon cilia forceps
Gordon forceps
Gordon reflex
Gordon splint
Gordon stethoscope
Gordon syndrome
Gordon technique
Gordon uterine forceps
Gordon uterine vulsellum
    forceps
Gordon-Bronstrom technique
Gordon-Taylor amputation

Gore-Tex artificial knee
    ligament
Gore-Tex AV fistula
Gore-Tex bifurcated vascular
    graft
Gore-Tex cardiovascular patch
Gore-Tex catheter
Gore-Tex cushion
Gore-Tex graft
Gore-Tex jump graft
Gore-Tex ligament
Gore-Tex patch
Gore-Tex prosthesis
Gore-Tex shunt
Gore-Tex soft-tissue patch
Gore-Tex surgical membrane
Gore-Tex tube
Gore-Tex vascular graft
Gore-Tex vascular implant
Gore-Tex vascular prosthesis
gorget
Gorland formula
Gorlin catheter
Gorlin pacing catheter
Gorney face-lift scissors
Gorney rhytidectomy scissors
Gorney scissors
Gorney septal scissors
Gorney turbinate scissors
Gorsch needle
Gorsch sigmoidoscope
gossamer silk sutures
Gosselin fracture
Gosset abdominal retractor
Gosset appendectomy retractor
Gosset retractor
Gosset self-retaining retractor
Gott butterfly heart valve
Gott cannula
Gott implant
Gott low-profile prosthesis
Gott mitral valve prosthesis
Gott prosthesis
Gott shunt
Gott tube
Gott valve
Gott-Daggett heart valve
    prosthesis

Gott-Daggett shunt
Gottschalk aspirator
Gottschalk middle ear aspirator
Gottschalk operation
Gottschalk saw
Gouffon hip pin
Gouffon hip pin system
gouge
    Abbott gouge
    Alexander bone gouge
    Alexander gouge
    Alexander mastoid bone
      gouge
    Alexander mastoid
      gouge
    Andrews gouge
    Andrews mastoid gouge
    annulus gouge
    antral gouge
    Army bone gouge
    Army pattern bone
      gouge
    arthroplasty gouge
    Aufranc arthroplasty
      gouge
    Aufranc gouge
    Ballenger gouge
    Bishop gouge
    Bishop mastoid gouge
    Boley gouge
    bone gouge
    Bowen gouge
    Campbell arthroplasty
      gouge
    Campbell gouge
    Capner gouge
    Cave gouge
    Cave scaphoid gouge
    Cobb gouge
    Compere gouge
    concave gouge
    Cooper gouge
    Crane gouge
    curved gouge
    Derlacki gouge
    Dix gouge
    Duray-Read gouge
    Dwyer gouge

gouge *continued*
    Faulkner antrum gouge
    Flanagan gouge
    Flanagan spinal fusion
      gouge
    Freer gouge
    Freer nasal gouge
    Guy gouge
    Guy model nasal gouge
    Heermann gouge
    Hibbs bone gouge
    Hibbs gouge
    hip gouge
    Hoen gouge
    Hoen lamina gouge
    Holmes gouge
    Hough gouge
    hump gouge
    Jewett gouge
    Kelley gouge
    Kezerian gouge
    Killian gouge
    Kuhnt gouge
    Lahey Clinic spinal
      fusion gouge
    Lahey gouge
    lamina gouge
    Lexer gouge
    Lillie gouge
    Lucas gouge
    Martin gouge
    mastoid gouge
    Metzenbaum gouge
    Meyerding gouge
    Moore gouge
    Moore spinal fusion
      gouge
    Murphy bone gouge
    Murphy gouge
    nasal gouge
    nasal hump gouge
    Nicola gouge
    Parkes gouge
    Parkes hump gouge
    Partsch gouge
    Pilling gouge
    Putti arthroplasty gouge
    Putti gouge

gouge *continued*

Read gouge
Rowen spinal fusion gouge
Rubin gouge
scaphoid gouge
Schuknecht gouge
septal gouge
Smith-Petersen arthroplasty gouge
Smith-Petersen gouge
spinal fusion gouge
spinal gouge
Stacke gouge
Stille gouge
Stille-pattern bone gouge
Swan gouge
swan-neck gouge
tissue gouge
Todd gouge
trough gouge
Troutman gouge
Troutman mastoid gouge
tubular gouge
Turner gouge
Turner spinal gouge
U.S. Army gouge
Walton foreign body gouge
Walton gouge
Watson-Jones bone gouge
Watson-Jones gouge
West bone gouge
West gouge
Zielke gouge
Zimmer gouge

Goulain mastopexy
Gould electromagnetic flowmeter
Gould intraocular implant lens
Gould lens
Gould PentaCath 5-lumen thermodilution catheter
Gould Statham pressure
Gould sutures
Goulet retractor

Gouley catheter
Gouley dilator
Gouley guide
Gouley sound
Gouley tunneled urethral sound
Gouley urethral sound
Goulian blade
Goulian knife
Goulian mammaplasty
Goulian procedure to harvest skin graft
gout
gouty arthritis
gouty tophus
Goutz catheter
Govons curet
Gowers maneuver
Gowers sign
Gowers tract
gown and bootees
gown change
gowning technique
Goyrand hernia
graafian cyst
graafian follicle
graafian ovules
graafian vesicle
Graber appliance
Graber-Duvernay hip procedure
Graber-Duvernay procedure
grabber
disk grabber
Gracey curet
gracilis muscle
gracilis muscle transposition
gracilis, musculus
grade
gradient
gradient coil
Gradle cilia forceps
Gradle corneal trephine
Gradle electrode
Gradle eyelid retractor
Gradle forceps
Gradle keratoplasty
Gradle needle electrode
Gradle operation

Gradle retractor
Gradle tonometer
Gradle trephine
gradual weightbearing
gradual withdrawal
graduated catheter
graduated compress
graduated pitcher
graduated sound
graduated tenotomy
graduated-sized catheter
Gradwohl sternal bone marrow
    aspirator
Graefe (also von Graefe)
Graefe cataract knife
Graefe cautery
Graefe cystitome
Graefe cystoscope
Graefe cystotome
Graefe disease
Graefe electric field
Graefe eye speculum
Graefe fixation forceps
Graefe flexible cystotome
Graefe forceps
Graefe hook
Graefe incision
Graefe iris forceps
Graefe iris needle
Graefe knife
Graefe knife-needle
Graefe muscle hook
Graefe needle
Graefe nonmagnetic fixation
    forceps
Graefe operation
Graefe scissors
Graefe sickle knife
Graefe sign
Graefe speculum
Graefe strabismus hook
Graefe test
Graefe tissue-grasping
    forceps
Graefenberg ring (also Gräfen-
    berg)
Graether buttonhook
Graether collar button

Graether collar buttonhook
Graether mushroom hook
Graether retractor
Grafco magnet
Gräfenberg ring (also Graefen-
    berg)
graft (see also *implant, patch,
    prosthesis, valve*)
    accordion graft
    acrylic graft
    activated graft
    Albee bone graft
    Albee graft
    albumin-coated vascular
        graft
    aldehyde-tanned bovine
        carotid artery graft
    allogeneic graft
    allograft
    aortic aneurysm graft
    aortocoronary bypass
        graft
    aortocoronary snake
        graft
    aortofemoral bypass graft
        (AFBG)
    aortohepatic arterial graft
    aortovein bypass graft
    arterial graft
    Augmen bone-grafting
        material
    autochthonous graft
    autodermic graft
    autoepidermic graft
    autogenous bone graft
    autogenous graft
    autogenous vein graft
    autograft
    autologous fat graft
    autologous graft
    autologous vein graft
    autoplastic graft
    AV Gore-Tex graft
    avascular graft
    B-B graft
    B-W graft
    Balnetar graft materials
    Banks bone graft

graft *continued*

Banks graft
Bard graft
Bard PTFE graft
Berens graft
bifurcated vascular graft
bifurcation graft
biograft
biograft umbilical
    prosthesis
Bionit vascular graft
BioPolyMeric vascular
    graft
Blair-Brown graft
Blair-Brown skin graft
bone graft
bone graft material
Bonfiglio bone graft
Boplant graft
bovine allograft
bovine graft
bovine heterograft
bovine pericardial heart
    valve xenograft
Boyd bone graft
Boyd graft
Braun graft
Braun skin graft
Braun-Wangensteen graft
brephoplastic graft
Brett bone graft
bypass graft
bypass vein graft
C-graft
cable graft
cadaveric graft
cadaveric homograft
Calcitite bone graft
    material
Campbell graft
cancellous bone graft
cancellous graft
Carpentier-Edwards
    xenograft
cartilage graft
Celestin graft material
celluloid graft material

graft *continued*

chessboard graft
chessboard skin graft
clothespin graft
Codivilla bone graft
Codivilla graft
collagen graft
composite graft
composite valve graft
corneal graft
coronary artery bypass
    graft (CABG)
cortical bone graft
cortical graft
corticocancellous graft
Cotton cartilage graft
Creech aortoiliac graft
Crescent graft
cross-leg bypass graft
cross-leg graft
crossover graft
Cryolife valvular graft
cryopreserved allograft
cutis graft
Dacron graft
Dacron graft clamp
Dacron knitted graft
Dacron onlay patch
    graft
Dacron patch graft
Dacron preclotted graft
Dacron tightly woven
    graft
Dacron tubular graft
Dacron velour graft
Dacron Weave Knit graft
Dardik biograft
Dardik graft
Dardik human graft
Dardik umbilical graft
Davis graft
de-aired graft
DeBakey graft
defatted skin graft
delayed graft
dermagraft
dermal graft

graft *continued*

Dermamesh graft
expander
dermic graft
diamond inlay bone graft
diced cartilage graft
Doherty graft
double-velour graft
double-velour knitted
graft
Douglas graft
Douglas mesh skin graft
Douglas skin graft
Dragstedt graft
Dragstedt skin graft
drums of skin graft
dual-onlay bone graft
dual-onlay graft
epidermic graft
Esser graft
fascial graft
fascicular graft
fat graft
fiberglass graft
filler graft
Forbes graft technique
free graft
full-thickness graft
glutaraldehyde-tanned
bovine carotid artery
graft
heterodermic graft
hyperplastic graft
iliac autograft
iliac graft
IMA graft
Impra bypass graft
Impra Flex vascular graft
Impra graft
Impra vascular graft
Impra vein graft
Inclan graft
inlay bone graft
inlay graft
Intact xenograft pros-
thetic valve
interbody graft tamp

graft *continued*

internal mammary artery
graft
internal thoracic artery
graft (ITA)
interposition Dacron
graft
interposition graft
intramedullary and
spongiosa graft
intramedullary bone graft
Ionescu-Shiley peri-
cardial valve graft
Ionescu-Shiley peri-
cardial xenograft
Ionescu-Shiley porcine
heterograft heart valve
island graft
isogeneic graft
isograft
isologous graft
isoplastic graft
ITA graft (internal
thoracic artery graft)
Ivalon graft
Ivalon sponge graft
Jeb graft
jump graft
Kebab graft
Kiel graft
knitted graft
knitted Teflon graft
Koenig graft
Krause-Wolfe graft
lamellar corneal graft
lamellar graft
latex sponge graft
lay-on graft
Lee graft
left internal mammary
artery graft (LIMA
graft)
LIMA graft (left internal
mammary artery graft)
living homograft
Lo-Por vascular graft
lyophilized graft

graft *continued*
    mandril graft
    Mangoldt epithelial graft
    Marlex graft
    Marlex mesh graft
    Marquez-Gomez conjunctival graft
    marsupial graft
    massive sliding graft
    McFarland tibia graft
    McMaster bone graft
    Meadox bifurcated graft
    Meadox Dardik biograft
    Meadox graft
    Meadox Microvel double-velour knitted Dacron arterial graft
    Meadox Microvel graft
    Meadox vascular graft
    Mediform dural graft
    Medi-graft vascular prosthesis
    medullary bone graft
    medullary graft
    Mersilene graft
    mesh graft
    mesh skin graft
    mesocaval H-graft shunt
    methyl methacrylate graft
    Meyerding bone graft
    Microknit vascular graft prothesis
    Microvel graft
    Millesi interfascicular grafts
    Milliknit graft
    Milliknit vascular graft prosthesis
    modified graft
    mucosal graft
    mucous membrane graft
    Mules graft
    muscle graft
    N-terface graft dressing
    nerve cable graft
    nerve graft
    Nicoll bone graft

graft *continued*
    nonpenetrating corneal graft
    nonvalved graft
    Ollier graft
    Ollier-Thiersch graft
    omental graft
    onlay bone graft
    onlay cortical graft
    onlay graft
    organ graft
    osseous graft
    osteoperiosteal bone graft
    osteoperiosteal graft
    Ostrup vascularized rib graft
    outer table graft
    Padgett graft
    Paladon graft
    Papineau bone graft
    Papineau cancellous graft
    paraffin graft
    partial-thickness graft
    patch graft
    patent graft
    Paufique graft knife
    pedicle graft
    peg bone graft
    peg graft
    penetrating corneal graft
    penetrating graft
    pericardial xenograft
    perichondrial graft
    Peri-Guard vascular graft
    periosteal graft
    Phemister graft
    Phemister onlay bone graft
    pigskin graft
    pinch graft
    pinch skin graft
    plasma TFE graft
    plasma TFE vascular graft
    Plexiglas graft

graft *continued*
- Plystan graft
- polyether graft material
- polyethylene graft
- polytetrafluoroethylene graft (PTFE)
- polyurethane graft
- polyvinyl graft
- porcine graft
- porcine heterograft
- porcine xenograft
- postage-stamp skin graft
- postauricular graft
- preclotted graft
- preputial island graft
- prop graft
- Proplast graft
- prosthetic graft
- prosthetic patch graft
- PTFE Gore-Tex graft
- PTFE graft
- Rastelli graft
- Rehne skin graft knife
- Reverdin graft
- Reverdin skin graft
- revision of graft
- rib graft
- ring graft
- rope graft
- rotational flap graft
- Russe bone graft
- Russe inlay bone graft
- saphenous graft
- saphenous vein bypass graft (SVBG)
- Sauvage arterial graft
- Sauvage Bionit graft
- Sauvage Dacron graft
- Sauvage graft
- Sauvage vein graft
- seamless arterial graft
- Seddon nerve graft
- seed graft
- segmental graft
- Shea vein graft scissors
- Sheen tip graft
- shell graft

graft *continued*
- sieve graft
- Silastic graft
- Silovi saphenous vein bypass graft
- Siloxane graft
- single-onlay cortical bone graft
- skin graft
- sleeve graft
- slice graft
- sliding inlay bone graft
- sliver bone graft
- snake graft
- Solvang graft
- Speed osteotomy and bone graft
- spinal graft tamper
- split graft
- split-skin graft
- split-thickness graft
- split-thickness skin graft
- sponge graft
- spongiosa bone graft
- spongiosa graft
- St. Jude composite valve graft
- stainless steel graft
- stent graft
- step graft
- straight graft
- straight tubular graft
- strut graft
- STSG (split-thickness skin graft)
- subdermal graft
- Supramid graft
- surrounding graft material
- SVBG (saphenous vein bypass grafting)
- swine xenograft
- syngeneic graft
- syngraft
- synthetic graft
- thick-split graft
- Thiersch graft

graft *continued*

    thin-split graft
    tube graft
    tunnel graft
    Wesolowski bypass graft
    Wesolowski Teflon graft
    white graft
    Wolfe graft
    Wolfe-Krause graft
graft blade plate
graft clamp
graft donor site
graft implantation
graft of fascia
graft of nerve
graft of organ
graft of tendon
graft rejection
graft tamp
graft thrombectomy
grafted kidney rejection
grafted skin
graft-enteric fistula
grafting
graft-seeker catheter
graft-seeking catheter
graft-versus-host disease (GVHD)
graft-versus-host reaction
Graham blunt hook
Graham cardiovascular scissors
Graham closure
Graham closure of ulcer
Graham elevator
Graham hook
Graham nerve hook
Graham omental patch
Graham operation
Graham patch
Graham pediatric scissors
Graham rib contractor
Graham scissors
Graham Steell murmur
Graham-Kerrison punch
Graham-Roscie operation
Gram cannula
Granberry decompressor
Grancher triad

grand multiparity
granddaughter cyst
Granger sign
Granger x-ray view
granny knot sutures
Grant abdominal aortic aneurysmal clamp
Grant aneurysmal clamp
Grant clamp
Grant gallbladder retractor
Grant holder
Grant needle holder
Grant operation
Grant retractor
Grant separator
Grantham electrode
Grantham lobotomy needle
Grantham needle
granular cell tumor
granulate
granulating wound
granulation
granulation tissue
granulation tube
granule
granuloma
granuloma pyogenicum
granulomatosis
granulomatous disease
granulomatous lesion
granulomatous lining
granulosa cell carcinoma
granulosa-theca cell tumor
granulosity
graph
graphic recording
Grapper instrument
Graseby pump
Graser diverticulum
Grashey position
grasp reflex
grasp response
grasp strength
grasped
grasping and cutting forceps
grasping biopsy forceps
grasping clamp
grasping forceps

grasping punch
grasping reflex
Grass pressure recording device
Grass-Cranley phleborrheogram
grating in joint
grating pain
grating sensation
grating sound
Gratiolet radiating fibers
grattage
grattage of conjunctiva
Graves Britetrac vaginal
   speculum
Graves scapula
Graves speculum
Graves vaginal speculum
gravid uterus
gravida (1, 2, 3, etc.)
gravitate
gravitating hemorrhage
gravitational line
gravitational shock
gravitational skin lines
gravity cystography
gravity displacement sterilizer
gravity drainage
gravity lumbar reduction (GLR)
gravity-free position
Gravlee umbilical gun
Gravlee washings
Gravlee-Jetz washer
Grawitz tumor
Gray clamp
Gray cystic duct forceps
Gray drill
Gray forceps
gray matter
Gray resectoscope
grayish tissue
grayline incision
gray-scale imaging
gray-scale ultrasonography
gray-scale ultrasound
Grayson ligament
Grayton corneal forceps
Grayton forceps
grease

grease gun injury
great adductor muscle
great anterior radicular artery
great auricular nerve
great cardiac vein
great cerebral vein
great cistern
Great Ormand Street tracheostomy
Great Ormand Street tube
great saphenous vein
great toe
great toe sign
great transverse commissure
great vessels
greater alar cartilage
greater arterial circle of iris
greater circle of iris
greater circulation
greater curvature
greater curvature banded
   gastroplasty
greater curvature of stomach
greater curvature ulcer
greater ischiatic notch
greater multangular bone
greater occipital nerve
greater omentum
greater palatine artery
greater palatine canal
greater palatine foramen
greater palatine nerve
greater pectoral muscle
greater pelvis
greater peritoneal sac
greater petrosal nerve
greater petrosal nerve hiatus
greater psoas muscle
greater rhomboid muscle
greater sacrosciatic notch
greater saphenous vein
greater saphenous vein ligation
   and stripping
greater sciatic foramen
greater sciatic notch
greater splanchnic nerve
greater superficial nerve

greater trochanter
greater trochanter muscle
greater tubercle
greater vestibular gland
greater zygomatic muscle
greatest angle of extension
greatest angle of flexion
greatest gluteal muscle
Greaves operation
Greck ileostomy bag
Greeley technique for gyneco-
    mastia reduction
Green automatic corneal
    trephine
green Bovie
green braided sutures
Green calipers
Green cataract knife
Green chalazion forceps
Green clamp
Green corneal curet
Green corneal dissector
Green curet
Green dissector
Green eye calipers
Green eye dissector
Green eye needle holder
Green eye spatula
Green eye speculum
Green fixation forceps
Green forceps
Green goiter retractor
Green holder
Green hook
Green knife
green laser
Green lens scoop
Green lid clamp
green monofilament polygly-
    conate sutures
Green mouth gag
Green needle holder
Green operation
Green pendulum scalpel
Green resectoscope
Green retractor
Green scapular procedure

Green scleral resection knife
Green scoop
Green shield
Green spatula
Green strabismus hook
Green tissue-grasping forceps
Green trephine
Green tucker
Green-Armytage cesarean
    section hemostat
Green-Armytage forceps
Green-Armytage operation
Green-Armytage reamer
Green-Armytage syringe
Green-Banks procedure
Greenberg Universal retractor
Greene endocervical curet
Greene endocervical uterine
    curet
Greene intraocular implant lens
Greene lens
Greene needle
Greene placental curet
Greene retractor
Greene sign
Greene tube-holding forceps
Greene uterine curet
Greenfield filter
Greenfield inferior vena caval
    filter
Greenfield needle
Greenfield vena caval filter
Green-Grice transfer
Greenhow incision
Greenhow-Rodman incision
Greenough microscope
Green-Sewall mouth gag
greenstick fracture
greenstick fracture splint
Greenville gastric bypass
Greenwald sound
Greenwood bipolar coagula-
    tion-suction forceps
Greenwood forceps
Greenwood trephine
Greer EZ Access drainage
Gregg cannula

Gregory baby profunda clamp
Gregory bulldog clamp
Gregory carotid bulldog
    clamp
Gregory clamp
Gregory external clamp
Gregory forceps
Gregory instruments for in situ
    saphenous vein bypass
Gregory Pell sectioning
    technique
Gregory stay sutures
Greiling gastroduodenal tube
Greiling tube
grenade-thrower fracture
grenz ray
Greulich-Pyle atlas
Greulich-Pyle bone age
Greville hot air bath
Grey Turner forceps
Grey Turner sign
Grice procedure for talipes
    valgus
Grice-Green arthrodesis of
    subtalar joint
Grice-Green operation
Grice-Green procedure for
    talipes valgus
grid
gridiron incision
Gridley intraocular lens
Grieshaber air pump
Grieshaber Balfour retractor
Grieshaber blade
Grieshaber corneal trephine
Grieshaber extractor
Grieshaber eye knife
Grieshaber eye needle
Grieshaber eye needle holder
Grieshaber forceps
Grieshaber holder
Grieshaber iris forceps
Grieshaber iris needle
Grieshaber keratome
Grieshaber knife
Grieshaber manipulator
Grieshaber needle
Grieshaber needle holder

Grieshaber retractor
Grieshaber trephine
Grieshaber vitrectomy tip
Grieshaber wire retractor
Griffen Roux-en-Y bypass
Griffin bandage lens dressing
Griffon tonsil scissors
Grillo patch
grimace test for knee pain
grimacing
Grimsdale operation
grind test
grinding test of Apley
grip strength
Gritti amputation
Gritti operation
grittiness
Gritti-Stokes amputation
gritty
gritty tumor
Groenholm lid retractor
Groenholm retractor
Groffman tracing
groin incision
groin puncture
Grollman catheter
Grollman pigtail catheter
grommet
        Silastic grommet
grommet drain tube
grommet tube
        blue Shepard grommet
        tube
        Shepard grommet tube
Grondahl-Finney esophago-
    gastroplasty
Grondahl-Finney operation
groove
groove sutures
grooved director
grooved director dilator
grooved eye gouge
grooved gorget
grooved piece
grooving reamer
Groshong catheter
Groshong double-lumen
    catheter

Groshong shunt
gross adenopathy
gross appearance
Gross clamp
Gross coarctation clamp
Gross coarctation occlusion
    clamp
Gross curet
gross deformity
gross description
Gross ductus spreader
Gross ear curet
Gross ear hook
Gross ear spoon
Gross ear spud
gross examination
Gross forceps
Gross hook
Gross operation
Gross patent ductus retractor
Gross probe
Gross retractor
Gross spatula
Gross spoon
Gross spreader
Gross spud
Gross spur crusher
gross tumor
Grosse-Kempf complete locking
    nail system
Grosse-Kempf dynamic locking
    nail system
Grosse-Kempf femoral nail
Grosse-Kempf locking nail
    system
Grosse-Kempf nail
Grosse-Kempf partial locking
    nail system
Grosse-Kempf static locking nail
    system
Grosse-Kempf tibial locking nail
    system
Grosse-Kempf tibial nail
grossly
Grossman operation
Grossman sign
Gross-Pomeranz-Watkins atrial
    retractor

Gross-Pomeranz-Watkins
    retractor
Grotting forceps
ground plate
grounding pad
Grover clamp
Grover meniscotome
Grover meniscus knife
growing tumor
growth
growth arrest
Gruber bougie
Gruber ear speculum
Gruber hernia
Gruber medicated bougie
Gruber speculum
Gruca hip reamer
Gruening eye magnet (also
    Grüning)
Gruening magnet (also
    *Grüning*)
Gruentzig (also Grüntzig)
Gruentzig 20-30 dilating
    catheter
Gruentzig arterial balloon
    catheter
Gruentzig balloon catheter
Gruentzig balloon catheter
    angioplasty
Gruentzig balloon dilator
Gruentzig catheter
Gruentzig coronary catheter
    dilating system
Gruentzig D dilating catheter
Gruentzig D-G dilating
    catheter
Gruentzig Dilaca catheter
Gruentzig dilatation of renal
    arteries
Gruentzig G dilating catheter
Gruentzig PTCA technique
Gruentzig S dilating catheter
Gruentzig steerable catheter
Gruentzig steerable system
Gruenwald dissecting forceps
Gruenwald dressing forceps
Gruenwald ear forceps
Gruenwald forceps

Gruenwald nasal forceps
Gruenwald nasal punch
Gruenwald nasal-cutting forceps
Gruenwald nasal-dressing
    forceps
Gruenwald neurosurgical
    rongeur
Gruenwald punch
Gruenwald retractor
Gruenwald rongeur
Gruenwald tissue forceps
Gruenwald-Bryant forceps
Gruenwald-Bryant nasal forceps
Gruenwald-Bryant nasal-cutting
    forceps
Gruenwald-Jansen forceps
Gruenwald-Love forceps
grumose (also grumous)
grumose material
grumous (also grumose)
grumous material
Grüning eye magnet (see
    *Gruening*)
grunting
grunting respirations
Grüntzig (see *Gruentzig*)
Gruppe forceps
Gruppe wire crimper
Gruppe wire prosthesis
Gruppe wire prosthesis-
    crimping forceps
Gruppe wire-crimping forceps
Grynfelt hernia
Grynfelt triangle
GSB knee prosthesis
GTF-A gastroscope
GU irrigant dressing
guaiac test
Guangzhou GD-1 prosthetic
    valve
guard
        Action Eyes and Albany
            eye guards
        BandageGuard half-leg
            protector
        CastGuard
        cervical drill guard

guard *continued*
    drill guard
    Fomon chisel guard
    Peri-Guard
    Peri-Guard vascular graft
    plastic mouth guard
    Ullrich drill guard
guarded chisel
guarded osteotome
guarded postoperative period
guarded prognosis
Guardian pacemaker
guarding
guarding and/or rebound
guarding and/or rigidity
guarding of muscle
guarding sign
gubernaculum
Gudden commissure
Gudden tract
Gudebrod sutures
Guedel airway
Guedel blade
Guedel laryngoscope
Guedel laryngoscope blade
Guedel rubber airway
Guepar (Group for Utilization
    and Study of Articular
    Prostheses)
Guepar hinge-knee prosthesis
Guepar knee prosthesis
Guepar prosthesis
Guepar total knee prosthesis
Guérin fold
Guérin fracture
Guérin lock
Guerrant-Cochran splint
Guggenheim adenoid forceps
Guggenheim fracture
Guggenheim scissors
Guglen hook
Guhl classification
Guibor canalicular tube
Guibor Expo eye bubble
Guibor Expo flat eye bandage
Guibor eye tube
Guibor Silastic intubation set

Guibor Silastic tube
Guibor tube
guide (see also *needle guide,*
      *saw guide*)
      acetabular guide
      ACL drill guide
      ACL guide
      ACS LIMA guide
      Acufex guide
      Adson drill guide
      Adson Gigli-saw guide
      Adson saw guide
      Adson-Shaefer dural
         guide
      AFB needle guide
         (aortofemoral bypass
         needle guide)
      Alvarado orthopedic
         guide
      Amplatz guide
      anterior femoral resec-
         tion guide
      AOR guide
      Arani guide
      Bailey Gigli-saw guide
      basal ganglia guide
      Béniqué catheter guide
      Blair Gigli-saw guide
      Blair saw guide
      Borchard bone wire
         guide
      bronchoscopic guide
      bronchoscopic instru-
         ment guide
      Brown-Roberts-Wells CT
         stereotaxic guide
         (BRW CT stereotaxic
         guide)
      BRW CT stereotaxic
         guide (Brown-Roberts-
         Wells CT stereotaxic
         guide)
      Caldwell guide
      calibrated guide pin
      calibrated-tip threaded
         guide pin
      cartilage guide

guide *continued*
      catheter guide
      Chamfer guide
      Cloward guide
      Cone guide
      Cooper basal ganglia
         guide
      Cooper guide
      Cooper nasal ganglia
         guide
      core wire guide
      Cor-Flex guide
      Cor-Flex wire guide
      Cottle bone guide
      Cottle cartilage guide
      Cottle guide
      Cottle knife guide
      cruciate ligament guide
      crus guide fork
      Cushing Gigli-saw
         guide
      Dap II biopsy needle
         guide
      Davis saw guide
      drill guide
      dural protector drill
         guide
      echo-guided ultrasound
      ERCP-guided biopsy
      Falope-ring guide kit
      femoral AP-sizing
         guide
      Ferciot wire guide
      filiform guide
      Fisher guide
      FL4 guide
      Flexguide intubation
         guide ·
      floppy-tipped guide
      Gabbay-Frater suture
         guide
      Galante hip guide
      Ghajar guide
      Gigli-saw guide
      Gouley guide
      Guyon catheter guide
      Harris hip guide

guide *continued*
     Harris-Galante hip guide
     Harrison guide
     Hewson ligament guide
     hip alignment guide
     Hi-Torque floppy guide
          catheter
     House guide
     House wire guide
     instrument guide
     Iowa needle guide
     Iowa trumpet forceps
          guide
     Iowa trumpet needle
          guide
     J-guide
     Joseph saw guide
     Kazanjian guide
     Kendrick Gigli-saw guide
     Kleegman needle guide
     Küntscher femur guide
          pin
     Lebsche wire saw guide
     Lumaguide infusion
          catheter
     Lunderquist guide
     Lunderquist-Ring torque
          guide
     mandrin guide
     Micro-Guide catheter
     Mueller catheter guide
     Mumford Gigli-saw guide
     nasal cartilage guide
     occlusal guide
     Pilotip catheter guide
     Poppen Gigli-saw guide
     Rand-Wells pallido-
          thalamectomy guide
     Raney Gigli-saw guide
     Rhinelander guide
     Richards adjustable-angle
          guide
     Richards barrel guide
     Richards calibrated-tip
          threaded guide
     Richards stationary-angle
          guide

guide *continued*
     Rosenburg drill guide
     Roth urethral suture
          guide
     saw guide
     scaphoid screw guide
     Schlesinger Gigli-saw
          guide
     Sheets lens guide
     stapes wire guide
     Stewart guide
     Stewart ligament guide
     Stille Gigli-saw guide
     strut guide
     Swan-Ganz guide wire
          TD catheter
     Teale lithotomy gorget
          guide
     telescoping guide
     tibial resection guide
     Todd-Heyer cannula
          guide
     Todd-Wells guide
     Todd-Wells stereotaxic
          guide
     torque guide
     trumpet needle guide
     vector guide to knee
          system from Dyonics
     Watson-Jones guide pin
     wave guide catheter
guide catheter
guide forceps
guide pin (see also *pin*)
     calibrated guide pin
     calibrated-tip threaded
          guide pin
     Küntscher femur guide
          pin
     Watson-Jones guide
          pin
guide sutures
guide wire (see also *wire*)
     ACS exchange guide
          wire
     ACS floppy-tip guide
          wire

guide wire *continued*

ACS gold-standard guide wire
ACS guide wire
ACS SOF-T guide wire
Amplatz Super Stiff guide wire
angiographic guide wire
Bentson floppy-tip guide wire
Bentson guide wire
Flex guide wire
flexible guide wire
flexible-J guide wire
floppy guide wire
floppy-tipped guide wire
high-torque guide wire
Hi-Per Flex guide wire
Hi-Torque Flex-T guide wire
Hi-Torque floppy guide wire
Hi-Torque intermediate guide wire
Hi-Torque standard guide wire
J-guide wire
J-tip guide wire
J-tipped exchange guide wire
Linx exchange guide wire
Lunderquist guide wire
Meditech guide wire
olives passed over guide wire
PDT guide wire
Puestow guide wire
Redifocus guide wire
Rosen guide wire
Schwarten guide wire
Simpson-Robert ACS guide wire
SOF-T guide wire
soft-tipped guide wire
Sones guide wire
SOS guide wire

guide wire *continued*

steerable guide wire
straight guide wire
TAD guide wire
Teflon-coated guide wire
transluminal coronary angioplasty guide wire
USCI guide wire
VeriFlex guide wire
Wholey guide wire
Wholey Hi-Torque floppy guide wire
Wholey Hi-Torque modified J-guide wire
Wholey Hi-Torque standard guide wire
guided transcutaneous biopsy
guided-needle aspiration cytology
guideline
guiding catheter
guiding sheath
Guild-Pratt rectal speculum
Guild-Pratt speculum
Guilford brace
Guilford ear scissors
Guilford sickle knife
Guilford stapedectomy
Guilford stapedectomy technique
Guilford-Schuknecht scissors
Guilford-Schuknecht wire-cutting scissors
Guilford-Wright instruments
Guilford-Wullstein instruments
Guilland sign
Guillian knife
guillotine

Ballenger-Sluder guillotine
Derra guillotine
Giertz rib guillotine
Goldman guillotine nerve knife
hemostatic tonsillar guillotine
Lilienthal guillotine

guillotine *continued*
    Lilienthal rib guillotine
    lingual guillotine
    Molt guillotine
    Molt-Storz guillotine
    Myles guillotine
    Olivecrona guillotine
      scissors
    Poppers tonsillar
      guillotine
    rib guillotine
    Sauer guillotine
    Sauerbruch rib guillotine
    Sluder guillotine
    Sluder tonsillar guillotine
    Sluder-Sauer guillotine
    Sluder-Sauer tonsil
      guillotine
    Storz guillotine
    tonsillar guillotine
    Van Osdel guillotine
guillotine amputation
guillotine amputation of
    appendix
guillotine amputation of cervix
guillotine incision
guillotine scissors
guillotine technique
Guisez tube
Guist enucleation hemostat
Guist enucleation scissors
Guist eye implant
Guist eye speculum
Guist fixation forceps
Guist forceps
Guist scissors
Guist speculum
Guist sphere eye implant
Guist sphere implant
Guist-Black eye speculum
Guist-Black speculum
Guiteras irrigation
Guiteras nozzle irrigator
Guiteras urethroscope
Guleke bone ronguer
Guleke-Stookey operation
Gull renal epistaxis

Gullstrand ophthalmoscope
Gullstrand slit lamp
gum lancet
gum line
gum scissors
gums
gun-barrel enterostomy
Gundelach punch
Gunderson conjunctival flap
Gunderson muscle forceps
Gunderson recession forceps
Gunn closing sign
Gunnar-Hey roller forceps
Gunning jaw splint
Gunning splint
gunshot wound
Gunston knee prosthesis
Gunter Von Noorden flap
Gunter Von Noorden incision
gurgling bowel sounds
gurgling rales
gurney
Gusberg cervical biopsy curet
Gusberg cervical cone curet
Gusberg curet
Gusberg endocervical biopsy
    curet
Gusberg endocervical biopsy
    punch
Gusberg endocervical curet
Gusberg hysterectomy clamp
Gusberg punch
Gusberg uterine forceps
Gussenbauer clamp
Gussenbauer operation
Gussenbauer sutures
gusset-type patch
gustatory anesthesia
Gustilo knee prosthesis
gut
gut and colon clamp
gut chromic sutures
gut plain sutures
gut sutures
gut wool
gut-associated lymphoid tissue
    (GALT)

Gutgeman auricular appendage clamp
Gutgeman clamp
Gutglass cervix hemostat
Gutglass cervix hemostatic forceps
Gutglass forceps
Guthrie fixation hook
Guthrie muscle
Guthrie skin hook
Gutierrez-Najar grasping forceps
Guttaform dental impression material
gutta-percha
gutter
gutter finger splint
gutter fracture
gutter splint
guttering of bone
Guttmann arthrodesis
Guttmann obstetrical retractor
Guttmann retractor
Guttmann speculum
Guttmann subtalar arthrodesis
Guttmann vaginal speculum
guttural pulse
guttural rales
guttural sound
Gutzeit operation
Guy gouge
Guy knife
Guy model nasal gouge
guy steadying sutures
guy sutures
Guyon amputation
Guyon bougie
Guyon canal
Guyon canal syndrome
Guyon catheter guide
Guyon clamp
Guyon curettage
Guyon dilator
Guyon exploratory bougie
Guyon kidney clamp
Guyon operation
Guyon sound

Guyon ureteral catheter
Guyon urethral sound
Guyon vessel clamp
Guyon-Béniqué sound
Guyon-Péan clamp
Guyon-Péan vessel clamp
Guyton electrode
Guyton forceps
Guyton operation
Guyton scissors
Guyton sutures
Guyton trephine
Guyton-Clark capsule fragment forceps
Guyton-Friedenwald sutures
Guyton-Lundsgaard sclerotome
Guyton-Maumenee speculum
Guyton-Noyes fixation forceps
Guyton-Noyes forceps
Guyton-Park eye speculum
Guyton-Park lid speculum
Guyton-Park speculum
Guzman-Blanco epiglottis retractor
GVHD (graft-versus-host disease)
Gwathmey ether hook
Gwathmey hook
Gwathmey oil-ether anesthesia
Gwathmey suction tube
Gwathmey-Yankauer ether inhaler
Gyn-A-Lite illuminator
Gyn-A-Lite speculum illuminator
gynecoid pelvis
gynecologic, gynecological
gynecological cryosurgery
gynecological examination
gynecological malignancy
gynecological procedure
gynecological surgery
gynecology
gynecology instrument set
gynecomastia
Gynefold pessary

Gynefold prolapse pessary
Gynefold retrodisplacement
    pessary
gynoplastics
gynoplasty
Gypsona cast material
Gypsona plaster dressing
gyre
gyrectomy
gyri (*sing.* gyrus)
gyri breves insulae
gyri cerebri
gyri insulae
gyri of cerebrum
gyri orbitales
gyri profundi cerebri
gyri temporales transversi
gyri transitivi cerebri
gyriform carcinoma
gyromagnetic ratio
gyrous area
gyrus (*pl.* gyri)
gyrus dentatus
gyrus fasciolaris
gyrus fornicatus
gyrus frontalis

gyrus fusiformis
gyrus geniculi
gyrus hippocampi
gyrus limbicus
gyrus lingualis
gyrus longus insulae
gyrus marginalis
gyrus of Broca
gyrus of insula
gyrus olfactorius lateralis of
    Retzius
gyrus olfactorius medialis of
    Retzius
gyrus paracentralis
gyrus parahippocampalis
gyrus paraterminalis
gyrus postcentralis
gyrus precentralis
gyrus rectus
gyrus subcallosus
gyrus supracallosus
gyrus supramarginalis
gyrus temporalis inferior
gyrus temporalis medius
gyrus temporalis superior
gyrus uncinatus

H-flap
H-flap incision
H-graft
H-H neonatal shunt for hydro-
    cephalus
H-incision
H-shaped anal anastomosis
H-shaped ileal pouch
Haab eye knife
Haab magnet
Haab needle
Haab reflex
Haab scleral resection knife
Haab-Grieshaber knife
Haag slit lamp
Haagensen staging of breast
    carcinoma (A, B, etc.)
Haagensen test
Haagensen triple biopsy of
    breast
Haag-Streit light
Haag-Streit microscope
Haag-Streit slit lamp
Haas dislocation operation
Haas operation
habenula
habenular commissure
Haberer abdominal spatula
Haberer gastrointestinal forceps
Haberer intestinal clamp
Haberer intestinal forceps
habitual abortion
habitual dislocation
habitual occlusion
habituation
Hachinski ischemic scale
Hacker hypospadias
Haddad-Riordan wrist
    arthrodesis

Haemolite autologous blood
    recovery system
Haemonetics bone marrow
    transplant system
Haemonetics cell saver
Haenig irrigating scissors
Haenig scissors
Haftelast self-adhering bandage
Hagar probe
Hagedorn cheiloplasty
Hagedorn needle
Hagedorn needle holder
Hagedorn operation
Hagedorn suture needle
Hagedorn-LeMesurier operation
Hagerty operation
Hagie hemostat
Hagie hip pin
Hagie pin
Hagie T-stack
Haglund deformity
Haglund scissors
Haglund speculum
Haglund spreader
Hagner bag
Hagner bag catheter
Hagner catheter
Hagner hemostatic bag
Hagner operation
Hagner urethral bag
Hague cataract lamp
Hague lamp
Hahn cannula
Hahn cleft
Hahn gastrotomy
Hahn operation
Haidinger brush
Haig Ferguson obstetrical
    forceps

Haight baby retractor
Haight operation
Haight periosteal elevator
Haight retractor
Haight rib spreader
Haight spreader
Haight-Finochietto retractor
Haight-Finochietto rib retractor
Haight-Finochietto spreader
Haik implant
Haimovici arteriotomy scissors
hair ball
hair clippers
hair follicle
hair transplant
hair-bearing area
hair-bearing graft
hairline
hairline of brow
hair-matrix carcinoma
hairpin loop
hairy nevus
hairy-cell leukemia
Haitz canaliculus punch
Hajek antral punch
Hajek antral punch forceps
Hajek antral retractor
Hajek antral rongeur
Hajek chisel
Hajek forceps
Hajek hammer
Hajek lip retractor
Hajek mallet
Hajek operation
Hajek punch
Hajek retractor
Hajek rongeur
Hajek septal chisel
Hajek sphenoid punch forceps
Hajek-Ballenger dissector
Hajek-Ballenger elevator
Hajek-Ballenger septal dissector
Hajek-Ballenger septal elevator
Hajek-Koffler bone punch
Hajek-Koffler forceps
Hajek-Koffler punch
Hajek-Koffler punch forceps

Hajek-Koffler sphenoidal punch
Hajek-Koffler sphenoidal punch
    forceps
Hajek-Skillern punch
Hajek-Tieck nasal speculum
Hakansson bone rongeur
Hakansson-Olivecrona rongeur
Hakim catheter
Hakim reservoir
Hakim shunt
Hakim tube
Hakim valve
Hakim-Cordis pump
Halberg forceps
Haldane tube
Hale forceps
Hale obstetrical forceps
half-axial projection
half-body irradiation
half-curved clamp
half-hitch knot
half-hitch sutures
half-moon retractor
half-ring leg splint
half-ring Thomas splint
half-shell cast
half-thickness
half-value
Hall air drill
Hall arthrotome
Hall band intrauterine device
Hall bur
Hall craniotome
Hall dermatome
Hall drill
Hall driver
Hall facet fusion
Hall in-and-out craniotome
Hall intrauterine device
Hall mastoid bur
Hall neurosurgical craniotome
Hall neurotome
Hall power drill
Hall prosthetic heart valve
Hall sagittal saw
Hall saw
Hall sign

Hall sternal saw
Hall surgical instruments
Halle chisel
Halle curet
Halle dura knife
Halle elevator
Halle ethmoidal curet
Halle infant speculum
Halle knife
Halle nasal elevator
Halle nasal speculum
Halle needle
Halle septal elevator
Halle septal needle
Halle sinus curet
Halle speculum
Halle vascular spatula
Haller circle
Haller layer of choroid
Halle-Tieck nasal speculum
Halle-Tieck speculum
Hall-Kaster disk prosthetic valve
Hall-Kaster heart valve
Hall-Kaster mitral valve
    prosthesis
Hall-Kaster tilting disk valve
    prosthesis
Hall-Osteon drill system
Hallpike maneuver
Hallpike-Dix maneuver
Hall-Serge aerotome
hallux
hallux abductus
hallux dolorosa
hallux extensus
hallux forceps
hallux malleus
hallux rigidus
hallux valgus
hallux varus
Hall-Zimmer saw
halo body cast
halo cast
halo nevus
halo ring
halo traction
halo vision

halo-femoral traction
halogen exam light
Halogen Lite set
halogen ophthalmoscope
halogen otoscope
halogenated agent
halo-pelvic traction
halothane anesthetic agent
halo-to-bale traction
Halpin operation
Halsey eye needle holder
Halsey forceps
Halsey nail scissors
Halsey needle
Halsey needle holder
Halsey Vital needle holder
Halsted clamp
Halsted curved mosquito
    forceps
Halsted forceps
Halsted hemostat
Halsted hemostatic forceps
Halsted incision
Halsted inguinal herniorrha-
    phy
Halsted interrupted mattress
    sutures
Halsted ligament
Halsted maneuver
Halsted mastectomy
Halsted mattress sutures
Halsted Micro-Line artery
    forceps
Halsted mosquito forceps
Halsted operation
Halsted radical mastectomy
Halsted sutures
Halsted-Bassini herniorrhaphy
Halsted-Ferguson operation
Halsted-Meyer incision
Halsted-Swanson tendon-
    passing forceps
Halsted-Willy Meyer incision
halter (see also *head halter*)
    Cerva Crane halter
    DePuy head halter
    Forrester head halter

halter *continued*
    Forrester-Brown head
      halter
    head halter (see separate
      listing)
    neck-wrap halter
    traction halter collar
    Tracto-Halter
    Zimfoam head halter
    Zimmer head halter
halter traction
hamartoma
hamartomatous gastric polyp
hamartomatous lesion
Hamas total wrist
Hamas upper limb prosthesis
hamate bone
Hamblin magnet
Hamby forceps
Hamby retractor
Hamby-Hibbs retractor
Hamilton bandage
Hamilton decompressor
Hamilton forceps
Hamilton tongue depressor
Hamis sutures
Hamm electrode
Hamm fulgurating electrode
Hamm resectoscope electrode
Hamman click
Hamman crunch
Hamman sign
hammer
    Bakelite hammer
    Baylor hammer
    Boxwood hammer
    Carroll aluminum
      hammer
    Chandler hammer
    Cloward hammer
    Crane hammer
    Déjérine-Davis percus-
      sion hammer
    Epstein hammer
    fiberhead hammer
    Gerzog hammer
    Hajek hammer

hammer *continued*
    Hibbs hammer
    House hammer
    House tapping hammer
    intranasal hammer
    Kirk orthopedic hammer
    Lucae bone hammer
    MacAusland bone
      hammer
    Meyerding aluminum
      hammer
    Neef hammer
    nylon head hammer
    percussion hammer
    Quisling hammer
    Rabiner neurological
      hammer
    Ralks hammer
    rawhide bone hammer
    reflex hammer
    rotatory hammer
    Rush hammer
    shatter hammer
    Smith-Petersen hammer
    standard pattern hammer
    stapes tapping hammer
    tack hammer
    tapping hammer
    vibratory hammer
    Wagner hammer
    White hammer
    Zeiss hammer lamp
hammer finger
hammer forceps
hammer nose
hammer toe
hammer toe correction
hammer toe correction with
    interphalangeal fusion
hammer toe repair
Hammersmith mitral prosthesis
Hammersmith prosthesis
hammock bandage
hammock dressing
hammock nephropexy
hammock pupil
hammocking

hammocking of posterior mitral
    leaflet
hammocking of valve
hammock-method nephropexy
Hammond blade
Hammond bunionectomy
Hammond operation
Hammond splint
Hammond winged retractor
    blade
Hamou hysteroscope
Hampton hump
Hampton line
Hampton small bowel operation
Hamrick elevator
Hamrick suction
Hamrick suction dissector
hamstring muscle
hamstring tendon
hamstrings
hamstrung knee
hamular notch
hamular process
Hanafee catheter
Hanafee catheter tip
Hancock amputation
Hancock aortic 242 prosthetic
    valve
Hancock aortic punch
Hancock aortic valve prosthesis
Hancock bioprosthetic valve
Hancock mitral valve prosthesis
Hancock operation
Hancock pericardial prosthetic
    valve
Hancock porcine heterograft
    heart valve
Hancock porcine heterograft
    valve
Hancock porcine valve
    prosthesis
Hancock porcine xenograft
Hancock valve
hand
        ape hand
        benediction hand
        bony overhand

hand *continued*
    clawhand
    cleft hand
    clubhand
    drop hand
    flat hand
    ghoul hand
    glass hand
    intrinsic minus hand
    Krukenberg hand
    lead hand
    lobster-claw hand
    mirror hand
    mitten hand
    Myobock artificial hand
    Neibauer hand
    opera-glass hand
    pawlike hand
    skeleton hand
    spade hand
    split hand
    trident hand
hand and arm scrub
hand brace
hand brush dispenser
hand cautery
hand chuck
hand cock-up sling
hand cock-up splint
hand drill
hand dynamometer
hand ear perforator
hand injection
hand nylon scrub brush
hand perforator
hand pump
hand retractor
hand saw
hand scrub
hand scrub brush
hand signal
hand splint
hand steadiness
hand strength test
hand surgery
hand surgery elevator
hand surgery instruments

hand surgery osteotome
hand table
hand trephine
hand tubing roller
hand-held exploring electrode
   probe
hand-held nebulizer
hand-held retractor
handicapped
Handi-hook
handle (see also *traction*
      *handle*)
   autopsy blade handle
   Bard-Parker knife handle
   Barton traction handle
   Beaver blade chuck
      handle
   Beaver blade handle
   Beaver chuck handle
   Beaver knife handle
   Beaver surgical blade
      handle
   Bill axis traction handle
   Bill traction handle
   Birt-A-Switch handle
   Bovie chuck-type handle
   bronchoscopic forceps
      handle
   Castroviejo-Kalt traction
      handle
   cautery handle
   chuck handle
   cord handle
   Cottle knife handle
   Cottle modified knife
      handle
   Cottle protected knife
      handle
   Dynagrip blade handle
   Dynagrip handle
   Farrior chuck handle
   forceps handle
   Gigli-saw handle
   hook-on battery handle
   hook-on laryngoscope
      handle
   House knife handle

handle *continued*
   interchangeable punch
      handle
   Jackson bronchoscopic
      forceps handle
   Jackson forceps handle
   Jackson Universal handle
   knife handle
   laryngoscope battery
      handle
   Luikart-Bill traction
      handle
   malleus handle
   obstetrical traction
      handle
   slotted handle
   Sluder Universal handle
   Strully Gigli-saw handle
   surgical knife handle
   T-handle
   traction handle
   Universal handle
   Universal handle for
      punch tips
   Universal handle with
      nasal-cutting tips
   Universal mirror handle
   Welch Allyn battery
      handle
   Welch Allyn cord handle
handle traction
handleless clamp
Handley incision
Handley operation
handpiece
   angle handpiece
   AVIT vitrectomy
      handpiece
   Chayes handpiece
   dental handpiece
   Emesco 9NS handpiece
   Emesco handpiece
   I-A handpiece (irrigating-
      aspirating handpiece)
   irrigating-aspirating
      handpiece (I-A
      handpiece)

handpiece *continued*
    Kerr handpiece
    Simcoe handpiece
Handtrol electrosurgical pencil
handwasher machine
Handy-Buck traction
Hanely-McDermott pelvimeter
Hanger prosthesis
hanging arm cast
hanging cast
hanging drop
hanging heart
hanging hip operation
hanging panniculus
hanging-drop technique
hanging-weight method for
   reducing dislocated
   shoulder
hangman's fracture
hangnail
Hank uterine dilator
Hank-Bradley uterine dilator
Hank-Dennen obstetrical
   forceps
Hanna splint
Hannahan bur
Hannahan forceps
Hannon curet
Hannon endometrial biopsy
   curet
Hannon endometrial curet
Hannover canal
Hansen-Street driver-extractor
Hansen-Street intramedullary
   nail
Hansen-Street intramedullary
   rod
Hansen-Street nail
Hansen-Street pin
Hansen-Street plate
Hanslik patellar prosthesis
haploscope
haptens
haptic area implant
haptic loop
haptics
haptocholangiostomy

Harada-Ito procedure
hard adhesions
hard cancer
hard cataract
hard indurated colon mass
hard lens
hard palate
hard subcutaneous node
hardening of arteries
hardening of artery walls
Hardesty hook
hardness
Hardy bivalve speculum
Hardy dissector
Hardy enucleator
Hardy implant fork
Hardy microbipolar forceps
Hardy microcuret
Hardy pituitary dissector
Hardy pituitary spoon
Hardy retractor
Hardy sellar punch
Hardy speculum
Hardy-Cushing speculum
Hardy-Duddy vaginal retractor
Hardy-Duddy weighted vaginal
   speculum
Hare splint device
Hare traction device
Hare traction splint
harelip
harelip forceps
harelip needle
harelip operation
harelip sutures
Hargin antrum trocar
Hargin trocar
Hark operation for talipes
   valgus
Harken auricular clamp
Harken cardiovascular forceps
Harken clamp
Harken erysiphake
Harken forceps
Harken heart needle
Harken needle
Harken prosthesis

Harken prosthetic valve
Harken retractor
Harken rib spreader
Harken spreader
Harken valve
Harken valvulotome
Harken-Cooley forceps
harlequin fetus
Harman approach
Harman bone graft
Harman deltoid procedure
Harman forceps
Harman incision
Harman operation
Harman technique
Harman-Fahey technique
harmonic suture
harmonious retinal correspon-
     dence
Harms forceps
Harms microtying forceps
Harms probe
Harms tying forceps
Harms-Tubingen forceps
Harms-Tubingen tying forceps
harness
Harold Crowe drill
Harold Crowe drill nail
Harold Hayes eustachian
     bougie
Harper cervical laminectomy
     punch
Harper periosteal elevator
Harper rongeur
harpoon
Harrah lung clamp
Harrington clamp
Harrington clamp forceps
Harrington deep surgical
     scissors
Harrington erysiphake
Harrington esophageal divertic-
     ulectomy
Harrington flat wrench
Harrington forceps
Harrington hook clamp
Harrington hook driver

Harrington instrumentation
Harrington operation
Harrington overlapping closure
Harrington retractor
Harrington rod
Harrington rod instrumentation
Harrington scissors
Harrington spinal elevator
Harrington spinal fusion
Harrington spinal instrumenta-
     tion
Harrington splanchnic retractor
Harrington strut
Harrington sutures
Harrington thoracic forceps
Harrington tonometer
Harrington-Carmalt clamp
Harrington-Mayo forceps
Harrington-Mayo rib shears
Harrington-Mayo scissors
Harrington-Mayo thoracic
     scissors
Harrington-Mayo tissue forceps
Harrington-Mixter clamp
Harrington-Mixter clamp
     forceps
Harrington-Mixter forceps
Harrington-Mixter thoracic
     forceps
Harrington-Pemberton retractor
Harrington-Pemberton sympa-
     thectomy retractor
Harris approach
Harris band
Harris broach
Harris catheter
Harris cement fixation system
Harris dissector
Harris drip
Harris forceps
Harris growth arrest line
Harris hip evaluation
Harris hip guide
Harris hip prosthesis
Harris hip screw
Harris implant
Harris incision

Harris intramedullary nail
Harris line
Harris nail
Harris operation
Harris precoat cemented hip
    prosthesis
Harris prosthesis
Harris punch
Harris reamer
Harris segregator
Harris separator
Harris sling
Harris suture-carrying forceps
Harris sutures
Harris tonsillar knife
Harris total hip
Harris total hip prosthesis
Harris trephine
Harris tube
Harris tube suction
Harris uterine injector (HUI)
Harris uterine injector catheter
Harris-Beath flatfoot procedure
Harris-Beath operation for
    talipes valgus
Harris-Beath technique
Harris-Beath x-ray view
Harris-Galante cup
Harris-Galante hip guide
Harris-Galante hip prosthesis
Harris-Galante porous metal hip
    prosthesis
Harris-Mueller procedure
Harris-Norton hip reamer
Harrison chalazion retractor
Harrison curet
Harrison groove
Harrison guide
Harrison implant
Harrison interlocked mesh
    dressing
Harrison interlocked mesh graft
Harrison interlocked mesh
    prosthesis
Harrison knife
Harrison prosthesis
Harrison retractor

Harrison scarifying curet
Harrison scissors
Harrison speculum
Harrison sulcus
Harrison suture-removing
    scissors
Harrison tucker
Harrison-Shea curet
Harris-Smith anterior interbody
    drill
harsh murmur
harsh respiration
Hart extension finger splint
Hart splint
Hartel technique
Hartley implant
Hartley mammary prosthesis
Hartley-Krause operation
Hartmann adenoidal curet
Hartmann alligator forceps
Hartmann bone rongeur
Hartmann catheter
Hartmann colostomy
Hartmann curet
Hartmann ear forceps
Hartmann ear rongeur
Hartmann ear-dressing forceps
Hartmann eustachian catheter
Hartmann forceps
Hartmann fossa
Hartmann hemostatic forceps
Hartmann knife
Hartmann mastoid rongeur
Hartmann mosquito forceps
Hartmann nasal speculum
Hartmann nasal-dressing
    forceps
Hartmann operation
Hartmann point
Hartmann pouch
Hartmann procedure
Hartmann punch
Hartmann resection
Hartmann rongeur
Hartmann solution
Hartmann speculum
Hartmann tonsillar dissector

Hartmann tonsillar punch
Hartmann tuning fork
Hartmann-Citelli alligator
     forceps
Hartmann-Citelli ear punch
Hartmann-Citelli ear punch
     forceps
Hartmann-Citelli forceps
Hartmann-Citelli punch
Hartmann-Dewaxer speculum
Hartmann-Gruenwald forceps
Hartmann-Gruenwald nasal-
     cutting forceps
Hartmann-Herzfeld ear forceps
Hartmann-Herzfeld ear rongeur
Hartmann-Herzfeld forceps
Hartmann-Herzfeld rongeur
Hartmann-Noyes nasal-dressing
     forceps
Hartmann-Proctor ear forceps
Hartstein iris cryoretractor
Hartstein retractor
Hartzler angioplasty balloon
Hartzler catheter
Hartzler dilatation catheter
Hartzler Micro catheter
Hartzler Micro II balloon for
     coronary angioplasty
Hartzler Micro II catheter
Hartzler Micro XT catheter
Hartzler rib retractor
Hartzler Ultra Lo-Profile catheter
Harvard manometer
Harvard PCA pump
Harvard pump
harvest
harvest organ
harvest tissue
harvesting an organ
Harvey Stone clamp
Harvey Stone hemostat
Harvey wire-cutting scissors
Hashimoto struma
Haslinger bronchoscope
Haslinger electroscope
Haslinger esophagoscope
Haslinger headrest

Haslinger laryngoscope
Haslinger palate retractor
Haslinger retractor
Haslinger tonsil hemostat
Haslinger tracheobroncho-
     esophagoscope
Haslinger tracheoscope
Haslinger uvula retractor
Hasner fold
Hasner lid
Hasner operation
Hasner valve
Hass hip osteotomy
Hass technique
Hassall-Henle wart
Hasson cannula
Hasson laparoscope
Hasson retractor
Hasson-Eder laparoscope
     cannula
Hastings procedure
Hatch catheter
Hatcher operation
Hatcher pin
hatchet
hatchet extractor
hatchet head deformity
Hatfield bone curet
Hatt golf-stick elevator
Hatt spoon
Haultaim operation
haunch bone
Hauser bunionectomy
Hauser heel cord procedure
Hauser knee procedure
Hauser operation
Hauser transplant
Hausmann vascular clamp
haustra (*sing.* haustrum)
haustra coli
haustral fold
haustral markings
haustral pattern
haustral segmentation
haustration
haustrum (*pl.* haustra)
Haven hook

Haven skin graft
Haverfield brain cannula
Haverfield cannula
Haverfield hemilaminectomy
　　retractor
Haverfield retractor
Haverfield-Scoville hemi-
　　laminectomy retractor
Haverfield-Scoville retractor
Haverhill clamp
Haverhill ear operation
haversian canal
haversian gland
haversian space
Havlicek spiral cannula
Havlicek trocar
hawk's beak elevator
Hawkins cervix conization
　　cautery
Hawkins forceps
Hawkins fracture
Hawkins needle
Hawkins sign
Hawks-Dennen forceps
Hawks-Dennen obstetrical
　　forceps
Hawley appliance
hay baler's fracture
Hayden curet
Hayden elevator
Hayden palate elevator
Hayden probe
Hayden tonsil curet
Hayem icterus
Hayes anterior resection clamp
Hayes anterior resection forceps
Hayes clamp
Hayes colon clamp
Hayes Martin forceps
Hayes phalangeal elevator
Hayes retractor
Hayes-Olivecrona forceps
Hayley table
Hayman dilator
Haynes cannula
Haynes operation
Haynes pin

Haynes-Griffin mandible splint
Haynes-Griffin splint
Hays hand retractor
Hayton-Williams forceps
Hayton-Williams mouth gag
hazard
hazard of surgery
hazardous waste
hazy
hazy urine
HBO (hyperbaric oxygen)
HCL (hard contact lens)
HD Canadian-type socket
HD2 prosthesis
HD2 total hip prosthesis
HEA (hemorrhages, exudates,
　　and aneurysms)
head and neck in extended
　　position
head brace
head circumference
head compression
head dependent position
head down presentation
head drape
head extended
head extension
head extractor
head fracture frame
head halter (see also *halter*)
　　DePuy head halter
　　Forrester head halter
　　Forrester-Brown head
　　　halter
　　Zimfoam head halter
　　Zimmer head halter
head halter traction
head harness
head holder (see also *holder*)
　　crown-of-thorns head
　　　holder
　　Derlacki-Juers head
　　　holder
　　Juers-Derlacki Universal
　　　head holder
　　Mayfield head holder
　　Veley head holder

head mirror
head of bed
head of femur
head of humerus
head of malleus
head of pancreas
head of radius
head of talus
head pain
head tilt
head trauma
head, eyes, ears, nose, and
    throat (HEENT)
headache
head-at-risk signs
headband (see *band*)
headband-and-mirror set
headgear
headhunter catheter
headhunter visceral angio-
    graphy catheter
headlight (see *light*)
head-low incision
headrest
       adjustable headrest
       Adson headrest
       Brown-Roberts-Wells
         headrest
       Craig headrest
       doughnut headrest
       Gardner headrest
       Gardner-Wells headrest
       Haslinger headrest
       horseshoe headrest
       Light headrest
       Light-Veley headrest
       Mayfield-Kees headrest
       Multipoise headrest
       neurosurgical headrest
       pin headrest
       pinion headrest
       Richards headrest
       Sam Roberts headrest
       Shea headrest
       Storz adjustable headrest
       Veley headrest
head-tilt method

heal spontaneously
healed by first intention
healed by second intention
healed fracture
healed scar
healing
healing biopsy incision
healing by first intention
healing by granulation
healing by second intention
healing by third intention
healing fracture
healing incision site
healing of fracture
healing per primam
healing per secundam inten-
    tionem
healing ridge
healing wound
Healon (sodium hyaluronate)
Healon irrigant
healthy tissue
healthy-appearing organ
Healy forceps
Healy gastrointestinal forceps
Healy intestinal forceps
Healy suture-removing forceps
Heaney bulldog-jaw needle
    holder
Heaney clamp
Heaney curet
Heaney forceps
Heaney hysterectomy forceps
Heaney hysterectomy retractor
Heaney needle holder
Heaney operation
Heaney retractor
Heaney sutures
Heaney uterine curet
Heaney vaginal hysterectomy
Heaney-Ballantine forceps
Heaney-Ballantine hysterectomy
    forceps
Heaney-Kantor forceps
Heaney-Kantor hysterectomy
    forceps
Heaney-Rezek forceps

Heaney-Rezek hysterectomy forceps
Heaney-Simon forceps
Heaney-Simon hysterectomy forceps
Heaney-Simon hysterectomy retractor
Heaney-Simon retractor
Heaney-Stumf forceps
hearing whistle
Hearn needle
heart action
heart attack
heart block
heart border
heart bypass
heart catheterization
heart chamber
heart conduction system
heart defect
heart disease
heart donor
heart failure
heart massage
heart monitor
heart murmur
heart muscle
heart needle
heart orifices
heart pacemaker
heart pacemaker leads
heart pain
heart prosthesis
heart rate
heart rhythm
heart shock
heart silhouette
heart size
heart sounds
heart surgery
heart tissue
heart tones
heart transplant
heart valve (see also *graft, implant, prosthesis, valve*)
    4-A Magovern heart valve

heart valve *continued*
    Abrams-Lucas flap heart valve
    auscultation sites of heart valves
    ball heart valve
    Beall heart valve
    bileaflet heart valve
    Biocor heart valve
    bioprosthetic heart valve
    Björk-Shiley heart valve
    bovine heart valve
    bovine pericardial heart valve xenograft
    Braunwald-Cutter caged-ball heart valve
    butterfly heart valve
    C-C heart valve (convexoconcave heart valve)
    caged-disk heart valve
    Cutter-Smeloff heart valve
    DeBakey heart valve
    Delrin heart valve
    Edwards heart valve
    Edwards-Duromedics bileaflet valve heart valve
    floating disk heart valve
    glutaraldehyde-tanned bovine heart valve
    glutaraldehyde-tanned porcine heart valve
    Gott butterfly heart valve
    Gott-Daggett heart valve prosthesis
    Hall prosthetic heart valve
    Hall-Kaster heart valve
    Hancock porcine heterograft heart valve
    Heimlich heart valve
    hingeless heart valve prosthesis
    Hufnagel caged-ball heart valve

heart valve *continued*
    Hufnagel disk heart valve
    Hufnagel disk heart valve prosthesis
    Ionescu-Shiley heart valve
    Ionescu-Shiley porcine heterograft heart valve
    Medtronic-Hall heart valve
    monocuspid tilting disk heart valve
    Omniscience heart valve
    pivotal disk heart valve
    porcine heart valve
    prosthetic heart valve
    Pyrolyte heart valve
    SCDK heart valve prosthesis
    SCDT heart valve prosthesis
    Shiley heart valve
    Silastic disk heart valve
    silicone ball heart valve
    Smeloff-Cutter heart valve prosthesis
    St. Jude Medical bileaflet heart valve
    St. Jude Medical prosthetic heart valve
    Starr Ball heart valve
    Starr-Edwards heart valve
    Sutter-Smeloff heart valve prosthesis
    three-legged cage heart valve
    tilting disk heart valve
    titanium ball heart valve
    titanium cage heart valve
    Wada hingeless heart valve prosthesis
    Wada monocuspid tilting disk heart valve
    xenograft heart valve
heart valve fixation
heart valve prosthesis

heartbeat
heart-lung bypass
heart-lung machine
heart-lung resuscitator
heart-lung transplant
heat cautery
heat pad
    Thermophore moist heat pad
heat radiation
heat sensation
heat therapy
heater probe unit (HPU)
Heath anterior chamber syringe
Heath chalazion curet
Heath chalazion forceps
Heath chalazion knife
Heath clip
Heath curet
Heath dilator
Heath dissector
Heath expressor
Heath forceps
Heath lid expressor
Heath operation
Heath punctum dilator
Heath scissors
Heath suture scissors
Heath suture-cutting scissors
Heath trephine flap dissector
heating pad
Heaton inguinal herniorrhaphy
Heaton operation
heave and lift
heavy cross-slot screwdriver
heavy elevator
heavy gauge sutures
heavy retention sutures
heavy silk retention sutures
heavy silk sutures
heavy twill belt
heavy weighted speculum
heavy wire sutures
heavy-angled scissors
heavy-ion mammography
Heberden anomaly
Heberden disease

Heberden nodes
hebosteotomy
hebotomy
Hebra blade
Hebra chalazion curet
Hebra corneal curet
Hebra fixation hook
Hedblom costal elevator
Hedblom elevator
Hedblom raspatory
Hedblom retractor
Hedblom rib retractor
hedger's cataract
heel and toe of anastomosis
heel bone
heel cord
heel cord lengthening
heel elevation
heel pad
heel spur
heel tendon
Heelbo decubitus elbow
    protector
Heelbo decubitus heel protector
Heelbo protector
heel-in-armpit method to
    reduce dislocated shoulder
heel-to-crown
HEENT (head, eyes, ears, nose,
    and throat)
Heermann alligator ear forceps
Heermann alligator forceps
Heermann chisel
Heermann ear forceps
Heermann forceps
Heermann gouge
Heermann incision
Heffernan speculum
Heffington lumbar seat
Heffington lumbar seat spinal
    surgery frame
Hefke-Turner sign
Hegar bougie
Hegar dilator
Hegar needle holder
Hegar operation
Hegar rectal dilator
Hegar sign

Hegar uterine dilator
Hegar-Baumgartner needle
Hegar-Baumgartner needle
    holder
Hegar-Goodell dilator
Hegar-Mayo-Seeley needle
    holder
Hegemann scissors
Hegenbarth clip
Hegenbarth clip forceps
Hegenbarth clip-applying
    forceps
Hegenbarth clip-removing
    forceps
Hegenbarth forceps
Hegenbarth-Adams clip
Hegenbarth-Michel clip-
    applying forceps
Heiberg-Esmarch maneuver
Heidelberg fixation forceps
Heidelberg-R surgical table
Heidenhain rods
Heifitz aneurysm clip
Heifitz clamp
Heifitz clip
Heifitz clip applier
Heifitz ingrown nail procedure
Heifitz operation
Heifitz retractor
Heifitz technique
Heifitz tongs
Heifitz traction tongs
height adjustment
Heile operation
Heimlich heart valve
Heimlich maneuver
Heimlich operation
Heimlich tube
Heimlich valve
Hein raspatory
Hein rongeur
Heine cyclodialysis
Heine operation
Heineke colon resection
Heineke operation
Heineke-Mikulicz gastroenteros-
    tomy
Heineke-Mikulicz herniorrhaphy

Heineke-Mikulicz hypospadias
    operation
Heineke-Mikulicz incision
Heineke-Mikulicz operation
Heineke-Mikulicz pyloroplasty
Heinig procedure
Heinkel sigmoidoscope
Heinkel-Semm dilator instru-
    ment
Heinkel-Semm laparoscopy
    instruments
Heishima balloon occluder
Heisrath operation
Heiss arterial forceps
Heiss artery
Heiss forceps
Heiss mastoid retractor
Heiss retractor
Heiss soft tissue retractor
Heister diverticulum
Heister fold
Heister mallet
Heister mouth gag
Heister valve
Heitz-Boyer clamp
Heitz-Boyer operation
Helanca prosthesis
Helanca seamless tube prosthe-
    sis
Helfrick anal retractor
Helfrick anal ring retractor
Helfrick retractor
helical axis of motion
helical catheter
helical fold
helical rim
helical sutures
helicinae penis, arteriae
helicine arteries of penis
helicis major, musculus
helicis minor, musculus
Heliodorus bandage
heliotrope eruption
Helistat sponge
helium anesthetic agent
helium-neon laser (He-Ne laser)
helix

Heller cardiomyotomy
Heller myotomy
Heller operation
Hellstrom pyeloplasty
Helmholtz coil
heloma
Helsper laryngectomy button
Helsper tracheostoma vent
Helweg tract
hemal node
hemangioma (*pl.* hemangiomas,
    hemangiomata)
hemangiopericytoma
hemangiosarcoma
hemapheresis
Hemaquet catheter introducer
Hemaquet introducer
Hemaquet sheath
Hemaquet sheath introducer
hemarthrosis
hemastick
hematocele
hematocrit
hematogenic shock
hematogenous contamination
hematogenous spread of cancer
hematologic disorder
hematoma
hematopoiesis
hematopoietic
hematopoietic gland
hematopoietic tissue
hematorrhea
hematuria
heme
Hemex prosthetic valve
hemiacidrin
hemianesthesia
hemianopia
hemianopsia
hemiatrophy
hemiazygos accessoria, vena
hemiazygos vein
hemiblock
hemibody irradiation
hemibody radiation therapy
hemic murmur

hemic systole
hemicolectomy
hemicorporectomy
hemicraniectomy
hemicylindrical bone graft
hemicylindrical graft
hemicystectomy
hemidecortication
hemidiaphragm
hemifacial atrophy
hemifacial hypertrophy
hemifacial spasm
hemigastrectomy
hemiglossectomy
hemihepatectomy
hemilaminectomy
hemilaminectomy blade
hemilaminectomy prong
hemilaminectomy retractor
hemilaryngectomy
hemi-LeFort fracture (I, II, etc.)
hemimandibulectomy
hemimastectomy
hemimaxillectomy
heminephrectomy
heminephroureterectomy
hemiparalysis
hemiparesis
hemipelvectomy
hemiphalangectomy
hemiplegia
hemiplegic
hemipylorectomy
hemisect
hemisection
hemisphere
hemisphere eye implant
hemisphere of brain
hemispherectomy
hemispheric functions
hemisphincter
hemithorax
hemithyroidectomy
hemitransfixion incision
hemivertebra
Hemmer connection sleeve
Hemmer connector flusher
Hemoccult

Hemoccult negative
Hemoccult positive
Hemoccult slide
hemoclip
hemoclip applier
hemoclip cartridge base
hemoclip clamp
hemoclip-applying forceps
HemoCue photometer
hemoculture
hemoculture negative
hemodialysis
hemodialysis tube
hemodialyzer
hemodynamic
hemodynamic collapse
hemodynamic instability
hemodynamic monitoring
hemodynamic support
hemoendothelial placenta
Hemofil
hemofiltration
hemoglobin
hemologic parameters
hemolymph glands
hemolysis test
hemolytic
hemolytic disease
hemolytic splenomegaly
hemolyzed serum
Hemopad
hemoperfusion
hemopneumothorax
hemoptysis
Hemopump
hemorrhage
hemorrhage per rhexis
hemorrhagenic
hemorrhagic
hemorrhagic condition
hemorrhagic shock
hemorrhea
hemorrhoid
hemorrhoid cryotherapy
hemorrhoid forceps
hemorrhoid infrared photo-
    coagulation
hemorrhoid laser excision

hemorrhoid sclerotherapy
hemorrhoid vaporization
hemorrhoidal
hemorrhoidal arteries
hemorrhoidal banding
hemorrhoidal clamp
hemorrhoidal forceps
hemorrhoidal ligator
hemorrhoidal needle
hemorrhoidal nerves
hemorrhoidal plexus
hemorrhoidal prolapse
hemorrhoidal skin tags
hemorrhoidal tags
hemorrhoidal veins
hemorrhoidal vessels
hemorrhoidectomy
hemorrhoidolysis
hemorrhoids
hemosiderin
hemospermia
hemostasis
hemostasis accomplished
hemostasis attained
hemostasis clip
hemostasis clip-applying
    forceps
hemostasis complete
hemostasis forceps
hemostasis obtained
hemostasis scalp clip
hemostasis secured
hemostasis silver clip
hemostat
    Adair hemostat
    Adson hemostat
    Allis hemostat
    angulated-vein hemostat
    Bardex hemostat
    Berne clips hemostat
    Block gastric hemostat
    Blohmka hemostat
    Blohmka tonsil hemostat
    Blotts hemostat
    Boettcher hemostat
    Bolder hemostat
    broadbill hemostat
    Brown-Buerger hemostat

hemostat *continued*
    bulldog hemostat
    Burre hemostat
    Carmalt hemostat
    Charnley-Barnes
      hemostat
    Coakley hemostat
    Coakley tonsil hemostat
    Colver tonsil hemostat
    Corboy hemostat
    Corwin hemostat
    Corwin tonsillar hemo-
      stat
    Crafoord hemostat
    Creevy-Bumpus hemo-
      stat
    Crile gall duct hemostat
    Crile hemostat
    curved hemostat
    Dandy hemostat
    Dandy scalp hemostat
    Davis hemostat
    Davis tonsillar hemostat
    Dean hemostat
    Dean tonsillar hemostat
    Deaver hemostat
    Dunhill hemostat
    fine-pointed hemostat
    Gant hemostat
    Gomco hemostat
    Guist enucleation
      hemostat
    Gutglass cervix hemostat
    Hagie hemostat
    Halsted hemostat
    Harvey Stone hemostat
    Haslinger tonsil hemostat
    Hopkins hemostat
    Hugh Young hemostat
    Jackson hemostat
    Jackson tracheal
      hemostat
    Judson-Bruce hemostat
    Kelly hemostat
    Kocher hemostat
    Kolodny hemostat
    Kolodny scalp hemostat
    Lewin tonsil hemostat

hemostat *continued*

Lewis hemostat
Lothrop hemostat
Lowsley hemostat
Maier hemostat
Maingot hemostat
Massachusetts hemostat
Mathrop hemostat
Mayfield aneurysmal
  hemostat
Mayo hemostat
Mayo-Ochsner hemostat
Mayo-Péan hemostat
McWhorter hemostat
McWhorter tonsillar
  hemostat
Meigs hemostat
Michel clip hemostat
microfibrillar collagen
  hemostat
Mixter hemostat
mosquito hemostat
Muck tonsillar hemostat
Nesbit hemostatic bag
NU-KNIT absorbable
  hemostat
Ochsner hemostat
Oxycel hemostat
Peat hemostat
Percy hemostat
Perdue hemostat
Perdue tonsillar hemostat
Providence Hospital
  hemostat
Raimondi hemostat
Rankin hemostat
Rankin-Crile hemostat
Rankin-Kelly hemostat
Richardson hemostat
Rochester-Carmalt
  hemostat
Rochester-Péan hemostat
Rumel bronchial
  hemostat
Sawtell hemostat
Sawtell-Davis hemostat
scalp hemostat

hemostat *continued*

Schnidt hemostat
Schnidt tonsillar hemo-
  stat
Shallcross hemostat
Shallcross tonsillar
  hemostat
Smedberg hemostat
Snyder hemostat
Spongostan hemostat
straight hemostat
tonsillar hemostat
tracheal hemostat
Weitlaner hemostat
Westphal hemostat
Woodward hemostat
hemostatic bag (see also *bag*)
Alcock hemostatic bag
Bardex hemostatic bag
Brodney hemostatic bag
coudé hemostatic bag
Emmet hemostatic bag
Foley hemostatic bag
Foley-Alcock hemostatic
  bag
Hagner hemostatic bag
Hendrickson hemostatic
  bag
Higgins hemostatic bag
Nesbit hemostatic bag
Pearman transurethral
  hemostatic bag
Pilcher hemostatic bag
short-tip hemostatic bag
Sones hemostatic bag
suprapubic hemostatic
  bag
two-way hemostatic bag
hemostatic catheter
hemostatic cervix forceps
hemostatic clamp
hemostatic clip
hemostatic forceps
hemostatic ligatures
hemostatic material
hemostatic neurosurgical
  forceps

hemostatic sutures
hemostatic thoracic clamp
hemostatic tissue forceps
hemostatic tonometer
hemostatic tonsillar forceps
hemostatic tonsillar guillotine
hemostatic tonsillectome
hemostatic tracheal forceps
hemothorax
Hemovac
Hemovac drain
Hemovac suction
Hemovac suction tube
Hemovac treatment unit
Hemovac tube
Hemovac unit
Henchke colpostat
Henderson approach
Henderson approximator
Henderson arthrodesis
Henderson chisel
Henderson graft
Henderson hip arthrodesis
Henderson lag screw
Henderson operation
Henderson reamer
Henderson retractor
Henderson technique
Hendren blade
Hendren cardiovascular forceps
Hendren clamp
Hendren ductus clamp
Hendren forceps
Hendren megaureter clamp
Hendren pediatric forceps
Hendren pediatric retractor
    blade
Hendren retractor blade
Hendren ureteral clamp
Hendrickson bag
Hendrickson drain
Hendrickson hemostatic bag
Hendrickson lithotrite
Hendrickson stone crusher
Hendrickson suprapubic drain
Hendry operation
He-Ne laser (helium-neon laser)

Henke forceps
Henke forceps tip
Henke punch forceps tip
Henke tonsillar dissector
Henke triangle
Henle ampulla
Henle fiber layer
Henle fissures
Henle glands
Henle ligament
Henle loop
Henle membrane
Henle sphincter
Henle spine
Henley dilator
Henley retractor
Henley subclavian artery clamp
Henley vascular clamp
Henner elevator
Henner endaural retractor
Henner retractor
Henner T-model endaural
    retractor
Henning cast spreader
Henning dilator
Henning plaster spreader
Henning sign
Henny rongeur
Henrotin forceps
Henrotin retractor
Henrotin speculum
Henrotin uterine vulsellum
    forceps
Henrotin vaginal speculum
Henrotin vulsellum forceps
Henry approach
Henry cilia forceps
Henry femoral herniorrhaphy
Henry hernia
Henry incision
Henry master knot
Henry operation
Henry repair of femoral hernia
Henry splenectomy
Henry technique
Henry-Geist operation
Henry-Geist spinal fusion

Henschke ovoid
Henschke-Mauch SNS knee
Henschke-Mauch SNS lower
    limb prosthesis
Henton hook
Henton needle
Henton suture hook
Henton suture needle
Henton tonsillar hook
Henton tonsillar suture hook
Henton tonsillar suture needle
Hepacon cannula
Hepacon catheter
Hepacon shunt
hepar
heparin
heparin lock
heparin lock introducer
heparin needle
heparin sodium
heparin well
heparin-bonded tube
heparinized
heparinized saline
heparinized solution infusion
hepatectomize
hepatectomy
hepatic
hepatic abscess
hepatic adenoma
hepatic architecture
hepatic artery
hepatic artery ligation
hepatic bed
hepatic blood flow
hepatic calculus
hepatic cecum
hepatic distention
hepatic diverticulum
hepatic duct
hepatic dullness
hepatic failure
hepatic fistula
hepatic flexure
hepatic fossa
hepatic hilum
hepatic ligament

hepatic lobe
hepatic lobectomy
hepatic necrosis
hepatic obstruction
hepatic outflow tract
hepatic plexus
hepatic radicals
hepatic resection
hepatic segments
hepatic triad
hepatic trinity
hepatic tumor
hepatic vein catheterization
hepatic veins
hepatic venous outflow
    obstruction
hepatic venous pressure
    gradient
hepatic web
hepatic web dilation
hepatica communis, arteria
hepatica propria, arteria
hepaticae, venae
hepaticocholangiocholecys-
    toenterostomy
hepaticocholangiogastrostomy
hepaticocholangiojejunostomy
hepaticocholedochostomy
hepaticocystoduodenostomy
hepaticodochotomy
hepaticoduodenostomy
hepaticoenterostomy
hepaticogastrostomy
hepaticojejunostomy
hepaticolenticular degeneration
hepaticolithectomy
hepaticolithotomy
hepaticolithotripsy
hepaticostomy
hepaticotomy
hepatic-renal angle
hepatitis
hepatization
hepatobiliary
hepatobiliary scan
hepatobiliary scintigraphy
hepatocele

hepatocellular
hepatocellular adenoma
hepatocholangiocystoduodenos-
    tomy
hepatocholangioduodenostomy
hepatocholangioenterostomy
hepatocholangiogastrostomy
hepatocholangiostomy
hepatocholedochostomy
hepatocirrhosis
hepatocolic ligament
hepatocystocolic ligament
hepatodiaphragmatic
    adhesions
hepatoduodenal
hepatoduodenal ligament
hepatoduodenal reflection
hepatoduodenostomy
hepatoenterostomy
hepatogastric
hepatogastric ligament
hepatogastroduodenal ligament
hepatogastrostomy
hepatogenic
hepatojejunostomy
hepatojugular
hepatojugular reflux
hepatolenticular disease
hepatolithectomy
hepatolithotomy
hepatoma
hepatomegalia
hepatomegaly
hepatopancreatic ampulla
hepatopancreatic fold
hepatopexy
hepatophrenic ligament
hepatoportoenterostomy
hepatoptosis
hepatorenal
hepatorenal angle
hepatorenal disease
hepatorenal ligament
hepatorenal pouch
hepatorrhaphy
hepatosplenomegaly
hepatostomy
hepatotomy

hepatoumbilical ligament
Hep-Lock
Herbert Adams clamp
Herbert bone screw
Herbert knee prosthesis
Herbert knife
Herbert operation
Herbert prosthesis
Herbert scaphoid bone screw
Herbert screw
Hercules scissors
Herculon suture material
Herculon sutures
Herczel dissector
Herczel elevator
Herczel periosteal elevator
Herczel raspatory
Herczel raspatory elevator
Herczel rib elevator
Herczel rib raspatory
hereditary disease
hereditary disorder
hereditary factors
hereditary predisposition
hereditary tendency
Herff clamp
Herff membrane-puncturing
    forceps
Herget biopsy forceps
Hering canal
Hering duct
Herman forceps
Herman-Taylor gastroscope
hermetically sealed pacemaker
Hermitex bandage
Herndon procedure
Herndon-Heyman operation for
    talipes valgus
Herndon-Heyman procedure
hernia (*pl.* herniae, hernias)
hernia adiposa
hernia en glissade
hernia foraminis ovalis
hernia par glissement
hernia pouch
hernia repair
hernia retractor
hernia sac

hernial
hernial aneurysm
hernial canal
hernial protrusion
hernial sac
herniary
herniated
herniated disk
herniated nucleus pulposus
herniation
herniation of brain
herniation of disk
herniation of muscle
herniation of nucleus pulposus
hernioappendectomy
hernioenterotomy
hernioid
herniolaparotomy
herniology
hernioplasty
herniopuncture
herniorrhaphy
herniorrhaphy incision
herniotome
herniotome knife
herniotomy
heroic measures
Herold-Torok technique
herpes
herpesvirus
herpetic
Herrick clamp
Herrick forceps
Herrick kidney clamp
Herrick kidney pedicle clamp
Herrick pedicle clamp
Herring tube
hersage
Hershey left ventricular assist
    device
Hertel bougie
Hertel bougie-urethrotome
Hertel exophthalmometer
Hertel forceps
Hertel kidney stone forceps
Hertel nephrostomy speculum
Hertel rigid dilator stone
    forceps

Hertel rigid kidney stone
    forceps
Hertel speculum
Hertel stone forceps
Hertel urethrotome
hertz units (Hz)
Hertzler baby retractor
Hertzler baby rib spreader
Hertzler rib retractor
Hertzler rib spreader
Hertzog intraocular lens
Hertzog lens
Herxheimer fibers
Herzfeld ear forceps
Herzfeld forceps
Herzmark hyperextension frame
Heschl gyrus
hesitancy
Hespan plasma volume
    expander
Hess capsule forceps
Hess capsule iris forceps
Hess expressor
Hess eyelid operation
Hess forceps
Hess iris forceps
Hess lens scoop
Hess lens spoon
Hess operation
Hess ptosis operation
Hess scoop
Hess spoon
Hess tonsil expressor
Hess-Barraquer forceps
Hess-Barraquer iris forceps
Hessburg intraocular lens
Hessburg needle
Hessburg trephine
Hessburg-Barron trephine
Hessburg-Barron vacuum
    trephine
Hesselbach hernia
Hesselbach ligament
Hesselbach triangle
Hesseltine clamp
Hesseltine umbiliclip
Hess-Gill eye forceps
Hess-Gill forceps

Hess-Gill iris forceps
Hess-Horwitz forceps
Hess-Horwitz iris forceps
hetastarch plasma expander
heteroautoplasty
heterochromic cataract
heterocladic anastomosis
heterodermic
heterogenous graft
heterograft
heterograft implant
heterograft valve
heterograft prosthesis
heterologous graft
heterologous tissue
heteronymous
hetero-osteoplasty
heteroplastic graft
heterotopic bone formation
heterotopic ossification
heterotopic pancreas
heterotopic pregnancy
heterotopic tissue
heterotopic transplant
heterotopic transplantation
heterotransplant
heterotransplantation
heterotrophs
Hetherington circular saw
Heubner artery
heurteloup leech
Heuter operation
Hevesy polyp forceps
Hewlett-Packard ear oximeter
Hewlett-Packard earlobe
     oximeter
Hewlett-Packard monitor
Hewlett-Packard transducer
Hewlett-Packard ultrasound
Hewson drill
Hewson ligament guide
Hewson passer
Hewson-Richards reamer
Hewy knife
hex screw (hexagon)
hexachlorophene
hexagon screw
hexagonal handle osteotome

hexagonal wrench
hexamethylenamine
hexapolar catheter
Hexcel cast
Hexcel cast dressing
Hexcel total condylar knee
     system prosthesis
Hexcelite cast
Hexcelite intermediate phase
     casting
Hexcelite long-arm cast
Hexcelite thermoplastic cast
hexhead bolt
hexhead nail
hexhead pin
hexhead screw
hexhead screwdriver
hexobarbital anesthetic agent
hexylcaine hydrochloride
     anesthetic agent
Hey amputation
Hey hernia
Hey internal derangement
Hey ligament
Hey operation
Hey saw
Hey skull saw
Heyer valve
Heyer-Pudenz valve
Heyer-Schulte biopsy clamp
Heyer-Schulte brain retractor
Heyer-Schulte breast implant
Heyer-Schulte breast prosthe-
     sis
Heyer-Schulte cerebrospinal
     fluid shunt system
Heyer-Schulte chin prosthe-
     sis
Heyer-Schulte clamp
Heyer-Schulte dural film
     sheeting
Heyer-Schulte hydrocephalus
     shunt instruments
Heyer-Schulte lens implant
Heyer-Schulte malar prosthesis
Heyer-Schulte mammary
     prosthesis
Heyer-Schulte microscope

Heyer-Schulte muscle biopsy clamp
Heyer-Schulte prosthesis
Heyer-Schulte Rayport muscle biopsy clamp
Heyer-Schulte retractor
Heyer-Schulte rhinoplasty implant
Heyer-Schulte shunt instruments
Heyer-Schulte shunt system
Heyer-Schulte silicone sphere
Heyer-Schulte subcutaneous tissue expander
Heyer-Schulte suction drain system
Heyer-Schulte testicular prosthesis
Heyer-Schulte tissue expander
Hey-Groves operation
Heyman capsule
Heyman clubfoot procedure
Heyman forceps
Heyman nasal forceps
Heyman nasal scissors
Heyman operation
Heyman operation for talipes equinovarus
Heyman procedure for genu recurvatum
Heyman septum-cutting rongeur
Heyman-Herndon operation
Heyman-Herndon release
Heyman-Herndon tarsometatarsal release for clubfoot
Heyman-Herndon-Strong technique
Heyman-Paparella angular scissors
Heyman-Paparella scissors
Heywood-Smith dressing forceps
Heywood-Smith sponge-holding forceps
HGM intravitreal laser
Hi Speed pulse lavage
hiatal
hiatal hernia
hiatal insufficiency
hiatopexy
hiatus
hiatus hernia
Hibbs approach
Hibbs arthrodesis
Hibbs biting forceps
Hibbs blade
Hibbs bone chisel
Hibbs bone curet
Hibbs bone gouge
Hibbs chisel
Hibbs chisel elevator
Hibbs clamp
Hibbs costal elevator
Hibbs curet
Hibbs elevator
Hibbs foot procedure
Hibbs forceps
Hibbs fracture appliance
Hibbs fracture frame
Hibbs frame
Hibbs gag
Hibbs gouge
Hibbs graft
Hibbs hammer
Hibbs hip arthrodesis
Hibbs laminectomy retractor
Hibbs mallet
Hibbs mouth gag
Hibbs onlay graft fusion of lumbar spine
Hibbs operation
Hibbs osteotome
Hibbs periosteal elevator
Hibbs retractor
Hibbs retractor blade
Hibbs self-retaining retractor
Hibbs spinal fusion
Hibbs spinal fusion chisel elevator
Hibbs spinal retractor blade
Hibbs sponge
Hibbs technique
Hibbs-Spratt curet
Hibbs-Spratt spinal fusion curet
hibernating myocardium
Hibiclens scrub
Hibiclens skin cleanser
Hibistat scrub

Hibitane tincture
Hickman catheter
Hickman indwelling catheter
Hickman indwelling right atrial
    catheter
Hickman line
Hickman Silastic semiperma-
    nent central line
Hickman-Broviac catheter
hickory-stick fracture
Hicks contraction
Hicks sign
Hicks version
HIDA scan
HIDA scan of gallbladder and
    liver
Hidalgo catheter
hidradenitis
hidradenitis suppurativa
hidradenoma
Hiebert esophageal suture
    spoon
Hiebert vascular dilator
Hierst perineoplasty
Hieshima coaxial catheter
Hiff operation
Higbee speculum
Higbee vaginal speculum
Higgenson syringe
Higgins bag
Higgins catheter
Higgins hemostatic bag
Higgins incision
Higgins operation
Higgins ureterointestinal
    anastomosis
Higgs spike operation for
    hammer toe correction
high forceps
high frequency
high incision
high ligation
high lithotomy
high occlusion
high operation for femoral
    hernia
high saphenous vein ligation
high small-bowel obstruction

high stirrups position
high subtotal gastrectomy
high voltage
high-amplitude shock wave
high-capacity drain
high-capacity silicone drain
high-dose chemotherapy
high-dose therapy
higher than head
higher than heart
higher than heart, legs elevated
highest intercostal artery
highest intercostal vein
high-fidelity catheter
high-flow cannula
high-flow catheter
high-forceps delivery
high-forceps operation
high-frequency cord
high-frequency focused
    transducer
high-grade obstruction
high-intensity light bundle
high-Knight brace
highly selective vagolysis
highly selective vagotomy
high-pitched
high-pitched bowel sounds
high-power field
high-pressure anesthesia
high-pressure chamber
high-resolution conventional
    static scanner
high-riding patella
high-risk needle (HR needle)
high-risk procedure
high-speed bur
high-speed drill
high-speed steel bur
high-speed wrist slip joint
high-torque guide wire
HIHA tendon implant
hila (*sing.* hilum)
hilar adenopathy
hilar dance
hilar fullness
hilar lymph nodes
hilar mass

hilar node
hilar plate
hilar prominence
hilar region
hilar shadow
hilar structure
Hildebrandt uterine hemostatic
    forceps
Hildreth cautery
Hildreth ocular cautery
Hildreth tip
Hildyard forceps
Hiles intraocular lens
Hiles lens
Hi-level bandage scissors
Hilgenreiner angle
Hilgenreiner brace
Hilgenreiner line
Hilgenreiner splint
Hilger facial nerve stimulator
Hilger nerve stimulator
Hilger stimulator
Hilger tracheal tube
Hilger tube
hili (*sing.* hilus)
Hill antireflux operation
Hill cluster harvest technique
Hill hiatal herniorrhaphy
Hill hiatus hernia operation
Hill hiatus herniorrhaphy
Hill median arcuate repair
Hill operation
Hill raspatory
Hill rectal retractor
Hill repair of hiatal hernia
Hill retractor
Hill sign
Hill stitch scissors
Hill suture
Hill-Allison operation
Hill-Ferguson rectal retractor
Hill-Ferguson retractor
Hillis eyelid retractor
Hillis lid retractor
Hillis perforator
Hillis retractor
Hill-Sachs lesion

Hi-Lo Jet tracheal tube
Hi-Lo tracheal tube
Hilsinger knife
Hilsinger tonsillar knife
Hilton muscle
hilum (*pl.* hila)
hilus (*pl.* hili)
hilus of ovary
Himmelstein pulmonary
    valvulotome
Himmelstein retractor
Himmelstein sternal retractor
Himmelstein valvulotome
hind kidney
hindbrain
Hinderer cartilage forceps
Hinderer cartilage-holding
    forceps
Hinderer malar prosthesis
Hinderer prosthesis
hindfoot
hindquarter amputation
Hines-Anderson pyelouretero-
    plasty
hinge
hinge joint
hinge position
hinge-axis movement
hinged articulation
hinged cast
hinged constrained knee
    prosthesis
hinged skin hook
hinged Thomas splint
hinged total knee prosthesis
hinged-leaflet aortic valve
hinged-leaflet vascular prosthe-
    sis
hinged-loop snare wire
hinge-knee prosthesis
hingeless heart valve prosthesis
hinging
Hinkle-James rectal speculum
Hinkle-James speculum
hip adduction
hip alignment guide
hip arthrodesis

hip arthroplasty
hip bone
hip cup prosthesis
hip dislocation
hip dysplasia
hip fixation
hip flange
hip flexion contracture
hip fracture
hip fusion
hip gouge
hip joint
hip musculature
hip nail
hip nailing
hip pin
hip pinning
hip pointer
hip prosthesis
HIP (homograft incus prosthesis)
hip replacement
hip retractor
hip ruler
hip screw
hip skid
hip spica
hip spica cast
hip spica dressing
Hi-Per Flex guide wire
hip-knee-ankle-foot orthosis (HKAFO)
Hippel (also von Hippel)
Hippel keratoplasty
Hippel operation
Hippel trephine
hippocampus
Hippocrates bandage
Hippocrates manipulation
hippocratic splash
hippocratic succussion
Hiram Kite three-part cast for clubfoot
Hirano bodies in hippocampus
Hirsch mucosal clamp
Hirschberg electromagnet
Hirschberg magnet

Hirschberg reflex
Hirschberg sign for pyramidal tract disease
Hirschfield eye light
Hirschman anoscope
Hirschman anoscope with obturator
Hirschman clamp
Hirschman forceps
Hirschman hemorrhoidal forceps
Hirschman hook
Hirschman intraocular implant lens
Hirschman iris hook
Hirschman jeweler's forceps
Hirschman lens
Hirschman lens forceps
Hirschman lens manipulator
Hirschman lens spatula
Hirschman proctoscope
Hirschman proctoscope with obturator
Hirschman retractor
Hirschman spatula
Hirschman speculum
Hirschman-Martin proctoscope
Hirschowitz fiberscope
Hirschowitz fiberscope gastroscope
Hirschowitz gastroduodenal scope
Hirschowitz gastroscope
Hirschsprung disease
Hirschtick splint
Hirschtick utility shoulder splint
Hirst forceps
Hirst operation
Hirst-Emmet obstetrical forceps
Hirst-Emmet placental forceps
hirudinization
His band
His bundle
His bundle electrogram
His bundle heart block
His bundle recording
His canal

*Hasson retractor*

His catheter
His perivascular space
His potential
His spindle
His-Haas operation
His-Haas procedure for long
    thoracic nerve palsy
His-Purkinje conduction
His-Purkinje system
Hiss bunionectomy
Histalog gastric analysis
His-Tawara bundle
His-Tawara node
Histoacryl adhesive
Histoacryl glue
Histoacryl glue adhesive
histocompatibility testing
histogram mode
histological diagnosis
histologically benign
histologically malignant
histologically normal
histopathologic
history and physical (H&P)
hitch
Hitchcock biceps procedure
Hitchcock procedure
Hi-Torque Flex-T guide wire
Hi-Torque floppy guide catheter
Hi-Torque floppy guide wire
Hi-Torque intermediate guide
    wire
Hi-Torque screw
Hi-Torque standard guide wire
Hitselberger sign
Hittorf tube
HKAFO (hip-knee-ankle-foot
    orthosis)
Hoaglund bone graft
Hoaglund graft
Hoaglund sign
hoarseness
hobnail liver
Hochenegg operation
hockey-stick elevator
hockey-stick incision
hockey-stick tricuspid valve

Hodge forceps
Hodge intestinal decompression
    tube
Hodge maneuver
Hodge obstetrical forceps
Hodge pessary
Hodgen apparatus
Hodgen splint
Hodgkin disease
Hodgson approach
Hodgson hypospadias repair
Hodgson spine fusion
Hodgson-Tuksu tumble flap
    hypospadias repair
Hodlick needle holder
Hodo-Kirklin incision
hoe
        excavator hoe
        Hough excavator hoe
        Hough hoe
        Hough-Saunders stapes
            hoe
        Joe's hoe
        middle ear hoe
        stapes hoe
hoe extractor
Hoehne sign
Hoen cannula
Hoen dural separator
Hoen elevator
Hoen explorer
Hoen forceps
Hoen gouge
Hoen grabber
Hoen hemilaminectomy
    retractor
Hoen hook
Hoen intervertebral disk
    rongeur
Hoen lamina gouge
Hoen laminectomy rongeur
Hoen laminectomy scissors
Hoen needle
Hoen nerve hook
Hoen periosteal elevator
Hoen periosteal raspatory
Hoen plate

Hoen raspatory
Hoen retractor
Hoen rongeur
Hoen scalp forceps
Hoen scalp retractor
Hoen scissors
Hoen separator
Hoen skull plate
Hoen ventricular cannula
Hoen ventricular needle
Hoesel needle holder
Hoff towel clamp
Hoffa fat
Hoffa operation
Hoffa tendon shortening
Hoffa-Lorenz operation
Hoffer intraocular implant
    lens
Hoffer knife
Hoffer lens
Hoffer procedure
Hoffer ridge of lens implant
Hoffmann biopsy punch
Hoffmann clamp
Hoffmann claw toe
Hoffmann duct
Hoffmann ear forceps
Hoffmann ear punch
Hoffmann ear punch forceps
Hoffmann ear rongeur
Hoffmann external fixation
    device
Hoffmann external fixation
    system
Hoffmann external fixator
Hoffmann eye implant
Hoffmann forceps
Hoffmann pin
Hoffmann punch
Hoffmann reconstruction of
    forefoot
Hoffmann scleral fixation
    pick
Hoffmann screw
Hoffmann sign
Hoffmann traction device
Hoffmann Vital external
    fixator

Hoffmann-Keller-Lapidus
    procedure
Hofmeister anastomosis
Hofmeister antecolic gastroje-
    junostomy
Hofmeister drainage bag
Hofmeister endometrial biopsy
    curet
Hofmeister gastrectomy
Hofmeister gastroenterostomy
Hofmeister operation
Hofmeister technique
Hofmeister-Billroth II gastrec-
    tomy
Hofmeister-Finsterer operation
Hofmeister-Polya operation
Hogan dacryocystostomy
Hogan keratoplasty
Hogan operation
Hogan test
Hoguet hernia repair
Hoguet maneuver
Hoguet operation
Hohl classification
Hohl fracture
Hohmann bunionectomy
Hohmann clamp
Hohmann operation
Hohmann osteotome
Hohmann retractor
Hohmann tennis elbow
    procedure
Hohn vessel dilator
Hoke arthrodesis of foot and
    ankle
Hoke flatfoot procedure
Hoke incision
Hoke operation
Hoke operation for talipes
    valgus
Hoke osteotome
Hoke spoon
Hoke technique
Hoke three-level incision
Hoke triple talus arthrodesis
Hoke-Bowen cement removal
    system
Hoke-Martin traction

Hoke-Roberts spoon
Hoku point
Hold-and-Hold immobilizer
Holden curet
Holden line
Holden uterine curet
holder (see also *head holder,*
      *needle holder*)
    Alabama-Green needle
      eye holder
    Alvarado surgical knee
      holder
    Andrews rigid chest
      support holder
    Anspach leg holder
    Arruga eye holder
    Baumgartner holder
    Bethea sheet holder
    blade holder
    bladebreaker holder
    bone-graft holder
    Boyce holder
    Bumgardner dental
      holder
    Bunt forceps holder
    Bunt instrument holder
    Castroviejo razor blade
      holder
    Chaffin-Pratt percolator
      hanger holder
    Circon leg holder
    Cottle instrument tray
      and spring holder
    Craig headrest holder
    Dees holder
    Derf holder
    Derlacki ossicle holder
    ear speculum holder
    Eber holder
    Ellis holder
    Eriksson-Paparella holder
    foot holder
    Furacin gauze holder
    Gifford holder
    Grant holder
    Green holder
    Grieshaber holder

holder *continued*
    head holder (see
      separate listing)
    House-Urban bone
      holder
    House-Urban holder
    House-Urban temporal
      bone holder
    instrument holder
    Jacobson holder
    Jarcho tenaculum holder
    Juers-Derlacki holder
    Lapides holder
    laryngoscope chest
      support holder
    laryngoscope holder
    leg holder
    Lenny Johnson surgical-
      assist knee holder
    Lewy chest holder
    Mathieu holder
    Mayo holder
    mirror holder
    Murray holder
    needle holder (see
      separate listing)
    prosthetic valve holder
    Quinn holder
    Reverdin holder
    Shea speculum holder
    speculum holder
    spring holder
    Steinmann holder
    Stephenson holder
    Surcan knee holder
    Surcan leg holder
    surgical-assist leg holder
    suture holder
    Swan needle eye holder
    Swiss blade holder
    temporal bone holder
    Tomac vest-style holder
    Vacutainer holder
    valve holder
    Weck instrument holder
    well-leg holder
    Wister forceps holder

holder *continued*
    Worcester instrument
      holder
    Young-Millin holder
hole punch set
Holinger anterior commissure
   laryngoscope
Holinger applicator
Holinger aspirating tube
Holinger bougie
Holinger bronchoscope
Holinger bronchoscopic magnet
Holinger bronchoscopic
   telescope
Holinger cannula
Holinger child esophagoscope
Holinger dissector
Holinger endarterectomy
   dissector
Holinger esophagoscope
Holinger forceps
Holinger hook-on folding
   laryngoscope
Holinger hourglass laryngo-
   scope
Holinger infant bronchoscope
Holinger infant esophagoscope
Holinger laryngeal dissector
Holinger laryngoscope
Holinger magnet
Holinger needle
Holinger scissors
Holinger slotted  laryngoscope
Holinger speculum
Holinger telescope
Holinger tube
Holinger-Garfield laryngoscope
Holinger-Hurst bougie
Holinger-Jackson bronchoscope
Hollande solution
Hollenhorst plaque
Holley table
Holley vascular stripper
Hollister bag
Hollister belt
Hollister catheter
Hollister circumcision device

Hollister clamp
Hollister colostomy bag
Hollister drainage bag
Hollister First Choice pouch
Hollister Holligard pouch
Hollister karaya 5 ostomy
   pouch
Hollister karaya seal pouch
Hollister laryngoscope
Hollister loop colostomy set
Hollister ostomy pouch
Hollister Premium pouch
Hollister self-adhesive catheter
Hollister tube
hollow
hollow cannula
hollow chisel
hollow lucite pessary
hollow organ
hollow sphere eye implant
hollow sphere implant
hollow sphere orbital implant
hollow sphere prosthesis
hollow viscus
hollow-fiber dialyzer
hollow-fiber hemodialyzer
hollow-object forceps
Holly elevator
Holman lung retractor
Holman retractor
Holman-Mathieu cannula
Holman-Mathieu salpingogra-
   phy cannula
Holmes chair
Holmes chisel
Holmes fixation forceps
Holmes forceps
Holmes gouge
Holmes nasopharyngoscope
Holmes operation
Holocaine anesthetic agent
holocrine gland
holosystolic murmur
Holscher nerve root retractor
Holscher root retractor
holster
Holt nail

Holt nail plate
Holt self-retaining catheter
Holter monitor
Holter pump
Holter pump clamp
Holter shunt
Holter tube
Holter tubing
Holter valve
Holter-Hausner catheter
Holth corneoscleral punch
Holth cystoscope
Holth cystotome
Holth forceps
Holth iridencleisis
Holth operation
Holth punch
Holth punch forceps
Holth punch sclerectomy
Holth sclerectomy
Holth sclerectomy punch
Holthouse hernia
Holth-Rubin punch
Holtz corneoscleral punch
Holtz curet
Holtz ear curet
Holtz endometrial curet
Holtzer stain
Holz procedure
Holzbach hysterectomy forceps
Holzbach retractor
Holzheimer mastoid retractor
Holzheimer retractor
Holzheimer skin retractor
Holzknecht stomach
Homans sign
homeograft
homeo-osteoplasty
homeostasis
Homer needle
Homerlok needle
homocladic anastomosis
homogeneity
homogeneous
homogeneous component
homogenous bone graft
homogenous graft

homogenous transplant
homograft
homograft cadaver
homograft graft
homograft implant
homograft prosthesis
homograft reaction
homograft rejection
homograft valve
homokeratoplasty
homologous
homologous graft
homoplastic
homoplastic graft
homoplasty
homotransplant
homotransplantation
Honan balloon
Honan cuff
Honan eye-pressure reducer
Honan manometer
Honan pressure reducer
hone
honeycomb cystitis
honeycomb lung
honeycomb pattern
Honore-Smathers tube
Hood dermatome
Hood dissector
Hood headlight
Hood operation
hooded transilluminator
Hood-Graves speculum
Hood-Graves vaginal speculum
Hood-Kirkland incision
hook (see also *buttonhook*)
    Adson angular hook
    Adson blunt dissecting
      hook
    Adson blunt hook
    Adson brain hook
    Adson dissecting hook
    Adson dissector hook
    Adson dural hook
    Adson hook
    Adson knot tier hook
    Adson sharp hook

hook *continued*

Allport hook
Allport incus hook
Angle vessel hook
APRL hooks (Army
    Prosthetics Research
    Laboratory hooks)
Army Prosthetics
    Research Laboratory
    hooks (APRL hooks)
Ashbell hook
attic hook
Aufranc hook
ball-end hook
Bane hook
Barr crypt hook
Barr fistula hook
Barr hook
Barsky hook
Barton hook
Bellucci hook
bent hook
Berens hook
Berens scleral hook
Bethune hook
Bethune nerve hook
bifid hook
Blair hook
blunt hook
blunt nerve hook
Boettcher hook
Boettcher tonsil hook
bone hook
Bonn hook
Bose hook
Bose tracheal hook
Boyes-Goodfellow hook
Bozeman hook
brain hook
Braun decapitation hook
Braun hook
Braun-Jardine-DeLee
    hook
Brown hook
Brown suture hook
Brown tissue hook
Buck hook

hook *continued*

buttonhook
calvarial hook
Carroll bone hook
Carroll hook
Carroll hook curet
Chernov hook
Chernov tracheostomy
    hook
Cloward dural hook
Cloward hook
coarctation hook
Collier-Martin hook
Colver examining
    retractor hook
Colver hook
compression hook
Converse hinged skin
    hook
Converse hook
Converse skin hook
cordotomy hook
corkscrew dural hook
corneal hook
Cottle double hook
Cottle hook
Cottle tenaculum hook
Cottle-Joseph hook
Crawford canaliculus
    hook
Crile hook
Crile nerve hook
Crile single hook
crochet hook
crura hook
crypt hook
Culler rectus muscle
    hook
curved hook
curved nerve hook
Cushing dural hook
Cushing hook
Daily fixation hook
Dandy hook
Dandy nerve hook
Davis hook
Day ear hook

hook *continued*

Day hook
DeBakey valve hook
decapitation hook
delicate skin hook
DePuy nerve hook
Dingman zygoma hook
dissecting hook
dissection hook
dissector hook
distraction hook
Dohlman hook
Dohlman incus hook
double hook
double-fixation hook
double-pronged hook
Doyen rib hook
Drews hook
Dudley hook
Dudley rectal tenaculum hook
Dudley tenaculum hook
Duplay hook
dural hook
ear hook
Edwards hook
Edwards rectal hook
Emmet tenaculum hook
Emmet uterine tenaculum hook
examining hook
extractor hook
eye fixation hook
eye hook
fenestration hook
Fenzel hook
fibroid hook
Fink hook
Fink muscle hook
Fisch dural hook
Fischl skin hook
fishhook
fistular hook
fixation hook
footplate hook
Frazier dural hook
Frazier hook

hook *continued*

Freer double-pronged hook
Freer hook
Freer skin hook
ganglion hook
Gass hook
Gass muscle hook
gasserian ganglion hook
Gillies hook
Gillies skin hook
Gillies zygomatic hook
Gillies-Dingman tenaculum hook
Goldman hook
Goldman Universal nerve hook
Goodhill hook
Graefe hook
Graefe muscle hook
Graefe strabismus hook
Graether buttonhook
Graether collar buttonhook
Graether mushroom hook
Graham blunt hook
Graham hook
Graham nerve hook
Green hook
Green strabismus hook
Gross ear hook
Gross hook
Guglen hook
Guthrie fixation hook
Guthrie skin hook
Gwathmey ether hook
Gwathmey hook
Handi-hook
Hardesty hook
Haven hook
Hebra fixation hook
Henton hook
Henton suture hook
Henton tonsillar hook
Henton tonsillar suture hook

hook *continued*

hinged skin hook
Hirschman hook
Hirschman iris hook
Hoen hook
Hoen nerve hook
Hough hook
House 90-degree hook
House crural hook
House footplate hook
House hook
House oval-window
  hook
House strut hook
Humby hook
incus hook
intracapsular lens
  expressor hook
iris hook
Jackson hook
Jackson tracheal hook
Jacobson hook
Jaeger hook
Jaeger strabismus hook
Jaffe hook
Jaffe iris hook
Jameson hook
Jameson muscle hook
Jameson strabismus
  hook
jaw hook
Johnson hook
Johnson skin hook
Jordan hook
Joseph hook
Joseph single-prong
  hook
Joseph skin hook
Juers hook
Keene compression
  hook
Kelly hook
Kelly tenaculum hook
Kilner hook
Kilner sharp hook
Kilner skin hook
Kimball hook

hook *continued*

Kimball nephrostomy
  hook
Kirby hook
Kirby intracapsular lens
  expressor hook
Kirby lens expressor
  hook
Kirby muscle hook
Kleinert-Kutz hook
Kleinert-Kutz skin hook
Klemme dura hook
Klemme hook
Knapp hook
Knapp iris hook
Knodt hook
Kobyashi hook
Krayenbuehl hook
Krayenbuehl vessel hook
Kuglen hook
Kuglen iris hook
Lahey Clinic dura hook
Lahey hook
Lange fistula hook
Leader hook
Leader vas hook
Leatherman child spinal
  hooks
lens expressor hook
lid hook
lid-retracting hook
ligature hook
Lillie attic hook
Lillie ear hook
Lillie hook
Linton hook
Linton vein hook
long blunt nerve hooks
long palate hook
Lordan hook
Lordan muscle-splitting
  hook
Loughnane hook
Lucae hook
Madden hook
Madden sympathectomy
  hook

Miya hook

hook *continued*

Malgaigne hook
Malis nerve hook
Manson hook
Marlen airing hook
Martin hook
Martin rectal hook
Maumenee iris hook
Mayo fibroid hook
Mayo hook
McIntyre irrigating iris
    hook
McMahon nephrostomy
    hook
McReynolds hook
Meyerding skin hook
microhook
microscopic hook
middle ear hook
Moe-style spinal hook
Moldestad vein hook
Muelly hook
Murphy hook
muscle hook
nasal hook
nasal polyp hook
Neivert hook
Neivert nasal polyp hook
Neivert polyp hook
nephrostomy hook
nerve hook
New hook
New tracheal hook
Newhart hook
Newhart incus hook
Newman hook
Nova hook
Nugent hook
O'Brien hook
obstetrical hook
O'Connor hook
O'Connor tenotomy
    hook
Osher-Fenzel hook
oval-window hook
Pajot hook
palate hook

hook *continued*

palate pusher hook
patellar hook
Peacock rhizotomy hook
Penn swivel hook
posterior palate hook
Praeger iris hook
Pratt crypt hook
Pratt hook
Pratt rectal hook
prostatic hook
Ramsbotham hook
rectal crypt hook
rectal hook
rectus muscle hook
Rizzuti lens hook
Robinson hook
Rolf muscle hook
Rosser crypt hook
Rosser hook
rubber-shod hook
Russian fixation hook
Sachs dural hook
Sachs hook
Sadler bone hook
Saunders-Paparella hook
Saunders-Paparella
    stapes hook
Scheer hook
Schnitman skin hook
Schuknecht footplate
    hook
Schuknecht hook
Schuknecht stapes hook
Schwartz expression
    hook
Schwartz hook
scleral hook
Scobee hook
Scobee muscle hook
Scobee oblique muscle
    hook
Scoville curved hook
Scoville curved nerve
    hook
Scoville hook
Scoville nerve hook

hook *continued*

Searcy fixation hook
Searcy hook
Selverstone cordotomy
   hook
Selverstone hook
Shambaugh endaural
   hook
Shambaugh fistula hook
Shambaugh hook
Shambaugh-Derlacki
   microhook
sharp hook
Shea footplate hook
Shea hook
Shutt hook
Simon fistula hook
Sinskey hook
Sisson hook
skin graft hook
skin hook
Sluder hook
Sluder sphenoidal hook
Smellie crochet hook
Smellie hook
Smellie obstetrical hook
Smith expressor hook
Smith hook
Smith lid hook
Smith lid-retracting hook
Smithwick blunt nerve
   hook
Smithwick buttonhook
Smithwick dissector
   hook
Smithwick hook
Smithwick nerve hook
Smithwick silk button-
   hook
Smithwick sympathec-
   tomy hook
Speare dural hook
spring hook
squint hook
St. Martin-Franceschetti
   secondary cataract
   hook

hook *continued*

Stallard scleral hook
stapes hook
Stevens hook
Stevens tenotomy hook
Stevens traction hook
Stewart crypt hook
Stewart hook
strabismus hook
straight dural hook
straight nerve hook
Strully dural twist hook
Strully hook
strut bar hook
strut hook
suture hook
swivel hook
sympathectomy hook
Tauber hook
tenaculum hook
Tennant iris hook
tenotomy hook
Tomas iris hook
Tomas suture hook
Tonnis dura hook
tonsillar hook
tonsillar suture hook
Torrence steel hook
tracheal hook
tracheostomy hook
tracheotomy hook
Trautman Locktite hook
two-prong dural hook
Tyrrell hook
Tyrrell iris hook
Tyrrell skin hook
Universal nerve hook
University of Kansas
   hook
Updegraff hook
uterine tenaculum hook
valve hook
vas hook
Volkmann bone hook
von Graefe (see *Graefe*)
Wagener ear hook
Walsh hook

hook *continued*
    Weary hook
    Weary nerve hook
    Weiss hook
    Welch Allyn hook
    Wiener corneal hook
    Wiener hook
    Wiener scleral hook
    Wiener suture hook
    Wilder hook
    Wilder lens hook
    Yankauer hook
    Zoellner hook
    Zoellner stapes hook
    zygoma hook
hook basket forceps
hook forceps
hook scissors
hook with spatula
hooked extractor
hooked intramedullary nails
hooked nail
hook-on battery handle
hook-on bronchoscope
hook-on folding laryngo-
    scope
hook-on laryngoscope handle
hook-type dermal curet
hook-type eye implant
hooped knee
Hooper deep surgery scissors
Hooper pediatric scissors
Hooper scissors
Hope bag
Hope murmur
Hope resuscitator
Hope sign
Hopkins aortic clamp
Hopkins aortic forceps
Hopkins aortic occlusion clamp
Hopkins arthroscope
Hopkins clamp
Hopkins dilator
Hopkins elevator
Hopkins endoscopy telescope
Hopkins forceps
Hopkins hemostat
Hopkins lens

Hopkins nasal endoscopy
    telescope
Hopkins operation
Hopkins pediatric telescope
Hopkins periosteal raspatory
Hopkins raspatory
Hopkins rod lens telescope
Hopkins sigmoidoscope
Hopkins telescope
Hopmann polyp
Hopp anterior commissure
    laryngoscope blade
Hopp blade
Hopp laryngoscope
Hopp laryngoscope blade
Hopp-Morrison laryngoscope
hordeolum
hordeolum eye implant
Horgan blade
Horgan center blade
Horgan operation
Horgan-Coryllos-Moure rib
    shears
Horgan-Wells rib shears
horizontal canal
horizontal fissure
horizontal folds
horizontal fracture
horizontal gastroplasty
horizontal incision
horizontal mattress sutures
horizontal maxillary fracture
horizontal overlap
horizontal plane
horizontal position
horizontal retractor
horizontal ring curet
horizontal sternotomy
horizontal sutures
horizontal tract
horizontal tube
horn
horn cells
horn of clitoris
horn of lateral ventricle
horn of spinal cord
horn of uterus
Horn sign

Horner muscle
Horner operation
Horner ptosis
Horner pupil
Horner-Trantas spots
hornpipe position
horsehair sutures
horseshoe abscess
horseshoe fistula
horseshoe flap
horseshoe headrest
horseshoe kidney
horseshoe magnet
horseshoe placenta
horseshoe pregnancy
horseshoe sutures
horseshoe tear
horseshoe tourniquet
horseshoe-shaped skin flap
Horsley anastomosis
Horsley bone knife
Horsley bone rongeur
Horsley bone wax
Horsley bone-cutting forceps
Horsley cranial rongeur
Horsley dural separator
Horsley elevator
Horsley forceps
Horsley gastrectomy
Horsley operation
Horsley pyloroplasty
Horsley rongeur
Horsley separator
Horsley sutures
Horsley trephine
Horsley wax
Horsley-Stille bone-cutting
    forceps
Horsley-Stille rib shears
Horton-Devine operation
Horvath operation
Horwitz-Adams ankle
    arthrodesis
Horwitz-Adams operation
hose
Hosemann choledochus
    forceps
Hosemann forceps

hose-pipe appearance of
    terminal ileum
Hosford dilator
Hosford eye dilator
Hosford foreign body spud
Hosford lacrimal dilator
Hosford spud
Hosford-Hicks forceps
Hosford-Hicks needle
Hosford-Hicks transfer forceps
hosiery
Hosmer Dorrance fracture
    bracing
Hosmer elbow prosthesis
hospital bucket
hospital course
hospitalization
hot biopsy
hot biopsy forceps
hot cathode tube
hot compress
hot cone
hot conization
hot defect
hot flexible forceps
hot gangrene
hot heel sign
hot infusion
hot knife
hot lesion
hot moist compresses
hot nodule
hot pack
hot patella sign
hot snare
hot spot
Hotchkiss operation
hot-cold lysis
hot-cold system
hot-cross-bun skull
hot-tipped catheter
hot-wire pneumotachometer
Hotz curet
Hotz ear applicator
Hotz ear curet
Hotz ear probe
Hotz entropion operation
Hotz probe

Hotz procedure
Hotz-Anagnostakis operation
Hough alligator forceps
Hough anterior crurotomy
    nipper
Hough auger
Hough bed
Hough crurotomy nipper
Hough drum scraper
Hough elevator
Hough excavator
Hough excavator hoe
Hough footplate auger
Hough footplate pick
Hough forceps
Hough gouge
Hough hoe
Hough hole
Hough hook
Hough knife
Hough operation
Hough osteotome
Hough oval-window excavator
Hough pick
Hough scissors
Hough spatula
Hough spatula elevator
Hough stapedectomy
Hough stapedial footplate auger
Hough tendon knife
Hough tympanoplasty knife
Hough whirlybird excavator
Houghland deformity
Hough-Rosen knife
Hough-Saunders stapes hoe
Houghton rongeur
Hough-Wullstein saw
hourglass anterior commissure
    laryngoscope
hourglass bladder
hourglass chest
hourglass deformity
hourglass gallbladder
hourglass murmur
hourglass stomach
Hourin needle
Hourin tonsil needle
hourly dose rate

House 90-degree hook
House adapter
House alligator crimper forceps
House alligator forceps
House alligator grasping forceps
House alligator scissors
House alligator-strut forceps
House angular knife
House blade
House block
House bur
House calipers
House calipers strut
House chisel
House crimper forceps
House crural hook
House cup forceps
House curet
House cutting block
House dissecting scissors
House dissector
House drum elevator
House elevator
House endaural elevator
House endolymphatic shunt
    tube
House endolymphatic shunt
    tube introducer
House excavator
House flap elevator
House footplate chisel
House footplate hook
House forceps
House Gelfoam pressure
    forceps
House Gimmick drum elevator
House Gimmick stapes elevator
House grasping forceps
House guide
House hammer
House hand-held retractor
House hook
House implant
House incudostapedial joint
    knife
House incus replacement
    prosthesis
House irrigator

House knife
House knife blade
House knife handle
House lancet
House lancet knife
House measuring rod
House Metzenbaum scissors
House myringotomy knife
House needle
House oiler tip
House oval-window hook
House pick
House piston
House pressure forceps
House prosthesis
House retractor
House rod
House scissors
House separator
House shunt
House shunt tube
House sickle knife
House speculum
house staff
House stainless steel mesh
    prosthesis
House stapedectomy
House stapes curet
House stapes elevator
House stapes needle
House stapes piston
House stapes speculum
House stapes wire prosthesis
House sterilizing box
House strut forceps
House strut hook
House suction adapter
House suction irrigator
House suction tube
House suction tube adapter
House suction-irrigator tube
House tapping hammer
House tube
House wire
House wire guide
House wire stapes prosthesis
House wire-fat prosthesis

House-Barbara needle
House-Barbara shattering
    needle
House-Bellucci alligator scissors
House-Bellucci scissors
House-Bellucci-Shambaugh
    alligator scissors
House-Bellucci-Shambaugh
    scissors
House-Derlacki chisel
House-Dieter eye forceps
House-Dieter malleus nipper
House-Dieter nipper
housemaid's knee
House-Paparella curet
House-Paparella stapes curet
Housepian clip-applying
    forceps
House-Radpour suction-irrigator
House-Rosen needle
House-Rosen utility knife
House-Stevenson suction-
    irrigator
House-Urban bone holder
House-Urban dissector
House-Urban ear marker
House-Urban gold ear marker
House-Urban holder
House-Urban marker
House-Urban middle fossa
    retractor
House-Urban oiler tip
House-Urban retractor
House-Urban rotary dissector
House-Urban temporal bone
    holder
House-Urban tip
House-Wullstein cup forceps
House-Wullstein ear forceps
House-Wullstein forceps
House-Wullstein oval cup
    forceps
Housset-Debray gastroscope
Houston halo
Houston halo cervical support
Houston halo traction
Houston muscle

Houston operation
Houston osteotomy
Houston shoulder arthrodesis
Houston valve
Hovanian procedure
Hoverbed
Hovius canal
Hovius circle
Hovius membrane
Hovius plexus
Howard abrader
Howard basket
Howard closing forceps
Howard forceps
Howard method
Howard spinal curet
Howard spiral dislodger
Howard stone basket
Howard stone dislodger
Howard technique
Howard tonsil forceps
Howard tonsil-ligating forceps
Howard-Flaherty spiral dis-
    lodger
Howard-Schatz laser technique
Howell coronary scissors
Howell tunable diaphragm
    stethoscope
Howmedica instruments
Howmedica Kinematic II total
    knee system
Howmedica knee system
Howmedica lag screw
Howmedica Luer screw
Howmedica orthopedic
    prosthesis
Howmedica PCA total hip
    system (porous coated
    anatomic total hip system)
Howmedica plate
Howmedica prosthesis
Howmedica screw
Howmedica surgical instru-
    ments
Howmedica total condylar knee
    replacement
Howmedica Universal total
    knee prosthesis

Howorth elevator
Howorth operation
Howorth osteotome
Howorth prosthesis
Howorth retractor
Howorth toothed retractor
Howse-Coventry hip apparatus
Howse-Coventry prosthesis
Howse-Coventry screw
Howship-Romberg sign
Hoxworth clip
Hoxworth forceps
Hoyer lift
Hoyer lift sling
Hoyt forceps
Hoyt hemostatic forceps
Hoytenberger tissue forceps
HPU (heater probe unit)
HR needle (high-risk needle)
Hruby contact implant
Hruby laser
Hruby lens
Hryntschak catheter
HSS knee prosthesis
hub saw
Hubbard bolt
Hubbard corneoscleral forceps
Hubbard electrode
Hubbard forceps
Hubbard plate
Hubbard tank
Hubbard tank hydrotherapy
Hubbard tub
Hubbell intraocular implant lens
Hubbell lens
Hubell meatoscope
Huber needle
Huber needle for translumbar
    aortogram
Huber procedure
Huchard sign
Huckstep intramedullary
    compression nail
Huckstep nail
Hudgins cannula
Hudgins salpingography
    cannula
Hudson all-clear nasal cannula

Hudson bone retractor
Hudson brace
Hudson brace with bur
Hudson brain forceps
Hudson bur
Hudson cerebellar attachment
Hudson cerebellar attachment
    drill
Hudson clamp
Hudson cranial bur
Hudson cranial rongeur
Hudson cranial rongeur forceps
Hudson double-ended elevator
Hudson dressing forceps
Hudson drill
Hudson elevator
Hudson forceps
Hudson line
Hudson Multi-Vent
Hudson retractor
Hudson rongeur
Hudson rongeur forceps
Hudson tissue-dressing for-
    ceps
Hudson-Jones knee cage brace
Hudson-Stähli line
Hueck ligament
Hueston finger amputation
Hueter bandage
Hueter maneuver
Hueter perineal dressing
Hueter sign
Hueter-Mayo operation
Huey scissors
Huey suture scissors
Huffman infant vaginoscope
Huffman speculum
Huffman vaginoscope
Huffman-Graves speculum
Huffman-Graves vaginal
    speculum
Huffman-Huber infant ure-
    throtome
Huffman-Huber infant vagino-
    scope
Huffman-Huber vaginoscope
Hufford esophagoscope
Hufnagel aortic clamp

Hufnagel ascending aortic
    clamp
Hufnagel caged-ball heart valve
Hufnagel clamp
Hufnagel commissurotomy
    knife
Hufnagel disk heart valve
Hufnagel disk heart valve
    prosthesis
Hufnagel forceps
Hufnagel implant
Hufnagel knife
Hufnagel mitral valve-holding
    forceps
Hufnagel needle holder
Hufnagel operation
Hufnagel prosthesis
Hufnagel prosthetic valve
Hufnagel valve
Hufnagel valve prosthesis
Hufnagel valve-holding clamp
Hufnagel-Ryder needle
    holder
Hu-Friedy dental bur
Huggins operation
Hugh Young adrenalectomy
Hugh Young hemostat
Hugh Young incision
Hugh Young pedicle clamp
Hughes eye implant
Hughes eye reconstruction
Hughes eyelid operation
Hughes implant
Hughes operation
Hughston button for meniscal
    repair
Hughston knee jerk test
Hughston knee view on x-ray
Hughston patellar procedure
Hughston patellar transplant
Hughston quadriceps recon-
    struction
Hughston technique
Hughston test
Hughston view
Huguier sinus
HUI (Harris uterine injection)
HUI catheter

HUI device for tubal lavage
Hulka cannula
Hulka tenaculum
Hulka uterine cannula
Hulka uterine manipulator
Hulka uterine tenaculum
Hulka-Kenwick forceps
Hulka-Kenwick uterine-
    manipulating forceps
human tissue polymer
human umbilical vein bypass
    graft (HUV bypass graft)
Humby hook
Humby knife
Humby operation
Hume clamp
humeral bone
humeral fracture
humeral head
humeral shaft
humeroradial
humeroradial articulation
humeroulnar
humeroulnar articulation
humeroulnar joint
humerus
humerus splint
HUMI cannula
HUMI cervical forceps skate
    flap
HUMI device for tubal lavage
HUMI injector
HUMI uterine manipulator
Hummelsheim operation
humor of eye
hump
hump forceps
hump gouge
Humphrey automatic refractor
Humphrey coronary sinus
    suction
Humphrey coronary sinus
    suction tube
Humphrey eye instruments
Humphrey lens analyzer
Humphrey overrefraction
    system

Humphrey perimeter
Humphrey vision analyzer
Humphries aortic clamp
Humphries clamp
Humphries reverse-curve aortic
    clamp
Humphry ligament
Hundley knee knife
hundredth-normal solution
Hunkeler lightweight intraocular
    lens implant
Hunner ulcer
Hunt bladder retractor
Hunt chalazion forceps
Hunt clamp
Hunt colostomy clamp
Hunt dissector
Hunt forceps
Hunt metal sound
Hunt method
Hunt needle
Hunt operation
Hunt reaction
Hunt retractor
Hunt sound
Hunt test
Hunt trocar
Hunter canal
Hunter curet
Hunter dural separator
Hunter gubernaculum
Hunter large uterine curet
Hunter ligament
Hunter operation
Hunter rod
Hunter separator
Hunter Silastic rod
Hunter splinter forceps
Hunter syndrome
Hunter tendon prosthesis
Hunter uterine curet
hunterian perforator
Hunter-Sessions balloon
Hunt-Hess neurological
    classification
Huntington chorea
Huntington operation

Huntington technique
Hunt-Lawrence pouch
Hunt-Yasargil pituitary forceps
Hupp retractor
Hupp tracheal retractor
Hurd bipolar diathermy
    electrode
Hurd bone forceps
Hurd dissector
Hurd electrode
Hurd elevator
Hurd forceps
Hurd pillar retractor
Hurd retractor
Hurd septal elevator
Hurd septal forceps
Hurd septum-cutting forceps
Hurd suture needle
Hurd tonsil dissector
Hurd tonsil elevator
Hurd tonsil knife
Hurdner tissue forceps
Hurd-Weder tonsil dissector
Hurler syndrome
Hurricaine local anesthetic
Hurst bougie
Hurst bullet-tip dilator
Hurst dilator
Hurst esophageal bougie
Hurst esophageal dilator
Hurst esophagus dilator
Hurst mercury bougie
Hurst mercury dilator
Hurst mercury-filled bougie
Hurst mercury-filled dilator
Hurst-Maloney dilator
Hurst-Tucker pneumatic dilator
Hurtig dilator
Hurwitz clamp
Hurwitz esophageal clamp
Hurwitz gastrostomy tube
Hurwitz intestinal clamp
Hurwitz thoracic trocar
Hurwitz trocar
Huschke auditory teeth
Huschke canal
Huschke foramen

Huschke ligament
Huschke valve
Huse cannula
Husen button for meniscal
    repair
Husks bone rongeur
Husks mastoid rongeur
Husks rongeur
Hutch bladder diverticulum
Hutch diverticulum
Hutch evacuator
Hutch operation
Hutchins biopsy needle
Hutchins needle
Hutchinson iris retractor
HUV bypass graft (human
    umbilical vein bypass graft)
Huxley respirator
Huzly applicator
Huzly aspirator
Huzly irrigator
Huzly tampon applicator
hyalin
hyaline cartilage
hyaline degeneration
hyalinization
hyaloid artery
hyaloid canal
hyaloid fossa
hyaloid membrane
hyaloid vessel
hyaloidea, arteria
hyaluronidase (Wydase)
Hyams catheter
Hyams clamp
Hyams conization technique
Hyams meatus clamp
Hyams operation
Hyams scleral knife
Hyams-Timberlake wire loop
    for electrode
Hybbinette-Eden operation
hybrid prosthesis
hydatid cyst
hydatid of Morgagni
hydatid pregnancy
hydatidiform mole

hydatidostomy
Hyde corneal forceps
Hyde "frog" irrigating cannula
Hyde shunt
hydraclip
hydraclip clamp
HydraCross TLC PTCA catheter
Hydragrip clamp
Hydragrip clamp insert
HydraPad
hydrarthrosis
hydrated pyelogram
hydration
hydration and turgor
hydraulic chair
hydraulic chair-table
hydraulic incontinent prosthesis
hydraulic knee
hydraulic pneumatic operator's
    stool
hydraulic stretcher
hydraulic table
hydraulic vein stripper
hydremic ascites
hydrocele
hydrocele colli
hydrocele feminae
hydrocele fluid
hydrocele of Nuck
hydrocele repair
hydrocele trocar
hydrocelectomy
hydrocephalus
hydrocephalus shunt
hydrocephalus shunt instru-
    ments
hydrocephalus shunt system
hydrochloric acid
hydrochloride
hydrochromotubation
Hydrocollator
Hydrocollator packs
Hydrocollator steam packs
hydrocortisone
Hydrocurve contact lens
Hydrocurve II intraocular lens
    implant

Hydroflex inflatable penile
    prosthesis
Hydroflex penile implant
Hydroflex penile implant rod
Hydroflex penile prosthesis
Hydroflex penile semirigid
    implant
hydrogen ion
hydrogen peroxide
Hydrojette aspirator
Hydron burn bandage
hydronephrosis
hydroperitoneum
hydropertubation
hydrophilic filter media
hydropic nephrosis
hydropigenous nephritis
hydropneumatic massage
hydrops
hydrops abdominis
hydrops fetalis
hydrops folliculi
hydrops of gallbladder
hydrops of pleura
hydrops spurius
hydrosalpinx
hydrosalpinx follicularis
hydrosalpinx simplex
hydrostatic bag
hydrostatic balloon
hydrostatic balloon catheter
hydrostatic bed
hydrostatic decompression
hydrostatic dilator
hydrostatic dissector
hydrostatic irrigator
hydrostatic pressure
hydrotherapy
hydrotherapy tank suit
hydrothorax
hydrotubation
hydroureter
hydroureteral nephrosis
hydroxide
hydroxyapatite ceramic material
hydroxyproline
hyfrecation

hyfrecator
hyfrecator-coagulator
Hyfrecutter
hygiene
hygienic practices
HygiNet elastic dressing retainer
HygiNet outer expandable
    netting
hygroma
hymen
hymenal
hymenal band
hymenal cyst
hymenal orifice
hymenal ring
hymenectomy
hymenoplasty
hymenorrhaphy
hymenotomy
Hynes pharyngoplasty
Hynes-Anderson dismembered
    pyeloplasty
hyoepiglottic ligament
hyoglossal membrane
hyoglossal muscle
hyoglossus, musculus
hyoid
hyoid bone
hyoid region
hyoid-cutting forceps
hyothyroid ligament
hyothyroid membrane
hyparterial bronchus
hypaxial muscle
hyperabduction maneuver
hyperactive bowel sounds
hyperactive carotid sinus reflex
hyperactive reflex
hyperactivity
hyperacute phase
hyperaerated chest
hyperalimentation
hyperalimentation catheter
hyperalimentation feeding
hyperalimentation fluid
hyperalimentation solution
hyperalimentation therapy

hyperalimentation tubing
hyperbaric
hyperbaric anesthesia
hyperbaric bed
hyperbaric chamber
hyperbaric oxygen
hyperbaric oxygen therapy
hyperbaric spinal anesthesia
hypercalcemia
hypercholesterolemic
    splenomegaly
Hyperclens soap
hyperechoic
hyperemesis gravidarum
hyperemia
hyperemic
hyperemic membranes
hyperextension
hyperextension brace
hyperextension fracture frame
hyperfunction
hyperfunctional
hyperirritability
hyperkeratotic lesion
hyperlucent lung
hypermastia
hypermature cataract
hypernephroma
hyperopia
hyperopic
hyperosmolar coma
hyperostosis
hyperoxaluria
hyperparathyroidism
hyperpathia
hyperphoria
hyperpituitarism
hyperplasia
hyperplastic
hyperplastic gastric polyp
hyperplastic graft
hyperplastic membrane
hyperplastic tissue
hyperreflexia
hyperreflexic bladder
hyperresonance to percussion
hypersecretion

hypersensitivity
hypersplenia
hypersplenism
hypertelorism
hypertension
hypertension and impotency
hypertensive
hypertensive arteriopathy
hypertensive arteriosclerosis
hypertensive heart disease
hypertensive lower esophageal
    sphincter
hypertensive pulmonary
    vascular disease
hypertensive therapy
hypertensive vascular disease
hyperthenar eminence
hyperthermia
hyperthyroid
hyperthyroidism
hypertonic
hypertonic bladder
hypertonic solution
hypertonic sphincter
hypertonic uterine dysfunction
hypertrophic
hypertrophic burn scar
hypertrophic cardiomyopathy
    (HCM)
hypertrophic cicatrix
hypertrophic gastritis
hypertrophic pyloric stenosis
hypertrophic scar
hypertrophic spur
hypertrophied
hypertropia
hyperventilate
hyperventilation
hyperventilation procedure
hypesthesia
hypesthesia and paralysis
hypnosis
hypnosis anesthesia
hypnotic agents
hypoactive bowel sounds
hypoactive bowel tones
hypoactive deep tendon
    reflexes

hypoactive movements
hypoactive reflex
hypobaric
hypobaric anesthesia
hypobaric spinal anesthesia
hypocalcemia
hypocalcification
hypochondriac region
hypochondriac region of
    abdomen
hypochondrium (*pl.* hypochon-
    dria)
hypocontractile
hypocystomy
hypocystotomy
hypodermatoclysis
hypodermatomy
hypodermic injection
hypodermic microscope
hypodermic needle
hypodermic syringe
hypodermic tablet
hypodermoclysis
hypoechoic
hypogastric arteries
hypogastric artery forceps
hypogastric branch of ilio-
    hypogastric nerve
hypogastric ganglion
hypogastric nerve
hypogastric plexus
hypogastric pressure
hypogastric region
hypogastric vein
hypogastric vessel
hypogastricus dexter, nervus
hypogastricus sinister, nervus
hypoglossal
hypoglossal canal
hypoglossal ganglion
hypoglossal nerve (cranial
    nerve XII)
hypoglossal nerve sign
hypoglossal-facial neuroanasto-
    mosis
hypoglossus, nervus
hypokalemia
hypokinesia

hypokinesis
hypolipoproteinemia
hypomastia
hypomastia with ptosis
hypomeric muscle
hyponychia
hypoparathyroidism
hypopharyngeal diverticulum
hypopharyngoscope
hypopharynx
hypophyseal forceps
hypophyseal fossa
hypophysection
hypophysectomy
hypophysectomy forceps
hypophysectomy instruments
hypophysis
hypopituitarism
hypoplasia
hypoplastic
hypoplastic heart
hypoplastic kidney
hypoplastic valve
hypopyon
hypopyon operation
hyporeflexic bladder
hypospadias
hypospadias operation
hypospadias repair
hypostatic ectasia
hypostatic splenization
hypotension
hypotensive
hypotensive agents
hypotensive anesthesia
hypothalamic
hypothalamic area
hypothalamic-pituitary-adrenal
    axis
hypothalamic-pituitary-ovarian
    axis
hypothalamic-pituitary-testicular
    axis
hypothalamotomy
hypothalamus
hypothenar
hypothenar eminence
hypothenar fascia

hypothenar muscles
hypothenar septum
hypothermal
hypothermia
hypothermia blanket
hypothermia cap
hypothermia mattress
hypothermic
hypothermic anesthesia
hypothermic mattress
hypothermic procedure
hypothermic surgery
hypothermic technique
hypothermy
hypothyroid ligament
hypothyroidism
hypotonic
hypotonic bladder
hypotonic colon
hypotonic duodenography
hypotony
hypotympanotomy
hypotympanum
hypovolemic shock
hypoxia
hypoxia and anoxia
Hyrtl anastomosis
Hyrtl loop
Hyrtl nerve
Hyrtl sphincter
Hyskon distending medium
Hyskon irrigation solution
Hyst T-tube
hysterectomy
hysterectomy clamp
hysterectomy forceps
hysterectomy knife
hysterectomy retractor
hysterectomy scissors
hysteresis of pacemaker
hysteresis rate of pacemaker
hysterocolpectomy
hysterocolposcope
hysteroflator
hysterogram
hysterography
hysterolysis
hysteromyomectomy

hysteromyotomy
hystero-oophorectomy
hysteropexy
hysteroplasty
hysterorrhaphy
hysterosalpingectomy
hysterosalpingogram (HSG)
hysterosalpingography
hysterosalpingography catheter
hysterosalpingo-oophorectomy
hysterosalpingorrhaphy
hysterosalpingostomy
hysteroscope
    ACMI hysteroscope
    Baggish hysteroscope
    Baloser hysteroscope
    Elmed hysteroscope
    examining hysteroscope
    fiberoptic hysteroscope

hysteroscope *continued*
    Hamou hysteroscope
    Hysteroser contact
      hysteroscope
    Storz hysteroscope
hysteroscope sheath
hysteroscopy
Hysteroser contact hystero-
    scope
Hysteroser contact hysteroscopy
    system
hysterotomy
hysterotrachelectomy
hysterotracheloplasty
hysterotrachelorrhaphy
hysterotrachelotomy
Hysterovac drain
Hysto-vac drain
Hz (hertz units)

I&A (irrigation and aspiration)
I&D (incision and drainage)
I&O (in and out; intake and output)
I-131 (radioactive iodine)
I-131 labeled hippuran
I-131 uptake
I-A handpiece (irrigating-aspirating handpiece)
I-A unit (irrigate-aspirate unit)
I-A Vitrophage
I-beam nail
I-Knife
I-Stat cautery
I-Temp cautery
IAB catheter (intra-aortic balloon catheter)
IABP (intra-aortic balloon pump)
Ialo photocoagulation
iatrogenic fracture
iatrogenic ureteral injury
iatrotechnique
IBD (inflammatory bowel disease)
IBF total knee instrumentation (Insall-Burstein-Freeman total knee instrumentation)
IBM blood cell processor
IBS (inflammatory bowel syndrome)
IC bed
IC stretcher
ICA (internal carotid artery)
ICAO (internal carotid artery occlusion)
ICCE (intracapsular cataract extraction)

ICD (intercanthal distance)
ice bag
ice ball
ice cap
ice chips
ice clot evacuator
ice pack
iced cystogram
iced saline
iced saline lavage
iced saline solution
ice-tong calipers
icing heart
ICLH (Imperial College, London Hospital)
ICLH apparatus
ICLH arthroplasty
ICLH staple system
ICP (intracranial pressure)
ICP catheter
ICP monitor
ICP Tele-Sensor
ICR (intracavitary radium)
ICS plate
icterus
ICU (intensive care unit)
IDD (intraluminal duodenal diverticulum)
Ideal arch wire
Ideal automatic tourniquet
identical pattern
identical plane dose
identifiable electrical activity
identification
identified and ligated
idiomuscular contractility

idiomuscular contraction
idionodal rhythm
idiopathic
idiopathic hypertrophic
    subaortic stenosis (IHSS)
idiopathic megacolon
idiopathic obstruction
idioventricular rhythm
IDIS angiography (intraopera-
    tive digital subtraction
    angiography)
I/E ratio (inspiratory/expiratory
    ratio)
IFC pheresis (intermittent-flow
    centrifugation pheresis)
Iglesias continuous-flow
    resectoscope
Iglesias dilator
Iglesias electrode
Iglesias evacuator
Iglesias fiberoptic resectoscope
Iglesias resectoscope
ignipuncture
IHSS (idiopathic hypertrophic
    subaortic stenosis)
II traction table
Ikegami video system
IKI catgut sutures
ILA stapling device
ILA surgical stapler
ILAC target
ileac, ileal
ileal arteries
ileal colostomy
ileal conduit
ileal inflow tract
ileal J-pouch
ileal loop
ileal loop stoma
ileal pouch-anal anastomosis
ileal pull-through operation
ileal pull-through procedure
ileal reservoir
ileal S-pouch
ileal stasis
ileal transverse colostomy
ileal varices
ileal veins

ileal W-pouch
ileectomy
ilei, arteriae
ileitis
ileoanal endorectal pull-through
    operation
ileoanal pouch
ileoanal pull-through procedure
ileoanal reservoir
ileoascending colostomy
ileobladder cystoscopy
ileobladderoscopy
ileocecal
ileocecal bladder
ileocecal bladder construction
ileocecal junction
ileocecal pouch
ileocecal valve
ileocecostomy
ileocecum
ileocolectomy
ileocolic
ileocolic artery
ileocolic fold
ileocolic intussusception
ileocolic lymph nodes
ileocolic plexus
ileocolic vein
ileocolica, arteria
ileocolica, vena
ileocolitis
ileocolitis ulcerosa chronica
ileocolostomy
ileocolotomy
ileocutaneous fistula
ileocystoplasty
ileocystostomy
ileoduodenotomy
ileoentectropy
ileoesophagostomy
ileofemoral deep vein thrombo-
    sis
ileogastric reflex
ileoileal anastomosis
ileoileal intussusception
ileoileostomy
ileojejunitis
ileoloopogram

ileoneocystostomy
ileopancreatostomy
ileopexy
ileoproctostomy
ileorectal
ileorectal anastomosis
ileorectostomy
ileorrhaphy
ileoscopy
ileosigmoid
ileosigmoid colostomy
ileosigmoid fistula
ileosigmoidostomy
ileostogram
ileostomy
ileostomy appliance
ileostomy bag
ileostomy closure
ileostomy effluent
ileostomy pouch
ileostomy sac
ileostomy stoma
ileostomy without colectomy
ileotomy
ileotransverse colostomy
ileotransverse colotomy
ileotransversostomy
ileoureterostomy
ileum
ileus
ileus following abdominal
    surgery
Ilfeld splint
Ilfeld-Gustafson splint
iliac
iliac artery
iliac autograft
iliac bifurcation
iliac bone
iliac chain
iliac clamp
iliac colon
iliac crest
iliac endarterectomy
iliac flexure
iliac flexure of colon
iliac forceps

iliac fossa
iliac graft
iliac lymph nodes
iliac muscle
iliac region
iliac spine
iliac vein
iliac vessels
iliaca communis, arteria
iliaca communis, vena
iliaca externa, arteria
iliaca externa, vena
iliaca interna, arteria
iliaca interna, vena
iliac-femoral, cannula
iliacus, musculus
Iliff blepharochalasis forceps
Iliff clamp
Iliff dacryoattachment for
    Stryker saw
Iliff exenteration
Iliff eyelid repair
Iliff lacrimal trephine
Iliff operation
Iliff procedure to correct ptosis
Iliff ptosis operation
Iliff trephine
Iliff-Haus operation
Iliff-Park speculum
ilioabdominal
iliococcygeal
iliococcygeal muscle
iliococcygeus, musculus
iliocolotomy
iliocostal muscle
iliocostal space
iliocostalis cervicis, musculus
iliocostalis lumborum, musculus
iliocostalis, musculus
iliocostalis thoracis, musculus
iliofemoral
iliofemoral ligament
iliofemoral triangle
iliohypogastric
iliohypogastric nerve
iliohypogastricus, nervus
ilioinguinal

ilioinguinal artery
ilioinguinal nerve
ilioinguinal vein
ilioinguinalis, nervus
iliolumbalis, arteria
iliolumbalis, vena
iliolumbar artery
iliolumbar vein
iliolumbocostoabdominal
iliopectineal
iliopectineal arch
iliopectineal bursa
iliopectineal eminence
iliopectineal line
iliopopliteal bypass
iliopsoas
iliopsoas bursa
iliopsoas muscle
iliopsoas, musculus
iliopsoas sign
iliopubic
iliosacral
iliosacral articulation
iliotibial
iliotibial band (ITB)
iliotibial tract
iliotrochanteric ligament
ilium
ilium bone
ilium crest
Ilizarov bone-lengthening
    technique
Ilizarov bone-straightening
    technique
Ilizarov fixator
Ilizarov leg-lengthening
    procedure
Ilizarov orthopedic method
Illinois needle
Illouz cannula
Illouz suction cannula
illuminated nasal speculum
illuminated probe
illuminated ureter probe
illumination probe
illuminator (see also *transillu-
    minator)*
        all-purpose transillumina-
        tor

illuminator *continued*
    Barkan illuminator
    Briggs transilluminator
    Bush ureteral illuminator
    Coldlite transilluminator
    endoilluminator
    Finnoff transilluminator
    Gyn-A-Lite illuminator
    Gyn-A-Lite speculum
        illuminator
    hooded transilluminator
    Lancaster transilluminator
    National transilluminator
    rotating transilluminator
    Shunn gun transillumina-
        tor
    slit illuminator
    speculum illuminator
    speculum transillumina-
        tor
    Tatum ureteral transillu-
        minator
    transilluminator
    ureteral illuminator
    Welch Allyn transillumi-
        nator
    Whitelite transillumina-
        tor
    Widner transilluminator
illuminator ear unit
illuminator head unit
illusion
ILS (intraluminal stapler)
IMA (internal mammary artery,
    inferior mesenteric artery)
IMA graft
IMAB (internal mammary artery
    bypass)
image acquisition time
image converter
image intensification
image intensifier
imager
imaginary line
imaging
imaging procedure
imaging staging
imaging system
imaging technique

Imatron C-100 system for heart studies
Imatron C-100 system for high-resolution body imaging
imbalance
imbricate
imbricated sutures
imbricating layer
imbricating stitch
imbricating sutures
imbrication
imbrication herniorrhaphy
IMED infusion device
IMED infusion pump
IMED pump
immature cataract
immature labor
immature ovarian teratoma
immeasurable fluid loss
immediate amputation
immediate fit prosthesis
immediate postoperative prosthesis (IPOP)
immediate postsurgical fitting (IPSF)
immediate transfer flap
immediate transfusion
immediately (stat)
Immergut suction tube
Immergut suction-coagulation tube
Immergut tube
immersion
imminent
imminent abortion
imminent death
immobile
immobilization
immobilization of joint
immobilize
immobilized extremity
immobilized in cast
immobilized in plaster cast
immobilized joint
immobilized knee
immobilizer
        C-splint immobilizer
        OEC knee immobilizer

immobilizer *continued*
        Tab-Strap knee immobilizer
        TCS knee immobilizer (tri-panel, convoluted, Y-strap knee immobilizer)
        Trimline knee immobilizer
        Zimmer Universal knee immobilizer with Zimfoam padding
immobilizing bandage
immobilizing dressing
immovable bandage
immovable joint
immune system
immunity
immunization
immunocompromised patient
immunodepressed patient
immunoelectro-osmophoresis
immunofiltration
immunofluorescent microscopy
immunoglobulin
immunologic, immunological
immunologic suppression
immunologic workup
immunoreactive
immunosuppressed patient
immunosuppressive therapy
immunotherapy
impacted
impacted calculus
impacted cerumen
impacted fecal material
impacted feces
impacted foreign body
impacted fracture
impacted molar
impacted stone
impacted stool
impacted teeth
impaction
impactor
impactor-extractor
impaired ability
impaired function
impaired sensation

impaired vision
impairment
Impala rubber band
impassable obstruction
impassable scar tissue
impassable stricture
impedance
impedance electrode
impedance plethysmography
    (IPG)
impediment
impending infarction
impending stroke
imperative
Imperator handpiece
Imperator oil
Imperator pressure oiler
Imperatori antral wash bottle
Imperatori forceps
Imperatori laryngeal forceps
Imperatori laryngeal speculum
imperceptible pulse
imperfect closure
imperforate
imperforate anus
imperforate hymen
impermeable
impermeable dressing
impermeable stricture
Impersol catheter
impervious
impinge
impingement
impingement syndrome
impinging on cortex
impinging on tumor
implant (see also *eye implant,
    graft, lens patch, prosthesis,
    valve*)
    3M mammary implant
    accordion implant
    acorn-shaped implant
    acrylic ball eye implant
    acrylic conformer eye
        implant
    acrylic eye implant
    acrylic implant

implant *continued*
    Acuflex intraocular lens
        implant
    adhesive silicone implant
    adjustable breast implant
    adrenal medullary
        implants
    AGC knee program
        implant
    alar-columella implant
    Allen eye implant
    Allen implant
    Allen orbital implant
    Allen Supramid implant
    Allen-Brailey intraocular
        lens implant
    Alpar implant
    Alpar intraocular lens
        implant
    AMO intraocular lens
        implant
    Anis Staple implant
        cataract lens
    AO/ASIF orthopedic
        implants
    Appolonio eye implant
    Appolonio implant
        cataract lens
    Arenberg-Denver inner-
        ear valve implant
    Arion implant
    Arruga eye implant
    Arruga implant
    Arruga movable eye
        implant
    Arruga-Moura-Brazil
        orbital implant
    artificial joint implant
    Ashworth-Blatt implant
    aspheric lens implant
    Azar Tripod eye implant
    Azar Tripod implant
        cataract lens
    Balnetar implant
    Bard implant
    Barkan implant
    Barraquer implant

implant *continued*

Beale intraocular implant lens

Bechert intraocular lens implant

Bechtol implant

Berens conical eye implant

Berens eye implant

Berens implant

Berens orbital implant

Berens pyramidal eye implant

Berens sphere eye implant

Berens-Rosa eye implant

Berens-Rosa scleral implant

Bietti eye implant

Bietti implant cataract lens

bilumen mammary implant

Binkhorst eye implant

Binkhorst implant

Binkhorst intraocular lens implant

Binkhorst lens implant

bioimplant

Blair-Brown implants

Boberg-Ans implant

Bonaccolto eye implant

bone implant

bovine implant

Boyd implant

Boyd intraocular implant lens

Branemark osseointegration implant

Braun implant

Brawner orbital implant

breast implant

Bron implant cataract lens

Brown-Dohlman corneal implant

implant *continued*

Brown-Dohlman eye implant

Brown-Dohlman implant

build-up eye implant

Bunker implant

Bunker intraocular implant lens

Byron intraocular implant lens

candle vaginal cesium implant

cardiovascular implant

carpal lunate implant

Carrion-Small penile implant

cartilage implant

Cartwright implant

Castroviejo implant

Celestin implant

celluloid implant

Chatzidakis implant

chessboard implant

chin implant

Choyce eye implant

Choyce implant

Choyce Mark eye implant

Clayman intraocular implant lens

Clayman lens implant

Coburn anterior chamber intraocular lens implant

Coburn Mark IX eye implant

cochlear implant

Cogan-Boberg-Ans lens implant

collagen implant

columella implant

condylar implant arthroplasty

conical eye implant

conical implant

contact shell implant

implant *continued*

conventional reform eye implant
conventional reform implant
conventional shell-type eye implant
Copeland intraocular lens implant
Copeland lens implant
Core-Vent implant
corneal eye implant
corneal implant
Corning implant
Cox-Uphoff implant
Cronin implant
Cronin mammary implant
curl-back shell eye implant
Custodis implant
custom-contoured implant
Cutler eye implant
Cutler implant
Dacron implant
Dannheim eye implant
Darin intraocular implant lens
DCS implant (dorsal column stimulator/ stimulation implant)
De Paco implant
DeBakey implant
defibrillator implant
dental implant
DePuy orthopedic implant
Dermostat implant
Dermostat orbital implant
DeWecker eye implant
Dickerson intraocular implant lens
Doherty eye implant
Doherty implant
Doherty sphere eye implant

implant *continued*

Doherty sphere implant
Donnheim implant
dorsal columella implant
dorsal column stimulator implant (DCS implant)
double-lumen breast implant
Dow Corning implant
Dragstedt implant
Drews intraocular implant lens
Duehr-Allen eye implant
Dulaney intraocular implant lens
dummy sources in cesium implant
dural implant
eccentric implantation
Edwards implant
Edwards Teflon intracardiac implant
Ehmke platinum Teflon implant
Eifrig intraocular implant lens
electrical implant
Ellingson intraocular implant lens
endometrial implants
endometriotic implant
endo-osseous dental implant
endo-osseous implant
Epstein lens implant
Esser implant
Ethrone implant
Ewald-Walker knee implant
Ewing eye implant
expandable breast implant
Extrafil breast implant
eye implant
eye sphere implant
fascia lata implant
Fechner intraocular implant lens

implant *continued*
Federov eye implant
Federov implant
Federov lens implant
Federov type I lens
implant
Federov type II lens
implant
fenestra implant
Ferguson implant
fetal substantia nigra
implants
Fibrel gelatin matrix
implant
finger joint implant
Finney penile implant
flexible Dualens implant
flexible rod penile
implant
Flexi-Flate II penile
implant
Flexi-Flate penile im-
plant
Flexi-rod II penile
implant
Fox eye implant
Fox eyelid implant
Fox implant
Fox sphere implant
free implant
Frey eye implant
front build-up eye
implant
full-thickness implant
Galin intraocular lens
implant
Garcia-Novito eye
implant
gel-filled implant
Gelfilm retinal orbital
implant
gel-saline mammary
implant
Gerow Small-Carrion
penile implant
Gillies implant
Gills intraocular implant
lens

implant *continued*
Gilmore intraocular
implant lens
glass sphere eye implant
glass sphere implant
gold eye implant
gold implant
gold sphere eye implant
Goldmann multi-
mirrored lens implant
Gore-Tex vascular
implant
Gott implant
Gould intraocular
implant lens
Greene intraocular
implant lens
Guist eye implant
Guist sphere eye implant
Guist sphere implant
Haik implant
haptic area implant
Hardy implant fork
Harris implant
Harrison implant
Hartley implant
hemisphere eye implant
heterograft implant
Heyer-Schulte breast
implant
Heyer-Schulte lens
implant
Heyer-Schulte rhino-
plasty implant
HIHA tendon implant
Hirschman intraocular
implant lens
Hoffer intraocular
implant lens
Hoffer ridge of lens
implant
Hoffmann eye implant
hollow sphere eye
implant
hollow sphere implant
hollow sphere orbital
implant
homograft implant

implant *continued*

hook-type eye implant
hordeolum eye implant
House implant
Hruby contact implant
Hubbell intraocular
    implant lens
Hufnagel implant
Hughes eye implant
Hughes implant
Hunkeler lightweight
    intraocular lens
    implant
Hydrocurve II intraocular
    lens implant
Hydroflex penile implant
Hydroflex penile
    semirigid implant
Implens intraocular
    implant lens
inflatable penile implant
Insall-Burstein intra-
    condylar knee implant
Intermedics intraocular
    lens implant
interstitial implant
intraocular lens implant
intraorbital implant
Ioptex laser intraocular
    lens implant
Iowa implant
Iowa orbital implant
iridium implant
iridium wire implant
iridocapsular implant
    cataract lens
Ivalon eye implant
Ivalon implant
Ivalon sponge implant
Jaffe ocular implant lens
joint implant
Jordan eye implant
Jordan implant
Keats intraocular implant
    lens
Kelman intraocular
    implant lens

implant *continued*

Keragen implant
King implant
King orbital implant
Koeppe gonioscopic lens
    implant
Koeppe intraocular lens
    implant
Kraff intraocular implant
    lens
Krasnov implant cataract
    lens
Kratz implant
Kratz intraocular implant
    lens
Kratz-Sinskey intraocular
    lens implant
Krause-Wolfe implant
Kryptok bifocal lens
    implant
Kwitko intraocular
    implant lens
Lacey total knee implant
Landegger orbital
    implant
LaPorte total toe implant
Lash-Loeffler implant
Leadbetter-Politano
    ureteral implant
    prosthesis
Lemoine eye implant
lens implant
Levitt eye implant
Levitt implant
Lifecath peritoneal
    implant
Lincoff eye implant
Lincoff implant
Little intraocular lens
    implant
Liverpool elbow implant
Lovac fundus contact
    lens implant
lucite eye implant
lucite implant
lucite sphere implant
lunate implant

implant *continued*

Lyda Ivalon-Lucite orbital implant
lymphoma implant
MacIntosh implant
magnetic eye implant
magnetic implant
mammary implant
Manschot intraocular implant lens
Marlex mesh implant
McCannel intraocular implant lens
McGhan breast implant
McGhan eye implant
McGhan implant
McIntyre intraocular implant lens
Medallion intraocular lens implant
Medical Optics eye implant
Medical Workshop intraocular lens implant
Melauskas orbital implant
Meme mammary implant
Mentor malleable semirigid penile implant
Mersilene implant
meshed ball implant
metal orthopedic implant
metallic implant
metastatic implant
Michelis intraocular implant lens
Microvel implant
middle ear implant
Miller-Galante total knee implant
Muhlberger implant
Muhlberger orbital implant
Muhlberger orbital implant prosthesis

implant *continued*

Mules eye implant
Mules implant
Mules sphere eye implant
Mules sphere implant
Naden-Rieth implant
Neer II total shoulder system implant
Nocito eye implant
Ollier-Thiersch implant
O'Malley self-adhering lens implant
orbital floor implant
orbital implant
ORC posterior chamber intraocular lens implant
orthotic attachment implant
osseous implant
Padgett implant
Panje implant
paraffin implant
patch implant
peanut eye implant
Pearce posterior chamber intraocular lens implant
Pearce vaulted-Y lens implant
pectoralis muscle implant
pedicle implant
penile implant
percutaneous dorsal column stimulator implant
permanent implant
pin implant
Pisces implant
plastic ball eye implant
plastic implant
plastic sphere eye implant
plastic sphere implant
Platina clip implant cataract lens

implant *continued*

Platina intraocular lens implant
Plexiglas eye implant
Plexiglas implant
Plystan implant
PMI implant
polyether implant material
polyethylene eye implant
polyethylene implant
polyethylene sphere implant
Polystan implant
polyurethane implant
polyvinyl implant
polyvinyl sponge implant
Porex Medpor implant
Porex PHA implant
Precision eye implant
Precision-Cosmet intraocular lens implant
press-fit implant
Proplast facial implant
Proplast implant
Proplast nasal implant
Proplast preformed implant
pyramidal eye implant
radiocarpal implant
radium implant
Radovan breast implant
Rastelli implant
Rayner-Choyce eye implant
reform eye implant
reform implant
removable implant
Reverdin implant
reverse-shape eye implant
reverse-shape implant
rhinoplasty implant
Ridley anterior chamber implant

implant *continued*

Ridley implant cataract lens
Ridley Mark II lens implant
Rodin implant
Rodin orbital implant
Rosa-Berens implant
Rosa-Berens orbital implant
Ruedemann eye implant
Ruiz plano fundus lens implant
SACH implant
Sauerbruch implant
Schachar implant cataract lens
Scharf implant cataract lens
Schepens hollow hemisphere implant
scleral buckle eye implant
scleral buckler implant
scleral eye implant
scleral implant
seed implant
semishell eye implant
semishell implant
serrefine implant
Shearing intraocular implant lens
shell eye implant
shell implant
shell-type eye implant
shell-type implant
Shepard intraocular lens implant
Sichel implant
Sichel movable implant
Sichel orbital implant
Silastic corneal implant
Silastic Cronin implant
Silastic eye implant
Silastic implant
Silastic scleral buckler implant

implant *continued*

Silastic silicone rubber implant
Silastic subdermal implant
silicone eye implant
silicone implant
silicone rod implant
silicone sponge implant
silicone-filled breast implant
Siloxane implant
Simcoe eye implant
Simcoe implant
Simcoe intraocular implant lens
Simcoe intraocular lens implant
Simcoe-Amo eye implant
Sinskey lens implant
Sled implant
Small-Carrion Silastic rod for penile implant
Smith intraocular implant lens
Smith orbital floor implant
Snellen eye implant
solid silicone with Supramid mesh implant
spermatocele implant
sphere eye implant
sphere implant
spherical eye implant
spherical implant
split-thickness implant
sponge implant
stainless steel implant
Stein intraocular implant lens
Stone eye implant
Stone implant
Straatsma intraocular implant lens
Strampelli implant

implant *continued*

Strampelli implant cataract lens
subdermal implant
submucosal implant
subperiosteal implant
superficial implant
Supramid implant
surface eye implant
surface implant
Surgibone implant
Surgicel implant
Surgitek Flexi-Flate II penile implant
Surgitek implant
Surgitek mammary implant
Swanson carpal lunate implant
Swanson carpal scaphoid implant
Swanson finger joint implant
Swanson great toe implant
Swanson hemi-implant
Swanson implant
Swanson radial head implant
Swanson radiocarpal implant
Swanson trapezium implant
Swanson ulnar head implant
Swanson wrist joint implant
Swiss MP joint implant
Syed template implant
Syed-Neblett implant
tantalum eye implant
tantalum implant
tantalum mesh implant
Techmedica implant system
Teflon implant
Teflon mesh implant

implant *continued*
    Teflon orbital floor
        implant
    tendon implant
    Tennant Anchorflex lens
        implant
    Tennant intraocular
        implant lens
    Tensilon implant
    testicular implant
    Tevdek implant
    Thiersch implant
    tire eye implant
    tire implant
    Townley implant
    trapezium implant
    Troncoso implant
    Troutman eye implant
    Troutman implant
    Troutman magnetic
        implant
    tunneled eye implant
    tunneled implant
    Ultex implant
    unicompartmental knee
        implant
    Unilab Surgibone
        surgical implant
    ureteral implant
    Uribe implant
    Uribe orbital implant
    Usher Marlex mesh
        implant
    VA magnetic implant
        (visual acuity magnetic
        implant)
    VA magnetic orbital
        implant (visual acuity
        magnetic orbital
        implant)
    Varigray implant
    Varigray lens implant
    Varilux implant
    Vitallium eye implant
    Vitallium implant
    Vivosil implant
    Volk conoid implant

implant *continued*
    Walter Reed implant
    Weavenit implant
    Weber hip implant
    Weber implant
    Weck-cel implant
    Wheeler eye implant
    Wheeler implant
    Wheeler sphere eye
        implant
    wire mesh eye implant
    wire mesh implant
    Wolfe implant
    Wolfe-Krause implant
    Zyderm collagen implant
    Zyderm implant
    Zyplast implant
implant arthroplasty
implant cataract lens
implant conformer
implant forceps
implant fork
implant lens
implant material
implant placement
implant surgery
implantable bone growth
    stimulator
implantable cardiac pulse
    generator
implantable defibrillator
implantable drug infusion pump
implantable pacemaker
implantation
implantation cyst
implantation of pacemaker
implantation of radioactive
    isotopes
implantation of radium
implantation of ureter into
    rectum
implantation technique
implanted electrode
implanted pacemaker
implanted pump
implanted sutures
implanted tube

implanting radioactive sources
implantodontics
implantodontist
Implast adhesive
Implast bone cement
implementation
Implens intraocular implant lens
Implens lens
implications
implied consent
implode
impotence
impotent
Impra bypass graft
Impra Flex vascular graft
Impra graft
Impra vascular graft
Impra vein graft
impregnated dressing
impregnated electrode
impregnated gauze
impression
impression tonometer
improper management
improved condition
improved Webb stripper
improvement
impulse
impulsion
impulsiveness
Imre canthoplasty
Imre flap operation
Imre keratoplasty
Imre lid operation
Imre operation
Imre treatment
IMV (intermittent mandatory
    ventilation)
IMVbird
in and out (I&O)
in ano
in extremis
in recto hernia
in situ
in situ bypass
in toto
in utero

inability
inaccessibility
inaction
inactivate
inactivating agent
inactive condition
inactive electrode
inactivity
inadequacy
inadequate blood flow
inadequate bowel prep
inadequate cardiac output
inadequate pelvis
inadequately sterilized instru-
    ments
Inahara shunt
Inahara-Pruitt vascular shunt
inborn error of metabolism
incandescent sheath
incapable
incapacitance
incapacitated
incapacitating
incapacity
incarcerated
incarcerated hernia
incarcerated omentum
incarcerated placenta
incarceration
InCare brace
incarnative
incentive inspirometry program
incentive spirometry
incessant movements
incidence
incident
incidental appendectomy
incidental finding
incidental murmur
incipient
incipient cataract
incipient gangrene
incisal surface of tooth
incise
incise and drain
incise drape
incised

incised wound
incision
    ab externo incision
    abdominal incision
    abdominothoracic
        incision
    Agnew-Verhoeff incision
    alar incision
    Alexander incision
    Amussat incision
    angular incision
    anterior pillar incision
    anterolateral thoracot-
        omy incision
    aortotomy incision
    apron U-shaped incision
    arcuate incision
    areolar incision
    arteriotomy incision
    Auvray incision
    backcut incision
    Bar incision
    Bardenheuer incision
    Battle incision
    Battle-Jalaguier-
        Kammerer incision
    bayonet incision
    belt-approach incision
    Bergmann incision
    Bergmann-Israel incision
    Bevan abdominal
        incision
    Bevan incision
    Bevan vertical elliptical
        skin incision of
        abdomen
    bivalved elliptical
        incision
    bivalved incision
    Blair incision
    Bosworth-Shawler
        incision
    bowling-pin incision
    Boyd incision
    Boyd posterior incision
    Brackin incision
    Brock incision

incision *continued*
    Brunner incision
    Bruser incision
    Bruser lateral incision
    Bruser skin incision
    Buck-Gramcko incision
    bur-hole incision
    buttonhole incision
    Caldwell-Luc incision
    Cave incision
    celiotomy incision
    cervical incision
    Chamberlain incision
    Cheatle-Henry incision
    Cherney abdominal
        incision
    Cherney incision
    Cherney-Winklesnit
        abdominal incision
    Chernez incision
    chevron incision
    Chiene incision
    choledochotomy incision
    Cincinnati incision
    circular guillotine
        incision
    circular incision
    circumareolar incision
    circumcisional incision
    circumcorneal incision
    circumferential incision
    circumferentiating skin
        incision
    circumlimbar incision
    circumoral incision
    circumscribing incision
    circum-umbilical incision
    classical incision
    clean and dry incision
    clitoral incision
    Clute incision
    Codman incision
    Coffey incision
    Cohen uterine incision
    collar incision
    confirmatory incision
    conjunctival incision

incision *continued*
  Conley incision
  Conley neck incision
  Conley radical neck
    incision
  Connell incision
  contraincision
  corneal incision
  corneoscleral incision
  corollary incision
  coronal incision
  cortical incision
  Cottle incision
  counterincision
  Courvoisier incision
  crease incision
  crescent incision
  crescent-shaped incision
  Crile incision
  crosshatch incision
  cross-shaped incision
  crucial incision
  cruciate incision
  Cubbins incision
  culdotomy incision
  curved incision
  curved periscapular
    incision
  curved-downward
    incision
  curvilinear incision
  curvilinear skin incision
  curving incision
  cutdown incision
  Czerny incision
  Davis-Geck incision
  Davis-Rockey incision
  de Quervain incision
    (also Quervain)
  Deaver incision
  Deaver skin incision
  deepened incision
  deltopectoral incision
  dorsal supine incision
  dorsolateral incision
  double-Y incision
  draining incisional
    site

incision *continued*
  dry incision
  Dührssen incision
  dumbbell incision
  dural incision
  Edebohls incision
  elliptical incision
  elliptical sagittal
    incision
  elongated S-incision
  Elsberg incision
  endaural incision
  enlarged incision
  enterotomy incision
  epigastric incision
  exploratory incision
  extraoral incision
  Falope-ring dual-incision
    instrument
  Falope-ring single-
    incision instrument
  Fergusson incision
  fishmouth incision
  flank incision
  flexed incision
  forequadrant incision
  Fowler angular incision
  Fowler incision
  Fowler-Weir incision
  frontotemporal craniot-
    omy incision
  Furniss incision
  Gaenslen incision
  Gatellier incision
  Gibson incision
  Gibson-Foley incision
  Gibson-Gibson posterior
    muscle-cutting incision
  Gillies incision
  Gilquist incision
  gingival incision
  gingivolabial incision
  Graefe incision
  grayline incision
  Greenhow incision
  Greenhow-Rodman
    incision
  gridiron incision

incision *continued*

groin incision
guillotine incision
Gunter Von Noorden
    incision
H-flap incision
H-incision
Halsted incision
Halsted-Meyer incision
Halsted-Willy Meyer
    incision
Handley incision
Harman incision
Harris incision
head-low incision
healing biopsy incision
healing incision site
Heermann incision
Heineke-Mikulicz
    incision
hemitransfixion incision
Henry incision
herniorrhaphy incision
Higgins incision
high incision
hockey-stick incision
hockey-stick "Rush"
    incision
Hodo-Kirklin incision
Hoke three-level incision
Hood-Kirkland incision
horizontal incision
Hugh Young incision
inframammary incision
infraorbital incision
infraumbilical incision
inguinal incision
initial incision
intercartilaginous incision
intestinal incision
intracapsular incision
intranasal intercartilagi-
    nous incision
inverted-T incision
inverted-U abdominal
    incision
J-shaped incision

incision *continued*

Jackson incision
Jalaguier incision
Joel-Cohen incision
Kammerer incision
Kammerer-Battle incision
Kehr incision
keratome incision
Kerr incision
Killian incision
Kocher biliary tract
    incision
Kocher collar incision
Kocher collar thyroidec-
    tomy incision
Kocher incision
Kocher modified-
    McBurney incision
L-curved incision
Lahey incision
lamellar incision
Lamm incision
Langenbeck incision
LaRoque herniorrhaphy
    incision
lateral flank incision
lateral incision
lateral rectus incision
lazy-H incision
lazy-S incision
lazy-Z incision
Lempert incision
Lempert incision for
    radical tympanoplasty
Leslie incision
Lilienthal incision
limbal incision
line incision
linear incision
linear skin incision
linear transverse incision
Linton incision
long oblique incision
longitudinal incision
longitudinal midline
    incision
Longuet incision

incision *continued*
   low incision
   low midline incision
   low transverse incision
   lower midline incision
   Ludloff incision
   lumboiliac incision
   Lyman incision
   Lynch incision
   MacFee incision
   Mackenrodt incision
   malar incision
   Manske-McCarroll-
     Swanson incision
   Martin incision
   Mason incision
   mastectomy incision
   Maylard incision
   Mayo-Robson incision
   McArthur incision
   McBurney gridiron
     incision
   McBurney incision
   McIndoe incision
   McKissock incision
   McLaughlin incision
   McMahon-Laird incision
   McVay incision
   medial incision
   medial parapatellar
     incision
   median appendectomy
     incision
   median incision
   median parapatellar
     incision
   median sternotomy
     incision
   Mercedes incision
   Meyer hockey-stick
     incision
   Meyer incision
   Meyer-Halsted incision
   midabdominal transverse
     incision
   midline abdominal
     incision

incision *continued*
   midline incision
   midline sternum-splitting
     incision
   midsternum splitting
     incision
   Mikulicz incision
   Morison incision
   Morris incision
   Moynihan incision
   Munro Kerr incision
   muscle-splitting incision
   myringotomy incision
   Nagamatsu incision
   nasal incision
   oblique incision
   oblique inguinal incision
   oblique relaxing incision
   Obwegeser incision
   Ollier incision
   omega-shaped incision
   operative incision
   orbicular incision
   original incision
   Orr incision
   oval incision
   paracostal incision
   parainguinal incision
   parallel incision
   paramedian appendec-
     tomy incision
   paramedian incision
   paramuscular incision
   parapatellar incision
   pararectus incision
   parasagittal incision
   parascapular incision
   paraumbilical incision
   paravaginal incision
   Parker incision
   parumbilical incision
   Péan incision
   penile-scrotal incision
   penoscrotal incision
   perianal incision
   periareolar incision
   perilimbal incision

incision *continued*

peripatellar incision
perirectal incision
periscapular incision
peritoneal incision
Perthes incision
Pfannenstiel incision
Phemister incision
planar incision
pleuropericardial incision
popliteal incision
postauricular incision
posterior incision
posterior stab incision
posterolateral incision
Pringle incision
proximal incision
puboxyphoid incision
puncture incision
pyelotomy incision
Quervain incision (also
   de Quervain)
racket incision
racquet incision
radial incision
Ragnault incision
Rambo endaural incision
rectus incision
rectus muscle-splitting
   incision
recumbent incision
relaxing incision
releasing incision
relief incision
Rethi incision
retroauricular incision
right rectus incision
right upper paramedian
   incision
rim incision
Risdon extraoral incision
Rockey-Davis appendec-
   tomy incision
Rockey-Davis incision
Rodman mastectomy
   incision
Rollet incision
Rosen incision

incision *continued*

Rosen incision knife
Roux-en-Y incision
Roux-en-Y jejunal loop
   incision
Rush incision
Russe incision
S-flap incision
S-shaped incision
saber incision
sabercut incision
saber-slash incision
salmon backcut incision
Salus incision
Sanders incision
saw incision
scalp incision
Schobinger incision
Schuchardt incision
scratch incision
scratch-type incision
scrotal incision
semicircular incision
semiflexed incision
semilunar incision
semishelving incision
serpentine incision
Shambaugh endaural
   incision
Shambaugh incision
sharp incision
Shea incision
Shea-Hough incision
shelving incision
shield incision
Shoepinger incision
shoulder-strap incision
Silovi incision
Simon incision
Singleton incision
sinuous incision
skin incision
skinfold incision
skinline incision
Skoog incision in palmar
   fasciectomy
Slaughter incision
Sloan abdominal incision

incision *continued*

Sloan incision
slot incision
slot-type rim incision
smile incision
smiling incision
Smith-Petersen incision
Souttar craniotomy incision
Souttar incision
Souttar skin incision
spiral incision
split incision
split-heel incision
St. Mark incision
stab incision
stab-wound incision
stellate incision
stepladder incision
Steri-stripped incision
sternal-splitting incision
Stewart incision
stocking-seam incision
straight incision
Strömbeck incision
Strömbeck mammaplasty incision
subcostal flank incision
subcostal incision
subinguinal incision
submammary incision
suboccipital incision
subtrochanteric incision
subumbilical incision
supracervical incision
suprapubic appendectomy incision
suprapubic incision
supraumbilical incision
surgical incision
Swan incision
T-incision
T-shaped incision
T-tube incision
temporal incision
Tenderfoot incision-making device

incision *continued*

tennis-racket incision
tepee incision
Thomas-Warren incision
thoracicoabdominal incision
thoracoabdominal incision
thoracotomy incision
Timbrall-Fisher incision
tracheal incision
transacromial incision
transaxillary incision
transection incision
transmeatal incision
transrectus incision
transverse abdominal incision
transverse appendectomy incision
transverse incision
trap incision
trapdoor incision
trifurcate incision
Turner-Warwick incision
U-shaped incision
Uchida incision
upper abdominal midline incision
upper midline incision
upward-gaze incision
utility-type incision
V-shaped incision
vermis incision
vertical bur-hole incision
vertical elliptical incision
vertical incision
vertical lateral parapatellar incision
vertical midline incision
Vischer incision
Vischer lumboiliac incision
von Graefe (see *Graef*)
von Langenbeck incision
Von Noorden incision
W-shaped incision

incision *continued*
    Ward-Hendrick incision
    Warren incision
    Watson-Jones incision
    Weber-Fergusson incision
    Weber-Fergusson-Longmire incision
    wedge incision
    Weir incision
    Wheeler incision
    Whipple incision
    wide skin incision
    Wies entropion incision
    Wilde incision
    Willy Meyer incision
    Wise breast incision
    xiphoid to os pubis incision
    xiphoid to umbilicus incision
    Y-incision
    York-Mason incision
    Y-shaped incision
    Y-type incision
    Z-flap incision
    Z-incision
    Z-plasty incision
    Z-shaped incision
    zigzag incision
incision and drainage (I&D)
incision and drainage of abscess
incision and drainage of bursa
incision and drainage of gland
incision and packing
incision and packing of wound
incision and removal of calculus
incision and resuture of wound
incision carried down
incision clean and dry
incision closed anatomically
incision closed in layers
incision closed musculofascially
incision curved downward
incision curved periscapularly
incision extended bilaterally
incision healed per primam intentionem
incision healed per secundam intentionem
incision into organ or tissue
incision line
incision of organ or tissue
incision retractor
incision scissors
incision site
incision widened
incisional
incisional biopsy
incisional hernia
incisional joint
incisional site draining
incisive
incisive canal
incisive foramen
incisive fossa
incisive muscle
incisive papilla
incisive sutures
incisivi labii inferioris, musculus
incisivi labii superioris, musculus
incisor
incisura (*pl.* incisurae)
incisura angularis ventriculi
incisura cardiaca ventriculi
incisurae helicis, musculus
Inclan graft
Inclan-Ober procedure
Inclan-Ober scapula procedure
inclination
inclination angle
inclined-plane elevator
inclusion
inclusion cyst
incompatibility
incompatible blood transfusion
incompatible bone marrow
incompetence
incompetent
incompetent aortic valve
incompetent atrioventricular valve
incompetent cervix
incompetent esophageal sphincter

incompetent foramen ovale
incompetent ileocecal valve
incompetent mitral valve
incompetent perforator
incompetent pulmonic valve
incompetent sphincter
incompetent tricuspid valve
incompetent valve
incompetent vein
incomplete
incomplete abortion
incomplete breech position
incomplete dislocation
incomplete fracture
incomplete hernia
incomplete left bundle branch
    block
incomplete paralysis
incomplete pregnancy
incomplete separation
incomplete thrombosis
inconclusive pattern
inconclusive pelvic exam
incongruous
Incono bag
inconsistency
incontinence
incontinence clamp
incontinence prosthesis
incontinent ileostomy
incontinent of feces
incontinent of stool
incontinent of urine
increment
incremental movement
incremental pacing
incubate
incubation
incubator
incudal fold
incudectomy
incudomalleal joint
incudomalleolar articulation
incudomalleolar joint
incudopexy
incudostapedial
incudostapedial articulation

incudostapedial joint
incudostapedial joint knife
incudostapedial knife
incudostapediopexy
incurvated
incus
incus bone
incus hook
incus replacement prosthesis
incus repositioning
indentation
independence
independent ambulation
index (*pl.* indices)
index finger
index of refraction
index of response
India rubber suture
Indian flap
Indian operation
Indian rhinoplasty
Indian rotation flap
Indian skin flap operation
Indiana conservative hip
Indiana reamer
indicated
indication
indicative of
indicator
indicator-dilution technique
indices (*sing.* index)
indicis proprius, musculus
indifferent electrode
indigo carmine dye
indirect ballottement
indirect contact with contami-
    nated instrument
indirect fracture
indirect fulguration
indirect hemagglutination
indirect hernia
indirect hernia sac
indirect infection
indirect inguinal hernia
indirect ophthalmoscope
indirect ophthalmoscopy
indirect reflex

indiscrete
indiscriminate lesion
indium scan
indium-64 scan
indium-111 scan
individual components
individual layers
individual therapy
individualized care
individualized transfusion
    therapy
individually clamped and
    coagulated
individually clamped and
    ligated
individually ligated
indolent radiation-induced
    rectal ulcer
Indong Oh prosthesis
induced abortion
induced anesthesia
induced change
induced delivery
induced labor
induced pneumothorax
induced sleep
induction
induction of anesthesia
induction of labor
inductive resistance
indurated
indurated mass
induration
induration and swelling
industrial accident
indwelling
indwelling catheter
indwelling catheter program
    (ICP)
indwelling stent
indwelling ureteral stent
inelastic
inevitable abortion
infant abdominal retractor
infant abduction splint
infant Ambu resuscitator
infant biopsy forceps

infant bougie
infant bronchoscope
infant catheter
infant cystoscope
infant dilator
infant electrotome
infant esophagoscope
infant eye speculum
infant eyelid retractor
infant feeding tube
infant female catheter
infant male catheter
infant rib retractor
infant rib shears
infant rib spreader
infant sound
infant telescope
infant urethral sound
infant urethrotome
infant vaginal speculum
infant vaginoscope
infant vascular clamp
infantile cataract
infantile condition
infantile hernia
infantile organ
infantometer
infarct
infarct-avid scintigraphy
infarctectomy
infarcted bowel
infarcted scar
infarcted transverse colon
infarction
infected case
infected incisional site
infected organ
infected wound
infecting organism
infection
infection complications
infection control
infection control program
infection prevention
infection route
infection spread
infectious disease

infectious etiology
infectious process
infective disorder
inferior
inferior alveolar artery
inferior alveolar nerve
inferior alveolar vein
inferior artery
inferior cardiac cervical nerve
inferior carotid triangle
inferior cerebellar arteries
inferior cerebellar veins
inferior cerebral veins
inferior clunial nerves
inferior constrictor pharyngeal
    muscle
inferior displacement
inferior duodenal fold
inferior duodenal recess
inferior epigastric artery
inferior fascia
inferior fissure
inferior flexure of duodenum
inferior frontal gyrus
inferior ganglion
inferior ganglion of vagus
inferior gemellus muscle
inferior gluteal artery
inferior gluteal nerve
inferior gluteal veins
inferior labial artery
inferior labial veins
inferior lacrimal canaliculus
inferior laryngeal artery
inferior laryngeal nerve
inferior laryngeal vein
inferior laryngotomy
inferior lateral cutaneous nerve
    of arm
inferior maxilla
inferior mesenteric artery (IMA)
inferior mesenteric ganglion
inferior nasal concha
inferior nerve
inferior oblique (IO)
inferior oblique muscle
inferior omental recess

inferior ophthalmic vein
inferior palpebral vein
inferior pancreaticoduodenal
    arteries
inferior parathyroid gland
inferior petrosal sinus
inferior phrenic arteries
inferior phrenic vein
inferior pole of thyroid
inferior posterior serratus
    muscle
inferior rectal artery
inferior rectal nerves
inferior rectal vein
inferior rectus (IR)
inferior root of ansa cervicalis
inferior sagittal sinus
inferior suprarenal artery
inferior tarsal muscle
inferior tarsus
inferior thyroid artery
inferior thyroid gland
inferior thyroid notch
inferior thyroid vein
inferior tracheotomy
inferior transverse ligament
inferior turbinate
inferior tympanic artery
inferior ulnar artery
inferior vein
inferior vena cava
inferior vena cava interruption
inferior venacavography
inferior vertebral notch
inferior vesical artery
inferior vessels
inferior wall
inferoapical defect
inferolateral
inferolateral aspect
inferomedian
inferonasally
inferoposterior
inferosuperior axial projection
inferosuperior projection
inferosuperior tangential
    projection

inferotemporal
infertility
infertility detection
infestation
infested material
infiltrate
infiltrated duct cell carcinoma
infiltrated with Xylocaine
infiltrating
infiltrating adenocarcinoma
infiltrating carcinoma
infiltrating ductal cell carcinoma
infiltrating glioma
infiltration
infiltration anesthesia
infiltrative process
inflamed
inflamed appendix
inflamed diverticulum
inflamed gallbladder
inflamed organ
inflammation
inflammation and swelling
inflammation of organ
inflammation of tissue
inflammatory bowel disease
    (IBD)
inflammatory bowel syndrome
    (IBS)
inflammatory change
inflammatory condition
inflammatory disease
inflammatory fibroid polyp
inflammatory fracture
inflammatory lesion
inflammatory mass
inflammatory pelvic disease
    (IPD)
inflammatory process
inflammatory reaction
inflammatory response
inflammatory tissue
inflatable
inflatable catheter
inflatable cuff
inflatable Foley bag catheter
inflatable mammary prosthesis

inflatable penile implant
inflatable penile prosthesis with
    reservoir
inflatable prosthesis
inflatable splint
inflatable tourniquet cuff
inflatable tracheal tube cuff
inflatable urinary incontinence
    prosthesis
inflated balloon
inflated eardrum
inflated tourniquet
inflation
inflation of bulb
inflation of tourniquet
inflator
inflow of arterial blood
inflow tract
influence
infolding
informed consent
infra-axillary
infracalcarine gyrus
infraclavicular
infraclavicular fossa
infraclavicular region
infraclavicular triangle
infracostal
infracted
infracted turbinate
infraction
infraction of turbinate
infracubital bypass
infraduction
infraglenoid
infrahepatic arteriography
infrahepatic arteriography and
    infusion
infrahepatic caval anastomosis
infrahyoid muscles
inframammary
inframammary crease
inframammary fold
inframammary incision
inframammary region
inframaxillary
infranodal extrasystole

infraoccipital nerve
infraorbital
infraorbital artery
infraorbital block
infraorbital branch of interior maxillary artery
infraorbital branch of maxillary nerve
infraorbital canal
infraorbital foramen
infraorbital incision
infraorbital nerve
infraorbital region
infraorbital sutures
infraorbitalis, arteria
infraorbitalis, nervus
infraorbitomeatal line
infrapatellar
infrapatellar fat pad
infrapatellar synovial fold
infrapiriform foramen
infrared microscope
infrared photocoagulation
infrared spectrophotometry
infrarenal node
infrascapular
infrascapular region
infrasonic frequency
infraspinatus
infraspinatus, musculus
infraspinatus reflex
infraspinatus tendon
infraspinous
infraspinous muscle
infrasternal
infrasternal angle of thorax
infratemporal fossa
infratemporal region
infratentorial
infratrochlear
infratrochlear branch of ophthalmic nerve
infratrochlear nerve
infratrochlearis, nervus
infraumbilical fold
infraumbilical incision
infrequent menstruation

infrequent pulse
infundibula (*sing.* infundibulum)
infundibula of kidney
infundibular forceps
infundibular punch
infundibular resection
infundibular rongeur
infundibular rongeur forceps
infundibular ventricular septal defect
infundibulectomy
infundibulectomy rongeur
infundibuliform
infundibuliform fascia
infundibulopelvic
infundibulopelvic ligament
infundibulum (*pl.* infundibula)
infundibulum of fallopian tube
infundibulum of heart
infundibulum of hypophysis
infundibulum of urinary bladder
infundibulum of uterine tube
Infusaid chemotherapy pump
Infusaid hepatic pump
Infusaid implantable drug delivery system
Infusaid infusion pump
Infusaid pump
Infusaid pump for drug infusion
infusate
Infuse-A-Port
infuser
infusing solutions
infusion
infusion cannula
infusion catheter
infusion chemotherapy
infusion device
infusion drip
infusion nephrotomography
infusion of antibiotics
infusion of chemotherapeutic agent
infusion pump
infusion pyelogram
infusion pyelography

infusion rate
infusion site
infusion technique
infusion tube
infusion-withdrawal pump
Ingals cannula
Ingals flexible silver cannula
Ingals nasal speculum
Ingals rectal injection cannula
Ingals speculum
Inge lamina spreader
Inge laminectomy retractor
Inge procedure
Inge retractor
Inge spreader
Ingersoll adenoid curet
Ingersoll curet
Ingersoll needle
Ingersoll tonsil needle
ingested
ingestion
ingestion of barium
ingestion of drugs
Inglis reconstruction
Inglis-Cooper technique
Inglis-Ranawat-Straub approach
Ingraham infant skull punch
Ingraham skull punch
Ingraham-Fowler clip-applying
    forceps
Ingraham-Fowler tantalum clip
Ingram catheter
Ingram operation for talipes
    equinovarus
Ingram operation for talipes
    valgus
Ingram procedure
Ingram regimen
Ingram technique
ingredient
ingress tube
ingrown hair
ingrown nail
ingrown toenail
ingrowth
inguinal
inguinal adenopathy

inguinal area
inguinal artery
inguinal canal
inguinal falx
inguinal fossa
inguinal hernia
inguinal hernia repair
inguinal herniorrhaphy
inguinal incision
inguinal ligament
inguinal lymph node
inguinal nerve
inguinal node dissection
inguinal nodes
inguinal reflex
inguinal region
inguinal ring
inguinal sphincter
inguinal triangle
inguinoabdominal
inguinocrural
inguinocrural hernia
inguinofemoral
inguinofemoral hernia
inguinolabial
inguinoproperitoneal
inguinoproperitoneal hernia
inguinoscrotal
inguinosuperficial
inguinosuperficial hernia
inhalant
inhalation
inhalation anesthesia
inhalation cannula
inhalation therapy
inhaled air
inherent risk
inherited abnormality
inherited disorder
inherited genetic defect
inherited tendency
inhibit blood clots
inhibit labor
inhibiting factor
inhibition
inhibition sign
inhibitor

inhibitory
initial diagnosis
initial dose
initial incision
initial therapy
initial treatment
initial venous shunt
initialization
initially
initiate therapy
initiation
injectable
injected
injecting contrast medium
injection
injection cannula
injection mass
injection needle
injection of air
injection of bursa
injection of contrast medium
injection of drug
injection of dye
injection of hemorrhoids
injection of radiopaque material
injection of varices
injection port
injector
injured limb
injured organ
injured patient
injured tissue
injury
injury site
inlay
inlay bone graft
inlay graft
inlay inguinal herniorrhaphy
inlet
inlet cannula
inlet forceps
inlet views
inner aspect
inner callus
inner canthus
inner core for outside housing
inner ear

inner ear ablation
inner hamstring
inner layer
inner pillar
inner quadrant
inner surface
inner table
inner table bones of skull
inner table frontal bone
inner table of skull
innermost intercostal muscles
innermost membrane of
    meninges
innervated muscles
innervation
innervation apraxia
innocent gallstone
innocent murmur
innocuous lump
innocuous tumor
Innomed bone curet
Innomed curet
innominate
innominate aneurysm
innominate artery
innominate bone
innominate endarterectomy
innominate osteotomy
innominate veins
Innovar anesthetic agent
innovation
Innovator Holter system
INO (internuclear ophthalmo-
    plegia)
inoculation
inoperable
inoperable cancer
inoperable carcinoma
inoperable condition
inoperable malignancy
inoperable patient
inoperable tumor
inorganic murmur
Inoue balloon catheter
inpatient surgery
input device
input frequency

input impedance
input shunt
input shunt incapacitance
input stage
input terminal
input voltage
inquiry
Inrad fine-needle prostate
　　aspiration kit
INRO surgical nail splint
Insall approach
Insall-Burstein arthroplasty
Insall-Burstein intracondylar
　　knee implant
Insall-Burstein knee prosthesis
Insall-Burstein prosthesis
Insall-Burstein total knee
　　prosthesis
Insall-Burstein total knee
　　replacement
Insall-Burstein total knee system
Insall-Burstein-Freeman total
　　knee
Insall-Hood posterior cruciate
　　reconstruction
insensible fluid output
insert mattress sutures
insert tube
inserted and positioned
inserter tack
insertion
insertion forceps
insertion of cannula
insertion of catheter
insertion of fixation device
insertion of metal plate
insertion of nail
insertion of pacemaker
insertion of pack
insertion of pin
insertion of prosthesis
insertion of radioactive material
insertion of radium
insertion of screw
insertion of T-tube
insertion of tampon
insertion of traction device

insertion of tube
insertion of vaginal pack
insertion of vascular prosthesis
insertion of wire
insertion tandem
inside diameter
insidious
inspected
inspection
inspection, palpation, percus-
　　sion, and auscultation
　　(IPPA)
inspersion
inspirated
inspiration
inspiratory
inspiratory dyspnea
inspiratory flow
inspiratory flow rate
inspiratory force
inspiratory murmur
inspiratory muscles
inspiratory pressure
inspiratory respiration
inspiratory sounds
inspiratory spasm
inspiratory stridor
inspiratory wheezing
inspiratory/expiratory ratio (I/E
　　ratio)
inspired oxygen
Inspiron device
inspissated
inspissated cerumen
inspissated feces
instability
instability of joint
Insta-clens handwasher
　　machine
installation
instant delivery
instantaneous axis of rotation
instantaneous pressure
Instastan
instep
instill
instill drops

instillation
instillation of anesthesia
instillation of contrast medium
instillation of diagnostic media
instillator
instinct
institution of therapy
instrument
instrument birth
instrument cradle
instrument cradling system
instrument guide
instrument holder
instrument marker
instrument polish
instrument rack
instrument roll
instrument set
instrument stand
instrument sterilizer
instrument sterilizing case
instrument table
instrument, sponge, and needle
    count
instrumental
instrumental compression
instrumental dilation
instrumentation
instrument-grasping forceps
instrument-handling forceps
insufficiency
insufflated peritoneal cavity
insufflation
insufflation anesthesia
insufflation device
insufflation of fallopian tubes
insufflation of lungs
insufflation of uterus
insufflator
        Buckstein colonic
            insufflator
        Buckstein insufflator
        colonic insufflator
        Dench insufflator
        Kidde insufflator
        Kidde tubal insufflator
        KLI insufflator

insufflator *continued*
        laparoscopy insufflator
        Neal insufflator
        Reuben insufflator
        tubal insufflator
        tube insufflator
        Venturi insufflator
        Weber colonic insufflator
        Weber insufflator
insular sclerosis
insular scotoma
insulated bayonet forceps
insulated forceps
insulated monopolar forceps
insulated suction tube
insulated tissue forceps
insulin
insulin pen pump
insurance
intact
intact anastomosis
intact bone structure
Intact catheter
intact hymen
intact motor tract
intact rib cage
intact skin sutures
intact tissues
intact tonsils
Intact xenograft prosthetic valve
intake
intake and output (I&O)
integral asepsis
integral dose
integral fiberoptic sheath
integrated electromyogram
integrated shape imaging
    system (ISIS)
integrating microscope
integration
integrity
InteguDerm dressing
integument
intense concentration
intensification factor
intensifying screen
intensity

intensive treatment
intent
intention
intentional replantation
interaction
interannular segment
interaortic balloon pump
interarterial fluid
interarticular cartilage
interarticular disk
interarytenoid muscle
interarytenoid notch
interatrial conduction delay
interatrial groove
interatrial septal defect
interatrial septum
interauditory canal tomogram
interauricular loop
interauricular septum
interbody circular rasp
interbody fusion
interbody fusion instruments
interbody fusion rasp
interbody graft tamp
interbody rasp
intercanthal distance (ICD)
intercanthic diameter
intercapillary nephrosclerosis
intercapital veins
intercapitales, venae
intercapitular vein of foot
intercapitular vein of hand
intercarotid ganglion
intercarpal articulation
intercarpal joint
intercartilaginous
intercartilaginous incision
intercartilaginous rim
intercavernous sinus
intercellular bridges
intercellular space
intercellular tissue space
interchangeable ear instruments
interchangeable forceps tips
interchangeable laryngeal
    forceps tips
interchangeable punch handle

interchondral articulation
interclavicular notch
intercondylar eminence
intercondylar fracture
intercondylar groove
intercondylar notch
intercondylar notch of femur
intercondylar process
interconnection
intercostal
intercostal anesthesia
intercostal arteries
intercostal articulation
intercostal block
intercostal catheter
intercostal drain
intercostal groove
intercostal margin
intercostal muscle
intercostal nerves
intercostal retraction
intercostal space
intercostal tenderness
intercostal trocar
intercostal tube
intercostal vein
intercostal vessels
intercostales anteriores, venae
intercostales externi, musculi
intercostales interni, musculi
intercostales, musculi
intercostales posteriores,
    arteriae
intercostales posteriores, venae
intercostalis superior dextra,
    vena
intercostalis superior sinistra,
    vena
intercostalis suprema, arteria
intercostalis suprema, vena
intercostobrachial nerves
intercostobrachiales, nervi
intercricothyroidotomy
intercricothyrotomy
interdental splint
interdental wire
interdermal buried sutures

interdigital
interdigital ligament
interdigital spaces
interdigitation
interelectrode distance
interface
interfacial surface tension
interfemoral
interference
interference microscope
interfering artifact
interhemispheric derivation
interilioabdominal amputation
interinnominoabdominal
    amputation
interior chest wall
interior maxillary branch of
    external carotid artery
interior mesogastric hernia
interior of tumor excavated
interlacing blood vessels
interlacing ligatures
interlaminar procedure
interlobar arteries
interlobar arteries of kidney
interlobar fissure
interlobar notch
interlobar veins
interlobar veins of kidney
interlobares renis, arteriae
interlobares renis, venae
interlobular arteries
interlobular arteries of kidney
interlobular arteries of liver
interlobular bile
interlobular veins of kidney
interlobular veins of liver
interlobulares hepatis, arteriae
interlobulares hepatis, venae
interlobulares renis, arteriae
interlobulares renis, venae
interlocked mesh prosthesis
interlocking ligatures
interlocking sound
interlocking sutures
interloop abscess
intermaxillary bone

intermaxillary fixation
intermaxillary sutures
intermaxillary traction
intermediary
intermediary amputation
intermediate
intermediate amputation
intermediate callus
intermediate dorsal cutaneous
    nerve
intermediate nerve
intermediate operation
intermediate supraclavicular
    nerves
intermediate tendon of dia-
    phragm
intermediate-weighted MR
    images
Intermedics APR universal hip
    system
Intermedics Cyberlith X
    multiprogrammable
    pacemaker
Intermedics intraocular lens
Intermedics intraocular lens
    implant
Intermedics intraocular radius
    gauge
Intermedics lithium-powered
    pacemaker
Intermedics pacemaker
Intermedics phaco and I-A kits
Intermedics pulse generator
Intermedics Quantum pace-
    maker
Intermedics Quantum program-
    mable pulse generator
Intermedics Quantum unipolar
    pacemaker
Intermedics Thinlith II pace-
    maker
intermedius, nervus
intermenstrual bleeding
intermenstrual pain
intermenstrual spotting
intermesenteric abscess
intermetacarpal articulation

intermetatarsal articulation
intermittent
intermittent claudication
intermittent mandatory ventilation (IMV)
intermittent pain
intermittent pneumatic compression (IPC)
intermittent positive pressure breathing (IPPB)
intermittent sutures
intermittent therapy
intermittent traction
intermuscular
intermuscular hernia
intermuscular septum
internal
internal abdominal ring
internal acoustic orifice
internal anal sphincter
internal anatomy
internal calcaneoastragaloid ligament
internal callus
internal capsule
internal carotid artery
internal carotid nerve
internal cerebral veins
internal crucial ligament
internal decompression trocar
internal derangement
internal ear
internal fibrocartilage
internal fistula
internal fixating device
internal fixation
internal fixation device
internal fixation of fracture
internal hemorrhage
internal hemorrhoidectomy
internal hemorrhoids
internal hernia
internal iliac artery
internal iliac vein
internal inguinal ring
internal intercostal muscles
internal intussusception

internal jugular vein
internal lateral ligament
internal mammary artery (IMA)
internal mammary artery bypass (IMAB)
internal mammary artery catheter
internal mammary artery graft
internal maxillary vein
internal monitor
internal oblique fascia
internal oblique muscle
internal obturator muscle
internal os
internal pillars
internal proctotomy
internal pudendal artery
internal pudendal vein
internal rectal sphincter
internal rotation
internal rotation contracture of hip
internal spermatic artery
internal spermatic fascia
internal spermatic vessels
internal sphincter
internal sphincterotomy
internal table
internal thoracic artery graft (ITA graft)
internal thyroarytenoid muscle
internal tibial torsion (ITT)
internal traction
internal urethral orifice
internal urethrotomy
internal vein stripper
internal vein stripping
internal version
internasal suture
International Federation of Gynecology and Obstetrics (FIGO)
international standard goniometer
internodal tract
internuclear ophthalmoplegia (INO)

interossea anterior, arteria
interossea communis, arteria
interossea posterior, arteria
interossea recurrens, arteria
interossei dorsales manus,
    musculi
interossei dorsales pedis,
    musculi
interossei palmares, musculi
interossei plantares, musculi
interosseous anterior nerve
interosseous artery
interosseous cartilage
interosseous cruris nerve
interosseous dorsalis nerve
interosseous knife
interosseous ligament
interosseous membrane
interosseous muscle
interosseous nerve
interosseous posterior nerve
interosseous talocalcaneal
    ligament
interosseous veins
interosseous wire fixation
interosseus anterior, nervus
interosseus cruris, nervus
interosseus dorsalis, nervus
interosseus posterior, nervus
interpalpebral
interpalpebral suture
interpalpebral zone
interparietal
interparietal bone
interparietal hernia
interparietal sulcus
interpedicular joint space
interpeduncular cistern
interpeduncular fossa
interpeduncular ganglion
interpelviabdominal amputation
interperiosteal fracture
interphalangeal
interphalangeal articulation
interphalangeal joint (IPJ)
interpleural space
interpolated flap

interpolation
Interpore
Interpore block
Interpore granule
Interpore porous hydroxy-
    apatite block
Interpore preshaped wedge
interposition arthroplasty
interposition Dacron graft
interposition graft
interposition of colon
interposition of graft
interposition of uterus
interposition operation
interposition uterine suspension
interpositional arthroplasty
interpretation
interpubic disk
interpupillary distance (IPD)
interpupillary line
interradicular alveoloplasty
interrupted black silk sutures
interrupted chromic catgut
    sutures
interrupted chromic sutures
interrupted cotton sutures
interrupted far-near sutures
interrupted fashion
interrupted fine silk sutures
interrupted Lembert sutures
interrupted mattress sutures
interrupted near-far sutures
interrupted plain catgut sutures
interrupted respiration
interrupted silk sutures
interrupted sutures
interrupted vertical mattress
    sutures
interruption
interscapular amputation
interscapular reflex
interscapular region
interscapulothoracic amputation
intersigmoid
intersigmoid hernia
intersigmoid recess
interspace

interspace narrowing
intersphincteric abscess
intersphincteric anal fistula
interspinal muscles
interspinal muscles of thorax
interspinales, musculi
interspinous pseudarthrosis
interstice
interstitial
interstitial atrophy
interstitial fibrosis
interstitial gland
interstitial hernia
interstitial implant
interstitial implantation
interstitial markings
interstitial pneumonia
interstitial radiation
interstitial spaces
interstitial therapy
interstitial tissues
Intertach pacemaker
intertarsal articulation
interthalamic commissure
interthoracoscapular amputation
intertragic notch
intertransversarii, musculi
intertransverse muscles
intertrochanteric crest
intertrochanteric fracture
intertrochanteric line
intertrochanteric plate
intertrochanteric ridge
intertuberal diameter
intertubercular groove
intertubular tissue
interureteric fold
interureteric ridge
intervaginal
interval
interval improvement
interval operation
intervening period
intervening tissues
intervention
interventional radiology
interventricular artery

interventricular cartilage
interventricular conduction
    defect
interventricular disk
interventricular fibrocartilage
interventricular foramen
interventricular ganglion
interventricular groove
interventricular heart block
interventricular notch
interventricular septal defect
    (IVSD)
interventricular septum
interventricular space
interventricular sulcus of heart
interventricular vein
intervertebral
intervertebral body
intervertebral curet
intervertebral disk
intervertebral disk forceps
intervertebral disk rongeur
intervertebral disk rongeur
    forceps
intervertebral punch
intervertebral vein
intervertebralis, vena
intervillous circulation
intervillous lacuna
interwoven bundle
intestinal
intestinal adhesions
intestinal anastomosis
intestinal anastomosis clamp
intestinal arteries
intestinal atony
intestinal atresia
intestinal bag
intestinal bleeding
intestinal bypass
intestinal calculus
intestinal clamp
intestinal contents
intestinal decompression
intestinal decompression trocar
intestinal diversion conduit
intestinal diverticulum

intestinal flora
intestinal fluid
intestinal forceps
intestinal glands
intestinal hernia
intestinal herniation
intestinal incision
intestinal infarction
intestinal intussusception
intestinal loop
intestinal lumen
intestinal motility disorder
intestinal mucosa
intestinal needle
intestinal obstruction
intestinal occlusion clamp
intestinal occlusion retractor
intestinal peritoneum
intestinal plication needle
intestinal polyp
intestinal prolapse
intestinal ring clamp
intestinal scissors
intestinal secretions
intestinal stasis
intestinal sutures
intestinal tissue-holding forceps
intestinal tract
intestinal trocar
intestinal tube
intestinal villi
intestinal web
intestinales, arteriae
intestine
intestinointestinal reflex
intima
intimal arteriosclerosis
intimal hyperplasia
intimal injury
intimal layer
intimal thickening
intimectomy
intimectomy knife
intolerable pain
intolerance
intoxication
intra vitam

intra-abdominal
intra-abdominal abscess
intra-abdominal adhesions
intra-abdominal contents
intra-abdominal exploration
intra-abdominal hemorrhage
intra-abdominal ileal reservoir
intra-abdominal laser procedure
intra-abdominal mass
intra-abdominal procedure
intra-abdominal surgery
intra-abdominal vasectomy
intra-abdominal viscera
intra-amniotic saline injection
intra-anal wart
intra-aortic
intra-aortic balloon
intra-aortic balloon assist device
intra-aortic balloon catheter
intra-aortic balloon counterpul-
    sation
intra-aortic balloon pump
    (IABP)
intra-aortic balloon pumping
    (IABP)
intra-arterial
intra-arterial cannula
intra-arterial chemotherapy
    catheter
intra-arterial digital subtraction
    angiography
intra-arterial injection
intra-articular arthrodesis
intra-articular fracture
Intra-Articular Surgical System
    cutter
intra-atrial baffle
intra-atrial conduction defect
intra-auricular muscle
intra-axial brain tumor
intracameral
intracapsular ankylosis
intracapsular cataract extraction
    (ICCE)
intracapsular fracture
intracapsular incision
intracapsular lens

intracapsular lens expressor
   hook
intracapsular lens extraction
intracapsular lens loupe
intracapsular lens spoon
intracapsular temporomandibular joint arthroplasty
intracapsularly
intracardiac cannula
intracardiac catheter
intracardiac injection
intracardiac needle holder
intracardiac patch
intracardiac patch prosthesis
intracardiac phonocardiography
intracardiac pressure
intracardiac retractor
intracardiac shunt
intracardiac vent
Intracath catheter
intracavernous injection
intracavitary application
intracavitary cesium therapy
intracavitary gynecologic
   applicator
intracavitary radiation
intracavitary radium (ICR)
intracavitary radium insertion
intracavitary therapy
intracellular fluid
intracerebral bleed
intracerebral electrode
intracerebral electroencephalogram
intracerebral hematoma
intracerebral hemorrhage
intracerebral inoculation
intracerebrovascular accident
intracervical bag
intracervical pack
intrachondrial bone
intracisternal puncture
intracondylar
Intracone intramedullary
   reaming system
intracordial Teflon injection set
intracoronary guiding catheter

intracoronary perfusion catheter
intracoronary thrombolysis
intracorporeal heart
intracranial aneursym
intracranial bruit
intracranial calcification
intracranial hemorrhage
intracranial hypertension
intracranial injury
intracranial lesion
intracranial metastasis
intracranial neoplasm
intracranial pressure (ICP)
intracranial pressure catheter
intracranial pressure catheter
   monitor
intracranial pressure monitor
   (ICP monitor)
intracranial pressure Tele-
   Sensor
intracranial tumor
intractable
intractable pain
intractable ulcer
intracutaneous injection
intracutaneous reaction
intracuticular
intracuticular nylon sutures
intracuticular sutures
intracystic
intradermal injection
intradermal mattress sutures
intradermal nevus
intradermal sutures
intraductal
intraductal carcinoma
intraepidermal carcinoma
intraepithelial neoplasia
intraepithelial vessels
intrafat
Intraflex intramedullary pins
intrafusal fibers
intragastric balloon
intragastric bubble
intragastric drip
intrahaustral contraction ring
intrahemispheric fissure

intrahepatic
intrahepatic abscess
intrahepatic atresia
intrahepatic AV fistula
intrahepatic biliary cystic
    dilation
intrahepatic biliary duct
intrahepatic block
intrahepatic cholangiojejunos-
    tomy
intrahepatic radicle
intrahepatic stone
intraligamentous ectopic
    pregancy
intraligamentous pregnancy
intralocular
intraluminal
intraluminal cyst
intraluminal duodenal diverticu-
    lum (IDD)
intraluminal filling defect
intraluminal gas
intraluminal mass
intraluminal pressure
intraluminal radiation therapy
intraluminal stone
intraluminal stripper
intraluminal tube
intraluminal tube prosthesis
intramaxillary fixation
Intramedic tubing
intramedullary
intramedullary and spongiosa
    graft
intramedullary anesthesia
intramedullary bar
intramedullary bone graft
intramedullary broach
intramedullary canal
intramedullary device
intramedullary drill
intramedullary fixation
intramedullary fixation device
intramedullary hemorrhage
intramedullary Küntscher nail
intramedullary nail
intramedullary nailing

intramedullary pin
intramedullary rod
intramedullary wire
intramesenteric abscess
intramucosal insert
intramural
intramural aneurysm
intramural artery
intramural colonic air
intramural diverticulum
intramural fibroid
intramural fistulous tract
intramural fixation
intramural leiomyomata
intramural pregnancy
intramuscular administration
intramuscular injection
Intran disposable intrauterine
    pressure measurement
    catheter
intranasal
intranasal anesthesia
intranasal antral speculum
intranasal application
intranasal block
intranasal bone lever
intranasal ethmoidectomy
intranasal hammer
intranasal intercartilaginous
    incision
intranasal packing
intranasal punch
intranasal saw
intranasal sinusotomy
intranasal splint
intranasal tube
intranuclear inclusion
intraocular
intraocular cannula
intraocular contents
intraocular forceps
intraocular hemorrhage
intraocular instruments
intraocular irrigating forceps
intraocular lens (IOL)
intraocular lens cannula
intraocular lens forceps

intraocular lens implant
intraocular muscles
intraocular pressure (IOP)
intraocular scissors
intraocular tension
Intra-Op autotransfusion system
intraoperative
intraoperative bleeding
intraoperative cholangiogram
intraoperative digital subtraction
    angiography (IDIS angi-
    ography)
intraoperative radiation
intraoral anesthesia
intraoral cancer
intraoral cone
intraoral lesion
intraoral projection
intraoral stent
intraoral wire
intraorbital implant
intraorbital tumor instruments
intraosseous anesthesia
intraosseous fixation
intraosseous therapy
intraosseous venography
intraparietal sulcus
intraparietal sulcus of Turner
intrapartum death
intrapartum hemorrhage
intrapelvic kidney pelvis
intrapelvic protrusion
intrapericardial aorticopulmo-
    nary shunt
intraperiosteal fracture
intraperitoneal adhesions
intraperitoneal air
intraperitoneal chemotherapy
intraperitoneal injection
intraperitoneal migration of
    pacemaker
intraperitoneal pregnancy
intraperitoneal transfusion
intraperitoneal viscus
intrapleural chemotherapy
intrapleural pneumonolysis
intrapleural sealed drainage unit

intrapulmonary hamartoma
intrapulmonary metastasis
intrapulmonary shunt
intrapulpal anesthesia
intrapyretic
intrarectal ultrasonography
intrarenal reflux
intrarenal vein
intraretinal microangiopathy
intraretinal microvascular
    abnormalities (IRMA)
intrascrotal pain
intraseptal alveoloplasty
Intrasil catheter
intraspinal anesthesia
intraspinal block
Intraspray lubricant
intratendinous
intrathecal
intrathecal contrast material
intrathecal injection
intrathecal space
intrathecally
intrathoracic gas volume
intrathoracic Nissen fundoplica-
    tion
intrathoracic pressure variations
intrathoracic stomach
intrathyroid cartilage
intratracheal anesthesia
intratracheal instillation
intratracheal tube
intratreatment
intratrochlear nerve
intrauterine amputation
intrauterine cannula
intrauterine catheter
intrauterine clotting
intrauterine contraceptive
    device (IUCD)
intrauterine curettage
intrauterine device (IUD) (see
    also *device*)
        Birnberg bow intrauter-
        ine device
        bow intrauterine device
        coil intrauterine device

intrauterine device (IUD)
*continued*
    Copper-7 intrauterine device
    Cu-7 intrauterine device
    Hall band intrauterine device
    Hall intrauterine device
    IUD bow
    IUD coil
    IUD string
    Lippes loop intrauterine device
    Margulies coil intrauterine device
    Margulies spiral intrauterine device
    Mazlin spring intrauterine device
    ParaGard intrauterine device
    Progestasert intrauterine device
    Saf-T-Coil intrauterine device
intrauterine fetus
intrauterine fracture
intrauterine gestation
intrauterine growth
intrauterine growth retardation (IUGR)
intrauterine pack
intrauterine pessary
intrauterine pregnancy
intrauterine pressure
intrauterine pressure catheter
intrauterine probe
intrauterine radium application
intrauterine transfusion
intravaginal therapy
intravascular
intravascular coagulation
intravascular coagulopathy
intravascular fluid
intravascular injection
intravascular mass
intravascular pressure

intravenous (IV)
intravenous administration
intravenous anesthesia
intravenous angiocardiography
intravenous bolus injection of contrast medium
intravenous catheter
intravenous cholangiogram (IVC)
intravenous cholangiography (IVC)
intravenous cholecystography
intravenous contrast material
intravenous dose
intravenous drip
intravenous feeding
intravenous fluid
intravenous infusion
intravenous injection
intravenous intubation
intravenous lead
intravenous line
intravenous needle
intravenous pacing catheter
intravenous Pitocin drip
intravenous pyelogram (IVP)
intravenous pyelography
intravenous regional anesthesia
intravenous tension
intravenous therapy
intravenous transfusion
intravenous tubing roller
intravenous urogram
intravenous urography
intraventricular
intraventricular conduction delay (IVCD)
intraventricular hemorrhage
intraventricular pressure
intravesical chemotherapy
intravesical prostatic tissue
intravesical space
intravitreal delivery
intravitreal laser
Intrel II spinal cord stimulation system
intrinsic

intrinsic defect
intrinsic factor
intrinsic mass
intrinsic minus hand
intrinsic pressure
intrinsicoid deflection
introduced
introducer (see also *sphere introducer*)
    Carter introducer sphere
    Carter sphere introducer
    catheter introducer
    Check-Flo introducer
    Cook introducer
    Cope needle introducer cannula
    Desilets-Hoffman catheter introducer
    Desilets-Hoffman introducer
    Desilets-Hoffman micropuncture introducer
    Desilets-Hoffman pacemaker introducer
    electrode introducer
    endolymphatic shunt tube introducer
    Eric Lloyd introducer
    eye sphere introducer
    Fergus percutaneous introducer kit
    French-Daid introducer
    Furlow introducer
    Hemaquet catheter introducer
    Hemaquet introducer
    Hemaquet sheath introducer
    heparin lock introducer
    House endolymphatic shunt tube introducer
    Littleford introducer
    Littleford-Spector introducer
    LPS Peel-Away introducer

introducer *continued*
    metallic sphere introducer
    Micropuncture Peel-Away introducer
    Mullins catheter introducer
    Mullins transseptal introducer
    Nottingham introducer
    peel-away introducer
    percutaneous lead introducer
    permanent lead introducer
    shunt-tube introducer
    sphere introducer
    subclavian introducer
    tube introducer
    Tuohy-Bost introducer
    Tuohy-Bost micropuncture introducer
    ventricular catheter introducer
introducer catheter
introducer for spheres
introducer sheath
introduction
introduction of radiopaque substance
introduction of radium
introitus
intromission
introverted
intrusion
intrusive surgery
intubate
intubated
intubation
intubation and suction
intubation anesthesia
intubation laryngoscope
intubation set
intubation tube
intubationist
intubator
intumescence

intumescent cataract
intussuscepted bowel
intussusception
intussusceptum
intussuscipiens
InVac
invading
invaginated
invaginated nipple
invaginated stump
invagination
invasion
invasive
invasive carcinoma
invasive lesion
invasive procedure
invasive technique
inverse symmetry
inversion
inversion ankle stress x-ray
inversion deformity
inversion operation
inversion position
inversion sprain
inversion time
inverted
inverted cone bur
inverted edge
inverted horseshoe flap
inverted jackknife position
inverted knot sutures
inverted sutures
inverted T-wave
inverted testis
inverted uterus
inverted V-sign
inverted-T fashion
inverted-T incision
inverted-U abdominal in-
    cision
inverter
        appendix inverter
        Barrett appendix inverter
        Barrett inverter
        Mayo-Boldt appendix
            inverter
        Mayo-Boldt inverter

inverter *continued*
        Mayo-Kelly appendix
            inverter
        Mayo-Kelly inverter
        Wangensteen tissue
            inverter
inverting appendiceal stump
inverting sutures
invertor
investigation
investing fascia
involuntary contraction
involuntary guarding
involuntary movement
involuntary muscle
involution
involution cyst
involution of uterus
involutional ovarian changes
involved site
involvement
involving
inward movement
inward rotation
IO (inferior oblique)
Ioban drape
Ioban antimicrobial incise drape
Ioban Steri-Drape
iodine
iodine catgut
iodine cup
iodized oil study
iodized surgical gut sutures
iodo prep
iodochromic catgut
iodoform gauze
iodoform gauze packer
iodoform gauze packing
iodohippurate sodium I-131
    renogram
Iodo-Niacin
iodophor solution
iodophor Steri-Drape
iodoventriculogram
iodoventriculography
iohexol contrast medium
iohexol CT scan

IOL (intraocular lens)
Iolab intraocular lens
Iolab lens
ion
ion laser
ion microscope
ion pump
ion therapy
Ionescu (also Jonnesco)
Ionescu operation
Ionescu sympathectomy
Ionescu tri-leaflet valve
    procedure
Ionescu valve
Ionescu-Shiley aortic valve
    prosthesis
Ionescu-Shiley bioprosthetic
    valve
Ionescu-Shiley bovine pericar-
    dial valve
Ionescu-Shiley heart valve
Ionescu-Shiley low-profile
    prosthetic valve
Ionescu-Shiley pericardial valve
    graft
Ionescu-Shiley pericardial
    xenograft
Ionescu-Shiley porcine hetero-
    graft heart valve
Ionescu-Shiley prosthesis
Ionescu-Shiley standard
    pericardial prosthetic
    valve
Ionescu-Shiley valve
ionic surgery
ionization
ionizing radiation
ionotherapy
iontophoresis
IOP (intraocular pressure)
IOptex laser intraocular lens
    implant
Iotrol study
Iowa forceps
Iowa hip component
Iowa hip evaluation
Iowa implant

Iowa membrane-puncturing
    forceps
Iowa needle guide
Iowa orbital implant
Iowa periosteal elevator
Iowa State fixation forceps
Iowa State forceps
Iowa total hip prosthesis
Iowa trumpet forceps guide
Iowa trumpet instrument
Iowa trumpet needle guide
Iowa University elevator
Iowa University periosteal
    elevator
IPC (intermittent pneumatic
    compression)
IPCO-Partridge defibrillator
IPD (inflammatory pelvic
    disease)
IPD (interpupillary distance)
IPG (impedance plethysmogra-
    phy)
IPJ (interphalangeal joint)
IPOP cast dressing (immediate
    postoperative prosthesis
    cast dressing)
IPPA (inspection, palpation,
    percussion, and ausculta-
    tion)
IPPB (intermittent positive
    pressure breathing)
IPSF (immediate postsurgical
    fitting)
ipsilateral
ipsilateral aspect
ipsilateral contraction
ipsilateral ear
ipsilateral mentalis muscle
ipsilateral nonreversed greater
    saphenous vein bypass
ipsilateral rhinorrhea
IR (inferior rectus)
Irex Exemplar ultrasound
iridectomesodialysis
iridectomize
iridectomy
iridectomy scissors

iridencleisis
iridesis
iridial folds
iridial tent
iridic muscles
iridium
iridium implant
iridium needle holder
iridium prosthesis
iridium wire implant
iridium-192 loaded stent
iridocapsular fixation lens
iridocapsular implant cataract
    lens
iridocapsular intraocular lens
iridocapsulectomy
iridocapsulotomy
iridocapsulotomy scissors
iridocorneal
iridocorneosclerectomy
iridocyclectomy
iridocystectomy
iridodesis
iridodialysis
iridolenticular
iridomesodialysis
iridoplasty
iridosclerotomy
iridostasis
iridotomy
iris
iris atrophy
iris bombé
iris ciliary body
iris contracture
iris crypt
iris dehiscence
iris dialysis
iris diastasis
iris disposable retractor
iris fixation intraocular lens
iris fixation lens
iris forceps
iris hernia
iris hook
iris inclusion operation
iris knife
iris knife-needle

iris microforceps
iris microscissors
iris miniature scissors
iris needle
iris pillars
iris pillars were reposited
iris plane intraocular lens
iris prolapse
iris protrusion
iris replacer
iris reposited
iris repositor
iris retractor
iris scissors
iris scraped free
iris spatula
iris stretching
iris stretching operation
iris transfixation
iritis
iritomy
IRMA (intraretinal microvascular
    abnormality)
Iron interne retractor
irradiance
irradiated cells
irradiated surgical defects
irradiation
irradiation and chemotherapy
irradiation and surgery
irradiation cataract
irradiation cystitis
irradiation effect
irradiation field
irradiation menses
irradiation process
irradiation pulse
irradiation rate
irradiation respirations
irradiation sterilization
irradiation therapy
irreducible
irreducible hernia
irregular amputated mucosal
    pattern
irregular bleeding
irregular calcification
irregular cervix

irregular contractions
irregular defects
irregular heart rhythm
irregular intervals
irregularity
irregularly irregular rhythm
irregularly shaped body
irresistible impulse
irreversible brain damage
irreversible coma
irreversible condition
irreversible disability
irreversible disorder
irrigate
irrigated bladder
irrigated with normal saline
    solution
irrigated with saline solution
irrigating bronchoscope
irrigating cannula
irrigating catheter
irrigating contact Goldmann
    lens
irrigating cord
irrigating curet
irrigating Dilaprobe
irrigating eye spatula
irrigating mushroom retractor
irrigating solution
irrigating tip
irrigating tube
irrigating uterine curet
irrigating valve
irrigating vectis
irrigating-aspirating handpiece
irrigating-aspirating tip
irrigation
irrigation and aspiration (I&A)
irrigation and curettage
irrigation catheter
irrigation fluid
irrigation of bladder
irrigation of nose
irrigation of sinuses
irrigation syringe
irrigation techniques
irrigation-aspiration core

irrigator
    anterior chamber
        irrigator
    antral irrigator
    B-H anterior chamber
        irrigator
    Barraquer irrigator
    Baumrucker irrigator
    Bishop-Harman anterior
        chamber irrigator
    Bishop-Harman irrigator
    Buie irrigator
    Buie rectal irrigator
    Carabelli irrigator
    Creevy irrigator
    DeVilbiss eye irrigator
    DeVilbiss irrigator
    Dougherty eye irrigator
    Dougherty irrigator
    eye irrigator
    Fink irrigator
    Fox irrigator
    Gibson eye irrigator
    Gibson irrigator
    Goldstein irrigator
    Guiteras nozzle irrigator
    House irrigator
    House suction irrigator
    House-Radpour suction-
        irrigator
    House-Stevenson
        suction-irrigator
    Huzly irrigator
    hydrostatic irrigator
    Kemp rectal irrigator
    Kurze suction-irrigator
    Lamb irrigator
    Lukens irrigator
    McKenna Tide-Ur-Ator
        irrigator
    Moncrieff irrigator
    Nezhat suction-irrigator
    ophthalmic irrigator
    Pediastrol self-irrigating
        bladder irrigator
    percolator irrigator
    rectal irrigator

irrigator *continued*
    Rollet irrigator
    Shambaugh irrigator
    Shea irrigator
    stainless irrigator
    suction-irrigator
    Sylva eye irrigator
    Sylva irrigator
    Thornwald irrigator
    Valentine irrigator
    Wells irrigator
irrigator-suction tube
irritability
irritable
irritable bladder
irritable bowel syndrome
irritable colon
irritable heart
irritable joint
irritable stricture
irritant
irritate
irritation
irritative lesion
irritative reaction
Irv ridge
Irvine corneal scissors
Irvine operation
Irvine probe-point scissors
Irvine scissors
Irvine viable organ-tissue transport system (IVOTTS)
Irvine-Gass syndrome
Irving operation
Irving sterilization operation
Irving technique of tubal ligation
Irving tubal ligation
Irwin operation
Irwin osteotomy
Irwin pelvic osteotomy
Irwin technique
IS joint knife (incudostapedial joint knife)
Isaacs aspiration syringe
Isaacs-Ludwig arteriole
ischemia

ischemic bowel
ischemic contracture
ischemic disease
ischemic necrosis
ischemic reflex
ischiadic nerve
ischiadicus, nervus
ischial
ischial bone
ischial brace
ischial ramus
ischial spines
ischial tuberosity
ischial weightbearing brace
ischial weightbearing leg brace
ischiatic
ischiatic hernia
ischiatic hernioplasty
ischiatic notch
ischiatic scoliosis
ischiectomy
ischioanal
ischiocapsular ligament
ischiocavernosus, musculus
ischiocavernous muscle
ischiococcygeal
ischiodymia
ischiofemoral
ischiofemoral arthrodesis
ischiogluteal
ischiohebotomy
ischiopubic
ischiopubic ramus
ischiopubiotomy
ischiorectal
ischiorectal abscess
ischiorectal fossa
ischiorectal hernia
ischiosacral
ischiovertebral
ischium
iseiconic lens
Isherwood position
Ishihara color test
Ishihara plate
Ishihara test chart book
Ishizuki hinge

ISIS (integrated shape imaging system)
island
island flap
island graft
island leg flap
island of Reil
island pedicle flaps
islands of Langerhans
islet cell tumor
islet structures
islets of Langerhans
isoantibody
isobaric anesthesia
isobaric spinal anesthesia
isobaric transition
isocentric oblique
isocentric technique
isodense with surrounding tissues
isodose curve
isodose shift method
isodosimetry
isoechoic
isoeffect curve
isoelectric electroencephalogram
isoelectric point
isoenzyme
isogeneic graft
isograft
isohydric cycle
isolate
isolated and tagged
isolated episode
isolated field
isolated heat perfusion
isolated infusion
isolated perfusion
isolated premature beats
isolation
isolation and asepsis
isolation and identification
isolation forceps
isologous graft
isometric transition
isoperistaltic

isoperistaltic anastomosis
isoperistaltic gastrojejunostomy
isoperistaltic jejunostomy
isoplastic graft
Isoproterenol
isotope bone scan
isotope calibrator
isotope scanning
isotope scanning studies
isotope studies
isotope therapy
isotopic pulse generator pacemaker
isotropic disk
Isovis wound protector
isovolumic contraction
Israel Benzedrine vaporizer
Israel blunt rake retractor
Israel decompressor
Israel depressor
Israel dissector
Israel nasal rasp
Israel operation
Israel rake retractor
Israel rasp
Israel raspatory
Israel retractor
Israel tonsillar dissector
Israel tube
isthmectomy
isthmica nodosa
isthmorrhaphy
isthmus
isthmus of fallopian tube
isthmus of uterus
isthmus tubae uterinae
Isuprel
ITA graft (internal thoracic artery graft)
Italian distant flap
Italian operation
Italian rhinoplasty
Itard catheter
ITB (iliotibial band)
ITT (internal tibial torsion)
IUCD (intrauterine contraceptive device)

IUD (intrauterine device) (see *intrauterine device*)
IUD bow
IUD coil
IUD dislodged
IUD spotting
IUD string
IUGR (intrauterine growth retardation)
IV (intravenous, intervertebral)
IV administration
IV administration of medication
IV anesthesia
IV angiocardiography
IV antibiotic
IV bolus injection of contrast medium
IV catheter
IV cholangiography
IV cocktail
IV contrast medium
IV discontinued
IV disk (intravertebral disk)
IV disk forceps (intravertebral disk forceps)
IV disk rongeur (intravertebral disk ronguer)
IV drip
IV feeding
IV hydration
IV infusion
IV line
IV needle
IV pyelogram
IV pyelography
IV stand
IV therapy
IV transfusion
IV urography
IVAC infusion pump
IVAC machine
IVAC pump
IVAC ventilator
IVAC volumetric infusion pump

Ivalon dressing
Ivalon eye implant
Ivalon graft
Ivalon implant
Ivalon material
Ivalon patch
Ivalon prosthesis
Ivalon rectopexy
Ivalon sponge
Ivalon sponge graft
Ivalon sponge implant
Ivalon sponge rectopexy
Ivalon sponge wrap
Ivalon sutures
Ivan laryngeal applicator
Ivar Parlmar reduction
IVC (intravenous cholangiogram, intravenous cholangiography)
IVCD (intraventricular conduction delay)
Iverson dermabrader
Ives anoscope
Ives proctoscope
Ives speculum
Ivinsco cervical dilator
Ivor Lewis esophagectomy
Ivor Lewis esophagogastrectomy
ivory bones
ivory exostosis
IVOTTS (Irvine viable organtissue transport system)
IVP (intravenous pyelogram)
IVSD (interventricular septal defect)
Ivy bleeding time
Ivy loop
Ivy loop wiring
Ivy mastoid rongeur
Ivy rongeur
Ivy wire
Ivy wire loops
Iwanoff retinal edema

J&J Band-Aid sterile drape
J&J dressing
J-Flex posterior chamber
    lens
J-guide
J-guide wire
J-junction
J-loop
J-loop ileostomy
J-loop posterior chamber lens
J-loop technique
J-point
J-point treadmill test
J-shaped anal anastomosis
J-shaped ileal pouch
J-shaped incision
J-shaped reservoir
J-stent
J-stripper
J-tip guide wire
J-tip wire
J-tipped exchange guide
    wire
J-tipped wire
J-Vac
J-Vac catheter
J-Vac closed wound drainage
J-Vac drain
J-Vac suction reservoir
J-wire
Jabaley-Stille Supercut scissors
Jaboulay amputation
Jaboulay button
Jaboulay gastroduodenostomy
Jaboulay operation
Jaboulay pyloroplasty
jacket
        body jacket
        Bonchek-Shiley cardiac
            jacket

jacket *continued*
    cuirass jacket
    Kalot jacket
    Kydex body jacket
    Minerva jacket
    Minerva plaster jacket
    Orthoplast jacket
    plaster-of-Paris jacket
    radix Raney jacket
    Raney flexion jacket
        brace
    Raney jacket
    Risser jacket
    Royalite body jacket
    Sayre jacket
    Von Lackum transection
        shift jacket brace
    Willock jacket
    Willock respiratory jacket
    Wilmington jacket
jacket-type chest dressing
jackknife position
Jackson alligator forceps
Jackson anterior commissure
    laryngoscope
Jackson applicator
Jackson atomizer
Jackson battery cord
Jackson biopsy forceps
Jackson bistoury
Jackson bone-extension clamp
Jackson bougie
Jackson bronchoscope
Jackson bronchoscopic forceps
    handle
Jackson bronchoscopic instru-
    ment
Jackson cane-shaped tube
Jackson clamp
Jackson dilator

Jackson double-ended retractor
Jackson elevator
Jackson esophageal bougie
Jackson esophagoscope
Jackson forceps
Jackson forceps handle
Jackson full-lumen esophago-
scope
Jackson full-lumen standard
bronchoscope
Jackson goiter retractor
Jackson hemostat
Jackson hemostatic forceps
Jackson hook
Jackson incision
Jackson infant biopsy forceps
Jackson infant forceps
Jackson intervertebral disk
rongeur
Jackson knife
Jackson laryngeal applicator
Jackson laryngeal applicator
forceps
Jackson laryngeal atomizer
Jackson laryngeal forceps
Jackson laryngeal instruments
Jackson laryngeal punch
forceps
Jackson laryngeal rotation
forceps
Jackson laryngectomy tube
Jackson laryngofissure forceps
Jackson laryngoscope
Jackson laryngostat
Jackson probe
Jackson punch
Jackson punch forceps
Jackson retractor
Jackson ring-rotation forceps
Jackson rotation forceps
Jackson scalpel
Jackson scissors
Jackson self-retaining goiter
retractor
Jackson shears
Jackson sliding laryngoscope
Jackson speculum

Jackson sponge carrier
Jackson square punch tip
Jackson standard full-lumen
esophagoscope
Jackson standard laryngoscope
Jackson tenaculum
Jackson tracheal bougie
Jackson tracheal forceps
Jackson tracheal hemostat
Jackson tracheal hemostatic
forceps
Jackson tracheal hook
Jackson tracheal knife
Jackson tracheal retractor
Jackson tracheal tenaculum
Jackson tracheal tube
Jackson tracheoscope
Jackson tracheotomic bistoury
Jackson tracheotomy set
Jackson tube
Jackson turbinate scissors
Jackson Universal handle
Jackson vaginal retractor
Jackson vaginal speculum
Jackson veil
Jackson-Babcock operation
Jackson-Moore shears
Jackson-Mosher dilator
Jackson-Plummer dilator
Jackson-Pratt catheter
Jackson-Pratt dissector
Jackson-Pratt drain
Jackson-Pratt reservoir
Jackson-Pratt suction drain
Jackson-Pratt suction reservoir
Jackson-Trousseau dilator
jackstone-type urinary bladder
stone
Jacob clamp
Jacob forceps
Jacob key
Jacob membrane
Jacob tenaculum
Jacob ulcer
Jacob uterine tenaculum
Jacob uterine vulsellum forceps
Jacob vulsellum forceps

Jacobaeus operation
Jacobaeus thoracoscope
Jacobaeus-Unverricht thoracoscope
Jacobs chuck
Jacobs chuck and key
Jacobs chuck drill
Jacobson anastomosis
Jacobson bulldog clamp
Jacobson clamp
Jacobson dressing forceps
Jacobson elevator
Jacobson endarterectomy spatula
Jacobson forceps
Jacobson goiter retractor
Jacobson hemostatic forceps
Jacobson holder
Jacobson hook
Jacobson knife
Jacobson knot tier
Jacobson microbulldog clamp
Jacobson microdressing forceps
Jacobson microscissors
Jacobson microsurgery instrument
Jacobson modified vessel clamp
Jacobson mosquito forceps
Jacobson needle holder
Jacobson nerve
Jacobson probe
Jacobson punch
Jacobson retinitis
Jacobson retractor
Jacobson scissors
Jacobson spatula
Jacobson spring-handled needle holder
Jacobson spring-handled scissors
Jacobson technique
Jacobson vessel clamp
Jacobson vessel punch
Jacobson Vital needle holder
Jacobson-Potts clamp
Jacobson-Potts vessel clamp
Jacobs-Palmer laparoscope

Jacquemier sign
Jacques stomach tube
Jaeger hook
Jaeger keratome
Jaeger keratome knife
Jaeger knife
Jaeger lid plate
Jaeger lid plate retractor
Jaeger lid retractor
Jaeger reading chart
Jaeger retractor
Jaeger strabismus hook
Jaeger-Whiteley catheter
Jaesche operation
Jaesche-Arlt operation
Jaffe bone disease
Jaffe disease
Jaffe hook
Jaffe iris hook
Jaffe lens
Jaffe lid retractor
Jaffe ocular implant lens
Jaffe scissors
Jaffe speculum
Jaffe wire lid retractor
Jahnke anastomosis clamp
Jahnke-Barron heart support net
Jahnke-Cook-Seeley clamp
Jahss osteotomy
Jaime operation
Jako biopsy
Jako facial nerve monitor
Jako knife
Jako laryngeal microforceps
Jako laryngeal microinstrument
Jako laryngeal microscissors
Jako laryngoscope
Jako monitor
Jako nerve monitor
Jako probe
Jako suction tube
Jako suspension otoscope
Jakob reverse pivot shift sign
Jakob technique
Jako-Pilling laryngoscope
Jalaguier cleft lip repair

Jalaguier incision
Jamar dynamometer
James accessory tract
James atrionodal bypass tract
James fibers
James intranodal tract
James wound-approximation
    forceps
Jameson calipers
Jameson dissecting scissors
Jameson eye calipers
Jameson forceps
Jameson hook
Jameson muscle clamp
Jameson muscle forceps
Jameson muscle hook
Jameson needle
Jameson needle holder
Jameson operation
Jameson recession forceps
Jameson strabismus hook
Jameson strabismus needle
Jameson tracheal muscle
    recession forceps
Jamison-Metzenbaum scissors
jamming injury
Jamshidi liver biopsy needle
Jamshidi muscle needle biopsy
Jamshidi needle
Jamshidi-Kormed bone marrow
    biopsy needle
Jancey nail fold removal
Janecki-Nelson technique
Janes fracture appliance
Janeway gastroscope
Janeway gastrostomy
Janeway lesion
Janeway sphygmomanometer
Janeway spots
Janko clamp
Jannetta aneurysm neck
    dissector
Jannetta bayonet forceps
Jannetta bayonet needle holder
Jannetta bayonet scissors
Jannetta dissector
Jannetta elevator

Jannetta forceps
Jannetta knife
Jannetta microbayonet forceps
Jannetta microneurosurgery
    instrument
Jannetta needle holder
Jannetta posterior fossa retractor
Jannetta retractor
Jannetta scissors
Jannetta sterilizing rack
Jannetta storage rack
Jannetta vascular decompres-
    sion of 5th nerve
Jannetta-Kurze dissecting
    scissors
Jannetta-Kurze scissors
Jansen bayonet forceps
Jansen bayonet nasal forceps
Jansen bayonet rongeur
Jansen bone curet
Jansen curet
Jansen disease
Jansen ear forceps
Jansen ear rongeur
Jansen forceps
Jansen mastoid raspatory
Jansen mastoid retractor
Jansen mastoid rongeur
Jansen mouth gag
Jansen nasal-dressing forceps
Jansen operation
Jansen periosteotome
Jansen raspatory
Jansen retractor
Jansen rongeur
Jansen scalp retractor
Jansen scissors
Jansen test
Jansen thumb forceps
Jansen-Cottle rongeur
Jansen-Gifford mastoid retractor
Jansen-Gifford retractor
Jansen-Gruenwald forceps
Jansen-Middleton forceps
Jansen-Middleton nasal-cutting
    forceps
Jansen-Middleton rongeur

Jansen-Middleton septal forceps
Jansen-Middleton septotomy
    forceps
Jansen-Middleton septum-
    cutting forceps
Jansen-Mueller forceps
Jansen-Newhart mastoid probe
Jansen-Newhart probe
Jansen-Struyken forceps
Jansen-Struyken septal forceps
Jansen-Wagner mastoid
    retractor
Jansen-Wagner retractor
Jansen-Zaufel bone rongeur
Jansen-Zaufel rongeur
Jantene operation
Japas foot procedure
Japas procedure
Jaquet apparatus
Jarcho cannula
Jarcho forceps
Jarcho self-retaining uterine
    cannula
Jarcho tenaculum
Jarcho tenaculum forceps
Jarcho tenaculum holder
Jarcho uterine tenaculum
    forceps
Jarit flat-top scissors
Jarit-Allis tissue forceps
Jarit-Crafoord forceps
Jarit-Kerrison laminectomy
    rongeur
Jarit-Liston bone-cutting
    forceps
Jarit-Pol suction tube
Jarit-Ruskin bone rongeur
Jarit-Yankauer suction tube
Jarjavay muscle
Jarvik-7 artificial heart
Jarvik-7 mechanical pump
Jarvis clamp
Jarvis forceps
Jarvis hemorrhoid forceps
Jarvis operation
Jarvis pile clamp
Jarvis snare
Jasbee esophagoscope

Jatene-Macchi prosthetic valve
jaundice
Javal ophthalmometer
Javerts placental forceps
Javerts polyp forceps
Javid bypass clamp
Javid bypass shunt
Javid bypass tube
Javid carotid artery bypass
    clamp
Javid carotid artery clamp
Javid catheter
Javid clamp
Javid endarterectomy shunt
Javid internal carotid shunt
Javid shunt
Javid tube
jaw
jaw fracture
jaw hook
jaw jerk reflex
jaw splint
jaw thrust maneuver
jawbone
jaw-neck resection
Jay cushion
Jayles forceps
Jay-Monnet acromioclavicular
    operation
Jazbi dissector
Jazbi nasal instrument set
Jazbi suction tonsillar dissector
Jazbi tonsil dissector
JB catheter
JB-1 catheter
J.E. Sheehan chisel
Jeanne sign
Jeanselme nodule
Jeb graft
Jebson-Taylor hand function
    test
Jefferson fracture
Jefferson retractor
jejunal
jejunal and ileal veins
jejunal arteries
jejunal bypass
jejunal diverticulum

jejunal feeding tube
jejunal interposition
jejunal limb
jejunal loop
jejunal mucosa
jejunal pouch
jejunal ulcer
jejunal veins
jejunal villi
jejunales, arteriae
jejunales et ilei, venae
jejunectomy
jejunitis
jejunocecostomy
jejunocholecystostomy
jejunocolic fistula
jejunocolostomy
jejunoileal bypass (JIB)
jejunoileitis
jejunoileostomy
jejunojejunostomy
jejunopexy
jejunoplasty
jejunorrhaphy
jejunostomy
jejunostomy tube
jejunotomy
jejunum
Jelco catheter
Jelco needle
Jelenko arch bar
Jelenko arch bar application
Jelenko bar
Jelenko splint
Jelks operation
jelly dressing
jelly-like mass
Jelm catheter
Jelm two-way catheter
Jenckel cholecystoduodenos-
    tomy
Jenckel method
Jendrassik maneuver
Jennings Loktite mouth gag
Jennings mouth gag
Jennings-Skillern mouth gag
Jenny mammary prosthesis
Jensen diamond polisher

Jensen forceps
Jensen intraocular lens forceps
Jensen lens forceps
Jensen operation
Jensen polisher
Jensen procedure muscles
Jensen scratcher
Jensen ties
Jensen transposition surgery for
    lateral rectus paresis
Jentzer trephine
Jerger tympanogram (types A,
    B, C)
Jergesen I-beam
Jergesen reamer
Jergesen tube
jerk test
jerking eye movements
jerking musculature
jerky movements
Jervey forceps
Jesberg aspirating tube
Jesberg bronchoscope
Jesberg clamp
Jesberg esophagoscope
Jesberg forceps
Jesberg grasping forceps
Jesberg infant bronchoscope
Jesberg scope
Jesberg tube
Jesberg upper esophagoscope
Jesionek lamp
Jesse-Stryker saw
jet douche
jet nebulizer
Jevity isotonic liquid nutrition
jeweler's bipolar forceps
jeweler's forceps
jeweler's microforceps
jeweler's pickup forceps
Jewett bar
Jewett bone extractor
Jewett brace
Jewett classification of bladder
    carcinoma
Jewett double-angle osteotomy
    plate
Jewett driver

Jewett electrode
Jewett fracture appliance
Jewett frame
Jewett gouge
Jewett hip nail
Jewett hyperextension brace
Jewett nail
Jewett nail instrument
Jewett nail overlay plate
Jewett operation
Jewett orthosis
Jewett pickup screw
Jewett plate
Jewett postfusion orthosis
Jewett prosthesis
Jewett reamer
Jewett screw
Jewett slotted plate
Jewett sound
Jewett urethral sound
JFB III endoscope
Jianu-Beck operation
jib
JIB (jejunoileal bypass)
jig
JL-4 catheter (Judkins left, 4 cm)
JL-5 catheter (Judkins left, 5 cm)
Jobe-Patt splint
Jobert de Lamballe operation
Jobert de Lamballe sutures
Jobert sutures
Jobson-Pynchon decompressor
Jobst boot
Jobst bra
Jobst compression unit
Jobst dressing
Jobst elastic stocking
Jobst extremity pump
Jobst mammary support
    dressing
Jobst stocking prosthesis
Jobst stockings
Jobst VPGS stockings
Jobst-Stride support stockings
Jobst-Stridette support stockings
jocked stand crutch
Jodd repair of postoperative
    ventral hernia

Joel-Baker anastomosis
Joel-Baker tube
Joel-Cohen abdominal incision
Joel-Cohen incision
Joe's hoe
Johannson lag screw
Johanson urethroplasty
John Green pendulum scalpel
John Wobig entropion repair
Johns Hopkins bulldog clamp
Johns Hopkins clamp
Johns Hopkins coarctation
    clamp
Johns Hopkins forceps
Johns Hopkins gallbladder
    forceps
Johns Hopkins gallbladder
    retractor
Johns Hopkins modified Potts
    clamp
Johns Hopkins needle holder
Johns Hopkins occluding
    forceps
Johns Hopkins retractor
Johns Hopkins stone basket
Johns Hopkins tube
Johnson basket
Johnson brain tumor forceps
Johnson erysiphake
Johnson esophagogastrostomy
Johnson forceps
Johnson hook
Johnson intestinal tube
Johnson knife
Johnson needle holder
Johnson position
Johnson prostatic needle holder
Johnson ptotic knife
Johnson retractor
Johnson screwdriver
Johnson skin hook
Johnson splint
Johnson stone basket
Johnson stone dislodger
Johnson technique
Johnson thoracic forceps
Johnson tonsillar punch
Johnson tube

Johnson twin-wire appliance
Johnson ureteral basket
Johnson ureteral stone basket
Johnson ventriculogram
    retractor
Johnson-Bell erysiphake
Johnson-Iowa total hip
Johnson-Johnson Press-Fit knee
    system
Johnson-Kerrison punch
Johnson-Spiegel procedure
Johnson-Tooke corneal knife
Johnson-Tooke knife
Johnston clamp
Johnston dilator
Johnston plug
joint
joint abnormality
joint ankylosis
joint arthroplasty
joint capsule
joint cartilage
joint click
joint crepitus
joint disease
joint dislocation
joint effusion
joint facet
joint fluid
joint fusion
joint implant
joint injury
joint instability
joint jack
joint knife
joint line
joint mice
joint motion
joint mouse
joint movement
joint pain
joint position
joint position sense
joint reconstruction
joint repair
joint replacement
joint rheumatoid arthritis

joint socket
joint space
joint stiffening
joint surface
joint swelling
joint tenderness
joint toilet
joint trauma
jointed vein stripper
joints of Luschka
joker (endarterectomy instru-
    ment)
joker dissector
joker elevator
Jolly dilator
Jolly prostatic scissors
Jolly test
Jolly uterine dilator
Jonas modification of Norwood
    procedure
Jonas penile prosthesis
Jonas silicone-silver penile
    prosthesis
Jonas silver penile prosthesis
Jonas-Graves speculum
Jonas-Graves vaginal
    speculum
Jonell countertraction metacar-
    pal splint
Jonell finger splint
Jonell splint
Jones adenoid curet
Jones ankle procedure
Jones bunionectomy
Jones canaliculus dilator
Jones clamp
Jones closure
Jones curet
Jones dilator
Jones dissecting scissors
Jones dressing
Jones forceps
Jones forearm splint
Jones fracture
Jones hammer toe operation
Jones hemostatic forceps
Jones IMA forceps

Jones knee procedure
Jones knife
Jones lacrimal canaliculus
    dilator
Jones metacarpal splint
Jones operation
Jones pin
Jones position
Jones punctum
Jones Pyrex tube
Jones repair
Jones repair of first toe
Jones retractor
Jones scissors
Jones splint
Jones suspension traction
Jones sutures
Jones tear duct tube
Jones technique
Jones tenodesis
Jones tenosuspension
Jones thoracic clamp
Jones toe procedure
Jones toe repair
Jones towel clamp
Jones towel forceps
Jones tube
Jones-Barnett technique
Jones-Brackett approach
Jonge position
Jonnesco (see *Ionescu*)
Jonnson maneuver
Joplin bunionectomy
Joplin forceps
Joplin operation
Joplin stripper
Joplin technique
Joplin tendon passer
Joplin toe prosthesis
Jordan bur
Jordan capsule knife
Jordan dilator
Jordan elevator
Jordan eye implant
Jordan hook
Jordan implant
Jordan knife

Jordan needle
Jordan perforating bur
Jordan stapedectomy knife
Jordan strut-measuring instru-
    ment
Jordan wire loop dilator
Jordan-Day bur
Jordan-Day cutting bur
Jordan-Day drill
Jordan-Day fenestration bur
Jordan-Day polishing bur
Jordan-Rosen curet
Jorgenson dissecting scissors
Jorgenson retractor
Jorgenson scissors
Jorgenson thoracic scissors
Joseph angular knife
Joseph button knife
Joseph button-end knife
Joseph chisel
Joseph clamp
Joseph double-edged knife
Joseph elevator
Joseph hook
Joseph knife
Joseph nasal knife
Joseph nasal rasp
Joseph nasal raspatory
Joseph nasal saw
Joseph nasal scissors
Joseph operation
Joseph perforator
Joseph periosteal elevator
Joseph periosteotome
Joseph periosteotome elevator
Joseph punch
Joseph rasp
Joseph raspatory
Joseph ruler
Joseph saw
Joseph saw guide
Joseph scissors
Joseph septal bar
Joseph septal clamp
Joseph septal fracture
    appliance
Joseph septal frame

Joseph serrated scissors
Joseph single-prong hook
Joseph skin hook
Joseph splint
Joseph tenaculum
Joseph-Killian elevator
Joseph-Maltz knife
Joseph-Maltz nasal saw
Joseph-Maltz saw
Joseph-Maltz scissors
Josephson catheter
joule unit
JP instruments (Jackson-Pratt)
JR-4 catheter (Judkins right, 4 cm)
JR-5 catheter (Judkins right, 5 cm)
JT interval
Judd cannula
Judd clamp
Judd female urethrocystoscope
Judd forceps
Judd hernia repair
Judd operation
Judd pyloroplasty
Judd strabismus forceps
Judd suture forceps
Judd trocar
Judd-Allis clamp
Judd-Allis forceps
Judd-Allis intestinal forceps
Judd-Allis tissue forceps
Judd-DeMartel forceps
Judd-DeMartel gallbladder forceps
Judd-Mason bladder retractor
Judd-Mason retractor
Judet approach
Judet arthrogram
Judet arthroplasty
Judet dissector
Judet femoral prosthetic head
Judet hip prosthesis
Judet hip x-ray view
Judet operation
Judet press-fit hip prosthesis
Judet prosthesis

Judet x-ray view
Judkins cardiac catheterization technique
Judkins catheter
Judkins coronary catheter (left/ right)
Judkins femoral catheterization technique
Judkins left coronary catheter
Judkins right coronary catheter
Judkins selective coronary arteriography
Judkins technique for coronary arteriogram
Judkins USCI catheter
Judkins-4 guiding catheter
Judson-Bruce hemostat
Juers crimper
Juers ear curet
Juers forceps
Juers hook
Juers-Derlacki holder
Juers-Derlacki Universal head holder
Juers-Lempert endaural rongeur
Juers-Lempert forceps
Juers-Lempert rongeur
Juers-Lempert rongeur forceps
Juevenelle clamp
jugal sutures
jugomaxillary
jugular
jugular arch
jugular bulb
jugular floor
jugular foramen
jugular ganglion
jugular gland
jugular lymph nodes
jugular nerve
jugular notch
jugular notch of sternum
jugular pulse
jugular sign
jugular trunk
jugular vein
jugular venous arch

jugular wall
jugularis anterior, vena
jugularis interna, vena
jugularis, nervus
jugulodigastric nodes
jugum
jugum forceps
Juhn trap
Juhn tympanocentesis trap
Julian forceps
Julian needle holder
Julian splenorenal forceps
Julian thoracic forceps
Julian thoracic hemostatic
     forceps
Julian Vital needle holder
Julian-Fildes clamp
jumbo biopsy forceps
jump facet
jump flap
jump graft
jump skin flap
jumper's knee
junction
junction obstruction
junctional
junctional arrhythmia
junctional cavity
junctional nevus
junctional pacemaker

junctional rhythm
junctional tachycardia
junctional tissue
juncturae tendineae
juncture
juncture stricture
Jung muscle
Jung-Schaffer lens
Junod boot
Jurasz forceps
Jurasz laryngeal forceps
Juri skin flap
Jutte tube
jutting mandible
juvenile melanoma
juvenile polyps
juvenile reflex
juxta-articular nodule
juxtaglomerular cell hyper-
     plasia
juxtaglomerular granules
juxtapapillary diverticulum
juxtapose
juxtaposition
juxtapyloric ulcer
juxtaregional lymph node
Juzo shrinker
Juzo stocking for throm-
     bophlebitis
Juzo stockings

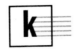

K-Cal calibration well
K-Cast
K-curette
K-Gar clamp
K-nail
K-pad hot pack
K-Pratt dilator
K-S adhesive needle holder
K-Simplex glue
K-Temp thermometer
K-Thermia blanket
K-Thermia equipment
K-Thermia OR cart
K-Thermia pad
K-wire (Kirschner wire)
Kader gastrostomy
Kader needle
Kader operation
Kader-Senn operation
KAFO (knee-ankle-foot
     orthosis)
Kager triangle
Kahler biopsy forceps
Kahler bronchial biopsy
     forceps
Kahler bronchial forceps
Kahler bronchoscopic forceps
Kahler bronchus-grasping
     forceps
Kahler forceps
Kahler laryngeal biopsy forceps
Kahler laryngeal forceps
Kahler polyp forceps
Kahn cannula
Kahn dilator
Kahn dissecting scissors
Kahn forceps
Kahn scissors
Kahn tenaculum

Kahn traction tenaculum
Kahn trigger cannula
Kahn uterine dilator
Kahn uterine trigger cannula
Kahn-Graves speculum
Kahn-Graves vaginal speculum
Kaiser speculum
Kajava classification of supernu-
     merary nipples and breasts
Kalamarides dural retractor
Kal-Dermic sutures
Kaliscinski ureteral procedure
Kall modification of Silverman
     needle
Kalman forceps
Kalman occluding forceps
Kalos pacemaker
Kalot jacket
Kalt capsule forceps
Kalt corneal needle
Kalt eye needle
Kalt eye needle holder
Kalt eye spoon
Kalt forceps
Kalt needle
Kalt needle holder
Kalt spoon
Kalt sutures
Kalt Vital needle holder
Kaltostat wound dressing
Kammerer incision
Kammerer-Battle incision
Kamp support
kanamycin solution
Kanavel brain-exploring
     cannula
Kanavel cannula
Kanavel cock-up splint
Kanavel conductor

Kanavel exploring cannula
Kanavel sign
Kanavel splint
Kane clamp
Kane umbilical clamp
Kane umbilical cord clamp
kangaroo ligature
kangaroo tendon
kangaroo tendon sutures
Kantor circumcision clamp
Kantor clamp
Kantor forceps
Kantor sign
Kantrex solution
Kantrowitz clamp
Kantrowitz dressing forceps
Kantrowitz forceps
Kantrowitz hemostatic clamp
Kantrowitz pacemaker
Kantrowitz thoracic clamp
Kantrowitz thoracic forceps
Kantrowitz tissue forceps
Kantrowitz vascular dissecting
    scissors
Kantrowitz vascular scissors
Kapel elbow procedure
Kapel technique
Kapetansky flap
Kaplan cold-punch resec-
    toscope
Kaplan needle
Kaplan resectoscope
Kaplan technique
Kaplan tracheostomy needle
Kaposi sarcoma
Kapp applying forceps
Kapp clamp
Kapp clip
Kapp microarterial clamp
Kapp-Beck bronchial clamp
Kapp-Beck clamp
Kapp-Beck coarctation clamp
Kapp-Beck colon clamp
Kapp-Beck forceps
Kapp-Beck serration
Kapp-Beck-Thomson clamp
Kappeler maneuver

Kara erysiphake
Kara needle
Karadanzic flap
Karamar-Mailatt tarsorrhaphy
    clamp
karaya adhesive
karaya adhesive appliance
karaya dressing
karaya electrode
karaya ring ileostomy appliance
karaya seal ileostomy appliance
karaya seal pouch
Karickhoff diagnostic lens
Karickhoff keratoscope
Karickhoff laser lens
Karickhoff lens
Karlin instrument
Karlin spinal table
Karmen catheter
Karmody venous scissors
Karnofsky tumor grading (1 to
    100)
Karp aortic punch
Karp aortic punch forceps
Karras angiography needle
Karras needle
Kartch pigtail probe
Kartchner carotid artery clamp
Kartchner carotid clamp
Kasai operation
Kasai portoenterostomy
Kasai procedure for biliary
    atresia
Kashiwagi calcaneal resection
Kashiwagi technique
Kaslow intestinal tube
Kaslow irrigation tube
Kaslow stomach tube
Kaslow tube
Kastec mitral valve prosthesis
Katena iris spatula
Katena trephine
Katena Vannas scissors
Katena-Ruby knife
Kates forefoot arthroplasty
Katon catheter
Katsch chisel

Katz-Berci optical stylet
Katz-Berci stylet
Katzeff cartilage scissors
Katzin corneal scissors
Katzin corneal transplant
scissors
Katzin scissors
Katzin transplant scissors
Katzin trephine
Katzin-Barraquer Colibri forceps
Katzin-Barraquer forceps
Katzin-Long balloon
Kaufer technique
Kaufer type II retractor
Kauffman sign
Kauffman test
Kaufman adapter
Kaufman clamp
Kaufman forceps
Kaufman incontinence proce-
dure
Kaufman incontinence prosthe-
sis
Kaufman insulated forceps
Kaufman kidney clamp
Kaufman operation
Kaufman penile prosthesis
Kaufman prosthesis
Kaufman syringe
Kaufman urinary incontinence
prosthesis
Kaufman vitrector
Kaufman vitreophage
Kay aortic clamp
Kay clamp
Kay tricuspid valvuloplasty
Kaycel towel
Kay-Cross oxygenator
Kaye antihelix operation
Kaye scissors
Kaye-Damus-Stansel operation
Kayess bandage scissors
Kay-Lambert clamp
Kay-Shiley disk prosthetic valve
Kay-Shiley disk valve prosthesis
Kay-Shiley mitral valve
Kay-Shiley valve prosthesis

Kay-Suzuki disk prosthesis
Kay-Suzuki disk valve prosthe-
sis
Kay-Suzuki valve prosthesis
Kazanjian bar
Kazanjian button
Kazanjian cutting forceps
Kazanjian forceps
Kazanjian guide
Kazanjian nasal forceps
Kazanjian nasal hump forceps
Kazanjian nasal hump-cutting
forceps
Kazanjian nasal-cutting forceps
Kazanjian operation
Kazanjian osteotome
Kazanjian scissors
Kazanjian shears
Kazanjian splint
Kazanjian T-bar
Kazanjian wire
Kazanjian-Cottle forceps
KCP phacoemulsifier
Kearney side-notch intraocular
lens
Kearns bag catheter
Kearns bladder dilator
Kearns dilator
Keates intraocular implant lens
Keates lens
Keating-Hart fulguration
Keating-Hart treatment
Kebab graft
KED (Kendrick extrication
device)
Keegan operation
keel
keel operation
keel stent
keeled chest
Keeler camera
Keeler cryophake
Keeler cryophake unit
Keeler cryoprosthesis
Keeler knife
Keeler loupe
Keeler ophthalmoscope

Keeler panoramic surgical
    telescope
Keeler polarizing ophthal-
    moscope
Keeley stripper
Keeley vein stripper
Keen operation
Keen point
Keen sign
Keene compression hook
Keene self-sealing sleeve and
    obturator
keeper tendon
Keer aneurysm clip
Kees aneurysm set
Kegel exercises
Kehr incision
Kehr operation
Kehr sign
Kehr T-tube
Kehr tube
Kehrer reflex
Keidel tube
Keisley sutures
Keith abdominal needle
Keith bundle
Keith drain
Keith needle
Keith node
Keith scissors
Keith-Flack node
Keith-Wagener hypertensive
    retinopathy classification
    (I-IV)
Keith-Wagener retinopathy
Keith-Wagener-Barker hyper-
    tensive classification (KWB
    classification)
Keitzer infant urethrotome
Keitzer urethrotome
Keizer everter
Keizer eye retractor
Keizer lid retractor
Keizer-Lancaster speculum
Kel retractor
Kelar microscope
kelectome

Kelikian knee surgery
Kelikian procedure
Kelikian tendon transfer
    procedure
Keller arthroplasty
Keller bunion osteotomy
Keller bunionectomy
Keller hallux rigidus operation
Keller hallux valgus operation
Keller operation
Keller osteotomy
Keller procedure
Keller-Blake half-ring leg splint
Keller-Blake splint
Kelley gouge
Kelling gastroscope
Kellman cystotome
Kellman instrument
Kellman irrigation-aspiration
    core
Kellman nose cone assembly
Kellman transducer assembly
Kellman-Elschnig cyclodialysis
    spatula
Kellogg decompressor
Kellogg-Speed operation
Kellogg-Speed spinal fusion
Kelly abdominal retractor
Kelly adenotome
Kelly artery forceps
Kelly clamp
Kelly combined packer and
    tucker
Kelly curet
Kelly cystoscope
Kelly dilator
Kelly dressing forceps
Kelly endoscope
Kelly fistula scissors
Kelly forceps
Kelly hemostat
Kelly hook
Kelly intestinal needle
Kelly needle
Kelly operation
Kelly orifice dilator
Kelly panendoscope

Kelly placenta forceps
Kelly plication suture
Kelly proctoscope
Kelly punch
Kelly rectal speculum
Kelly retractor
Kelly scissors
Kelly sigmoidoscope
Kelly speculum
Kelly sphincteroscope
Kelly sutures
Kelly technique
Kelly tenaculum hook
Kelly tissue forceps
Kelly tube
Kelly tucker
Kelly urethral forceps
Kelly urinary incontinence
    operation
Kelly uterine dilator
Kelly uterine scissors
Kelly uterine tenaculum
Kelly-Deming operation
Kelly-Descemet membrane
    punch
Kelly-Descemet punch
Kelly-Gray curet
Kelly-Gray uterine curet
Kelly-Gray uterine forceps
Kelly-Kennedy operation
Kelly-Kennedy sutures
Kelly-Kennedy vaginal plication
Kelly-Littauer stitch scissors
Kelly-Murphy forceps
Kelly-Murphy hemostatic
    forceps
Kelly-Murphy hemostatic
    uterine vulsellum forceps
Kelly-Rankin forceps
Kelly-Sims retractor
Kelly-Sims vaginal retractor
Kelly-Stoeckel operation
Kelman anterior chamber
    intraocular lens
Kelman cannula
Kelman cryostylet
Kelman cyclodialysis

Kelman cystotome
Kelman dipstick
Kelman extractor
Kelman forceps
Kelman intraocular implant lens
Kelman irrigation-aspiration tip
Kelman irrigator forceps
Kelman keratome
Kelman lens
Kelman Multiflex II intraocular
    lens
Kelman needle
Kelman Omnifit II intraocular
    lens
Kelman phacoemulsification
    (KPE)
Kelman Quadraflex anterior
    chamber intraocular lens
Kelman retractor
Kelman speculum
Kelman-McPherson forceps
Kelman-McPherson microtying
    forceps
Kelman-McPherson tissue
    forceps
keloid
keloid formation
keloid of cornea
keloplasty
kelotomy
Kelsey clamp
Kelsey pile clamp
Kelvin pacemaker
Kelvin scale
Kemp rectal irrigator
Kemp trocar
Ken driver
Ken driver-extractor
Ken nail
Ken plate
Ken screwdriver
Ken sliding nail
Kenalog
Kendrick extrication device
    (KED)
Kendrick Gigli-saw guide
Kendrick technique

Kennan cervical punch
Kennedy bar
Kennedy forceps
Kennedy ligament augmenta-
    tion device (Kennedy LAD)
Kennedy urinary incontinence
    operation
Kennedy uterine vulsellum
    forceps
Kennedy-Cornwell bladder
    evacuator
Kennedy-Losee modification
Kennerdell-Maroon dissector
Kennerdell-Maroon orbital
    retractor set
Kennerdell-Maroon orbital
    tumor instruments
Kenny-Howard splint
Kensey atherectomy catheter
Kent bundle
Kent forceps
Kent-His bundle
Keofeed feeding tube
Keragen implant
keratectomy
keratin pearl
keratinized cell
keratocyst
keratolens
keratoleptynsis
keratome
    Agnew keratome
    Atkinson keratome
    Beaver blade keratome
    Beaver keratome
    Berens keratome
    Castro-Martinez kera-
        tome
    Castroviejo keratome
    Czermak keratome
    Daily keratome
    electromicrokeratome
    Fink-Rowland keratome
    Fuchs keratome
    Grieshaber keratome
    Jaeger keratome
    Kelman keratome

keratome *continued*
    Kirby keratome
    Lancaster keratome
    Landolt keratome
    Lichtenberg keratome
    McCaslin keratome
    McReynolds keratome
    McReynolds pterygium
        keratome
    McReynolds-Castroviejo
        keratome
    pterygium keratome
    Rowland keratome
    Wiener keratome
keratome blade
keratome incision
keratometer
    OV-1 surgical keratome-
        ter
    Terry keratometer
keratomileusis
keratopathy
keratoplasty scissors
keratoprosthesis
keratoscope
    Bright-Ring keratoscope
    Karickhoff keratoscope
    photokeratoscope
keratosis (*pl.* keratoses)
keratotic lesion
keratotomy
keratotomy forceps
keratotomy knife
Kerckring folds
Kerckring nodule
Kerckring valve
Kerlix bandage
Kerlix conforming bandage
    dressing
Kerlix dressing
Kerlix fluff
Kerlix gauze
Kerlix gauze roll
Kerlix rolls
Kern bag
Kern bone clamp
Kern bone-holding clamp

Kern bone-holding forceps
Kern clamp
Kern forceps
Kernan-Jackson bronchoscope
Kernan-Jackson coagulating
    bronchoscope
Kern-Lane bone-holding forceps
Kernohan grading of malignant
    astrocytoma of spinal cord
Kernohan notch
Kerr abduction splint
Kerr cesarean section
Kerr clip
Kerr drill
Kerr electrotorque motor
Kerr hand drill
Kerr handpiece
Kerr incision
Kerr motor
Kerr rongeur
Kerr sign
Kerr splint
Kerrison forceps
Kerrison laminectomy rongeur
Kerrison mastoid rongeur
Kerrison punch
Kerrison retractor
Kerrison rongeur
Kerrison technique
Kerrison-Costen ear rongeur
Kerrison-Ferris Smith rongeur
Kerrison-Rhoton punch
Kerrison-Rhoton sella punch
Kerrison-Spurling rongeur
Kesilar cannula
Kessel plate
Kessel-Bonney extension
    osteotomy
Kessler operation
Kessler prosthesis
Kessler stitch
Kessler suture repair of tendon
Kessler sutures
Kessler upper limb prosthesis
Kestenbach-Anderson proce-
    dure
Kestenbaum eye procedure

Kestler ambulatory head
    traction
Ketaject
Ketalar
ketamine hydrochloride
    anesthetic agent
ketone bodies
Kevlar material
Kevorkian biopsy punch
Kevorkian curet
Kevorkian endocervical curet
Kevorkian forceps
Kevorkian punch biopsy
Kevorkian-Younge biopsy curet
Kevorkian-Younge biopsy
    forceps
Kevorkian-Younge cervical
    biopsy forceps
Kevorkian-Younge curet
Kevorkian-Younge endocervical
    biopsy curet
Kevorkian-Younge forceps
Kevorkian-Younge uterine
    biopsy forceps
key
key chuck
Key knee arthrodesis
Key operation
Key periosteal elevator
key pinch
key point
Key-Conwell classification of
    pelvic fracture
Keyes bone-splitting chisel
Keyes chisel
Keyes cutaneous punch
Keyes dermal punch
Keyes lithotrite
Keyes punch
Keyes skin punch
Keyes-Ultzmann syringe tube
Keyes-Ultzmann-Luer cannula
key-free compression hip screw
    fixation
key-free compression screw
keyhole laminectomy
keyhole pupil

key-in-lock maneuver
key-in-lock rotation
Key-Schmidt method
Keys-Kirschner traction
key-slot patella tendon transfer
keystone ligament
Keystone viewer
Kezerian chisel
Kezerian curet
Kezerian gouge
Kezerian osteotome
Khodadad clamp
Khodadad clip
Khodadad microclip forceps
Kibrick test for infertility
Kibrick-Isojima test for infertility
kick bucket
kick count
Kickaldy-Willis hip arthrodesis
Kidd trocar
Kidd tube
Kidde atomizer
Kidde Flex-i-Tip
Kidde insufflator
Kidde nebulizer
Kidde tourniquet cuff
Kidde tubal insufflator
Kidde uterine cannula
Kidde-Robbins tourniquet
Kidner operation
Kidner podiatric procedure
Kidner removal of accessory
    navicular bone
Kidner technique
kidney
kidney biopsy
kidney clamp
kidney failure
kidney function
kidney hilus
kidney impairment
kidney injury
kidney internal splint/stent
    catheter (KISS catheter)
kidney pedicle clamp
kidney pelvectomy

kidney pelvis
kidney perfused and cooled
kidney perfusion pump
kidney position
kidney punch
kidney recipient
kidney rest
kidney retractor
kidney scan
kidney shadow
kidney stone
kidney stone forceps
kidney suture needle
kidney tissue
kidney transplant
kidney-elevating forceps
kidneys, ureters, bladder
    (KUB)
Kiefer clamp
Kiel classification of lymphoma
Kiel classification of non-
    Hodgkin lymphoma
Kiel graft
Kielland (also Kjelland)
Kielland blade
Kielland forceps
Kielland obstetrical forceps
Kielland operation
Kielland rotation
Kielland-Luikart forceps
Kielland-Luikart obstetrical
    forceps
Kienböck disease
Kienböck dislocation
Kiene bone tamp
Kiernan space
Kiesselbach area
Kiesselbach plexus
Kiesselbach triangle
Kifa catheter
Kifa clip
Killian antrum cannula
Killian bronchoscope
Killian cannula
Killian chisel
Killian cutting forceps tip

Killian double-articulated
    forceps tip
Killian double-ended elevator
Killian elevator
Killian forceps
Killian forceps tip
Killian frontal sinus chisel
Killian frontal sinus operation
Killian gouge
Killian incision
Killian knife
Killian nasal speculum
Killian operation
Killian rectal speculum
Killian rongeur
Killian septal compression
    forceps
Killian septal elevator
Killian septal forceps
Killian septal speculum
Killian speculum
Killian suction tube
Killian suspension apparatus
Killian tonsil knife
Killian tube
Killian washing tube
Killian-Claus chisel
Killian-Eicken cannula
Killian-Freer operation
Killian-Jameson forceps
Killian-King goiter retractor
Killian-King retractor
Killian-Reinhard chisel
Killip classification of heart
    disease (I, II, etc.)
Killip wire
Kilner chisel
Kilner elevator
Kilner hook
Kilner mouth gag
Kilner needle holder
Kilner operation
Kilner retractor
Kilner scissors
Kilner sharp hook
Kilner skin hook
Kilner suture carrier

Kilner-Dott mouth gag
Kilner-Doughty mouth gag
Kilner-Doughty plate
kilogram
Kimball catheter
Kimball hook
Kimball nephrostomy hook
Kimberly sign
Kimpton spreader
Kimpton vein spreader
Kimpton-Brown tube
Kimray thermodilution
Kimray-Greenfield antiembolus
    filter
Kimray-Greenfield filter
Kimray-Greenfield vena caval
    filter
Kimura platinum spatula
Kimura spatula
KinAir bed
Kindt artery clamp
Kindt carotid artery clamp
Kindt clamp
Kinematic II total knee prosthe-
    sis
Kinematic II total knee system
Kinematic prosthesis
Kinematic rotating-hinge knee
    prosthesis
kineplastic
kineplastic amputation
kineplasty
kinesthetic disorder
kinetic
kinetic continuous passive
    motion device
kinetic CPM device
KinetiX ventilation monitor
kinetocardiogram
kinetocardiography
Kinetron
King brace
King catheter
King goiter retractor
King goiter self-retaining
    retractor
King guiding catheter

King hip fusion procedure
King implant
King multipurpose catheter
King multipurpose coronary
    graft catheter
King needle
King of Hearts Holter monitor
King operation
King orbital implant
King punch
King retractor
King suture needle
King tissue forceps
King traction
King trephine
King vocal cord operation
King-Hurd dissector
King-Hurd retractor
King-Hurd tonsil dissector
King-Prince forceps
King-Prince recession forceps
King-Richards operation
Kingsley forceps
Kingsley splint
King-Steelquist technique
kinked aorta
kinking of duct
kinking of graft
kinking of ureter
kink-resistant catheter
kink-resistant peritoneal
    catheter
Kinney-Brown AC splint
Kinsella elevator
Kinsella periosteal elevator
Kinsella-Buie clamp
Kinsella-Buie lung clamp
kiotome
kiotomy
KIP laser
Kirby cataract extraction
Kirby cataract knife
Kirby corneoscleral forceps
Kirby expressor
Kirby fixation forceps
Kirby flat zonule separator
Kirby forceps

Kirby hook
Kirby hook expressor
Kirby intracapsular expressor
    with curved zonular sepa-
    rator
Kirby intracapsular lens
    expressor
Kirby intracapsular lens
    expressor hook
Kirby intracapsular lens forceps
Kirby intracapsular lens loupe
Kirby intracapsular lens
    separator
Kirby intracapsular lens spoon
Kirby intracapsular scoop
Kirby iris forceps
Kirby iris spatula
Kirby keratome
Kirby knife
Kirby lens dislocator
Kirby lens expressor
Kirby lens expressor hook
Kirby lens forceps
Kirby lens loop
Kirby lens spoon
Kirby lid retractor
Kirby loop
Kirby muscle hook
Kirby operation
Kirby retractor
Kirby scissors
Kirby separator
Kirby sliding technique
Kirby spatula
Kirby spoon
Kirby sutures
Kirby tissue forceps
Kirby-Arthus fixation forceps
Kirby-Bracken iris forceps
Kirchner diverticulum
Kirchner retractor
Kirchner wire
Kirk amputation
Kirk mallet
Kirk orthopedic hammer
Kirk technique
Kirkaldy-Willis hip arthrodesis

Kirkaldy-Willis operation
Kirkheim-Storz urethrotome
Kirkland curet
Kirkland knife
Kirkland retractor
Kirklin atrial retractor
Kirklin fence
Kirkpatrick forceps
Kirkpatrick tonsil forceps
Kirmisson elevator
Kirmisson operation
Kirmisson periosteal elevator
Kirmisson raspatory
Kirmisson respirator
Kirner deformity
Kirschner abdominal retractor
Kirschner abdominal self-
    retaining retractor
Kirschner apparatus
Kirschner bone drill
Kirschner bow
Kirschner hip replacement
    system
Kirschner interlocking intramed-
    ullary nail
Kirschner operation
Kirschner sutures
Kirschner TOD plate
Kirschner total hip replacement
Kirschner total shoulder
    prosthesis
Kirschner traction
Kirschner traction apparatus
Kirschner wire (K-wire)
Kirschner wire drill
Kirschner wire splint
Kirschner wire spreader
Kirschner wire tightener
Kirschner wire traction
Kirschner wire traction bow
Kirwin cystoscope
KISS catheter (kidney internal
    splint/stent catheter)
kissing balloon
kissing balloon technique
kissing spine syndrome
kissing ulcer

Kistner button
Kistner dissector
Kistner plastic tube
Kistner probe
Kistner tracheostomy tube
Kistner tube
Kitchen postpartum gauze
    packer
Kite cast
Kite corrective cast
Kitlowski operation
Kitner clamp
Kitner dissector
Kitner forceps
Kitner instrument
Kitner retractor
Kitner sponge
Kitner thyroid-packing forceps
Kiwisch bandage
KJ (knee jerk)
Kjelland (see *Kielland*)
Klaar headlight
Klaff septal speculum
Klaff speculum
Klatskin cholangiocarcinoma
Klatskin liver biopsy needle
Klatskin needle
Klatskin tumor
Klause antrum punch
Klause-Carmody antrum punch
Klebanoff common duct bougie
Klebanoff common duct sound
Klebanoff gallstone scoop
Klebanoff scoop
Kleegman cannula
Kleegman dilator
Kleegman needle guide
KleenSpec disposable laryngo-
    scope
KleenSpec disposable sigmoido-
    scope
KleenSpec disposable speculum
KleenSpec forceps
KleenSpec laryngoscope
KleenSpec otoscope adapter
KleenSpec otoscope tip
KleenSpec sigmoidoscope

KleenSpec speculum
KleenSpec vaginal speculum
Kleesattel elevator
Kleesattel raspatory
Kleiger closure
Klein punch
Kleinert fingertip
Kleinert operation
Kleinert rubber-band splint
Kleinert sutures
Kleinert technique
Kleinert tendon passer
Kleinert volar pedicle procedure
Kleinert volar pedicle splint
Kleinert volar V-Y plasty
Kleinert-Kutz bone rongeur
Kleinert-Kutz bone-cutting forceps
Kleinert-Kutz clamp
Kleinert-Kutz dissector
Kleinert-Kutz elevator
Kleinert-Kutz hook
Kleinert-Kutz skin hook
Kleinert-Kutz tendon retriever
Kleinert-Kutz tendon retriever forceps
Kleinert-Ragdell retractor
Kleinsasser laryngeal microscissors
Kleinsasser laryngeal microsurgery instruments
Kleinsasser laryngoscope
Kleinsasser operating laryngoscope
Kleinschmidt appendectomy clamp
Kleinschmidt technique
Klein-Tolentino ring
Klemm sign
Klemme appendectomy retractor
Klemme dura hook
Klemme gasserian ganglion retractor
Klemme hook
Klemme laminectomy retractor

Klemme locked intramedullary nail
Klemme nail
Klemme retractor
Klenzak brace
Klenzak orthosis
Klenzak splint
KLI bipolar forceps
KLI dual control assembly
KLI electrosurgery system
KLI Falope-ring instrument system
KLI forceps
KLI insufflator
KLI laparoscopy console
KLI monopolar forceps
Klima-Rosegger trocar
Kling adhesive dressing
Kling bandage
Kling cervical brace
Kling conform dressing
Kling dressing
Kling elastic
Kling elastic gauze
Kling gauze
Kling gauze dressing
Kling-Richards operation
Klinkenberg-Loth scissors
Kloehn headgear
Klondike bed
Kloti cutter
Kloti vitreous cutter
Klumpke paralysis
Klute clamp
Knapp cataract knife
Knapp cystotome
Knapp eye speculum
Knapp flap operation
Knapp forceps
Knapp hook
Knapp iris hook
Knapp iris knife needle
Knapp iris repositor
Knapp iris scissors
Knapp iris spatula
Knapp knife
Knapp knife-needle

Knapp lacrimal sac retractor
Knapp lens scoop
Knapp lid operation
Knapp needle
Knapp operation
Knapp probe
Knapp pterygium operation
Knapp retractor
Knapp scissors
Knapp scoop
Knapp spatula
Knapp speculum
Knapp spoon
Knapp trachoma forceps
Knapp-Imre lid operation
Knapp-Wheeler-Reese operation
Knapt scissors
knee action
knee bend
knee bone
knee cap
knee immobilized
knee jerk (KJ)
knee joint
knee ligament
knee motion
knee orthosis
knee plate
knee prosthesis
knee replacement
knee retractor
knee splint
knee stiffness
knee support
knee swelling
knee-ankle-foot orthosis
    (KAFO)
knee-chest position
knee-elbow position
kneeling-squatting position
Knee-Pak
knife (see also *scalpel*)
    Abraham knife
    Abraham tonsil knife
    abscess knife
    acetabular knife
    Acufex drawknife

knife *continued*
    Adson blunt knife
    Adson dural knife
    Adson knife
    Adson sharp knife
    Agnew canaliculus knife
    Agnew knife
    Alcon I-knife
    Alcon surgical knife
    Alexander otoplasty
        knife
    Allen-Barkan knife
    Allen-Hanbury knife
    Amenabar knife
    amputating knife
    amputation knife
    angle knife
    angular knife
    antral knife
    appendotome knife
    arachnoid knife
    Arbuckle antral knife
    Armour dural knife
    Armour knife
    Atkins knife
    Atkins tonsil knife
    Atkinson eye knife
    Austin dental knife
    Austin dissection knife
    Austin knife
    Austin sickle knife
    Ayerst knife
    Ayre cone knife
    Ayre knife
    Ayre-Scott knife
    back-cutting knife
    Bailey-Glover-O'Neill
        commissurotomy knife
    Bailey-Glover-O'Neill
        knife
    Bailey-Morse knife
    Ballenger cartilage knife
    Ballenger knife
    Ballenger mucosa knife
    Ballenger nose knife
    Ballenger septal knife
    Ballenger swivel knife

knife *continued*
   banana knife
   Banner enucleation knife
   Bard-Parker knife
   Bard-Parker surgical knife
   Barkan goniotomy knife
   Barkan knife
   Barker Vacu-tome knife
   Barnhill adenoid knife
   Baron ear knife
   Baron knife
   Barraquer corneal knife
   Barraquer knife
   Barrett knife
   Barrett uterine knife
   Barth mastoid knife
   Beard cataract knife
   Beard knife
   Beard lid knife
   Beaver blade cataract knife
   Beaver blade discission knife
   Beaver cataract knife blade
   Beaver discission knife blade
   Beaver knife
   Beck knife
   Beck-Schenck tonsil knife
   Beer canaliculus knife
   Beer cataract knife
   Beer knife
   Bellucci knife
   Berens corneal knife
   Berens knife
   Berens sclerotomy knife
   Billeau ear knife
   Bircher meniscus knife
   bistoury knife
   Bizzarri-Guiffrida knife
   bladebreaker knife
   Blair cleft palate knife
   Blair knife
   Blair-Brown knife

knife *continued*
   Blair-Brown skin graft knife
   Blake knife
   Bodian discission knife
   Bonta knife
   Bonta mastectomy knife
   Bosher commissurotomy knife
   Bosher knife
   Bovie knife
   Bowman eye knife
   brain knife
   Brock commissurotomy knife
   Brock knife
   Brophy bistoury knife
   Brophy cleft palate knife
   Brophy knife
   Brown cleft palate knife
   Brown knife
   Brun bone knife
   Buck dissecting knife
   Buck ear knife
   Buck knife
   Buck myringotome knife
   Buck myringotomy knife
   Bucy cordotomy knife
   Bucy knife
   Burford-Lebsche knife
   button knife
   button-end knife
   button-nosed knife
   Caltagirone knife
   Caltagirone skin graft knife
   canal knife
   canaliculus knife
   Canfield knife
   Canfield tonsil knife
   Carpenter knife
   Carpenter tonsil knife
   Carter knife
   cartilage knife
   Castroviejo bladebreaker knife
   Castroviejo knife

knife *continued*
- Castroviejo ophthalmic knife
- Castroviejo-Wheeler discission knife
- cataract knife
- catlin amputating knife
- cautery knife
- Cave cartilage knife
- Cave knife
- cervical cordotomy knife
- cervical knife
- chalazion knife
- circle knife
- cirsotome knife
- cleft palate knife
- coagulating knife
- Cobbett knife
- cold knife
- cold-cone knife
- Collin amputating knife
- Collings knife
- Colver knife
- commissurotomy knife
- cone biopsy knife
- Cone knife
- conization knife
- Converse knife
- cordotomy knife
- corneal knife
- Cornman dissecting knife
- Cottle double-edged knife
- Cottle knife
- Cottle nasal knife
- Crescent plaster knife
- Crile cleft palate knife
- Crile knife
- Cronin palate knife
- Crosby knife
- crypt knife
- Culbertson canal knife
- Curdy knife
- Curdy sclerotome knife
- Curran eye knife
- curved knife

knife *continued*
- Cushing dural hook knife
- Cushing dural knife
- Cushing knife
- Cusick eye knife
- cutting Bovie knife
- Czermak eye knife
- Daily eye knife
- Davidoff cordotomy knife
- Davidoff knife
- Daviel chalazion knife
- Daviel knife
- Davis knife
- Davis tonsillar knife
- Day knife
- Day tonsillar knife
- Dean curved eye knife
- Dean iris knife
- Dean knife
- Dean needle knife
- Dean tonsillar knife
- deep knife
- DeLee knife
- Dench knife
- dental knife
- DePalma knife
- Derf ear knife
- Derlacki capsule knife
- Derlacki knife
- Dermot-Pierse ball-tipped knife
- Derra commissurotomy knife
- Derra knife
- D'Errico knife
- Desmarres knife
- Desmarres paracentesis knife
- Deutschman cataract knife
- Deutschman knife
- Devonshire knife
- diamond knife
- diathermia knife
- Dieffenbach knife

knife *continued*

Dintenfass ear knife
Dintenfass-Chapman knife
discission knife
double-edged knife
double-ended flap knife
Douglas knife
Down epiphyseal knife
Downing cartilage knife
Downing knife
drum elevator knife
Dupuytren knife
dural hook knife
dural knife
ear knife
electric knife
electrocautery knife
electrosurgical cutting knife
electrosurgical knife
Elschnig cataract knife
Elschnig knife
Elschnig pterygium knife
embryotomy knife
endotherm knife
Equen-Neuffer knife
Equen-Neuffer laryngeal knife
Eves tonsillar knife
expansile knife
eye knife
facial nerve knife
Farrior knife
Farrior-McHugh knife
Fergusson bone knife
Ferris Smith knife
Ferris-Robb knife
Ferris-Robb tonsil knife
Fine-Gill corneal knife
Fisher knife
Fisher tonsil knife
fistular knife
fistulotome knife
flap knife
Fletcher knife
Fletcher tonsil knife

knife *continued*

Fomon double-edged knife
Fomon knife
Frazier cordotomy knife
Frazier knife
Freer knife
Freer mucosa knife
Freer septal knife
Freer-Ingal septal knife
Freer-Ingal submucous knife
Freiberg cartilage knife
Freiberg knife
Friesner ear knife
Friesner knife
Gamma knife
Gamon eye knife
Gandhi knife
ganglion knife
Garrison knife
Gerzog ear knife
Gerzog knife
Gerzog-Ralks ear knife
Gerzog-Ralks knife
Gill corneal knife
Gill knife
Girard-Swan knife-needle
Glasscock-House knife
glaucoma knife
Goldman guillotine nerve knife
Goldman knife
Goldman serrated knife
Goldman-Fox knife
goniotomy knife
Goode knife
Goodhill knife
Goodhill-Down knife
Goodyear knife
Goodyear tonsillar knife
Goulian knife
Graefe (also *von Graefe*)
Graefe cataract knife
Graefe knife
Graefe knife-needle

knife *continued*
    Graefe sickle knife
    Green cataract knife
    Green knife
    Green scleral resection
        knife
    Grieshaber eye knife
    Grieshaber knife
    Grover meniscus knife
    Guilford sickle knife
    Guillian knife
    Guy knife
    Haab eye knife
    Haab scleral resection
        knife
    Haab-Grieshaber knife
    Halle dural knife
    Halle knife
    Harris tonsillar knife
    Harrison knife
    Hartmann knife
    Heath chalazion knife
    Herbert knife
    herniotome knife
    Hewy knife
    Hilsinger knife
    Hilsinger tonsillar knife
    Hoffer knife
    Horsley bone knife
    hot knife
    Hough knife
    Hough tendon knife
    Hough tympanoplasty
        knife
    Hough-Rosen knife
    House angular knife
    House incudostapedial
        joint knife
    House knife
    House lancet knife
    House myringotomy
        knife
    House sickle knife
    House-Rosen utility knife
    Hufnagel commis-
        surotomy knife
    Hufnagel knife

knife *continued*
    Humby knife
    Hundley knee knife
    Hurd tonsil knife
    Hyams scleral knife
    hysterectomy knife
    I-Knife
    incudostapedial joint
        knife
    incudostapedial knife
    interosseous knife
    intimectomy knife
    iris knife
    IS joint knife (incudo-
        stapedial joint knife)
    jackknife position
    Jackson knife
    Jackson tracheal knife
    Jacobson knife
    Jaeger keratome knife
    Jaeger knife
    Jako knife
    Jannetta knife
    Johnson knife
    Johnson ptotic knife
    Johnson-Tooke corneal
        knife
    Johnson-Tooke knife
    joint knife
    Jones knife
    Jordan capsule knife
    Jordan knife
    Jordan stapedectomy
        knife
    Joseph angular knife
    Joseph button knife
    Joseph button-end knife
    Joseph double-edged
        knife
    Joseph knife
    Joseph nasal knife
    Joseph-Maltz knife
    Katena-Ruby knife
    Keeler knife
    keratotomy knife
    Killian knife
    Killian tonsil knife

knife *continued*

Kirby cataract knife
Kirby knife
Kirkland knife
Knapp cataract knife
Knapp knife
Knapp knife-needle
Koos vessel knife
Kratz-Ziegler knife
Krause ear knife
Kreissl knife
Kreissl meatotomy knife
Krull acetabular knife
Krull knife
Kyle crypt knife
Kyle knife
Ladd knife
lamina knife
Lancaster eye knife
Lancaster knife
lancet knife
Landolt eye knife
Lang knife
Langenbeck flap knife
Langenbeck knife
Langenbeck resection
    knife
Lanigan cartilage knife
laparotrachelotomy knife
laryngeal knife
Lebsche knife
Lebsche sternal knife
Lebsche thoracic knife
Lee knife
Lee-Cohen knife
Leland knife
Leland tonsillar knife
Lempert knife
Lempert paracentesis
    knife
lenticular knife
lid knife
Lieb-Guerry eye knife
ligature knife
Lillie knife
Lillie tonsillar knife
Lister knife

knife *continued*

Liston amputating knife
Liston knife
Lothrop knife
Lothrop tonsillar knife
Lowe-Breck cartilage
    knife
Lowe-Breck knife
Lowe-Breck meniscec-
    tomy knife
Lowell glaucoma knife
Lowell knife
Lundsgaard knife
Lundsgaard-Burch knife
Lynch knife
Lynch tonsillar knife
MacCallum knife
Machemer sclerotomy
    knife
MacKenty cleft palate
    knife
MacKenty knife
Magielski canal knife
Maltz angle knife
Maltz cartilage knife
Maltz knife
Mandelbaum ear knife
Marcks knife
Martinez knife-dissector
mastectomy knife
mastoid knife
Maumenee eye knife
Mayo knife
McCabe canal knife
McCabe dissector knife
McCabe flap knife-
    dissector
McCarthy diathermic
    knife
McCaslin knife-needle
McCaslin needle-knife
McHugh facial nerve
    knife
McHugh flap knife
McHugh knife
McKeever cartilage knife
McKeever knife

knife *continued*
- McMurray knife
- McPherson-Wheeler iris microknife
- McPherson-Wheeler knife
- McPherson-Ziegler iris knife
- McPherson-Ziegler knife
- McPherson-Ziegler microknife
- McReynolds knife
- McReynolds pterygium knife
- McReynolds-Castroviejo pterygium knife
- Mead lancet knife
- meatotomy knife
- meniscal knife
- meniscectomy knife
- Mercer cartilage knife
- Merrifield knife
- Metzenbaum knife
- Metzenbaum septum knife
- Metzger infant knife
- Meyhoeffer eye knife
- Meyhoeffer knife
- microblade knife
- microvessel knife
- middle ear canal knife
- middle ear capsule knife
- middle ear knife
- Miller tonsillar knife
- Millette tonsil knife
- Millette-Tydings knife
- Mitchell knife
- mitral knife
- mitral stenosis knife
- Moebius cataract knife
- Moebius knife
- Monocorps milium knife
- Moorehead ear knife
- Moorehead knife
- Mori knife
- mucosa knife
- mucus knife

knife *continued*
- Murphy knife
- Murphy plaster knife
- myelotomy knife
- myringoplasty knife
- myringotome knife
- myringotomy knife
- nasal knife
- nasal swivel knife
- needle-knife
- Neff meniscus knife
- Neivert knife
- Nelson Rocker knife
- Neoflex bendable knife
- Neoflex electrocautery knife
- NeoKnife
- neurosurgical knife
- Newman knife
- Niedner knife
- Nunez-Nunez knife
- Nunez-Nunez mitral stenosis knife
- obtuse-angle knife
- O'Connor hex probe knife
- O'Connor left-curve knife
- O'Connor meniscotomy knife
- O'Connor probe knife
- O'Connor retrograde knife
- O'Connor right-curve knife
- O'Connor straight knife
- Oertli knife
- Oertli razor bladebreaker knife
- Olivecrona trigeminus knife
- O'Malley knife
- operating knife
- ophthalmic knife
- Oretorp meniscectomy knife
- oval knife
- Pace hysterectomy knife

knife *continued*

Pace knife
Page knife
Page tonsillar knife
Paparella knife
paracentesis knife
Parker knife
Parker knife-needle
Parker serrated discission knife
Paton corneal knife
Paton knife
Paufique corneal knife
Paufique graft knife
Paufique knife
Paufique lamellar knife
phalangeal knife
Philadelphia tonsil knife
pituitary capsulectomy knife
plaster cast knife
plaster knife
Politzer angular ear knife
Politzer ear knife
Politzer knife
Politzer-Ralks knife
Pope rectal knife
Potter knife
Potts expansile knife
Potts knife
Prince knife
pterygium knife
ptosis knife
pull knife
pulmonary valve knife
Ralks ear knife
Ralks knife
Ramsbotham knife
Rayport dural knife
Rayport knife
Reese knife
Reese ptosis knife
Rehne skin graft knife
Reiner ear knife
Reiner knife
retrograde knife
reversible knife

knife *continued*

Richardson right-angle ear knife
Richardson right-angle knife
Ridlon knife
Ridlon plaster knife
Rish knife
Rizzuti scleral knife
Rizzuti-Spizziri knife
Robb knife
Robb tonsillar knife
Robertson knife
Robertson tonsillar knife
Robinson flap knife
Rochester knife
Rochester mitral stenosis knife
roller knife
Rosen incision knife
Rosen knife
Rowland eye knife
Royce ear knife
Royce knife
ruby knife
Salenius meniscus knife
sapphire knife
Sato corneal knife
Sato eye knife
Sato knife
Scheer knife
Scheie goniopuncture knife
Scheie goniotomy knife
Scheie knife
Scholl knife
Scholl meniscus knife
Schuknecht knife
Schuknecht roller knife
Schultze embryotomy knife
Schultze knife
Schwartz cordotomy knife
Schwartz knife
scimitar-blade knife
sclerotomy knife

knife *continued*

Seiler conization knife
Seiler knife
Seiler tonsillar knife
Sellor knife
semilunar cartilage knife
septal knife
serrated knife
Sexton bayonet ear knife
Sexton ear knife
Sexton knife
Shaffer eye knife
Shambaugh knife
Shambaugh-Derlacki knife
Shambaugh-Lempert knife
Sharpoint knife
Sharpoint microsurgical knife
Sharpoint slit knife
Shaw knife
Shea knife
Sheehy canal knife
Sheehy knife
Sheehy-House knife
Sherman knife
Sichel iris knife
Sichel knife
sickle knife
sickle middle-ear knife
sickle tonsillar knife
sickle-shaped House knife
sickle-shaped knife
Silver knife
Sims knife
skin graft knife
skin knife
skiving knife
Sluder knife
Sluder tonsillar knife
Smillie cartilage knife
Smillie knife
Smillie meniscus knife
Smith cataract knife
Smith cordotomy knife

knife *continued*

Smith knife
Smith-Fisher cataract knife
Smith-Fisher knife
Smith-Green cataract knife
Smith-Green knife
Somers tonsillar knife
Speed-Sprague knife
sphenoidal knife
Spizziri knife
stapedectomy knife
stapedius tendon knife
Stecher arachnoid knife
sternal knife
Stern-McCarthy knife
Stevens eye knife
Stevens tissue knife
Stewart cartilage knife
Stewart knife
stiletto knife
Stilli knife
Storz folding-handle ear knife
Storz knife
Storz-Duredge cataract knife
straight cutting knife
Strayer knife
submucous knife
suction knife
Suker knife
Swan knife-needle
Swanson knife
swivel knife
sword knife
Tabb ear knife
Tabb knife
Tabb myringoplasty knife
Taylor knife
tenotomy knife
Thiersch knife
Thiersch skin graft knife
Thomas knife

knife *continued*

Thorpe foreign body knife
Tobold knife
tonsillar knife
Tooke knife
tracheal bronchial knife
tracheal knife
Troutman corneal knife
Tubby knife
turbinate knife
twin knife
Tydings knife
Tydings tonsil knife
tympanoplastic knife
tympanoplasty knife
Ullrich uterine knife
U.S. Army-pattern knife
uterine knife
Vacu-tome knife
valvotomy knife
Van Osdel tonsillar knife
Vannas abscess knife
Vannas knife
Vaughan abscess knife
vessel knife
Victor blood lancet knife
Virchow brain knife
Virchow knife
Virchow skin graft knife
vitreous knife
von Graefe (see *Graef*)
Walker-Lee eye knife
Walton ear knife
Walton knife
Watson skin-grafting knife
Weber canaliculus knife
Weber eye knife
Weber knife
Webster knife
Webster skin graft knife
Weck knife
Weck-blade knife
Weiss eye knife
Weiss-pattern knife
Weitter plaster knife

knife *continued*

Wheeler discission knife
Wheeler knife
Wheeler malleable-shape knife
whirlybird knife
Wiener eye knife
Wilder eye knife
Wolf chisel knife
Wolf draw knife
Wolf meniscal knife
Woodruff spatula knife
Wullstein ear knife
Wullstein knife
X-Acto utility knife
Yamanda myelotomy knife
Yankauer salpingeal knife
Yasargil arachnoid knife
Yasargil knife
Yazujian eye knife
Ziegler eye needle-knife
Ziegler iris knife
Ziegler iris knife-needle
Ziegler knife
Ziegler knife-needle
Ziegler needle-knife
knife and scissors dissection
knife blade
knife conization
knife electrode
knife handle
knife-needle
Knight brace
Knight forceps
Knight nasal forceps
Knight nasal scissors
Knight nasal septum-cutting forceps
Knight needle
Knight polyp forceps
Knight scissors
Knight septum-cutting forceps
Knight turbinate forceps
Knighton hemilaminectomy self-retaining retractor

Knighton-Kerrison punch
Knight-Sluder forceps
Knight-Taylor orthosis
Knight-Taylor thoracolumbo-
    sacral orthosis
knitted Dacron arterial graft
knitted graft
knitted Teflon graft
knitted Teflon prosthesis
knitted vascular prosthesis
knobby process
knocked-down shoulder
knock-knee
Knodt distraction rod
Knodt hook
Knodt rod
Knodt rod fusion of spine
Knolle cannula
Knolle cystitome
Knolle intraocular lens
Knolle irrigating loop with
    I&A tip
Knolle lens
Knolle lens speculum
Knolle polisher
Knolle posterior capsule
    polisher
Knolle-Kelman cystitome
Knolle-Pearce cannula
Knolle-Pearce lens loop
knot
    Adson knot tier
    barrel knot sutures
    bench knot pusher-tier
    clove-hitch knot
    double knot
    friction knot
    granny knot
    half-hitch knot
    Henry master knot
    inverted knot sutures
    Jacobson knot tier
    master knot of Henry
    reef knot
    sailor's knot
    single-handed knot
        sutures

knot *continued*
    slip-knot tie
    square knot
    stay knot
    surgeon's knot
    surgical knot
    syncytial knot
knot formation
knot of Henry
knot pusher-tier
knot tier
knot tying
knot-holding forceps
Knowles bandage scissors
Knowles pin
Knowles pin nail
Knowles scissors
knuckle
knuckle of bowel
knuckle of choroid
knuckle of colon
knuckle of tube
knuckle pad
knuckle-binder splint
knurled CD rod (Cotrel-
    Dubousset rod)
knurled Cotrel-Dubousset
    rod
Koagamin dressing
Kobak needle
Kobelt tube
Koby cataract
Kobyashi hook
Koch ileostomy
Koch node
Koch shoulder reduction
Kocher approach
Kocher artery forceps
Kocher biliary tract incision
Kocher bladder retractor
Kocher brain spoon
Kocher bronchocele sound
Kocher clamp
Kocher collar incision
Kocher collar thyroidectomy
    incision
Kocher dilatation ulcer

Kocher dissector
Kocher elevator
Kocher forceps
Kocher fracture
Kocher fracture of capitellum
Kocher gallbladder retractor
Kocher goiter dissector
Kocher goiter self-retaining
    retractor
Kocher hemostat
Kocher incision
Kocher intestinal clamp
Kocher intestinal forceps
Kocher kidney-elevating forceps
Kocher maneuver
Kocher Micro-Line intestinal
    forceps
Kocher operation
Kocher periosteal dissector
Kocher periosteal elevator
Kocher point
Kocher raspatory
Kocher reflex
Kocher retractor
Kocher scissors
Kocher shoulder reduction
Kocher sound
Kocher spoon
Kocher ulcer
Kocher-Crotti goiter retractor
Kocher-Crotti goiter self-
    retaining retractor
Kocher-Crotti retractor
kocherization
Kocher-McFarland approach
Kocher-McFarland arthroplasty
    approach
Kocher-Ochsner hemostatic
    forceps
Kocher-Osborn hip arthroplasty
Koch-Mason dressing
Kock continent ileostomy
Kock ileal reservoir
Kock operation
Kock pouch
Kock pouch modified proce-
    dure
Kock reservoir

Kock reservoir ileostomy
Kocks operation for uterine
    prolapse
Koeberlé forceps
Koeberlé operation
Koenig (also *König*)
Koenig disease
Koenig elevator
Koenig graft
Koenig nail-splitting scissors
Koenig operation
Koenig raspatory
Koenig retractor
Koenig rod
Koenig technique
Koenig vascular forceps
Koenig-Schaefer approach
Koenig-Wittek operation
Koeppe goniolens
Koeppe gonioscope
Koeppe gonioscopic lens
    implant
Koeppe intraocular lens implant
Koeppe lens
Koeppe nodule
Koerner flap
Koerte (also *Körte*)
Koerte gallstone forceps
Koerte retractor
Koerte-Ballance operation
Koester nodule
Koffler forceps
Koffler operation
Koffler septum bone forceps
Koffler septum forceps
Koffler-Lillie forceps
Koffler-Lillie septum forceps
Kogan endospeculum
Kogan endospeculum forceps
Kogan speculum
Kohler disease
Kohlman dilator
Kohlman urethral dilator
Kohlrausch folds
Kohlrausch veins
Kohn needle
koilocytotic
Kokowicz raspatory

Kolb bronchus forceps
Kolb forceps
Kolb trocar
Kolle-Lexer operation
Koln clip
Kolodny clamp
Kolodny forceps
Kolodny hemostat
Kolodny scalp hemostat
Kolomnin operation
Kompak sphygmomanometer
Kondoleon operation
König (see *Koenig*)
Kono operation
Kono patch enlargement of
    ascending aorta
Konon aortic valve replacement
Kontron balloon
Kontron intra-aortic balloon
Koontz hernia needle
Koos vessel knife
Kopan needle
Kopetzky bur
Kopetzky sinus bur
Koplik sign
Koplik spot
Korányi auscultation
Korányi percussion
Korányi sign
Kormed disposable liver biopsy
    needle
Kormed needle
Korotkoff method
Korotkoff sound
Körte (see *Koerte*)
Kortzeborn hand procedure
Kos attic cannula
Kos cannula
Koteline bifocal lens
Kotex pad
Kowa automatic fundus lens
Kowa camera
Kowa fundus camera
Kowa hand camera
Kowa hand-held slit lamp
Kowa Optimed camera
Kowa retinal camera

Kowa slit lamp
Kowalzig operation
Koylon foam rubber dressing
Koyter muscle
Kozlinski retractor
Kozlowski tube
KPE (Kelman phacoemulsifica-
    tion)
Kraff intraocular implant lens
Kramer bivalve ear speculum
Kramer ear speculum
Kramer forceps
Kramer speculum
Kramer syringe
Kramer telescope
Kramer-Craig-Noel osteotomy
Kraske operation
Kraske position
Krasky retractor
Krasnov implant cataract lens
Krasnov lens
Kratz implant
Kratz intraocular implant lens
Kratz lens
Kratz polisher
Kratz posterior chamber
    intraocular lens
Kratz scratcher
Kratz-Jensen polisher
Kratz-Jensen scratcher
Kratz-Johnson intraocular
    lens
Kratz-Sinskey intraocular lens
    implant
Kratz-Ziegler knife
Kraupa operation
Krause biopsy forceps
Krause cannula
Krause ear knife
Krause ear snare
Krause forceps
Krause forceps tip
Krause gland
Krause nasal snare
Krause operation
Krause punch
Krause punch forceps tip

Krause snare
Krause through-cutting forceps
    tip
Krause transverse suture
Krause trocar
Krause Universal forceps
Krause ventricle
Krause-Wolfe graft
Krause-Wolfe implant
Krause-Wolfe operation
Krause-Wolfe prosthesis
Krayenbuehl hook
Krayenbuehl vessel hook
Kreibig operation
Kreiker blepharochalasis
Kreiker operation
Kreischer bone chisel
Kreischer chisel
Kreiselman incubator
Kreiselman packer
Kreiselman resuscitator
Kreiselman unit
Kreissl knife
Kreissl meatotomy knife
Krentz photogastroscope
Kretschmer retractor
Kreuscher bunionectomy
Kreuscher operation
Kreuscher scissors
Kreutzmann cannula
Kreutzmann trocar
Krieberg operation
Krimer operation
Kristeller retractor
Kristeller speculum
Kristeller technique
Kristeller vaginal speculum
Kristiansen screw
Kroener fimbriectomy
Kroener operation
Kromayer lamp
Kromayer mercury vapor
    light
Kron bile duct dilator
Kron dilator
Kron gall duct dilator
Kron gall duct probe
Kron probe

Kronecker needle
Kronendonk pin
Kroner apparatus
Kroner tubal ligation
Kronfeld electrode
Kronfeld eyelid retractor
Kronfeld forceps
Kronfeld micropin forceps
Kronfeld pin
Kronfeld retractor
Kronfeld suture forceps
Krönig area
Krönig cesarean section
Krönig isthmus
Krönig percussion
Krönlein hemostatic forceps
Krönlein hernia
Krönlein operation
Krönlein-Berke operation
Krönlein-Berke retractor
Kronner external fixator
Kronner skeletal fixation
Krukenberg amputation
Krukenberg arm
Krukenberg hand
Krukenberg operation
Krukenberg procedure
Krukenberg spindle
Krukenberg tumor
Krukenberg veins
Krull acetabular knife
Krull knife
Krupin glaucoma valve
Krupin valve
Krupin-Denver eye valve
Krwawicz cataract extractor
Krwawicz cataract lens
Krwawicz cryoextractor
Kry-Med 300 cryoprobe
Kryostik
Kryptok bifocal lens
Kryptok bifocals lens implant
krypton laser
K/S-Allis forceps
KSO brace
KUB (kidneys, ureters, bladder)
KUB x-ray
Kudo hinge

Kuettner technique
Kugel anastomosis
Kugel artery
Kugelberg-Welander disease
Kuglen hook
Kuglen iris hook
Kuglen lens manipulator
Kuglen retractor
Kuhlman brace
Kuhlman cast cutter
Kuhlman Kast Kutter
Kuhlman cervical traction
Kuhlman traction
Kuhn mask
Kuhn tube
Kuhnt capsule forceps
Kuhnt dacryostomy
Kuhnt eyelid operation
Kuhnt fixation forceps
Kuhnt forceps
Kuhnt gouge
Kuhnt intermediary tissue
Kuhnt operation
Kuhnt postcentral vein
Kuhnt tarsectomy
Kuhnt-Helmbold operation
Kuhnt-Szymanowski eyelid
    operation
Kuhnt-Szymanowski operation
Kuhnt-Thorpe operation
Kulenkampff anesthesia
Kulvin-Kalt forceps
Kulvin-Kalt iris forceps
Kumar applicator
Kumar-Cowell-Ramsey tech-
    nique
Küntscher cloverleaf nail
Küntscher driver
Küntscher femur guide pin
Küntscher intramedullary nail
Küntscher nail
Küntscher nail driver
Küntscher nail extender
Küntscher nail instrument
Küntscher nail set
Küntscher pin
Küntscher reamer

Küntscher rod
Kuntscher shaft reamer
Küntscher traction apparatus
Küntscher-Hudson brace
Kurlander orthopedic wrench
Kurosaka bone screw
Kurosaka cannulated screw
Kurosaka extremity screw
Kurosaka interference fixation
    screw
Kurten stripper
Kurten vein stripper
Kurten wire brush
Kurzbauer position
Kurze dissecting scissors
Kurze dissector
Kurze forceps
Kurze microbiopsy forceps
Kurze microdissector
Kurze micrograsping forceps
Kurze microneurosurgery
    instrument
Kurze microscissors
Kurze pickup forceps
Kurze scissors
Kurze suction-irrigator
Kurze suction-irrigator tube
Kushner-Tandatnick curet
Kushner-Tandatnick endo-
    metrial biopsy
Kushner-Tandatnick endo-
    metrial biopsy curet
Kussmaul breathing
Kussmaul pulse
Kussmaul respirations
Kussmaul sign
Küster hernia
Küster operation
Küstner operation
Küstner sign
Küstner sutures
Küstner uterine tenaculum
    forceps
Kutler amputation
Kutler fingertip
Kutler V-Y flaps
Kutzmann clamp

KWB classification (Keith-Wagener-Barker hypertensive classification)

Kwitko intraocular implant lens

Kydex body jacket

Kydex brace

Kyle applicator

Kyle crypt knife

Kyle ear applicator

Kyle knife

Kyle nasal speculum

Kyle speculum

kymogram

kymograph chart

kymography

Kyoto-Barrett-Boyes perfusion technique

kyphectomy

Kypher sutures

kyphoscoliosis

kyphosis

kyphotic

kyphotic angle

kyphotic pelvis

l or L (liter)
L-curved incision
L-osteotomy
L-plasty repair
L-plate
L-R shunt
L-shaped elevator
L-transposition of great arteries
    (levotransposition of great
    arteries)
L-type capsulotomy
L-type nose-bridge prosthesis
LA/Ao ratio (left atrial/aortic)
Labbé operation
Labbé triangle
Labbé vein
labia (*sing.* labium)
labia major
labia majora
labia minor
labia minora
labial
labial arteries
labial bar
labial flange
labial fold
labial frenum
labial hernia
labial nerves
labial region
labial splint
labial swelling
labial veins
labiales anteriores, nervi
labiales anteriores, venae
labiales inferiores, venae
labiales posteriores, nervi
labiales posteriores, venae
labialis inferior, arteria

labialis superior, arteria
labialis superior, vena
labiectomy
labiodental sulcus
labioglossopharyngeal nerve
labioplasty
labioscrotal swelling
labiotenaculum
labium (*pl.* labia)
labor augmentation
labor pain
labor terminated
Laborde dilator
Laborde forceps
Laborde tracheal dilator
labored breathing
labored respiration
labrum
labyrinth
labyrinth curet
labyrinth membrane
labyrinth of brain
labyrinthectomy
labyrinthi, arteriae
labyrinthi, venae
labyrinthine arteries
labyrinthine function
labyrinthine symptoms
labyrinthine veins
labyrinthotomy
LAC (long-arm cast)
LaCarrere electrode
LaCarrere electrodiaphake
LaCarrere operation
lace sutures
lacerable
lacerated
lacerated perineum
lacerated tendon

635

lacerated wound
laceration
laceration of organ
Lacey condylar total knee
    system
Lacey prosthesis
Lacey rotating hinge
Lacey total knee implant
Lachman maneuver
Lachman tear
Lachman-MacIntosh test
lachrymal (see *lacrimal*)
lacidem sutures
laciniate ligament
lacrimal apparatus
lacrimal artery
lacrimal bone
lacrimal canal
lacrimal canaliculus
lacrimal cannula
lacrimal caruncle
lacrimal chisel
lacrimal crest
lacrimal dilator
lacrimal duct
lacrimal duct probe
lacrimal gland
lacrimal needle
lacrimal nerve
lacrimal papilla
lacrimal probe
lacrimal punctum
lacrimal retractor
lacrimal sac
lacrimal sac retractor
lacrimal sound
lacrimal syringe
lacrimal trephine
lacrimal tube
lacrimal veins
lacrimalis, arteria
lacrimalis, nervus
lacrimalis, vena
lacrimation
lacrimoconchal suture
lacrimoethmoidal suture
lacrimomaxillary suture

lacrimonasal duct
lacrimoturbinal suture
lactate solution
lactated Ringer solution
lactating breast
lactation
lacteal
lacteal cataract
lactic acid
lactiferous duct
lacuna (*pl.* lacunae)
lacuna magna
lacuna musculorum
lacuna vasorum
lacunae of Morgagni
lacunar
lacunar infarct
lacunar infarction
lacunar ligament
LAD (left anterior descending
    artery, ligament augmenta-
    tion device)
Ladd band
Ladd calipers
Ladd clamp
Ladd elevator
Ladd intracranial pressure
    sensor
Ladd knife
Ladd lid clamp
Ladd operation
Ladd pressure monitor
Ladd procedure for malrotation
    of bowel
Ladd raspatory
Laennec cirrhosis
Laennec sign
Laerdal resuscitator
LaForce adenotome
LaForce adenotome blade
LaForce hemostatic tonsillec-
    tome
LaForce knife spud
LaForce spud
LaForce tonometer
LaForce tonsillectome
LaForce tonsillectomy

LaForce-Grieshaber adenotome
LaForce-Stevenson adenotome
LaForce-Storz adenotome
LAG (lymphangiogram)
lag screw
lag technique
lag time
Lagleyze eyelid operation
Lagleyze needle
Lagleyze-Trantas operation
lagophthalmos
Lagrange eye scissors
Lagrange modification of Arruga
    operation
Lagrange modification of Berens
    operation
Lagrange operation
Lagrange scissors
Lagrange sclerectomy
Lagrange-Letoumel hip socket
    prosthesis
Lahey (see also *Lahey Clinic*)
Lahey bag
Lahey carrier
Lahey catheter
Lahey clamp
Lahey Clinic (see also *Lahey*)
Lahey Clinic dura hook
Lahey Clinic instruments
Lahey Clinic osteotome
Lahey Clinic rectal scissors
Lahey Clinic retractor
Lahey Clinic spinal fusion
    gouge
Lahey dissecting scissors
Lahey drain
Lahey forceps
Lahey gall duct forceps
Lahey goiter retractor
Lahey goiter tenaculum
Lahey gouge
Lahey hemostatic forceps
Lahey hook
Lahey incision
Lahey ligature carrier
Lahey needle
Lahey operation

Lahey osteotome
Lahey retractor
Lahey scissors
Lahey sutures
Lahey tenaculum
Lahey thoracic clamp
Lahey thoracic forceps
Lahey thyroid retractor
Lahey thyroid scissors
Lahey thyroid tenaculum
Lahey thyroid traction forceps
Lahey thyroid traction vulsellum
    forceps
Lahey trephine
Lahey tube
Lahey Y-tube
Lahey-Babcock forceps
Lahey-Metzenbaum dissecting
    scissors
Lahey-Péan forceps
Lahey-Sweet dissecting forceps
LAI knee prosthesis
Laidley cystoscope
Laing concentric hip cup
Laing plate
Laird cyclodialysis spatula
Laird spatula
Laird-McMahon anorectoplasty
Lairmonth procedure
laissez-faire lid operation
Lakeside scissors
Lalonde tendon approximator
Lam modification of Jones
    procedure
Lam operation
Lamaze childbirth technique
Lamaze method of childbirth
Lamb cannula
Lamb irrigator
Lamb transfer
Lambda Omni Stanicor pace-
    maker
Lambda pacemaker
lambda wave
lambdoid suture
lambdoid suture line
Lambert aortic clamp

Lambert chalazion forceps
Lambert forceps
Lambert-Berry raspatory
Lambert-Berry rib raspatory
Lambert-Kay aorta clamp
Lambert-Kay clamp
Lambert-Kay vascular clamp
Lambert-Lowman bone clamp
Lambert-Lowman clamp
Lambotte bone-holding forceps
Lambotte chisel
Lambotte clamp
Lambotte elevator
Lambotte forceps
Lambotte osteotome
Lambotte rasp
Lambotte raspatory
Lambotte splitting chisel
Lambotte-Henderson osteotome
Lambrinudi operation
Lambrinudi operation for talipes
    equinovarus
Lambrinudi splint
Lambrinudi triple arthrodesis
lamella (*pl.* lamellae)
lamellar bone
lamellar cataract
lamellar corneal graft
lamellar graft
lamellar incision
lamellar keratoplasty
lamellated bone
Lamicel
lamina (*pl.* laminae)
lamina affixa
lamina cribrosa
lamina dissector
lamina elevator
lamina externa
lamina gouge
lamina interna
lamina knife
lamina propria
lamina spread
lamina spreader
lamina superficialis fasciae
    cervicalis

laminar
laminar air flow
laminar flow
laminaria
laminaria insertion
laminaria seaweed obstetrical
    dilator
laminaria tent
laminate induration
laminectomy
laminectomy chisel
laminectomy frame
laminectomy instrument
laminectomy punch
laminectomy raspatory
laminectomy retractor
laminectomy retractor blade
laminectomy rongeur
laminectomy scissors
laminectomy self-retaining
    retractor
laminectomy shears
Laminex needle
laminogram
laminogram examination
laminograph
laminography
laminotomy
Lamis patella clamp
Lamm incision
Lamont elevator
Lamont nasal rasp
Lamont nasal raspatory
Lamont nasal saw
Lamont rasp
Lamont saw
lamp (see also *light, slit lamp*)
    all-purpose lamp
    Beck bull's eye lamp
    binocular slit lamp
    Birch-Hirschfield lamp
    bull's eye lamp
    capsular floor lamp
    carbon arc lamp
    cataract lamp
    Duke-Elder lamp
    Eldridge-Green lamp

lamp *continued*
    electric head lamp
    Gullstrand slit lamp
    Haag slit lamp
    Haag-Streit slit lamp
    Hague cataract lamp
    Hague lamp
    Jesionek lamp
    Kowa hand-held lamp
    Kowa slit lamp
    Kromayer lamp
    Lampert excavator
    Minin lamp
    ophthalmic lamp
    quartz lamp
    quartz mercury ultraviolet lamp
    Reichert slit lamp
    Shahan ophthalmic lamp
    slit lamp
    Smith head lamp
    Smith-Fisher cataract lamp
    Thorpe slit lamp
    tungsten arc lamp
    Universal lamp
    Wood lamp
    Zeiss hammer lamp
    Zeiss slit lamp
    Zoalite lamp
Lancaster eye knife
Lancaster eye magnet
Lancaster eye speculum
Lancaster keratome
Lancaster knife
Lancaster lid speculum
Lancaster magnet
Lancaster operation
Lancaster sclerotome
Lancaster speculum
Lancaster transilluminator
Lancaster-O'Connor forceps
Lancaster-O'Connor speculum
lance (see also *lancet*)
    Rolf lance
    Sharpoint V-lance blade

Lanceford porous metal hip prosthesis
lancet (see also *lance, lancet knife*)
    abscess lancet
    acne lancet
    gingival lancet
    gum lancet
    House lancet
    laryngeal lancet
    spring lancet
lancet knife (see also *lance, lancet*)
    House lancet knife
    Victor blood lancet knife
lancet-shaped biopsy forceps
Lanchner operation
lancinating
lancinating pain
Lancisi muscle
Lancisi nerve
Lancisi sign
Landau dilator
Landau pelvic access trocar
Landau trocar
Landegger orbital implant
Landers contact lens
Landers vitrectomy ring
Landers-Foulk lens
landmark
landmark preserved
Landolt bodies
Landolt enucleation scissors
Landolt eye knife
Landolt eyelid reconstruction
Landolt keratome
Landolt operation
Landolt pituitary speculum
Landolt ring
Landsmeer ligaments
Landström muscle
Landzert fossa
Lane band
Lane bone-holding clamp
Lane bone-holding forceps
Lane catheter
Lane clamp

Lane cleft palate needle
Lane dissector
Lane elevator
Lane forceps
Lane gastroenterostomy clamp
Lane intestinal clamp
Lane intestinal forceps
Lane mouth gag
Lane needle
Lane operation
Lane periosteal elevator
Lane periosteal raspatory
Lane plate for long-bone
    fixation
Lane raspatory
Lane rectal catheter
Lane retractor
Lane rongeur
Lane screwdriver
Lane suture needle
Lane towel clamp
Lane ureteral meatotomy
    electrode
Lane-Lannelongue operation
Lang dissector
Lang eye speculum
Lang knife
Lang scoop
Lang speculum
Lang sutures
Lange antrum punch
Lange approximation forceps
Lange fistula hook
Lange metatarsus varus
    procedure
Lange mouth gag
Lange operation
Lange position
Lange punch
Lange retractor
Lange skin-fold calipers
Lange speculum
Lange tendon lengthening
Lange tendon repair
Lange-Converse rongeur
Langenbeck amputation
Langenbeck bone-holding
    forceps

Langenbeck elevator
Langenbeck flap
Langenbeck flap knife
Langenbeck forceps
Langenbeck incision
Langenbeck knife
Langenbeck metacarpal saw
Langenbeck needle holder
Langenbeck operation
Langenbeck pedicle mucoperi-
    osteal flap
Langenbeck periosteal elevator
Langenbeck periosteal raspatory
Langenbeck raspatory
Langenbeck resection knife
Langenbeck retractor
Langenbeck saw
Langenbeck-Cushing vein
    retractor
Langenbeck-O'Brien raspatory
Langenbeck-Ryder needle
    holder
Langenskiold fusion of growth
    plate
Langenskiold hip osteotomy
Langenskiold technique
Langer axillary arch
Langer lines
Langer muscle
Langerhans island
Lange-Wilde snare
Langley nerves
Lanigan cartilage knife
Lannelongue operation
Lannu anterior chamber lens
Lanz low-pressure cuff endotra-
    cheal tube
Lanz operation
Lanz point
Lanz tracheostomy tube
Lanz tube
lap count
lap pack
lap pad
lap sheet
lap sponge
lap tapes
laparectomy

laparoaminoscopy
laparocele
laparocholecystotomy
laparocolectomy
laparocolostomy
laparocolotomy
laparocystectomy
laparocystidotomy
laparoenterostomy
laparoenterotomy
laparogastroscopy
laparogastrostomy
laparogastrotomy
laparohepatotomy
laparohysterosalpingo-
    oophorectomy
laparoileotomy
laparomyomectomy
laparonephrectomy
laparorrhaphy
laparoscope
    ACMI laparoscope
    Eder laparoscope
    Frangenheim laparo-
       scope
    Hasson laparoscope
    Hasson-Eder laparoscope
       cannula
    Jacobs-Palmer laparo-
       scope
    Lent laparoscope
    Lent photo-laparoscope
    Sharplav laparoscope
    Stoltz laparoscope
    Storz laparoscope
    Wolf laparoscope
laparoscope instrument
laparoscope lens warmer
laparoscopic cannula
laparoscopic forceps
laparoscopic sterilization
laparoscopic trocar
laparoscopic trocar sleeve
laparoscopic tubal ligation
laparoscopic tubal sterilization
laparoscopy
laparoscopy cannula
laparoscopy dilation instrument

laparoscopy insufflator
laparosplenectomy
laparosplenotomy
laparotome
laparotomy
laparotomy pack
laparotomy pad
laparotomy sponge
laparotrachelotomy
laparotrachelotomy knife
laparotyphlotomy
Lapides catheter
Lapides collecting bag
Lapides elastic belt
Lapides holder
Lapides needle
Lapides needle holder
Lapides procedure
Lapides tube
Lapides urological procedure
Lapidus bed
Lapidus bunionectomy
Lapidus technique
Laplace forceps
Laplace liver retractor
Laplace retractor
LaPorte total toe implant
Lapwall laparotomy sponge
Lapwall sponge
Lapwall wound protector
lardaceous organ
lardaceous tissue
Lardennois button
large bowel
large bowel curet
Large clamp
large for gestational age
    (LGA)
large intestine
large loop electrode
large physiological cup
Large self-retaining retactor
Large vena caval clamp
large-bore bile duct
    endoprosthesis
large-bore cannula
large-bore catheter
large-bore gastric lavage tube

large-bore needle
large-bowel obstruction
large-diameter bougie
large-droplet fatty liver
large-loop electrode
large-lumen catheter
large-particle biopsy
Larkin position
Larmon forefoot arthroplasty
LaRocca lacrimal tube
LaRocca tube
LaRoque hernia repair
LaRoque herniorrhaphy
LaRoque herniorrhaphy incision
LaRoque sutures
LaRoque-Branson hernia repair
Laroyenne operation
Larrey amputation
Larrey bandage
Larrey dressing
Larrey operation
Larrey point
Larrey space
Larry director
Larry grooved director
Larry probe
Larry rectal director
Larry rectal probe
Larsen tendon forceps
Larson anterior cruciate
    augmentation
Larson hip evaluation
Larson syndrome
laryngea inferior, arteria
laryngea inferior, vena
laryngea superior, arteria
laryngea superior, vena
laryngeal
laryngeal adhesion
laryngeal aditus
laryngeal applicator
laryngeal artery
laryngeal atomizer
laryngeal biopsy forceps
laryngeal block
laryngeal cannula
laryngeal carcinoma
laryngeal cartilage

laryngeal commissure
laryngeal crisis
laryngeal curet forceps
laryngeal dilator
laryngeal dissector
laryngeal drop operation
laryngeal enterotome
laryngeal forceps
laryngeal forceps tip
laryngeal knife
laryngeal lancet
laryngeal mirror
laryngeal mucosa
laryngeal nerve
laryngeal plexus
laryngeal pouch
laryngeal probe
laryngeal prominence
laryngeal prosthesis
laryngeal punch
laryngeal punch forceps
laryngeal reconstruction
laryngeal reflex
laryngeal retractor
laryngeal rotation forceps
laryngeal saw
laryngeal scissors
laryngeal sinus
laryngeal snare
laryngeal speculum
laryngeal sponging forceps
laryngeal stenosis
laryngeal stridor
laryngeal swab
laryngeal syringe
laryngeal tube
laryngeal vein
laryngeal ventricle
laryngeal web
laryngectomy
laryngectomy clamp
laryngectomy saw
laryngectomy tube
laryngeus inferior, nervus
laryngeus recurrens, nervus
laryngeus superior, nervus
laryngocentesis
laryngoesophagectomy

laryngofissure
laryngofissure forceps
laryngofissure profilometer
laryngofissure retractor
laryngofissure saw
laryngofissure scissors
laryngofissure shears
laryngogram
laryngography
laryngology
laryngopharyngeal reflex
laryngopharyngectomy
laryngopharyngoesophagec-
    tomy
laryngoplasty
laryngorrhaphy
laryngoscope
    adult laryngoscope
    adult reverse-bevel
        laryngoscope
    Albert-Andrews laryngo-
        scope
    Andrews laryngoscope
    anesthetist's folding
        laryngoscope
    anterior commissure
        laryngoscope
    Atkins-Tucker laryngo-
        scope
    Atkins-Tucker shadow-
        free laryngoscope
    Bizzarri-Guiffrida
        laryngoscope
    Briggs laryngoscope
    Broyles anterior commis-
        sure laryngoscope
    Broyles laryngoscope
    Burton laryngoscope
    Chevalier Jackson
        laryngoscope
    Clerf laryngoscope
    commissure laryngo-
        scope
    Dedo laryngoscope
    Dedo-Jako microlaryngo-
        scope
    Dedo-Pilling laryngo-
        scope

laryngoscope *continued*
    direct laryngoscope
    disposable laryngoscope
    dual distal-lighted
        laryngoscope
    ESI laryngoscope
    fiberoptic laryngoscope
    Fink laryngoscope
    Finnoff laryngoscope
    Flagg laryngoscope
    folding laryngoscope
    Foregger laryngoscope
    Fragen anterior commis-
        sure microlaryngo-
        scope
    Garfield-Holinger
        laryngoscope
    Guedel laryngoscope
    Haslinger laryngoscope
    Holinger anterior
        commissure laryngo-
        scope
    Holinger hook-on
        folding laryngoscope
    Holinger hourglass
        laryngoscope
    Holinger laryngoscope
    Holinger slotted  laryn-
        goscope
    Holinger-Garfield
        laryngoscope
    Hollister laryngoscope
    hook-on folding laryngo-
        scope
    Hopp laryngoscope
    Hopp-Morrison laryngo-
        scope
    hourglass anterior
        commissure laryngo-
        scope
    intubation laryngoscope
    Jackson anterior commis-
        sure laryngoscope
    Jackson laryngoscope
    Jackson sliding laryngo-
        scope
    Jackson standard
        laryngoscope

laryngoscope *continued*
  Jako laryngoscope
  Jako-Pilling laryngoscope
  KleenSpec disposable
    laryngoscope
  KleenSpec laryngoscope
  Kleinsasser laryngoscope
  Kleinsasser operating
    laryngoscope
  Lewy laryngoscope
  Lundy laryngoscope
  Lynch laryngoscope
  Lynch suspension
    laryngoscope
  Machida fiberoptic
    laryngoscope
  Machida laryngoscope
  MacIntosh laryngoscope
  Magill laryngoscope
  Miller laryngoscope
  mirror laryngoscope
  multipurpose laryngo-
    scope
  optical laryngoscope
  polio laryngoscope
  reverse-bevel laryngo-
    scope
  rhinolaryngoscope
  Roberts laryngoscope
  Roberts self-retaining
    laryngoscope
  rotating laryngoscope
  Rusch laryngoscope
  Sam Roberts laryngo-
    scope
  Sam Roberts self-
    retaining laryngoscope
  Sanders intubation
    laryngoscope
  Sanders laryngoscope
  self-retaining laryngo-
    scope
  shadow-free laryngo-
    scope
  Siker laryngoscope
  sliding laryngoscope
  slotted laryngoscope
  standard laryngoscope

laryngoscope *continued*
  Storz anterior commis-
    sure laryngoscope
  Storz infection ventilation
    laryngoscope
  Storz-Hopkins laryngo-
    scope
  straight-blade laryngo-
    scope
  suspension laryngoscope
  Tucker laryngoscope
  Tucker-Jako laryngo-
    scope
  wasp-waist laryngoscope
  Welch Allyn Kleenspec
    laryngoscope
  Welch Allyn laryngo-
    scope
  Wis-Foregger laryngo-
    scope
  Wis-Hipple laryngoscope
  Yankauer laryngoscope
laryngoscope battery handle
laryngoscope blade
laryngoscope chest support
  holder
laryngoscope folding blade
laryngoscope holder
laryngoscopic visualization
laryngoscopy
laryngospasm
laryngostat
    Jackson laryngostat
laryngostomy
laryngotomy
laryngotracheobronchoscopy
laryngotracheoscopy
laryngotracheostomy
laryngotracheotomy
larynx
larynx inspected
Lasag lens
Lasag Micropter II laser
Lasègue maneuver
Lasègue sign
laser
    ablative laser therapy
    AMO laser

laser *continued*
- argon laser
- argon-krypton laser
- Biophysic Medical laser
- Britt argon laser
- carbon dioxide laser
- Cilco laser
- CO2 laser
- Coherent argon laser
- Coherent radiation argon laser
- Coherent system of CO2 surgical laser
- Cooper argon laser
- CooperVision argon laser
- CooperVision laser
- dye laser
- endoscopic laser cautery
- Erbium-YAG laser
- ExciMed 200 ultraviolet laser surgery
- excimer cool laser
- excimer laser
- gas laser
- green laser
- helium-neon laser
- hemorrhoid laser excision
- He-Ne laser (helium-neon beam)
- HGM intravitreal laser
- Howard-Schatz laser technique
- Hruby laser
- intravitreal laser
- ion laser
- KIP laser
- krypton laser
- Lasag Micropter II laser
- Lasertek laser
- Lasertek YAG laser
- LASTAC laser system
- Mainster retina laser lens
- Marquette 3-channel laser Holter
- MCM smart Laser
- Meditec laser

laser *continued*
- Mira laser
- Nd:YAG laser
- neodymium laser
- Ophthalas laser
- pulsed angiolaser
- Q-switched YAG laser system
- red laser
- ruby laser
- Schatz laser technique
- Sharplan CO2 laser
- Sharplan laser
- SITE argon laser
- SITE laser
- smart laser
- Spectra-Physics argon laser
- Spectra-Physics microsurgical laser
- stereotactic laser
- surgical laser
- tunable dye laser
- Visulas Nd:YAG laser
- Xanar 20 Amulase CO2 laser
- YAG laser (yttrium-aluminum-garnet laser)
- yttrium-aluminum-garnet laser (YAG laser)
- Zeiss laser

laser ablation
laser angioplasty
laser balloon
laser beam
laser catheter
laser conization
laser endarterectomy
laser excision
laser flow cytometer
laser hemorrhoidectomy
laser intraocular lens IOPtex
laser laparoscopy
laser microprobe
laser microscope
laser microsurgery
laser photoablation
laser photocoagulation

laser probe
laser procedure
laser radiation
laser recanalization
laser speckle
laser therapy
laser tip
laser treatment
laser vaporization
laser-balloon angioplasty
laser-balloon procedure
Laserdish pacing lead
Laserflex intraocular lens
laseroscopy
Laserpor pacing lead
LaserSonics EndoBlade
LaserSonics Nd:YAG LaserBlade
    scalpel
LaserSonics SurgiBlade
Lasertek laser
Lasertek YAG laser
LASH (left anterior superior
    hemiblock)
Lash hysterectomy
Lash operation
lash reflex
Lash technique
Lash-Loeffler implant
Lash-Masler penile prosthesis
Lash-Moser prosthesis
lasing medium
Lassoe hand surgery
Lassoe wire
last menstrual period
LASTAC coronary angioplasty
LASTAC laser system
Latarjet nerve
Latarjet vein
latch key lid
late abortion
late decelerations
late phase reaction
latency
latency period
latent cancer
latent pacemaker
latent period
lateral

lateral abdominal region
lateral ampullary nerve
lateral anterior position
lateral anterior x-ray position
lateral aperture
lateral approach
lateral aspect
lateral band
lateral border
lateral canal
lateral canthus
lateral cerebral fissure
lateral cerebral sulcus
lateral circumflex femoral
    artery
lateral collateral ligaments
lateral column
lateral compartment
lateral condyle
lateral condyle bone
lateral constriction phenomenon
lateral conus
lateral cricoarytenoid muscle
lateral crus
lateral curvature of spine
lateral cutaneous nerve
lateral decubitus position
lateral displacement
lateral dorsal cutaneous nerve
lateral electrical spine stimula-
    tion (LESS)
lateral epicondyle
lateral extension
lateral femoral cutaneous nerve
lateral field
lateral film
lateral flank incision
lateral foramen
lateral fornix
lateral geniculate body
lateral gutter
lateral hemispheres
lateral incision
lateral inferior genicular artery
lateral inguinal fossa
lateral internal pelvic reservoir
lateral lacunae of cranial dura
    mater

lateral ligament
lateral lithotomy
lateral lobes of prostate
lateral malleolus
lateral mamillary nucleus of
    Rose
lateral mass
lateral meniscus
lateral nystagmus
lateral oblique fascia
lateral osteotomy
lateral palpebral arteries
lateral pancreaticojejunostomy
lateral plantar artery
lateral plantar nerve
lateral position
lateral posterior nasal arteries
lateral presentation
lateral process
lateral projection
lateral prone position
lateral pterygoid muscle
lateral pterygoid nerve
lateral rectus (LR)
lateral rectus incision
lateral rectus position
lateral recumbent position
lateral region
lateral retractor
lateral sacral arteries
lateral sacral veins
lateral sinus
lateral striate arteries
lateral sulcus
lateral superior genicular artery
lateral supraclavicular nerves
lateral surface
lateral tarsal arteries
lateral thoracic artery
lateral thoracic vein
lateral thorax
lateral to the incision
lateral umbilical folds
lateral ventricle
lateral ventricle horn
lateral version of uterus
lateral views
lateral wall

lateral x-ray view
lateralization
lateralizing
lateral-lateral pouch
laterally reflected
laterocollateral ligament
lateromedial oblique projection
lateropharyngeal space
latex bag
latex band
latex catheter
latex drain
latex prosthesis
latex sponge graft
latex tube
Lathbury applicator
latissimus dorsi muscle
latissimus dorsi, musculus
Latram mastectomy procedure
Latrobe retractor
lats (slang for latissimus)
lattice degeneration
lattice retinal degeneration
Latzko cesarean section
Latzko closure
Latzko colpocleisis
Latzko fistula repair
Latzko operation
Latzko radical hysterectomy
Latzko repair of vesicovaginal
    fistula
Lauenstein procedure
Lauenstein wrist procedure
Lauenstein x-ray projection
Lauer forceps
Laufe aspirating curet
Laufe cervical dilator
Laufe forceps
Laufe obstetrical forceps
Laufe retractor
Laufe uterine polyp forceps
Laufe-Barton-Kielland obstetri-
    cal forceps
Laufe-Barton-Kielland-Piper
    obstetrical forceps
Laufe-Novak diagnostic curet
Laufe-Piper forceps
Laufe-Piper obstetrical forceps

Laufe-Piper uterine polyp
    forceps
Laufe-Randall curet
Lauge-Hansen ankle classifica-
    tion
Laugier hernia
Launois-Cléret deformity
Laurens operation
Laurens-Alcatel nuclear pow-
    ered pacemaker
lavage
lavage and suction
lavage of bronchi
lavage of joint
lavage of pleura
lavage of sinus
lavage of stomach
lavaged with sterile saline
laveur
Law position
Lawford speculum
Lawrence deep forceps
Lawrence forceps
Lawrence position
Laws gastroplasty
Lawson operation
Lawson-Thornton plate
Lawton forceps
Lawton microneedle holder
Lawton scissors
Lawton-Balfour self-retaining
    retractor
Lawton-Schubert biopsy for-
    ceps
Lawton-Wittner cervical biopsy
    forceps
layer of tissue
layered
layered closure
Layman decompressor
Layman-Storz snare
lay-on graft
lazy bowel
lazy-H incision
lazy-S incision
lazy-Z incision
LCA (left coronary artery)

LCP disease (Legg-Calvé-Perthes
    disease)
LCS total knee system
LCS with Porocoat total knee
    system
LCX, LCx (left circumflex artery)
LDA stapler
LDF stapler
LDS applier
LDS clip
LDS instrument
LDS stapler
Leach-Igou osteotomy
Leach-Igou step-cut medial
    osteotomy
lead
lead apron
lead artifact
lead hand
lead line
lead placement
lead shield
lead strip
Leadbetter epiphysis
Leadbetter maneuver
Leadbetter operation
Leadbetter-Politano operation
Leadbetter-Politano ureteral
    implant prosthesis
Leadbetter-Politano ureteral
    reimplantation
Leadbetter-Politano uretero-
    neocystotomy
Leadbetter-Politano uretero-
    vesical reimplantation
Leadbetter-Politano uretero-
    vesicoplasty
Leader forceps
Leader hook
Leader vas hook
Leader vas isolation forceps
Leader-Kohlman dilator
lead-filled head mallet
lead-filled mallet
lead-pipe colon
lead-pipe fracture
leads

lead-shot tie sutures
leaf (*pl.* leaves)
leaflet
leaflet prolapse
leaflet retractor
leaflet thickening
leaflet tip
leaflike villi
Leahey marginal chalazion
   forceps
Leahey operation
leak
leakage of fluid
leaking about shunt site
leaking aneurysm
leaky valve
leapfrog position
least gluteal muscle
Leasure aspirator
Leasure tracheal retractor
Leasure tuning fork
leather bottle stomach
leather restraint
Leather valve cutter
Leather venous valvulotome
Leather-Carmody scissors
Leatherman child spinal hooks
Leatherman trochanteric
   retractor
leaves (*sing.* leaf)
leaves of broad ligament
leaves of dura
leaves of mesentery
LeBerne treatment table
Leboyer delivery technique
Lebsche chisel
Lebsche forceps
Lebsche knife
Lebsche punch
Lebsche raspatory
Lebsche rongeur
Lebsche shears
Lebsche sternal knife
Lebsche thoracic knife
Lebsche wire saw guide
lecithin/sphingomyelin ratio
   (L/S ratio)

LeCocq brace
lecture-scope
LeDentu sutures
Ledhey forceps
LeDran sutures
LeDuc-Camey ileocolostomy
LeDuc-Camey ileocystoplasty
Lee delicate hemostatic forceps
Lee double-ended retractor
Lee graft
Lee knife
Lee microvascular clamp
Lee needle
Lee technique
leech
leeching
Lee-Cohen elevator
Lee-Cohen knife
Lees arterial forceps
Lees clamp
Lees nontraumatic forceps
Lees vascular clamp
Leff stethoscope
Lefferts forceps
LeFort amputation
LeFort bougie
LeFort catheter
LeFort colpocleisis
LeFort dilator
LeFort filiform bougie
LeFort follower
LeFort fracture (I, II, or III)
LeFort male catheter
LeFort operation
LeFort osteotomy
LeFort sound
LeFort sutures
LeFort urethral catheter
LeFort urethral sound
LeFort urethral speculum
LeFort uterine prolapse repair
LeFort I apertognathia repair
LeFort I maxillary reconstruction
LeFort-Wehrbein-Duplay
   hypospadias repair
left anterior descending artery
   (LAD)

left atrium
left atrium to distal arterial
    aortic bypass
left axis deviation
left bundle branch block
left cardiac catheterization
left colic artery
left colic vein
left colon
left colonic flexure
left coronary angiogram
left coronary artery
left coronary cinearteriogram
left decubitus position
left deviation
left diaphragm
left dorsoanterior
left dorsoposterior
left fifth intercostal space
left gastric artery
left gastric vein
laft gastroepiploic artery
left gastroepiploic vein
left gutter
left heart bypass
left hemicolectomy
left hepatic duct
left hilum
left hypogastric nerve
left inferior pulmonary vein
left intercostal space
left internal mammary artery
    graft (LIMA graft)
left lateral
left lateral bending
left lateral decubitus position
left lateral position
left lateral projection
left lateral region
left lobe
left lower lobe (LLL)
left lower quadrant (LLQ)
left main bronchus
left mentoanterior position
    (LMA position)
left mentoposterior position
    (LMP position)

left mentotransverse position
    (LMT position)
left occipitoanterior position
    (LOA position)
left occipitoposterior position
    (LOP position)
left occipitotransverse position
    (LOT position)
left organ
left posterior oblique
left pulmonary artery
left radical groin dissection
left region
left rhomboid muscle
left rotation
left sacroanterior position (LSA
    position)
left sacroposterior position (LSP
    position)
left scapuloanterior position
    (LScA position)
left scapuloposterior position
    (LScP position)
left segmental colectomy
left shift
left superficial temporal artery
    to middle cerebral artery
    anastomosis
left superior pulmonary vein
left suprarenal vein
left testicular vein
left umbilical vein
left upper lobe (LUL)
left upper lobe bronchus
left upper quadrant (LUQ)
left venous angle
left ventricle
left ventricular
left ventricular assist device
    (LVAD)
left ventricular cineangiogram
left ventricular clamp catheter
left ventricular end-diastolic
    pressure
left ventricular inflow tract
left ventricular outflow tract
left-curved scissors

left-handed
left-sided
left-to-right shunt
left-to-right subtotal pancreatec-
    tomy
leg brace
leg cast
leg elevation
leg extension splint
leg flap
leg holder
leg motion
leg raising
leg rigidly extended
leg roll
leg splint
Legat point
leg-block anesthesia
Legen self-retaining retractor
Legend pacemaker
Legg operation
Legg osteotome
Legg-Calvé-Perthes disease (LCP
    disease)
Legg-Perthes disease
leggings
leg-holding device
leg-length discrepancy
leg-length measurement
Legueu kidney retractor
Legueu retractor
Lehman catheter
Lehman syringe
Lehman ventriculography
    catheter
Leigh capsule forceps
Leigh forceps
Leigh zonule lens stripper
Leighton needle
Leinbach olecranon screw
Leinbach osteotome
Leinbach prosthesis
Leinbach screw
leiomyoma (*pl.* leiomyomas,
    leiomyomata)
leiomyomata uteri
leiomyosarcoma

Leios pacemaker
Leiske intraocular lens
Leiske lens
Leiske Optiflex lens
Leiske Physioflex intraocular
    lens
Leiter cystoscope
Leiter tube
Leitz microscope
Lejeune applicator
Lejeune forceps
Lejeune scissors
Lejeune thoracic forceps
Leksell bone rongeur
Leksell cardiovascular rongeur
Leksell director
Leksell forceps
Leksell frame
Leksell punch
Leksell rongeur
Leksell stereotaxic frame
Leksell sternal approximator
Leksell sternal spreader
Leksell trephine
Leksell-Stille thoracic-cardio-
    vascular rongeur
Leland knife
Leland tonsillar knife
Leland-Jones clamp
Leland-Jones forceps
Leland-Jones peripheral
    vascular clamp
Leland-Jones vascular clamp
Lell esophagoscope
Lell laryngofissure saw
Lell saw
Lell tube
LeMaitre valvulotome
Lembert sutures
Lem-Blay circumcision clamp
Lem-Blay clamp
LeMesurier operation
LeMesurier rectangular flap
Lemmon blade
Lemmon contractor
Lemmon intimal dissector
Lemmon needle holder

Lemmon rib approximator
Lemmon rib spreader
Lemmon self-retaining sternal
    retractor
Lemmon sternal approximator
Lemmon sternal elevator
Lemmon sternal retractor
Lemmon sternal spreader
Lemmon-Russian forceps
Lemoine eye implant
Lemoine forceps
Lemoine-Searcy anchor
Lemole atrial valve self-retaining
    retractor
lemon sign
lemon squeezer obstetrical
    elevator
Lempert bone rongeur
Lempert bur
Lempert curet
Lempert elevator
Lempert endaural rongeur
Lempert evacuator
Lempert excavator
Lempert extractor
Lempert fenestration
Lempert forceps
Lempert incision
Lempert incision for radical
    tympanoplasty
Lempert instrument
Lempert knife
Lempert malleus cutter
Lempert malleus punch
Lempert operation
Lempert paracentesis knife
Lempert perforator
Lempert procedure
Lempert punch
Lempert retractor
Lempert rongeur
Lempert rongeur forceps
Lempert sutures
Lempert-Colver retractor
Lempert-Colver speculum
Lempka stripper
Lempka vein stripper

Lenart-Kullman technique
length
lengthening
lengthening of bone
lengthening of tendon
lengthwise
Lennander operation
Lennarson suction tube
Lennarson tube
Lennhoff sign
Lenny Johnson surgical-assist
    knee holder
Lenox Hill brace
Lenox Hill knee brace
Lenox Hill knee orthosis
Lenox Hill Spectralite knee
    brace
lens (*pl.* lenses)
    Abraham iridectomy lens
    Abraham lens
    achromatic lens
    ACMI microlens
    acrylic lens
    Acuflex intraocular lens
        implant
    adherent lens
    AIRLens contact lens
    Alcon intraocular lens
    Alcon lens
    Allen-Brailey intraocular
        lens implant
    Alpar intraocular lens
        implant
    Alpar lens
    American intraocular lens
    American Medical Optics
        intraocular lens
    AMO intraocular lens
        implant
    angled-vision lens system
    Anis posterior chamber
        capsule intraocular
        lens
    Anis Staple implant
        cataract lens
    anterior chamber
        intraocular lens

lens (lenses) *continued*
    Appolionio implant
       cataract lens
    Appolionio lens
    Aquaflex contact lens
    aspheric lens implant
    Azar flexible loop
       anterior chamber
       intraocular lens
    Azar Tripod implant
       cataract lens
    Azar Tripod lens
    Bagolini lens
    Barkan goniolens
    Barkan goniotomy lens
    Barkan lens
    Barnes-Hind lens
    Baron lens
    Bausch-Lomb lens
    Beale intraocular implant
       lens
    Beale lens
    Bechert intraocular lens
       implant
    biconcave lens
    biconvex lens
    bicylindrical lens
    Bietti implant cataract
       lens
    Bietti lens
    bifocal lens
    Binkhorst intraocular
       lens implant
    Binkhorst lens
    Binkhorst lens implant
    Bi-Soft contact lens
    bispherical lens
    Bitoric lens
    Boberg-Ans lens
    Boyd intraocular implant
       lens
    Boyd lens
    Bron implant cataract
       lens
    Brücke lens
    Bunker intraocular
       implant lens

lens (lenses) *continued*
    Bunker lens
    Byron intraocular
       implant lens
    Byron lens
    Cardona lens
    cataract lens
    Charles intraocular
       lens
    Charles lens
    Choyce anterior chamber
       lens
    Choyce implant cataract
       lens
    Choyce lens
    Choyce-Tennant lens
    Cilco intraocular lens
    Cilco lens
    Clayman intraocular
       implant lens
    Clayman lens
    Clayman lens implant
    Clayman-Kelman lens
    Coburn anterior chamber
       intraocular lens
       implant
    Coburn intraocular lens
    Coburn lens
    Cogan-Boberg-Ans lens
       implant
    Comberg contact lens
    concave lens
    concavoconcave lens
    concavoconvex lens
    conoid lens
    contact lens
    converging lens
    convex lens
    convexity of lens
    convexoconcave lens
    Cooper lens
    CooperVision J-loop
       intraocular lens
    Copeland intraocular
       lens implant
    Copeland lens
    Copeland lens implant

lens (lenses) *continued*

Copeland radial pan-
chamber intraocular
lens
coquille plano lens
Cosmet lens
Crookes lens
crystalline lens
cylindrical lens
Danker-Wohlk contact
lens
Darin intraocular implant
lens
Darin lens
decentered lens
Dickerson intraocular
implant lens
Dickerson lens
dispersing lens
Drews intraocular
implant lens
Drews lens
Dulaney intraocular
implant lens
Dulaney lens
Dura-T contact lens
Durasoft lens
ectopia of lens
Eifrig intraocular implant
lens
Eifrig lens
elevating lens
Ellingson intraocular
implant lens
Ellingson lens
Epstein lens implant
express lens
expressor lens
Ezvue violet haptic one-
piece lens
Fechner intraocular
implant lens
Fechner lens
Federov lens implant
Federov type I lens
implant
Federov type II lens
implant

lens (lenses) *continued*

fiberoptic lens
flexible Dualens implant
Flexlens
FormFlex intraocular
lens
FormFlex lens
Foroblique lens
Frenzel lenses
Fresnel lens
Galin intraocular lens
implant
Galin lens
Gills intraocular implant
lens
Gills lens
Gilmore intraocular
implant lens
Gilmore lens
Goldmann goniolens
Goldmann lens
Goldmann multi-
mirrored lens implant
goniolens
gonioscopy lens
Gould intraocular
implant lens
Gould lens
Greene intraocular
implant lens
Greene lens
Gridley intraocular
lens
hard lens
HCL (hard contact lens)
Hertzog intraocular lens
Hertzog lens
Hessburg intraocular
lens
Heyer-Schulte lens
implant
Hiles intraocular lens
Hiles lens
Hirschman intraocular
implant lens
Hirschman lens
Hoffer intraocular
implant lens

lens (lenses) *continued*
  Hoffer lens
  Hopkins lens
  Hruby lens
  Hubbell intraocular
    implant lens
  Hubbell lens
  Hunkeler lightweight
    intraocular lens
    implant
  Hydrocurve contact lens
  Hydrocurve II intraocular
    lens implant
  implant cataract lens
  implant lens
  Implens intraocular
    implant lens
  Implens lens
  Intermedics intraocular
    lens
  Intermedics intraocular
    lens implant
  intracapsular lens
  intraocular lens (IOL)
  intraocular lens implant
  IOL (intraocular lens)
  Iolab intraocular lens
  Iolab lens
  IOptex laser intraocular
    lens implant
  iridocapsular fixation
    lens
  iridocapsular implant
    cataract lens
  iridocapsular intraocular
    lens
  iris fixation intraocular
    lens
  iris fixation lens
  iris plane intraocular lens
  irrigating contact
    Goldmann lens
  iseikonic lens
  J-Flex posterior chamber
    lens
  J-loop posterior chamber
    lens

lens (lenses) *continued*
  Jaffe lens
  Jaffe ocular implant
    lens
  Jensen lens forceps
  Jung-Schaffer lens
  Karickhoff diagnostic
    lens
  Karickhoff laser lens
  Karickhoff lens
  Kearney side-notch
    intraocular lens
  Keates intraocular
    implant lens
  Keates lens
  Kelman anterior chamber
    intraocular lens
  Kelman intraocular
    implant lens
  Kelman lens
  Kelman Multiflex II
    intraocular lens
  Kelman Omnifit II
    intraocular lens
  Kelman Quadraflex
    anterior chamber
    intraocular lens
  keratolens
  Knolle intraocular lens
  Knolle lens
  Koeppe goniolens
  Koeppe gonioscopic lens
    implant
  Koeppe intraocular lens
    implant
  Koeppe lens
  Koteline bifocal lens
  Kowa automatic fundus
    lens
  Kraff intraocular implant
    lens
  Krasnov implant cataract
    lens
  Krasnov lens
  Kratz intraocular implant
    lens
  Kratz lens

lens (lenses) *continued*

Kratz posterior chamber intraocular lens
Kratz-Johnson intraocular lens
Kratz-Sinskey intraocular lens implant
Krwawicz cataract lens
Kryptok bifocal lens
Kryptok bifocal lens implant
Kuglen lens manipulator
Kwitko intraocular implant lens
Landers contact lens
Landers-Foulk lens
Lannu anterior chamber lens
Lasag lens
laser intraocular lens IOPtex
Laserflex intraocular lens
Leiske intraocular lens
Leiske lens
Leiske Optiflex lens
Leiske Physioflex intraocular lens
Lieb-Guerry cataract lens
Liteflex intraocular lens
Liteflex lens
Little intraocular lens implant
Little lens
loop lens
Lovac fundus contact lens implant
Machemer lens
Mainster retina laser lens
Manschot intraocular implant lens
Manschot lens
McCannel intraocular implant lens
McCannel lens
McGhan intraocular lens

lens (lenses) *continued*

McGhan lens
McGhan-3M intraocular lens
McIntyre intraocular implant lens
McIntyre lens
McLean prism contact lens
McPherson lens forceps
Medallion intraocular lens implant
Medallion lens
Medical Workshop intraocular lens implant
Medicornea Kratz-type intraocular lens
meniscal lens
Michelis intraocular implant lens
Michelis lens
Nova Curve lens
O'Malley self-adhering lens implant
Omnifit intraocular lens
open lens
Optiflex intraocular lens
Optiflex lens
ORC anterior chamber intraocular lens
ORC posterior chamber intraocular lens implant
Osher lens
Pannu intraocular lens
Pearce posterior chamber intraocular lens implant
Pearce Tripod lens
Pearce vaulted-Y lens implant
periscopic lens
Pharmacia intraocular lens
plano lens

lens (lenses) *continued*
    planoconcave lens
    planoconvex lens
    plastic lens
    Platina clip implant
      cataract lens
    Platina clip lens
    Platina intraocular lens
      implant
    posterior chamber
      intraocular lens
    Precision-Cosmet
      intraocular lens
      implant
    Prokop intraocular
      lens
    Prokop lens
    prosthetic lens
    punktal lens
    retroscopic lens
    Ridley implant cataract
      lens
    Ridley lens
    Ridley Mark II lens
      implant
    right-angle lens
    Ritch lens
    Rodenstock lens
    Ruiz plano fundus lens
      implant
    Sauflon contact lens
    Schachar implant cataract
      lens
    Schachar lens
    Scharf implant cataract
      lens
    Scharf lens
    sclerosed lens
    semiflexible intraocular
      lens
    Severin intraocular lens
    Severin lens
    Shearing intraocular
      implant lens
    Shearing lens

lens (lenses) *continued*
    Sheets intraocular lens
    Sheets lens
    Shepard intraocular lens
      implant
    Shepard lens
    Shepard-Reinstein
      intraocular lens
    Simcoe anterior chamber
      lens
    Simcoe intraocular
      implant lens
    Simcoe intraocular lens
      implant
    Simcoe lens
    Simcoe posterior
      chamber lens
    Sinskey blue loop
      intraocular lens
    Sinskey intraocular
      lens
    Sinskey lens
    Sinskey lens implant
    Sinskey posterior
      chamber intraocular
      lens
    Sinskey posterior
      chamber lens
    Smith intraocular implant
      lens
    Smith lens
    Soflens contact lens
    soft lens
    Softcon contact lens
    Softcon lens
    Soper cone hard contact
      lens
    Sputnik-Federov lens
    Stableflex lens
    Stein intraocular implant
      lens
    Stein lens
    Stokes lens

lens (lenses) *continued*
Straatsma intraocular
implant lens
Straatsma lens
Strampelli implant
cataract lens
Strampelli lens
Surefit anterior chamber
intraocular lens
Surgidev intraocular lens
Surgidev lens
T-contact lens
T-lens
Tennant Anchorflex
anterior chamber
intraocular lens
Tennant Anchorflex lens
implant
Tennant intraocular
implant lens
Tennant lens
Thorpe plastic lens
three-mirror contact lens
Tolentino lens
toric lens
Ultex bifocal lens
Ultex lens
Varigray lens implant
Vest lens
Volk conoid ophthalmic
lens
Volk Pan retinal lens
Ward-Lempert lens
Wesley Jessen lens
Worst intraocular lens
Worst lens
Worst Medallion lens
Zeiss aspheric lens
lens cannula
lens capsule
lens delivered by tumbling
procedure
lens delivered intracapsularly
lens elevated
lens expressor (see also
*expressor*)
Arruga lens expressor

lens expressor *continued*
Berens lens expressor
intracapsular lens
expressor
Kirby intracapsular lens
expressor
Kirby lens expressor
Medallion lens expressor
Smith lens expressor
lens expressor hook
lens extracted
lens extraction
lens forceps
lens implant
lens implant forceps
lens loupe (see also *loop, loupe*)
Adler lens loupe
Amenabar lens loupe
Arlt lens loupe
Beebe lens loupe
Berens lens loupe
Callahan lens loupe
Daviel lens loupe
intracapsular lens loupe
Kirby intracapsular lens
loupe
Mark lens loupe
New Orleans lens loupe
Troutman lens loupe
Weber-Elschnig lens
loupe
Zeiss lens loupe
lens manipulator
lens opacification
lens opacity
lens prism
lens scoop
lens spatula
lens spoon
lens system
Lent laparoscope
Lent photolaparoscope
Lente silver nitrate probe
lenticular
lenticular bone
lenticular cataract
lenticular degeneration

lenticular knife
lenticular process
lenticular process of incus
Lentulo drill
Lentulo spiral drill
Lentz tracheotomy tube
Leo Schwartz sponge-holding
    forceps
Leonard deep forceps
Leonard forceps
Leonard tube
Leonard-George position
Leone eye procedure
Leopold operation
L'Episcopo operation
L'Episcopo-Zachary shoulder
    procedure
Lepley-Ernst tube
leptomeningeal
leptomeninges
Leptos pacemaker
Lere bone mill
Leri sign
Leriche forceps
Leriche hemostatic forceps
Leriche operation
Leriche tissue forceps
Lerman hinge brace
Lermoyez nasal punch
Lermoyez punch
Leroy catheter
LeRoy clip
LeRoy disposable scalp clip
LeRoy scalp clip-applying
    forceps
LES (lower esophageal sphinc-
    ter)
Leser-Trelat sign
Lesgaft hernia
Lesgaft space
Lesgaft triangle
lesion
lesion milked out
lesion of organ
lesion of tissue
lesion resected
Leslie incision

Leslie-Ryan approach
L'Esperance erysiphake
L'Esperance needle
Lespinasse sutures
LESS (lateral electrical spine
    stimulation)
lesser alar cartilage
lesser arterial circle of iris
lesser circle of iris
lesser curvature
lesser curvature of stomach
lesser curvature ulcer
lesser multangular bone
lesser occipital nerve
lesser omentum
lesser ovarian vein
lesser palantine arteries
lesser palatine canal
lesser palatine foramen
lesser palatine nerves
lesser pancreas
lesser peritoneal sac
lesser petrosal nerve
lesser petrosal nerve hiatus
lesser sciatic foramen
lesser sciatic notch
lesser trochanter
lesser tubercle
lesser zygomatic muscle
Lester fixation forceps
Lester forceps
Lester Jones operation
Lester Martin modification of
    Duhamel procedure
Lester-Burch eye speculum
lethal damage
lethal injury
Letournel approach
Letournel fracture plate
leucotomy (see *leukotomy*)
Leukofix surgical tape
Leukofix tape
Leukoflex surgical tape
Leukoflex tape
leukoma
leukonychia
leukoplakia

Leukopor surgical tape
Leukopor tape
leukorrhea
Leukos pacemaker
Leukosilk surgical tape
Leukosilk tape
leukotome
    Bailey leukotome
    Dorsey leukotome
    Dorsey transorbital
      leukotome
    Freeman leukotome
    Freeman transorbital
      leukotome
    Lewis leukotome
    Love leukotome
    McKenzie leukotome
leukotomy
Levant dislodger
Levant stone dislodger
Levant stone dislodger basket
levator
levator anguli oris, musculus
levator ani muscle
levator ani, musculus
levator aponeurosis
levator check ligament
levator glandulae thyroideae,
    musculus
levator hernia
levator labii superioris alaeque
    nasi, musculus
levator labii superioris, muscu-
    lus
levator muscle
levator nerve
levator palpebrae superioris,
    musculus
levator prostatae, musculus
levator resection
levator scapulae, musculus
levator sling
levator span
levator veli palatini, musculus
levatores costarum, musculi
levatores prostatae, musculi
LeVeen catheter
LeVeen dialysis shunt

LeVeen endarterectomy
LeVeen peritoneal shunt
LeVeen peritoneovenous shunt
LeVeen shunt
LeVeen valve
level of anesthesia
level of awareness
level of consciousness
level of pain
Levenson tissue forceps
lever
    Austin Moore-Murphy
      bone lever
    bone lever
    cantilever
    Cottle bone lever
    intranasal bone lever
    Murphy bone lever
lever pessary
leverage fracture
lever-type screwdriver
Levin duodenal tube
Levin electrode
Levin tube
Levin tube catheter
Levin-Davol tube
Levine foreign body spud
Levine gradation of cardiac
    murmurs (grades 1-6)
Levine hip dislocation operation
Levine shunt
Levine sign
Levis splint
Levitt eye implant
Levitt implant
levocardia
levocardiogram
levoduction of eye
levogram
levophase of angiogram
Levora fixation forceps
levorotatory
levorotatory scoliosis
levotransposition
levotransposition of great
    arteries (L-transposition of
    great arteries)
Levret forceps

Levy mold orthotics
Levy perineal retractor
Lewicky instrument
Lewicky needle
Lewin baseball finger splint
Lewin bone clamp
Lewin bone-holding clamp
Lewin bone-holding forceps
Lewin bunion dissector
Lewin clamp
Lewin dissector
Lewin forceps
Lewin sesamoidectomy
    dissector
Lewin splint
Lewin tonsil hemostat
Lewin tonsil screw
Lewin-Stern finger splint
Lewin-Stern thumb splint
Lewis cystometer
Lewis decompressor
Lewis forceps
Lewis hemostat
Lewis intramedullary device
Lewis lead on ECG
Lewis lens scoop
Lewis leukotome
Lewis loupe
Lewis mouth gag
Lewis nasal raspatory
Lewis periosteal elevator
Lewis position
Lewis rasp
Lewis raspatory
Lewis retractor
Lewis scoop
Lewis septal forceps
Lewis snare
Lewis suspension device
Lewis tongue depressor
Lewis tonsillar hemostatic
    forceps
Lewis tonsillar snare
Lewis tube
Lewis uvula retractor
Lewis-Chekofsky femur
    resection
Lewkowitz forceps

Lewkowitz lithotomy forceps
Lewy bodies
Lewy chest holder
Lewy laryngoscope
Lewy suspension apparatus
Lewy-Rubin needle
Lexan head
Lexer chisel
Lexer dissecting scissors
Lexer gouge
Lexer operation
Lexer osteotome
Lexer scissors
Lexer tissue forceps
Lex-Ton lumbar laminectomy
    frame
Leydig drain
Leyla footplate
Leyla retractor
Leyla-Yasargil retractor
Leyro-Diaz forceps
LFA (low-friction arthroplasty)
LGA (large for gestational age)
Lich operation
lichenified lesions
Lich-Gregoire repair in kidney
    transplant surgery
Lichtenberg carbide-jaw needle
    holder
Lichtenberg keratome
Lichtenberg needle holder
Lichtenberg trephine
Lichtenstein herniorrhaphy
Lichtenstein inguinal hernia
    repair
Lichtwicz antral needle
Lichtwicz antral trephine
Lichtwicz antral trocar
Lichtwicz needle
Lichtwicz trocar
lid block anesthesia
lid clamp
lid dermabrader
lid elevator
lid everter (see also *everter*)
        Berens lid everter
        Walker lid everter
lid expressor

lid forceps
lid hook
lid knife
lid lag
lid margin
lid operation
lid plasty
lid plate
lid ptosis
lid ptosis operation
lid reflex
lid retractor
lid scalpel
lid speculum
lid surgery
lid suture operation
Liddle aorta clamp
lid-fracturing blepharoplasty
Lidge reducer sleeve
lidocaine drip
lidocaine hydrochloride
    anesthetic agent
lidocaine jelly
lid-retracting hook
Lieb-Guerry cataract lens
Lieb-Guerry eye knife
Lieb-Guerry forceps
Lieberkühn crypts
Lieberkühn follicles
Lieberkühn gland
Lieberman abrader
Lieberman forceps
Lieberman proctoscope
Lieberman sigmoidoscope
Lieberman sigmoidoscope with
    swinging window
Lieberman suturing forceps
Lieberman tying forceps
Liebermeister groove
Liebolt arthrodesis
Liebolt operation
lien
lien accessorius
lien mobilis
lienal
lienal artery
lienal vein

lienalis, arteria
lienalis, vena
lienculus
lienectomy
lienocolic
lienopancreatic
lienophrenic
lienorenal
lienorenal ligament
Lieppman cystitome
Life Care Pump
Life Suit
Lifecath catheter
Lifecath peritoneal implant
lifeless body
lifeline necklace
Lifemed cannula
Lifepak defibrillator
life-saving suction tube
life-saving tube
life-support measure
life-sustaining measure
life-sustaining procedure
life-threatening condition
lift sheet
lift-and-cut biopsy
Liga surgical clip
Ligaclip
ligament
ligament augmentation
ligament augmentation device
    (LAD)
ligament of Henry
ligament of incus
ligament of knee
ligament of lens
ligament of malleus
ligament of Struthers
ligament of Toldt
ligament of Treitz
ligament of Wrisburg
ligament reflecting edge
ligament shelving edge
ligamenta (sing. ligamentum)
ligamenta flava forceps
ligamental mucosa
ligamenti teretis uteri, arteria

ligamentous
ligamentous ankylosis
ligamentous calcification
ligamentous falx
ligamentous instability
ligamentous joint
ligamentous strain
ligamentous structure
ligamentum (*pl.* ligamenta)
ligamentum teres
ligamentum teres femoris
ligamentum venosum
ligamentum-grasping forceps
ligand adhesive
Ligapak suture
ligate
ligated and amputated
ligated and retracted
ligated and sectioned
ligated and transected
ligated with silk
ligated with transfixion suture
ligation
ligation and stripping
ligation of artery
ligation of bleeders
ligation of vas deferens
ligation of vein
ligation of vessels
ligation sutures
ligator
    hemorrhoidal ligator
    McGivney ligator
    Rudd Clinic hemor-
      rhoidal ligator
    Rudd Clinic ligator
    Salvatore ligator
ligature (see also *suture*)
    catgut ligature
    chain ligature
    chromic ligature
    elastic ligature
    elastic-thread ligature
    encircling tape ligature
    Erichsen ligature
    free ligature
    hemostatic ligature

ligature *continued*
    interlacing ligature
    interlocking ligature
    kangaroo ligature
    McGraw elastic ligature
    Mersilene tape ligature
    occluding ligature
    portligature
    Potts ligature
    provisional ligature
    proximal ligature
    pursestring ligature
    soluble ligature
    suboccluding ligature
    suture ligature
    tape ligature
    terminal ligature
    wire ligature
ligature carrier (see also *carrier,*
    *ligature passer*)
    Braun ligature carrier
    Deschamps ligature
      carrier
    Favoloro ligature carrier
    Fitzwater ligature car-
      rier
    Lahey ligature carrier
    Madden ligature carrier
    Tauber ligature carrier
    Wangensteen ligature
      carrier
    Young ligature carrier
ligature forceps
ligature hook
ligature knife
ligature needle
ligature passer (see also *passer,*
    *ligature carrier*)
    O'Donahue ligature
      passer
    Yankauer ligature passer
ligature set
ligature sutures
ligature wire
ligature-carrying aneurysm
    forceps
ligature-carrying forceps

light (see also *lamp*)
ACMI fiberoptic light source
AFI coaxial headlight system
Bernstein light
Birch-Hirschfield light
black light
Burton black light
Burton Fresnel floor light
carbon arc light
Clar-73 headlight
Co-Axa Lite light
coaxial headlight
Denecke headlight
direct-focus headlight
dual-beam fiberoptic light source
Duke-Elder ultraviolet light
Eldridge-Green color vision light
examining light
fiberoptic cold light source
fiberoptic headlight
fiberoptic light
Finsen carbon arc light
Finsen-Reya light
flashlight
Fresnel floor light
Glolite infrared light
Good-Lite super head-light
gooseneck light
Haag-Streit light
Halogen exam light
headlight
Hirschfield eye light
Hood headlight
Klaar headlight
Kromayer mercury vapor light
Lumiwand light
Minilux headlight
Minin light
Murphy light

light *continued*
neurosurgical light
overhead light
Simpson light
Spot-quartz light
Storz headlight
Storz-Denecke headlight
surgeon's headlight
Tyndall light
uviol light
Wehmerlite IV-A headlight
Wood black light
Wood light
light amplification
light and accommodation
light carrier
light coagulation for retinal detachment
light cross-slot screwdriver
Light headrest
light microscope
lighted retractor
lightning cataract
Light-Veley (also Dr. Light-Veley)
Light-Veley apparatus
Light-Veley bur
Light-Veley cranial drill
Light-Veley drill
Light-Veley headrest
lignocaine anesthetic agent
Lilienthal bullet probe
Lilienthal guillotine
Lilienthal incision
Lilienthal probe
Lilienthal rib guillotine
Lilienthal rib spreader
Lilienthal spreader
Lilienthal-Sauerbruch retractor
Lilienthal-Sauerbruch rib spreader
Liliequist membrane
Lillehei forceps
Lillehei pacemaker
Lillehei retractor

Lillehei valve forceps
Lillehei valve prosthesis
Lillehei valve-grasping forceps
Lillehei-Cruz-Kaster prosthesis
Lillehei-Kaster aortic valve
    prosthesis
Lillehei-Kaster mitral valve
    prosthesis
Lillehei-Kaster pivoting-disk
    prosthetic valve
Lillehei-Kaster prosthesis
Lillehei-Warden catheter
Lillie alligator scissors
Lillie antral trocar
Lillie attic cannula
Lillie attic hook
Lillie cannula
Lillie ear hook
Lillie forceps
Lillie frontal sinus probe
Lillie gouge
Lillie hook
Lillie intestinal forceps
Lillie knife
Lillie nasal speculum
Lillie probe
Lillie retractor
Lillie rongeur
Lillie scissors
Lillie sinus bone-nibbling
    rongeur
Lillie speculum
Lillie tissue-holding forceps
Lillie tonsillar knife
Lillie tonsillar scissors
Lillie trocar
Lillie-Killian forceps
Lillie-Killian septal bone
    forceps
Lillie-White tenaculum
LIMA graft (left internal
    mammary artery graft)
limb
limb girdle
limb lead
limb salvage
limb splint

limbal groove
limbal incision
limbal sutures
Limberg flap
limb-girdle dystrophy
limbic lobe
limbic suture
limbic system
limb-threatening problem
limbus (pl. limbi)
limbus corneae
limitation of motion (LOM)
limitation of surgery
limited joint motion
limited joint movement
limited prognosis
limited range of motion
limited straight-leg raising
limiting plate
limp
Lincoff eye implant
Lincoff implant
Lincoff operation
Lincoff Silastic sponge
Lincoln cardiovascular scis-
    sors
Lincoln deep scissors
Lincoln pediatric scissors
Lincoln scissors
Lincoln-Metzenbaum scissors
Lindbergh pump
Lindblom position
Linde cryogenic probe
Linde walker
Lindeman bur
Lindeman cannula
Lindeman hysteroflator
Lindeman knee procedure
Lindeman needle
Lindeman procedure
Lindeman-Silverstein tube
Linder sign
Lindesmith operation
Lindholm anatomical tracheal
    tube
Lindholm operation
Lindholm tracheal tube

Lindley carbide-jaw needle
   holder
Lindley needle holder
Lindner anastomosis clamp
Lindner corneoscleral sutures
Lindner cyclodialysis spatula
Lindner cyclodialysis spoon
Lindner operation
Lindner sclerotomy
Lindner spatula
Lindsay nail
Lindsay operation
line incision
line of demarcation
line of fracture
line of occlusion
line of Ogston
line of Toldt
line of Zahn
linea alba
linea alba cervicalis
linea aspera
linea corneae senilis
linea glutea
linea semilunaris
linea terminalis pelvis
lineage
linear
linear amputation
linear array scanner
linear atrophy
linear cautery
linear defect
linear density
linear depression
linear erosion
linear fracture
linear groove
linear incision
linear marking
linear opacification
linear osteotomy
linear polyethylene sutures
linear raphe
linear scarring
linear skin incision
linear skin lesion

linear skull fracture
linear stapler
linear stapling device
linear strand
linear transverse incision
linear ulcer
linen sutures
linen thread sutures
liner
lines of expression
lingual
lingual arch
lingual artery
lingual bar
lingual block
lingual flange
lingual forceps
lingual frenum
lingual ganglion
lingual gland
lingual guillotine
lingual gyrus
lingual hemorrhoid
lingual nerve
lingual occlusion
lingual papillae
lingual spatula
lingual splint
lingual sulcus
lingual surface of tooth
lingual thyroid
lingual tongue flap
lingual tonsillectome
lingual tonsillectomy
lingual tonsils
lingual vein
lingualis, arteria
lingualis, nervus
lingualis, vena
lingula (*pl.* lingulae)
lingular bronchus
lingular segment
lingulectomy
linguofacial trunk
lining
lining anesthesia
lining of organ

PIC line - percutaneous intravenous central
     catheter

linitis plastica
Link approximator
Link boutonnière finger splint
Link rotating total knee system
Link total hip
Linnartz clamp
Linnartz forceps
Linnartz intestinal clamp
Linnartz stomach clamp
Linn-Graefe iris forceps
Linscheid tendon transfer
lint
Linton clamp
Linton elastic hose
Linton flap
Linton hook
Linton incision
Linton operation
Linton radical vein ligation
Linton retractor
Linton shunt
Linton splanchnic retractor
Linton stocking
Linton subfascial ligation
Linton tourniquet
Linton tourniquet clamp
Linton tube
Linton vein hook
Linton vein stripper
Linton vein stripping
Linton-Blakemore needle
Linton-Nachlas tube
Linton-Talbott operation
Linx exchange guide wire
lion-jaw bone-holding forceps
lion-jaw clamp
lion-jaw forceps
lion-jaw tenaculum
Liotta-BioImplant prosthetic
    valve
lip adhesion operation
lip clamp
lip flap
lip line
lip movements
lip of cervix
lip of mouth

lip reflex
lip region
lip retractor
lip sclerotomy
lip shave
lip sutures
lip traction bow
lip tumor
lip vermilion
lipectomy
lipocele
lipodissector
lipoid granuloma
lipoid hyperplasia
lipoid material
lipoid nephrosis
lipoma (*pl.* lipomas, lipomata)
lipomatous
lipomatous ileocecal valve
lipomatous lesion
lipomatous-like tissue
liposarcoma
Lippes intrauterine loop
Lippes loop intrauterine device
    (Lippes loop IUD)
lipping
Lippman hip prosthesis
Lippy incus prosthesis
Lipschwitz needle
Lipscomb orthopedic procedure
Lipscomb-Henderson-Elkins
    technique
Lipsett operation
Lipsett scissors
liquefaction
liquefaction of fat
liquefaction of vitreous
liquefactive
liquid biopsy
liquid conductor Bovie
liquid intake
liquid nitrogen
Lisch nodules
Lisfranc amputation
Lisfranc ankle dislocation
Lisfranc foot fracture
Lisfranc fracture

Lisfranc joint
Lisfranc ligament
Lisfranc operation
Lissauer paralysis
Lissauer tract
Lissauer zone
List needle
Lister bandage scissors
Lister conjunctival forceps
Lister dressing
Lister forceps
Lister knife
Lister scissors
Lister tubercle
Lister-Burch eye speculum
Lister-Burch speculum
Liston amputating knife
Liston bone-cutting forceps
Liston forceps
Liston knife
Liston operation
Liston rongeur
Liston scissors
Liston shears
Liston splint
Liston-Key Horsley rib shears
Liston-Littauer bone-cutting
    forceps
Liston-Ruskin bone-cutting
    rongeur
Liston-Ruskin shears
Liston-Stille forceps
Lite hip cast
Lite-Beam splinting system
Liteflex intraocular lens
Liteflex lens
liter (l or L)
lith II pacemaker
lithiasis
lithium pacemaker
lithium-powered pacemaker
lithocenosis
lithoclast
lithocystotomy
lithodialysis
litholabe
litholapaxy

litholysis
litholyte
litholytic
lithometer
lithomyl
lithonephria
lithonephritis
lithonephrotomy
lithoscope
Lithostart nonimmersion
    lithotriptor
lithotome
lithotomist
lithotomy
lithotomy forceps
lithotomy position
lithotomy-Trendelenburg
    position
lithotony
lithotresis
lithotripsy
lithotripter (see *lithotriptor*)
lithotriptic
lithotriptor
    American endoscopy
        mechanical lithotriptor
    Candela laser lithotriptor
    Circon-ACMI electrohy-
        draulic lithotriptor
    Dornier gallstone
        lithotriptor
    Dornier lithotriptor
    Dornier waterbath
        lithotriptor
    electrohydraulic lithotrip-
        tor
    EPL (extracorporeal
        piezoelectric lithotrip-
        tor)
    extracorporeal piezoelec-
        tric lithotriptor
    Lithostart nonimmersion
        lithotriptor
    Olympus lithotriptor
    Technomed Sonolith
        3000 lithotriptor
    ultrasonic lithotriptor

STS: Medstone

lithotriptor *continued*
    Wilson-Cook mechanical
      lithotriptor
lithotriptor machine
lithotriptoscope
    Ravich lithotriptoscope
    Ravich lithotriptoscope
      with Luer lock
lithotriptoscopy
lithotrite
    Alcock lithotrite
    Alcock-Hendrickson
      lithotrite
    Bigelow lithotrite
    Hendrickson lithotrite
    Keyes lithotrite
    Löwenstein lithotrite
    Lowsley lithotrite
    Ravich lithotrite
    Reliquet lithotrite
    Teevan lithotrite
    Thompson lithotrite
lithotrity
Litt forceps
Littauer cilia forceps
Littauer ear-dressing forceps
Littauer forceps
Littauer nasal-dressing forceps
Littauer rongeur
Littauer scissors
Littauer stitch scissors
Littauer suture scissors
Littaur-Liston bone-cutting
    forceps
Littauer-Liston forceps
Littauer-West cutting forceps
litter
little finger
Little intraocular lens implant
Little Leaguer's elbow
Little Leaguer's shoulder
Little lens
Little retractor
little toe
Littleford introducer
Littleford-Spector introducer
Littler carrying scissors

Littler operation
Littler procedure
Littler scissors
Littler-Cooley technique
Littler-Eaton reconstruction
Littlewood amputation
Littlewood operation
Littman Class II pediatric
    stethoscope
Littre glands
Littre hernia
Littre operation
Littre sutures
Littre-Richter hernia
Litwak cannula
Litwak left atrial-aortic bypass
Litwak mitral valve scissors
Litwak scissors
Litwak utility scissors
Litwin dissecting scissors
Litwin scissors
live birth
live splint
liveborn infant
Lively splint
liver
liver bed
liver biopsy
liver biopsy needle
liver biopsy set
liver cell adenoma
liver damage
liver death
liver donation
liver edge
liver enlargement
liver failure
liver flap
liver flap sign
liver function
liver involvement
liver nodule
liver recipient
liver retractor
liver scan
liver scintiphoto
liver shadow

liver shock
liver span
liver tender
liver transplant
liver tumor
liver, kidneys, and spleen (LKS)
liver, spleen, and kidneys (LSK)
liver, spleen, and kidneys not
    enlarged
liver-holding clamp
liver-spleen scan
Livermore trocar
Liverpool elbow implant
Liverpool knee prosthesis
livid cyanosis
lividity
Livierato reflex
Livierato sign
living homograft
living suture
living-related donor
Livingston bar
Livingston forceps
Livingston triangle
livor mortis
Lizar operation
LKS (liver, kidneys, and spleen)
LLC (long-leg cast)
LLL (left lower lobe)
Llobera fixation forceps
Llobera forceps
Lloyd catheter
Lloyd esophagoscopic catheter
Lloyd tube
Lloyd-Davis clamp
Lloyd-Davis operation
Lloyd-Davis sigmoidoscope
Lloyd-Davis stirrups
Lloyd-Roberts clubfoot proce-
    dure
Lloyd-Roberts osteotomy
Lloyd-Roberts-Lettin technique
LLQ (left lower quadrant)
LMA position (left men-
    toanterior position)
LMP position (left mentopos-
    terior position)

LMT position (left men-
    totranverse position)
LOA position (left occipi-
    toanterior position)
load-bearing
loading applicator
loading dose
load-sharing
lobar
lobar atelectasis
lobar atrophy
lobar emphysema
lobar hyperplasia
lobar pneumonia
lobar sclerosis
lobe
lobe enlargement
lobe of brain
lobe of liver
lobe of lung
lobe of pituitary gland
lobe of prostate
lobe of thyroid gland
lobectomy
lobectomy forceps
lobectomy of lung
lobectomy of prostate
lobectomy of thyroid
lobectomy scissors
lobectomy tourniquet
lobed placenta
lobe-grasping forceps
lobe-holding forceps
Lobell splinter forceps
Lobenstein-Tarnier forceps
lobotomy
lobotomy electrode
lobotomy needle
lobotomy of brain
Lobstein ganglion
lobster-claw deformity
lobster-claw foot
lobster-claw hand
lobster-claw operation
lobster-tail catheter
lobular
lobular architecture of liver

lobular carcinoma
lobular patches of atelectasis
lobular pattern
lobulate
lobulated contour
lobulated kidney
lobulated mass
lobulated tumor mass
lobulation
lobule
lobulette
lobulus (*pl.* lobuli)
local anesthesia
local disease
local excision
local field block
local flap
local infection
local infiltration
local instillation
local involvement
local irradiation
local lesion
local metastasis
local radiation therapy
local reaction
local recurrence
local recurrence of carcinoma
Localio sacral tumor procedure
localization
localization films
localized
localized advancement flap
localized cancer
localized defect
localized lesion
localized mass
localized neurological sign
localized pain
localized plaque formation
localized radiotherapy
localized sepsis
localized signs of weakness
localized tenderness
localizer cast
localizing electrode
localizing neurological sign

localizing sign
locally advanced condition
location
locator (see also *metal locator, magnet*)
    Berman locator device
    Berman metal locator
    Berman-Moorhead locator
    Berman-Moorhead metal locator
    electroacoustic locator
    Kirby lens dislocator
    metal locator
    nerve locator
    Porex nerve locator
lochia
lochia alba
lochia cruenta
lochia purulenta
lochia rubra
lochia sanguinolenta
loci (*sing.* locus)
lock finger
lock knee
lock needle
lock stitch
lock sutures
Locke bone clamp
locked joint
locked knee
locked sutures
locking clamp
locking of joint
locking prosthesis
locking running sutures
locking stitch
locking sutures
lockjaw
Locklin stitch scissors
lock-stitch sutures
Lockwood clamp
Lockwood forceps
Lockwood intestinal forceps
Lockwood ligament
Lockwood tendon
Lockwood-Allis forceps

Lockwood-Allis intestinal
    forceps
locomotion
locomotor
locomotor ataxia
loculate
loculated abscess
loculated effusion
loculated emphysema
loculated empyema
loculated fluid
loculated pleural effusion
locus (*pl.* loci)
lodged
Loeffler (also Löffler)
Loeffler sutures
Loening stomach tube
Loetwig ganglion
Loewi suspension device
Löffler (see *Loeffler*)
Lofstrand brace
Lofstrand crutches
Logan bow support
Logan box
Logan dissector
Logan elevator
Logan lacrimal sac self-retaining
    retractor
Logan lip traction bow
Logan retractor
Logan traction bow
loge de Guyon ulnar nerve
    block
Logracino bunionectomy
Löhlein diameter
Löhlein operation
loin
Lok-it screwdriver
Lok-screw double-slot screw-
    driver
Lok-screw screwdriver
lollipop bite-block
LOM (limitation of motion)
Lombard mastoid rongeur
Lombard rongeur
Lombard-Beyer forceps
Lombard-Beyer rongeur

Lombard-Beyer rongeur forceps
Lombard-Boies rongeur
Londermann corneal trephine
Londermann operation
London College foil carrier
London elbow hinge
London forceps
London prosthesis
London retractor
London tissue forceps
London total elbow
long abductor muscle
long abductor tendon
long adductor muscle
long axis of kidney
long axis scan
long axis view
long blunt nerve hook
long bone
long bone fracture
long bone survey
long ciliary arteries
long ciliary nerves
long extensor muscle
long external lateral ligament
long fibular muscle
long flexor muscle
Long forceps
long gyrus of insula
Long hysterectomy forceps
long intestinal tube
Long Island College Hospital
    placenta forceps
Long Island forceps
long levator muscle
long limb gastric bypass
long muscle
long needle
long nerve of Bell
long oblique incision
long palate hook
long palmar muscle
long periosteal elevator
long peroneal muscle
long philtrum
long plantar ligament
long posterior ciliary artery

long posterior ciliary axis
long process of incus
long radial extensor muscle
long rectangular flap
long rotator muscles
long scissors
Long stitch scissors
long thoracic nerve
long tract
long-arm cast (LAC)
long-armed cast
Longdwel catheter
Longdwel catheter needle
Longdwel needle
Longdwel Teflon catheter
long-handle curet
Longhem prosthesis
longissimus capitis, musculus
longissimus cervicis, musculus
longissimus colli, musculus
longissimus muscle
longissimus, musculus
longissimus thoracis, musculus
longitudinal
longitudinal arch
longitudinal arch supports
longitudinal arteriogram
longitudinal axis
longitudinal bundle
longitudinal cerebral fissure
longitudinal cystotomy
longitudinal diameter
longitudinal esophageal
   stricture
longitudinal fissure of cerebrum
longitudinal fold of duodenum
longitudinal fracture
longitudinal incision
longitudinal ligament
longitudinal medial bundle
longitudinal midline incision
longitudinal muscle
longitudinal myotomy
longitudinal nerves
longitudinal plane
longitudinal presentation
longitudinal sinus

longitudinal sulcus
longitudinal suture of palate
longitudinal sutures
longitudinalis superior linguae,
   musculus
longitudinally
long-leg brace
long-leg cast (LLC)
Longmire anastomosis
Longmire operation
Longmire valvulotome
Longmire-Mueller curved
   valvulotome
long-nose retriever snare
long-standing condition
long-term treatment
long-tract sign
Longuet incision
Longuet operation
longus capitis, musculus
longus colli, musculus
long-wave irradiation
Look coaxial flexible disposable
   cannula
Loomis ring
loop (see also *loupe*)
   afferent loop
   air-filled loop
   alpha loop
   alpha sigmoid loop
   Axenfeld loop
   Beck loop
   Billeau ear loop
   Billeau loop
   Billeau Teflon-coated
    loop
   bowel loop
   Bricker loop
   Bush stabilized cutting
    loop
   C-loop of duodenum
   Cannon endarterectomy
    loop
   capillary loop
   Clayman-Knolle lens
    loop
   closed loop

loop *continued*
- colonic loop
- colostomy loop
- contiguous loop
- Cordonnier ureteroileal loop
- cutting loop
- diathermic loop
- double-reverse alpha sigmoid loop
- duodenal loop
- ear loop
- efferent loop
- endarterectomy loop
- foreign body loop
- Gamma transverse colon loop
- Gerdy interauricular loop
- hairpin loop
- haptic loop
- Henle loop
- Hyrtl loop
- ileal loop
- interauricular loop
- intestinal loop
- Ivy loop
- Ivy wire loop
- J-loop
- jejunal loop
- Kirby lens loop
- Kirby loop
- Knolle-Pearce lens loop
- Lippes intrauterine loop
- Lippes loop (intrauterine device)
- maxi-vessel loop
- Meyer loop
- N-loop
- N-shaped sigmoid loop
- P-loop
- peduncular loop
- platinum loop
- prosthetic loop
- puborectalis loop
- re-entrant loop
- resectoscope cutting loop

loop *continued*
- rubber vessel loop
- Sarns safety loop
- scoops and loops
- sentinel loop
- sigmoid loop
- Silastic loop
- snare loop
- Stoerck loop
- subclavian loop
- T-loop
- terminal ileal loop
- thyroid loop
- tripronged loop
- twisted wire loop
- ureteroileal loop
- vascular loop
- vector loop
- ventricular loop
- Vesi-loop
- vessel loop
- Vieussens loop
- Wilder lens loop

loop choledochojejunostomy
loop colostomy
loop colostomy set
loop diuretics
loop electrode
loop esophagojejunostomy
loop gastrojejunostomy
loop jejunostomy
loop of bowel
loop of suture material
loop of Vieussens
loop ostomy bridge
loop retractor
loop sutures
looped cautery
loopogram
loopography
loops of redundant colon
loop-type snare forceps
loop-type stone-crushing forceps
Loopuyt needle
loose bodies
loose body forceps

loose connective tissue
loose fracture
loose knee procedure
loose shoulder
loosely approximated
loosely closed
loosening of prosthetic joint
Looser lines
Looser zone
lop ear
LOP position (left occipito-
   posterior position)
Lopez-Enriquez operation
Lo-Por arterial prosthesis
Lo-Por vascular graft
Lo-Pro tracheal tube
Lo-Profile balloon catheter
Lo-Profile II balloon catheter
Lo-Profile steerable dilatation
   catheter
Lord hemorrhoidectomy
Lord hydrocelectomy
Lord operation
Lord press-fit hip prosthesis
Lordan chalazion forceps
Lordan forceps
Lordan hook
Lordan muscle-splitting hook
Lord-Blakemore tube
lordoscoliosis
lordosis
lordotic curve
lordotic projection
lordotic view
Lore forceps
Lore suction tip-holding forceps
Lore suction tube-holding
   forceps
Lore tube
Lore-Lawrence tube
Lorenz bandage scissors
Lorenz brace
Lorenz needle holder
Lorenz operation
Lorenz osteotomy
Lorenz position
Lorenz sign

Lorenz tube
Lorenzo bone fixation screw
Lorenzo reamer
Lorenzo screw
Lorenzo SMO prosthesis
Lorenz-Rees nasal rasp
Loreta operation
Lorfan anesthesia
Lorfan anesthetic agent
Lorie antral trephine
Lorie retractor
Lorie tonsillar suture instrument
Lorie trephine
Loring ophthalmoscope
Lorna nonperforating towel
   clamp
Lorus knee orthosis
Losee knee reconstruction
Losee maneuver
losing
loss
Lossen operation
LOT position (left occipitotrans-
   verse position)
Lotheissen femoral hernia repair
Lotheissen hernia repair
Lotheissen herniorrhaphy
Lotheissen operation
Lotheissen-McVay operation
Lothrop dissector
Lothrop forceps
Lothrop hemostat
Lothrop knife
Lothrop ligature forceps
Lothrop retractor
Lothrop tonsillar knife
Lothrop uvula retractor
Lottes intramedullary nail
Lottes nail
Lottes operation
Lottes pin
Lottes reamer
Lottes reduction technique
Lottes rod
Lottes triflange intramedullary
   nail
loud piping rales

loud systolic murmur
loudness
Loughnane hook
Louis angle
Lounsbury curet
Lounsbury placenta curet
loupe (see also *lens loupe, loop*)
    Adler lens loupe
    Amenabar lens loupe
    Arlt lens loupe
    Arlt loupe
    Bausch-Lomb loupe
    Beebe binocular loupe
    Beebe lens loupe
    Beebe loupe
    Berens lens loupe
    Berens loupe
    binocular loupe
    binocular prism loupe
    binocular surgical loupe
    Callahan lens loupe
    corneal loupe
    Daviel lens loupe
    Daviel loupe
    Dualoupe
    ear loupe
    eye loupe
    intracapsular lens loupe
    Keeler loupe
    Kirby intracapsular lens
      loupe
    lens loupe
    Lewis loupe
    magnifying loupe
    Mark lens loupe
    McKenzie leukotomy
      loupe
    New Orleans Eye and
      Ear loupe
    New Orleans lens loupe
    New Orleans loupe
    plastic Berger eye loupe
    Storz binocular loupe
    Storz binocular prism
      loupe
    surgical loupe
    Troutman lens loupe

loupe *continued*
    Weber-Elschnig lens
      loupe
    Weber-Elschnig loupe
    Wilder loupe
    Zeiss lens loupe
Lovac fundus contact lens
    implant
Love leukotome
Love nasal splint
Love nerve retractor
Love retractor
Love splint
Love uvula retractor
Love-Adson elevator
Love-Adson periosteal elevator
Love-Gruenwald cranial rongeur
Love-Gruenwald forceps
Love-Gruenwald pituitary
    rongeur
Love-Gruenwald rongeur
Love-Kerrison forceps
Love-Kerrison rongeur
Lovelace bladder forceps
Lovelace forceps
Lovelace gallbladder trocar
Lovelace hemostatic forceps
Lovelace thyroid traction
    vulsellum forceps
Lovset maneuver
low anterior resection
low back
low birth weight
low cervical cesarean section
low cesarean section
Low Dye strapping
Low Dye taping technique for
    plantar fasciitis
low forceps
low frequency
low grade
low incision
low intermittent suction
low level
low ligation
low midline incision
low risk

low small-bowel obstruction
low spinal anesthesia
low stirrups
low threshold
low tracheotomy
low transverse incision
low viscosity cement (LVC)
low voltage
low-back pain
Löw-Beer forceps
Löw-Beer position
Löw-Beer projection
Löw-Beer view
low-dose therapy
Lowe ring
Lowe-Breck cartilage knife
Lowe-Breck elbow prosthesis
Lowe-Breck knife
Lowe-Breck meniscectomy
    knife
Lowell glaucoma knife
Lowell knife
Lowell pleural needle
Löwenberg forceps
Löwenstein lithotrite
Löwenstein operation
lower abdomen
lower abdominal organ
lower airway obstruction
lower back
lower esophageal sphincter
    (LES)
lower extremity
lower eyelid
Lower forceps
lower fragment
Lower gall duct forceps
lower GI procedure
lower GI series
lower jaw
Lower lateral forceps
Lower lateral scissors
lower lid
lower limb
lower lip
lower lobe
lower lobe of lung
lower mantle

lower margin of field
lower midline incision
lower operation for femoral
    hernia
lower panendoscopy
lower pole
lower teeth
Lower trocar
lower uterine segment
lower uterine segment cesarean
    section
Lower-Shumway cardiac
    transplant
lowest splanchnic nerve
low-forceps delivery
low-forceps operation
low-friction arthroplasty (LFA)
Lowis IV disk rongeur forceps
Lowis periosteal elevator
low-level echo enhancement
Lowman bone clamp
Lowman bone-holding clamp
Lowman clamp
Lowman flatfoot procedure
Lowman forceps
Lowman hand retractor
Lowman rongeur
Lowman sling procedure
Lowman-Gerster bone clamp
Lown cardioverter
Lown technique
low-pitched bowel sounds
low-profile prosthesis
low-profile valve prosthesis
low-riding patella
Lowsley forceps
Lowsley grasping forceps
Lowsley hemostat
Lowsley lithotrite
Lowsley needle
Lowsley nephropexy
Lowsley operation
Lowsley prostate retractor
Lowsley prostatic lobe-holding
    forceps
Lowsley prostatic traction
Lowsley prostatic tractor
Lowsley retractor

Lowsley ribbon-gut needle
Lowsley stone crusher
Lowsley tractor
Lowsley urethroscope
Lowsley-Luc forceps
Lowsley-Peterson cystoscope
Lowsley-Peterson endoscope
Lowsman operation for talipes
    valgus
low-tension pulse
loxotomy
LPS balloon
LPS catheter
LPS Peel-Away introducer
LR (lateral rectus)
L/S ratio (lecithin/sphingomye-
    lin ratio)
LSA position (left sacroanterior
    position)
LScA position (left scapulo-
    anterior position)
LScP position (left scapulopos-
    terior position)
LSK (liver, spleen, and kidneys)
LSP position (left sacroposterior
    position)
LSU reciprocation-gait orthosis
    brace
Lubafax dressing
Lubraseptic
lubricant
lubricating jelly
lubrication
Luc ethmoid forceps
Luc forceps
Luc operation
Luc septum forceps
Luc septum-cutting forceps
Lucae bayonet
Lucae bone hammer
Lucae dressing forceps
Lucae ear speculum
Lucae forceps
Lucae hook
Lucae mallet
Lucae mastoid mallet
Lucae probe

Lucas chisel
Lucas curet
Lucas gouge
Lucas-Cottrell operation
Lucas-Cottrell osteotomy
Lucas-Murray knee arthrodesis
Lucas-Murray operation
Lucchese mitral valve dilator
lucency
lucent calculi
lucent defect
lucent line
lucinate ligament
lucite
lucite eye implant
lucite implant
lucite pessary
lucite sphere implant
Luck bone drill
Luck bone saw
Luck drill
Luck fasciotome
Luck hallux valgus procedure
Luck operation
Luck procedure for Dupuytren
    contracture release
Luck saw
Luck-Bishop saw
Luckett operation
Luco operation
Ludloff bunionectomy
Ludloff hallux valgus procedure
Ludloff incision
Ludloff operation
Ludloff osteotomy
Ludloff sign
Ludwig angle
Ludwig applicator
Ludwig ganglion
Ludwig sinus applicator
Luedde exophthalmometer
Luedde measurement
Luedde transparent rule
Luer bone curet
Luer bone rongeur
Luer curet
Luer forceps

Luer gallstone scoop
Luer hemorrhoidal forceps
Luer needle
Luer reconstruction plate
Luer retractor
Luer rongeur
Luer scoop
Luer speculum
Luer suction cannula adapter
Luer syringe
Luer tip cap
Luer tip syringe
Luer tracheal cannula
Luer tracheal double-ended
   retractor
Luer tracheal tube
Luer tube
Luer-Friedman bone rongeur
Luer-Hartmann rongeur
Luer-Koerte scoop
Luer-Liston-Wheeling rongeur
Luer-Lok catheter connection
Luer-Lok pump
Luer-Lok syringe
Luer-Whiting forceps
Luer-Whiting mastoid rongeur
Luethy-Beck needle holder
lugged plate
Lugol iodine preparation
Lugol solution
lugolized
Luhr fixation system
Luhr mandibular plate
Luhr maxillofacial system
Luikart forceps
Luikart Iconoclast blunt
   dissection instrument
Luikart obstetrical forceps
Luikart-Bill traction handle
Luikart-Kielland forceps
Luikart-McLean forceps
Luikart-Simpson forceps
Lukens aspirator
Lukens bone wax dressing
Lukens cannula
Lukens catgut sutures
Lukens collector
Lukens enterotome

Lukens enterotomy
Lukens irrigator
Lukens retractor
Lukens suction tube
Lukens thymus retractor
Lukens tracheal double-ended
   retractor
LUL (left upper lobe)
Lulu clamp
Lumaguide infusion catheter
lumbales, arteriae
lumbales, nervi
lumbales, venae
lumbalis ascendens, vena
lumbalis ima, arteria
lumbar
lumbar aortogram
lumbar aortography
lumbar aortography needle
lumbar arteries
lumbar colotomy
lumbar curvature
lumbar curve
lumbar epidural anesthesia
lumbar flexure
lumbar hemilaminectomy
lumbar hernia
lumbar laminectomy
lumbar lordotic curve
lumbar lymph nodes
lumbar musculature
lumbar myelogram
lumbar nephrotomy
lumbar nerve block
lumbar nerves
lumbar plexus
lumbar puncture
lumbar puncture needle
lumbar reflex
lumbar region
lumbar scoliosis
lumbar splanchnic nerves
lumbar spine
lumbar spur
lumbar spurring
lumbar subarachnoid catheter
lumbar suture
lumbar sympathectomy

lumbar veins
lumbar vertebrae
lumbarization
lumbocolostomy
lumbocolotomy
lumbocostoabdominal triangle
lumbodorsal
lumbodorsal fascia
lumboiliac incision
lumboinguinal nerve
lumboperitoneal shunt
lumbosacral belt
lumbosacral curve
lumbosacral disk protrusion
lumbosacral fusion
lumbosacral joint
lumbosacral projection
lumbosacral series
lumbosacral spine
lumbosacral sprain
lumbosacral strain
lumbosacral support
lumbosacral trunk
lumbotomy retractor
lumbrical bar
lumbrical muscles
lumbricales manus, musculi
lumbricales, musculi
lumbricales pedis, musculi
Lumelec catheter
lumen (*pl.* lumina)
lumen finder
       Carabelli lumen finder
       full-view lumen finder
lumen of appendix
lumen of artery
lumen of bowel
lumen of bronchial artery
lumen of gut
lumen of vein
lumiform splint
lumina (*sing.* lumen)
LUMINA-operating telescope
LUMINA-SL telescope
luminal defect
luminal irregularity
luminal narrowing

luminous intensity
luminous ophthalmoscope
luminous rays
Lumiwand light
lump
lump kidney
lumpectomy
lunar hymen
lunate bone
lunate dislocation
lunate fracture
lunate implant
Lund operation
Lund-Browder burn chart
Lunderquist guide
Lunderquist guide wire
Lunderquist wire
Lunderquist working wire
Lunderquist-Ring torque guide
Lundquist nephrostomy wire
Lundsgaard blade
Lundsgaard knife
Lundsgaard rasp
Lundsgaard sclerotome
Lundsgaard-Burch corneal
    raspatory
Lundsgaard-Burch knife
Lundsgaard-Burch rasp
Lundsgaard-Burch sclerotome
Lundy laryngoscope
Lundy needle
Lundy-Irving needle
lung
lung abscess
lung base
lung biopsy
lung brushings
lung calculus
lung cancer
lung carcinoma
lung clamp
lung elasticity
lung exclusion clamp
lung fields
lung forceps
lung function studies
lung hilus

lung infarct
lung infiltrate
lung lingula
lung markings
lung metastasis
lung parenchyma
lung resection
lung retractor
lung scan
lung scissors
lung tissue
lung tourniquet
lung washings
lung-grasping forceps
lungs clear to percussion and
    auscultation
lunula
Luongo cannula
Luongo curet
Luongo elevator
Luongo hand retractor
Luongo instruments
Luongo needle
Luongo retractor
Luongo sphenoid irrigating
    cannula
LUQ (left upper quadrant)
Luque instrumentation
Luque rod
Luque rod fixation
Luque segmental spinal
    instrumentation
Luque wire
Luschka crypt
Luschka foramen
Luschka ganglion
Luschka joints
Luschka laryngeal cartilage
Luschka muscles
Luschka nerve
Luschka tonsil
Lusskin drill
lutein cells
luteinize
Luther-Peter retractor
Lutkens sphincter
Lutz forceps

Lutz septal forceps
Lutz septal ridge forceps
Lutz septal ridge-cutting
    forceps
luxation
Luxtec fiberoptic system
luxus heart
Luys segregator
Luys separator
LV apex cannula (left ventricu-
    lar apex cannula)
LVAD (left ventricular assist
    device)
LVC cement (low viscosity
    cement)
LVEDP (left ventricular end-
    diastolic pressure)
Lyda Ivalon-Lucite orbital
    implant
Lyman incision
Lyman Smith brace
Lyman Smith traction
lymph
lymph cells
lymph channel
lymph circulation
lymph dialysis
lymph gland
lymph involvement
lymph node
lymph node adenopathy
lymph node classification
lymph node disease
lymph node dissection
lymph node enlargement
lymph node involvement
lymph node irradiation
lymph node metastasis
lymph node resection
lymph node system
lymph node–bearing tissue
lymph nodule
lymph space
lymph system
lymph vessel
lymphadenectomy
lymphadenoid tissue

lymphadenopathy
lymphadenotomy
lymphangiectasis
lymphangiectomy
lymphangiogram (LAG)
lymphangiography
lymphangioma
lymphangioplasty
lymphangiorrhaphy
lymphangiotomy
lymphangitic metastasis
lymphatic
lymphatic chain
lymphatic channel
lymphatic drainage
lymphatic duct
lymphatic fluid
lymphatic involvement
lymphatic metastasis
lymphatic nodules
lymphatic obstruction
lymphatic sinuses
lymphatic spread
lymphatic system
lymphatic tissue
lymphatic trunk
lymphatic vessels
lymphaticostomy
lymphatics
lymphedema
lymphocyte
lymphoid
lymphoid hyperplasia
lymphoid irradiation
lymphoid mass
lymphoid polyp
lymphoid tissue
lymphoma
lymphoma implant
lymphomatoid granuloma
lymphomatous infiltrate
lymphosarcoma
lymphosarcomatous nodule
lymphoscintigraphy
Lynch curet
Lynch dissector

Lynch electrode
Lynch forceps
Lynch frontal sinus exploration
Lynch incision
Lynch knife
Lynch laryngeal dissector
Lynch laryngoscope
Lynch operation
Lynch scissors
Lynch sinusectomy
Lynch spatula
Lynch splint
Lynch suspension
Lynch suspension apparatus
Lynch suspension laryngoscope
Lynch tonsillar dissector
Lynch tonsillar knife
Lynco arch support
Lynn Achilles-tendon proce-
    dure
LYOFOAM dressing
LYOFOAM wound dressing
Lyon forceps
Lyon tube
Lyon-Horgan operation
lyophilized graft
lyophilized pigskin
lyre of uterus
lyre of vagina
lyre-shaped finger
lyse
lysed
lysed adhesions
lysis
lysis of adhesions
lysis time
Lyster tube
Lyster water bag
lytic area
lytic bone lesion
lytic defect
lytic disease
lytic lesion
Lytle metacarpal splint
Lytle splint
Lytle sutures

M Beaver blade
M-A tube (Miller-Abbott tube)
M-blade
M-bur (M-1, M-2, etc.)
M-pattern
ma (milliamperes)
Mac (see also *Mc*)
MAC (monitored anesthesia
    care)
MacAusland bone hammer
MacAusland chisel
MacAusland dissector
MacAusland elbow arthroplasty
MacAusland mallet
MacAusland muscle retractor
MacAusland operation
MacAusland reamer
MacAusland retractor
MacAusland skid
MacAusland-Kelly retractor
MacCallum knife
MacCallum patch
MacCarty procedure
MacDonald clamp
MacDonald dissector
MacDonald periosteal elevator
macerated
macerated fetus
maceration
Macewen drill
Macewen herniorrhaphy
Macewen operation
Macewen osteotomy
Macewen saw
Macewen sign
Macewen-Shands osteotomy for
    coxa vara
MacFee incision

MacFee neck flap
MacGregor conjunctival forceps
MacGregor forceps
MacGregor osteotome
Machek operation
Machek ptosis operation
Machek-Blaskovics operation
Machek-Gifford operation
Machemer calipers
Machemer cutter
Machemer lens
Machemer sclerotomy knife
Machemer VISC (vitreous
    infusion suction cutter)
Machemer vitreous cutter
Machemer vitreous infusion
    suction cutter (Machemer
    VISC)
Machida bronchoscope
Machida FDS (fiberduodeno-
    scope)
Machida fiberduodenoscope
    (FDS)
Machida fiberoptic laryngo-
    scope
Machida laryngoscope
MacIntosh blade
MacIntosh blade anesthesia
MacIntosh implant
MacIntosh knee prosthesis
MacIntosh laryngoscope
MacIntosh operation
MacIntosh over-the-top
    reconstruction of knee
MacIntosh prosthesis
MacIntosh sign
MacIntosh tibial plateau
    prosthesis

MacIntosh tibial prosthesis
Mack ear plugs
Mack tonometer
Mack tonsillectome
MacKay contour retractor
MacKay contour self-retaining
    retractor
MacKay retractor
MacKay-Marg tonometer
Mack-Brunswick operation
Mackenrodt incision
Mackenrodt operation
MacKenty antral tube
MacKenty cleft palate knife
MacKenty elevator
MacKenty forceps
MacKenty knife
MacKenty periosteal elevator
MacKenty punch
MacKenty scissors
MacKenty septal elevator
MacKenty sphenoid punch
MacKenty tissue forceps
MacKenty tube
Mackenzie (see also *McKenzie*)
Mackenzie amputation
Mackenzie point
Mackid operation
Mackler esophageal tube
Mackler intraluminal tube
    prosthesis
Mackler tube
Mackler tube prosthesis
Maclay scissors
Maclay tonsillar scissors
MacNab-Dall spinal fusion
Macon Hospital speculum
macrodactyly
macrodontia
Macrofit hip prosthesis
macrogenia
macrophage
macroscopic
macroscopic anatomy
macrosomia
macrosomic baby
MacroVac

macula (*pl.* maculae)
macula degeneration
macula retinoscope
macula-off retinal detachment
macular change
macular degeneration
macular fan
macular star
Madayag needle
Madden clamp
Madden dissector
Madden forceps
Madden herniorrhaphy
Madden hook
Madden incisional hernior-
    rhaphy
Madden intestinal clamp
Madden ligature carrier
Madden sympathectomy hook
Madden technique
Madden-Potts forceps
Maddox needle
Maddox pliers
Maddox rod
Madelung deformity
Madlener operation
Madlener sterilization
Madoff suction tube
Madonna fingers
Madreporic femoral component
Madsen Tympan-O-Scope
Madura foot
Maestro pacemaker
Magendie foramen
Magielski canal knife
Magielski cautery
Magielski chisel
Magielski curet
Magielski electrocoagulator
Magielski elevator
Magielski forceps
Magielski needle
Magielski tonsil forceps
Magielski-Heermann forceps
Magill band
Magill catheter-introducing
    forceps

Magill forceps
Magill laryngoscope
Magill tube
Magitot keratoplasty
Magitot operation
magneprobe
magnesium tuning forks
magnet (see also *locator, metal locator*)
    Alnico magneprobe magnet
    Atlas-Storz eye magnet
    Berman magnet
    Bonaccolto magnet
    bronchoscopic magnet
    Bronson magnet
    Cody magnetic probe
    Coronet magnet
    cryomagnet
    electromagnet
    endoscopic magnet
    Equen magnet
    Equen stomach magnet
    eye magnet
    Firlene eye magnet
    Grafco magnet
    Gruening (also Grüning)
    Gruening eye magnet
    Gruening magnet
    Grüning (also Gruening)
    Grüning eye magnet
    Grüning magnet
    Haab magnet
    Hamblin magnet
    Hirschberg electromagnet
    Hirschberg magnet
    Holinger bronchoscopic magnet
    Holinger magnet
    horseshoe magnet
    Lancaster eye magnet
    Lancaster magnet
    Mag-Optin eye magnet
    Mellinger magnet
    Mueller giant eye magnet

magnet *continued*
    needle magnet
    permanent magnet
    Ralks eye magnet
    Ralks magnet
    stomach magnet
    Storz magnet
    Sweet electric magnet
    Sweet eye magnet
    Sweet magnet
    temporary magnet
    Wildgen-Reck magnet
magnet operation
magnetic cup
magnetic extraction
magnetic eye implant
magnetic field
magnetic implant
magnetic resonance imaging (MRI)
magnetoencephalography
magnetogyric ratio
Magnetriever ureteral stent retriever
Magnevist
magnification
magnifier
    Coil magnifier
    endomagnifier
    Storz adjustable magnifier
    Storz endomagnifier
    Storz-Bruenings ear magnifier
    Zeiss binocular head magnifier
magnifying loupe
magnitude shunt
magnum foramen
Magnum Oto-Tool system
Magnus operation
Magnuson abduction humerus splint
Magnuson arthroplasty
Magnuson circular twin saw
Magnuson operation

Magnuson patellar procedure
Magnuson reduction technique
Magnuson saw
Magnuson single circular saw
Magnuson splint
Magnuson strut
Magnuson transplantation of
    subscapularis tendon
Magnuson twist drill
Magnuson valve
Magnuson valve prosthesis
Magnuson-Cromie prosthesis
Magnuson-Cromie valve
    prosthesis
Magnuson-Stack arthroplasty
Magnuson-Stack shoulder
    arthroplasty
Magnuson-Stack shoulder
    arthrotomy
Mag-Optin eye magnet
Magovern ball-valve mallet
Magovern ball-valve prosthesis
Magovern-Cromie ball-cage
    prosthetic valve
Magovern-Cromie prosthesis
Magovern-Cromie valve
    prosthesis
Magpi hypospadias repair
Magpi technique
Maguire-Harvey cutter
Maguire-Harvey vitreous
    cutter
Mahaim bundle in heart
Mahler sign
Mahoney dilator
Mahoney intranasal antral
    speculum
Mahoney speculum
Mahorner retractor
Mahorner thyroid retractor
Mahorner-Mead operation
Mahurkar catheter
Mahurkar dual-lumen catheter
Mahurkar dual-lumen dialysis
    catheter
Mahurkar dual-lumen femoral
    catheter

Maier dressing forceps
Maier forceps
Maier hemostat
Maier uterine-dressing forceps
Mailith pacemaker
Mailler colon forceps
Mailler cut-off forceps
Mailler intestinal forceps
Mailler rectal forceps
main bronchus
main pancreatic duct (MPD)
main pulmonary artery
main renal vein
main stem bronchus
Maingot clamp
Maingot hemostat
Maingot hysterectomy forceps
Maingot operation
Mainster retina laser lens
mainstream
maintenance chemotherapy
maintenance dialysis
maintenance dose
maintenance level
maintenance therapy
Mainz pouch urinary reservoir
Mainz urinary reservoir pouch
Mair operation
Maison retractor
Maisonneuve amputation
Maisonneuve bandage
Maisonneuve fracture
Maisonneuve sign
Maisonneuve urethrotome
Majewsky operation
major airway
major amputation
major connector bar
major fracture
major motor group
major operation
major palatine artery
major surgery
major trauma
Makkas operation
malacotomy
maladie-de-Roger

maladjustment
malalignment
malar arch
malar area
malar bone
malar elevator
malar eminence
malar incision
malar process
malar prosthesis
Malawer fibular resection
Malbec operation
Malbran operation
maldevelopment
male castration
male catheterization
male reproductive organs
Malecot 2-wing catheter
Malecot 2-wing drain
Malecot 4-wing catheter
Malecot 4-wing drain
Malecot catheter
Malecot drain
Malecot gastrostomy tube
Malecot suprapubic cystostomy
    catheter
Malecot tube
Malecot urethral catheter
malformation
malformed fetus
malfunction
Malgaigne amputation
Malgaigne apparatus
Malgaigne clamp
Malgaigne fracture
Malgaigne hook
Malgaigne luxation
malignancy
malignant
malignant disease
malignant fibrous histiocytoma
malignant growth
malignant hyperthermia
malignant lymphoma
malignant melanoma
malignant mesenchymal
    tumor
malignant neoplasm

malignant polyp
malignant process
malignant tumor
malignant ulcer
Maliniac nasal raspatory
Maliniac nasal retractor
Maliniac rasp
Maliniac retractor
Malis angled-up bipolar forceps
Malis coagulator
Malis electrocautery
Malis elevator
Malis forceps
Malis microcuret
Malis microdissector
Malis needle holder
Malis nerve hook
Malis neurological scissors
Malis retractor
Malis scissors
Malis titanium microsurgical
    forceps
malleable
malleable blade retractor
malleable copper retractor
malleable plate
malleable probe
malleable retractor
malleable rod
malleable scoop
malleable screw
malleable spatula
malleable stainless steel
    retractor
malleo-incudal joint
malleolar artery
malleolar folds
malleolar fracture
malleolar plexus
malleolaris anterior medialis,
    arteria
malleolus (*pl.* malleoli)
malleolus muscle
malleotomy
Malleotrain active ankle support
Malleotrain ankle sleeve
mallet
    aluminum mallet

mallet *continued*
Bakelite mallet
Bergman mallet
Blount mallet
Boxwood mallet
Brahms mallet toe
    procedure
bronze mallet
Brown mallet
cervical mallet
Chandler mallet
Children's Hospital
    mallet
combination mallet
Cooper mallet
Cottle mallet
Crane mallet
Delrin face mallet
fibermallet
Gerzog mallet
Gerzog mastoid mallet
Hajek mallet
Heister mallet
Hibbs mallet
Kirk mallet
lead-filled head mallet
lead-filled mallet
Lucae mallet
Lucae mastoid mallet
MacAusland mallet
Magovern ball-valve
    mallet
Meyerding mallet
Meyerding solid alumi-
    num mallet
Newhart mallet
nylon head mallet
Ombrédanne mallet
orthopedic mallet
plastic mallet
Ralks mallet
Richards combination
    mallet
Rush pin lead-filled head
    mallet with extractor
small brass mallet
small head mallet

mallet *continued*
Smith-Petersen mallet
standard pattern mallet
steel mallet
Stille mallet
White mallet
mallet finger
mallet fracture
mallet toe
malleus
malleus bone
malleus cutter
malleus forceps
malleus handle
malleus nipper
malleus punch
Mallinckrodt angiographic
    catheter
Mallinckrodt catheter
Mallor pacemaker
Mallory-Head hip component
Mallory-Head hip program
Mallory-Head hip prosthesis
Mallory-Weiss mucosal tear
Mallory-Weiss tear
Malm-Himmelstein pulmonary
    valvulotome
Malm-Himmelstein valvulotome
malocclusion
malodorous
malodorous discharge
malomaxillary suture
Maloney bougie
Maloney catheter
Maloney dilator
Maloney esophageal dilator
Maloney mercury bougie
Maloney mercury-filled dilator
Maloney mercury-filled
    esophageal dilator
Maloney tapered bougie
Maloney tapered-tip dilator
maloplasty
Malpighi vesicles
malpighian bodies
malpighian capsule
malposition

malrotation
malsensing pacemaker
Malstrom extraction
Malt technique in liver trans-
    plantation
maltreatment
Maltz angle knife
Maltz bayonet saw
Maltz cartilage knife
Maltz knife
Maltz nasal saw
Maltz needle
Maltz rasp
Maltz raspatory
Maltz retractor
Maltz saw
Maltz-Anderson nasal rasp
Maltz-Lipsett nasal rasp
Maltz-Lipsett rasp
Maltz-Lipsett raspatory
Maltzman needle
malum
malunion
malunion of fracture
malunited fracture
mamilla (*pl.* mamillae)
mamillary process
mamillary sutures
mamilliplasty
mamma
mammaplasty
mammary
mammary abscess
mammary artery
mammary body
mammary duct
mammary fold
mammary glands
mammary implant
mammary involvement
mammary prosthesis
mammary ptosis procedure
mammary region
mammary souffle
mammary support dressing
mammary vein

mammary vessels
mammectomy
mammiform
Mammo-lock needle
mammogram
mammogram lesion
mammography
mammoplasia
mammoplasty (mammaplasty
    preferred)
mammotomy
Manan needle
Manchester colporrhaphy
Manchester operation
Manchester repair
Manchester uterine suspension
Manchester-Donald-Fothergill
    operation
Manchu cotton dressing
Mandelbaum cannula
Mandelbaum catheter
Mandelbaum ear knife
mandible
mandible splint
mandibular
mandibular arch
mandibular arch bar
mandibular artery
mandibular articulation
mandibular block
mandibular bone
mandibular dentitional odontec-
    tomy
mandibular foramen
mandibular fossa
mandibular hemisection
mandibular lymph nodes
mandibular nerve
mandibular notch
mandibular port
mandibular prosthesis
mandibular protraction
mandibular ramus
mandibular recontouring
    alveolectomy
mandibular ridge

mandibular teeth
mandibularis, nervus
mandibulectomy
mandril graft
mandrin
mandrin dilator
mandrin guide
maneuver
Mangoldt epithelial graft
Manhattan Eye and Ear corneal
    dissector
Manhattan Eye and Ear probe
Manhattan Eye and Ear spat
Manhattan Eye and Ear suture
    forceps
Manhurkar catheter
Mani catheter
Mani cerebral catheter
manifest deviation
manifestation
manipulation
manipulation of fracture
manipulation of joint
manipulation of muscle
manipulation of prosthetic
    device
Mankin procedure
Mann forceps
Mann technique
Mann-Bollman fistula
Mann-DuVries technique
Manning forceps
Manning retractor
Mannis suture probe
mannitol
Mannkopf sign
Mann-Williamson operation
Mann-Williamson ulcer
manometer (see also *sphygmo-*
    *manometer*)
        Harvard manometer
        Honan manometer
        rhinomanometer
        Riva-Rocci manometer
        sphygmomanometer (see
            separate listing)
        spinal manometer

manometer *continued*
        standby Baumanometer
        strain-gauge manometer
manometric pressure
manometry
manoptoscope
Manschot intraocular implant
    lens
Manschot lens
Mansfield balloon
Mansfield balloon catheter
Mansfield dilatation balloon
    catheter
Mansfield forceps
Manske-McCarroll-Swanson
    incision
Manson hook
Manson-Aebli scissors
Mantelow transfer
Mantisol drain
mantle
mantle block
mantle field
mantle radiation treatment
mantle technique
mantle therapy
Mantz dilator
Mantz rectal dilator
manual core endarterectomy
manual delivery of placenta
manual dermatome
manual injection
manual inspection
manual manipulation
manual palpation
manual positioning
manual reduction of dislocation
manual reduction of fracture
manual removal of placenta
manual resuscitation bag
manual traction
manually
manubriogladiolar junction
manubrium
manubrium of malleus
many-tailed bandage
many-tailed dressing

MAP (mean arterial pressure;
   motor nerve action
   potential)
map-guided endocardial
   resection surgery
Maquet endoscopy table
Maquet knee operation
Maquet procedure
Maquet table
Maquet tibial procedure
Marafioti-Westin rod
Marax bronchodilator
Marble bone pin
marble bones
marbleized
Marcaine hydrochloride
   anesthetic agent
march foot
march fracture
March-Barton forceps
Marchetti operation
Marcks knife
Marcks operation
Marckwald operation
Marcuse forceps
Marcuse tube clamp
Marcy operation
Marfan epigastric puncture
margin of field
margin of wound
marginal
marginal artery
marginal chalazion forceps
marginal clamp
marginal fracture
marginal portion
marginal sinus
marginal ulcer
Margulies coil intrauterine
   device
Margulies spiral intrauterine
   device
marian lithotomy
Marin bur
Marin operation
Marin reamer
Marion drain

Marion screw
Mario-Stone staple
Marjolin ulcer
Mark II total knee replacement
   system
Mark III halo
Mark IV nasogastric tube
Mark IV repair
Mark lens loupe
marked narrowing
markedly comminuted
markedly dilated
markedly enlarged
marker (see also *scleral marker*)
   Amsler chart marker
   Amsler scleral marker
   cookie cutter areolar
      marker
   D'Assumpcao rhytido-
      plasty marker
   diamond green marker
   E-rosette cell marker
   ear marker
   Etch-Master instrument
      marker
   Freeman cookie-cutter
      areolar marker
   Gass scleral marker
   genetic markers
   gold ear marker
   Gonin-Amsler marker
   Gonin-Amsler scleral
      marker
   House-Urban ear marker
   House-Urban gold ear
      marker
   House-Urban marker
   instrument marker
   nipple marker
   scleral marker (see
      separate listing)
marker transit studies
Markham-Meyerding retractor
marking pen
marking pencil
markings
Markley retractor

Marks-Bayne technique
Markwalder bone rongeur
Markwalder forceps
Marlen airing hook
Marlen belt
Marlen clamp
Marlen gas relief pouch
Marlen ileostomy bag
Marlen Odor-Ban pouch
Marlen Solo ileostomy pouch
Marlen weightless bag
Marlen zip-closed pouch
Marlex atraumatic obstetrical
    tenaculum
Marlex atraumatic tenaculum
Marlex band
Marlex bandage
Marlex graft
Marlex mesh
Marlex mesh abdominal
    rectopexy
Marlex mesh graft
Marlex mesh implant
Marlex mesh prosthesis
Marlex mesh rectopexy
Marlex mesh sling
Marlex prosthesis
Marlex screen
Marlex sheet
Marlex sponge
Marlex sutures
Marlex tenaculum
Marmor knee prosthesis
Marmor procedure
Marmor prosthesis
Marmor tibial prosthesis
Marmor total knee prosthesis
Maroon lip curet
Maroon-Jannetta neurodissector
Marquardt bone rongeur
Marquette 3-channel laser
    Holter
Marquez-Gomez conjunctival
    graft
marrow
marrow cavity
marrow depression

marrow embolism
marrow injection
marrow nailing
marrow space
marrow spoon
marrow-lymph gland
Marsan belt
Marsan Loop-Loc colostomy bag
    system
Marshall knee procedure
Marshall meniscectomy
Marshall oblique vein
Marshall V-sutures
Marshall vein
Marshall-Marchetti operation
Marshall-Marchetti repair
Marshall-Marchetti-Krantz
    operation
Marshall-Marchetti-Krantz
    uterine suspension
Marshik forceps
Marshik tonsillar forceps
Marshik tonsil-seizing forceps
Marstock apparatus
marsupial flap
marsupial graft
marsupial notch
marsupial skin flap
marsupialization
marsupialization of abscess
marsupialization of cyst
marsupialization of lesion
Martaugh flusher
Martel clamp
Martin abdominal retractor
Martin anoplasty
Martin bandage
Martin cartilage clamp
Martin cartilage scissors
Martin clamp
Martin dermal curet
Martin drainage tube
Martin forceps
Martin gouge
Martin hook
Martin incision
Martin laryngectomy tube

Martin lip retractor
Martin muscle clamp
Martin nasopharyngeal biopsy
    forceps
Martin needle
Martin operation
Martin palate retractor
Martin pelvimeter
Martin probe
Martin rectal hook
Martin rectal speculum
Martin reduction technique
Martin retractor
Martin rubber dressing
Martin scissors
Martin screw
Martin screw for hip fracture
Martin snare
Martin speculum
Martin stripper
Martin technique
Martin throat scissors
Martin thumb forceps
Martin tissue forceps
Martin tube
Martin uterine tenaculum
    forceps
Martin wire cutter
Martin-Davy rectal speculum
Martin-Davy speculum
Martinez knife-dissector
Martini bone cutter
Martinotti cells
Martius operation
Martius-Harris operation
Martorell ulcer
Marwedel gastrostomy
Marwedel operation
Marx needle
Maryan biopsy punch forceps
Maryan forceps
mashed
mask
masked fat
Mason clamp
Mason gastroplasty
Mason incision

Mason operation
Mason splint
Mason suction tube
Mason vascular clamp
Mason vertical-banded gastro-
    plasty
Mason-Allen splint
Mason-Allen Universal hand
    splint
Mason-Allen Universal sling
Mason-Auvard speculum
Mason-Auvard weighted vaginal
    speculum
Mason-Judd retractor
Mason-Judd self-retaining
    retractor
mass
Massachusetts General Hospital
    (see *MGH*)
Massachusetts hemostat
massage
masseter muscle
masseter, musculus
masseteric area
masseteric artery
masseteric nerve
masseteric reflex
masseteric space
masseteric vein
masseterica, arteria
massetericus, nervus
Massie driver
Massie extractor
Massie II nail system
Massie inserter
Massie nail
Massie screwdriver
massive
massive ascites
massive bleeding
massive collapse
massive dose
massive dose technique
massive heart attack
massive hemorrhage
massive infection
massive involvement

massive radiation
massive sliding graft
massive sliding nails
massive transfusion protocol
massive transfusions
massive tumor
Masson fascial needle
Masson fascial stripper
Masson needle
Masson needle holder
Masson-Luethy needle holder
Masson-Mayo-Hegar needle
    holder
MAST (military antishock
    trousers)
MAST suit
mastadenoma
mastalgia
mastectomy
mastectomy incision
mastectomy knife
mastectomy scar
mastectomy support
master knot of Henry
Master screwdriver
Master-Allen syndrome
Masters intestinal clamp
Masterson clamp
Masterson hysterectomy forceps
Masters-Schwartz intestinal
    clamp
Masters-Schwartz liver clamp
masthelcosis
masticating surface
masticatory movements
masticatory muscle
Mastin clamp
Mastin muscle clamp
mastitis
Mastner median episiotomy and
    repair
mastocarcinoma
mastochondroma
mastodynia
mastogram
mastography
mastoid

mastoid air cells
mastoid antrotomy
mastoid antrum
mastoid bone
mastoid bone bur
mastoid bur
mastoid canaliculi
mastoid catheter
mastoid cavity
mastoid chisel
mastoid curet
mastoid dressing
mastoid emissary vein
mastoid fontanelle
mastoid fossa
mastoid gouge
mastoid knife
mastoid mallet
mastoid notch
mastoid obliteration operation
mastoid operation
mastoid packer
mastoid probe
mastoid process
mastoid raspatory
mastoid retractor
mastoid rongeur
mastoid rongeur forceps
mastoid search
mastoid searcher
mastoid self-retaining retractor
mastoid suction tube
mastoid sutures
mastoid wall
mastoidectomy
mastoidotomy
mastoidotympanectomy
mastoid-retaining retractor
mastoncus
mastopathia
mastopathia cystica
mastopathy
mastopexy
mastoplastia
mastoplasty
mastoptosis
mastorrhagia

mastorrhaphy
mastoscirrhus
mastosis
mastostomy
mastotomy
MAT (multifocal atrial tachy-
    cardia)
Matas aneurysmoplasty
Matas band
Matas operation
Matchett prosthesis
Matchett-Brown femoral head
    replacement
Matchett-Brown hip arthroplasty
Matchett-Brown hip prosthesis
matching donor
maternal bleed
maternal placenta
Mathews drill
Mathews forceps
Mathews osteotome
Mathews rectal speculum
Mathews speculum
Mathieu double-ended retractor
Mathieu forceps
Mathieu holder
Mathieu needle holder
Mathieu raspatory
Mathieu retractor
Mathieu tongue-seizing forceps
Mathieu urethral forceps
Mathieu-Hevesy needle holder
Mathieu-Kocher needle holder
Mathieu-Ryder needle holder
Mathieu-Stille needle holder
Mathrop hemostat
Mathys cementless prosthesis
matricectomy
matrix (*pl.* matrices)
matrix band
matrix calculus
matrix cells
matrix vesicles
Matsner episiotomy
Matsner median episiotomy
    repair
Matson elevator

Matson operation
Matson periosteal elevator
Matson raspatory
Matson rib elevator
Matson rib spreader
Matson rib stripper
Matson stripper
Matson-Alexander elevator
Matson-Alexander rib elevator
Matson-Alexander rib stripper
Matson-Mead apicolysis
    retractor
Matson-Mead periosteal stripper
Matson-Mead stripper
matted node
Mattis corneal scissors
Mattis scissors
Mattison-Upshaw retractor
Mattox aortic clamp
Mattox maneuver
mattress sutures
maturation
mature bone
mature cataract
mature cell
mature ovum
mature placenta
mature stump
maturity
Matzenauer speculum
Matzner tube
Mauck operation
Mauksch operation
Maumenee capsule forceps
Maumenee corneal forceps
Maumenee cross-action capsule
    forceps
Maumenee erysiphake
Maumenee eye knife
Maumenee forceps
Maumenee iris hook
Maumenee straight-action
    capsule forceps
Maumenee tissue forceps
Maumenee trephine
Maumenee-Barraquer vitreous
    sweep spatula

Maumenee-Colibri forceps
Maumenee-Goldberg operation
Maumenee-Park erysiphake
Maumenee-Park eye speculum
Maumenee-Park lid speculum
Maunder oral screw gag
Maunoir hydrocele
Maunoir iris scissors
Maunoir scissors
Maunsell sutures
Maunsell-Weir operation
Mauriceau maneuver
Mauriceau method
Mauriceau-Levret maneuver
Mauriceau-Smellie maneuver
Mauriceau-Smellie-Veit maneu-
    ver
Max Fine forceps
Max Fine tying forceps
Max forceps
Maxam sutures
MaxCast
MaxCast tape
Maxi-Driver
Maxilith pacemaker
maxilla (*pl.* maxillae)
maxillares, venae
maxillaris, arteria
maxillaris, nervus
maxillary
maxillary alveolectomy
maxillary alveoloplasty
maxillary anchorage
maxillary antrotomy
maxillary antrum
maxillary artery
maxillary articulation
maxillary bone
maxillary crest
maxillary dental prosthesis
maxillary excision
maxillary fracture
maxillary nerve
maxillary protraction
maxillary recontouring alveolec-
    tomy
maxillary ridge

maxillary sinus cannula
maxillary sinuses
maxillary sinusotomy
maxillary teeth
maxillary torus
maxillary tubercles
maxillary tuberosity
maxillary veins
maxillectomy
maxillofacial
maxillofacial prosthesis
maxillofacial region
maxillomandibular traction
maxillotomy
maximal
maximal intensity
maximal tension skin lines
Maxi-Myst vaporizer
maximum
maximum breathing capacity
maximum dimension
maximum dosage
maximum pressure
maxi-vessel loops
Maxon absorbable suture
Maxon sutures
Maxur operation
May chair
May kidney clamp
May ophthalmoscope
May sign
May stand
Maydl colostomy
Maydl hernia
Maydl operation
Mayer nasal splint
Mayer pessary
Mayer position
Mayer reflex
Mayer speculum
Mayer splint
Mayer trapezius transfer
Mayer vaginal speculum
Mayfield aneurysm clip
Mayfield aneurysm forceps
Mayfield aneurysm hemostat
Mayfield applying forceps

Mayfield bayonet osteotome
Mayfield bone rongeur
Mayfield brain spatula
Mayfield clip
Mayfield curet
Mayfield forceps
Mayfield head holder
Mayfield osteotome
Mayfield overhead table
Mayfield retractor
Mayfield skull clamp
Mayfield spatula
Mayfield spinal curet
Mayfield table
Mayfield-Kees headrest
May-Harrington forceps
Maylard incision
Mayo abdominal retractor
Mayo bone-cutting forceps
Mayo bunion deformity
    procedure
Mayo bunion repair
Mayo bunionectomy
Mayo cannula
Mayo carrier
Mayo clamp
Mayo common duct probe
Mayo common duct scoop
Mayo common duct spoon
Mayo cystic duct scoop
Mayo dissecting scissors
Mayo elbow prosthesis
Mayo fibroid hook
Mayo forceps
Mayo gallstone scoop
Mayo gastrojejunostomy
Mayo hammer toe correction
Mayo hemostat
Mayo herniorrhaphy
Mayo holder
Mayo hook
Mayo hysterectomy
Mayo instrument table
Mayo kidney clamp
Mayo knife
Mayo linen sutures
Mayo needle

Mayo needle holder
Mayo operation
Mayo probe
Mayo pyloric vein
Mayo retractor
Mayo sacroiliac belt
Mayo scissors
Mayo scoop
Mayo stand
Mayo stripper
Mayo sutures
Mayo tissue forceps
Mayo trocar-point needle
Mayo ureter isolation forceps
Mayo uterine scissors
Mayo vein stripper
Mayo vessel clamp
Mayo-Adams appendectomy
    retractor
Mayo-Adams retractor
Mayo-Adams self-retaining
    retractor
Mayo-Adson self-retaining
    retractor
Mayo-Blake forceps
Mayo-Blake gallstone forceps
Mayo-Boldt appendix inverter
Mayo-Boldt inverter
Mayo-Collins double-ended
    retractor
Mayo-Collins retractor
Mayo-Fueth operation
Mayo-Guyon clamp
Mayo-Guyon vessel clamp
Mayo-Harrington dissecting
    scissors
Mayo-Harrington forceps
Mayo-Harrington scissors
Mayo-Hegar curved-jaw needle
    holder
Mayo-Hegar needle holder
Mayo-Kelly appendix inverter
Mayo-Kelly inverter
Mayo-Lovelace clamp
Mayo-Lovelace crusher
Mayo-Lovelace retractor
Mayo-Lovelace spur crusher

Mayo-Myers external vein stripper
Mayo-Myers stripper
Mayo-New scissors
Mayo-Noble dissecting scissors
Mayo-Noble scissors
Mayo-Ochsner cannula
Mayo-Ochsner forceps
Mayo-Ochsner hemostat
Mayo-Ochsner suction trocar cannula
Mayo-Ochsner trocar
Mayo-Péan forceps
Mayo-Péan hemostat
Mayo-Polya gastric resection
Mayo-Potts dissecting scissors
Mayo-Potts scissors
Mayo-Robson forceps
Mayo-Robson gallstone scoop
Mayo-Robson gastrointestinal forceps
Mayo-Robson incision
Mayo-Robson intestinal clamp
Mayo-Robson intestinal forceps
Mayo-Robson operation
Mayo-Robson position
Mayo-Robson scoop
Mayo-Russian forceps
Mayo-Russian gastrointestinal forceps
Mayo-Simpson retractor
Mayo-Sims dissecting scissors
Mayo-Sims scissors
Mayo-Stille dissecting scissors
Mayo-Stille scissors
Mayo-Ward hysterectomy
Mays operation
Mazas hinge elbow
Mazet knee disarticulation
Mazlin spring intrauterine device (spring IUD)
mazopexy
Mazur ankle-rating system
Mazur operation
MB band
Mc (see also *Mac*)
mc (millicuries)

MCA (middle cerebral artery)
McAllister needle holder
McAllister scissors
McArdle sign
McArdle syndrome
McArthur incision
McArthur method
McArthur operation
McAtee apparatus
McAtee compression screw device
McAtee olecranon device
McAtee screw
McAtee-Tharias-Blazina arthroplasty
McBride bunion repair
McBride bunionectomy
McBride cup
McBride operation
McBride plate
McBride prosthesis
McBride tripod-pin traction
McBride-Akin operation
McBride-Moore prosthesis
McBurney fenestrated retractor
McBurney incision
McBurney operation
McBurney point
McBurney retractor
McBurney sign
McCabe canal knife
McCabe crurotomy saw
McCabe dissector knife
McCabe elevator
McCabe facial nerve dissector
McCabe flap knife dissector
McCabe rasp
McCaffrey positioner
McCall operation
McCall-Schumann operation
McCannel intraocular implant lens
McCannel lens
McCannel sutures
McCarey-Kaufman solution
McCarroll operation
McCarroll osteotomy hip

McCarthy bladder evacuator
McCarthy catheter
McCarthy coagulation electrode
McCarthy cystoscope
McCarthy diathermic knife
McCarthy electrode
McCarthy electrotome
McCarthy evacuator
McCarthy forceps
McCarthy fulguration electrode
McCarthy miniature electrotome
McCarthy miniature resec-
    toscope
McCarthy miniature telescope
McCarthy panendoscope
McCarthy resectoscope
McCarthy telescope
McCarthy visual hemostatic
    forceps
McCarthy-Alcock forceps
McCarthy-Alcock hemostatic
    forceps
McCarthy-Campbell cystoscope
McCarthy-Peterson cystoscope
McCash procedure for
    Dupuytren contracture
McCash-Randall operation
McCaskey antral curet
McCaskey catheter
McCaskey curet
McCaslin keratome
McCaslin knife-needle
McCaslin needle-knife
McCauley operation for talipes
    equinovarus
McClamary elevator
McCleery-Miller anastomosis
McCleery-Miller clamp
McCleery-Miller intestinal
    anastomosis clamp
McCleery-Miller intestinal clamp
McClintock placenta forceps
McClure eye scissors
McClure iris scissors
McClure scissors
McCollum tube
McConnell knee technique

McCort sign
McCoy forceps
McCoy septal forceps
McCoy septum-cutting forceps
McCrae dilator
McCrea cystoscope
McCrea infant sound
McCrea sound
McCullough externofrontal
    retractor
McCullough forceps
McCullough retractor
McCullough suture forceps
McCullough suture-tying
    forceps
McCullough utility forceps
McCurdy needle
McCurdy staphylorrhaphy
    needle
McCutchen hip
McDavid knee brace
McDermott clip
McDermott extractor
McDonald cerclage
McDonald cervical cerclage
McDonald clamp
McDonald operation
McDonald pelvimetry
McDowell mouth gag
McDowell needle
McDowell operation
McDowell reflex
McElroy curet
McElroy instrument
McElveney procedure
McElveney punch
McEvedy operation
McFadden aneurysm clip
McFadden clip
McFadden Vari-Angle aneurysm
    system
McFarland tibia graft
McFarland-Osborne approach
McGannon eye retractor
McGannon forceps
McGannon iris retractor
McGannon lens forceps

McGannon retractor
McGavic operation
McGaw volumetric pump
McGee crimper
McGee forceps
McGee operation
McGee piston
McGee splint
McGee stainless piston
McGee wire-closure forceps
McGee wire-crimper forceps
McGee-Caparosa wire crimper
McGee-Paparella wire-crimping
    forceps
McGee-Priest forceps
McGee-Priest wire-crimping
    forceps
McGee-Priest-Paparella closure
    forceps
McGee-Priest-Paparella crimper-
    forceps
McGhan breast implant
McGhan breast prosthesis
McGhan eye implant
McGhan implant
McGhan intraocular lens
McGhan lens
McGhan Magna-Site tissue
    expander
McGhan MicroTorque perma-
    nent eyelining machine
McGhan mini-motor rotary bur
    machine
McGhan plastic surgical needle
McGhan-3M intraocular lens
McGill forceps
McGill operation
McGill retractor
McGivney hemorrhoidal forceps
McGivney ligator
McGoey-Evans acetabular cup
McGoey-Evans cup
McGoon cannula
McGoon coronary perfusion
    catheter
McGowan needle
McGowan-Keeley tube

McGravey forceps
McGravey tissue forceps
McGraw elastic ligature
McGraw sutures
McGregor forceps
McGregor forehead flap
McGregor line
McGregor needle
McGuire clamp
McGuire corneal scissors
McGuire forceps
McGuire operation
McGuire rib spreader
McGuire scissors
McGuire urinal
McHenry forceps
McHenry scissors
McHenry tonsillar artery forceps
McHugh facial nerve knife
McHugh flap knife
McHugh knife
McHugh speculum
McIndoe cartilage scissors
McIndoe chisel
McIndoe colpocleisis
McIndoe dressing forceps
McIndoe elevator
McIndoe forceps
McIndoe incision
McIndoe nipple placement in
    reduction mammaplasty
McIndoe operation
McIndoe orthopedic procedure
McIndoe osteotome
McIndoe rasp
McIndoe retractor
McIndoe scissors
McIndoe vaginal reconstruction
McIntire aspiration-irrigation
    system
McIntire needle
McIntire splint
McIntosh double-lumen catheter
McIntosh forceps
McIntosh suture-holding forceps
McIntyre aspirating unit
McIntyre aspiration needle

McIntyre cannula
McIntyre cystitome
McIntyre intracapsular lens
    extraction
McIntyre intraocular implant
    lens
McIntyre irrigating iris hook
McIntyre irrigating unit
McIntyre irrigation needle
McIntyre lens
McIver catheter
McIver nephrostomy catheter
McIver nephrostomy tube
McIvor mouth gag
McKay ear forceps
McKay forceps
McKee brace
McKee hinge elbow
McKee prosthesis
McKee table
McKee-Farrar acetabular cup
McKee-Farrar cup
McKee-Farrar hip prosthesis
McKee-Farrar rasp
McKee-Farrar total hip arthro-
    plasty
McKee-Farrar total hip prosthe-
    sis
McKeever arthrodesis
McKeever bunionectomy
McKeever cartilage knife
McKeever clavicle procedure
McKeever foot procedure
McKeever knee prosthesis
McKeever knife
McKeever operation
McKeever patella cap prosthesis
McKeever patella prosthesis
McKeever prosthesis
McKeever Vitallium cap
    prosthesis
McKenna Tide-Ur-Ator evacu-
    ator
McKenna Tide-Ur-Ator irrigator
McKenzie (see also *Mackenzie*)
McKenzie brain clip-applying
    forceps

McKenzie bur
McKenzie clamp
McKenzie clip
McKenzie clip rack
McKenzie drill
McKenzie enlarging bur
McKenzie forceps
McKenzie grasping forceps
McKenzie leukotome
McKenzie leukotomy loupe
McKenzie operation
McKenzie perforating twist
    drill
McKenzie perforator
McKenzie perforator drill
McKenzie silver brain clip
McKenzie sphenoid punch
McKesson mouth gag
McKesson mouth probe
McKesson mouth tube
McKesson pneumothorax
    apparatus
McKesson restrictor
McKibbin splint
McKinney eye speculum
McKinney fixation ring
McKinney speculum
McKinty rasp
McKissock incision
McKissock keyhole areolar
    template
McKissock mammaplasty
McKissock mastectomy
McKissock operation
McKissock pedicle flap tech-
    nique
McKissock reduction mamma-
    plasty
McKissock sutures
MCL (medial collateral liga-
    ment)
McLaughlin extractor
McLaughlin incision
McLaughlin nail
McLaughlin operation
McLaughlin plate
McLaughlin screw

McLaughlin speculum
McLaughlin tarsorrhaphy
McLaughlin tendon rupture
    repair
McLaughlin Vitallium nail
McLean capsule forceps
McLean capsulotomy scissors
McLean clamp
McLean corneoscleral sutures
McLean forceps
McLean operation
McLean ophthalmological
    forceps
McLean prism contact lens
McLean scissors
McLean tonometer
McLean-Tucker obstetrical
    forceps
McLean-Tucker-Kielland obstet-
    rical forceps
McLean-Tucker-Luikart obstetri-
    cal forceps
McLight PCL brace
MCM smart Laser
McMahon nephrostomy hook
McMahon-Laird incision
McMaster bone graft
McMurray femoral neck
    osteotomy
McMurray knife
McMurray maneuver
McMurray sign
McMurray test
McNaught keel
McNaught keel laryngeal
    prosthesis
McNaught prosthesis
McNealey visceral retractor
McNealey-Glassman clamp
McNealey-Glassman-Babcock
    forceps
McNealey-Glassman-Babcock
    viscera-holding forceps
McNealey-Glassman-Babcock
    visceral forceps
McNealey-Glassman-Mixter
    clamp

McNealey-Glassman-Mixter
    forceps
McNealey-Glassman-Mixter
    ligature-carrying aneurysm
    forceps
McNeill-Chamberlain ster-
    notomy
McNeill-Goldmann blepharostat
McNeill-Goldmann blepharostat
    ring
McNeill-Goldmann ring
McNeill-Goldmann scleral ring
McNutt driver
McNutt extractor
MCP (metacarpophalangeal)
McPheeters table
McPherson angled forceps
McPherson corneal forceps
McPherson eye speculum
McPherson forceps
McPherson iris spatula
McPherson lens forceps
McPherson needle holder
McPherson scissors
McPherson spatula
McPherson speculum
McPherson suturing forceps
McPherson tying forceps
McPherson-Castroviejo corneal
    microscissors
McPherson-Castroviejo scissors
McPherson-Pierse forceps
McPherson-Vannas  iris
    microscissors
McPherson-Vannas iris scissors
McPherson-Vannas scissors
McPherson-Westcott conjuncti-
    val scissors
McPherson-Westcott stitch
    scissors
McPherson-Wheeler blade
McPherson-Wheeler iris
    microknife
McPherson-Wheeler knife
McPherson-Ziegler iris knife
McPherson-Ziegler knife
McPherson-Ziegler microknife

McQuigg clamp
McQuigg forceps
McQuigg-Mixter bronchial forceps
McQuigg-Mixter forceps
McReynolds calcaneus procedure
McReynolds driver
McReynolds driver-extractor
McReynolds extractor
McReynolds eye spatula
McReynolds hook
McReynolds keratome
McReynolds knife
McReynolds operation
McReynolds pterygium keratome
McReynolds pterygium knife
McReynolds pterygium operation
McReynolds pterygium scissors
McReynolds pterygium transplant
McReynolds scissors
McReynolds spatula
McReynolds transplant of pterygium
McReynolds-Castroviejo keratome
McReynolds-Castroviejo pterygium knife
McRoberts maneuver
McVay hernia repair
McVay hernioplasty
McVay herniorrhaphy
McVay incision
McVay operation
McWhinnie dissector
McWhinnie electrode
McWhirter mastectomy
McWhorter hemostat
McWhorter tonsillar forceps
McWhorter tonsillar hemostat
MD brace (Medical Design brace)
Mead bone rongeur
Mead lancet knife

Mead mallet
Mead mastoid rongeur
Mead rongeur
Meadox bifurcated graft
Meadox Dardik biograft
Meadox graft
Meadox ICP monitor
Meadox Microvel double-velour knitted Dacron arterial graft
Meadox Microvel graft
Meadox woven velour prosthesis
Meadox-Cooley woven low-porosity vascular prosthesis
mean arterial pressure (MAP)
mean circulation time
mean pressure
Means-Lernan mediastinal crunch
measure
measurement
measuring rod
Measuroll sutures
meat forceps
meatal
meatal clamp
meatal dilator
meatal incision
meatal sound
meatal stenosis
meat-grasping forceps
meatoantrotomy
meatoplasty
meatoscope
   Hubell meatoscope
meatotome
    Bunge meatotome
    Dreisse meatotome
    electric meatotome
    Ellik meatotome
    Otis meatotome
    Riba electric ureteral meatotome
    ureteral meatotome
meatotomy
meatotomy electrode
meatotomy knife

meatus
meatus acustici externi, nervus
meatus clamp
mechanic's waste dressing
mechanical axis
mechanical axis cord
mechanical biliary obstruction
mechanical block
mechanical bowel obstruction
mechanical device
mechanical duct obstruction
mechanical extrahepatic
    obstruction
mechanical finger
mechanical finger forceps
mechanical forceps
mechanical heart
mechanical ileus
mechanical insulin pump
mechanical intestinal obstruc-
    tion
mechanical lithotripsy
mechanical obstruction
mechanical respirator
mechanical scanner
mechanical small-bowel
    obstruction
mechanical stimulation
mechanical stimulus
mechanical styptic
mechanical ventilation
mechanical ventilator
mechanism
mechanogastrography
Meckel band
Meckel cavity
Meckel diverticulectomy
Meckel diverticulum
Meckel ganglion
Meckel ganglionectomy
Meckel operation
Meckel rod
Meckel scan
meckelectomy
meconium
meconium aspiration
meconium aspirator

meconium discharge
meconium fluid
meconium ileus
meconium plug
meconium-stained amniotic
    fluid
Mecring cementless acetabulum
    system
Mecron cannulated cancellous
    screw
Mecron titanium Voorhoeve
    sheath
Medallion intraocular lens
    implant
Medallion lens
Medallion lens expressor
Medcor pacemaker
Meddox vascular graft
Medi bandage scissors
Medi vascular stockings
media (*sing.* medium)
medial
medial angle
medial anterior malleolus artery
medial aperture
medial aspect
medial bicipital sulcus
medial border
medial capsule
medial circumflex femoral
    artery
medial collateral ligament
    (MCL)
medial compartment
medial condyle
medial crus
medial cutaneous nerve
medial deviation
medial dorsal cutaneous nerve
medial eminence
medial epicondyle
medial flap
medial foramen
medial incision
medial inferior genicular artery
medial inguinal fossa
medial joint level

medial ligament
medial lobule
medial longitudinal fasciculus
medial malleolus
medial meniscectomy
medial meniscus
medial muscle
medial nerve
medial osteotomy
medial palpebral arteries
medial palpebral ligament
medial parapatellar incision
medial plantar artery
medial plantar nerve
medial plateau of tibia
medial portion
medial protrusion
medial pterygoid muscle
medial pterygoid nerve
medial pterygoid plate
medial puboprostatic ligaments
medial rectus
medial superior genicular artery
medial supraclavicular nerves
medial surface
medial talocalcaneal ligament
medial tarsal arteries
medial umbilical fold
medial wall
medialize
medially
medially reflected
median antebrachial vein
median appendectomy incision
median arcuate ligament
median artery
median aspect
median basilic vein
median cephalic vein
median cubital vein
median episiotomy
median fissure
median furrow of prostate
median harelip
median incision
median laryngotomy
median line

median lithotomy
median nerve
median palatine suture
median parapatellar incision
median plane
median raphe
median sacral artery
median section
median sternotomy
median sternotomy incision
median sulcus
median umbilical fold
median vein
mediana antebrachii, vena
mediana, arteria
mediana basilica, vena
mediana cephalica, vena
mediana cubiti, vena
median-sagittal plane
medianus, nervus
mediastinal
mediastinal cannula
mediastinal catheter
mediastinal cavity
mediastinal drain
mediastinal mass
mediastinal node biopsy
mediastinal organ
mediastinal pleura
mediastinal plexus
mediastinal shadow
mediastinal shift
mediastinal sump connector
mediastinal sump filter
mediastinal thickening
mediastinal tumor
mediastinal tumor excision
mediastinal veins
mediastinal widening
mediastinales, venae
mediastinitis
mediastinoscope
    Carlens fiberoptic
       mediastinoscope
    Carlens mediastinoscope
mediastinoscopic
mediastinoscopy

mediastinotomy
mediastinum
mediate amputation
Medical Design brace (MD brace)
Medical Optics eye implant
Medical Workshop intraocular lens implant
medicated bougie
medication
Medici aerosol adhesive tape remover dressing
medicine cup
medicine glass
Medi-Clens handwasher machine
Medicon contractor
Medicon forceps
Medicon rib retractor
Medicon spreader
Medicon wire-twister forceps
Medicon-Jackson forceps
Medicon-Jackson rectal forceps
Medicon-Packer mosquito forceps
Medicopaste
Medicornea Kratz intraocular lens
Medicus bed
Medicut cannula
Medicut catheter
Medicut intravenous needle
Medicut needle
Mediform dural graft
Mediform dural substitute
Medi-graft vascular prosthesis
Medina catheter
Medina ileostomy catheter
Medina ileostomy catheter tube
Meding tonsil enucleator
Meding tonsil enucleator tonometer
Meding tonsil enucleator tonsillectome
Medinvent vascular stent
mediocarpal articulation

mediocollateral ligament of knee
mediolateral episiotomy
mediolateral lithotomy
mediolateral projection
mediolateral view
mediotarsal amputation
Mediplast
MediPort implanted vascular device
MediPort machine
MediPort-DL double-lumen catheter
Medi-quet surgical tourniquet
Mediscus low-air-loss bed
Medistat hemostatic sponge
Medi-Strumpf elastic stockings
Meditape
Meditec laser
Meditech arterial dilatation catheter
Meditech balloon catheter
Meditech bipolar probe
Meditech catheter
Meditech guide wire
Meditech Mansfield dilating catheter
Meditech steerable catheter
Meditron bipolar generator with irrigation
medium (*pl.* media)
medium chromic sutures
medium forceps
medium screwdriver
Med-Neb respirator
Medoc-Celestin endoprosthesis
Medoc-Celestin pulsion tube
Medrad angiographic injectors
Medrad catheter
Medrad injector
Medrafil sutures
Medrafil wire sutures
Medtel pacemaker
Medtronic Activitrax pacemaker
Medtronic aortic punch
Medtronic balloon catheter
Medtronic Byrel-SX pacemaker

Medtronic corkscrew electrode
    pacemaker
Medtronic Cyberlith pacemaker
Medtronic demand pacemaker
Medtronic external/internal
    pacemaker
Medtronic Hancock aortic
    punch
Medtronic Hancock valve
Medtronic INTACT porcine
    bioprosthesis valve
Medtronic pacemaker
Medtronic Pacette pacemaker
Medtronic prosthetic valve
Medtronic Pulsor Intrasound
    pain reliever
Medtronic Symbios pacemaker
Medtronic-Alcatel pacemaker
Medtronic-Hall heart valve
Medtronic-Hall monocuspid
    tilting-disk valve
Medtronic-Hall tilting-disk valve
    prosthesis
Medtronic-Laurens-Alcatel
    pacemaker
Medtronic-Zyrel pacemaker
medulla (*pl.* medullae)
medulla oblongata
medulla spinalis
medullary
medullary bone graft
medullary callus
medullary canal
medullary canal reamer
medullary carcinoma
medullary cavity
medullary cells
medullary fold
medullary graft
medullary nail
medullary nailing
medullary pin
medullary segment
medullary tube
medullated fibers and sheaths
medullated nerve
medullectomy

medulloblastoma
medusa
Medx camera
Medx scanner
Meek clavicle sling
Meek operation
Meeker forceps
Meeker gallbladder forceps
Meeker gallstone clamps
Meeker hemostatic forceps
Meek-Wall dermatome
Meek-Wall microdermatome
meerschaum probe
Mega prosthesis
megacolon
megalogastria
megaureter clamp
megavolt therapy
meibomian cyst
meibomian expressor forceps
meibomian foramen
meibomian forceps
meibomian glands
Meigs curet
Meigs endometrial curet
Meigs hemostat
Meigs operation
Meigs radical hysterectomy
Meigs retractor
Meigs sutures
Meissner corpuscles
Meissner ganglion
Meissner plexus
melanin-pigmented cells
melanocytic nevus
melanocytoma
melanoderma
melanoleukoderma colli
melanoma
melanosis
melanotic
melanotic carcinoma
melanotic whitlow
Melauskas orbital implant
Melco suction
melena
Meleney synergistic gangrene

Meleney ulcer
melenic stool
Meller lacrimal sac retractor
Meller operation
Meller retractor
Meller spatula
Meller speculum
Mellinger eye speculum
Mellinger magnet
Mellinger speculum
melonoplasty
meloplasty
Meltzer adenoid punch
Meltzer adenoid punch forceps
Meltzer anesthesia
Meltzer nasopharyngoscope
Meltzer punch
Meltzer sign
membrana
membrana adventitia
membrana tympani
membrane
membrane of brain
membrane of cervix uteri
membrane of Demours
membrane of Descemet
membrane of joint
membrane of meninges
membrane of tympanum
membrane oxygenator
membrane rupture
membrane-puncturing forceps
membranectomy
membranous
membranous canal
membranous cataract
membranous labyrinth
membranous lining
membranous tissue
membranous tube
membranous urethra
membranous ventricular septal
    defect
membranous wall
Meme breast prosthesis
Meme mammary implant
Mendel dorsal reflex of foot

Mendel ligature forceps
Mendel-Bekhterev sign
Mendez ultrasonic cystotome
Mendez-Schubert aorta punch
Menelaus triple arthrodesis
Menetrier disease
Menge operation
Menge pessary
Menge stem pessary
Mengert index
Mengert membrane-puncturing
    forceps
Menghini liver biopsy needle
Menghini needle
Menghini percutaneous liver
    biopsy
Meniere disease
meningea anterior, arteria
meningea media, arteria
meningea posterior, arteria
meningeae mediae, venae
meningeae, venae
meningeal adhesions
meningeal arteries
meningeal hemorrhage
meningeal nerve
meningeal veins
meningeal vessels
meningeorrhaphy
meninges
meningioma
meningitis
meningocele
meningococci
meninx
meniscal
meniscal bone
meniscal clamp
meniscal fluid
meniscal knife
meniscal lens
meniscal retractor
meniscal sign
meniscal tear
meniscectomy
meniscectomy knife
meniscectomy probe

meniscectomy scissors
meniscofemoral ligament
meniscoresis
meniscotome
    Bowen-Grover meniscotome
    Dyonics meniscotome
    Grover meniscotome
    Ruuska meniscotome
    Smillie meniscotome
    Storz meniscotome
meniscotome power unit
meniscotome sheath
meniscus
meniscus of acromioclavicular
    joint
meniscus of knee
meniscus of temporomaxillary
    joint
Mennen plate
menometrorrhagia
menorrhagia
menorrhea
Menson-Scheck hanging-hip
    procedure
menstrual extraction
mental artery
mental foramen
mental nerve
mentalis, arteria
mentalis, musculus
mentalis, nervus
mentoanterior
mento-occipital diameter
mentoparietal diameter
mentoplasty
mentoplasty augmentation
mentoposterior
Mentor bladder pacemaker
Mentor cautery
Mentor inflatable penile
    prosthesis
Mentor malleable semirigid
    penile implant
Mentor penile prosthesis with
    rear-tip extender
Mentor Resi prosthesis

Mentor Self-Cath penile
    prosthesis
Mentor wet-field coagulator
Mentor wet-field cordless
    coagulator
Mentor wet-field hemostatic
    eraser
mentotransverse
meperidine anesthetic agent
mepivacaine hydrochloride
    anesthetic agent
meprobamate
mEq (milliequivalents)
Mercedes incision
Mercedes tip cannula
Mercer cartilage knife
Mercier catheter
Mercier operation
Mercier sound
Merck respirator
Mercurio position
mercury cell-powered pace-
    maker
mercury-containing balloon
mercury-filled bougie
mercury-filled dilator
mercury-filled esophageal
    bougie
mercury-in-Silastic strain gauge
mercury-weighted bougie
mercury-weighted dilator
mercury-weighted tube
meridional aberration
meridional section
Merindino operation
Merkel cell carcinoma of
    buttock
Merkel disk
Merkel muscle
Merlin stone forceps
Merlis obstetrical excavator
Mermingas operation
Merocel nasal packing
Merocel sponge
merocrine gland
Merrill Supramid suturing
    technique

Merrill-Levassier retractor
Mers suture
Mersilene band
Mersilene dressing
Mersilene gauze
Mersilene graft
Mersilene implant
Mersilene mesh
Mersilene mesh dressing
Mersilene prosthesis
Mersilene sutures
Mersilene tape
Mersilene tape ligature
Merthiolate dressing
Merz hysterectomy forceps
mesangial matrix
mesencephalic flexure
mesencephalic tractotomy
mesencephalon
mesencephalotomy
mesenchymal
mesenchymal mixed tumor
mesenchymal tissue
mesenchymal tumor
mesenchyme
mesenterectomy
mesenteric
mesenteric adhesions
mesenteric artery
mesenteric attachments
mesenteric cyst
mesenteric fistula
mesenteric ganglion
mesenteric hernia
mesenteric infarction
mesenteric inferior artery
mesenteric lymph nodes
mesenteric node
mesenteric stranding
mesenteric superior artery
mesenteric superior vein
mesenteric thrombosis
mesenteric triangle
mesenteric vascular lesion
mesenteric vein
mesenterica inferior, arteria
mesenterica superior, arteria

mesenterica superior, vena
mesenteriopexy
mesenteriorrhaphy
mesenteriplication
mesentery
mesentorrhaphy
mesh
    Dacron mesh
    Dexon mesh
    Douglas mesh skin graft
    fine-mesh dressing
    fine-mesh gauze
    Harrison interlocked
      mesh prosthesis
    House stainless steel
      mesh prosthesis
    Marlex mesh
    Mersilene mesh
    Mylar mesh
    Ortho-Mesh
    polyglycolic acid mesh
    polypropylene mesh
    skin mesh
    stainless steel mesh
    steel mesh
    Supramid mesh implant
    synthetic mesh
    Tanner-Vandeput mesh
    tantalum mesh
    Teflon mesh
    titanium mesh
    Usher Marlex mesh
    Vitallium mesh
    wire mesh graft
    wire mesh prosthesis
mesh graft
mesh prosthesis
mesh skin graft
mesh sutures
meshed ball implant
meshwork
mesial
mesial occlusion
mesial surface
mesoappendicitis
mesoappendix
mesobi-ileal shunt

mesocaval anastomosis
mesocaval H-graft shunt
mesocaval interposition shunt
mesocaval shunt
mesocecum
mesocolic
mesocolic band
mesocolic hernia
mesocolic lymph nodes
mesocolic shelf
mesocolon
mesocolopexy
mesocoloplication
mesocuneiform bone
mesodermal segment
mesodermal tumor
mesogastrium
mesolateral fold
mesonephric drain
mesonephric duct
mesonephric fold
mesopexy
mesorectum
mesorrhaphy
mesosalpinx
mesosigmoid
mesosigmoidopexy
mesothelial cells
mesothelioma
mesothenar muscle
mesouterine fold
mesovarium
Messner plate
Meta MV cardiac pacemaker
metabolic bone disease
metabolic calculus
metabolic disturbance
metabolic rate
metabolic stone
metabolism
metacarpal
metacarpal arteries
metacarpal bones
metacarpal double-ended
   retractor
metacarpal epiphyseal centers
metacarpal fracture

metacarpal head
metacarpal of wrist
metacarpal saw
metacarpal splint
metacarpal veins
metacarpeae dorsales, arteriae
metacarpeae dorsales, venae
metacarpeae palmares, arteriae
metacarpeae palmares, venae
metacarpectomy
metacarpocarpal articulations
metacarpophalangeal (MCP)
metacarpophalangeal articulation
metacarpophalangeal joint
metal applicator
metal band
metal band sutures
metal cannula
metal catheter
metal clamp
metal clip
metal connector
metal electrode
metal irrigating tip
metal locator (see also *locator,
   magnet*)
      Berman metal locator
      Berman-Moorhead metal
         locator
metal nail
metal needle
metal olive
metal orthopedic implant
metal pin
metal plate
metal prosthesis
metal rod
metal ruler
metal screw
metal sound
metal splint
metal suction connector
metal syringe
Metaline dressing
metallic clamp
metallic fixation device

metallic foreign body (MFB)
metallic fragment
metallic implant
metallic sphere introducer
metallic-tip cannula
metal-tipped cannula
metal-weighted Silastic feeding tube
metaphyseal flair
metaphysis
metaplastic polyp
Metaport catheter
metaraminol
metastasis (*pl.* metastases)
metastatic
metastatic cancer
metastatic carcinoma
metastatic disease
metastatic focus
metastatic implant
metastatic involvement
metastatic lesion
metastatic node
metastatic site
metastatic spread
metastatic tumor
metatarsal
metatarsal arteries
metatarsal bone
metatarsal cuneiform exostosis
metatarsal cuneiform joint
metatarsal fracture
metatarsal head
metatarsal osteotomy
metatarsal splint
metatarsal veins
metatarseae dorsales, arteriae
metatarseae dorsales, venae
metatarseae plantares, arteriae
metatarseae plantares, venae
metatarsectomy
metatarsophalangeal (MTP)
metatarsophalangeal articulations
metatarsophalangeal joint
metatarsus

metatarsus abductus
metatarsus adductus
metatarsus equinus
metatarsus primus varus
Metcalf spring drop brace
Metcher eye speculum
Metcher speculum
meter
method
Methodist suction tube
methohexital sodium anesthetic agent
methoxyflurane anesthetic agent
methyl methacrylate
methyl methacrylate adhesive
methyl methacrylate bone cement
methyl methacrylate cement
methyl methacrylate glue
methyl methacrylate graft
methylene blue dye
methylene blue insufflation
meticulous
metopic suture
Metras catheter
metric ophthalmoscopy
metric system
metrizamide cisternogram
metrizamide myelography
metro catheter
metroplasty
metrorrhagia
mets (slang for metastases)
Mett tube
Metycaine hydrochloride anesthetic agent
Metzenbaum baby tonsillar scissors
Metzenbaum chisel
Metzenbaum dissecting scissors
Metzenbaum dressing scissors
Metzenbaum forceps
Metzenbaum gouge
Metzenbaum knife
Metzenbaum needle holder
Metzenbaum scissors

Metzenbaum septum knife
Metzenbaum tonsillar forceps
Metzenbaum tonsillar scissors
Metzenbaum-Lipsett plastic
  scissors
Metzenbaum-Lipsett scissors
Metzenbaum-Tydings forceps
Metzger infant knife
Meyer cervical orthosis
Meyer cyclodiathermy needle
Meyer hockey-stick incision
Meyer incision
Meyer light pipe
Meyer line
Meyer loop
Meyer mastectomy
Meyer needle
Meyer operation
Meyer sinus
Meyerding aluminum hammer
Meyerding bone graft
Meyerding bone skid
Meyerding chisel
Meyerding curet
Meyerding double-ended
  retractor with skin hook
Meyerding facet eroder
Meyerding finger retractor
Meyerding gouge
Meyerding laminectomy self-
  retaining retractor
Meyerding mallet
Meyerding nail
Meyerding osteotome
Meyerding prosthesis
Meyerding retractor
Meyerding saw-toothed curet
Meyerding skid
Meyerding skin hook
Meyerding solid aluminum
  mallet
Meyerding-Deaver retractor
Meyer-Halsted incision
Meyers hip procedure
Meyer-Schwickerath operation
Meyers-McKeever avulsion
  fracture classification

Meyerson sign
Meyhoeffer chalazion curet
Meyhoeffer curet
Meyhoeffer eye knife
Meyhoeffer knife
Meynet bundle
Meynet commissure
Meynet decussation
Meynet nodes
Meynet nodosities
Meynet tract
MFB (metallic foreign body)
MGH (Massachusetts General
  Hospital)
MGH elevator
MGH forceps
MGH glenoid punch
MGH knee prosthesis
MGH needle holder
MGH osteotome
MGH periosteal elevator
MGH vulsellum forceps
MI (myocardial infarct; myocar-
  dial infarction)
Miami fracture brace
Micasloc porous knee system
Mich compression arthrodesis
Michael Reese prosthesis
Michael Reese shoulder
  prosthesis
Michel aortic clamp
Michel clamp
Michel clip
Michel clip hemostat
Michel clip-applying forceps
Michel deformity
Michel forceps
Michel rhinoscopic mirror
Michel scalp clip
Michel suture clip
Michel tissue forceps
Michel trephine
Michel wound clip
Michelis intraocular implant lens
Michelis lens
Michelson bronchoscope
Michelson infant bronchoscope

Michigan forceps
Michigan intestinal forceps
Mick applicator
Micrins forceps
Micrins needle holder
Micro SI Holter system
microadenoma
Micro-Aire bone saw
Micro-Aire drill
Micro-Aire instruments
Micro-Aire osteotome
Micro-Aire pulse lavage system
microanastomosis
microanastomosis approximator
microanastomosis clip
microanastomosis clip approxi-
    mator
microaneurysm
microangiopathy
microarterial clamp
microarterial clamp applier
microballoon probe
microbayonet forceps
microbayonet rasp
microbayonet scoop
microbial action
microbiology
microbiopsy forceps
microbipolar forceps
microblade knife
microbone curet
microbrenner
microbronchoscopic tissue
    forceps
microbulldog clamp
microcautery unit
microcellular organism
microcephaly
microcirculation
microclamp
microclamp clip
microclamp forceps
microclip
microclip applier
microclip forceps
microcolon
microcrimped prosthesis

microcuret
microcurie
microdermatome
microdissector
Microdon dressing
microdressing forceps
microelectrode
microelectrode technique
microembolic disease
microextractor forceps
microfibrillar collagen hemo-
    stat
Microfoam dressing
Microfoam surgical tape
microforceps
microgastria
Micro-Glide exchange wire
micrognathia
micrograph
Micro-Guide catheter
microhook
microinvasive carcinoma
microinvasive catheter
Microknit arterial prosthesis
Microknit vascular graft
    prosthesis
microlaryngeal instruments
Micro-Line artery forceps
Microlith P pacemaker
microlithiasis
Microloc knee system
micromanometer-tip catheter
micromembranous stethoscope
micromike
micromoles
micromyelia
micron needle
microneedle
microneedle holder
microneedle holder forceps
microneurosurgery
microneurosurgery forceps
micropannus
microphone
microphthalmus
micropin
micropin forceps

micropoint cautery
micropoint needle
Micropore hypoallergenic tape
Micropore surgical tape
    dressing
Micropore tape
microprobe
microprobe surgical tape
Micropuncture Peel-Away
    introducer
microradiography
microraspatory
microroentgenography
microrongeur
microscissors
microscope
        AFI Micros 5 microscope
            system
        aural microscope
        Barraquer-Zeiss micro-
            scope
        beta ray microscope
        binocular microscope
        biomicroscope
        capillary microscope
        centrifuge microscope
        Codman-Mentor micro-
            scope
        Cohan microscope
        Cohan-Barraquer
            microscope
        color contrast micro-
            scope
        compound microscope
        Contraves microscope
        corneal microscope
        coupling microscope
        darkfield microscope
        Derlacki-Shambaugh
            microscope
        electron microscope
        epic microscope
        epimicroscope
        fluorescence microscope
        fluorescent microscope
        Greenough microscope
        Haag-Streit microscope

microscope *continued*
    Heyer-Schulte micro-
        scope
    hypodermic microscope
    infrared microscope
    integrating microscope
    interference microscope
    ion microscope
    Kelar microscope
    laser microscope
    Leitz microscope
    light microscope
    Neibauer-Kleinert
        microscope
    Olympus microscope
    Omni operating micro-
        scope
    opaque microscope
    operating microscope
    operation microscope
        drape
    OPMI operating micro-
        scope
    OPMI-6 operating
        microscope
    otomicroscope
    phase microscope
    phase-contrast micro-
        scope
    photon microscope
    polarizing microscope
    projector x-ray micro-
        scope
    rectified microscope
    rectified polarizing
        microscope
    reflecting microscope
    Rheinberg microscope
    scanning electron
        microscope
    schlieren microscope
    Shambaugh operating
        microscope
    Shambaugh-Derlacki
        microscope
    simple microscope
    slit-lamp microscope

microscope *continued*
    specular microscope
    Storz-Urban surgical
      microscope
    stroboscopic microscope
    surgical microscope
    television microscope
    trinocular microscope
    ultramicroscope
    ultrasonic microscope
    ultraviolet microscope
    Weck ceiling-mount
      operating microscope
    Weck operating micro-
      scope
    Weck-cel operating
      microscope
    Wild operating micro-
      scope
    Wild surgical microscope
    x-ray microscope
    Yasargil microscope
    Yasargil surgical
      microscope
    Zeiss diploscope
      microscope
    Zeiss microscope
    Zeiss operating micro-
      scope
    Zeiss OPMI operating
      microscope
    Zeiss OPMI-6 operating
      microscope
    Zeiss-Cohan-Barraquer
      microscope
microscope eyepiece
microscopic hook
microscopic scissors
microscopy
microsection
Micro-Sharp blade
MicroSkin urostomy pouch
microsponge
microstomia
microsurgery
microsurgery biopsy forceps
microsurgery dissector

microsurgery needle holder
microsurgery retractor
microsurgical scissors
microsurgical spatula
microsuture forceps
microsuture-tying forceps
Microtek drill system
Micro-Temp pad
Micro-Temp pump
Microthin P2 pacemaker
microtia
microtip bipolar forceps
microtissue forceps
microtome
Micro-Tracer portable ECG
microtying eye forceps
microtying forceps
microutility forceps
MicroVac
microvascular abnormalities
microvascular clamp
microvascular forceps
microvascular needle holder
microvascular neurosurgery
microvascular scissors
Microvasic Rigiflex balloon
Microvasive sclerotherapy
    needle
Microvel graft
Microvel implant
Microvel prosthesis
microvessel knife
microvit scissors
microvitreoretinal blade (MVR)
microvolt
microwave
microwave diathermy
Microwec scissors
micturition
micturition bag
micturition reflex
midabdominal transverse
    incision
midabdominal wall
Midas Rex drill
Midas Rex pneumatic tool
midaxillary line

midbody
midbrain
midcarpal disarticulation of
    wrist
midcarpal joint
midcervical apophyseal joint
midcostal line
midcycle phase
Middeldorpf splint
mid-depth
middle cardiac cervical nerve
middle cardiac vein
middle cerebral artery (MCA)
middle cerebral peduncle
middle cervical ganglion
middle clunial nerves
middle colic artery
middle colic vein
middle collateral artery
middle constrictor pharyngeal
    muscle
middle ear
middle ear arrow-tube
middle ear aspirator
middle ear canal knife
middle ear capsule knife
middle ear chisel
middle ear curet
middle ear elevator
middle ear excavator
middle ear forceps
middle ear hoe
middle ear hook
middle ear implant
middle ear knife
middle ear ring curet
middle ear strut forceps
middle ear suction cannula
middle extrahepatic bile duct
middle finger
middle fossa
middle frontal gyrus
middle genicular artery
middle gluteal muscle
middle lobe
middle lobe bronchus
middle lobe of prostate

middle meatus
middle meningeal artery
middle meningeal veins
middle palatine suture
middle palmar space
middle portion
middle rectal artery
middle rectal vein
middle scalene muscle
middle suprarenal artery
middle temporal artery
middle temporal vein
middle thyroid vein
middle turbinate
middle umbilical fold
middle umbilical ligament
middle vesical artery
middle-ear dermoid cyst of
    ovary
Middleton adenoid curet
Middleton curet
Middleton line
midesophageal diverticulum
midexpiratory flow rate
midfemoral block
midflow rate
midforceps
midforceps delivery
midforceps operation
midgut ischemia
midline
midline abdominal crease
midline abdominal incision
midline episiotomy
midline incision
midline scar
midline sternum-splitting
    incision
midline structures
midline tumor
midlung field
midoccipital electrode
midpelvic anteroposterior
    diameter
midpelvic diameter
midpenile hypospadias
midplane

midpoint
midportion
midsacral region
midsagittal plane
midsection
midshaft of bone
midsigmoid colon
midsternal line
midsternum-splitting incision
midstream aortogram catheter
midsystolic buckling
midsystolic closure of aortic
    valve
midtarsal
midtemporal area
midtemporal focus
midtemporal spiking
midthigh
midtibial perforator
midtransverse colon
midtrimester bleeding
Miescher tube
Miescher tubule
migrating
migration
migratory cells
migratory deep vein throm-
    bophlebitis
Mik (see *Mikulicz*)
mika operation
Mikhail bone block
Mikros pacemaker
Mikro-tip angiocatheter
Mikulicz angle
Mikulicz clamp
Mikulicz colostomy
Mikulicz crusher
Mikulicz drain
Mikulicz enterectomy
Mikulicz forceps
Mikulicz gastrectomy
Mikulicz gastrotomy
Mikulicz incision
Mikulicz operation
Mikulicz pack
Mikulicz pad
Mikulicz peritoneal clamp

Mikulicz peritoneal forceps
Mikulicz pharyngoesophageal
    reconstruction
Mikulicz pyloroplasty
Mikulicz retractor
Mikulicz tarsectomy
Mikulicz tonsillar forceps
Mikulicz-Vladimiroff operation
Milan uterine curet
Milch operation
Milch ulna procedure
mild chromic sutures
mild concussion
mild to moderate pain
mild trabeculation
Miles abdominoperineal
    resection
Miles antral curet
Miles clamp
Miles clip
Miles nasal punch
Miles operation
Miles proctosigmoidectomy
Miles rectal clamp
Miles retractor
Miles skin clip
Miles Teflon clip
Miles vena cava clip
Milex forceps
Milex pessary
Milex retractor
Milex spatula
miliary
miliary aneurysm
miliary embolism
milieu
military antishock trousers
    (MAST)
milium (*pl.* milia)
milk ducts
milk lines
milked out
milked superiorly
milking
milkmaid's elbow dislocation
milkman's syndrome
milky ascites

milky fluid
milky urine
Millar catheter
Millar catheter-tipped transducer
Millar micromanometer catheter
Millar pigtail angiographic
    catheter
Millard cheiloplasty
Millard forehead flap
Millard island flap
Millard operation
Millard rotation-advancement
    operation
Millard rotation-advancement
    technique
Millen retropubic prostatectomy
Millen technique
Millender arthroplasty
Millender-Nalebuff wrist
    arthrodesis
Miller bayonet forceps
Miller curet
Miller dilator
Miller dissecting scissors
Miller flatfoot procedure
Miller forceps
Miller laryngoscope
Miller operation
Miller operation for talipes
    valgus
Miller position
Miller raspatory
Miller rectal forceps
Miller rectal scissors
Miller retractor
Miller scissors
Miller speculum
Miller syndrome
Miller technique
Miller tonsillar dissector
Miller tonsillar knife
Miller tube
Miller vaginal speculum
Miller-Abbott catheter
Miller-Abbott double-channel
    intestinal tube
Miller-Abbott intestinal tube
Miller-Abbott tube (M-A tube)

Miller-Apexo elevator
Miller-Galante hip prosthesis
Miller-Galante porous Tivanium
    total knee system
Miller-Galante total knee
    implant
Miller-Senn double-ended
    retractor
Miller-Senn retractor
Miller-vac drain
Millesi interfascicular grafts
Millette tonsil knife
Millette-Tydings knife
mill-house murmur
milliamperes (ma)
millicuries (mc)
milliequivalents (mEq)
Milligan double-ended dissector
Milligan self-retaining retractor
Milligan speculum
milligrams (mg)
millijoules (mJ)
Milliknit arterial prosthesis
Milliknit graft
Milliknit vascular graft prosthe-
    sis
milliliters (ml)
millimeter ruler
millimeters (mm)
millimoles (mM)
Millin bladder retractor
Millin capsule forceps
Millin capsule-grasping forceps
Millin clamp
Millin forceps
Millin lobe-grasping forceps
Millin operation
Millin retractor
Millin retropubic bladder
    retractor
Millin self-retaining retractor
Millin suction tube
Millin T-shaped angled forceps
Millin T-shaped forceps
Millin tube
Millin-Bacon bladder self-
    retaining retractor
Millin-Bacon retractor

Millin-Bacon spreader
milliner's needle
millinery bag
Millin-Read operation
Millipore filter
Millipore sutures
milliseconds (msec)
millivolts (mV)
Mill-Rose biopsy forceps
Mill-Rose cytology brush
Mill-Rose esophageal injector
Mill-Rose injector
Mill-Rose instrument cleaner
Mills arteriotomy scissors
Mills cautery
Mills forceps
Mills tissue forceps
Mills valvulotome
Miltex retractor
Miltex rib spreader
Milton-Adams suspension
Milwaukee brace
Milwaukee orthosis
Milwaukee scoliosis brace
Milwaukee shoulder
Mimer room
Mimer table
Miner osteotome
Minerva cast
Minerva jacket
Minerva plaster collar
Minerva plaster jacket
Mingazzini-Foerster operation
Mini Stryker power drill
miniature
miniature electrotome
miniature forceps
miniature intestinal forceps
miniature scissors
miniature sound
Minibird II
Minicath
Minidialyzer
mini-dose
mini-driver instruments
minilaparotomy
Minilith pacemaker
Minilux headlight

minimal
minimal assistance
minimal bleeding
minimal blood loss
minimal extensibility
minimal tension skin lines
mini-micro forceps
minimum
mini-Mustardé procedure
Minin lamp
miniphage
Mini-Profile dilatation catheter
MiniSnyder Hemovac
Mini-Ullrich bone clamp
Minix pacemaker
mink encephalopathy
Minkowski method
Minnesota four-lumen tube
Minnesota Mining and Manufac-
    turing Company
    (3M dressing)
Minnesota retractor
Minnesota tube
minor amputation
minor connector bar
minor discomfort
minor fissure
minor laceration
minor operation
minor procedure
Minor sign
minor surgery
minor surgery scissors
minor vessel
minor wound
Minos air drill
Minotaur labyrinth
Minsky circle
Minsky operation
minute anatomy
minute bleeding mucosal ulcer
Miochol
Mira cautery
Mira diathermy
Mira drill
Mira laser
Mira photocoagulator
Mira reamer

Mira scissors
Mira tip eye cautery
Mira unit
Mira-Charnley reamer
Mirault operation
Mirault-Brown-Blair operation
mirror
> Boilo head mirror
> Boilo laryngeal mirror
> diagnostic mirror
> Everclear laryngeal mirror
> head mirror
> headband-and-mirror set
> laryngeal mirror
> Michel rhinoscopic mirror
> pharyngeal mirror
> Purkinje-Sanson mirror images
> rhinoscopic mirror
> three-mirror contact lens
> Universal mirror handle

mirror cannula
mirror focus
mirror hand
mirror holder
mirror image
mirror laryngoscope
mirroring of extremities
miscarriage
Mischler reservoir
Mischler shunt
Mischler valve
Mischler-Pudenz shunt
Miskimon cerebellar self-retaining retractor
mismatched marrow
missed abortion
mist
mist therapy
Mistogen nebulizer
Mistogen passover humidifier
Mital elbow release
Mitchel aortotomy clamp
Mitchel-Adam multipurpose clamp

Mitchell basket
Mitchell bunionectomy
Mitchell distal osteotomy
Mitchell knife
Mitchell operation
Mitchell osteotomy
Mitchell stone basket
Mitchell-Clark hernia repair
Mitchell-Diamond biopsy forceps
Mitchell-Diamond forceps
mitigate
Mitner rotary bone rasp
mitral annuloplasty
mitral commissurotomy
mitral dilator
mitral forceps
mitral insufficiency
mitral knife
mitral regurgitation
mitral stenosis knife
mitral valve
mitral valve commissurotomy
mitral valve dilator
mitral valve fusion
mitral valve leaflet tip
mitral valve prosthesis
mitral valve replacement
mitral valve retractor
mitral valve ring
mitral valve spreader
mitral valve-hinging operation
mitral valve-holding forceps
mitral valvotomy
mitral valvulotomy
Mitroflow pericardial prosthetic valve
Mitrothin P2 pacemaker
Mitsubishi angioscope
Mitsubishi angioscopic catheter
mitten hand
mitten pattern
Mittlemeir broach
Mittlemeir ceramic hip prosthesis
Mittlemeir ceramic total hip
Mittlemeir femoral prosthesis

Mityvac vacuum extraction
    delivery
mixed abscess
mixed amputation
mixed anesthesia
mixed cataract
mixed condition
mixed glands
mixed hemorrhoids
mixed joint
mixed lesion
mixed nerve
mixed rhythm
mixed tumor
mixed-cholesterol gallstone
MixEvac bone cement mixer
Mixter clamp
Mixter common duct dilaprobe
Mixter dilating probe
Mixter dilator
Mixter forceps
Mixter full-curve forceps
Mixter gall duct forceps
Mixter gallbladder forceps
Mixter gallstone forceps
Mixter general operating
    scissors
Mixter hemostat
Mixter irrigating probe
Mixter needle
Mixter probe
Mixter punch
Mixter right-angle clamp
Mixter scissors
Mixter tube
Mixter-McQuigg forceps
Mixter-O'Shaugnessy dissecting
    and ligature forceps
Mixter-Paul hemostatic forceps
Mixtner catheter
mixture
Mizzy needle
mJ (millijoule)
MLT tube
mm (millimeters)
mM (millimoles)
MM band

mm Hg (millimeters of mercury)
mM/L (millimoles per liter)
MMM (3M; Minnesota Mining
    and Manufacturing
    Company)
MMM drape (3M drape)
MMM dressing (3M dressing)
MMM Vi-Drape (3M Vi-Drape)
Moberg advancement pedicle
Moberg arthrodesis
Moberg chisel
Moberg forceps
Moberg osteotome
Moberg procedure
Moberg retractor
mobile
mobile cecum
mobile gallbladder
mobile kidney
mobile mass
mobile testicle
mobile wad compartment of
    forearm
mobility
mobilization
mobilize
mobilized cecum
mobilized uterus
mobilizer
        Derlacki mobilizer
        Derlacki-Hough mobil-
            izer
        ear mobilizer
        Valtchev uterine
            mobilizer
Mobin-Uddin filter
Mobin-Uddin umbrella filter
Mobin-Uddin vena caval filter
Mobitz heart block
Mobitz I AV heart block
Mobitz I block
Mobitz II AV heart block
Mobitz II block
Möbius (see *Moebius*)
Mobley-Webster needle holder
modality
mode

moderate
moderate contractions
moderate narrowing
moderate pain
moderate shift
moderate voltage
moderately differentiated
    adenoma
modification
modified
modified flap operation
modified graft
modified operation
modified position
modified procedure
modified prosthesis
modified radical mastectomy
modified radical mastoidectomy
modified reconstruction
modified shunt
modified surgical procedure
modified technique
modify
modular knee prosthesis
modular prosthesis
modulation
module
Moe impactor
Moe intertrochanteric plate
Moe nails
Moe plate
Moe procedure
Moe spinal fusion
Moe-style spinal hook
Moebius (also Mobius)
Moebius cataract knife
Moebius knife
Moebius sign
Moehle corneal forceps
Moehle forceps
Moehle scissors
Moersch bronchoscope
Moersch bronchoscopic
    specimen forceps
Moersch cardiospasm dilator
Moersch electrode
Moersch esophagoscope

Moersch forceps
Mogen circumcision clamp
Mohr clamp
Mohr splint
Mohrenheim fossa
Mohs chemotherapy
Mohs excision of basal cell
    carcinoma
Mohs micrographic che-
    mosurgery
Mohs procedure
Mohs surgery
Mohs technique
moist compress
moist dressing
moist gangrene
moist heat
moist lap packs
moist rales
moist tape
moistened tape
molal solution
molar
molar pregnancy
mold
mold arthroplasty
molded splint
molded Teflon
molder's sign
Moldestad vein hook
molding
molding of head
mole
molecular
molecule
moleskin
moleskin and felt scissors
moleskin bandage
moleskin traction
moleskin traction hitch dressing
Molesworth elbow procedure
Molesworth-Campbell approach
Moll glands
Mollison mastoid rongeur
Mollison retractor
Mollison self-retaining retractor
Mollo boots

Molnar disk
Molt curet
Molt dissector
Molt elevator
Molt forceps
Molt guillotine
Molt mouth gag
Molt mouth prop
Molt periosteal elevator
Molt-Storz guillotine
Molt-Storz tonsillectome
molybdenum
molybdenum radiation therapy
Momberg tourniquet
Momberg tube
Monaghan respirator
Monaghan ventilator
Monaldi drain
Monaldi operation
monarticular
monaural hearing
Mönckeberg arteriosclerosis
Mönckeberg degeneration
Mönckeberg sclerosis
Moncrieff cannula
Moncrieff discission
Moncrieff irrigator
Moncrieff operation
Monel metal radium applicator
monitor
    Accucap CO2/O2
      monitor
    Accucom cardiac output
      monitor
    Accutorr monitor
    ambulatory Holter
      monitor
    apnea monitor
    Arrhythmia Net arrhyth-
      mia monitor
    Baim-Turi monitor
    CA monitor  (cardiac-
      apnea monitor)
    cardiac-apnea monitor
      (CA monitor)
    cardiac monitor
    CardioDiary heart
      monitor

monitor *continued*
    continuous Holter
      monitor
    Cosman monitor
    Dinamap blood pressure
      monitor
    Dinamap monitor
    Doplette monitor
    Doppler monitor
    Doppler-Cavin monitor
    Doptone monitor
    electrocardiographic
      monitor
    Electrodyne cardiac
      monitor
    Endotek urodynamic
      monitor
    facial nerve monitor
    fetal monitor
    fluoroscopic monitor
    Hawksley blood pressure
      monitor
    heart monitor
    Hewlett-Packard
      monitor
    Holter monitor
    internal monitor
    MAC (monitored
      anesthesia care)
    Meadox ICP monitor
    nerve monitor
    Ohio Vortex respiration
      monitor
    Ohmeda 6200 CO2
      monitor
    Pressure Sense
      monitor
    Pressurometer blood
      pressure monitor
    PSA-1 monitor
    pulse monitor
    telemetry monitor
    Tri-Met apnea monitor
    Ultra COM monitor
monitored
monitored anesthesia care
    (MAC)
monitored bed

monitoring
monitoring cannula
monitoring lines
Moniz sign
Monk hip prosthesis
Monk orthopedic procedure
Monks operation
Monks-Esser flap
Monks-Esser island flap
monoarticular
monochromatic radiation
Monocorps milium knife
monocular bandage
monocular dressing
monocular eye dressing
monocular patch
monocular rotations
monocular vision
monocuspid tilting disk heart
    valve
monofilament clear sutures
monofilament green sutures
monofilament nylon sutures
monofilament stainless steel
    wire
monofilament sutures
monofilament wire
monofilament wire sutures
Monoject sphygmomanometer
Monoject suction tube
monomanual delivery
monomer suction biopsy tube
monopolar cautery
monopolar coagulating forceps
monopolar connection cord
monopolar electrocoagulation
monopolar forceps
monopolar insulated forceps
Monorail angioplasty catheter
monorail technique
Monosmith nasal speculum
monostrut valve
monosynaptic reflex
Monro bursa
Monro foramen
Monro line
Monro sulcus

Monro-Richter line
mons pubis
monster rongeur
montage
Montague abrader
Montague proctoscope
Montague sigmoidoscope
Montefiore tracheal tube
Montefiore tube
Monteggia dislocation
Monteggia fracture
Monteggia fracture-dislocation
Montenovesi cranial rongeur
    forceps
Montenovesi rongeur
Montercaux ankle fracture
Montevideo units (uterine
    contractions)
Montgomery glands
Montgomery speculum
Montgomery strap dressing
Montgomery straps
Montgomery T-piece tube
Montgomery T-tube
Montgomery tape
Montgomery tracheal cannula
    system
Montgomery vaginal speculum
Montgomery-Bernstine specu-
    lum
Monticelli-Spinelli external
    fixation system
Moody forceps
moon boot
Moon rectal retractor
moon-shaped face
moon-shaped facies
Moore adjustable nails
Moore approach
Moore bone reamer
Moore bone retractor
Moore button
Moore chisel
Moore direction finder
Moore drill
Moore driver
Moore elevator

Moore extractor
Moore forceps
Moore fracture
Moore gallbladder spoon
Moore gallstone scoop
Moore gouge
Moore hip prosthesis
Moore hip-locking prosthesis
Moore hollow chisel
Moore humeral head procedure
Moore measuring rod
Moore nail
Moore nail set
Moore operation
Moore osteotomy
Moore pin
Moore plate
Moore prosthesis
Moore prosthesis extractor
Moore prosthesis mortising
    chisel
Moore prosthesis rasp
Moore rasp
Moore raspatory
Moore reamer
Moore retractor
Moore rod
Moore scoop
Moore self-locking prosthesis
Moore shoulder procedure
Moore spinal fusion gouge
Moore spoon
Moore template
Moore thoracoscope
Moore tracheostomy buttons
Moore tube
Moore-Blount driver
Moore-Blount extractor
Moore-Blount plate
Moore-Blount screwdriver
Moore-Corradi operation
Moorehead cheek retractor
Moorehead clamp
Moorehead dental retractor
Moorehead dissector
Moorehead ear knife
Moorehead elevator

Moorehead knife
Moorehead lid clamp
Moorehead periosteotome
Moorehead retractor
Moorhead pressure anesthesia
    unit
Moorhead suction anesthesia
    unit
mooring fibers
mop-end tear
Morand foot
Morax keratoplasty
Morax operation
morbid obesity
morbidly obese
morcellation
morcellation operation
morcellement
morcellement nephrectomy
morcellement operation
morcellization
Morch respirator
Morch swivel tracheostomy
    tube
Morch tracheostomy tube
Morch tube
Morch ventilator
Morel ear
Morel-Fatio blepharoplasty
Moren-Moretz vena caval clip
Moreno clamp
Morestin operation
Moretz clip
Moretz prosthesis
Morgagni appendix
Morgagni column
Morgagni foramen
Morgagni hernia
Morgagni nodules
Morgagni sphere
Morgagni ventricle
morgagnian cataract
morgagnian cyst
Morgan pelvic support
Morgenstein blunt forceps
Mori knife
moribund

Morison incision
Morison method
Morison pouch
Moritz-Schmidt forceps
Moritz-Schmidt laryngeal
    forceps
Morley peritoneocutaneous
    reflex
morphine anesthetic agent
morphine sulfate
morphologic
morphologic feature
morphology
Morquio sign
Morrey total elbow
Morris aortic clamp
Morris biphase screw
Morris cannula
Morris catheter
Morris defibrillator
Morris drain
Morris incision
Morris retractor
Morris splint
Morris taper
Morrison toe flap
Morrison-Hurd dissector
Morrison-Hurd pillar retractor
Morrison-Hurd retractor
Morrison-Hurd tonsillar
    dissector
morsal teeth
Morsch-Retec respirator
Morsch-Retec respirator tube
Morse aortic scissors
Morse blade
Morse retractor
Morse scissors
Morse sternal spreader
Morse taper
Morse-Andrews suction tube
Morse-Ferguson suction tube
morselize
morselized
morselizer
Morson forceps
mortality

mortar kidney
mortise
mortise of joint
mortise x-ray view
mortising chisel
Morton bandage
Morton dislodger
Morton foot
Morton neuroma
Morton ophthalmoscope
Morton stone dislodger
Morton toe
mosaic
mosaic development
mosaic duodenal mucosal
    pattern
mosaicism
mosaicism of cervix
Moschcowitz enterocele repair
Moschcowitz hernia repair
Moschcowitz operation
Mosetig-Moorhof bone wax
Mosher bag
Mosher cardiospasm dilator
Mosher curet
Mosher drain
Mosher esophagoscope
Mosher esophagoscope tube
Mosher ethmoid curet
Mosher ethmoid punch
Mosher ethmoid punch forceps
Mosher forceps
Mosher lifesaver tube
Mosher lifesaving tube
Mosher operation
Mosher punch
Mosher retractor
Mosher speculum
Mosher suction tube
Mosher tube
Mosher-Toti operation
Moskowitz procedure
Mosley anterior shoulder repair
Mosley shoulder repair
Mosley stone crusher
mosquito clamp
mosquito forceps

mosquito hemostat
mosquito hemostatic forceps
mosquito lid clamp
Moss gastrostomy tube
Moss Mark IV gastrostomy tube
Moss Mark IV nasal tube
Moss tube
Motais operation
mother cell
mother cyst
mother-daughter endoscope
mother-to-infant transmission
motile organism
motility
motion
motor activity
motor and sensory function
motor center
motor defect
motor development
motor function
motor nerve
motor nerve action potential
    (MAP)
motor neuron
motor oil peritoneal fluid
motor power and coordination
motor reflexes
motor skills
Mott double-ended retractor
Mott retractor
mottled appearance
mottled area
mottled calcification
mottled in appearance
mottling
mottling of extremities
Moult curet
Mouly reduction mammaplasty
Mount forceps
Mount intervertebral disk
    rongeur forceps
Mount laminectomy rongeur
Mount-Mayfield forceps
Mount-Olivecrona forceps
Mouradian humeral fixation
    device system

Moure esophagoscope
Moure-Coryllos rib shears
mouse-tooth clamp
mouse-tooth forceps
Mousseau-Barbin prosthetic
    tube
mouth gag (see also *gag*)
    Boyle-Davis mouth gag
    Brophy mouth gag
    Collis mouth gag
    Crowe-Davis mouth gag
    Dann-Jennings mouth
        gag
    Davis mouth gag
    Davis-Crowe mouth gag
    Denhardt mouth gag
    Denhardt-Dingman
        mouth gag
    Dingman mouth gag
    Dingman-Denhardt
        mouth gag
    Dott mouth gag
    Dott-Kilner mouth gag
    Doyen mouth gag
    Doyen-Jansen mouth gag
    Ferguson mouth gag
    Ferguson-Ackland mouth
        gag
    Ferguson-Brophy mouth
        gag
    Ferguson-Gwathmey
        mouth gag
    Frohm mouth gag
    Fulton mouth gag
    Green mouth gag
    Green-Sewall mouth gag
    Hayton-Williams mouth
        gag
    Heister mouth gag
    Hibbs mouth gag
    Jansen mouth gag
    Jennings Loktite mouth
        gag
    Jennings mouth gag
    Jennings-Skillern mouth
        gag
    Kilner mouth gag

mouth gag *continued*
    Kilner-Dott mouth gag
    Kilner-Doughty mouth gag
    Lane mouth gag
    Lange mouth gag
    Lewis mouth gag
    McDowell mouth gag
    McIvor mouth gag
    McKesson mouth gag
    Molt mouth gag
    Negus mouth gag
    Newkirk mouth gag
    oral screw mouth gag
    oral speculum mouth gag
    Proetz mouth gag
    Proetz-Jansen mouth gag
    Pynchon mouth gag
    Ralks-Davis mouth gag
    Roser mouth gag
    side mouth gag
    Sluder mouth gag
    Sluder-Ferguson mouth gag
    Sluder-Jansen mouth gag
    Sydenham mouth gag
    Wesson mouth gag
    Whitehead mouth gag
    Wolf mouth gag
mouth-to-mouth resuscitation
movable
movable kidney
move normally
moved and positioned
movement
moving strip x-ray technique
moxa
moxibustion
Moynihan bile duct probe
Moynihan clamp
Moynihan clip
Moynihan forceps
Moynihan gall duct forceps
Moynihan gallstone probe
Moynihan gallstone scoop
Moynihan gastrojejunostomy

Moynihan incision
Moynihan intestinal operation
Moynihan operation
Moynihan position
Moynihan probe
Moynihan respirator
Moynihan scoop
Moynihan towel clamp
Moynihan-Navratil forceps
Moynihan-Navratil speculum
Mozart Gold instruments
MPC scissors
MPD (main pancreatic duct)
MPF catheter
MRI (magnetic resonance imaging)
MRI scan
msec (milliseconds)
MSRs (muscles, strength, reflexes)
MTBE (methyl tert-butyl ether)
MTP (metatarsophalangeal)
mucinous adenoma
mucinous carcinoma
mucinous tumor
Muck forceps
Muck tonsillar forceps
Muck tonsillar hemostat
mucobuccal fold
mucocele
mucociliary blanket
mucoclasis
mucocutaneous
mucocutaneous border
mucocutaneous hemorrhoid
mucocutaneous junction
mucocutaneous wart
mucoepidermoid carcinoma
mucogingival junction
mucoid discharge
mucoid impaction
mucoid material
mucoid secretion
mucolabial fold
mucoperichondrium
mucoperiosteal elevator
mucoperiosteal flap

mucoperiosteal flap operation
mucoperiosteal flap trimming
mucoperiosteal implant
    placement
mucoperiosteum
mucopurulent
mucopurulent discharge
mucorrhea
mucosa
mucosa elevator
mucosa knife
mucosa speculum
mucosal
mucosal abnormality
mucosal cuff
mucosal folds
mucosal graft
mucosal guideline pattern
mucosal hernia
mucosal island
mucosal pattern
mucosal proctectomy and
    ileoanal pull-through
mucosal sleeve resection
mucosal suspensory ligament
mucosal tear
mucosa-to-mucosa closure
mucosectomy
mucoserous cells
mucoserous otitis media
mucosis
mucosis otitis
mucotome
        Norelco mucotome
mucous (adjective)
mucous discharge
mucous fistula
mucous fluid
mucous glands
mucous lake of stomach
mucous membrane graft
mucous membranes
mucous plug
mucous polyp
mucous stool
mucous thread
mucous tissue

mucus (noun)
mucus forceps
mucus knife
mucus-secreting gland
Muehr craniotome
Mueller (also Müller)
Mueller bur
Mueller catheter guide
Mueller cautery
Mueller cesarean section
Mueller clamp
Mueller curet
Mueller Currentrol cautery
Mueller Duo-Lock hip prosthe-
    sis
Mueller duct
Mueller electric trephine
Mueller electronic tonometer
Mueller fibers
Mueller forceps
Mueller giant eye magnet
Mueller hip plate
Mueller hip prosthesis
Mueller hip system
Mueller lacrimal sac retractor
Mueller maneuver
Mueller micrograin prosthesis
Mueller muscle
Mueller needle
Mueller operation
Mueller osteotomy
Mueller pediatric clamp
Mueller prosthesis
Mueller retractor
Mueller round Gigli saw
Mueller saw
Mueller scissors
Mueller sclerectomy
Mueller shield
Mueller sign
Mueller speculum
Mueller stapling system
Mueller suction tube
Mueller technique
Mueller tongue blade
Mueller tonometer
Mueller total hip

Mueller trephine
Mueller vaginal hysterectomy
Mueller vena caval clamp
Mueller-Balfour retractor
Mueller-Balfour self-retaining
    retractor
Mueller-Charnley total hip
    prosthesis
Mueller-Dammann pulmonary
    artery banding
Mueller-Frazier suction tube
Mueller-Frazier tube
Mueller-Hillis maneuver
Mueller-LaForce adenotome
Mueller-Markham patent ductus
    forceps
Mueller-Poole suction tube
Mueller-Poole tube
Mueller-Pynchon suction tube
Mueller-Pynchon tube
Mueller-Yankauer suction tube
Mueller-Yankauer tube
Muelly hook
Muenster cast
Muer anoscope
Muer proctoscope
MUGA (multiple gated acquisi-
    tion)
MUGA cardiac blood pool scan
MUGA scan
MUGA test
Muhlberger implant
Muhlberger orbital implant
Muhlberger orbital implant
    prosthesis
Muir cautery clamp
Muir clamp
Muir hemorrhoidal forceps
Muir rectal cautery clamp
mulberry calculus
mulberry cell
mulberry fat
mulberry gallstone
Mulder sign
Muldoon dilator
Muldoon lacrimal dilator
Muldoon lacrimal probe

Muldoon lid retractor
Muldoon meibomian forceps
Muldoon tube
Mules eye implant
Mules graft
Mules implant
Mules operation
Mules prosthesis
Mules scoop
Mules sphere eye implant
Mules sphere implant
Mulholland sphincterotomy
Müller (see *Mueller*)
müllerian duct
müllerian tumor
Mulligan cervical biopsy
    punch
Mulligan dissector
Mulligan prosthesis
Mulligan Silastic prosthesis
Mullins blade
Mullins blade and balloon
    septostomy
Mullins blade technique
Mullins catheter introducer
Mullins decompressor
Mullins sheath
Mullins transseptal atrial
    septostomy
Mullins transseptal catheter
Mullins transseptal introducer
Mullins transseptal sheath
multangular bone
multangulum majus
multiacinar
multiaxial joint
Multiclip
Multiclip disposable ligating clip
    device
Multicor Gamma pacemaker
Multicor II pacemaker
multicuspid teeth
multidisciplinary team
multielectrode impedance
    catheter
multifaceted
multifidi, musculi

multifidus muscle
multifilament sutures
multifilament wire
multifocal
multifocal atrial tachycardia
    (MAT)
multifocal contractions
multifocal heartbeats
multihit injury
multiholed tube
multilead electrode
multilesion angioplasty
multilevel spinal fusion
Multilith pacemaker
multilobed placenta
multilobular cyst
Multi-Lock knee brace
multilocular
multilocular cyst
multiloculated
multilumen catheter
multilumen probe
Multi-Med triple-lumen catheter
Multi-Med triple-lumen infusion
    catheter
multinodular
multinodular goiter
multiparity
multiparous female
multiple
multiple amputation
multiple apertures
multiple biopsies
multiple births
multiple fasciotomies
multiple foci
multiple fractures
multiple fragmentations
multiple gated acquisition
    (MUGA)
multiple metastases
multiple pregnancies
multiple resectoscope
multiple surgical excisions
multiple tenotomies
multiple trauma
multiple washings

multiple-action rongeur
multiple-lumen tube
multiple-point electrode
multiple-stage omphalocele
    repair
multiplier
Multipoise headrest
multipolar impedance catheter
multiprogrammable pacemaker
multipurpose ball electrode
multipurpose catheter
multipurpose clamp
multipurpose forceps
multipurpose instruments
multipurpose laryngoscope
multirooted tooth
multiseptate gallbladder
multisided Z-plasty closure
Multistim electrode catheter
multistrand sutures
multisystem trauma
Mumford arthroscopy
Mumford clavicle resection
Mumford Gigli-saw guide
Mumford operation
Mumford-Neer procedure
mummified fetus
mummified pulp
mummylike wrap
Munchen endometrial biopsy
    curet
Mundie forceps
Mundie placenta forceps
Munnell operation
Munro abscess
Munro brain scissors
Munro Kerr cesarean section
Munro Kerr incision
Munro Kerr maneuver
Munro microabscess
Munro point
Munro retractor
Munro scissors
Munro self-retaining retractor
Munson sign
Munster cast
mural aneurysm

mural kidney
mural pregnancy
Murdock eye speculum
Murdock speculum
Murdock-Wiener eye speculum
Murdock-Wiener speculum
Murless fetal head extractor
Murless head extractor
Murless head extractor forceps
Murless vector head extractor
murmur
Murphy approach
Murphy ball reamer
Murphy bone gouge
Murphy bone lever
Murphy bone skid
Murphy brace
Murphy button
Murphy chisel
Murphy common duct dilator
Murphy dilator
Murphy drip tube
Murphy endotracheal tube
Murphy forceps
Murphy gallbladder retractor
Murphy gouge
Murphy hook
Murphy intestinal needle
Murphy kidney punch
Murphy knife
Murphy light
Murphy method
Murphy needle
Murphy percussion
Murphy plaster knife
Murphy punch
Murphy rake retractor
Murphy reamer
Murphy retractor
Murphy scissors
Murphy sign
Murphy tonsillar forceps
Murphy treatment
Murphy tube
Murphy-Balfour center blade
Murphy-Balfour retractor
Murphy-Lane bone skid

Murphy-Lane skid
Murphy-Péan hemostatic
    forceps
Murray forceps
Murray holder
Murray knee prosthesis
Murray operation
Murray-Thomas arm splint
Murtagh self-retaining infant
    scalp retractor
muscle
muscle advancement technique
muscle atrophy
muscle biopsy clamp
muscle bleeding points
muscle bulk
muscle bundle
muscle clamp
muscle contraction
muscle control
muscle coordination
muscle cramp
muscle fiber
muscle fixation
muscle flap
muscle forceps
muscle function
muscle graft
muscle guarding
muscle hook
muscle injuries
muscle mass
muscle pain
muscle pedicle
muscle prosthesis
muscle repair
muscle repositioning
muscle response
muscle rupture
muscle sense
muscle stamp
muscle status
muscle stimulation
muscle strain
muscle tension
muscle testing
muscle tightness

muscle tissue
muscle tone
muscle tonicity
muscle transfer
muscle tumor
muscles, strength, reflexes
   (MSRs)
muscle-splitting incision
muscular
muscular aches
muscular artifact
muscular atrophy
muscular attachment
muscular contraction
muscular control
muscular defect
muscular disease
muscular layer
muscular pain
muscular paralysis
muscular reflex
muscular relaxation
muscular rigidity
muscular senses
muscular spasm
muscular strabismus
muscular structure
muscular system
muscular tension
muscular tissues
muscular tone
muscular trabeculation
muscular tremors
muscular twitching
muscular veins
muscular ventricular septal
   defect
muscular wall
muscular weakness
musculature
musculoaponeurotic system
musculocartilaginous structure
musculocutaneous
musculocutaneous amputa-
   tion
musculocutaneous artery
musculocutaneous flap
musculocutaneous nerve

musculocutaneous vein
musculocutaneus, nervus
musculofascial layers
musculofascial structures
musculofascial wall
musculofascially
musculophrenic artery
musculophrenic veins
musculophrenica, arteria
musculophrenicae, venae
musculoplasty
musculoskeletal
musculoskeletal disorder
musculoskeletal evaluation
musculoskeletal tissue
musculospiral nerve
musculotendinous cuff
musculus (*pl.* musculi) (see
   specific musculi)
Museholdt forceps
Museux forceps
Museux uterine vulsellum
   forceps
Museux-Collins uterine vulsellum forceps
mush clamp
mush heart
mushroom catheter
mushroom overlap of pars
   interarticularis
mushrooming
mushroom-type plate
Musial tissue forceps
musical bowel sounds
musical murmur
Musken tonometer
muslin dressing
Musset sign
mustache dressing
Mustard atrial baffle repair
Mustard flap otoplasty
Mustard iliopsoas transfer
Mustard intra-atrial operation
Mustard operation
mustard plaster
mustard poultice
Mustard transposition of great
   arteries

Mustard transposition of great
    vessels
Mustardé four-flap epicanthal
    repair
Mustardé otoplasty
Mustardé procedure
Mustardé sutures
Mustardé-Furnas otoplasty
mutation
mutilation
mV (millivolts)
MVR (microvitreoretinal)
MVR blade
MVR plate
myalgia
mycotic aneurysm
mydriatic eye drops
mydriatic pupils
mydriatic rigidity
myectomy
myelin globules
myelin kidney
myelin sheath
myelinated nerve fibers
myeloblastoma
myelocytoma
myelogenous callus
myelogenous disease
myelogram
myelography
myeloid cell
myeloid leukemia
myeloid metaplasia
myeloid tissue
myeloid/erythroid ratio
myeloma
myeloparalysis
myelopathic muscular atrophy
myelopathy
myelosuppressed
myelotomy
myelotomy knife
myenteric plexus
Myers intraluminal stripper
Myers knee retractor
Myers punch
Myers retractor

Myers stripper
Myers vein stripper
Myerson antrum trocar
Myerson electrode
Myerson forceps
Myerson miniature laryngeal
    biopsy forceps
Myerson punch
Myerson saw
Myerson sign
Myerson snout
Myerson trocar
Myerson-Moncrieff cannula
Mylar catheter
Mylar mesh
Mylar sheeting
Myles adenotome
Myles antral curet
Myles cannula
Myles clamp
Myles curet
Myles forceps
Myles guillotine
Myles guillotine adenotome
Myles hemorrhoidal clamp
Myles hemorrhoidal forceps
Myles nasal punch
Myles nasal speculum
Myles nasal-cutting forceps
Myles punch
Myles sinus antral cannula
Myles snare
Myles speculum
Myles tonsillectome
Myles tonsillectome snare
Myles-Ray speculum
mylohyoid
mylohyoid line
mylohyoid muscle
mylohyoid nerve
mylohyoid region
mylohyoid ridge
mylohyoideus, musculus
mylohyoideus, nervus
mylopharyngeal muscle
myoblastoma
Myobock artificial hand

myocardial
myocardial clamp
myocardial conduction defect
myocardial contusion
myocardial damage
myocardial dilator
myocardial disease
myocardial electrode
myocardial fibers
myocardial fibrosis
myocardial hypertrophy
myocardial infarct (MI)
myocardial infarction (MI)
myocardial insufficiency
myocardial ischemia
myocardial necrosis
myocardial perfusion
myocardial revascularization
myocardial scar
myocardial tumors
myocardiectomy
myocardiopathy
myocardiorrhaphy
myocardiotomy
myocardium
myocardosis
myocervical collar
myochromic
myoclasis
myoclonal antibodies
myoclonic jerk
myoclonic seizure
myoclonus
myocontrol signals
Myocure blade
myocutaneous flap
myoelectric control prosthesis
myofascial
myography
myoid cells
myoma (*pl.* myomas, myomata)
myomalacia cordis
myomata uteri
myomatectomy
myomectomy
myometrial
myometrium

myomotomy
myonephropexy
myoneural junction
myoneurectomy
myoneuroma
myoneurosis
myopathy
myopectoral inhibition of
    pacemaker
myopia
myopic
myoplastic
myoplasty
myopotential
myorrhaphy
myostasis
Myostim unit
myotasis
myotatic contraction
myotatic reflex
myotenontoplasty
myotenotomy
myotome
myotome distribution of nerve
myotomy
myotonia
myotonic cataract
myotonic discharges
myotonic reflexes
myotonic response
myovascular
Myrhaug procedure
myringectomy
myringodectomy
myringoplasty
myringoplasty knife
myringostapediopexy
myringotome
    Buck myringotome
myringotome knife
myringotomy
myringotomy drain tube
myringotomy incision
myringotomy knife
myringotomy tube
myringotomy with insertion of
    polyethylene collar buttons

Myrtle leaf probe
myxoid cyst
myxoid cystoma
myxoma
myxomatosis

myxomatous tissue
myxomembranous
    colitis
myxoneurosis
myxosarcoma

N-loop
N-shaped sigmoid loop
N-terface graft dressing
Nabatoff stripper
Nabatoff vein stripper
Naboth cysts
Naboth follicles
Naboth glands
Naboth vesicles
nabothian cyst
nabothian follicle
nabothian gland
Nachlas tube
Nachlas-Linton tube
Naclerio diaphragm retractor
Nadbath akinesia
Naden-Rieth femoral prosthetic
    head
Naden-Rieth implant
Naden-Rieth prosthesis
nadir
Naffziger operation
Naffziger-Poppen-Craig orbital
    decompression
Nagamatsu incision
Nagel scissors
Nägele obliquity
Nägele pelvis
Nägeli maneuver
Nahai tensor fascia lata
    flap
Nahigian butterfly flap
Nahigian Z-plasty
nail
        adjustable nail
        Augustine boat nail
        Augustine nail
        Badgley nail
        Barr nail

nail *continued*
    boat nail
    Brooker-Wills interlock-
      ing nail
    Burgess nail
    Calandruccio nail
    cannulated nail
    clincher nail
    cloverleaf nail
    condylocephalic nail
    Coventry nail
    Curry hip nail
    Delitala T-nail
    DePuy nail
    Deyerle nail
    diamond nail
    Dooley nail
    eggshell nail
    Ender intramedullary nail
    Ender nail
    Engel-May nail
    Fenton nail
    fingernail
    four-flanged nail
    fracture nail
    Gamma locking nail for
      hip
    Gissane spike nail
    Grosse-Kempf nail
    hangnail
    Hansen-Street intra-
      medullary nail
    Hansen-Street nail
    Harold Crowe drill nail
    Harris intramedullary nail
    Harris nail
    hexhead nail
    hip nail
    Holt nail

nail *continued*
  hooked intramedullary
    nail
  hooked nail
  Huckstep intramedullary
    compression nail
  Huckstep nail
  I-beam nail
  ingrown nail
  intramedullary Küntscher
    nail
  intramedullary nail
  Jewett hip nail
  Jewett nail
  K-nail
  Ken nail
  Ken sliding nail
  Kirschner interlocking
    intramedullary nail
  Klemme locked intra-
    medullary nail
  Klemme nail
  Knowles pin nail
  Küntscher cloverleaf nail
  Küntscher intramedullary
    nail
  Küntscher nail
  Lindsay nail
  Lottes intramedullary nail
  Lottes nail
  Lottes triflange intra-
    medullary nail
  Massie nail
  massive sliding nail
  McLaughlin nail
  McLaughlin Vitallium nail
  medullary nail
  metal nail
  Meyerding nail
  Moe nail
  Moore adjustable nail
  Moore nail
  nested nails
  Neufeld nail
  noncannulated nail
  Norman tibial nail
  Nylok self-locking nail

nail *continued*
  osteotomy nail
  Pidcock nail
  Pugh nail
  Redler nail
  Richards nail
  Rush intramedullary nail
  Rush nail
  Russell-Taylor interlock-
    ing nail
  Russell-Taylor nail
  Russell-Taylor tibial
    interlocking nail
  Sampson nail
  Schneider intramedullary
    nail
  Schneider medullary nail
  Schneider nail
  self-adjusting nail
  self-broaching nail
  sliding nail
  Slocum-Smith-Petersen
    nail
  Smillie nail
  Smith-Petersen cannu-
    lated nail
  Smith-Petersen nail
  Staples osteotomy nail
  Steinmann nail
  Street diamond-shaped
    nail
  Street nail
  Synphes nail
  Temple University nail
  Terry nail
  Thatcher nail
  Thornton nail
  three-flanged nail
  Tiemann nail
  toenail
  triflange intramedullary
    nail
  triflange nail
  V-medullary nail
  Venable-Stuck nail
  Vesely nail
  Vesely-Street nail

nail *continued*
    Vitallium nail
    Watson-Jones nail
    Webb nail
    Webb stove nail
    Williams nail
    Z-fixation nail
    Zickel intramedullary
        nail
    Zickel nail
    Zimmer intramedullary
        nail
    Zimmer nail
    Zimmer telescoping nail
nail bed
nail cutter
nail extension
nail fold
nail injury
nail lunula
nail matrix
nail nipper (see also *nipper*)
    Turnbull nail nipper
nail plate (see also *plate*)
    Holt nail plate
    Neufeld femoral nail
        plate
nail-extracting forceps
nailing
nailing of bone
nailing of hip
nail-patella syndrome
Nakayama instruments
Nalebuff wrist arthrodesis
Nalline
nanocurie (nCi)
nanogram (ng)
nanoliter (nl)
nanometer (nm)
nanomole
nanopascal
nape
naphthalinic cataract
napkin-ring annular lesion
napkin-ring defect
napkin-ring lesion
Napoleon Bonaparte sign

Narath omentopexy
Narath operation
narcosis
narcotic agent
narcotic antagonist
narcotic drug
narcotic effect
naris (*pl.* nares)
narrow cone
narrow duodenal opening
narrow elevator
narrow retractor
narrow rim
narrow-angle glaucoma
narrowed blood vessel
narrowed duct
narrowed valve
narrowing
narrowing and lipping
nasal
nasal airway
nasal airway obstruction
nasal alligator forceps
nasal aperture
nasal applicator
nasal arteries
nasal bistoury
nasal bone
nasal bone crusher
nasal bone forceps
nasal border
nasal bridge
nasal canal
nasal cannula
nasal canthus
nasal capsule
nasal cartilage
nasal cartilage guide
nasal cartilage-cutting board
nasal cartilage-holding forceps
nasal catheter
nasal cavity
nasal chamber
nasal chisel
nasal chisel-osteotome
nasal concha
nasal congestion

nasal contour
nasal crest
nasal culture
nasal curet
nasal cutting forceps
nasal dilator
nasal discharge
nasal dissector
nasal dome cartilage
nasal dorsal-angled scissors
nasal douche
nasal drainage
nasal drip pad
nasal duct
nasal elevator
nasal eminence
nasal endoscopy telescope
nasal feeding
nasal flaring
nasal forceps
nasal fossa
nasal fracture
nasal gavage
nasal gouge
nasal hemorrhage
nasal hook
nasal hump gouge
nasal hump forceps
nasal hump-cutting forceps
nasal incision
nasal insertion forceps
nasal instruments
nasal intubation
nasal knife
nasal lower lateral forceps
nasal meatus
nasal mucosa
nasal muscle
nasal needle
nasal needle holder
nasal needle holder forceps
nasal notch of maxilla
nasal obstruction
nasal osteotome
nasal packing
nasal pancreatogram
nasal passage

nasal plastic instruments
nasal polyp
nasal polyp forceps
nasal polyp hook
nasal polypectomy
nasal polypus forceps
nasal probe
nasal punch
nasal pyramid
nasal rasp
nasal reconstruction
nasal reflex
nasal retractor
nasal ridge
nasal rongeur
nasal saw
nasal saw blade
nasal scissors
nasal septal forceps
nasal septoplasty
nasal septum
nasal septum reconstruction
   (NSR)
nasal sill
nasal sinus
nasal smear
nasal snare
nasal speculum
nasal spine
nasal splint
nasal spur
nasal stent cutter
nasal strut
nasal suction cup
nasal suction tip
nasal suction tube
nasal suture needle
nasal suture
nasal swivel knife
nasal tampon
nasal tenaculum
nasal trephine
nasal truss
nasal tube
nasal turbinate
nasal vein
nasal venule

nasal vestibule
nasal washings
nasal-cutting forceps
nasal-cutting tip
nasal-dressing forceps
nasales externae, venae
nasales posteriores, laterales et
    septi, arteriae
nasal-grasping forceps
nasalis, musculus
nasal-packing forceps
Nashold electrode
nasoantral window
nasobiliary catheter
nasobiliary catheter cholangio-
    gram
nasobiliary drainage
nasobiliary pigtail catheter
    placement
nasobiliary tube
nasociliaris, nervus
nasociliary branches of ophthal-
    mic nerve
nasociliary nerve
nasoduodenal feeding tube
nasoendotracheal anesthesia
nasoendotracheal intubation
nasoesophageal feeding tube
nasofrontal suture
nasofrontal vein
nasofrontalis, vena
nasogastric
nasogastric aspirate
nasogastric drainage
nasogastric feeding tube
nasogastric intubation
nasogastric suction
nasogastric tube
nasograph
nasojejunal feeding tube
nasolabial
nasolabial crease
nasolabial droop
nasolabial fold
nasolabial junction
nasolabial reflex
nasolacrimal canal
nasolacrimal duct

nasolacrimal sac
nasolacrimal tube
nasomandibular fixation
nasomaxillary fracture
nasomaxillary suture
nasomental reflex
nasopalatine injection
nasopalatine nerve
nasopalatine plexus of
    Woodruff
nasopalatine recess
nasopalatinus, nervus
nasopancreatic drainage
nasopharyngeal applicator
nasopharyngeal area
nasopharyngeal biopsy
    forceps
nasopharyngeal pack
nasopharyngeal retractor
nasopharyngeal speculum
nasopharyngeal sponge
nasopharyngeal tube
nasopharyngoscope
    ACMI nasopharyngo-
        scope
    Broyles nasopharyngo-
        scope
    Holmes nasopharyngo-
        scope
    Meltzer nasopharyngo-
        scope
    Yankauer nasopharyngo-
        scope
nasopharynx
nasoseptal deviation
nasoseptal reconstruction
nasotracheal catheter
nasotracheal intubation
nasotracheal intubation
    anesthesia
nasotracheal suctioning
nasotracheal tube
nasoturbinal concha
Nassif parascapular flap
natal cleft
natatory ligament
Natelson tube
Nathan pacemaker

Natick standing-pull test
National cautery
National cautery electrode
National coagulator
National cystoscope
National general-purpose
    cystoscope
National instruments
National proctoscope
National speculum
National transilluminator
native valve
natural amputation
natural bypass
natural joint
natural line
natural pacemaker
natural skin lines
natural sutures
natural teeth
Natural-Loc acetabular cup
    prosthesis
Natural-Loc RM acetabular cups
Natural-Y breast prosthesis
Naugh os calcis apparatus
    tractor
Naughton protocol
Nauheim carbonated bath
nausea
nauseated
navel
navicular
navicular arthritis
navicular bone
navicular fossa
navicular fossa of male urethra
navicular fracture
navicular pad
navicular projection
naviculocapitate
Navratil stirrups
NB (newborn)
NBIH catheter
nCi (nanocurie)
Nd:YAG laser
Neal cannula
Neal catheter

Neal catheter trocar
Neal fallopian cannula
Neal insufflator
Neal-Robertson litter
near-and-far sutures
near-edge of incision
near-far sutures
near-miss
near-term gestation
Nebinger-Praun operation
nebulized solution
nebulizer
neck dissection
neck extension position
neck flexion
neck fracture
neck lift
neck of femur
neck of organ or structure
neck sign
neck vein distention
neck veins
neck wound
neck-shaft angle
neck-wrap halter
necrosectomy
necrosis (*pl.* necroses)
necrotic
necrotic debris
necrotic pulp
necrotic tissue
necrotic ulceration
necrotizing
necrotomy
NED (no evidence of disease)
needle (see also *suture needle*)
    abdominal needle
    Abrams needle
    abscission needle
    Acland needle
    ACS needle
    active length needle
    Addix needle
    Adson aneurysm needle
    Adson needle
    Adson scalp needle
    Adson suture needle

needle *continued*

Adson-Murphy needle
Adson-Murphy trocar
    point needle
advancement needle
Agnew needle
Agnew tattooing needle
Alabama-Green needle
    eye holder
Alexander needle
Alexander tonsil needle
Altmann needle
AMC needle
Amplatz angiography
    needle
Amplatz needle
Amsler needle
Anchor needle sterilizing
    box
Anchor surgical needle
anesthesia block needle
aneurysm needle
aneurysmal needle
angiography needle
angular needle
antral needle
antrum-exploring needle
aorta vent needle
aortic root perfusion
    needle
aortic vent needle
aortogram needle
aortography needle
Arkan sharpening-stone
    needle
arterial blood needle
arterial needle
arteriogram needle
aspirating needle
aspiration biopsy needle
aspiration needle
Atkinson needle
Atkinson retrobulbar
    needle
Atraloc needle
atraumatic needle
atraumatic suture needle

needle *continued*

Austin needle
B&D needle
B-D bone marrow
    biopsy needle
B-D needle
B-D spinal needle
Babcock needle
Ballade needle
Barbara needle
Barker needle
Barraquer needle
Barraquer-Vogt needle
Barrett hebosteotomy
    needle
Barrett needle
Becton-Dickinson
    Teflon-sheathed
    needle
Beeth needle
Bengash-type needle
bent needle
Berbecker needle
Beyer needle
Beyer paracentesis
    needle
Bierman needle
biopsy needle
bipolar needle
Birtcher electrosurgical
    needle
Black-Decker needle
Blackmon needle
Blair-Brown needle
block anesthesia needle
blunt needle
bone marrow needle
Bonney needle
Bonney suture needle
boomerang bladder
    needle
Bovie needle
Bowman cataract needle
Bowman iris needle
Bowman needle
brain biopsy needle
Braun needle

needle *continued*
- Brockenbrough needle
- Brophy needle
- Brophy-Deschamps needle
- Brown needle
- Brown staphylorrhaphy needle
- Brughleman needle
- Buerger needle
- Buncke quartz needle
- Bunnell needle
- Bunnell tendon needle
- butterfly IV needle
- butterfly needle
- BV-2 needle
- Calhoun needle
- Calhoun-Merz needle
- Campbell needle
- Campbell ventricular needle
- cardioplegic needle
- Carlens needle
- Carpule needle
- Carroll needle
- Castroviejo needle
- cataract needle
- cataract-aspirating needle
- catheter needle
- caudal needle
- cerebral angiography needle
- cervical needle
- cervix suture needle
- Charles needle
- Charles vacuuming needle
- Charlton antrum needle
- Charlton needle
- Chiba eye needle
- Chiba needle
- Childs-Phillips intestinal plication needle
- Childs-Phillips needle
- Childs-Phillips plication needle
- Cibis ski needle

needle *continued*
- Clagett needle
- cleft palate needle
- Cloquet needle
- Cobb-Ragde needle
- Colver needle
- Colver tonsil needle
- Concept Multi-Liner lining needle
- cone biopsy needle
- Cone needle
- Cone ventricular needle
- Conrad-Crosby biopsy needle
- Conrad-Crosby needle
- Control-Release needle
- Cooley aortic vent needle
- Cooper chemopallidectomy needle
- Cooper needle
- Cope biopsy needle
- Cope needle
- Cope pleural biopsy needle
- Cope thoracentesis needle
- copper-clad steel needle
- corneal needle
- corneal suture needle
- Coston iris needle
- couching needle
- Cournand arterial needle
- Cournand needle
- Cournand-Grino angiography needle
- Cournand-Grino needle
- Craig needle
- Crawford fascial needle
- Crawford needle
- Cross needle trocar
- CTX needle
- CU-8 needle
- Culp biopsy needle
- Curry needle
- curved needle
- curved suture needle

needle *continued*
Cushing needle
cutting needle
cyclodiathermy needle
D-Tach needle
dacryocystorhinostomy
    needle
Daily cataract needle
Damshek needle
Dandy needle
Dandy ventricular needle
Dandy-Cairns brain
    needle
Dandy-Cairns ventricular
    needle
Davis knife-needle
Davis needle
Davis tonsillar needle
Dean iris knife-needle
Dean needle
Dean-Senturia needle
DeBakey needle
debridement needle
Dees needle
Dees suture needle
Deknatel K-needle
Deknatel needle
Denis Browne needle
Deschamps ligature
    needle
Deschamps needle
Deschamps-Navratil
    ligature needle
Deschamps-Navratil
    needle
desiccation needle
desiccation-fulguration
    needle
Desmarres needle
Desmarres paracentesis
    needle
Devonshire needle
diamond-point suture
    needle
diathermic needle
Dingman needle
Dingman passing needle

needle *continued*
discission needle
diskographic needle
Dix needle
DLP cardioplegic needle
docking needle
Docktor needle
Dorsey needle
Dos Santos aortography
    needle
Dos Santos lumbar
    aortography needle
double-barreled needle
Douglas suture needle
Doyen needle
Drapier needle
Drews lavage needle
Dupuy-Dutemps needle
Dupuy-Weiss needle
Durham needle
DuVries needle
Dyonics needle scope
    arthroscope
E-Z-EM Cut biopsy
    needle
egress needle
Emmet needle
Emmet-Murphy needle
epilation needle
Epstein needle
Estridge ventricular
    needle
exploring needle
extrusion needle
eye needle
eyed needle
eyed suture needle
eyeless atraumatic suture
    needle
eyeless needle
eyeless suture needle
fascia needle
Federspiel needle
Fein needle
Ferguson needle
Ferguson suture needle
fine needle

needle *continued*

Finochietto needle
Fischer needle
Fischer pneumothoracic needle
Fisher eye needle
Fisher needle
fishhook needle
fistular needle
flat spatula needle
* flexible injection needle
Floyd needle
Flute needle
Flynt needle
Foltz needle
Frackelton needle
Francke needle
Frankfeldt hemorrhoidal needle
Frankfeldt needle
Franklin-Silverman biopsy needle
Franklin-Silverman needle
Frazier needle
Frazier ventricular needle
Frederick needle
Frederick pneumothorax needle
Freenseen liver biopsy needle
French needle
French-eye needle
Gallie fascia needle
Gallie needle
ganglion injection needle
Gardner needle
Gardner suture needle
gastrointestinal needle
GC needle (general closure needle)
general closure needle
Geuder corneal needle
Geuder keratoplasty needle
Gill needle
Gillmore needle

needle *continued*

Girard needle
Girard-Swan knife-needle
Goldbacher needle
Gordh needle
Gorsch needle
Graefe iris needle
Graefe knife-needle
Graefe needle
Grantham lobotomy needle
Grantham needle
Greene needle
Greenfield needle
Grieshaber eye needle
Grieshaber iris needle
Grieshaber needle
Haab needle
Hagedorn needle
Hagedorn suture needle
Halle needle
Halle septal needle
Halsey needle
harelip needle
Harken heart needle
Harken needle
Hawkins needle
Hearn needle
heart needle
Hegar-Baumgartner needle
hemorrhoidal needle
Henton needle
Henton suture needle
Henton tonsillar suture needle
heparin needle
Hessberg needle
high-risk needle
Hoen needle
Hoen ventricular needle
Holinger needle
Homer needle
Homerlok needle
Hosford-Hicks needle

needle *continued*

Hourin needle
Hourin tonsil needle
House needle
House stapes needle
House-Barbara needle
House-Barbara shattering
  needle
House-Rosen needle
HR needle (high-risk
  needle)
Huber needle
Hunt needle
Hurd suture needle
Hutchins biopsy needle
Hutchins needle
hypodermic needle
Illinois needle
Ingersoll needle
Ingersoll tonsil needle
injection needle
intestinal needle
intestinal plication
  needle
intravenous needle (IV
  needle)
iris knife-needle
iris needle
IV needle (intravenous
  needle)
Jameson needle
Jameson strabismus
  needle
Jamshidi liver biopsy
  needle
Jamshidi needle
Jamshidi-Kormed bone
  marrow biopsy needle
Jelco needle
Jordan needle
Kader needle
Kall modification of
  Silverman needle
Kalt corneal needle
Kalt eye needle
Kalt needle
Kaplan needle

needle *continued*

Kaplan tracheostomy
  needle
Kara needle
Karras angiography
  needle
Karras needle
Keith abdominal needle
Keith needle
Kelly intestinal needle
Kelly needle
Kelman needle
kidney suture needle
King needle
King suture needle
Klatskin liver biopsy
  needle
Klatskin needle
Knapp iris knife-needle
Knapp knife-needle
Knapp needle
knife-needle
Knight needle
Kobak needle
Kohn needle
Koontz hernia needle
Kopan needle
Kormed disposable liver
  biopsy needle
Kormed needle
Kronecker needle
lacrimal needle
Lagleyze needle
Lahey needle
Laminex needle
Lane cleft palate needle
Lane needle
Lane suture needle
Lapides needle
large-bore needle
Lee needle
Leighton needle
L'Esperance needle
Lewicky needle
Lewy-Rubin needle
Lichtwicz antral needle
Lichtwicz needle

needle *continued*
  ligature needle
  Lindeman needle
  Linton-Blakemore needle
  Lipschwitz needle
  List needle
  liver biopsy needle
  lobotomy needle
  lock needle
  long needle
  Longdwel catheter
    needle
  Longdwel needle
  Loopuyt needle
  Lowell pleural needle
  Lowsley needle
  Lowsley ribbon-gut
    needle
  Luer needle
  lumbar aortography
    needle
  lumbar puncture needle
  Lundy needle
  Lundy-Irving needle
  Luongo needle
  Madayag needle
  Maddox needle
  Magielski needle
  Maltz needle
  Maltzman needle
  Mammo-lock needle
  Manan needle
  Martin needle
  Marx needle
  Masson fascial needle
  Masson needle
  Mayo needle
  Mayo trocar-point needle
  McCaslin knife-needle
  McCurdy needle
  McCurdy staphylor-
    rhaphy needle
  McDowell needle
  McGhan plastic surgical
    needle
  McGowan needle
  McGregor needle

needle *continued*
  McIntire needle
  McIntyre aspiration
    needle
  McIntyre irrigation
    needle
  Medicut intravenous
    needle
  Medicut needle
  Menghini liver biopsy
    needle
  Menghini needle
  metal needle
  Meyer cyclodiathermy
    needle
  Meyer needle
  micron needle
  microneedle
  micropoint needle
  Microvasive sclerother-
    apy needle
  milliner's needle
  Mixter needle
  Mizzy needle
  Mueller needle
  Murphy intestinal needle
  Murphy needle
  nasal needle
  nasal suture needle
  Nelson ligature needle
  Nelson needle
  New needle
  Newman needle
  Newman rectal injection
    needle
  Noci stimuli needle
  noncutting needle
  noncutting suture needle
  Nordenstrom biopsy
    needle
  O'Brien airway needle
  obstetrical anesthesia
    needle
  obstetrical block
    anesthesia needle
  Op-Pneu laparoscopy
    needle

needle *continued*

Overholt needle
Pace ventricular needle
Page needle
Palmer-Drapier needle
palpating needle
Paparella needle
paracentesis needle
Parhad needle
Parhad-Poppen needle
Parker knife-needle
Parker needle
Penfield biopsy needle
Penfield needle
PercuCut biopsy needle
percutaneous needle
Pereyra needle
pericardiocentesis
    needle
Pitkin needle
pleural biopsy needle
plication needle
pneumoperitoneum
    needle
pneumothorax injection
    needle
pneumothorax needle
pop-off needle
Poppen needle
Poppen ventricular
    needle
Potter needle
Potts needle
Potts-Cournand angiogra-
    phy needle
Potts-Cournand needle
Presbyterian Hospital
    needle
prostatic biopsy needle
pudendal needle
puncture needle
Quantico needle
quartz needle
radium needle
rectal injection needle
rectal needle
renal needle

needle *continued*

retrobulbar prosthesis
    needle
Retter needle
Reverdin needle
Reverdin suturing needle
reverse-cutting needle
rib needle
ribbon gut needle
Rider-Moeller needle
Riedel needle
Riley needle
Robb needle
Roberts needle
Rochester needle
root needle
Rosen needle
Rosenthal needle
Roser needle
Ross needle
Rotex II biopsy needle
Rotex needle
round needle
Rubin needle
Ruskin antral needle
Ruskin needle
Sabreloc needle
Sabreloc spatula needle
Sachs needle
Salah needle
Salah sternal needle
Sanders-Brown needle
Sanders-Brown-Shaw
    needle
Sarot needle
Saunders needle
Saunders-Paparella
    needle
scalpene needle
Scheer needle
Scheie cataract needle
Scheie cataract-aspirating
    needle
Scheie needle
Schuknecht needle
scleral spatula needle
sclerotherapy needle

needle *continued*

Scoville needle
Scoville ventricular
  needle
Seldinger needle
septal needle
Seraflo A-V fistula needle
  set
seton needle
Shambaugh needle
shattering needle
Sheldon-Spatz needle
Sheldon-Swann needle
Shirodkar needle
short needle
side-cutting spatulated
  needle
side-flattened needle
Silverman biopsy needle
Silverman needle
Silverman-Boeker
  needle
Simcoe needle
Sims needle
Singer needle
ski needle
skinny Chiba needle
skinny needle
Sluder needle
Smiley-Williams needle
spatula-split needle
sphenopalatine needle
spinal needle
Spinelli biopsy needle
spring-eye needle
spring-hook wire needle
stab needle
Stamey needle
staphylorrhaphy needle
sternal needle
sternal puncture needle
Stille-Mayo-Hegar
  needle
Stille-Seldinger needle
Stocker cyclodiathermy
  puncture needle
Stocker needle
stop needle

needle *continued*

Storz aspiration biopsy
  needle
Storz flexible injection
  needle
Storz needle cannula
strabismus needle
straight needle
straight suture needle
Strauss needle
Sturmdorf cervical
  needle
Sturmdorf needle
Sturmdorf pedicle
  needle
suction biopsy needle
surgeon's regular needle
surgical needle
Sutton needle
suture needle
suture-release needle
suturing needle
swaged needle
swaged-on needle
Swan knife-needle
Swann-Sheldon needle
Swedgeon already-
  threaded needle
taper needle
Tapercut needle
tapered needle
taper-point needle
taper-point suture needle
tattooing needle
Tauber needle
Teflon needle
Teflon-covered needle
Terry-Mayo needle
THI needle
thin-walled needle
tissue desiccation needle
titanium needle
Titus needle
Todd needle
tonsillar needle
tonsillar suture needle
Travenol biopsy needle
Travenol needle

needle *continued*

    Travert needle
    triple-lumen needle
    trocar needle
    Troutman needle
    Tru-Cut biopsy needle
    Tru-Cut liver biopsy
       needle
    Tru-Cut needle
    Tuohy aortography
       needle
    Tuohy needle
    Tuohy spinal needle
    Turkel liver biopsy
       needle
    Turkel needle
    Turner-Warwick needle
    University of Illinois
       marrow needle
    University of Illinois
       needle
    Updegraff cleft palate
       needle
    Updegraff needle
    uterine needle
    Vacutainer needle
    vacuuming needle
    Veenema-Gusberg
       needle
    Veirs needle
    venipuncture needle
    venous needle
    venting aortic Bengash
       needle
    ventricular needle
    Veress needle
    Veress spring-loaded
       laparoscopy needle
    Veress-Frangenheim
       needle
    Vicat needle
    Vim needle
    Vim-Silverman
       needle
    Visi-Black needle
    Visi-Black surgical
       needle
    Visitec needle

needle *continued*

    Visitec retrobulbar
       needle
    Vogt-Barraquer eye
       needle
    von Graefe iris needle
    von Graefe knife-needle
    von Graefe needle
    Voorhees needle
    Walker needle
    Wang needle
    Wangensteen needle
    Ward-French needle
    Watson-Williams
       needle
    wedge-line needle
    Weeks needle
    Weiss needle
    Welsh olive-tipped
       needle
    Wertheim-Navratil
       needle
    Westerman-Jansen
       needle
    whirlybird needle
    Wiener eye needle
    Wolf antral needle
    Wolf-Veress needle
    Wood needle
    Wooten eye needle
    Wright fascia needle
    Wright needle
    Wright-Crawford
       needle
    Yankauer needle
    Yankauer septal needle
    Yankauer suture needle
    Ziegler iris knife-needle
    Ziegler knife-needle
    Ziegler needle
    Zoellner needle
needle aspiration
needle aspiration biopsy
needle biopsy
needle count
needle electrode
needle extension
needle forceps

needle guide (see also *guide*)
    AFB needle guide
      (aortofemoral bypass
      needle guide)
    Dap II biopsy needle
      guide
    Iowa needle guide
    Iowa trumpet needle
      guide
    Kleegman needle guide
    trumpet needle guide
needle holder (see also *holder*)
    Abbey needle holder
    Adaptic needle holder
    adhesive needle holder
    Adson needle holder
    Aesculap needle holder
    Alabama-Green needle
      holder
    Anchor spring-suture
      needle holder
    angled needle holder
    angular needle holder
    angulated-needle holder
    Anis microsurgical
      needle holder
    Arruga needle holder
    Axhausen needle holder
    Ayers cardiovascular
      needle holder
    Ayers needle holder
    baby needle holder
    Barraquer microneedle
      holder
    Barraquer needle
      holder
    Baum needle holder
    Baum tonsil needle
      holder
    Baumgartner needle
      holder
    Baum-Metzenbaum
      needle holder
    bayonet needle holder
    Berens needle holder
    Berry sternal needle
      holder

needle holder *continued*
    Blair-Brown needle
      holder
    boomerang needle
      holder
    Boyce needle holder
    Boynton needle holder
    Bozeman needle holder
    Bozeman-Finochietto
      needle holder
    Bozeman-Wertheim
      needle holder
    Brown needle holder
    carbide-jaw needle
      holder
    cardiovascular thoracic
      needle holder
    Carroll needle holder
    Castroviejo microneedle
      holder
    Castroviejo needle
      holder
    Castroviejo Vital needle
      holder
    Castroviejo-Barraquer
      needle holder
    Castroviejo-Green needle
      holder
    Castroviejo-Kalt needle
      holder
    Castroviejo-Troutman
      needle holder
    Cohan needle holder
    Collier eye needle holder
    Collier needle holder
    combination forceps/
      needle holder
    combined needle holder
      and scissors
    Converse needle holder
    Converse-Gillies needle
      holder
    Cooley microvascular
      needle holder
    Cooley needle holder
    Cooley Vital microvascu-
      lar needle holder

needle holder *continued*

Corboy needle holder
Cottle needle holder
Crile needle holder
Crile-Murray needle holder
Crile-Wood needle holder
Crile-Wood Vital needle holder
curved needle holder
Davis needle holder
DeBakey cardiovascular needle holder
DeBakey needle holder
DeBakey Vital needle holder
Derf needle holder
Derf Vital needle holder
diamond needle holder
Doyen needle holder
dry needle holder
Eber needle holder
Eiselberg-Mathieu needle holder
Ellis eye needle holder
Ellis Vital needle holder
Elschnig needle holder
Ermold needle holder
eye needle holder
Ferris Smith needle holder
Finochietto needle holder
Finochietto Vital needle holder
Foster needle holder
Foster-Gillies needle holder
French-eye needle holder
French-eye Vital needle holder
Furlow needle holder
Gardner needle holder
Giannini needle holder
Gifford needle holder

needle holder *continued*

Gill needle holder
Gillies needle holder
Gillies-Sheehan needle holder
Grant needle holder
Green eye needle holder
Green needle holder
Grieshaber eye needle holder
Grieshaber needle holder
Hagedorn needle holder
Halsey eye needle holder
Halsey needle holder
Halsey Vital needle holder
Heaney bulldog-jaw needle holder
Heaney needle holder
Hegar needle holder
Hegar-Baumgartner needle holder
Hegar-Mayo-Seeley needle holder
Hodlick needle holder
Hoesel needle holder
Hufnagel needle holder
Hufnagel-Ryder needle holder
intracardiac needle holder
iridium needle holder
Jacobson needle holder
Jacobson spring-handled needle holder
Jacobson Vital needle holder
Jameson needle holder
Jannetta bayonet needle holder
Jannetta needle holder
Johns Hopkins needle holder
Johnson needle holder
Johnson prostatic needle holder
Julian needle holder

needle holder *continued*
Julian Vital needle
holder
K-S adhesive needle
holder
Kalt eye needle holder
Kalt needle holder
Kalt Vital needle holder
Kilner needle holder
Langenbeck needle
holder
Langenbeck-Ryder
needle holder
Lapides needle holder
Lawton microneedle
holder
Lemmon needle holder
Lichtenberg carbide-jaw
needle holder
Lichtenberg needle
holder
Lindley carbide-jaw
needle holder
Lindley needle holder
Lorenz needle holder
Luethy-Beck needle
holder
Malis needle holder
Masson needle holder
Masson-Luethy needle
holder
Masson-Mayo-Hegar
needle holder
Mathieu needle holder
Mathieu-Hevesy needle
holder
Mathieu-Kocher needle
holder
Mathieu-Ryder needle
holder
Mathieu-Stille needle
holder
Mayo needle holder
Mayo-Hegar curved-jaw
needle holder
Mayo-Hegar needle
holder

needle holder *continued*
McAllister needle holder
McPherson needle
holder
Metzenbaum needle
holder
MGH needle holder
Micrins needle holder
microneedle holder
microsurgery needle
holder
microvascular needle
holder
Mobley-Webster needle
holder
nasal needle holder
needle holder
Neivert needle holder
Neivert-Neivert needle
holder
neurosurgical needle
holder
New Orleans needle
holder
O'Brien needle holder
Olsen-Hegar needle
holder
Par-Style needle holder
Paton needle holder
Pilling vascular needle
holder
Pittman needle holder
plastic needle holder
Potts-Smith needle
holder
prostatic needle holder
Quinn needle holder
Randall-Brown needle
holder
Ravich needle holder
Register needle holder
Rienhoff needle holder
Rochester needle holder
Roger needle holder
Ryder needle holder
Sarot cardiovascular
needle holder

needle holder *continued*
- Sarot needle holder
- Sarot petit point needle holder
- Sarot thoracic needle holder
- spring-handled needle holder
- Stevens needle holder
- Stevenson needle holder
- Stille-French needle holder
- Stille-Mathieu needle holder
- Stille-Metzenbaum needle holder
- Storz-Castroviejo needle holder
- Stratte needle holder
- suture needle holder
- Swan eye needle holder
- taper-point needle holder
- TC needle holder
- Tennant needle holder
- Tilderquist eye needle holder
- Tilderquist needle holder
- Toennis needle holder
- tonsillar needle holder
- Troutman needle holder
- Troutman-Barraquer needle holder
- Twisk needle holder
- vascular needle holder
- Vital Cooley microvascular needle holder
- Vital intracardiac needle holder
- Vital needle holder
- Vital Ryder microvascular needle holder
- Voohr needle holder
- Wagner needle holder
- Wangensteen needle holder
- Webster needle holder

needle holder *continued*
- Wertheim needle holder
- Widia needle holder
- wire needle holder
- wire-twister needle holder
- Yasargil needle holder
- Young needle holder
- Young-Millin needle holder
- Zweifel needle holder

needle holder forceps
needle magnet
needle marks
needle puncture
needle site
needle stick
needle-knife
needle-knife sphincterotome
needle-nosed pliers
needlepoint electrocautery
needles-and-pins sensation
needling
needling of cataract
needling of lens
Neef hammer
Neer acromioplasty
Neer classification of shoulder fractures
Neer hemiarthroplasty
Neer I shoulder joint prosthesis
Neer II proximal humerus prosthesis
Neer II shoulder joint prosthesis
Neer II shoulder prosthesis
Neer II shoulder replacement
Neer II total shoulder system implant
Neer prosthesis
Neer resection of acromion
Neer shoulder prosthesis
Neer shoulder replacement prosthesis
Neff meniscus knife
negative biopsy
negative bone scan

negative culture
negative findings
negative pressure
negative reaction
negative results
negligible blood loss
Negus bronchoscope
Negus forceps
Negus mouth gag
Negus-Broyles bronchoscope
Negus-Green forceps
Neibauer hand
Neibauer hand prosthesis
Neibauer prosthesis
Neibauer-Cutter operation
Neibauer-Glynn procedure
Neibauer-King open reduction
Neibauer-Kleinert microscope
Neil-Moore electrode
Neivert double-ended retractor
Neivert hook
Neivert knife
Neivert nasal polyp hook
Neivert needle holder
Neivert polyp hook
Neivert retractor
Neivert snare
Neivert tonsillar snare
Neivert-Eves snare
Neivert-Neivert needle holder
Nélaton ankle dislocation
Nélaton bullet probe
Nélaton catheter
Nélaton dislocation
Nélaton dislocation of ankle
Nélaton fold
Nélaton line
Nélaton operation
Nélaton rubber tube drain
Nélaton sphincter
Nelson first-rib raspatory
Nelson forceps
Nelson general operating
    scissors
Nelson ligature needle
Nelson lung-dissecting forceps
Nelson needle

Nelson retractor
Nelson rib self-retaining
    retractor
Nelson rib spreader
Nelson rib stripper
Nelson Rocker knife
Nelson scissors
Nelson thoracic scissors
Nelson thoracic trocar
Nelson tissue forceps
Nelson trocar
Nelson uterine scissors
Nelson-Bethune rib shears
Nelson-Martin forceps
Nelson-Metzenbaum scissors
Nelson-Roberts stripper
Nembutal anesthetic agent
neocystostomy
neodymium laser
Neoflex bendable knife
Neoflex electrocautery knife
NeoKnife cautery
NeoKnife electrosurgical
    instrument
Neo-Med cautery
neonatal death
neonate
neoplasm
neoplastic
neoplastic disease
neoplastic disorder
neoplastic fracture
neoplastic growth
neoplastic lesion
neoplastic polyp
neoplasty
neoprene dressing
neoprene orthosis
neoprene sleeves
neoprene splint
neoprene support
Neos pacemaker
neosalpingostomy
neostigmine
neostomy
Neo-Synephrine
neo-ureterocystotomy

neovascular
neovascular glaucoma
neovascularization
nephralgia
nephrectomy
nephritic calculus
nephritis
nephroarteriolar sclerosis
nephroblastoma
nephrocapsectomy
nephrocolic ligament
nephrocolopexy
nephrocystanastomosis
nephrogenic ascites
nephrogenic tissue
nephrogram
nephrography
nephrolithiasis
nephrolithotomy
nephrolithotomy forceps
nephrolithotripsy
nephrolumbar ganglion
nephrolysis
nephroma
nephro-omentopexy
nephropathic cardiopathy
nephropathy
nephropexy
nephrophthisis
nephroplasty
nephroptosis
nephropyelolithotomy
nephropyeloplasty
nephropyeloureterostomy
nephrorrhagia
nephrorrhaphy
nephrosclerosis
nephroscope
    Berci-Shore nephroscope
    percutaneous nephro-
      scope
    Storz nephroscope
nephroscopy
nephrosis
nephrosonephritis
nephrosplenopexy
Nephross dialyzer

nephrostomy
nephrostomy catheter
nephrostomy clamp
nephrostomy hook
nephrostomy speculum
nephrostomy tube
nephrotic syndrome
nephrotome plate
nephrotomogram
nephrotomography
nephrotomy
nephrotoxic
nephrotoxicity
nephroureterectomy
nephroureterocystectomy
NER (no evidence of recur-
    rence)
NERD (no evidence of recur-
    rent disease)
nerve
nerve accommodation
nerve action potential
nerve activity
nerve avulsion
nerve block
nerve block anesthesia
nerve bundle
nerve cable graft
nerve cell
nerve cell body
nerve cell fibers
nerve center
nerve compression
nerve cuff
nerve damage
nerve deafness
nerve decompression
nerve deficit
nerve dissection
nerve distribution
nerve endings
nerve entrapment
nerve evulsion
nerve fibers
nerve graft
nerve hook
nerve impingement

nerve implantation
nerve impulse
nerve injury
nerve involvement
nerve locator
nerve monitor
nerve of Grassi
nerve of Latarjet
nerve of pterygoid canal
nerve of Wrisberg
nerve protector
nerve receptors
nerve retractor
nerve root
nerve root laminectomy
    dissector
nerve rootlet
nerve signal
nerve sign
nerve stimulant
nerve stimulation
nerve stimulator (see also
    *stimulator*)
    ACUTENS transcutane-
      ous nerve stimulator
    Concept nerve stimulator
    TCNS (transcutaneous
      nerve stimulator)
    TENS (terminal electrode
      nerve stimulator)
    terminal electrode nerve
      stimulator (TENS)
    TNS (transcutaneous
      nerve stimulator)
    transcutaneous electrical
      nerve stimulator
      (TENS)
    transcutaneous nerve
      stimulator (TCNS, TNS)
nerve sutures
nerve tabes
nerve tissue
nerve tumor
nerve-blocking anesthesia
nervous system
nervous tissues
nervus (*pl.* nervi) (see specific
    nervi)

Nesacaine-CE anesthetic
    agent
Nesbit cystoscope
Nesbit electrotome
Nesbit hemostatic bag
Nesbit operation
Nesbit resection of prostate
Nesbit snare
Nesta stitch sutures
nested nails
nested trocar
net shunt
Nettleship dilator
Nettleship iris repositor
Nettleship-Wilder dilator
Nettleship-Wilder lacrimal
    dilator
Neubauer cannula
Neubauer forceps
Neubauer scissors
Neubauer vitreous micro-
    extractor forceps
Neubeiser splint
Neuber drainage tube
Neuber operation
Neuber tube
Neufeld driver
Neufeld femoral nail plate
Neufeld nail
Neufeld pin
Neufeld plate
Neufeld rolling traction
Neufeld screw
Neufeld tractor
Neumann scissors
Neurain drill
Neurairtome drill
neural
neural apraxia
neural arch defect
neural atrophy
neural canal
neural deafness
neural discharge
neural fold
neural foramen
neural impulse
neural parenchyma

neural pathway
neural prosthesis
neural retinal layer
neural stimuli
neural transmitter
neural tube
neural tube defect
neuraxis irradiation
neurectasia
neurectomy
neurenteric cyst
neurexeresis
neurilemma
neurilemoma
neurinoma
neuroacanthocytosis
neuroanastomosis
neuroblastoma
neurocirculatory asthenia
neurocutaneous syndrome
neurodiagnostic scanner
neuroectodermal tumor
neuroemergency
neuroencephalomyelopathy
neuroepithelial cells
neuroepithelioma
neurofibrillary tangles
neurofibroma
neurofibromatosis
neuroforamina
neurogenic
neuroglia
neurohypophysectomy
neurolemma
neurolemmoma
neuroleptic medication
neurologic, neurological
neurological assessment
neurological complications
neurological defect
neurological deficit
neurological disease
neurological disorder
neurological disturbance
neurological dysfunction
neurological emergency
neurological examination

neurological function
neurological impairment
neurological instability
Neurological Institute elevator
Neurological Institute periosteal
    elevator
neurological scissors
neurological sign
neurological survey
neurological sutures
neurological symptoms
neurological syndrome
neurological trauma
neurologically intact
neurolysis
neuroma
neuromuscular
neuromuscular blocking agents
neuromuscular control
neuromuscular disorder
neuromuscular firing
neuromuscular junction
neuromyography
neuron
neuropathy
neurophysiology
neuroplasty
neuroretinopathy
neurorrhaphy
neurosarcokleisis
NeuroSectOR
NeuroSectOR ultrasound
neurosensory cells
neurosurgery
neurosurgical bur
neurosurgical connector
neurosurgical dissector
neurosurgical dressing forceps
neurosurgical elevator
neurosurgical forceps
neurosurgical headrest
neurosurgical intervention
neurosurgical knife
neurosurgical ligature forceps
neurosurgical light
neurosurgical needle holder
neurosurgical tissue forceps

neurosutures
neurotome
    aponeurotome
    Bradford enucleation
      neurotome
    enucleation neurotome
    Hall neurotome
neurotomy
neurotonic reaction
neurotony
neurotoxic drug
Neuro-Trace instrument
neurotransmitters
neurotripsy
neurotropic
neurotropic atrophy
neurovascular bundle
neurovascular compromise
neutral electrode
neutral position
neutral reaction
neutralization
neutralizing
neutron beam therapy
neutron radiation
neutropenic patient
Neviaser clavicle procedure
Neviaser operation
Neville tracheal prosthesis
Neville tracheobronchial
    prosthesis
Nevins forceps
Nevins tissue forceps
nevoid lesion
nevoid pigmentation
nevus (*pl.* nevi)
nevus cell
Nevyas cystitome
Nevyas drape retractor
New biopsy forceps
new bone formation
New electrode
New England Baptist acetabular
    cup
New England Baptist arthro-
    plasty
New forceps

new growth
New hook
New needle
New Orleans endarterectomy
    stripper
New Orleans Eye and Ear
    forceps
New Orleans Eye and Ear loupe
New Orleans forceps
New Orleans lens loupe
New Orleans loupe
New Orleans needle holder
New Orleans stripper
New scissors
New tissue forceps
New tracheal hook
New tracheal retractor
New tube
New York Eye and Ear cannula
New York Eye and Ear fixation
    forceps
New York Eye and Ear forceps
New York Heart Association
    classification of heart
    disease (I-IV)
New York Hospital electrode
New York Hospital retractor
New York Hospital suction
    tube
New York speculum
newborn (NB)
newborn eyelid retractor
Newell lid retractor
Newhart hook
Newhart incus hook
Newhart mallet
Newington orthosis
Newington plate
Newkirk mouth gag
New-Lambotte osteotome
Newman forceps
Newman hook
Newman knife
Newman needle
Newman plate
Newman proctoscope
Newman rectal injection needle

Nichols prep

Newman tenaculum
Newman tenaculum forceps
Newman uterine tenaculum
Newman uterine tenaculum
    forceps
Newton disk
Newton total ankle system
Newvicon vacuum tube
Nezhat suction-irrigator
ng (nanogram)
NG (nasogastric)
NG aspirate
NG tube
niche
Nichol clamp
Nichol procedure
Nichol rongeur
Nichol speculum
Nichol vaginal suspension
    procedure
Nicholas medial compartment
    reconstruction
Nickel-Perry technique
nicking
Nicola clamp
Nicola gouge
Nicola microforceps
Nicola operation for shoulder
    dislocation
Nicola pituitary rongeur
Nicola raspatory
Nicola shoulder arthroplasty
Nicoll bone graft
Nicoll plate
nidus
Niedner anastomosis clamp
Niedner clamp
Niedner dissecting forceps
Niedner forceps
Niedner knife
Niedner pulmonic clamp
Niedner valvulotome
Niemann splenomegaly
night splint
NightBird nasal CPAP
nightstick fracture
NIH catheter

NIH left ventriculography
    catheter
NIH mitral valve forceps
NIH mitral valve-grasping
    forceps
Nikon camera
Nimbus Hemopump cardiac
    assist device
Nimeh method
ninth cranial nerve (IX)
nipper (see also *nail nipper*)
        anterior crurotomy
            nipper
        crural nipper
        crurotomy nipper
        cuticle nipper
        Dieter nipper
        Dieter-House nipper
        Hough anterior
            crurotomy nipper
        Hough crurotomy nipper
        House-Dieter malleus
            nipper
        House-Dieter nipper
        malleus nipper
        Turnbull nail nipper
        Turnbull nipper
        Wister nipper
nipping at arteriovenous
    crossings
nipple
nipple discharge
nipple everted
nipple marker
nipple plasty
nipple retraction
nipple shadow
nipple site
nipple transposition
nipple valve
nippled stoma
Nipride (sodium nitroprusside)
Niro arch bars
Niro wire-twister forceps
Nirschl fasciotomy
Nirschl procedure
Nirschl technique

Nisbet fixation forceps
Nisentil anesthetic agent
Nissen antireflux operation
Nissen cystic forceps
Nissen forceps
Nissen fundoplication
Nissen fundoplication wrap
Nissen gall duct forceps
Nissen gastrectomy
Nissen hiatal hernia repair
Nissen operation
Nissen procedure
Nissen rib spreader
Nissen sutures
Nissen 360-degree transabdominal fundoplication
Nissen 360-degree wrap fundoplication
nitrogen
nitrous oxide anesthetic agent
Nizetic operation
nl (nanoliter)
nm (nanometer)
no appreciable change
no evidence of disease (NED)
no evidence of recurrence (NER)
no evidence of recurrent disease (NERD)
no line of demarcation
no significant change
no-absorption anesthesia
Nobis aortic occluder
Noble bowel plication
Noble forceps
Noble iris forceps
Noble operation
Noble position
Noble procedure for volvulus
Noble scissors
Noble small bowel plication
Noblock retractor
Noci stimuli needle
Nocito eye implant
nodal arrhythmia
nodal beat
nodal bigeminy

nodal rhythmia
nodal tachycardia
nodal tissue
nodding
node
node dissection
nodose
nodosity
nodoventricular bypass tract
nodular
nodular density
nodular goiter
nodular lesion
nodular liver
nodular thyroid
nodular tumor
nodularity
nodulation
nodule
Noel-Thompson operation
Noiles prosthesis
Noland-Budd cervical curet
Noland-Budd curet
no-loop gastrojejunostomy
non sequitur
nonabsorbable surgical sutures
nonabsorbable sutures
nonabsorbent material
nonaddictive painkillers
nonadhering dressing
nonadhesive dressing
nonbiological signal
noncalcified stone
noncannulated nail
noncaseating granuloma
noncemented component
noncemented prosthesis
noncirrhotic liver
noncommunicating hydrocele
noncompetitive pacemaker
noncompliance
noncompliant patient
nonconductor
nonconstrained knee prosthesis
Non-Contact tonometer
noncontributory history

noncrushing bowel clamp
noncrushing clamp
noncrushing forceps
noncrushing intestinal clamp
noncrushing liver-holding
    clamp
noncrushing pickup forceps
noncrushing tissue-holding
    forceps
noncrushing vascular clamp
noncutting needle
noncutting suture needle
nondeciduous placenta
nondescent of cecum
nondialysis time
nondirective therapy
nondisplaced crack fracture
nondisplaced fracture
nondominant
nonepithelial tumor
noneverting sutures
nonfade scope
nonfenestrated forceps
nonfiberoptic bronchoscopy
nonfilamented form
nonfunctional
nonfunctioning
nonhealing
nonhinged constrained knee
    prosthesis
non-Hodgkin lymphoma
noninflammatory
noninvasive lesion
noninvasive pacemaker
    programming
noninvasive procedure
noninvasive temporary pace-
    maker
noninversion
nonirritating diet
nonlocalized inflammation
nonmagnetic dressing forceps
nonmagnetic forceps
nonmagnetic tissue forceps
nonmalignant tissue
nonmarginal syndesmophytes
nonmarital introitus

nonocclusive mesenteric
    thrombosis
nonpenetrating corneal graft
nonpenetrating keratoplasty
nonpenetrating wound
nonperforating
nonperforating towel clamp
nonpitting edema
nonproductive cough
nonradiating
nonradiating pain
nonradioactive metal pellets
nonrebreathing anesthesia
nonrebreathing valve
nonslipping forceps
nonspecific
nonspecific change
nonspecific gas pattern
nonsterile technique
nonstress test (NST)
nonstriated muscle
nonsynovial joint
nontoothed forceps
nontoxic goiter
nontraumatic cardiac tampo-
    nade
nontraumatizing forceps
nontraumatizing viscera forceps
nonunion
nonunion of fracture
nonvalved graft
nonviable
nonviable scar
nonviable tissue
nonweightbearing (NWB)
nonweightbearing brace
Noon AV fistula clamp
noose sutures
Nordenstrom biopsy needle
Nordson debrider
Norelco mucotome
normal caliber duct
normal condition
normal saline
normal vital sign
normal-appearing mucosa
normally

Norman tibial bolt
Norman tibial nail
Norman tibial pin
normoactive bowel sounds
normoactive bowel tones
normoactive reflexes
normoblast
normocephalic
normophysiological reflexes
Northbent scissors
Northbent suture scissors
North-South retractor
Norton adjustable cup reamer
Norton ball reamer
Norton operation
Norton-Latzko extraperitoneal
    cesarean section
Norwich approach
Norwood forceps
Norwood operation for
    hypoplastic left-sided heart
Norwood rectal snare
Norwood snare
Norwood univentricular heart
    procedure
nosebleed
nose-bridge prosthesis
nosocomial infection
nostril
nostril elevator
notch
notched rotation osteotomy
notched ruler
notched wave
notching of pulmonic valve
notchplasty
Noto dressing forceps
Noto sponge-holding forceps
no-touch technique
Nott speculum
Nott-Guttmann speculum
Nott-Guttmann vaginal specu-
    lum
Nottingham introducer
Nourse syringe
Nova Curve lens
Nova hook

Nova II pacemaker
Novacor LVAD (Novacor left
    ventricular assist device)
Novacor left ventricular assist
    device
Novacor pump
Novafon sound massager
Novak biopsy curet
Novak curet
Novak fixation forceps
Novak uterine suction curet
Novak-Schoeckaert endometrial
    biopsy curet
Novocain anesthetic agent
Novofil sutures
noxious stimulus
Noyes anterior cruciate recon-
    struction
Noyes forceps
Noyes iridectomy scissors
Noyes iris scissors
Noyes nasal-dressing forceps
Noyes punch
Noyes rongeur
Noyes scissors
Noyes speculum
Noyes-Shambaugh alligator
    scissors
Noyes-Shambaugh scissors
NPO (nothing by mouth)
NSR (nasal septal reconstruc-
    tion)
NST (nonstress test)
nuchal cord
nuchal flexure
nuchal ligament
nuchal line
nuchal region
nuchal ridge
nuchal rigidity
nuchofrontal projection
Nuck canal
Nuck diverticulum
Nuck hydrocele
nuclear bleeding scan
nuclear cataract
nuclear imaging

nuclear medicine
nuclear membrane
nuclear pacemaker
nuclear powered pacemaker
nuclear probe
nuclear scanner
nuclei
nucleic acid
nucleoli
nucleotide
Nucleotome diskectomy
    instruments
nucleus
nucleus lateralis of Le Gros
    Clark
nucleus of Gudden
nucleus of Luys
nucleus of Perlia
nucleus of Rose
nucleus pulposus
nuclide
Nuform gauze
Nu-Gauze dressing
Nu-Gauze packing material
Nu-Gauze sponge
Nugent aspirator
Nugent erysiphake
Nugent forceps
Nugent hook
Nugent soft cataract aspirator
Nugent utility forceps
Nugent-Gradle stitch scissors
Nugent-Green-Dimitry erysi-
    phake
Nugowski forceps
Nu-Hope ileostomy pouch
Nuk nipple
NU-KNIT absorbable hemostat
NuKO knee orthosis
nulligravida
Nulling pattern on x-ray
nullipara
nulliparous introitus
nulliparous patient
numbing
numbness

numerous
Nunez approximator
Nunez clamp
Nunez tube
Nunez-Nunez knife
Nunez-Nunez mitral stenosis
    knife
Nupercaine hydrochloride
    anesthetic agent
nursemaid's elbow
nursing care
nursing procedure
Nurulon sutures
Nussbaum clamp
Nussbaum intestinal clamp
Nussbaum intestinal forceps
Nussbaum narcosis
nutcracker esophagus
nutcracker's syndrome
nutmeg liver
Nutraflex Poole tube
Nutricath catheter
nutriciae humeri, arteriae
nutrient arteries of humerus
Nuttall operation
Nuttall retractor
Nu-wrap rolls dressing
NWB (nonweightbearing)
Nycore angiography catheter
Nycore catheter
Nyhus-Nelson gastric decom-
    pression tube
Nyhus-Nelson jejunal feeding
    tube
Nylen-Bárány maneuver
Nylok bolt
Nylok self-locking nail
nylon hand scrub brush
nylon head hammer
nylon head mallet
nylon monofilament sutures
nylon retention sutures
nylon scrub brush
nylon sutures
nylon vascular prosthesis
nystagmograph

# O

OA (occipital artery)
oat cell carcinoma
O'Beirne sphincter
O'Beirne tube
Ober operation
Ober sign
Ober tendon passer
Ober-Barr brachioradialis
	transfer
Oberhill obstetrical forceps
Oberhill retractor
Oberhill self-retaining retractor
Oberst operation
Ober-Young operation
obese abdomen
obliqua atrii sinistri, vena
oblique
oblique amputation
oblique arytenoid muscle
oblique astigmatism
oblique bandage
oblique conus
oblique diameter
oblique film
oblique fissure
oblique fracture
oblique hernia
oblique incision
oblique inguinal hernia
oblique inguinal incision
oblique lateral projection
oblique muscle
oblique popliteal ligament
oblique position
oblique presentation
oblique projection
oblique ramus sliding
	osteotomy
oblique relaxing incision

oblique sinus of pericardium
oblique spot view
oblique study
oblique tendon
oblique vein
oblique view
obliquely contracted pelvis
obliquity
obliquity reflex
obliquus auriculae, musculus
obliquus capitis inferior,
	musculus
obliquus capitis superior,
	musculus
obliquus externus abdominis,
	musculus
obliquus inferior bulbi, muscu-
	lus
obliquus internus abdominis,
	musculus
obliquus, musculus
obliquus superior bulbi,
	musculus
obliterate
obliterated
obliterating
obliteration
obliterative vascular disease
O'Brien airway needle
O'Brien akinesia
O'Brien block
O'Brien cataract
O'Brien forceps
O'Brien foreign body spud
O'Brien hook
O'Brien needle holder
O'Brien rib retractor
O'Brien rongeur
O'Brien spatula

O'Brien suture scissors
O'Brien-Elschnig forceps
obscure
obscured
observation
observed value
obstetric, obstetrical
obstetrical analgesia
obstetrical anesthesia
obstetrical anesthesia needle
obstetrical binder
obstetrical block anesthesia
    needle
obstetrical delivery
obstetrical double-armed
    sutures
obstetrical forceps
obstetrical history
obstetrical hook
obstetrical hysterectomy
obstetrical infection
obstetrical instruments
obstetrical position
obstetrical retractor
obstetrical spoon
obstetrical stirrups
obstetrical surgery
obstetrical traction handle
obstetrical ultrasonography
obstetrics instrument set
obstipated
obstipation
obstructed airway
obstructed labor
obstructed nares
obstructed shunt
obstructed testis
obstructed tube
obstructing
obstructing adhesions
obstructing airway
obstructing lesion
obstructing mass
obstruction
obstructive airway defect
obstructive airway disease
obstructive defect

obstructive disease
obstructive lesion
obstructive problem
obstructive site
obstructive symptoms
obtain (attain)
obtained (attained)
obtunded
obtundity
obturating embolus
obturator
    accessory obturator
    Alcock obturator
    Alcock-Timberlake
        obturator
    atraumatic distending
        obturator
    Beall mitral obturator
    blunt obturator
    concave sheath and
        obturator
    convex sheath and
        obturator
    Cripps obturator
    cystoscope obturator
    deflecting obturator
    Ellik-Shaw obturator
    eyed obturator
    Keene self-sealing sleeve
        and obturator
    Rumel tourniquet eyed
        obturator
    Storz atraumatic distend-
        ing obturator
    Storz deflecting obturator
    Timberlake obturator
    tracheal tube with
        obturator
    ureteral catheter
        obturator
obturator artery
obturator crest
obturator cystoscope
obturator deflecting resecto-
    scope
obturator fascia
obturator foramen

obturator fossa
obturator hernia
obturator membrane
obturator muscle
obturator nerve
obturator resectoscope
obturator sign
obturator test
obturator urethroscope
obturator veins
obturatoria accessoria, arteria
obturatoria, arteria
obturatoriae, venae
obturatorius externus, musculus
obturatorius internus, musculus
obturatorius, nervus
obtuse
obtuse angle
obtuse-angle knife
obviate
Obwegeser channel retractor
Obwegeser incision
Obwegeser osteotomy
Obwegeser periosteal elevator
Obwegeser periosteal retractor
Obwegeser retractor
Obwegeser sagittal mandibular
    osteotomy
Obwegeser splitting chisel
Obwegeser stripper
occasional
occipital artery
occipital bone
occipital crest
occipital diploic vein
occipital emissary vein
occipital foramen
occipital fracture
occipital lobe
occipital muscle
occipital nerve
occipital protuberance
occipital region
occipital segment
occipital sinus
occipital spur
occipital suture

occipital triangle
occipital vein
occipitalis, arteria
occipitalis major, nervus
occipitalis minor, nervus
occipitalis tertius, nervus
occipitalis, vena
occipitoanterior position
occipitoatlantal articulation
occipitofrontal circumference
occipitofrontal diameter
occipitofrontal muscle
occipitofrontalis, musculus
occipitomastoid suture
occipitomastoid suture lines
occipitomental diameter
occipitoparietal suture
occipitoposterior position
occipitosacral position
occipitosphenoidal suture
occipitotemporal convolution
occipitotransverse position
occiput posterior
occlude
occluded blood vessel
occluded duct
occluded fistula
occluded intracranial vessel
occluder
        aorta occluder
        aortic occluder
        eye occluder
        Florester vascular
            occluder
        Heishima balloon
            occluder
        Nobis aortic occluder
occluding clamp
occluding forceps
occluding fracture frame
occluding ligature
occlusal contact
occlusal guide
occlusal harmony
occlusal level
occlusal mold
occlusal pattern

occlusal position
occlusal pressure
occlusal rest bar
occlusal surface
occlusion
occlusion catheter
occlusion clamp
occlusion forceps
occlusion multipurpose clamp
occlusive
occlusive balloon
occlusive disease
occlusive dressing
occlusive ileus
occult
occult blood
occult cancer
occult compression injury
occult fracture
occult infection
occult lesion
occurrence
occurring
OCG (oral cholecystogram)
Ochsenbein gingivectomy
Ochsner artery clamp
Ochsner artery forceps
Ochsner clamp
Ochsner ether inhaler
Ochsner flexible spiral gallstone
    probe
Ochsner forceps
Ochsner gallbladder trocar
Ochsner gallbladder tube
Ochsner gallstone probe
Ochsner hemostat
Ochsner malleable retractor
Ochsner muscle
Ochsner position
Ochsner probe
Ochsner retractor
Ochsner ring
Ochsner scissors
Ochsner thoracic clamp
Ochsner treatment
Ochsner trocar
Ochsner tube

Ochsner-DeBakey crusher
Ochsner-DeBakey spur crusher
Ochsner-Favoloro self-retaining
    retractor
Ockerblad clamp
Ockerblad forceps
Ockerblad ureter technique
OCL (Orthopedic Casting
    Laboratory)
OCL bowel prep
OCL splinting and casting
    system
o'clock position (1 through 12)
O'Connell suture
O'Connor biopsy forceps
O'Connor clamp
O'Connor depressor
O'Connor double-edge curet
O'Connor eye forceps
O'Connor finger cup
O'Connor forceps
O'Connor grasping forceps
O'Connor hex probe knife
O'Connor hook
O'Connor hook scissors
O'Connor left-curve knife
O'Connor lid clamp
O'Connor meniscotomy knife
O'Connor operating arthroscope
O'Connor operating scope
O'Connor operation
O'Connor probe knife
O'Connor retractor
O'Connor retrograde knife
O'Connor right-curve knife
O'Connor sheath
O'Connor straight knife
O'Connor tenotomy hook
O'Connor-Elschnig fixation
    forceps
O'Connor-O'Sullivan retractor
O'Connor-O'Sullivan self-
    retaining retractor
O'Connor-Peter operation
ocrylate
ocular adnexa
ocular ballottement

ocular cautery
ocular cup
ocular fundi
ocular globe
ocular muscle
ocular nerve
ocular pressure
ocular prosthesis
ocular refraction
ocular region
ocular tendon
ocular tension
ocular tremor
ocular vesicle
oculogram
oculomotor nerve (cranial
    nerve III)
oculomotor nerve sign
oculomotor sulcus
oculomotorius, nervus
ocutome
ocutome vitrector
ocutome vitreous blade
Oddi muscle
Oddi sphincter
Odland ankle prosthesis
Odman-Ledin catheter
O'Donaghue knee splint
O'Donaghue splint
O'Donaghue stirrup splint
O'Donahue ligature passer
O'Donahue suture passer
O'Donoghue cotton cast
O'Donoghue dressing
O'Donoghue facetectomy
O'Donoghue operation
O'Donoghue procedure
O'Donoghue triad
odontectomy
odontexesis
odontogenic tumor
odontoid process
odontoma
odontoplasty
odontoscopy
odontotomy
O'Dwyer intubation

O'Dwyer intubation tube
OEC forearm splint
OEC hip prosthesis
OEC knee immobilizer
OEC wrist splint
Oertli knife
Oertli lid retractor
Oertli razor bladebreaker knife
Oertli sutures
OES colonoscope
Oettingen abdominal retractor
Oettingen abdominal self-
    retaining retractor
off-center
offset hand retractor
offset hinge prosthesis
offset reamer
offset reverse dome bunion-
    ectomy (ORD bunionec-
    tomy)
O'Gawa irrigating cannula
O'Gawa-Castroviejo forceps
Ogden classification of fractures
Ogilvie femoral herniorrhaphy
Ogilvie herniorrhaphy
Ogilvie operation
Ogston operation
Ogston-Luc operation
Ogura cartilage forceps
Ogura forceps
Ogura fossa
Ogura operation
Ogura saw
Ogura technique
Ogura tissue forceps
Oh femoral component
OH pressurizer (Oxy-Hood
    pressurizer)
O'Hanlon forceps
O'Hanlon gastrointestinal clamp
O'Hanlon intestinal clamp
O'Hanlon-Poole tube
O'Hara forceps
O'Hara operation
O'Harris-Petruso cup
O'Harris-Petruso ring
OHD (organic heart disease)

Ohio Bubble humidifier
Ohio critical care ventilator
Ohio Hope resuscitator
Ohio resuscitation unit
Ohio Vortex respiration monitor
Ohmeda 6200 CO2 monitor
ohmmeter
oiled silk dressing
oiled silk sutures
oiler tip
ointment
ointment box
Olbert balloon catheter
Olbert balloon dilatation
    catheter
old fracture
old infarct
old scarring
Oldberg brain retractor
Oldberg dissector
Oldberg forceps
Oldberg intervertebral disk
    rongeur
Oldberg pituitary rongeur
Oldberg retractor
Oldberg rongeur
O'Leary gastroplasty
olecranon
olecranon bursa
olecranon fossa
olecranon ligament
olecranon process
olecranon spur
oleoarthrosis
oleothorax
olfactorii, nervi
olfactory
olfactory bulb
olfactory glands
olfactory membrane
olfactory nerve (cranial nerve I)
olfactory nerve sign
olfactory tract
oligoclonal band
olisthetic vertebra
olivary catheter
olivary dilator

olive
    expandable olive
    metal olive
    palpable pyloric olive
    Sippy dilating olive
olive dilator
olive ring
olive tip
olive wire
Olivecrona aneurysm clamp
Olivecrona aneurysm clip
Olivecrona aneurysm forceps
Olivecrona brain spatula
Olivecrona clip
Olivecrona clip-applying
    forceps
Olivecrona dissector
Olivecrona double-ended
    dissector
Olivecrona dura scissors
Olivecrona endaural rongeur
Olivecrona forceps
Olivecrona guillotine scissors
Olivecrona mastoid rongeur
Olivecrona rongeur
Olivecrona saw
Olivecrona scissors
Olivecrona silver clip
Olivecrona spatula
Olivecrona trigeminus knife
Olivecrona-Stille dissector
Olivecrona-Toennis clip-
    applying forceps
Oliver retractor
Oliver scalp retractor
olives passed over guide wire
olive-tip, olive-tipped
olive-tipped bougie
olive-tipped stripper
olivocerebellar tract
olivocochlear bundle of
    Rasmussen
olivopontocerebellar atrophy
Ollier graft
Ollier incision
Ollier layer
Ollier operation

Ollier raspatory
Ollier retractor
Ollier-Murphy approach in hip
    arthroplasty
Ollier-Thiersch graft
Ollier-Thiersch implant
Ollier-Thiersch operation
Ollier-Thiersch prosthesis
Olliger splint
Olschevksy tube
Olsen-Hegar needle holder
Olshausen operation
Olshausen sign
Olympic mask
Olympus alligator-jaw endo-
    scopic forceps
Olympus angioscope
Olympus basket-type endo-
    scopic forceps
Olympus biopsy forceps
Olympus bronchoscope
Olympus choledochofiberscope
Olympus colonoscope
Olympus cystoscope
Olympus duodenofiberscope
Olympus duodenoscope
Olympus endoscope
Olympus endoscopic biopsy
    forceps
Olympus esophagofiberscope
Olympus esophagoscope
Olympus FBK 13 endoscopic
    biopsy forceps
Olympus fiberoptic broncho-
    scope
Olympus fiberoptic sigmoido-
    scope
Olympus fiberscope
Olympus flexible ENT scope
Olympus flexible sigmoido-
    scope
Olympus gastrocamera
Olympus gastroscope
Olympus GIF-XQ fiberoptic
    instrument
Olympus heat probe
Olympus hot biopsy forceps

Olympus lithotriptor
Olympus magnetic extractor
    forceps
Olympus microscope
Olympus minisnare forceps
Olympus monopolar cannula
Olympus needle-knife papillo-
    tome
Olympus operating camera
Olympus panendoscope
Olympus pelican-type endo-
    scopic forceps
Olympus rat-tooth endoscopic
    forceps
Olympus rubber-tip endoscopic
    forceps
Olympus scope
Olympus shark-tooth endo-
    scopic forceps
Olympus sigmoidoscope
Olympus sphincterotome
Olympus tripod-type endo-
    scopic forceps
Olympus ureterorenofiberscope
Olympus W-shaped endoscopic
    forceps
Olympus-Iglesias system
O'Malley knife
O'Malley ocutome
O'Malley self-adhering lens
    implant
O'Malley-Heinz cutter
Ombrédanne forceps
Ombrédanne mallet
Ombrédanne operation
Omega compression hip screw
    system
Omega screw
omega-shaped incision
omental
omental adhesions
omental adhesive band
omental band
omental bursa
omental cake
omental cyst
omental enterocleisis

omental graft
omental hernia
omental recess
omental studding
omentectomy
omentofixation
omentopexy
omentoplasty
omentorrhaphy
omentosplenopexy
omentotomy
omentum
omentum majus
omentum minus
omentumectomy
Omer sternoclavicular dislocation
Omer technique
Omer-Capen carpectomy
Ommaya cerebrospinal fluid reservoir
Ommaya intraventricular reservoir system
Ommaya reservoir
Ommaya reservoir prosthesis
Ommaya reservoir transensor
Ommaya shunt
Ommaya tube
Omni catheter
Omni knee brace
Omni operating microscope
Omni plate CHS system (compression hip screw system)
Omni retractor
Omni-Atricor pacemaker
Omnicarbon prosthetic valve
Omnicor pacemaker
Omnicor programmer
Omni-Ectocor pacemaker
Omnifit intraocular lens
Omniflex balloon catheter
Omni-Flow infusion system
Omni-Orthocor pacemaker
Omni-Park eyelid speculum
OmniPhase semirigid penile prosthesis

Omniscience heart valve
Omniscience prosthetic valve
Omniscience tilting-disk valve
Omni-Stanicor pacemaker
Omni-Theta pacemaker
Omnivac splint
Omni-Ventricor pacemaker
omoclavicular triangle
omohyoid muscle
omohyoideus, musculus
omphalectomy
omphalelcosis
omphalic
omphalocele
omphalomesenteric duct
omphalomesenteric veins
omphalomesenteric vessels
omphalospinous line
omphalotomy
oncogenic virus
oncologic anatomy
oncotic pressure
oncotomy
One Time skin stapler
One Time staple remover
on-edge mattress sutures
one-horn bridge
O'Neill cardiac clamp
O'Neill clamp
O'Neill scissors
one-piece ostomy pouch
one-sheet pack
one-sixth molar lactate solution
one-snip punctum operation
one-stage operation
one-stage pancreatoduodenectomy
one-vessel angioplasty
ongoing surveillance
onlay bone graft
onlay bone patch
onlay cortical graft
onlay Dacron prosthesis
onlay graft
onset
on-table angiogram
onychauxis

onychectomy
onychia
onychocryptosis
onychogryphosis
onychomycosis
onychoplasty
onychorrhexis
onychotomy
oophorectomy
oophoretic cyst
oophorocystectomy
oophorohysterectomy
oophoropexy
oophoroplasty
oophorrhaphy
oophorosalpingectomy
oophorostomy
oophorotomy
oothecectomy
ooze
oozing
opacification
opacifying
opacity
opaque
opaque arthrography
opaque calculus
opaque material
opaque medium
opaque microscope
opaque shadows
open airway
open amputation
open anesthesia
open biopsy
open bite
open dislocation
open drainage
open drop anesthesia
open endotracheal inhalation
    anesthesia
open fistula
open fracture
open heart
open heart surgery
open inhalation anesthesia

open lens
open mitral commissurotomy
open oblique osteotomy
open operation
open perineal biopsy
open reduction
open reduction and fixation
open reduction and internal
    fixation (ORIF)
open reduction of dislocation
open reduction of fracture
open reduction of fracture-
    dislocation
open reduction with internal
    fixation (ORIF)
open technique
open thimble splint
open valvulotomy
open wound
open-angle glaucoma
open-end aspirating tube
open-end ostomy pouch
opening ABD wedge bunionec-
    tomy
opening snap
opening wedge
opening wedge osteotomy
open-patch technique
open-sky technique
open-sky vitrectomy
opera-glass hand
operable
operable cancer
operable case
operating esophagoscope
operating gastroscope
operating knife
operating microscope
operating otoscope
operating room (OR)
operating room supervisor
operating scissors
operating scope
operating suite
operating table
operating telescope

operating voltage
operation
operation drape
operation microscope drape
operative
operative amputation
operative damage
operative delivery
operative field
operative findings
operative incision
operative intervention
operative procedure
operative repair
operative scar
operative site
operative suite
operative surgery
operative therapy
operative wound
operator's stool
opercular fold
operculectomy
operculum (*pl.* opercula)
Ophthaine anesthetic agent
Ophthalas laser
ophthalmectomy
ophthalmia
ophthalmic artery
ophthalmic calipers
ophthalmic cautery
ophthalmic cautery electrode
ophthalmic cup
ophthalmic irrigator
ophthalmic knife
ophthalmic lamp
ophthalmic nerve
ophthalmic ointment
ophthalmic pick
ophthalmic plexus
ophthalmic recurrent nerve
ophthalmic sable brush
ophthalmic tumor
ophthalmic ultrasonography
ophthalmic vein
ophthalmic vesicle

ophthalmica, arteria
ophthalmica inferior, vena
ophthalmica superior, vena
ophthalmicus, nervus
ophthalmodynamometer
    Bailliart ophthalmo-
        dynamometer
    dial-type ophthalmo-
        dynamometer
    Dynoptor ophthalmo-
        dynamometer
    electronic ophthalmo-
        dynamometer
    Reichert ophthalmo-
        dynamometer
    suction ophthalmo-
        dynamometer
ophthalmodynamometry
ophthalmomeningea, vena
ophthalmomeningeal vein
ophthalmometer
ophthalmoplegia
ophthalmoscope
    auto-ophthalmoscope
    binocular ophthalmo-
        scope
    direct ophthalmoscope
    Friedenwald ophthalmo-
        scope
    Ful-Vue ophthalmoscope
    ghost ophthalmoscope
    Gullstrand ophthalmo-
        scope
    halogen ophthalmoscope
    indirect ophthalmoscope
    Keeler ophthalmoscope
    Keeler polarizing
        ophthalmoscope
    Loring ophthalmoscope
    luminous ophthalmo-
        scope
    May ophthalmoscope
    Morton ophthalmoscope
    Propper ophthalmoscope
    reflecting ophthalmo-
        scope

ophthalmoscope *continued*
    Reichert Ful-Vue
      ophthalmoscope
    Schepens binocular
      indirect ophthalmo-
      scope
    Schepens indirect
      ophthalmoscope
    Schepens ophthalmo-
      scope
    Welch Allyn ophthalmo-
      scope
    Zeiss-Opton ophthalmo-
      scope
ophthalmoscope camera
ophthalmoscopic examination
ophthalmoscopy
ophthalmotomy
opisthotonos position
OPMI operating microscope
OPMI-6 operating microscope
Oppenheim brace
Oppenheimer splint
Op-Pneu laparoscopy needle
opponens digiti minimi manus,
    musculus
opponens pollicis, musculus
opponens splint
opponensplasty
opposing margin
opposing muscle
opposing portal
opposing vocal cord
opposite side
oppressive pain
Opraflex drape
Opraflex incise drape
Op-Site dressing
Op-Site occlusive dressing
Optacon
Op-Temp cautery
optic, optical
optic axis
optic canal
optic center
optic chiasm
optic commissure

optic cup
optic disk
optic foramen
optic ganglion
optic iridectomy
optic nerve (cranial nerve II)
optic papilla
optic radiation
optic recess
optic tract
optic vesicle
optical biopsy forceps
optical cavity
optical density
optical esophagoscope
optical iridectomy
optical laryngoscope
optical stylet
opticociliary neurectomy
opticociliary neurotomy
opticociliary vessels
opticomalacia
opticostriate region
opticus, nervus
Opti-Fix acetabular component
Opti-Fix femoral component
Opti-Fix porous coated hip
    system
Opti-Fix titanium hip system
Optiflex intraocular lens
Optiflex lens
Optima bipolar pulse generator
Optima pacemaker
Optima pulse generator
optimal diastolic pressure
optimal dose
optimum
option
optional
Optiscope angioscope
Optiscope catheter
OR (operating room)
OR cart
ora
ora serrata
oral agent
oral analgesic

oral anesthesia
oral antibiotic
oral cancer
oral cavity
oral cholecystogram
oral contents
oral contraceptive
oral dose
oral drug
oral endotracheal tube
oral fistula
oral forceps
oral intubation
oral mucosa
oral panendoscope
oral passages
oral restorative surgery
oral rongeur forceps
oral route
oral screw mouth gag
oral screw tongue depressor
oral secretions
oral speculum mouth gag
oral surgery
oral surgery rongeur
oral temperature
oral tissues
oral urogram
oral urography
Orandi blade
Orban curet
orbicular alignment
orbicular incision
orbicular muscle
orbicular ring
orbicularis block
orbicularis oculi, musculus
orbicularis oris, musculus
orbit
orbital abscess
orbital akinesia
orbital bone
orbital canal
orbital cavity
orbital contents
orbital enucleation compressor
orbital exenteration

orbital fissure
orbital fistula
orbital floor
orbital floor implant
orbital floor prosthesis
orbital fracture reduction
orbital implant
orbital margin
orbital muscle
orbital operculum
orbital plate
orbital projections
orbital prosthesis
orbital retractor
orbital ridge
orbital rim
orbital septum
orbitalis, musculus
orbitomeatal plane
orbitopathy
orbitotomy
ORC anterior chamber intra-
    ocular lens
ORC posterior chamber
    intraocular lens implant
orchectomy (orchiectomy
    preferred)
orchidectomy
orchidoepididymectomy
orchidopexy
orchidoplasty
orchidorrhaphy
orchidotomy
orchiectomy
orchiopexy
orchioplasty
orchiorrhaphy
orchiotomy
orchipexy
orchiplasty
orchotomy
ORD bunionectomy (offset
    reverse dome bunionec-
    tomy)
Ord operation
orderly
Oregon prosthesis

Oregon tunneler
Oretorp meniscectomy knife
organ
organ bank
organ donation
organ donor
organ exenteration
organ failure
organ graft
organ of Corti
organ of Zuckerkandl
organ rejection
organ sharing
organ source
organ transplant
organ viability
organic disease
organic disorder
organic dysfunction
organic heart disease (OHD)
organic lesion
organic murmur
organic origin
organic pain
organic stricture
organically impaired brain
    function
organism
organizing hemorrhagic cyst
organizing thrombus
organoid
organomegaly
organoscopy
Orgen SpF spinal bone growth
    stimulator
orientation
ORIF (open reduction and
    internal fixation)
orifice
origin
original incision
original tumor site
originating infection
Orion pacemaker
Oris pin
Orlon vascular prosthesis
oroantral fistula

orocutaneous fistula
orogastric tube
oronasal fistula
oropharyngeal airway
oropharyngeal carcinoma
oropharyngeal pack
oropharynx
oropharynx pack
orotracheal intubation
orotracheal tube
Orr forceps
Orr gall duct forceps
Orr incision
Orr method
Orr technique
Orr treatment
Orr-Loygue proctopexy
Orr-Loygue transabdominal
    proctopexy
Orsi-Grocco method
Orthair bunionectomy instru-
    ments
Orthair orthopedic instruments
Orthair oscillating saw
Orthairtome II drill
Ortho All-Flex diaphragm
Ortho Tech cock-up wrist splint
orthocardiac reflex
Orthocor II pacemaker
orthodontic appliance
orthodontic band
Orthofix external fixation device
Orthoflex dressing
Orthoflex elastic plaster
    bandage
Orthofuse implantable growth
    stimulator
OrthoGen bone growth
    stimulator
orthognathic surgery
Ortho-last splint
Ortholav irrigation and suction
    device
Ortholoc IM instrumentation
Ortholoc prosthesis
Orthomedics brace
Ortho-Mesh

Ortho-Mold spinal brace
OrthoPak bone growth stimula-
    tor
orthopedic
orthopedic drill
orthopedic hardware
orthopedic mallet
orthopedic strap clavicle splint
orthopedic surgery
orthopedic table
orthopedic wrench
orthopelvimetry
Orthoplast dressing
Orthoplast fracture brace
Orthoplast jacket
orthoplastic rhinoplasty
orthopnea
orthopnea position
orthoroentgenogram
orthoroentgenography
orthosis
orthostatic
orthostatic drainage
orthostatic dyspnea
orthostatic hypotension
orthostatic lines
orthostatic tachycardia
orthotherapy
orthotic
orthotic attachment implant
orthotic device
orthotonos position
orthotopic cardiac transplant
orthotopic liver transplantation
orthotopic transplant
orthotopic transplantation
Orthotron machine
Ortolani click
Ortved dislodger
os (*pl.* ossa)
os calcis
os cuboideum
os epitympanicum
os ethmoidale
os frontale
os hyoideum
os interparietale

os lacrimale
os lunatum
os magnum
os mastoideum
os nasale
os occipitale
os odontoideum
os orbiculare
os palatinum
os parietale
os penis
os pubis
os pubis spline
os sphenoidale
os temporale
os trigonum
os triquetrum
os unguis
os uteri
os vesalianum pedis
os zygomaticum
Osbon ErecAid system
Osbon technique for impotence
Osborne lesion of elbow
Osborne ligament
Osborne operation
Osborne osteotomy plate
Osborne-Cotterill elbow
    procedure
oscillating nystagmus
oscillating saw
oscillating sternotomy saw
oscillation
oscillatory saw
oscillometrics
oscillometry
Oscor pacemaker
Osgood operation
Osgood supracondylar
    osteotomy of femur
Osgood-Schlatter disease
O'Shaughnessy clamp
O'Shaughnessy forceps
Osher lens
Osher lid retractor
Osher-Fenzel hook
Osler nodes

Osler triad
osmolarity of blood
Osmond-Clarke foot procedure
Osmond-Clarke shoulder
    operation
osmosis
osmostat
osmotic pressure
osseointegration process
osseotendinous
osseous
osseous abnormality
osseous graft
osseous implant
osseous labyrinth
osseous metastasis
osseous portion
osseous spiral lamina
osseous structures
osseous tissue
ossicle
ossicle-holding forceps
ossicular chain
ossicular chain replacement
    prosthesis
ossicular replacement prosthesis
ossiculectomy
ossiculotomy
ossification
ossification centers
ossified edge
Ossof-Sisson surgical stent
ostectomy
ostectomy plate
osteoarthritic changes
osteoarthritic lipping
osteoarthrotomy
osteoblastic lesion
osteocartilaginous body
osteocartilaginous growth
osteochondral exostosis
osteochondral junction
osteochondrodystrophy
osteochondrosis
osteoclasis
osteoclast
    Collin osteoclast

osteoclast *continued*
        Phelps-Gocht osteo-
            clast
        Rizzoli osteoclast
osteoclasty
osteodensitometry
OsteoGen
OsteoGen bone growth
    stimulator
osteogenesis
osteogenic
osteoid
osteological preparation
osteolysis
osteolytic calvarial lesion
osteoma
osteomalacia
osteomeatal sinus tract
Osteone air drill
Osteonics femoral component
Osteonics hip prosthesis
Osteonics prosthesis
Osteonics system
osteoperiosteal bone graft
osteoperiosteal graft
osteophyte
osteophyte elevator
osteophyte formation
osteoplastic amputation
osteoplastic craniotomy
osteoplastic flap
osteoplastic flap clamp
osteoplastic frontal sinus
    operation
osteoplastic necrotomy
osteoplastic rhinoplasty
osteoplasty
osteoporotic compression
    fracture
osteorrhaphy
osteospongioma
Osteostim apparatus
Osteostim electrical bone
    growth stimulator
Osteostim prosthesis
osteosuture
osteosynthesis

osteotome (see also *periosteo-tome*)

A-O osteotome
alar osteotome
Alexander costal periosteotome
Alexander osteotome
Alexander perforating osteotome
Alexander periosteo-tome
Alexander-Farabeuf costal periosteotome
Alexander-Farabeuf periosteotome
Amico osteotome
Anderson-Neivert osteotome
Andrews osteotome
Army osteotome
Army-pattern osteotome
articular osteotome
articulation osteotome
baby costal periosteo-tome
Bakelite-handled osteotome
Ballenger periosteotome
Barsky osteotome
bayonet osteotome
beat-up osteotome
Blount osteotome
Blount scoliosis osteo-tome
Bowen osteotome
Box osteotome
Brophy periosteotome
Brown periosteotome
Buck osteotome
Campbell osteotome
Carroll osteotome
Carroll-Legg osteotome
Carroll-Smith-Petersen osteotome
Cavin osteotome
Cherry osteotome
chisel-osteotome

osteotome *continued*

Cinelli guarded osteo-tome
Cinelli osteotome
Clayton osteotome
Cloward osteotome
Cloward spinal fusion osteotome
Cobb osteotome
Compere osteotome
Converse guarded osteotome
Converse osteotome
costal periosteotome
Cottle chisel osteotome
Cottle osteotome
Cottle-Medicon osteo-tome
Crane osteotome
Cross osteotome
crossbar chisel-osteo-tome
Dautrey osteotome
Dautrey-Munro osteo-tome
Dean periosteotome
Dileant osteotome
Dingman osteotome
Duray-Read osteotome
Duray-Ward osteotome
Epstein osteotome
Ferris Smith-Lyman periosteotome
Fomon osteotome
Fomon periosteotome
Frazier osteotome
Freer periosteotome
French-pattern osteo-tome
guarded osteotome
hand surgery osteotome
hexagonal handle osteotome
Hibbs osteotome
Hohmann osteotome
Hoke osteotome
Hough osteotome

osteotome *continued*

Howorth osteotome
Jansen periosteotome
Joseph periosteotome
Kazanjian osteotome
Kezerian osteotome
Lahey Clinic osteotome
Lahey osteotome
Lambotte osteotome
Lambotte-Henderson
   osteotome
Legg osteotome
Leinbach osteotome
Lexer osteotome
MacGregor osteotome
Mathews osteotome
Mayfield bayonet
   osteotome
Mayfield osteotome
McIndoe osteotome
Meyerding osteotome
MGH osteotome
Micro-Aire osteotome
Miner osteotome
Moberg osteotome
Moorehead periosteo-
   tome
nasal chisel-osteo-
   tome
nasal osteotome
New-Lambotte osteo-
   tome
Parkes osteotome
perforating osteotome
periosteotome
Potts periosteotome
Read osteotome
Rish osteotome
Roos osteotome
rotosteotome
Rowland osteotome
Rubin osteotome
scoliosis osteotome
Sheehan osteotome
Shepard osteotome
Silver osteotome
Simmons osteotome
single-guarded osteo-
   tome

osteotome *continued*

slotting-bur osteotome
Smith-Petersen osteo-
   tome
Speer periosteotome
spinal fusion osteotome
Stille osteotome
Stille-pattern osteotome
Stryker impact osteotome
Swiss-pattern osteotome
thin osteotome
U.S. Army osteotome
U.S. Army-pattern
   osteotome
Vaughan periosteotome
vomer osteotome
West osteotome
West-Beck periosteo-
   tome
Wood osteotome
osteotomized
osteotomy
osteotomy nail
osteotomy pin
osteotomy plate
osteotribe (see *rasp*)
osteotripsy
osteotrite
ostial
Ostic plaster dressing
ostium (*pl.* ostia)
ostomy
ostomy appliance
ostomy bag
Ostrom antral punch
Ostrom antrum punch-tip
   forceps
Ostrom forceps
Ostrom nose punch
Ostrom punch
Ostrum punch forceps
Ostrup vascularized rib graft
O'Sullivan operation
O'Sullivan retractor
O'Sullivan-O'Connor abdominal
   retractor
O'Sullivan-O'Connor retractor
O'Sullivan-O'Connor self-
   retaining retractor

O'Sullivan-O'Connor specu-
lum
O'Sullivan-O'Connor vaginal
retractor
O'Sullivan-O'Connor vaginal
speculum
Oswestry staples
Osypka atrial lead
otectomy
otic depression
otic ganglion
otic shunt
Otis bougie à boule
Otis bougie à boule dilator
Otis bulb cystoscope
Otis meatotome
Otis proctoscope
Otis prostatic urethral sound
Otis urethral sound
Otis urethrotome
Otis urological bougie
Otis-Brown cystoscope
otitis externa
otitis interna
otitis media
Otlinger technique
otogenous
otogenous pyemia
Oto-Microscope
Oto-mid permanent ventilation
tube
otonecrectomy
otopexy
otopharyngeal tube
otoplasty
otosclerectomy
otoscleronectomy
otosclerosis
otosclerotic fixation
otosclerotic process
otoscope
Bruening otoscope
Bruening pneumatic
otoscope
Brunton otoscope
diagnostic otoscope
fiberoptic otoscope
halogen otoscope

otoscope *continued*
Jako suspension
otoscope
operating otoscope
pneumatic otoscope
Politzer otoscope
Siegle otoscope
Welch Allyn otoscope
otoscopic examination
otoscopy
ototome drill
Ottenheimer common duct
dilator
Ottenheimer dilator
Otto Barkan Bident retractor
Otto forceps
Otto pelvis
Ottoback knee prosthesis
Ouchterlony technique
outcome
outcropping of lesions
outer aspect
outer border
outer canthus
outer convexity
outer interrupted silk sutures
outer layer
outer rim
outer surface
outer table bones of skull
outer table graft
outer table of frontal bone
outer table of skull
Outerbridge ridge
Outerbridge scale
Outerbridge uterine dilator
outermost
outermost covering
outermost layer
outflow
outflow cardiac patch
outflow tract
outfolding
outfracture
outgoing
outlay operation
outlet
outlet cannula

outlet forceps
outlet forceps delivery
outlet narrowing
outlet obstruction
outlet occlusion
outline
outlining
out-of-body surgery
outpatient
output
output device
outrigger splint
outrigger wrist splint
outside diameter
outward movement
outward rotation
OV-1 surgical keratometer
ova (*sing.* ovum)
oval amputation
oval cup forceps
oval esophagoscope
oval incision
oval knife
oval niche
oval speculum
oval window
oval-form colonic groove
oval-shaped
oval-window curet
oval-window excavator
oval-window hook
ovarian
ovarian abscess
ovarian artery
ovarian calculus
ovarian cancer
ovarian carcinoma
ovarian cycle
ovarian cyst
ovarian cystectomy
ovarian duct
ovarian fimbria
ovarian follicle
ovarian fossa
ovarian hernia
ovarian ligament
ovarian mass
ovarian plexus

ovarian pregnancy
ovarian stroma
ovarian trocar
ovarian tube
ovarian tumor
ovarian vein
ovarica, arteria
ovarica dextra, vena
ovarica sinistra, vena
ovariectomy
ovarioabdominal pregnancy
ovariocentesis
ovariosalpingectomy
ovary
overall alignment
overall assessment
overall size
over-and-out cheek flap
over-and-over sutures
over-and-over whip sutures
overdevelopment
overdistention
overdosage
overdose
overdosed patient
overdosing
overdrive atrial pacing
overexposure
overflow outlet
overgrafting
overgrowth
overhang
Overhauser effect on x-ray
overhead fracture frame
overhead light
overheated
Overholt double-ended elevator
Overholt elevator
Overholt forceps
Overholt needle
Overholt operation
Overholt periosteal elevator
Overholt raspatory
Overholt retractor
Overholt spreader
Overholt thoracic forceps
Overholt-Finochietto rib
     spreader

Overholt-Geissendoerfer
    dissecting forceps
Overholt-Jackson bronchoscope
Overholt-Mixter dissecting
    forceps
overlap
overlapping closure
overlapping sutures
overlay
overload
overlying
overlying skin
overriding aorta
overripe cataract
oversensing pacemaker
oversew
oversewn
overstimulation
Overstreet endometrial polyp
    forceps
Overstreet forceps
Overstreet polyp forceps
over-the-top cruciate repair
Overton shunt
Overton spinal fusion
overtransfusion
overture
overuse
oviduct
oviductal pregnancy
ovoid
        Delclos ovoid
        Henschke ovoid
ovoid outline
ovoid packing
ovoid radium application
ovulating
ovulation cycle
ovulatory menstruation
ovule
ovum (*pl.* ova)
ovum forceps
Owen catheter
Owen cloth dressing
Owen gauze dressing
Owen operation
Owen position

Owen rayon gauze
Owen sutures
Owen view
Oxaine anesthetic agent
oxethazaine anesthetic agent
Oxford operation
Oxford total knee prosthesis
Oxford tube
oximetric catheter
oximetry catheter
Oxycel cautery
Oxycel cotton
Oxycel dressing
Oxycel gauze
Oxycel hemostat
Oxycel pack
oxygen
oxygen cisternography
oxygenated blood
oxygenated hemoglobin
oxygenation
oxygenator
        Bentley oxygenator
        bubble oxygenator
        bubble trap pump
          oxygenator
        Capiox II oxygenator
        DeBakey heart pump
          oxygenator
        disk oxygenator
        film oxygenator
        Kay-Cross oxygenator
        membrane oxygenator
        Oxy-Hood oxygenator
        pump oxygenator
        rotating disk oxygen-
          ator
        Sci-Med oxygenator
        screen oxygenator
        Shiley oxygenator
oxygenator pump
oxygen-starved tissue
Oxy-Hood oxygenator
Oxy-Hood pressurizer
oxyquinoline dressing
oxytocin
Oyloidin sutures

P&A (percussion and auscultation)
P-loop
PA (posteroanterior; pulmonary
   artery)
PA and lateral projections
   (posteroanterior)
PA banding (pulmonary artery
   banding)
PA film (posteroanterior film)
PA lordotic projection
   (posteroanterior lordotic
   projection)
PA position (posteroanterior
   position)
PA projection (posteroanterior
   projection)
PA view (posteroanterior view)
PABP (pulmonary artery
   balloon pump)
PAC (premature atrial contrac-
   tion)
pacchionian foramen
pacchionian glands
Pace hysterectomy knife
Pace knife
Pace periosteal elevator
Pace ventricular needle
pacemaker
   AA1 single-chamber
      pacemaker
   AAI pacemaker
   AAIR pacemaker
   AAT pacemaker
   Accufix pacemaker
   Acculith pacemaker
   Activitrax pacemaker
   Activitrax single-chamber
      responsive pacemaker

pacemaker *continued*
   Activitrax variable-rate
      pacemaker
   activity-sensing pace-
      maker
   AEC pacemaker
   Aequitron pacemaker
   AFP pacemaker
   AICD pacemaker
   AID-B pacemaker
   Alcatel pacemaker
   American Optic
      R-inhibited pacemaker
   American Optical
      Cardiocare pace-
      maker
   Amtech-Killeen pace-
      maker
   AOO pacemaker
   Arco atomic pacemaker
   Arco lithium pace-
      maker
   Arco pacemaker
   artificial pacemaker
   Arzco pacemaker
   Astra pacemaker
   ASVIP pacemaker
   asynchronous mode
      pacemaker
   asynchronous pace-
      maker
   asynchronous ventricular
      VOO pacemaker
   atrial pacemaker
   atrial synchronous
      ventricular-inhibited
      pacemaker
   atrial tracking pace-
      maker

pacemaker *continued*

atrial triggered ventricular-inhibited pacemaker

Atricor Cordis pacemaker

atrioventricular junctional pacemaker (AV junctional pacemaker)

atrioventricular sequential demand pacemaker (AV sequential demand pacemaker)

Atricor pacemaker

atrioventricular sequential pacemaker (AV sequentialpacemaker)

Aurora dual-chamber pacemaker

Autima II dual-chamber cardiac pacemaker

Autima II pacemaker

AV junctional pacemaker (atrioventricular junctional pacemaker)

AV sequential demand pacemaker (atrioventricular sequential demand pacemaker)

AV sequential pacemaker (atrioventricular sequential pacemaker)

AV synchronous pacemaker (atrioventricular synchronous pacemaker)

Avius sequential pacemaker

Basix pacemaker

Betacel-Biotronik pacemaker

bifocal demand pacemaker

Biotronik demand pacemaker

Biotronik pacemaker

bipolar Medtronic pacemaker

pacemaker *continued*

bipolar pacemaker

bipolar temporary pacemaker catheter

bladder pacemaker

burst pacemaker

Byrel pacemaker

cardiac pacemaker

Cardio-Pace Medical Durapulse pacemaker

Chardack Medtronic pacemaker

Chardack pacemaker

Chardack-Greatbatch pacemaker

Chorus pacemaker

Chronocor IV external pacemaker

cilium pacemaker

Classix pacemaker

Command PS pacemaker

committed mode pacemaker

Cook pacemaker

cor pacemaker

Coratomic pacemaker

Coratomic R-wave inhibited pacemaker

Cordis Atricor pacemaker

Cordis Chronocor pacemaker

Cordis Ectocor pacemaker

Cordis fixed-rate pacemaker

Cordis Gemini pacemaker

Cordis Multicor pacemaker

Cordis Omni Stanicor Theta transvenous pacemaker

Cordis Omnicor Stanicor pacemaker

Cordis pacemaker

Cordis Sequicor pacemaker

pacemaker *continued*

Cordis Ventricor pacemaker
Cosmos pacemaker
Cosmos pulse-generator pacemaker
CPI Astra pacemaker
CPI Maxilith pacemaker
CPI Microthin pacemaker
CPI Minilith pacemaker
CPI pacemaker
CPI Ultra II pacemaker
cross-talk pacemaker
Cyberlith demand pacemaker
Cyberlith pacemaker
CyberTach pacemaker
Daig pacemaker
DDD pacemaker (dual-sensing, -pacing, -mode)
DDI mode pacemaker
Delta pacemaker
demand pacemaker
Devices, Ltd., pacemaker
Diplos pacemaker
dual-chamber AV sequential pacemaker
dual-chamber pacemaker
dual-pass pacemaker
Durapulse pacemaker
DVI pacemaker
Ectocor pacemaker
ectopic atrial pacemaker
ectopic pacemaker
Ela pacemaker
Elecath pacemaker
electric cardiac pacemaker
Electrodyne pacemaker
Elema pacemaker
Elema-Schonander pacemaker
Elevath pacemaker

pacemaker *continued*

Elgiloy lead-tip pacemaker
Elgiloy pacemaker
Encor pacemaker
endocardial bipolar pacemaker
endocardial pacemaker
Enertrax pacemaker
epicardial pacemaker
escape pacemaker
external asynchronous pacemaker
external demand pacemaker
external pacemaker
external transthoracic pacemaker
external-internal pacemaker
externally controlled noninvasive programmed stimulation pacemaker
Fast-Pass lead pacemaker
fixed-rate asynchronous atrial pacemaker
fixed-rate asynchronous ventricular pacemaker
fixed-rate pacemaker
fully automatic pacemaker
fully automatic, atrioventricular universal dual-channel pacemaker
Galaxy pacemaker
GE pacemaker
Gemini pacemaker
General Electric pacemaker
Genisis dual-chamber pacemaker
Genisis pacemaker
Guardian pacemaker

pacemaker *continued*
    heart pacemaker
    hermetically sealed
        pacemaker
    implantable pacemaker
    implanted pacemaker
    Intermedics Cyberlith X
        multiprogrammable
        pacemaker
    Intermedics lithium-
        powered pacemaker
    Intermedics pacemaker
    Intermedics Quantum
        pacemaker
    Intermedics Quantum
        unipolar pacemaker
    Intermedics Thinlith II
        pacemaker
    Intertach pacemaker
    isotopic pulse generator
        pacemaker
    junctional pacemaker
    Kalos pacemaker
    Kantrowitz pacemaker
    Kelvin pacemaker
    Lambda Omni Stanicor
        pacemaker
    Lambda pacemaker
    latent pacemaker
    Laurens-Alcatel nuclear
        powered pacemaker
    Legend pacemaker
    Leios pacemaker
    Leptos pacemaker
    Leukos pacemaker
    Lillehei pacemaker
    lith II pacemaker
    lithium pacemaker
    lithium-powered
        pacemaker
    Maestro pacemaker
    Mailith pacemaker
    Mallor pacemaker
    malsensing pacemaker
    Maxilith pacemaker
    Medcor pacemaker
    Medtel pacemaker
    Medtronic Activitrax
        pacemaker

pacemaker *continued*
    Medtronic Byrel-SX
        pacemaker
    Medtronic corkscrew
        electrode pace-
        maker
    Medtronic Cyberlith
        pacemaker
    Medtronic demand
        pacemaker
    Medtronic external/
        internal pacemaker
    Medtronic pacemaker
    Medtronic Pacette
        pacemaker
    Medtronic Symbios
        pacemaker
    Medtronic-Alcatel
        pacemaker
    Medtronic-Laurens-
        Alcatel pacemaker
    Medtronic-Zyrel pace-
        maker
    Mentor bladder pace-
        maker
    mercury cell-powered
        pacemaker
    Meta MV cardiac
        pacemaker
    Microlith P pacemaker
    Microthin P2 pace-
        maker
    Mikros pacemaker
    Minilith pacemaker
    Minix pacemaker
    Mitrothin P2 pace-
        maker
    Multicor Gamma
        pacemaker
    Multicor II pacemaker
    Multilith pacemaker
    multiprogrammable
        pacemaker
    Nathan pacemaker
    natural pacemaker
    Neos pacemaker
    noncompetitive pace-
        maker
    Nova II pacemaker

pacemaker *continued*

nuclear pacemaker
nuclear powered pacemaker
Omni-Atricor pacemaker
Omnicor pacemaker
Omni-Ectocor pacemaker
Omni-Orthocor pacemaker
Omni-Stanicor pacemaker
Omni-Theta pacemaker
Omni-Ventricor pacemaker
Optima pacemaker
Orion pacemaker
Orthocor II pacemaker
Oscor pacemaker
oversensing pacemaker
Pacesetter pacemaker
Pacesetter Synchrony pacemaker
Pacette pacemaker
Pasar pacemaker
Pasar tachycardia reversion pacemaker
Pasys pacemaker
permanent myocardial pacemaker
permanent pacemaker
permanent rate-responsive pacemaker
permanent transvenous pacemaker
permanent ventricular pacemaker
Permathane Pacesetter lead pacemaker
Phoenix single-chamber pacemaker
physiologic pacemaker
Pinnacle pacemaker
PolyFlex implantable pacing lead pacemaker
PolyFlex lead pacemaker
Prima pacemaker
Prism-CL pacemaker

pacemaker *continued*

Programalith A-V pacemaker
Programalith II pacemaker
Programalith III pacemaker
Programalith pacemaker
programmable pacemaker
Programmer III pacemaker
Prolith pacemaker
Pulsar NI pacemaker
Quantum pacemaker
R-synchronous VVT pacemaker
radiofrequency pacemaker
rate-responsive pacemaker
rescuing pacemaker
respiratory-dependent pacemaker
reversion pacemaker
RS4 pacemaker
Schaldach electrode pacemaker
Schuletz pacemaker
screw-in lead pacemaker
Seecor pacemaker
Sensolog pacemaker
Sensor Kelvin pacemaker
sensor-based single-chamber pacemaker
Sequicor II pacemaker
Sequicor III pacemaker
Sequicor pacemaker
Shaldach pacemaker
shifting pacemaker
Siemens-Elema multi-programmable pacemaker
Siemens-Elema pacemaker
Siemens-Pacesetter pacemaker

pacemaker *continued*

single-chamber pace-
maker
single-pass pacemaker
sinus node pacemaker
sinus pacemaker
Sorin pacemaker
Spectraflex pacemaker
Spectrax bipolar
pacemaker
Spectrax pacemaker
Spectrax programmable
Medtronic pacemaker
standby pacemaker
Stanicor Gamma
pacemaker
Stanicor Lambda demand
pacemaker
Stanicor pacemaker
Starr-Edwards hermeti-
cally sealed pacemaker
Starr-Edwards pacemaker
Symbios dual-chamber
pacemaker
Symbios pacemaker
synchronous burst
pacemaker
synchronous mode
pacemaker
synchronous pacemaker
Synchrony pacemaker
tachycardia-terminating
pacemaker
Tachylog pacemaker
Telectronics pacemaker
temporary pacemaker
temporary transvenous
pacemaker
Thermos pacemaker
Thinlith II pacemaker
tined lead pacemaker
transcutaneous pace-
maker
transpericardial pace-
maker
transthoracic pacemaker
transvenous catheter
pacemaker

pacemaker *continued*

transvenous pacemaker
transvenous ventricular
demand pacemaker
Trios M pacemaker
Ultra pacemaker
Unilith pacemaker
unipolar atrial pace-
maker
unipolar atrioventricular
pacemaker
unipolar pacemaker
unipolar sequential
pacemaker
USCI Vario permanent
pacemaker
variable rate pacemaker
VAT pacemaker
VDD pacemaker
Ventak AICD pacemaker
Ventricor pacemaker
ventricular demand
pacemaker
ventricular pacemaker
ventricular-suppressed
pacemaker
ventricular-triggered
pacemaker
Versatrax cardiac
pacemaker
Versatrax II pacemaker
Versatrax pacemaker
Vicor pacemaker
Vista pacemaker
Vitatrax II pacemaker
Vitatron pacemaker
Vivalith-10 pacemaker
Vivatron pacemaker
VVI bipolar Programalith
pacemaker
VVI pacemaker
VVI single-chamber
pacemaker
VVI/AAI pacemaker
VVIR single-chamber
rate-adaptive pace-
maker
VVT pacemaker

pacemaker *continued*
    wandering atrial pace-
      maker (WAP)
    wandering pacemaker
    Xyrel pacemaker
    Xyticon 5950 bipolar
      demand pacemaker
    Zitron pacemaker
    Zoll NTP pacemaker
    Zoll pacemaker
pacemaker battery
pacemaker catheter
pacemaker electrode
pacemaker generator
pacemaker lead
pacemaker lead attachment
pacemaker pocket
pacemaker pouch
pacemaker programmer
pacemaker rhythm
Paceport catheter
Pace-Potts forceps
Pacer-Tracer
Pacesetter arthroscopy system
Pacesetter pacemaker
Pacesetter programmable pulse
    generator
Pacesetter Synchrony pace-
    maker
Pacette pacemaker
Pach-Pen tonometer
pachyonychia
Paci operation
pacifico cannula
pacifico catheter
pacing
pacing and sensing
pacing catheter
pacing electrode
pacing electrode wire
pacing impulse
pacing system
pacing technique
pacing wire
pacing wire electrode
pacinian corpuscles
pack
    Adaptic gauze pack

pack *continued*
  Bellows pack
  beta-lactose pack
  cold pack
  dry pack
  film pack
  finger-cot pack
  full pack
  gas pack
  Gelfoam pack
  hot pack
  Hydrocollator pack
  Hydrocollator steam
    pack
  ice pack
  intracervical pack
  intrauterine pack
  K-pad hot pack
  lap pack
  laparotomy pack
  Mikulicz pack
  moist lap pack
  nasopharyngeal pack
  one-sheet pack
  oropharyngeal pack
  oropharynx pack
  Oxycel pack
  partial pack
  pharyngeal pack
  salt pack
  Sultrin impregnated
    vaginal pack
  Thermaphore hot pack
  three-quarters pack
  vaginal pack
  Vag-Pack
  wet pack
  wet-sheet pack
  Zephiran pack
packaged irrigating solution
packed cell volume
packed red blood cells
packed with gauze
packer (see also *gauze packer*)
  Allport gauze packer
  Allport packer
  Bernay gauze packer
  Bernay uterine packer

packer *continued*
- gauze packer
- iodoform gauze packer
- Kelly combined packer and tucker
- Kitchen postpartum gauze packer
- Kreiselman packer
- mastoid packer
- Woodson dura separator and packer

Packer mosquito forceps

packing (see also *gauze packing*)
- Adaptic gauze packing
- Brodhead uterine gauze packing
- dry packing
- gauze packing
- Gelfoam packing
- intranasal packing
- iodoform gauze packing
- Merocel nasal packing
- nasal packing
- Nu-Gauze packing
- ovoid packing
- polyurethane packing
- Pope Merocel ear packing
- transvenous packing
- vaginal packing
- Vaseline petrolatum packing

Packo pars plana cannula

PAD (percutaneous automated diskectomy)

pad
- ABD pad
- abdominal fat pad
- abdominal pad
- Action OR table pad
- antimesenteric fat pad
- Aquamatic K-Pad
- Aquapad heating pad
- Bardeen pad
- buccal fat pad
- Casco heating pad

pad *continued*
- chair pad
- disposable electrode pad
- Dycen pad
- electrode pad
- electrosurgical dispersive pad
- epaulet shoulder pad
- eye heating pad
- eye pad
- fat pad
- felt pad
- felt-gauze pad
- gauze pad
- grounding pad
- heating pad
- heel pad
- Hemopad
- HydraPad
- infrapatellar fat pad
- K-pad
- K-Thermia pad
- knuckle pad
- Kotex pad
- lap pad
- laparotomy pad
- Micro-Temp pad
- Mikulicz pad
- nasal drip pad
- navicular pad
- Passavant pad
- periarterial pad
- pericardial fat pad
- perineal pad
- peripad
- prep pad
- Proneze pad
- Proplast pad
- protective eye pad
- retropatellar fat pad
- retrosternal fat pad
- Sensor Pad
- Spence gel mattress pad
- Steri-pads dressing
- Surgi-Pad combined dressing
- Telfa pad

pad *continued*
    Thermophore moist heat pad
    thumb pad
    underpad
    vaginal pad
    volar pad
pad electrode
pad sign
padded clamp
padded knee supports
padded splint
padding
paddle
    cardioversion paddle
    compression paddle
    defibrillation paddle
paddy bear cast
Padgett blade
Padgett dermatome
Padgett graft
Padgett implant
Padgett prosthesis
Padgett shark-mouth cannula
Padgett-Concorde suction cannula
Padgett-Hood dermatome
Padgett-Hood electrodermatome
PAFD (percutaneous abscess and fluid drainage)
Page forceps
Page knife
Page needle
Page procedure
Page tonsillar forceps
Page tonsillar knife
Pagenstecher linen thread sutures
Pagenstecher operation
Pagenstecher scoop
Pagenstecher sutures
Paget disease
PAIC (procedures, alternatives, indications, complications)
painful
painless
painted area

paint-gun injury
paired vertebral arches
Pajot hook
Pajot maneuver
Palacos bone cement
Palacos cement
Paladon graft
Paladon prosthesis
palatal bar
palatal linguoplate
palatal pushback
palatal pushback operation
palatal reflex
palatal shelves
palate
palate elevator
palate hook
palate lengthening
palate pusher hook
palate retractor
palatina ascendens, arteria
palatina descendens, arteria
palatina externa, vena
palatina major, arteria
palatinae minores, arterae
palatine
palatine aponeurosis
palatine arch
palatine artery
palatine block anesthesia
palatine bones
palatine durum
palatine folds
palatine foramen
palatine nerve
palatine notch
palatine process
palatine protuberance
palatine raphe
palatine reflex
palatine spine
palatine suture
palatine tonsil
palatine uvula
palatine vein
palatine velum
palatini minores, nervi

palatinus major, nervus
palatoethmoid suture
palatoethmoidal suture
palatoglossal arch
palatoglossal muscle
palatoglossus, musculus
palatography
palatomaxillary suture
palatopharyngeal fold
palatopharyngeal muscle
palatopharyngeus, musculus
palatoplasty
palatorrhaphy
Palfyn sutures
Pallab finger splint
palliate
palliation
palliative
palliative operation
palliative procedure
palliative surgery
pallid
pallid and shocky
pallidectomy
pallidoansection
pallidoansotomy
pallidotomy
pallidum
pallor
palm
palma manus
Palma operation
palmar aponeurosis
palmar contraction
palmar digital arteries
palmar digital nerves
palmar digital veins
palmar erythema
palmar fascia
palmar interosseous muscle
palmar ligaments
palmar metacarpal arteries
palmar metacarpal veins
palmar muscle
palmar space
palmar splint
palmaris brevis, musculus

palmaris longus, musculus
palmate folds
Palmaz stent
Palmaz vascular stent
Palmer biopsy drill forceps
Palmer biopsy forceps
Palmer dilator
Palmer uterine dilator
Palmer-Drapier needle
Palmer-Widen operation
palpability of pulses
palpable adenopathy
palpable mass
palpable organ
palpable pulse
palpable pyloric olive
palpable thrill
palpably enlarged organ
palpated
palpating finger
palpating needle
palpation
palpation probe
palpator
    Farrior blunt palpator
palpatory percussion
palpebra (*pl.* palpebrae)
palpebral
palpebral arteries
palpebral commissure
palpebral fissure
palpebral fold
palpebral furrow
palpebral raphe
palpebral region
palpebral veins
palpebrales inferiores, venae
palpebrales laterales, arteriae
palpebrales mediales, arteriae
palpebrales superiores, venae
palpebrales, venae
palpebronasal fold
palpitations
Palumbo dynamic patellar brace
Palumbo knee brace
Palumbo sleeve
PAM (potential acuity meter)

pampiniform plexus
pampiniform vein
pan splint
Panas operation
Panas ptosis correction technique
Pancoast operation
Pancoast sutures
Pancoast tumor
pancolectomy
pancreas
pancreas divisum
pancreatectomy
pancreatic
pancreatic abscess
pancreatic ascites
pancreatic calculus
pancreatic cutaneous fistula
pancreatic cyst
pancreatic duct
pancreatic duct stent
pancreatic hamartoma
pancreatic islet cell tumor
pancreatic pseudocyst
pancreatic ranula
pancreatic tissue
pancreatic veins
pancreaticae, venae
pancreaticobiliary ductal junction
pancreaticobiliary ductography
pancreaticobiliary operation
pancreaticobiliary sphincter
pancreaticobiliary tract
pancreaticocystoduodenostomy
pancreaticocystoenterostomy
pancreaticocystogastrostomy
pancreaticocystojejunostomy
pancreaticocystostomy
pancreaticoduodenal arteries
pancreaticoduodenal veins
pancreaticoduodenales inferiores, arteriae
pancreaticoduodenales, venae
pancreaticoduodenales superiores, arteriae
pancreaticoduodenectomy

pancreaticoduodenostomy
pancreaticoenterostomy
pancreaticogastric folds
pancreaticogastrostomy
pancreaticoileostomy
pancreaticojejunostomy
pancreaticopleural fistula
pancreaticosplenic ligament
pancreaticosplenic lymph node
pancreaticosplenic omentum
pancreatoduodenectomy
pancreatoduodenectomy bypass
pancreatoduodenostomy
pancreatoenterostomy
pancreatogram
pancreatography
pancreatolithectomy
pancreatolithotomy
pancreatomy
pancreatotomy
pancreectomy
pancreolithotomy
pancreoprivic
pan-culture
panendography
panendoscope
panendoscope electrode
panendoscopy
Pang forceps
Pang technique
panhysterectomy
panhystero-oophorectomy
panhysterosalpingectomy
panhysterosalpingo-oophorectomy
Panje implant
Panje prosthesis
Panje voice box
Panje voice button
Panje voice button laryngeal prosthesis
Panje voice valve
panmural
panniculectomy
panniculotomy
panniculus (*pl.* panniculi)
panniculus adiposus

panniculus carnosus
Pannu intraocular lens
pannus
pan-oral radiography
panoramic radiograph
panoramic view
Panorex films
Panorex x-ray
Panoview arthroscope
panproctocolectomy
Pansch fissure
pan-sensitive
pantaloon embolism
pantaloon hernia
pantaloon inguinal hernia
pantaloon operation
pantomographic view
pantomography
pantoscope
pants-over-vest hernia repair
pants-over-vest herniorrhaphy
pants-over-vest repair
pants-over-vest sutures
panty cast
panus
Panvue scope
Panzer gallbladder scissors
Panzer scissors
Pap smear
Papanicolaou smear
Paparella calipers
Paparella catheter
Paparella curet
Paparella elevator
Paparella fenestrometer
Paparella knife
Paparella needle
Paparella otologic surgery
    elevator
Paparella pick
Paparella polyethylene tube
Paparella retractor
Paparella scissors
Paparella self-retaining retractor
Paparella tube
Paparella wire-cutting scissors
Paparella-McCabe crurotomy
    saw

papaverine hydrochloride
paper drape
paper tape
paper-doll fetus
papilla (*pl.* papillae)
papilla drain
papilla of Vater
papillares, musculi
papillary
papillary adenoma
papillary carcinoma
papillary duct
papillary muscles
papillary stenosis
papillary tumor
papillate
papillation
papillectomy
papilloma (*pl.* papillomas,
    papillomata)
papilloma forceps
papillomatous goiter
papillosphincterotomy
papillotome
        Classen-Demling
            papillotome
        Erlangen papillotome
        Olympus needle-knife
            papillotome
papillotomy
Papineau bone graft
Papineau cancellous graft
Papineau sequestrectomy and
    curettage
papulous vaginitis
papyraceous fetus
papyraceous layer
Paquelin cautery
PAR (procedures, alternatives,
    risks)
par glissement hernia
PAR room (postanesthesia
    recovery room)
para (1, 2, 3, etc.)
parabola of urinary stream
paracentesis (*pl* paracenteses)
paracentesis abdominis
paracentesis capitis

paracentesis cordis
paracentesis knife
paracentesis needle
paracentesis pericardii
paracentesis pulmonis
paracentesis thoracis
paracentesis vesicae
paracentetic
paracentral lobule
paracervical anesthetic
paracervical block anesthesia
paracervix
parachute mitral valve
parachute valve
Paracine dressing
paracolic abscess
paracolic gutter
paracolon
paracorporeal heart
paracostal incision
paradental pyorrhea
paradox
paradoxical contraction
paradoxical effect
paradoxical pulse
paraduodenal
paraduodenal fold
paraduodenal hernia
paraesophageal
paraesophageal hernia
paraesophageal hiatal hernia
paraesophageal varices
parafascicular thalamotomy
    (PFT)
paraffin
paraffin block
paraffin dressing
paraffin graft
paraffin implant
paraffin prosthesis
paraganglioma
ParaGard intrauterine device
parahiatal hernia
parahippocampal gyrus
paraileostomal hernia
parainguinal incision
paraldehyde
parallax

parallel
parallel incision
parallel jaw clip
parallel loop electrode
parallel opposing tangential
    fields
parallel plate dialyzer
parallel plate hemodialyzer
parallel to wound edges
parallel-jaw spring clip
parallel-transverse incision
paralunate dislocation
paralysis
paralytic
paralytic colonic obstruction
paralytic ileus
paralytic intestinal obstruction
paralyzed limb
paramedial sulcus
paramedian appendectomy
    incision
paramedian incision
paramediastinal shadow
paramesonephric duct
parameter
parametrial
parametrial curettage
parametrial fixation
parametrial mass
parametrial thickening
parametric hematocele
parametrium
parametrium clamp
parametrium forceps
paramuscular incision
paranasal sinuses
paranephric fat body
paraneural anesthesia
paraneural block
paraoperative
parapatellar
parapatellar incision
paraperitoneal
paraperitoneal hernia
paraperitoneal nephrectomy
parapharyngeal lymph nodes
paraphimosis
paraplegia

pararectal abscess
pararectus incision
pararenal fat
parasaccular
parasaccular hernia
parasacral anesthesia
parasacral block
parasagittal
parasagittal incision
parasagittal lesion
parasagittal meningioma
parascapular incision
parasites
parasitic cyst
parasol tube
paraspinal muscles
paraspinal thrust
paraspinous fascia
paraspinous muscles
paraspinous musculature
parasternal
parasternal lymph nodes
parasternal tissue
parastomal hernia
parasympathetic nerve
parasympathetic system
parasymphyseal
parasystole
parathyroid gland
parathyroidectomy
paratracheal nodes
paratrooper fracture
paratubular adhesions
paraumbilical hernia
paraumbilical incision
paraumbilical veins
paraumbilicales, venae
paraurethral duct
paraurethral glands
paraurethral suspension
parauterine adhesions
paravaginal abscess
paravaginal hysterectomy
paravaginal incision
paraventricular veins
paravertebral anesthesia
paravertebral block
paravertebral mass

paravertebral muscle spasm
paravertebral musculature
paravertebral thoracoplasty
paravesical fossa
paravesical pouch
paravesical space
parchment heart
parchment induration
Pardos scissors
Paré sutures
pared with motor saw
Parel-Crock cutter
Parel-Crock vitreous cutter
parenchyma
parenchyma infiltration
parenchyma testis
parenchymal
parenchymal density
parenchymal infiltrate
parenchymal scarring
parenchymal softening
parenchymal tissue
parenchymatous
parenchymatous carcinoma
parenchymatous change
parenchymatous goiter
parenchymatous implantation
parenchymatous injection
parenchymatous tissue
parenteral administration
parenteral alimentation
parenteral hyperalimentation
paresis
paresthesia
Parhad needle
Parhad-Poppen needle
Parham band
Parham-Martin band
Parham-Martin bone clamp
Parham-Martin bone-holding
    clamp
Parham-Martin clamp
Parham-Martin ronguer
paries (pl. parietes)
parietal
parietal area
parietal bone
parietal diameter

parietal emissary vein
parietal hernia
parietal lamina
parietal lobe
parietal peritoneum
parietal pleura
parietal pregnancy
parietal presentation
parietal shunt
parietal suture
parietes (*sing.* paries)
parietocolic fold
parietography
parietomastoid suture
parieto-occipital fissure
parieto-occipital region
parieto-occipital suture
parieto-orbital projection
parietoperitoneal fold
parietotemporal region
Park aneurysm
Park blade
Park blade septostomy
Park eye speculum
Parke-Davis splint
Parker clamp
Parker double-ended retractor
Parker fixation forceps
Parker incision
Parker knife
Parker knife-needle
Parker needle
Parker retractor
Parker serrated discission knife
Parker-Heath cautery
Parker-Heath eye syringe
Parker-Kerr basting stitch
Parker-Kerr clamp
Parker-Kerr end-to-end entero-
    enterostomy
Parker-Kerr enteroenterostomy
Parker-Kerr forceps
Parker-Kerr operation
Parker-Kerr sutures
Parker-Mott double-ended
    retractor
Parker-Mott retractor
Parkes gouge

Parkes hump gouge
Parkes nasal raspatory
Parkes nasal retractor
Parkes operation
Parkes osteotome
Parkes rasp
Park-Guyton eye speculum
Park-Guyton-Callahan eye
    speculum
Parkhill operation
Parkland resuscitation
Parkland tubal ligation
Park-Maumenee eye speculum
Park-Maumenee lid speculum
Parks fistulotomy
Parks ileoanal anastomosis
Parks ileoanal reservoir
Parks ileostomy pouch
Parks partial sphincterotomy
Parks retractor
Parks sphincterotomy
Parks transanal anastomosis
Parma band
Parona space
paronychia
paroophoritic cyst
parosteal
parosteal osteosarcoma
parotid
parotid capsule
parotid duct
parotid gland
parotid lymph node
parotid notch
parotid plexus
parotid tumor
parotid veins
parotideae, venae
parotidectomy
parotiditis
parotidoscirrhus
parotitis
parous
parous cervix
parous introitus
parovarian
parovarian cyst
paroxysm

paroxysmal
Parrish procedure
Parrot atrophy of newborn
Parrot node
Parrot sign
parrot-beak basket
parrot-beak basket biter
parrot-beak flap
parrot-beak meniscus tear
parrot-beak shape of distal
    esophagus
parry fracture
pars (*pl.* partes)
pars defect
pars plana
pars pylorica
pars superior duodeni
Parsonnet dilator
Parsonnet pouch
Parsonnet probe
Par-Style needle holder
partes (*sing.* pars)
partial
partial amputation
partial anesthesia
partial bowel obstruction
partial breech delivery
partial breech extraction
partial bypass
partial excision
partial ileal bypass
partial impairment
partial occlusion clamp
partial occlusion forceps
partial ossicular reconstructive/
    replacement prosthesis
    (PORP)
partial pack
partial paralysis
partial plate
partial pressure
partial rebreathing anesthesia
partial resection
partial union of fracture
partial weightbearing (PWB)
partially

partially occluding clamp
partial-thickness graft
particle
particulate contaminants
particulate material
particulate matter
Partipilo clamp
Partipilo gastrostomy
partitioning
Partsch chisel
Partsch gouge
Partsch operation
parumbilical
parumbilical hernia
parumbilical incision
PASA (proximal articular set
    angle)
Pasar pacemaker
Pasar tachycardia reversion
    pacemaker
PASG (pneumatic antishock
    garment)
passage
passage of blood
passage of catheter
passage of clots
passage of flatus
passage of instrument
passage of meconium
passage of sound
passage of stone
passage of tissue
passageway
Passavant bar
Passavant cushion
Passavant pad
Passavant ridge
passed per mucosa
passed with difficulty
passed with ease
passed without difficulty
passer (see also *ligature passer,*
    *tendon passer*)
      Brand tendon passer
      Bunnell tendon passer
      Dingman wire passer

passer *continued*
   Gallie tendon passer
   Hewson passer
   Joplin tendon passer
   Kleinert tendon passer
   Ober tendon passer
   O'Donahue ligature
      passer
   O'Donahue suture passer
   Schnidt passer
   Yankauer ligature passer
passing
passive
passive contraction
passive exercise
passive flexion
passive joint movement
passive placement
passive relaxation
passive stretching
passive tremor
passively flexed
Passow chisel
past history
paste
paste plate
Pastia sign
Pasys pacemaker
patch (see also *graft, implant,
   prosthesis*)
   autologous pericardial
      patch
   cardiac patch
   Carrel patch
   colic patch
   colonic patch
   cotton-wool patch
   Dacron patch
   Dacron Sauvage patch
   Donaldson eye patch
   Edwards patch
   epidural blood patch
   eye patch
   felt patch
   Gore-Tex cardiovascular
      patch
   Gore-Tex patch

patch *continued*
   Gore-Tex soft-tissue
      patch
   Graham omental patch
   Graham patch
   Grillo patch
   gusset-type patch
   intracardiac patch
   Ivalon patch
   MacCallum patch
   monocular patch
   onlay bone patch
   outflow cardiac patch
   pericardial patch
   Peyer patch
   shagreen patch
   Silastic patch
   smoker's patch
   Teflon felt patch
   Teflon intracardiac patch
   Teflon patch
   Thal gastric patch
   transannular patch
   velour patch
   white patch
patch angioplasty
patch booster
patch closure of defect
patch dressing
patch implant
patch procedure for Peyronie
   disease
patch prosthesis
patch-graft angioplasty
patch-reinforced mattress suture
patchy area
patchy infiltrate
patchy ulceration
patella
patella alta
patella apprehension test
patella baja
patella bone
patella cap prosthesis
patella compression test
Patella disease (pyloric stenosis)
patella dislocation

patellapexy
patellaplasty
patellar button
patellar chondromalacia
patellar clamp
patellar dome
patellar facet cartilage
patellar fold
patellar hook
patellar ligament
patellar prosthesis
patellar reflex
patellar retinaculum
patellar synovial fold
patellar tendon
patellar tendon-bearing cast
    (PTB)
patellar tendon-bearing walking
    cast (PTB walker)
patellar tracking
patellectomy
patelloadductor reflex
patellofemoral articulation
patellofemoral prosthesis
patency
patency of veins
patent
patent canal of Nuck
patent duct
patent ductus
patent ductus arteriosus (PDA)
patent ductus arteriosus ligation
patent ductus clamp
patent ductus forceps
patent ductus retractor
patent fallopian tube
patent graft
patent lumen
patent opening
patent orifice
patent tube
Paterson cannula
Paterson forceps
Paterson laryngeal forceps
Paterson long-shank brain clip
Paterson nodules
Paterson pseudarthrosis of tibia

Patey axillary node dissection
Patey fracture
Patey mastectomy
Patey operation
pathfinder
Pathfinder catheter
pathologic, pathological
pathologic amputation
pathologic change
pathologic classification
pathologic compression fracture
pathologic condition
pathologic disease
pathologic dislocation
pathologic fracture
pathologic histology
pathologic organism
pathologic perforation
pathologic process
pathologic reflex
pathologic rigidity
pathologic specimen
pathologic stool
pathologic tissue examination
pathologist
pathology
pathology and staging
pathway
patient
patient electrode
patient plate
patient-controlled analgesia
patient-controlled analgesia
    administered epidurally
    (PCAE)
Paton corneal dissector
Paton corneal forceps
Paton corneal knife
Paton corneal transplant
    forceps
Paton corneal trephine
Paton forceps
Paton knife
Paton needle holder
Paton spatula
Paton transplant spatula
Paton trephine

Patrick maneuver
Patrick sign
Patrick test
Patrick trigger area
Patten Bottom Perthes brace
pattern
Patterson forceps
Patterson operation
Patterson trocar
Pattey modified radical mastec-
	tomy
patties
Patton bur
Patton cannula
Patton dilator
Patton nasal speculum
Patton speculum
patulent
patulous
Pauchet gastrectomy
paucity
paucity of findings
Paufique blade
Paufique corneal knife
Paufique corneal trephine
Paufique detached retina
	operation
Paufique forceps
Paufique graft knife
Paufique keratoplasty
Paufique knife
Paufique lamellar knife
Paufique operation
Paufique suture forceps
Paufique synechotomy
Paufique trephine
Paul condom bag
Paul drainage tube
Paul lacrimal sac retractor
Paul retractor
Paul-Mikulicz operation
Paul-Mikulicz resection
Paul-Mixter tube
Paulson knee retractor
Pauwels adduction osteotomy
Pauwels angle
Pauwels fracture

Pauwels fracture forceps
Pauwels fracture of proximal
	femoral neck
Pauwels fracture operation
Pauwels osteotomy
Pauwels Y-osteotomy
pavement cells
pavilion of oviduct
paving-stone degeneration
Pavlik harness
Pavlik hip harness
Pavulon anesthesia
paw pigmentation
Pawlik triangle
pawlike hand
Payne jejunoileostomy
Payne operation
Payne-DeWind jejunoileal
	bypass
Payne-Ochsner arterial for-
	ceps
Payne-Ochsner forceps
Payne-Péan arterial forceps
Payne-Péan forceps
Payne-Rankin arterial forceps
Payne-Rankin forceps
Payr clamp
Payr forceps
Payr gastrectomy
Payr gastrointestinal clamp
Payr pylorus clamp
Payr pylorus forceps
Payr resection clamp
Payr retractor
PBI (penile pressure/brachial
	pressure index)
PCA (porous coated anatomic)
PCA hip
PCA knee
PCA knee prosthesis
PCA primary total knee system
PCA reconstructive system
PCA total hip system
PCA total knee replacement
PCAE (patient-controlled
	analgesia administered
	epidurally)

PCNL (percutaneous nephros-
    tolithotomy)
PCO (polycystic ovary)
PCW (pulmonary capillary
    wedge)
PDA (patent ductus arteriosus)
PDA (posterior descending
    artery)
PDS sutures (polydioxanone
    sutures)
PDS Vicryl sutures
PDT guide wire
PDT guiding catheter
PE Plus II balloon dilatation
    catheter
PE Plus II peripheral balloon
    catheter
PE tube (polyethylene tube;
    pressure equalization tube)
Peabody bunionectomy
Peabody classification of foot
    and ankle paralysis
Peabody foot procedure
Peabody splint
Peabody tibialis tendon transfer
Peabody-Mitchell bunionectomy
peacock dressing
Peacock rhizotomy hook
peak expiratory flow
peak-and-trough levels
peaked pupil
peak-to-peak deflection
peak-to-peak systolic gradient
Péan amputation
Péan clamp
Péan forceps
Péan GI forceps
Péan hemostatic clamp
Péan hemostatic forceps
Péan hysterectomy
Péan hysterectomy clamp
Péan hysterectomy forceps
Péan incision
Péan operation
Péan position
Péan scissors
Péan sponge forceps

Péan-Billroth I gastrectomy
peanut dissector
peanut eye implant
peanut forceps
peanut sponge
peanut sponge-holding forceps
peanut-fenestrated forceps
peanut-grasping forceps
PEAP (positive end-airway
    pressure)
peapod chisel
peapod intervertebral disk
    forceps
peapod intervertebral disk
    rongeur
peapod rongeur
Pearce posterior chamber
    intraocular lens implant
Pearce Tripod lens
Pearce vaulted-Y lens implant
Pearlcast polymer plaster
    bandage
pearly nodule
Pearman penile Silastic prosthe-
    sis
Pearman transurethral he-
    mostatic bag
Pearsall Chinese twisted sutures
Pearsall silk sutures
pear-shaped bur
pear-shaped fluted bag
pear-shaped heart
Pearson attachment to Thomas
    splint
Pearson clavicle attachment
    splint
Pearson position
Pease bone drill
Pease-Thomson traction bow
Peat hemostat
peau d'orange
Peck chisel
Peck scissors
Peck-Vienna nasal speculum
pectate line
pectenotomy
pectinate

pectinate ligament
pectinate line
pectinate muscles
pectinati, musculi
pectineal
pectineal crural hernia
pectineal fascia
pectineal hernia
pectineal ligament
pectineal line
pectineal muscle
pectineus, musculus
pectoral
pectoral fascia
pectoral fremitus
pectoral girdle
pectoral groove
pectoral muscles
pectoral nerve
pectoral reflex
pectoral regions
pectoralis major, musculus
pectoralis minor, musculus
pectoralis muscle implant
pectoralis, nervus
pectus carinatum
pectus deformity
pectus excavatum
pectus gallinatum
pectus recurvatum
pedal edema
pedal pulse
Pederson speculum
Pederson vaginal speculum
Pediastrol self-irrigating bladder
    irrigator
pediatric balloon catheter
pediatric bone rongeur
pediatric bridge
pediatric bronchoscope
pediatric bulldog clamp
pediatric catheter
pediatric endoscope
pediatric esophagoscope
pediatric feeding tube
pediatric Foley catheter
pediatric forceps

pediatric nasogastric tube
pediatric scissors
pediatric self-retaining retractor
pediatric surgery
pediatric telescope
pediatric vascular clamp
pedicle
pedicle clamp
pedicle flap
pedicle graft
pedicle implant
pedicle intact
pedicle mucoperiosteal flap
pedicle of lung
pedicle of spleen
pedicle prosthesis
pedicle stump
pedicled cyst
pedicleized
pediculated cells
pedography
peduncle
peduncular loop
pedunculated
pedunculated adenoma
pedunculated fibroid
pedunculated growth
pedunculated lesion
pedunculated nodule
pedunculated polyp
pedunculotomy
peek-and-see method
peel
peel off
Peel Pak bag
peel-away catheter
peel-away introducer
peel-away sheath
peel-off catheter
PEEP (positive end-expiratory
    phase/pressure)
Peers towel clamp
Peet forceps
Peet lighted splanchnic retractor
Peet mosquito forceps
Peet nasal rasp
Peet operation

Peet splinter forceps
Peet technique for leg constrictures
peg bone graft
peg cells
peg graft
PEG (percutaneous endoscopic gastrostomy; polyethylene glycol)
PEG lavage (polyethylene glycol lavage)
PEG procedure (percutaneous endoscopic gastrostomy procedure)
PEG self-adhesive elastic dressing (polyethylene glycol self-adhesive elastic dressing)
PEG tube (percutaneous endoscopic gastrostomy tube)
peg-and-socket hammer toe repair
peg-top prosthesis
Pehr abduction splint
Peiper-Beyer bone rongeur
Peiper-Beyer laminectomy rongeur
Pelger-Huët anomaly
Pelite liner
Pelkmann sponge forceps
Pelkmann uterine forceps
Pelkmann uterine-dressing forceps
pellucidum septum
Pelton Localite
pelvectomy
pelvic
pelvic adhesions
pelvic aneurysm
pelvic bone
pelvic canal
pelvic cavity
pelvic clamp
pelvic colon
pelvic colon of Waldeyer
pelvic deformities
pelvic diameter

pelvic diaphragm
pelvic drainage
pelvic endometriosis
pelvic examination
pelvic exenteration
pelvic floor
pelvic fossa
pelvic fracture
pelvic girdle
pelvic gutter
pelvic inflammatory disease (PID)
pelvic inlet
pelvic irradiation
pelvic laparoscopy
pelvic laparotomy
pelvic lymph node
pelvic malignancy
pelvic mass
pelvic measurements
pelvic metastases
pelvic muscular support
pelvic musculature
pelvic node
pelvic obliquity
pelvic organ exenteration
pelvic organs
pelvic osteotomy
pelvic outlet
pelvic peritoneal cavity
pelvic peritoneum
pelvic peritonitis
pelvic plexus
pelvic presentation
pelvic relaxation
pelvic ring fractures
pelvic scanography
pelvic sling
pelvic splanchnic nerves
pelvic splint
pelvic steal test
pelvic strait
pelvic support
pelvic tilt
pelvic traction
pelvic ultrasound
pelvic version
pelvic viscera

pelvic wall
pelvic washings
pelvic-femoral angle
pelvifemoral
pelvifixation
pelvilithotomy
pelvimeter
    Collin pelvimeter
    Collyer pelvimeter
    DeLee pelvimeter
    DeLee-Breisky pelvimeter
    Douglas pelvimeter
    Hanely-McDermott pelvimeter
    Martin pelvimeter
    Pilling-Douglas pelvimeter
    Schneider pelvimeter
pelvimetry
pelvimetry study
pelvioileoneocystostomy
pelviolithotomy
pelvioneostomy
pelvioplasty
pelvioprostatic capsule
pelvioscopy
pelviostomy
pelviotomy
pelviradiography
pelvirectal
pelvirectal anesthesia
pelvis (*pl.* pelves)
pelvisacral
pelviscope
pelvisection
pelviureteroplasty
pelvoscopy
Pemberton clamp
Pemberton forceps
Pemberton osteotomy
Pemberton retractor
Pemberton sigmoid anastomosis clamp
Pemberton sigmoid clamp
Pemberton spur crusher
Pemberton spur-crushing clamp

Pemco prosthetic valve
Pemco pump
Pemco valve prosthesis
Penberthy double-action aspirator
pencil
    Amoils cryopencil
    Blaisdell skin pencil
    caustic pencil
    cautery pencil
    cryopencil
    disposable electrosurgical pencil
    electrosurgical pencil
    Handtrol electrosurgical pencil
    skin pencil
    Wallach pencil cryosurgical device
    Wallach pencil
    Weck electrosurgery pencil
pencil Doppler probe
pencil dosimeter
pencil-probe Doppler
pencil-shaped stools
pending
pendular movement
pendulous
pendulous abdomen
pendulous breasts
pendulous urethra
pendulum rhythm
pendulum scalpel
penectomy
penetrability
penetrating abdominal trauma
penetrating corneal graft
penetrating drill
penetrating graft
penetrating keratoplasty
penetrating trauma
penetrating ulcer
penetrating wound
penetration fracture
penetrator
Penfield biopsy needle

*Percuflex (per Spell)*

Penfield clip
Penfield dissector
Penfield elevator
Penfield forceps
Penfield needle
Penfield neurodissector
Penfield retractor
Penfield silver clip
Penfield suture forceps
penile brachial pressure index
penile clamp
penile discharge
penile epispadias
penile implant
penile induration
penile injury
penile lesion
penile plethysmography
penile pneumoplethysmography
penile pressure/brachial
    pressure index (PBI)
penile prosthesis
penile prosthesis cylinders
penile reconstruction
penile reflex
penile shaft
penile sheath
penile skin
penile wart
penile-scrotal incision
penis
penis clamp
penlight cautery
Penn drill
Penn scissors
Penn State artificial heart
Penn swivel hook
Penn trocar
Penn tuning fork
Penn umbilical scissors
pennate muscles
penniform muscle
Pennington clamp
Pennington elevator
Pennington forceps
Pennington hemostatic forceps
Pennington rectal speculum
Pennington septum elevator

Pennington speculum
Pennington tissue-grasping
    forceps
penoplasty
penoscrotal hypospadias
penoscrotal incision
Penrose drain
Penrose seton
Penrose tourniquet
Penrose tube
pentalogy of Fallot
Pentax bronchoscope
Pentax colonofiberscope
Pentax fiberoptic sigmoido-
    scope
Pentax flexible sigmoido-
    scope
Pentax gastroscope
Pentax side-viewing endoscope
pentazocine
Penthrane anesthetic agent
pentobarbital anesthetic agent
Pentothal anesthetic agent
peptic
peptic gland
peptic stricture
peptic ulcer
peptic ulcer disease (PUD)
per contiguum
per continuum
PER fracture (pronation,
    external rotation fracture)
per high power field
per mucosa
per os (p.o., PO, or po)
per primam healing
per primam intentionem
per rectum
per secundam healing
per secundam intentionem
per urethram
per vaginam
Percaine anesthetic agent
percardiectomy
percent
percentage
Percival gastric balloon
percolator irrigator

*Per-Close*

Percor dual-lumen intra-aortic
balloon catheter
Percor intra-aortic balloon
catheter
Percor-DL catheter (dual-lumen
catheter)
Percor-Stat intra-aortic balloon
Percor-Stat-DL catheter (dual-
lumen catheter)
perc-q-cath
PercuCut biopsy needle
percussible
percussion
percussion and auscultation
(P&A)
percussion hammer
percussion note
percussion of bone
percussion sound
percussion wave
percutaneous
percutaneous abscess and fluid
drainage (PAFD)
percutaneous antegrade biliary
drainage
percutaneous antegrade
pyelography
percutaneous antegrade
urography
percutaneous aortic val-
vuloplasty (PAV)
percutaneous arteriogram
percutaneous arteriography
percutaneous aspiration
percutaneous automated
diskectomy (PAD)
percutaneous balloon aortic
valvuloplasty
percutaneous balloon dilation
percutaneous balloon val-
vuloplasty
percutaneous biopsy
percutaneous carotid arteriography (PCA)
percutaneous catheter
percutaneous catheter cecostomy

percutaneous catheter commissurotomy
percutaneous catheterization
percutaneous cholangiogram
percutaneous cholangiography
percutaneous cordotomy
percutaneous diskectomy
percutaneous dorsal column
stimulator implant
percutaneous endoscopic
gastrostomy (PEG)
percutaneous exposure
percutaneous femoral arteriogram
percutaneous femoral-femoral
cardiopulmonary bypass
percutaneous gastrostomy
percutaneous hepatobiliary
cholangiography
percutaneous intra-aortic
balloon counterpulsation
catheter (PIBC catheter)
percutaneous Judkins technique
percutaneous laser angioplasty
percutaneous lead introducer
percutaneous mitral balloon
valvotomy (PMV)
percutaneous mitral balloon
valvuloplasty
percutaneous mitral valvotomy
percutaneous needle
percutaneous nephroscope
percutaneous nephrosto-
lithotomy (PCNL)
percutaneous nephrostomy
percutaneous pinning
percutaneous puncture
percutaneous route
percutaneous splenoportal
venography
percutaneous stent
percutaneous stone manipulation
percutaneous subclavian-
subclavian bypass
percutaneous transfemoral
arteriography

percutaneous transfemoral
technique
percutaneous transhepatic
biliary drainage catheter
percutaneous transhepatic
cholangiogram
percutaneous transhepatic
cholangiography (PTC)
percutaneous transhepatic
decompression (PTD)
percutaneous transhepatic
drainage (PTD)
percutaneous transhepatic
pigtail catheter
percutaneous transhepatic
portography
percutaneous transjugular
approach
percutaneous translumbar
aortography
percutaneous transluminal
angioplasty (PTA, PTLA)
percutaneous transluminal
atherectomy
percutaneous transluminal
balloon dilatation (PTBD)
percutaneous transluminal
coronary angioplasty
(PTCA)
percutaneous transluminal renal
angioplasty (PTRA)
percutaneous transtracheal
bronchography
percutaneous transvenous mitral
commissurotomy
percutaneous ultrasonic
lithotripsy
percutaneous vasectomy
percutaneously
Percy cautery
Percy clamp
Percy forceps
Percy hemostat
Percy intestinal forceps
Percy retractor
Percy tissue forceps
Percy-Wolfson gallbladder
forceps

Percy-Wolfson gallbladder
retractor
Percy-Wolfson retractor
Perdue hemostat
Perdue tonsillar hemostat
Perdue tonsillar hemostat
forceps
Perell fetoscope
Pereyra bladder neck suspension
Pereyra bladder suspension
Pereyra cannula
Pereyra needle
Pereyra operation
Pereyra paraurethral suspension
Pereyra vesicourethral suspension
perforantes, arteriae
perforantes, venae
perforated acid peptic ulcer
perforated appendix
perforated diverticulum
perforated eardrum
perforated gallbladder
perforated ulcer
perforated viscus
perforating appendicitis
perforating arteries
perforating bur
perforating drill
perforating forceps
perforating fracture
perforating osteotome
perforating twist drill
perforating ulcer
perforating vein
perforating wound
perforation
perforative
perforative appendicitis
perforator
    Acra-Cut cranial perfora-
    tor
    Amnihook perforator
    amniotic membrane
    perforator
    antral perforator

perforator *continued*
    Baylor amniotic perforator
    Bishop antrum perforator
    Bishop perforator
    Blot perforator
    Chapman-Dintenfass perforator
    cranial perforator
    cranial twist drill perforator
    Cushing cranial perforator
    Cushing perforator
    DeLee-Perce perforator
    D'Errico perforator
    Friesner ear perforator
    hand ear perforator
    hand perforator
    Hillis perforator
    hunterian perforator
    incompetent perforator
    Joseph perforator
    Lempert perforator
    McKenzie perforator
    midtibial perforator
    Politzer ear perforator
    Royce perforator
    Smellie obstetrical perforator
    Smellie perforator
    Smith perforator
    Stein membrane perforator
    Stein perforator
    Stryker perforator
    Thornwald perforator
    tibial perforator
    tympanum perforator
    Wellaminski antral perforator
    Wellaminski perforator
    Williams ear perforator
    Williams perforator
    Wilson amniotic perforator
perforator and tributaries
perforators tied

performance
Performance surgical instruments
performed in routine fashion
perfunctory
perfusate
perfusion
perfusion cannula
perfusion catheter
perfusion defect
perfusion lung scan
perfusion of coronary artery
perfusion pressure
perfusion rate
perfusion scan
perfusion study
perfusion technique
perialveolar wiring
periampullary diverticulum
periampullary tumor
perianal
perianal abscess
perianal hematoma
perianal incision
perianal maceration
perianal reflex
perianal skin
perianal skin tag
perianal wart
periaortic chain
periaortic irradiation
periaortic lymph node
periaortic nodes
periapical abscess
periapical curettage
periapical lesion
periareolar
periareolar incision
periarterial pad
periarterial sympathectomy
periarticular calcification
periarticular fracture
periarticular soft tissues
peribronchial cuffing
peribronchial markings
pericallosal artery
pericallosal veins
pericapillary cells

pericardectomy
pericardiac veins
pericardiaceae, venae
pericardiacophrenic artery
pericardiacophrenic veins
pericardiacophrenica, arteria
pericardiacophrenicae, venae
pericardial
pericardial baffle
pericardial cavity
pericardial effusion
pericardial fat pad
pericardial fluid
pericardial fusion
pericardial murmur
pericardial patch
pericardial peel
pericardial pleura
pericardial puncture
pericardial raspatory
pericardial recess
pericardial rub
pericardial rupture
pericardial sac
pericardial sling
pericardial space
pericardial tumor
pericardial xenograft
pericardicentesis
pericardiectomy
pericardiocentesis
pericardiocentesis needle
pericardiolysis
pericardiomediastinitis
pericardioplasty
pericardiorrhaphy
pericardiostomy
pericardiotomy
pericardium
pericardotomy
pericaval
pericecal abscess
pericholecystic abscess
pericholecystic adhesions
pericholecystic edema
perichondrial elevator
perichondrial graft

pericolic abscess
pericolonic abscess
pericolonic penetration
pericortical clamp
pericostal suture
peridectomy
peridental
peridental membrane
peridural anesthesia
Peries medicated hygienic wipe
    dressing
perigastric
perigastric adhesions
perigastric lymph nodes
Peri-Guard
Peri-Guard vascular graft
perihernial
perihilar area
perihilar mass
perihilar scarring
peri-infarction block
peri-infarction conduction
    defect
perilimbal
perilimbal incision
perilobar pancreatitis
perilobular duct
perilunate dislocation
perilunate fracture
perilymph
perilymph fluid
perilymphatic fistula (PLF)
perimeter
perimetry
perinatal
perinatal injury
perineal
perineal area
perineal artery
perineal bandage
perineal biopsy
perineal body
perineal dissection
perineal fascia
perineal hernia
perineal hypospadias
perineal lithotomy

perineal mass
perineal needle biopsy
perineal nerve
perineal pad
perineal prostatectomy
perineal prostatectomy retractor
perineal reflection
perineal region
perineal retractor
perineal section
perineal self-retaining retractor
perineal sheet
perineal sinus
perineal skin tag
perineal space
perineal support
perineal support sutures
perineal tear
perineal tissue
perineales, nervi
perinealis, arteria
perineocele
perineoplasty
perineorrhaphy
perineotomy
perinephric
perinephric abscess
perinephric air injection
perinephric capsule
perinephric fascia
perinephric fat
perineum
perineural anesthesia
perineural block
perineurium
perinuclear cataract
periocular
periodic dilatation
periodic slowing
periodontal
periodontal anesthesia
periodontal ligament
periodontal probe
perioperative
periorbital ecchymosis
periorbital edema
periorbital hematoma

periorbital soft tissue
periorbital swelling
periosteal
periosteal band
periosteal bone
periosteal cyst
periosteal elevator (see also
    *elevator*)
    Adson periosteal elevator
    Allis periosteal elevator
    Aufranc periosteal
        elevator
    beat-up periosteal
        elevator
    Behrend periosteal
        elevator
    Bethune periosteal
        elevator
    blunt periosteal elevator
    Bowen periosteal
        elevator
    Bristow periosteal
        elevator
    Brophy periosteal
        elevator
    Buck periosteal elevator
    Cameron periosteal
        elevator
    Cameron-Haight
        periosteal elevator
    Campbell periosteal
        elevator
    Carroll periosteal
        elevator
    Carroll-Legg periosteal
        elevator
    Cheyne periosteal
        elevator
    Cloward periosteal
        elevator
    Cobb periosteal elevator
    Converse periosteal
        elevator
    Coryllos periosteal
        elevator
    Coryllos-Doyen perios-
        teal elevator

periosteal elevator *continued*
- costal periosteal elevator
- Cottle periosteal elevator
- Crego periosteal elevator
- curved periosteal elevator
- Cushing periosteal elevator
- Cushing-Hopkins periosteal elevator
- Davidson periosteal elevator
- Davidson-Sauerbruch-Doyen periosteal elevator
- Davis periosteal elevator
- D'Errico periosteal elevator
- Dingman periosteal elevator
- double-ended periosteal elevator
- Doyen periosteal elevator
- Dunning periosteal elevator
- Farabeuf periosteal elevator
- Federspiel periosteal elevator
- Fiske periosteal elevator
- Fomon periosteal elevator
- Freer periosteal elevator
- Goodwillie periosteal elevator
- Haight periosteal elevator
- Harper periosteal elevator
- Herczel periosteal elevator
- Hibbs periosteal elevator
- Hoen periosteal elevator
- Iowa periosteal elevator
- Iowa University periosteal elevator

periosteal elevator *continued*
- Joseph periosteal elevator
- Key periosteal elevator
- Kinsella periosteal elevator
- Kirmisson periosteal elevator
- Kocher periosteal elevator
- Lane periosteal elevator
- Langenbeck periosteal elevator
- Lewis periosteal elevator
- long periosteal elevator
- Love-Adson periosteal elevator
- Lowis periosteal elevator
- MacDonald periosteal elevator
- MacKenty periosteal elevator
- Matson periosteal elevator
- MGH periosteal elevator
- Molt periosteal elevator
- mucoperiosteal elevator
- Neurological Institute periosteal elevator
- Obwegeser periosteal elevator
- Overholt periosteal elevator
- Pace periosteal elevator
- periosteal elevator
- Poppen periosteal elevator
- Raney periosteal elevator
- Read periosteal elevator
- Roberts-Gill periosteal elevator
- Sayre periosteal elevator
- Scott-McCracken periosteal elevator
- Sedillot periosteal elevator

periosteal elevator *continued*
    Sewall mucoperiosteal elevator
    Spurling periosteal elevator
    Steele periosteal elevator
    Stille periosteal elevator
    Tenzel periosteal elevator
    Turner periosteal elevator
    von Langenbeck periosteal elevator
    Willauer-Gibbon periosteal elevator
    Yankauer periosteal elevator
periosteal fibroma
periosteal flap
periosteal flaps raised
periosteal ganglion
periosteal graft
periosteal implantation
periosteal level
periosteal membranous lining
periosteal raspatory
periosteal stripping
periosteal thickening
periosteoplastic amputation
periosteorrhaphy
periosteotome
    Alexander costal periosteotome
    Alexander periosteotome
    Alexander-Farabeuf costal periosteotome
    Alexander-Farabeuf periosteotome
    baby costal periosteotome
    Ballenger periosteotome
    Brophy periosteotome
    Brown periosteotome
    costal periosteotome
    Dean periosteotome
    Ferris Smith-Lyman periosteotome

periosteotome *continued*
    Fomon periosteotome
    Freer periosteotome
    Jansen periosteotome
    Joseph periosteotome
    Moorehead periosteotome
    Potts periosteotome
    Speer periosteotome
    Vaughan periosteotome
    West-Beck periosteotome
periosteotomy
periosteum
periosteum elevator
periosteum sheath
periosteum stripper
peripad
peripalpebral
peripapillary retinal edema
peripapillary scotoma
Peri-Patch peritoneal catheter extension set
peripatellar incision
peripatellar pain
peripelvic cyst
peripheral
peripheral artery bypass
peripheral atherectomy catheter
peripheral blood
peripheral blood vessel forceps
peripheral blood vessels
peripheral cataract
peripheral circulation
peripheral fields
peripheral iridectomy
peripheral iridectomy forceps
peripheral iridotomy
peripheral laser angioplasty (PLA)
peripheral long-line catheter
peripheral mass
peripheral nerve repair
peripheral nerve stimulation
peripheral nerves
peripheral nervous system
peripheral neuropathy

peripheral perfusion
peripheral pulses
peripheral reflex
peripheral vascular clamp
peripheral vascular disease
peripheral vascular forceps
peripheral vascular surgery
peripheral vessel
peripheral vision
peripherally inserted central
    catheter (PICC)
periphery
periportal carcinoma
periportal cirrhosis
periportal sinusoidal dilatation
perirectal
perirectal abscess
perirectal incision
perirectal incision and drainage
perirenal fascia
perirenal fat
perirenal space
perirenal tissues
periscapular incision
periscleral space
periscopic lens
perisinusoidal space
perispinal area
perispondylitis
peristalsis
peristaltic
peristaltic activity
peristaltic anastomosis
peristaltic motion
peristaltic movement
peristaltic rushes
peristaltic sounds
peristaltic unrest
peristaltic valve
peristaltic wave
perisylvian
peritectomy
perithelium
peritomist
peritomy
peritoneal
peritoneal abscess

peritoneal attachments
peritoneal autoplasty
peritoneal band
peritoneal button
peritoneal catheter
peritoneal cavity
peritoneal clamp
peritoneal closure
peritoneal dialysis
peritoneal dialysis catheter
peritoneal drainage
peritoneal floor
peritoneal fluid
peritoneal incision
peritoneal insertion of shunt
peritoneal lavage
peritoneal membrane
peritoneal mouse
peritoneal puncture
peritoneal reflection
peritoneal sac
peritoneal shunt
peritoneal sign
peritoneal space
peritoneal studding
peritoneal surface
peritoneal tap
peritoneal-atrial shunt
peritonealization
peritonealize
peritoneal-venous shunt
peritoneocaval shunt
peritoneocentesis
peritoneoclysis
peritoneocutaneous reflex
peritoneography
peritoneointestinal reflex
peritoneopericardial hernia
peritoneoplasty
peritoneoscope
        Photo-Flash peritoneo-
            scope
        Storz peritoneoscope
peritoneoscopy
peritoneoscopy examination
peritoneotomy
peritoneovenous

peritoneovenous shunt
peritoneum
peritonization
peritonize
peritonsillar
peritonsillar abscess
peritonsillar cellulitis
peritonsillar tags
periumbilical
periungual desquamation
periungual wart
periurethral
periurethral duct carcinoma
periurethral tissues
perivascular cells
perivascular lymph spaces
perivascular space
periventricular white matter
perivesical abscess
perivesical fascia
perivesical hernia
PERK protocol (prospective
    evaluation of radial
    keratotomy protocol)
Perkins elevator
Perkins retractor
Perkins tonometer
Perkins traction
Perkins tractor
Per-Lee middle ear tubes
Per-Lee myringotomy tubes
Per-Lee ventilating tubes
Perlmann tumor of kidney
Perlon sutures
Perma-Cath catheter
Perma-Cath drain
Perma-Hand braided silk
    sutures
Perma-Hand silk sutures
Perma-Hand sutures
permanent
permanent callus
permanent colostomy
permanent damage
permanent demand ventricular
    pacing system
permanent end colostomy

permanent ileostomy
permanent implant
permanent lead introducer
permanent loop ileostomy
permanent magnet
permanent myocardial pace-
    maker
permanent pacemaker
permanent paralysis
permanent rate-responsive
    pacemaker
permanent remission
permanent stoma
permanent stricture
permanent transvenous
    pacemaker
permanent ventricular pace-
    maker
Permathane Pacesetter lead
    pacemaker
permeability
permeable
permeation analgesia
permeation anesthesia
permissible
permission
permit
peronea, arteria
peroneae, venae
peroneal
peroneal artery
peroneal muscle
peroneal nerve
peroneal retinaculum
peroneal sheath
peroneal sign
peroneal sulcus
peroneal tendon
peroneal tendon sheath
peroneal tubercle
peroneal veins
peroneal vessels
peroneus brevis, musculus
peroneus communis, nervus
peroneus longus, musculus
peroneus profundus, nervus
peroneus superficialis, nervus

peroneus tertius, musculus
peroral
peroral endoscopy
peroral esophageal prosthesis
peroral gastroscope
peroral pneumocolon double-
    contrast follow-through
peroral retrograde pancreati-
    cobiliary ductography
peroxide
perpendicular
perpendicular plate of ethmoid
perpetual arrhythmia
Perras mammary prosthesis
Perritt fixation forceps
Perritt forceps
PERRLA (pupils equal, round,
    react to light and accom-
    modation)
Perry bag
Perry forceps
Perry ileostomy bag
Perry procedure for genu
    recurvatum
Perry-O'Brien-Hodgson
    technique
perseverance
perseverate
perseveration
persistence
persistent
Personna surgical blade
perspective
Per-Stat-DL catheter
Perthes incision
pertinent findings
pertrochanteric fracture
pertubation
pervasive
pervenous catheter
pes abductus
pes cavus
pes equinus
pes planus
pes valgus
pes varus
pessary
        Albert Smith pessary

pessary *continued*
    Blair modification of
        Gellhorn pessary
    blue ring pessary
    Chambers doughnut
        pessary
    Chambers pessary
    cup pessary
    diaphragm pessary
    doughnut pessary
    Dutch pessary
    Emmert-Gellhorn
        pessary
    Findley folding pessary
    Gariel pessary
    Gehrung pessary
    Gellhorn pessary
    globe prolapsus pessary
    Gynefold pessary
    Gynefold prolapse
        pessary
    Gynefold retrodisplace-
        ment pessary
    Hodge pessary
    hollow lucite pessary
    intrauterine pessary
    lever pessary
    lucite pessary
    Mayer pessary
    Menge pessary
    Menge stem pessary
    Milex pessary
    Plexiglas pessary
    Prochownik pessary
    prolapse ring pessary
    prolapsus pessary
    red pessary
    retrodisplaced pessary
    retroversion pessary
    ring pessary
    safety pessary
    Smith pessary
    Smith-Hodge pessary
    stem pessary
    White foam pessary
    Wylie pessary
    Wylie stem pessary
    Zwanck pessary

pessary *continued*
    Zwanck radium pessary
pessary doughnut
PET (positron emission
    tomography)
PET balloon
PET scanning
petechia (*pl.* petechiae)
petechial hemorrhage
Peter operation
Peter-Bishop forceps
Peters tissue forceps
Petersen bag
Petersen lithotomy
Petersen operation (GI)
Petersen rectal bag
Peterson cervical collar
Peterson operation (gyn)
Petit canal
Petit hernia
Petit ligament
▸ Petit sutures
Petrie spica cast
petrobasilar suture
petrolatum
petrolatum dressing
petrolatum gauze
petrolatum gauze dressing
petrolatum-impregnated gauze
petrosal ganglion
petrosal nerve
petrosal sinuses
petrosphenobasilar suture
petrosphenoid
petrosphenoidal syndrome
petrospheno-occipital suture of
    Gruber
petrosquamosal
petrosquamous
petrosquamous sutures
petrosus major, nervus
petrosus minor, nervus
petrosus profundus, nervus
petrotympanic fissure
petrous
petrous apices
petrous bone
petrous pyramid

petrous pyramid air cells
petrous ridge
petrous tips
PETT (positron emission
    transaxial/transverse
    tomography)
Petz clamp
Petz clip
Peyer patch
Peyer plaque
Peyman vitrectomy unit
Peyman vitrector
Peyman vitreophage unit
Peyman vitreous-grasping
    forceps
Peyman-Green vitreous forceps
Peyronie-like plaque
Peyrot thorax
Peyton brain spatula
Pezzar tube
Pezzer (see also *de Pezzer*)
Pezzer catheter
Pezzer drain
Pezzer mushroom-tipped
    catheter
Pezzer suprapubic cystostomy
    catheter
Pfannenstiel incision
Pfau atticus punch
Pfau forceps
Pfau punch
PFC component (Press-Fit
    condylar component)
Pfeiffer procedure
PFFD (proximal focal femoral
    deficiency)
Pfister stone basket
Pfister-Schwartz basket forceps
Pfister-Schwartz stone basket
Pfizer scan
Pfluger tube
PFT (parafascicular thalamot-
    omy)
PFTE shunt (polyfluorotetraeth-
    ylene shunt)
PGIA instrument
pH
pH probe

phacocystectomy
phacoemulsification
phacoemulsifier-aspirator
phacoemulsifier-extractor
phacoerysis
phacolysis
phakodialysis spatula
phakofragmatome
phalangeal articulation
phalangeal bone
phalangeal forceps
phalangeal fracture
phalangeal knife
phalangeal set
phalangeal tuft
phalangectomy
phalanges (*sing*. phalanx)
phalangization
phalangophalangeal amputa-
    tion
phalanx (*pl*. phalanges)
phalanx distalis
phalanx media
phalanx proximalis
Phalen maneuver
Phalen sign
Phalen sign for carpal tunnel
Phalen test
phallectomy
phallic
phalloplasty
phallotomy
phallus
Phaneuf artery forceps
Phaneuf clamp
Phaneuf forceps
Phaneuf maneuver
Phaneuf uterine artery forceps
Phaneuf vaginal forceps
Phaneuf-Graves operation
phantom clamp
phantom limb
phantom limb pain
phantom pregnancy
Pharmacia intraocular lens
Pharmaseal catheter
Pharmaseal drain
pharyngea ascendens, arteria

pharyngeae, venae
pharyngeal aperture
pharyngeal artery
pharyngeal branch of internal
    maxillary artery
pharyngeal bursa
pharyngeal constrictor muscle
pharyngeal flap
pharyngeal flap operation
pharyngeal flap palatoplasty
pharyngeal hemisphincter
pharyngeal insufflation anesthe-
    sia
pharyngeal lymph node
pharyngeal mirror
pharyngeal orifice
pharyngeal ostium
pharyngeal pack
pharyngeal plexus
pharyngeal pouch
pharyngeal raphe
pharyngeal recess
pharyngeal reflex
pharyngeal speculum
pharyngeal tonsil
pharyngeal tube
pharyngeal tubercle
pharyngeal veins
pharyngectomy
pharyngobasilar fascia
pharyngoepiglottic fold
pharyngoesophageal diverticu-
    lectomy
pharyngoesophageal diverticu-
    lum
pharyngoesophageal recon-
    struction
pharyngoesophageal sphincter
pharyngogram
pharyngolaryngectomy
pharyngopalatine arch
pharyngopalatine muscle
pharyngopalatinus, musculus
pharyngoplasty
pharyngorrhaphy
pharyngoscope
    ACMI nasopharyngo-
        scope

pharyngoscope *continued*
    Berci-Ward laryngo-
      pharyngoscope
    Broyles nasopharyngo-
      scope
    Holmes nasopharyngo-
      scope
    hypopharyngoscope
    Meltzer nasopharyngo-
      scope
    Storz laryngopharyngo-
      scope
    Yankauer nasopharyngo-
      scope
pharyngoscopy
pharyngotomy
pharyngotympanic tube
pharynx
phase
phase microscope
phase-contrast microscope
phasic activity
Pheasant elbow
Pheasant elbow dislocation
    operation
Pheasant technique
Pheifer-Young retractor
Phelps brace
Phelps gracilis test
Phelps operation
Phelps operation for talipes
    equinovarus
Phelps splint
Phelps-Baker gracilis test
Phelps-Gocht osteoclast
Phemister approach
Phemister elevator
Phemister graft
Phemister incision
Phemister onlay bone graft
Phemister operation
Phemister punch
Phemister rasp
Phemister raspatory
Phemister reamer
phenol
phenol neurolysis
phenomenon

phenopeel
phenylalanine mustard
pheochromocytoma
pheresis
Philadelphia cocktail
Philadelphia collar
Philadelphia collar cervical
    support
Philadelphia tonsil knife
Philips endorectal transducer
Philips endovaginal trans-
    ducer
Philips ultrasound machine
Phillips bougie
Phillips catheter
Phillips clamp
Phillips dilator
Phillips fixation forceps
Phillips forceps
Phillips muscle
Phillips recessed head screw
Phillips rectal clamp
Phillips screw
Phillips screwdriver
Phillips urethral catheter
philtral roll
philtrum
phimosis
phimosis forceps
phimosis vaginalis
Phipps forceps
pHisoDerm
pHisoHex
phlebectomy
phlebitic induration
phlebogram
phlebography
phlebolith
phlebolithiasis
phleboplasty
phleborrhagia
phleborrhaphy
phleborrheogram (PRG)
phleborrheograph
phleborrheography
phlebosclerosis
phlebothrombosis
phlebotome

phlebotomy
phlegm
phlegmon
phlegmonous
phlegmonous mass
Phoenix outrigger system
Phoenix single-chamber
    pacemaker
Phoenix total hip prosthesis
phonating edge
phonating structure
phonoangiography
phonocardiogram
phonocardiogram study
phonocardiography
phonocatheterization
Phoropter
Phoropter retractor
phosphatase
phosphate scan
photic stimulation
photoablation
photochemotherapy
photocoagulation
photocoagulator (see also
    coagulator)
        American Optical
            photocoagulator
        argon laser photocoagu-
            lator
        Coherent argon laser
            photocoagulator
        Mira photocoagulator
        xenon arc photocoagula-
            tor
        xenon photocoagulator
        Zeiss photocoagulator
photoculdoscope
Photo-Flash peritoneoscope
photofluorographic examination
photogastroscope
photographic radiometer
photokeratoscope
photometer
photon beam densitometry
photon microscope
photon-deficient lesion

photo-ophthalmia
photo-strobe
phototherapy
phrenemphraxis
phrenic
phrenic arteries
phrenic avulsion
phrenic evulsion
phrenic ganglion
phrenic lymph node
phrenic nerve
phrenic nerve stimulation
phrenic retractor
phrenic surface of spleen
phrenic veins
phrenicae inferiores, arteriae
phrenicae inferiores, venae
phrenicae superiores, arteriae
phrenicectomized
phrenicectomy
phrenicectomy forceps
phrenici accessorii, nervi
phreniclasia
phreniclasis
phrenicoabdominal nerves
phrenicocolic ligament
phrenicoesophageal ligament
phrenicoexeresis
phrenicolienal ligament
phreniconeurectomy
phrenicosplenic ligament
phrenicostomy
phrenicotomy
phrenicotripsy
phrenicus, nervus
phrenoesophageal ligament
phrenopericardial angle
phrenoplegia
phrygian cap
phrygian cap deformity
phrygian cap of gallbladder
Phynox clip
Phynox cobalt alloy clip
physeal plate
physical
physical sign
physical therapy (PT)

physically
physican's pickup forceps
physician's splinter forceps
Physick operation
Physick pouch
physiologic, physiological
physiologic pacemaker
physiologic curettement
physiology
physiotherapy
phytobezoar
PI surgical stapler
pia mater
PIBC catheter (percutaneous
    intra-aortic balloon
    counterpulsation catheter)
PICA (posterior inferior
    cerebellar artery)
PICA (posterior inferior
    communicating artery)
PICC (peripherally inserted
    central catheter)
pick
        Austin pick
        Bellucci pick
        Burch fixation pick
        Burch ophthalmic pick
        Burch pick
        Crane pick
        Drews pick
        Farrior anterior footplate
            pick
        Farrior footplate pick
        Farrior oval-window pick
        Farrior posterior
            footplate pick
        footplate pick
        Hoffmann scleral fixation
            pick
        Hough footplate pick
        Hough pick
        House pick
        ophthalmic pick
        Paparella pick
        Rhein pick
        right-angle pick
        Rosen pick
        Saunders-Paparella pick

pick   *continued*
        Scheer pick
        Schuknecht pick
        Shea pick
        slightly curved ear pick
        slightly curved pick
        small pick
        stapes pick
        strut pick
        Trent eye pick
        Wells pick
        Wells scleral suture pick
pick chisel
pick up (verb)
Picker Vanguard deep therapy
    unit
Pico operation
Picot retractor
Picot speculum
Picot vaginal speculum
Picot weighted speculum
pickup (noun, adj.)
pickup forceps
pickup noncrushing forceps
pickup screw
PID (pelvic inflammatory
    disease)
Pidcock nail
Pidcock pin
piecemeal
piecemeal removal
Piedmont all-cotton elastic
    dressing
Piedmont fracture of radius
Pier abduction splint
Pierce antral trocar
Pierce antral wash tube
Pierce attic cannula
Pierce cannula
Pierce cheek retractor
Pierce dissector
Pierce double-ended elevator
Pierce elevator
Pierce mastoid rongeur
Pierce raspatory
Pierce retractor
Pierce rongeur
Pierce saccade

Pierce submucous dissector
Pierce syringe
Pierce trocar
Pierce tube
Pierce washing tube
Pierce-Donachy ventricular
    assist device
Pierce-O'Connor operation
piercing instrument
Pierre Robin micrognathia
Pierrot-Murphy ankle procedure
Pierse Colibri forceps
Pierse corneal forceps
Pierse forceps
Pierse-Hoskins forceps
Pierson attachment
Pierson traction
Piezolith-EPL
Piffard curet
Piffard dermal curet
Piffard placental curet
pigeon breast deformity
pigeon toe
piggyback heart transplant
piggyback IV fluid
piggyback mammary prosthesis
piggyback probe
piggybacking
pigment
pigmentary
pigmentation
pigmented gallstone
pigmented lesion
pigmented nevus
pigment-laden
pigskin graft
pigtail catheter
pigtail nephrostomy drain
pigtail probe
pigtail stent
Pilcher bag
Pilcher bag catheter
Pilcher catheter
Pilcher hemostatic bag
Pilcher hemostatic suprapubic
    bag
pile clamp

pile forceps
pillar
pillar and dissector
pillar cells
pillar forceps
pillar of diaphragm
pillar of fornix
pillar projection
pillar retractor
pillar-grasping forceps
Pillet hand prosthesis
Pilling bronchoscope
Pilling clamp
Pilling duralite tracheal tube
Pilling forceps
Pilling gouge
Pilling shears
Pilling stethoscope
Pilling sutures
Pilling tracheostomy tube
Pilling tube
Pilling vascular needle holder
Pilling Wolvek sternal approxi-
    mator
Pilling-Douglas pelvimeter
Pilling-Favoloro retractor
Pilling-Liston bone utility
    forceps
Pilling-Ruskin rongeur
pillion fracture
pillow
pillow sign
pillow splint
pilocarpine
pilojection
pilonidal cyst
pilonidal cystectomy
pilonidal cystectomy and
    sinusectomy
pilonidal dimple
pilonidal sinus
pilosebaceous opening
pilosebaceous unit
pilot drill
piloting trocar
Pilotip catheter
Pilotip catheter guide

pin (see also *guide pin*)
    Ace pin
    ASIF screw pin
    Asnis pin
    Austin Moore pin
    Barr pin
    beaded hip pin
    Böhler pin
    Bohlman pin
    Breck pin
    calibrated guide pin
    calibrated-tip threaded
      guide pin
    Clerf-Arrowsmith pin
      closer
    Clerf-Arrowsmith safety
      pin closure
    cloverleaf pin
    Compere pin
    Compere threaded pin
    Conley pin
    Craig pin
    Crowe-tip pin
    Crutchfield skull-tip pin
    Davis pin
    Delitala T-pin
    Denham pin
    DePuy pin
    Deyerle pin
    duodenal pin
    Ender pin
    Fahey hip pin
    Fahey pin
    Fahey-Compere pin
    fixation pin
    Furniss-Clute pin
    Gouffon hip pin
    guide pin
    Hagie hip pin
    Hagie pin
    Hansen-Street pin
    Hatcher pin
    Haynes pin
    Hegge pin
    hexhead pin
    hip pin
    Hoffmann pin

pin *continued*
    intramedullary pin
    Jones pin
    Knowles pin
    Kronendonk pin
    Kronfeld pin
    Küntscher femur guide
      pin
    Küntscher pin
    Lottes pin
    Marble bone pin
    medullary pin
    metal pin
    micropin
    Moore pin
    Neufeld pin
    Norman tibial pin
    Oris pin
    osteotomy pin
    Pidcock pin
    pinion pin
    Pischel micropin
    Pischel pin
    Pugh hip pin
    Rhinelander pin
    Riordan pin
    Roger Anderson pin
    Rush intramedullary
      pin
    Rush pin
    Rush safety pin
    safety pin
    Sage pin
    Schneider pin
    Schneider self-broaching
      pin
    Schweitzer pin
    self-broaching pin
    self-tapering pin
    Shantz pin
    Shriners pin
    skeletal pin
    SMo Moore pin
    Smillie pin
    Smith-Petersen fracture
      pin
    Smith-Petersen pin

pin *continued*
 spring pin
 Stader pin
 Steinmann calibrated pin
 Steinmann pin
 Street medullary pin
 Street pin
 threaded pin
 tibial pin
 trochanteric pin
 Turner hip pin
 Turner pin
 Venable-Stuck fracture pin
 Venable-Stuck pin
 von Saal medullary pin
 von Saal pin
 Walker pin
 Watson-Jones guide pin
 Webb pin
 Zimfoam pin
 Zimmer pin
pin cutter
pin headrest
pin implant
pin sutures
pin tract
pin tract sinus
Pinard fetoscope
Pinard sign
pin-bending forceps
pincers
pinch forceps
pinch graft
pinch nose strut
pinch skin graft
pinchcock clamp
pinchcock mechanism
pinched nerve
pinching pain
pin-cushion distortion
pineal body
pineal calcification
pineal gland
pinealectomy
pinealoma
pinealotomy

ping-pong fracture
pinhole
pinion headrest
pinion pin
pink
pink twisted cotton sutures
pinkish
pinky compression procedure
 (lens implant surgery)
pinna
Pinnacle pacemaker
pinnectomy
pinned
pinning
pinning operation
pinpoint os
pinpoint pupils
pinprick
pinprick analgesia
pins-and-needles sensation
Pinto distractor
pin-tract infection
pinwheel exam
pinwheel hypesthesia
PIP (pressure inversion point)
Pipelle endometrial suction
 curet
Piper forceps
Piper lateral wall retractor
Piper obstetrical forceps
piperocaine hydrochloride
 anesthetic agent
pipette
PIPIDA hepatobiliary scanning
 agent
piping rales
Pipkin fracture
Pirie bone
piriform aperture wiring
piriform crest
piriform fossa
piriform muscle
piriform opening
piriform process
piriform recess
piriform sills
piriform sinus

piriformis, musculus
Pirogoff amputation
Pirogoff angle
Pirogoff operation
Pirquet decompressor
Pisces device
Pisces implant
Pischel electrode
Pischel elevator
Pischel forceps
Pischel micropin
Pischel pin
Pischel scleral ruler
pisiform bone
pisihamate ligament
pisitriquetral joint
pisometacarpal ligament
pistol-shot pulse
piston
piston prosthesis
piston sign
piston strut
pistoning movement
piston-type prosthesis
Pitanguy demarcator
Pitanguy fat
Pitanguy forceps
Pitanguy mammaplasty
Pitanguy reduction mamma-
    plasty
Pitha forceps
Pitha urethral forceps
Pitkin dermatome
Pitkin needle
Pitkin syringe
Pitocin augmentation of labor
Pitocin drip
Pitot tube
Pitt tracheostomy tube
pitting edema
Pittman needle holder
Pittsburgh triangular frame
pituitary
pituitary ablation
pituitary adenoma
pituitary body
pituitary capsulectomy

pituitary capsulectomy knife
pituitary curet
pituitary disorder
pituitary elevator
pituitary forceps
pituitary fossa
pituitary gland
pituitary growth hormone
pituitary lesion
pituitary rongeur
pituitary rongeur forceps
pituitary stalk
pituitary tumor
pituitectomy
Pituitrin uterine injection
pivot aneurysm clip applier
pivot joint
pivot microanastomosis clip
    applier
pivotal disk heart valve
PLA (peripheral laser
    angioplasty)
placed in position
placed in traction
placement
placenta
placenta accreta
placenta bipartita
placenta clamp
placenta curet
placenta delivered
placenta expelled
placenta extracted
placenta forceps
placenta intact
placenta previa
placenta previa forceps
placenta reflexa
placenta removed
placenta retained
placenta scan
placental bruit
placental circulation
placental dysfunction
placental dystocia
placental forceps
placental fragment

placental growth hormone
placental index
placental insufficiency
placental membrane
placental presentation
placental septum
placental site
placental tissue
placental transfusion
placental villi
placentogram
placentography
Placido disk
placing of clamp
plafond
plain catgut sutures
plain film
plain films of abdomen
plain forceps
plain gauze
plain gauze ABD
plain gut sutures
plain interrupted sutures
plain pattern plate
plain screwdriver
plain sutures
plain thumb forceps
plain tie
plain tissue forceps
plain view
plain wire speculum
plain x-ray
planar image
planar incision
plane
plane configuration
Plange spud
planigram
planimetry
planned
planning
plano lens
plano T-bandage
planoconcave
planoconcave lens
planoconvex
planoconvex lens

planographic examination
planovalgus deformity
planovalgus feet
plant
plantar
plantar arch
plantar artery
plantar aspect
plantar aspect of foot
plantar axial x-ray
plantar calcaneal spur
plantar calcaneocuboid
    ligament
plantar digital arteries
plantar digital nerves
plantar digital veins
plantar fascia
plantar fasciotomy
plantar fasciitis
plantar flexion
plantar flexors
plantar interosseous muscles
plantar ligaments
plantar metatarsal arteries
plantar metatarsal vein
plantar muscle
plantar nerve
plantar reflex
plantar response
plantar surface
plantar verruca
plantar view
plantar wart
plantar-flexed metatarsal
plantaris lateralis, arteria
plantaris lateralis, nervus
plantaris medialis, arteria
plantaris, musculus
plaque
plaquing
plasm
plasma
plasma exchange
plasma expander
plasma protein fraction
plasma scalpel
plasma TFE graft

plasma TFE vascular graft
plasma transfusion
plasma volume expander
Plasmalyte
plasmapheresis
plasmid-carrying cell
plaster
plaster bandage
plaster boot
plaster cast
plaster cast cutter
plaster cast knife
plaster dressing
plaster knife
plaster pants dressing
plaster pants prosthesis
plaster saw
plaster shears
plaster spline
plaster splint
plaster-of-Paris cast
plaster-of-Paris dressing
plaster-of-Paris jacket
plaster-of-Paris scissors
Plastibell circumcision
Plastibell clamp
plastic achillotenotomy
plastic Adzef sheet
plastic and reconstructive
    surgery
plastic ball
plastic ball eye implant
plastic Berger eye loupe
plastic bridge colostomy pouch
plastic cannula
plastic catheter
plastic closure
plastic conformer
plastic construction
plastic crown
plastic curet
plastic drape
plastic dressing
plastic eye knife box
plastic floor reaction orthosis
plastic implant
plastic induration

plastic lens
plastic membrane
plastic motor
plastic mouth guard
plastic needle holder
plastic operation
plastic reconstruction
plastic repair
plastic revision
plastic scissors
plastic Silastic
plastic sphere eye implant
plastic sphere implant
plastic splint
plastic suction tip
plastic surgery
plastic surgery elevator
plastic surgery scissors
plastic sutures
plastic syringe
plastic tube
Plasticor torque-type prosthesis
Plasti-Pore ossicular replace-
    ment prosthesis
Plasti-Pore strut
Plasti-Pore total ossicular
    replacement prosthesis
    (Plasti-Pore TORP)
Plasti-Pore TORP (Plasti-Pore
    total ossicular replacement
    prosthesis)
plastisol
Plastizote collar
Plastizote neck collar
Plastizote orthotic device
Plastizote plate
Plastogel
plasty
plate (see also *nail plate*)
        AIO compression plate
        anal plate
        anchor plate
        AO compression plate
        AO plate
        AOI compression
            plate
        ASIF plate

plate *continued*

Babcock plate
Badgley plate
Bagby compression plate
Bagby plate
Batchelor plate
bent blade plate
blade plate
Blount blade plate
Blount plate
bone plate
bony plate
Bosworth plate
breast plate
Brophy plate
Burns plate
buttress plate
Champy bone plate
cloverleaf plate
coaptation plate
cobra plate
cobra-head plate
Collison plate
compression plate
compression screw plate
condylar blade plate
cribriform plate
Davis tooth plate
DCFAO plate
DCP plate (dynamic
    compression plate)
dental plate
DePuy plate
Deyerle plate
disposable ground plate
dorsal plate
double-angled blade
    plate
dural plate
dynamic compression
    plate (DCP)
Eggers bone plate
Eggers plate
Elliot femoral condyle
    blade plate
Elliot femoral condyle
    plate

plate *continued*

Elliot plate
Ellis plate
endplate
endplate of vertebrae
epiphyseal plate
femoral condyle plate
femoral plate
finger plate
flat plate
flat plate of abdomen
Foley plate
footplate
gait plate
Gelfilm plate
graft blade plate
ground plate
growth plate
Hansen-Street plate
hilar plate
Hoen plate
Hoen skull plate
Holt nail plate
Howmedica plate
Hubbard plate
ICS plate
intertrochanteric plate
Ishihara plate
Jaeger lid plate
Jewett double-angle
    osteotomy plate
Jewett nail overlay plate
Jewett plate
Jewett slotted plate
Ken plate
Kessel plate
Kilner-Doughty plate
Kirschner TOD plate
knee plate
L-plate
Laing plate
Lawson-Thornton plate
Letournel fracture plate
Leyla footplate
lid plate
limiting plate
Luer reconstruction plate

plate 833

plate *continued*
- lugged plate
- Luhr mandibular plate
- malleable plate
- McBride plate
- McLaughlin plate
- medial pterygoid plate
- Mennen plate
- Messner plate
- metal plate
- Moe intertrochanteric plate
- Moe plate
- Moore plate
- Moore-Blount plate
- Mueller hip plate
- mushroom-type plate
- MVR plate
- nail plate
- nephrotome plate
- Neufeld femoral nail plate
- Neufeld plate
- Newington plate
- Newman plate
- Nicoll plate
- Omni plate CHS system (compression hip screw system)
- orbital plate
- Osborne osteotomy plate
- ostectomy plate
- osteotomy plate
- palatal linguoplate
- partial plate
- paste plate
- patient plate
- perpendicular plate of ethmoid
- physeal plate
- plain pattern plate
- Plastizote plate
- polyethylene plate
- pterygoid plate
- Pugh plate
- Rhinelander plate
- Richards hip screw plate

plate *continued*
- Richards side plate
- Schuknecht footplate hook
- Schweitzer spring plate
- screw plate
- self-compressing plate
- semitubular plate
- Senn bone plate
- serpentine bone plate
- serpentine plate
- Shelton plate
- Sherman bone plate
- Sherman plate
- side plate
- Silastic plate
- six-hole stainless steel plate
- skull plate
- slide plate
- slotted plate
- Smith-Petersen plate
- SMo plate
- spinal fusion plate
- spring plate
- stapes footplate
- steel plate
- Steffee plate
- suction plate
- supracondylar plate
- Synthes plate
- Synthes metallic plate
- T-plate
- tantalum plate
- tarsal plate
- Teflon plate
- Temple University plate
- Thornton plate
- Thornton side plate
- tibial fixation plate
- tibial relocation plate
- TOD plate (titanium optimized design plate)
- trochanteric plate
- V-blade plate

plate *continued*
- V-type intertrochanteric plate
- Venable bone plate
- Venable plate
- vertebral endplate
- Vitallium plate
- volar plate
- VSP plate
- vulcanite dental plate
- Wainwright osteotomy plate
- Wenger slotted plate
- Whitman plate
- Wiener gold plate
- Wilson plate
- Wright knee plate
- Wright plate
- Wurzburg plate
- Y-bone plate
- Y-plate
- Yaeger lid plate
- Z-plate
- Zimmer femoral condyle blade plate
- Zimmer hip plate
- Zuelzer hook plate
- Zuelzer plate

plateau fracture
plateau joint surface
plateaued
plateauing
platelet
plates and screws
platform forceps
platform lift
platform system
platform walker
Platina clip implant cataract lens
Platina clip lens
Platina intraocular lens implant
plating
platinum
platinum blade electrode
platinum conjunctival smear spatula
platinum filter
platinum iridium capsule

platinum loop
platinum material
platinum spatula
Platou osteotomy
platysma
platysma muscle
platysmal reflex
Playfair uterine caustic applicator
pleating
pledget
pledget dressing
pledget sponge
pledget sutures
pledgeted Ethibond sutures
pledgeted sutures
Plenk-Matson rasp
Plenk-Matson raspatory
plesiosectional tomography
plethoric dysmenorrhea
plethysmogram
plethysmography
pleura
pleuracentesis
pleuracotomy
pleural abrasion
pleural adhesion
pleural biopsy
pleural biopsy needle
pleural biopsy punch
pleural bleb
pleural cavity
pleural cupola
pleural dissector
pleural effusion
pleural fibrosis
pleural fluid
pleural fremitus
pleural friction rub
pleural lavage
pleural mass
pleural metastasis
pleural peel
pleural plaquing
pleural pleurisy
pleural poudrage
pleural rale
pleural reaction

pleural rub
pleural sac
pleural scarring
pleural shock
pleural space
pleural suction tube
pleural surface
pleural symphysis
pleural thickening
pleural tube
pleural villi
pleuralized
pleurectomy
pleurectomy forceps
Pleur-Evac autotransfusion
    system
Pleur-Evac suction
Pleur-Evac suction tube
Pleur-Evac tube
pleurocentesis
pleurodesis
pleuroesophageal muscle
pleuroesophageus, musculus
pleurolysis
pleuroparietopexy
pleuropericardial incision
pleuropericardial murmur
pleuropericardial window
pleuroperitoneal canal
pleuroperitoneal hernia
pleuropexy
pleuropneumonolysis
pleuropulmonary congestion
pleurotomy
Pleurovac chest catheter
plexectomy
plexiform neuroma
Plexiglas eye implant
Plexiglas graft
Plexiglas implant
Plexiglas pessary
Plexiglas prosthesis
Plexiglas splint
plexus (*pl.* plexus, plexuses)
plexus anesthesia
plexus of Santorini
plexus pampiniformis
Pley capsule forceps

Pley forceps
PLF (perilymphatic fistula)
pliable
pliable paraffin
plica (*pl.* plicae)
plica duodenalis
plica duodenojejunalis
plica duodenomesocolica
plica epigastrica
plica gastropancreatica
plica ileocecalis
plica paraduodenalis
plica semilunaris
plica umbilicalis
plicae (*sing.* plica)
plicated tongue
plicating sutures
plication
plication needle
plication of bowel
plication sutures
plicecotomy
plicotomy
pliers
        crown-crimping pliers
        dental pliers
        fisherman's pliers
        Maddox pliers
        needle-nosed pliers
        Power Grip pliers
        Risley pliers
        root pliers
        slip joint pliers
        Swan-Jacob goniotomy
            pliers
        vice-grip pliers
PLIF procedure (posterior
    lumbar interbody fusion
    procedure)
plombage
Plondke uterine-elevating
    forceps
plug
        Air-Lon decannulation
            plug
        Air-Lon plug
        Alcock catheter plug
        Alcock plug

plug *continued*
    bile plug
    Biomet plug
    bone plug
    catheter plug
    choanal plug
    Corner plug
    cotton plug
    decannulation plug
    Diomet plug
    Dittrich plug
    Doc's ear plug
    Dohlman plug
    fibrin plug
    gastrostomy plug
    glass vaginal plug
    Johnston plug
    Mack ear plug
    meconium plug
    mucus plug
    Reich-Nechtow plug
    Seidel plug
    Sims plug
    Teflon Bardic plug
plugged
plugged tube
plugging
plumb line sign
plumb line test
Plummer bag
Plummer bougie
Plummer dilator
Plummer esophageal dilator
Plummer water-filled pneumatic
    esophageal dilator
Plummer-Vinson apparatus
Plummer-Vinson applicator
Plummer-Vinson dilator
Plummer-Vinson radium
    applicator
plural pregnancy
Plystan graft
Plystan implant
Plystan prosthesis
PMH scissors
PMI (point of maximal
    impulse)

PMI implant
PMMA (polymethyl meth-
    acrylate)
PMMA bone cement
PMT AccuSpan tissue expander
PMT tissue expander
pneumatic
pneumatic antishock garment
    (PASG)
pneumatic antishock trousers
pneumatic bag
pneumatic bag esophageal
    dilatation
pneumatic balloon catheter
pneumatic balloon catheter
    dilation
pneumatic balloon dilator
pneumatic compression
pneumatic compression
    stockings
pneumatic cuff
pneumatic dilator
pneumatic otoscope
pneumatic retinopexy
pneumatic space
pneumatic splint
pneumatic tonometer
pneumatic tourniquet
pneumatonographer
pneumatonometer
pneumectomy
pneumoarthrogram
pneumocentesis
pneumocisternogram
pneumocisternography
pneumoencephalogram
pneumoencephalography
pneumogastric nerve
pneumogram
pneumography
pneumogynogram
pneumogynography
pneumohydraulic infusion
    system
pneumolysis
pneumomediastinogram
pneumomediastinography

pneumonectomy
pneumonocentesis
pneumonolysis
pneumonopexy
pneumonoresection
pneumonorrhaphy
pneumonotomy
pneumoperitoneum
pneumoperitoneum needle
pneumopexy
pneumoresection
pneumotachometer
pneumothorax
pneumothorax apparatus (see
   also *apparatus*)
      Davidson pneumothorax
        apparatus
      McKesson pneumothorax
        apparatus
pneumothorax injection needle
pneumothorax needle
pneumoventriculogram
pneumoventriculography
pneuPAC resuscitator
pneuPAC ventilator
p.o., PO, or po (by mouth, per
   os)
pocket chamber
pocket of pus
pocket operation
pocket probe
Pocket-Dop II
podalic version
point
point electrode
point forceps
point of election
point of maximal impulse (PMI)
point tenderness
pointed pinna
pointed scissors
pointed-tip electrode
pointer
pointing
poison
poker spine
Poland classification of fractures

polar cataract
polar presentation
polarity
polarization
polarizing microscope
Polar-Mate bipolar microcoagu-
   lator
Polaroid camera
Polaroid film
pole
pole of kidney
Poliak eye retractor
policeman's heel
polio laryngoscope
Polisar-Lyons tube
polisher
polishing brush
polishing bur
polishing disk
Politano-Leadbetter operation
Politzer air bag
Politzer angular ear knife
Politzer bag
Politzer ear knife
Politzer ear perforator
Politzer ear speculum
Politzer knife
Politzer operation
Politzer otoscope
Politzer speculum
politzerization
Politzer-Ralks knife
Polk goniometer
Polk sponge forceps
Polley-Bickel trephine
Polli surgical garments
pollicis brevis, musculus
pollicis longus, musculus
pollicization
Pollock amputation
Pollock double corneal for-
   ceps
Pollock forceps
Pollock operation
Pollock punch
polly-beak deformity of nose
pollywogs

poly-1-hydroxyethyl meth-
   acrylate
Polya anastomosis
Polya gastrectomy
Polya gastroenterostomy
Polya gastrojejunostomy
Polya operation
Polya technique
polyacetyl
Polyak operation
polyamide sutures
polyaxial joint
polycentric knee prosthesis
polycentric prosthesis
polycycloidal tomography
polycystic disease
polycystic kidney
polycystic liver
polycystic ovary (PCO)
polycystic renal disease
Polydek sutures
polydioxanone sutures (PDS)
polyester
polyester fiber sutures
polyester sutures
polyester-reinforced Dacron
   tape
polyether graft material
polyether implant material
polyether prosthesis material
polyethylene
polyethylene ball
polyethylene cannula
polyethylene catheter
polyethylene cement
polyethylene collar button
polyethylene drain
polyethylene drainage tube
polyethylene eye implant
polyethylene glycol lavage
polyethylene graft
polyethylene implant
polyethylene plate
polyethylene prosthesis
polyethylene snare
polyethylene sphere implant
polyethylene stent

polyethylene strut
polyethylene sutures
polyethylene talar prosthesis
polyethylene tube
polyethylene vein stripper
polyfilament sutures
PolyFlex implantable pacing
   lead pacemaker
PolyFlex lead
PolyFlex lead pacemaker
PolyFlex traction dressing
polyfluorotetraethylene shunt
   (PFTE shunt)
polyglycolic acid
polyglycolic acid mesh
polyglycolic sutures
polylobar liver
polymer
polymeric carbon
polymerization
polymethyl methacrylate
   (PMMA)
polymorphic
polymorphonuclear cell
polymorphous
polymyxin
polyneuritis
polyneuropathy
polyolefin elastomer
polyp
polyp forceps
polyp grasper
polyp snare
polyp stalk
polypectomy
polyphasic wave
polypoid
polypoid adenoma
polypoid lesion
polypoid mass
polypoid polyp
polypoid tissue
polyposis
polyposis coli
polyposis gastrica
polyposis intestinalis
polyposis ventriculi

polypotome
polypotrite
polypous endocarditis
polypous gastritis
polypropylene
polypropylene braid
polypropylene button sutures
polypropylene mesh
polypropylene sutures
polypus
polypus forceps
polyradicular joint disease
polyscope
Polysporin ointment
Polystan catheter
Polystan implant
Polystan perfusion cannula
Polystan shunt
Polystan venous return catheter
polystyrene foam
polysulfone
polytef
polytetrafluoroethylene
polytetrafluoroethylene graft
    (PTFE graft)
Polytrac Gomez retractor
Polytrac retractor
polyunguia
polyurethane
polyurethane foam embolus
polyurethane graft
polyurethane implant
polyurethane packing
polyurethane prosthesis
polyuria
polyvinyl alcohol
polyvinyl alcohol splint
polyvinyl alcohol splinting
    material
polyvinyl alcohol sponge
polyvinyl catheter
polyvinyl curet
polyvinyl drain
polyvinyl graft
polyvinyl implant
polyvinyl prosthesis
polyvinyl sponge

polyvinyl sponge implant
polyvinyl tube
polyvinyl tubing
Pomeranz aortic clamp
Pomeranz retractor
Pomeroy ear syringe
Pomeroy manner
Pomeroy operation
Pomeroy salpingectomy
Pomeroy sterilization
Pomeroy syringe
Pomeroy tubal ligation
Poncet operation
pond fracture
Pond splint
Ponka anesthetic technique
Ponka herniorrhaphy
Ponka local anesthesia tech-
    nique
pons (*pl.* pontes)
pons cerebelli
pons hepatis
pons oblongata
pons tarini
pons varolii
Ponseti splint
Ponsky-Gauderer PEG proce-
    dure
Ponsky-Gauderer PEG tube
pontes (*sing.* pons)
pontile hemianesthesia
pontine
pontine angle
pontine flexure
pontine lesions
pontine tumor
Pontocaine anesthetic agent
pontoon
Pool Pfeiffer self-locking clip
pool sucker
Poole abdominal suction tube
Poole suction tip
Poole suction tube
Poole trocar
Poole tube
pooling
poorly defined

poorly differentiated
poorly visualized
POP bandage (plaster-of-Paris bandage)
pop scar
Pope halo dressing
Pope Merocel ear packing
Pope Merocel ear wick
Pope rectal knife
poplitea, arteria
poplitea, vena
popliteal aneurysm
popliteal artery
popliteal bypass
popliteal cyst
popliteal entrapment
popliteal fossa
popliteal incision
popliteal lymph node
popliteal muscle
popliteal nerve
popliteal notch
popliteal pulse
popliteal space
popliteal vein
popliteus, musculus
pop-off needle
pop-off sutures
Poppen clamp
Poppen coagulator
Poppen elevator
Poppen fashion
Poppen forceps
Poppen Gigli-saw guide
Poppen intervertebral disk rongeur
Poppen needle
Poppen periosteal elevator
Poppen pituitary rongeur
Poppen rongeur
Poppen scissors
Poppen suction tube
Poppen ventricular needle
Poppen-Blalock carotid artery clamp
Poppen-Blalock clamp
Poppen-Blalock-Salibi clamp

Poppen-Gelpi laminectomy self-retaining retractor
Poppers tonsillar guillotine
poppet
poppet valve
porcelain gallbladder
porcelain inlay
porcine graft
porcine heart valve
porcine heterograft
porcine heterograft prosthesis
porcine valve
porcine xenograft
porencephalic cyst
pores
Porex Medpor implant
Porex nerve locator
Porex PHA implant
Porex tissue expander
Porges stone dislodger
Porocoat material
porokeratosis
poroplastic splint
porosis
porotic
porotomy
porous bones
porous coat cup for Richards hip prosthesis
porous coated anatomic knee prosthesis (PCA knee prosthesis)
porous ingrowth
porous materials
porous prosthetic materials
PORP (partial ossicular reconstructive/replacement prosthesis)
Porro cesarean hysterectomy
Porro cesarean section
Porro hysterectomy
Porro operation
Porro-Veit operation
port of entry
port wine mark
porta
porta hepatis

Popovich

porta hepatis plexus
porta lienis
Porta Pulse 3 defibrillator
portable
portable aspirator
portable dialysis system
portable dialysis unit
portable film
portable respirator
portable suction aspirator
port-A-Cath
portacaval
portacaval anastomosis
portacaval shunt
portacaval transposition
portacid
portae, vena
portal
portal block
portal cannula
portal catheter
portal circulation
portal decompression
portal fissure
portal hypertension
portal obstruction
portal shunt
portal sinus
portal system
portal systemic anastomosis
portal to systemic venous shunt
portal triad
portal vascular bed
portal vein
portal vein thrombosis
portal venography
portal venous system
portal-systemic shunt
portarenal shunt
Porter duodenal forceps
Porter forceps
Porter-Richardson-Vainio elbow
    synovectomy
Portex cannula
Portex speaking tube
Portex tracheostomy
Portex tracheostomy tube

Portex tube
portio
portio and stroma
portligature
Portmann interposition opera-
    tion
Portmann retractor
Portmann speculum
Portnoy catheter
Portnoy ventricular cannula
Portnoy ventricular-end shunt
portoenterostomy
portogram
portograph
Porto-lift
portopulmonary shunt
portorenal shunt
portosystemic anastomosis
portosystemic encephalopathy
portosystemic shunt
portosystemic vascular shunt
Porto-vac catheter
Porto-vac suction tube
Porzett splint
Posey belt
Posey restraint
Posey sling
Posey support
position
    Adams position
    adduction position
    Albers-Schoenberg
        position
    Albert position
    anatomical position
    antero-oblique position
    anteverted position
    arm extension position
    beach-chair position
    Blackett-Healy position
    Bonner position
    Boyce position
    Bozeman position
    Brickner position
    brow-down position
    brow-up position
    Buie position

position *continued*
    Caldwell position
    calibrated position
    Camp-Coventry position
    Casselberry position
    chest position
    claw-toe position
    Cleaves position
    coiled position
    craniocaudad position
    cross-table lateral
      position
    decortical position
    decubitus position
    Depage position
    dextroposition
    dorsal decubitus position
    dorsal elevated position
    dorsal inertia position
    dorsal lithotomy position
    dorsal position
    dorsal recumbent
      position
    dorsal rigid position
    dorsodecubitus position
    dorsorecumbent position
    dorsosacral position
    dorsosupine position
    Duncan position
    Edebohls position
    Elliot position
    English position
    erect position
    eversion position
    extended position
    extreme Trendelenburg
      position
    face-down position
    Feist-Mankin position
    fetal position
    Fick position
    figure-four position
    flexion position
    Fowler position
    fracture position
    frog-legged position
    froglike position

position *continued*
    frontoanterior position
    frontotransverse position
    Fuchs position
    functional position
    Gaynor-Hart position
    genucubital position
    genufacial position
    genupectoral position
    Grashey position
    gravity-free position
    head dependent position
    high stirrups position
    hinge position
    horizontal position
    hornpipe position
    incomplete breech
      position
    inversion position
    inverted jackknife
      position
    Isherwood position
    jackknife position
    Johnson position
    joint position
    Jones position
    Jonge position
    juxtaposition
    kidney position
    knee-chest position
    knee-elbow position
    kneeling-squatting
      position
    Kraske position
    Kurzbauer position
    Lange position
    Larkin position
    lateral anterior position
    lateral decubitus position
    lateral position
    lateral prone position
    lateral rectus position
    lateral recumbent
      position
    Law position
    Lawrence position
    leapfrog position

position *continued*
    left decubitus position
    left lateral decubitus position
    left lateral position
    left mentoanterior position (LMA position)
    left mentoposterior position (LMP position)
    left mentotransverse position (LMT position)
    left occipitoanterior position (LOA position)
    left occipitoposterior position (LOP position)
    left occipitotransverse position (LOT position)
    left sacroanterior position (LSA position)
    left sacroposterior position (LSP position)
    left scapuloanterior position (LScA position)
    left scapuloposterior position (LScP position)
    Leonard-George position
    Lewis position
    Lindblom position
    lithotomy position
    lithotomy-Trendelenburg position
    LMA position (left mentoanterior position)
    LMP position (left mentoposterior position)

position *continued*
    LMT position (left mentotransverse position)
    LOA position (left occipitoanterior position)
    LOP position (left occipitoposterior position)
    Lorenz position
    LOT position (left occipitotransverse position)
    Low-Beers position
    LSA position (left sacroanterior position)
    LScA position (left scapuloanterior position)
    LScP position (left scapuloposterior position)
    LSP position (left sacroposterior position)
    malposition
    Mayer position
    Mayo-Robson position
    Mercurio position
    Miller position
    modified position
    Moynihan position
    neck extension position
    neutral position
    Noble position
    oblique position
    obstetrical position
    occipitoanterior position
    occipitoposterior position
    occipitosacral position
    occipitotransverse position
    occlusal position
    Ochsner position

position *continued*

    o'clock position
       (1 through 12)
    orthopnea position
    orthotonos position
    Owen position
    PA position (postero-
       anterior position)
    Péan position
    Pearson position
    posteroanterior position
       (PA position)
    postreduction position
    Proetz position
    prone jackknife posi-
       tion
    prone position
    recumbent position
    rest position
    reverse Trendelenburg
       position
    reverse Waters x-ray
       position
    right antero-oblique
       position
    right decubitus position
    right lateral position
    right mentoanterior
       position (RMA
       position)
    right mentoposterior
       position (RMP
       position)
    right mentotransverse
       position (RMT
       position)
    right occipitoanterior
       position (ROA
       position)
    right occipitoposterior
       position (ROP
       position)
    right occipitotransverse
       position (ROT
       position)
    right sacroanterior
       position (RSA position)

position *continued*

    right sacroposterior
       position (RSP posi-
       tion)
    right scapuloanterior
       position (RScA
       position)
    right scapuloposterior
       position (RScP
       position)
    right upper quadrant
       position (RUQ
       position)
    RMA position (right
       mentoanterior
       position)
    RMP position (right
       mentoposterior
       position)
    RMT position (right
       mentotransverse
       position)
    ROA position (right
       occipitoanterior
       position)
    Robson position
    ROP position (right
       occipitoposterior
       position)
    Rose head-extension
       position
    Rose position
    ROT position (right
       occipitotransverse
       position)
    RSA position (right
       sacroanterior posi-
       tion)
    RSP position (right
       sacroposterior
       position)
    RScA position (right
       scapuloanterior
       position)
    RScP position (right
       scapuloposterior
       position)

position *continued*

RUQ position (right upper quadrant position)
SA position (sacro-anterior position)
sacroanterior position (SA position)
sacrodextra anterior position
sacrodextra posterior position
sacroposterior position (SP position)
sacrotransverse position
Samuel position
scapuloanterior position
scapuloposterior position
Schuller position
scultetus position
semibarber position
semierect position
semi-Fowler position
semiprone position
semireclining position
semirecumbent position
semiupright position
Settegast position
shock position
shoe-and-stocking position
Simon position
Sims position
sitting position
ski position
SP position (sacro-posterior position)
Staunig position
Stecher position
steep Trendelenburg position
Stenver position
Stern position
superimposition
supine position
Tarrant position
Taylor position

position *continued*

Titterington semiaxial position
tonsil position
Towne position
Trendelenburg position
Twining position
upright position
usual anatomic position
Valentine position
Walcher position
Waters position
Waters-Waldron position
Wigby-Taylor position
Williams position
Wolfenden position
Zanelli position
positioned and draped
positioner
acetabular cup positioner
cup positioner
McCaffrey positioner
series II acetabular cup positioner
Vac-Pac positioner
positioning
positioning of patient
positive airway pressure
positive bowel sounds
positive charge
positive culture
positive end-airway pressure (PEAP)
positive end-expiratory phase (PEEP)
positive end-expiratory pressure (PEEP)
positive finding
positive maneuver
positive node
positive pressure
positive reaction
positive result
positive torsion
positive x-ray finding
Positran technique
positrocephalogram

positrocephalography
Positrol catheter
Positrol USCI catheter
positron
positron computed tomography
positron emission tomography
    (PET)
Posner gonioprism
Posner procedure
possible diagnosis
post C-section
Post forceps
Post trocar and washing
    cannula
Post washing cannula
postabortal infection
postacute phase
postage-stamp skin graft
postanal gut
postanal pit
postanal repair
postanesthesia
postanesthesia recovery room
    (PAR room)
postangioplasty angiogram
postaural approach
postauricular
postauricular approach
postauricular area
postauricular graft
postauricular incision
postauricular sulcus
postaxial muscle
postbulbar diverticula
postbulbar duodenal ulcer
postbulbar ulcer
postcannulation
postcardinal veins
postcardiotomy
postcardiotomy intra-aortic
    balloon pumping
postcaval
postcaval shunt
postcaval ureter
postcentral gyrus
postcentral vein
postcerebrovascular accident

postcesarean section
postcholecystectomy syndrome
postcoital bleeding
postcommissurotomy syndrome
postcricoid region
postcricoid space
postcricoid web
postcystoscopy
postdelivery
posterior
posterior abdominal wall
posterior ampullary nerve
posterior annular ligament
posterior approach
posterior aspect
posterior auricular branch of
    external carotid artery
posterior auricular muscle
posterior auricular nerve
posterior auricular vein
posterior bone block
posterior bow femoral fracture
posterior canal separator
posterior capsule
posterior cecal artery
posterior cerebral artery
posterior cervical lip
posterior chamber
posterior chamber intraocular
    lens
posterior circumflex humeral
    artery
posterior colporrhaphy
posterior column
posterior commissure
posterior communicating artery
posterior conjunctival arteries
posterior cricoarytenoid muscle
posterior cruciate ligament
posterior cutaneous femoral
    nerve
posterior cutaneous nerve
posterior descending artery
    (PDA)
posterior ethmoidal branch of
    ophthalmic artery
posterior ethmoidal nerve

posterior exenteration
posterior facial vein
posterior false ligament
posterior forceps
posterior fossa
posterior fossa retractor
posterior horn
posterior impaction
posterior incision
posterior infarction
posterior inferior cerebellar
    artery (PICA)
posterior inferior communicat-
    ing artery (PICA)
posterior intercostal arteries
posterior intercostal veins
posterior internal orbital canal
posterior interosseous artery
posterior interosseous nerve
posterior interventricular
posterior iridodialysis
posterior jejunostomy
posterior labial hernia
posterior labial nerves
posterior labial veins
posterior lamina
posterior leaf of broad ligament
posterior ligament
posterior lumbar interbody
    fusion (PLIF)
posterior median fissure
posterior median sulcus
posterior meningeal artery
posterior nephrectomy
posterior nerve root
posterior occlusion
posterior palate hook
posterior palatine sutures
posterior pelvic exenteration
posterior pillar
posterior rectopexy
posterior rectus sheath
posterior rhizotomy
posterior scalene muscle
posterior scrotal nerves
posterior scrotal veins
posterior segment

posterior septal space
posterior spinal artery
posterior splint
posterior stab incision
posterior subcapsular cataract
    (PSC)
posterior sulcus
posterior superior alveolar
    artery
posterior table
posterior talocalcaneal ligament
posterior temporal diploic vein
posterior tibial artery
posterior tibial muscle
posterior tibial nerve
posterior tibial recurrent artery
posterior tibial vein
posterior tibial tendon
posterior tympanic artery
posterior urethroscope
posterior vagal trunk
posterior vaginal hernia
posterior vein of left ventricle
posterior ventriculi sinistri
    cordis, vena
posterior view
posterior vitrectomy
posterior wall
posteriorly
posteroanterior (PA)
posteroanterior film
posteroanterior lordotic
    projection
posteroanterior position
posteroanterior study
posteroanterior view
posteroanterior x-ray view
posteroinferior aspect
posterointermediate sulcus
posterolateral
posterolateral aspect
posterolateral flap
posterolateral fontanelle
posterolateral incision
posterolateral infarction
posterolateral sclerosis
posterolateral sulcus

posteromedial aspect
posteromedian lobule
posterosuperior iliac spine
posterotemporal region
posterotransverse diameter
postevacuation film
postexchange bilirubin
postexcitation wave
postextraction bleeding
postfistula placement
postganglionic neuron
postglomerular arteriole
Post-Harrington erysiphake
postinfarction ventriculoseptal
    defect
postinflammatory polyp
postirradiation
postischemic stenosis
postlaryngectomy
postlaser conization
postlaser edema
postligation
postlumbar puncture
postmastectomy
postmenopausal
postmortem
postmyocardial infarction
postnasal applicator
postnasal balloon
postnasal bleeding
postnasal discharge
postnasal dressing
postnasal drip
postnasal sponge forceps
postnasal tube
postnecrotic tissue
postoperative
postoperative abscess
postoperative adhesions
postoperative care
postoperative change
postoperative complication
postoperative condition
postoperative course
postoperative discomfort
postoperative followup
postoperative ileus

postoperative infection
postoperative pain
postoperative progress
postoperative reaction
postoperative recovery
postoperative relief
postoperative shock
postoperative status
postoperative vomiting
postoperative withdrawal
postoperative wound infection
postorbital pain
postpartum
postpartum sterilization
postperfusion syndrome
postpericardiotomy syndrome
postpharyngeal abscess
postplaced sutures
postpoliomyelitic contracture
postponed labor
postprandial
postprandial distention
postprandial pain
postradiation
postreduction films
postreduction position
postreduction status
postrenal
postseizure
postsplenectomy
postsplenic
poststyloid space
postsurgery exercises
postsurgical course
postsurgical followup
postsurgical recurrent ulcer
post-term birth
post-transfusion
post-trauma
post-traumatic
post-TUR clamp
post-TUR irrigation clamp
post-TUR irrigation control
    clamp
postural changes
postural drainage
postural fixation test

postural hypertension
postural hypotension
postural tone
postural version
posture
posturing
postvoiding cystogram
postvoiding cystography
postvoiding film
postvoiding residual (PVR)
Potain apparatus
Potain aspirating trocar
Potain aspirator
Potain sign
Potain trocar
potential
potential acuity meter (PAM)
potential cautery
potentially
Potenza finger arthrodesis
Poth operation
Pott abscess
Pott eversion osteotomy
Pott fracture
Pott paraplegia
Pott puffy tumor
Pott splint
Pott tibial osteotomy
Potter classification of polycys-
    tic kidney
Potter knee arthrodesis
Potter knife
Potter needle
Potter sponge forceps
Potter tonsillar forceps
Potter version
Potter-Bucky diaphragm
Potts 60-degree angled
    scissors
Potts anastomosis
Potts aortic clamp
Potts aortic-pulmonary artery
    anastomosis
Potts bronchial forceps
Potts bulldog forceps
Potts cardiovascular clamp
Potts clamp

Potts coarctation clamp
Potts coarctation forceps
Potts dilator
Potts dissector
Potts divisional clamp
Potts ductus clamp
Potts elevator
Potts expansile dilator
Potts expansile knife
Potts expansile valvulotome
Potts fixation forceps
Potts forceps
Potts infant rib shears
Potts knife
Potts ligature
Potts needle
Potts operation
Potts patent ductus clamp
Potts patent ductus forceps
Potts periosteotome
Potts rib shears
Potts scissors
Potts shears
Potts shunt
Potts tenaculum
Potts tenotomy scissors
Potts thumb forceps
Potts tie sutures
Potts valvulotome
Potts vascular scissors
Potts-Cournand angiography
    needle
Potts-Cournand needle
Potts-De Martel scissors
Potts-Neidner clamp
Potts-Niedner aorta clamp
Potts-Riker dilator
Potts-Riker valvulotome
Potts-Satinsky clamp
Potts-Smith aortic clamp
Potts-Smith aortic occlusion
    clamp
Potts-Smith cardiovascular
    scissors
Potts-Smith forceps
Potts-Smith needle holder
Potts-Smith operation

Potts-Smith scissors
Potts-Smith side-to-side
    anastomosis
Potts-Smith tenaculum
Potts-Smith tissue forceps
Potts-Smith vascular scissors
Potts-Smith-Gibson operation
Potts-Yasargil scissors
pouch
        anopouch
        Bard Extra Ileo B pouch
        Bard ostomy pouch
        Bard pouch
        blind upper esophageal
            pouch
        Bongort ostomy pouch
        branchial pouch
        Broca pouch
        Cardio-Cool myocardial
            protection pouch
        closed-end ostomy
            pouch
        Coloplast colostomy
            pouch
        Coloplast flange pouch
        Coloplast pouch
        Coloset ostomy pouch
        colostomy pouch
        continent ileal pouch
        Cymed Micro skin
            pouch
        Dansac ileal pouch
        Dansac karaya seal
            pouch
        Dansac ostomy pouch
        dartos pouch
        Dennis-Brown pouch
        Douglas pouch
        drainable ostomy pouch
        gastric pouch
        H-shaped ileal pouch
        Hartmann pouch
        hepatorenal pouch
        hernia pouch
        Hollister First Choice
            pouch
        Hollister Holligard pouch

pouch *continued*
    Hollister karaya 5 ostomy
        pouch
    Hollister karaya seal
        pouch
    Hollister ostomy pouch
    Hollister Premium pouch
    Hunt-Lawrence pouch
    ileal J-pouch
    ileal S-pouch
    ileal W-pouch
    ileoanal pouch
    ileocecal pouch
    ileostomy pouch
    J-shaped ileal pouch
    jejunal pouch
    karaya seal pouch
    Kock pouch
    laryngeal pouch
    lateral-lateral pouch
    Mainz urinary reservoir
        pouch
    Marlen gas relief pouch
    Marlen Odor-Ban pouch
    Marlen Solo ileostomy
        pouch
    Marlen zip-closed pouch
    MicroSkin urostomy
        pouch
    Morison pouch
    Nu-Hope ileostomy
        pouch
    one-piece ostomy pouch
    open-end ostomy pouch
    pacemaker pouch
    paravesical pouch
    Parks ileostomy pouch
    Parsonnet pouch
    pharyngeal pouch
    Physick pouch
    plastic bridge colostomy
        pouch
    Prussak pouch
    Rathke pouch
    rectal pouch
    rectouterine pouch
    rectovaginal pouch

pouch *continued*
- rectovesical pouch
- renal pouch
- S-shaped ileal pouch
- S-shaped pouch
- side-to-side jejunal pouch
- Silon pouch chimney
- Squibb Sur-Fit ostomy pouch
- suprapatellar pouch
- Sur-Fit Mini pouch
- terminal ileal pouch
- three-loop ileal pouch
- two-piece ostomy pouch
- United Max-E pouch
- United Surgical Bongort Lifestyle pouch
- United Surgical Feather-lite ileostomy pouch
- United Surgical Shear Plus pouch
- United Surgical Soft & Secure pouch
- urostomy pouch
- vallecular pouch
- vesicouterine pouch
- VPI nonadhesive pouch
- W-shaped ileal pouch
- W-shaped pouch
- Willis pouch
- Zenker pouch

pouch of Douglas
pouch of Hartmann
pouch of Morison
pouch of Munro
pouched ileostomy
pouchitis
pouchography
poudrage
Poulard entropion
Poulard operation
Poulard-Pochissov operation
pounds of traction
Poupart inguinal ligament
Poupart ligament
Poupart ligament shelving edge

Poupart line
Pousson pigtail catheter
Poutasse clamp
Poutasse forceps
Poutasse renal artery forceps
powder
powder blower
power cord
Power Grip pliers
power injection
Power operation
Power Play knee brace
Pozzi operation
Pozzi tenaculum
Pozzi tenaculum forceps
PPD dialyzer
PPG (polypropylene glycol)
PPG probe
PPG-AFO brace (ankle-foot orthosis brace)
PPG-TLSO brace (thoracolumbar standing orthosis brace)
PPT orthotic device
Praeger iris hook
Prague maneuver
Prall urethral sound
pramoxine hydrochloride anesthetic agent
Pratt anoscope
Pratt antrum curet
Pratt bivalve retractor
Pratt crypt hook
Pratt curet
Pratt dilator
Pratt director
Pratt ethmoid curet
Pratt forceps
Pratt hook
Pratt nasal curet
Pratt probe
Pratt proctoscope
Pratt rectal dilator
Pratt rectal director
Pratt rectal hook
Pratt rectal probe
Pratt rectal scissors

Pratt rectal speculum
Pratt scissors
Pratt sigmoid speculum
Pratt sound
Pratt speculum
Pratt T-shaped hemostatic
    forceps
Pratt uterine dilator
Pratt-Sims closure
Pratt-Smith forceps
Pratt-Smith tissue-grasping
    forceps
Pravay syringe
preampullary portion of bile
    duct
preauricular radiation therapy
preaxial muscle
precancerous lesion
precancerous polyp
precannulation antibiotic
precapillary anastomosis
precardinal veins
precatheterization
precaution
precautionary measure
precentral gyrus
precipitate
precipitated by
precipitating cause
precipitation
precipitin tube
precipitous
Precise disposable skin stapler
Precision eye implant
Precision-Cosmet intraocular
    lens implant
preclotted graft
Precoat Plus total hip
precordial region
precornified cell
precostal anastomosis
precursor
precursor lesion
precut sphincterotome
precut sutures
predetermined
prediastolic murmur

predicted
predicting
predisposing cause
predisposition
predominance
predominant
pre-eclampsia of pregnancy
pre-eclamptic toxemia
Preefer eye speculum
pre-ejection time
pre-evacuation film
pre-existing
preference
preferred
prefollicle cells
preformed catheter
preformed Cordis catheter
prefrontal lobotomy
prefrontal region
preganglionic cells
preganglionic neurons
preglomerular arteriole
pregnancy
pregnant
prehepatic coma
prehepatic edema
preinsular gyri
preinvasive carcinoma
prelaryngeal node
preliminary film
preliminary impression
preliminary iridectomy
preliminary studies
preload
premalignant lesion
premature atrial contraction
    (PAC)
premature beat
premature birth
premature closure of valve
premature contraction
premature delivery
premature labor
premature rupture of mem-
    branes (PROM)
premature separation of
    placenta

premature ventricular contraction (PVC)
prematurely
premaxilla
premaxillary suture
premedicate
premedicated patient
premedication
premenarche
premenopausal
premenstrual
Premier total hip system
premolar teeth
premolars
premonitory contraction
premonitory pain
premorbid
premotor area
premotor neuron
prenatal course
prenatal development
prenatal diagnosis
preoccipital notch
preoperative
preoperative care
preoperative checklist
preoperative evaluation
preoperative hair clippers
preoperative orders
preoperative sedation
preoperative therapy
preoral gut
prep and drape
prep for delivery
prep pad
prepackaged medication
prepapillary bile duct
preparation
preparation and draping
preparatory
prepared and draped in routine
manner
prepatellar bursa
preperitoneal bleeder
preperitoneal fat
preperitoneal space
preplaced sutures

Prepodyne scrub
preponderance
prepped and draped
prepped and draped in routine
manner
Preptic dressing
prepubic
prepubic fascia
prepuce
prepuce forceps
prepuce of penis
preputial
preputial gland
preputial island graft
preputial space
preputiotomy
prepyloric
prepyloric atresia
prepyloric gastric ulcer
prepyloric sphincter
prepyloric ulcer
prepyloric vein
prepylorica, vena
prerectal lithotomy
prereduction film
presacral
presacral anesthesia
presacral block
presacral fascia
presacral insufflation
presacral neurectomy
presacral rectopexy
presacral space
Presbyterian Hospital clamp
Presbyterian Hospital elevator
Presbyterian Hospital forceps
Presbyterian Hospital needle
Presbyterian Hospital occluding
clamp
Presbyterian Hospital T-clamp
presection sutures
presence of infection
presenile sclerosis
present illness
preservation
preserved
preserving

preshaped catheter
Preshaw clamp
presplenic fold
Press-Fit condylar component
    (PFC component)
Press-Fit condylar knee system
Press-Fit condylar total knee
    system
press-fit implant
press-fit prosthesis
Presso-Elastic dressing
Pressoplast compression
    dressing
Presso-Superior dressing
pressure
pressure anesthesia
pressure applied
pressure atrophy
pressure bandage
pressure changes
pressure cuff
pressure dressing
pressure elevator
pressure equalization tube
pressure forceps
pressure fracture
pressure gauge
pressure gradient
pressure inversion point (PIP)
pressure maintained
pressure monitoring
pressure point
pressure pump
pressure sensation
Pressure Sense monitor
pressure transducer
pressure urgency
pressure velocity (PV)
Pressurometer blood pressure
    monitor
presternal notch
Preston dynamometer
Preston ligamentum flavum
    forceps
Preston pinch gauge
prestyloid space
presumed consent

presumptive
presumptive diagnosis
presystolic murmur
preternatural anus
prethreaded Teflon pledget
pretibial edema
pretibial fever
pretracheal fascia
pretracheal node
pretransplant surgery
pretreatment evaluation
prevacuum sterilizer
prevalence
preventricular artery
preventricular stenosis
prevertebral fascia level
prevertebral ganglia
prevesical space
prevesical space of Retzius
prevesicle space
previous
previously
PRG (phleborrheogram)
Pribram suction tube
Price muscle biopsy clamp
Price operation
Price-Thomas bronchial clamp
Price-Thomas bronchial forceps
Price-Thomas clamp
Price-Thomas forceps
Price-Thomas rib stripper
Priessnitz bandage
Priessnitz compress
Priessnitz dressing
Priestly catheter
prilocaine hydrochloride
    anesthetic agent
Prima pacemaker
PrimaCast
Primaderm dressing
primarily
primary
primary amputation
primary anastomosis
primary brain tumor
primary carcinoma
primary closure

primary colostomy
primary hemorrhage
primary intra-axial brain tumor
primary nerve repair
primary palate
primary procedure
primary suture line
primary sutures
primary union
Primbs suturing forceps
prime mover
prime site
primed
priming of artificial kidney
priming of pump
priming solution
primip (primipara)
primipara
primiparous patient
primitive dislocation
primitive gut
Prince advancement forceps
Prince cautery
Prince clamp
Prince eye cautery
Prince forceps
Prince knife
Prince muscle forceps
Prince rongeur
Prince scissors
Prince tonsillar scissors
Prince trachoma forceps
Prince ureteropelvioplasty
Prince-Potts scissors
Prince-Potts tonsillar scissors
princeps pollicis, arteria
principal artery of thumb
principle
Pringle clamp
Pringle incision
Pringle maneuver
Printz anesthesia unit
Printz suction
Prinzmetal angina
prior to admission
prior to birth
prior to delivery

prior to discharge
prior to examination
prior to surgery
prior to x-ray
prism
prism diopters
Prism-CL pacemaker
Pristine gloves
Pritchard arthroplasty
Pritchard cannula
Pritchard speculum
Pritchard syringe
Pritchard-Walker elbow hinge
Pritikin punch
Pritikin scleral punch
private
privileges
prizefighter's ear
p.r.n., prn, PRN (whenever
    necessary)
probability
probang
probe (see also *cryoprobe*)
        8-channel cross-sectional
            anal sphincter probe
        Alnico magneprobe
            magnet
        Amoils cryoprobe
        Amussat probe
        Anel lacrimal probe
        angled probe
        Arbuckle probe
        Arbuckle sinus probe
        Arndorfer esophageal
            motility probe
        back-stop laser probe
        Bakes probe
        Barr fistula probe
        Barr probe
        Becker probe
        Beckman probe
        Bermen-Werner probe
        bicap probe
        biliary balloon probe
        biometry probe
        biplane sector probe
        bipolar probe

probe *continued*

- blood-flow probe
- blunt probe
- Bowman lacrimal probe
- Bowman probe
- Brackett dental probe
- Brackett probe
- brain probe
- Bresgen probe
- Bresgen sinus probe
- Brock probe
- Brodie fistula probe
- Brodie probe
- bronchoscopic probe
- Bruel-Kjaer transvaginal ultrasound probe
- Brymill cryoprobe
- Buck ear probe
- Buck probe
- Buie fistula probe
- Buie probe
- bullet probe
- Bunnell dissecting probe
- Bunnell forwarding probe
- Bunnell probe
- canaliculus probe
- cardiac probe
- cataract probe
- Chandler V-pacing probe
- Cherry brain probe
- Cherry probe
- Circon-ACMI electro-hydraulic lithotriptor probe
- Coakley nasal probe
- Coakley probe
- Cody magnetic probe
- common duct probe
- continuously perfused probe
- Cooper cryoprobe
- Crawford canaliculus probe
- cryogenic probe
- cryoprobe

probe *continued*

- Desjardins gallstone probe
- Desjardins probe
- Dilaprobe
- dilating probe
- dilator probe
- disposable probe
- dissecting probe
- dissection probe
- Dix spud probe
- Doppler flow probe
- Doppler probe
- double-end probe
- drum probe
- ear probe
- Earle probe
- Earle rectal probe
- echocardiographic probe
- electric probe
- electrohydraulic litho-triptor probe
- electromagnetic flow probe
- Ellis probe
- Emmet probe
- Emmet uterine probe
- endocervical probe
- endoscopic bicap probe
- endoscopic heat probe
- Esmarch probe
- Esmarch tin bullet probe
- eustachian probe
- eyed probe
- Fenger gall duct probe
- Fenger gallbladder probe
- Fenger gallstone probe
- Fenger probe
- Fenger spiral gallstone probe
- Ferguson probe
- fiberoptic probe
- filiform bougie probe
- Fish antral probe
- Fish sinus probe
- fistular probe
- flexible probe

probe *continued*

- flow probe
- Fluhrer rectal probe
- Fogarty biliary balloon probe
- Fogarty biliary probe
- Fogarty probe
- foreign body probe
- forwarding probe
- Fraenkel sinus probe
- fragmentation probe
- French-pattern lacrimal probe
- Fresgen frontal sinus probe
- Frigitronics cryoprobe
- Frigitronics probe
- frontal sinus probe
- gall duct probe
- gallstone probe
- galvanic probe
- Gant probe
- Geldmacher tendon-passing probe
- Gilmore probe
- Girard probe
- Girdner probe
- Gross probe
- Hagar probe
- hand-held exploring electrode probe
- Harms probe
- Hayden probe
- Hotz ear probe
- Hotz probe
- illuminated probe
- illuminated ureter probe
- illumination probe
- intrauterine probe
- irrigating Dilaprobe
- Jackson probe
- Jacobson probe
- Jako probe
- Jansen-Newhart mastoid probe
- Jansen-Newhart probe
- Kartch pigtail probe

probe *continued*

- Kistner probe
- Knapp probe
- Kron gall duct probe
- Kron probe
- Kry-Med 300 cryoprobe
- lacrimal duct probe
- lacrimal probe
- Larry probe
- Larry rectal probe
- laryngeal probe
- laser microprobe
- laser probe
- Lente silver nitrate probe
- Lilienthal bullet probe
- Lilienthal probe
- Lillie frontal sinus probe
- Lillie probe
- Linde cryogenic probe
- Lucae probe
- magneprobe
- malleable probe
- Manhattan Eye and Ear probe
- Mannis suture probe
- Martin probe
- mastoid probe
- Mayo common duct probe
- Mayo probe
- McKesson mouth probe
- Meditech bipolar probe
- meerschaum probe
- meniscectomy probe
- microballoon probe
- microprobe
- Mixter common duct Dilaprobe
- Mixter dilating probe
- Mixter irrigating probe
- Mixter probe
- Moynihan bile duct probe
- Moynihan gallstone probe
- Moynihan probe
- Muldoon lacrimal probe

probe *continued*

multilumen probe
Myrtle leaf probe
nasal probe
Nélaton bullet probe
nuclear probe
Ochsner flexible spiral gallstone probe
Ochsner gallstone probe
Ochsner probe
Olympus heat probe
palpation probe
Parsonnet probe
pencil Doppler probe
pencil-probe Doppler
periodontal probe
pH probe
piggyback probe
pigtail probe
pocket probe
PPG probe
Pratt probe
Pratt rectal probe
Quickert probe
Quickert-Dryden probe
Radiometer probe
rectal probe
Richards probe
Rockey dilating probe
Rockey probe
Rolf lacrimal probe
Rosen ear probe
Rosen endaural probe
Rosen probe
Rubinstein cryoprobe
salpingeal probe
Sandhill probe
Sarns temperature probe
scissors probe
Sheer probe
Shirodkar probe
silver probe
Simpson lacrimal probe
Sims probe
Sims uterine probe
sinus probe
Skillern probe

probe *continued*

Skillern sinus probe
Skillern sphenoid probe
Spencer labyrinth exploration probe
Spencer probe
sphenoidal probe
Spiesman fistula probe
spiral probe
Storz-Bowman lacrimal probe
suction probe
tactile probe
Teflon probe
telephone probe
temperature probe
Theobald probe
Theobald sinus probe
thermistor probe
tin-bullet probe
transesophageal probe
tulip probe
uterine probe
vacuum intrauterine probe
Versadopp Doppler probe
vertebrated probe
Vibrodilator probe
Wasko common duct probe
Wasko probe
water probe
Weaver sinus probe
Welch Allyn probe
whalebone eustachian probe
whirlybird probe
Williams lacrimal probe
Williams probe
wire probe
Worst pigtail probe
Worst probe
Yankauer probe
Yankauer salpingeal probe
Yellow Springs probe

probe *continued*
> Yeoman probe
> Ziegler lacrimal probe
> Ziegler needle probe
> Ziegler probe

probe catheter
probe catheterization
probe dilator
probed
probe-point scissors
Probetron readings for radium inserts
probing
probing catheter
probing of lacrimonasal duct
probing of wound
problem
procaine hydrochloride anesthetic agent
procedure
procedure drape
procedures, alternatives, indications, complications (PAIC)
procedures, alternatives, risks (PAR)
procerus muscle
procerus, musculus
process
processing
processus vaginalis
Prochownik pessary
procidentia
procidentia of uterus
proctalgia
proctalgia fugax
proctectasia
proctectomy
Procter-Livingston endoprosthesis
Procter-Livingston tube
procteurynter
procteurysis
proctoclysis
proctococcypexy
proctocolectomy
proctocolonoscopy
proctocystoplasty

proctocystotomy
Proctodone
proctoelytroplasty
proctologic, proctological
proctologic ball electrode
proctologic biopsy forceps
proctologic cotton carrier
proctological forceps
proctological grasping forceps
proctological polyp forceps
proctology
proctolysis
proctoperineoplasty
proctoperineorrhaphy
proctopexy
proctoplasty
proctoptosis
Proctor cheek retractor
Proctor elevator
Proctor mucosal elevator
Proctor phrenectomy forceps
Proctor phrenicectomy forceps
Proctor retractor
Proctor suction tube
proctorrhaphy
proctoscope
> ACMI proctoscope
> Bacon proctoscope
> Bodenheimer proctoscope
> Boehm proctoscope
> Brinkerhoff proctoscope
> Buie-Hirschman proctoscope
> Fansler proctoscope
> Gabriel proctoscope
> Goldbacher proctoscope
> Hirschman proctoscope
> Hirschman-Martin proctoscope
> Ives proctoscope
> Kelly proctoscope
> Lieberman proctoscope
> Montague proctoscope
> Muer proctoscope
> National proctoscope
> Newman proctoscope

proctoscope *continued*
    Otis proctoscope
    Pratt proctoscope
    Pruitt proctoscope
    rotating speculum
        proctoscope
    Sims proctoscope
    Sklar proctoscope
    Strauss proctoscope
    Turell proctoscope
    Tuttle proctoscope
    Vernon-David procto-
        scope
    Welch Allyn proctoscope
    Yeoman proctoscope
proctoscopic air
proctoscopic examination
proctoscopic fulguration
    electrode
proctoscopic speculum
proctoscopy
proctosigmoidectomy
proctosigmoiditis
proctosigmoidopexy
proctosigmoidoscope
    ACMI fiberoptic procto-
        sigmoidoscope
    ACMI proctosigmoido-
        scope
    fiberoptic procto-
        sigmoidoscope
proctosigmoidoscopic evalua-
    tion
proctosigmoidoscopic examina-
    tion
proctosigmoidoscopy
proctostenosis
proctostomy
proctotome
proctotomy
proctovalvotomy
procurement
prodromal labor
producing
production
productive
products of conception

Proetz atomizer
Proetz decompressor
Proetz displacement syringe
Proetz mouth gag
Proetz position
Proetz tongue depressor
Proetz-Jansen mouth gag
profile
Profile Plus catheter
Profile Plus dilatation catheter
profilometer
    Cottle profilometer
    laryngofissure profilome-
        ter
    Straith profilometer
Proflex dilatation catheter
profunda brachii, arteria
profunda clitoridis, arteria
profunda clitoridis, venae
profunda Dacron patchplasty
profunda endarterectomy
profunda femoris, arteria
profunda femoris, vena
profunda linguae, arteria
profunda linguae, vena
profunda penis, arteria
profundae penis, venae
profundaplasty
profundus function
profundus muscle
profundus tendon
profuse bleeding
profuse hemorrhage
profuse menstruation
profuse sweating
profusion
Progestasert intrauterine device
progestational
prognathia
prognathic mandible
prognathism
prognosis
prognostic factors
prognostic indicators
program
Programalith A-V pacemaker
Programalith II pacemaker

Programalith III pacemaker
Programalith III pulse generator
Programalith pacemaker
programmable pacemaker
programmed
programmer
Programmer III pacemaker
programming
progress
progressed
progressing
progression
progressive
progressive condition
progressive disease
progressive enlargement
progressive failure
progressive loss
progressive paralysis
progressive relaxation
progressive symptoms
project
project sites of heart
projectile
projecting
projection
projector x-ray microscope
Prokop intraocular lens
Prokop lens
prolabium
prolactin
prolapse
prolapse of Morgagni
prolapse ring pessary
prolapsed fibroid
prolapsed hemorrhoid
prolapsed rectum
prolapsed stoma
prolapsed vaginal wall
prolapsed valve
prolapsing internal hemorrhoid
prolapsus
prolapsus ani
prolapsus pessary
prolapsus recti
Prolene sutures
proliferating

proliferation
proliferative
proliferative endometrium
proliferative phase of wound
    healing
proliferative retinopathy
    photocoagulation (PRP)
Prolith pacemaker
prolong
prolongation
prolonged
prolonging
PROM (premature rupture of
    membranes)
Pro-Med compressed air
    system
prominence
prominent
promontory
promontory of tympanum
prompt emptying
prompt excretion of dye
prompt surgical closure
promptly
pronation
pronation and supination
pronation sign
pronation, external rotation
    fracture (PER fracture)
pronator drift
pronator muscle
pronator quadratus, musculus
pronator teres, musculus
prone
prone jackknife position
prone position
prone rectus test
Proneze pad
Proneze pillow
prong
pronged retractor
pronounced
pronouncement
prop graft
propagated contractions
proparacaine hydrochloride
    anesthetic agent

proper alignment and apposition of fracture
proper hepatic artery
proper lamina
proper ligament
proper membrane
proper palmar digital arteries
proper palmar digital nerves
proper plantar digital arteries
proper plantar digital nerves
proper sterilization procedure
properitoneal
properitoneal fat
properitoneal hernia
properly
properties
prophylactic cholecystectomy
prophylactic course
prophylactic therapy
prophylaxis
Proplast facial implant
Proplast graft
Proplast implant
Proplast nasal implant
Proplast pad
Proplast pants
Proplast preformed implant
Proplast prosthesis
Proplast staples
Proplast washer
proportional
proportions
proposed treatment
propoxycaine hydrochloride anesthetic agent
propoxyphene
Propper ophthalmoscope
Propper retinoscope
propranolol hydrochloride
proprioception
proprioceptive
proptosed
proptosis
propulsion
propylene dressing
proscribe
prospective

prospective evaluation of radial keratotomy protocol (PERK protocol)
prostaglandin suppository
prostate
prostate gland
prostatectomy
prostatectomy bag
prostatic biopsy needle
prostatic biopsy set
prostatic cancer
prostatic capsule
prostatic catheter
prostatic cavity
prostatic dissector
prostatic diverticulum
prostatic driver
prostatic duct
prostatic enlargement
prostatic enucleator
prostatic forceps
prostatic fossa
prostatic fraction
prostatic ganglion
prostatic hook
prostatic hypertrophy
prostatic lobe
prostatic lobe forceps
prostatic lobe-holding forceps
prostatic needle holder
prostatic plexus
prostatic punch
prostatic retractor
prostatic scissors
prostatic sinus
prostatic tissue
prostatic tractor
prostatic trocar
prostatic urethra
prostatic utricle
prostatic vesicle
prostaticovesical plexus
prostaticovesiculectomy
prostatism
prostatitis
prostatocystotomy
prostatolithotomy

prostatoseminovesiculectomy
prostatotomy
prostatovesicular junction
prostatovesiculectomy
prosthesis (*pl.* prostheses) (see also *graft, implant, patch, valve*)
    4-A Magovern prosthesis
    4-A Magovern valve prosthesis
    A-Turner prosthesis
    accordion prosthesis
    Ace Kyle prosthesis
    Acrax prosthesis
    acrylic bar prosthesis
    acrylic prosthesis
    Adrian-Flat prosthesis
    Akiyama prosthesis
    Alivium prosthesis
    Aljan prosthesis
    Allen-Brown prosthesis
    Allo-Pro prosthesis
    Alvarez prosthesis
    Alvarez valve prosthesis
    AMC wrist prosthesis
    American Medical Systems inflatable penile prosthesis
    AML orthopedic prosthesis
    AMS Hydroflex penile prosthesis
    AMS inflatable penile prosthesis
    AMS malleable penile prosthesis
    AMS semirigid penile prosthesis
    Anametric knee prosthesis
    Anametric prosthesis
    Anatomique osteal prosthesis
    Anderson columella prosthesis
    Angelchik antireflux prosthesis

prosthesis *continued*
    Angelchik prosthesis
    ankle prosthesis
    anti-incontinence penile prosthesis
    antireflux prosthesis
    aortic valve prosthesis
    aortofemoral prosthesis
    Arizona condylar tibial plateau prosthesis
    Armstrong-Schuknecht stapes prosthesis
    arterial prosthesis
    Ashley breast prosthesis
    Ashworth Dow Corning prosthesis
    Atkinson endoprosthesis
    Attenborough knee prosthesis
    Aufranc hip prosthesis
    Aufranc-Turner cemented hip prosthesis
    Aufranc-Turner hip prosthesis
    Austin Moore hip prosthesis
    Austin Moore prosthesis
    Autophor femoral prosthesis
    ball-and-cage valve prosthesis
    ball-cage prosthesis
    ball-type prosthesis
    ball-valve prosthesis
    Balnetar prosthesis
    Bard prosthesis
    Barnard mitral valve prosthesis
    Bateman bipolar cup hip prosthesis
    Bateman finger joint prosthesis
    Bateman prosthesis

prosthesis *continued*
  Bateman Universal
    proximal femur
    prosthesis (UPF
    prosthesis)
  Bateman UPF prosthesis
    (Universal proximal
    femur prosthesis)
  BDH hip prosthesis
  Beall disk valve prosthe-
    sis
  Beall mitral valve
    prosthesis
  Bechtol cemented hip
    prosthesis
  Bechtol glenohumeral
    joint prosthesis
  Bechtol hip prosthesis
  Bechtol prosthesis
  Becker mammary
    prosthesis
  Bentall cardiovascular
    prosthesis
  Berens prosthesis
  Bias hip prosthesis
  Bias porous metal hip
    prosthesis
  Bi-Centric endo-
    prosthesis
  bifurcated aortofemoral
    prosthesis
  bifurcated seamless
    prosthesis
  bifurcation prosthesis
  bileaflet prosthesis
  biliary duct prosthesis
  biliary endoprosthesis
  bilioduodenal prosthesis
  biograft umbilical
    prosthesis
  Bio-Groove total hip
    prosthesis
  biometric prosthesis
  Bionit II vascular
    prosthesis
  Bionit prosthesis
  Bionit vascular prosthesis

prosthesis *continued*
  bioprosthesis
  bipolar cup hip prosthe-
    sis
  bipolar prosthesis
  Bivona low-resistance
    voice prosthesis
  Bivona voice prosthesis
  Björk-Shiley aortic valve
    prosthesis
  Björk-Shiley mitral valve
    prosthesis
  Björk-Shiley prosthesis
  Björk-Shiley valve
    prosthesis
  Blair-Brown prosthesis
  Blazina prosthesis
  Bock prosthesis
  bone prosthesis
  bovine pericardial
    prosthesis
  bovine prosthesis
  Boyne dental prosthesis
  Braun prosthesis
  Braunwald prosthesis
  Braunwald-Cutter ball-
    valve prosthesis
  Braunwald-Cutter
    prosthesis
  Braun-Wangensteen
    prosthesis
  breast prosthesis
  Bridge prosthesis
  Brigham total knee
    prosthesis
  Buchholz knee prosthe-
    sis
  Buchholz prosthesis
  Buchholz total hip
    prosthesis
  Byers prosthesis
  bypass prosthesis
  CAD hip prosthesis
  CAD prosthesis
  Caffiniere prosthesis
  caged-ball valve prosthe-
    sis

prosthesis *continued*
Calnan-Nicole prosthesis
Capetown prosthesis
Cardona eye prosthesis
carpal prosthesis
Carpentier annuloplasty ring prosthesis
Carpentier-Edwards aortic valve prosthesis
Carpentier-Edwards bioprosthesis
Carpentier-Edwards valve prosthesis
Carpentier-Rhone-Poulenc mitral rings prosthesis
Carrion penile prosthesis
cartilage prosthesis
Cartwright heart prosthesis
Cartwright valve prosthesis
Cartwright vascular prosthesis
Cathcart endoprosthesis
Catterall prosthesis
Causse-Shea prosthesis
Celestin prosthesis
celluloid prosthesis
ceramic hip prosthesis
Cervital partial ossicular replacement prosthesis (Cervital PORP)
Cervital PORP (Cervital partial ossicular replacement prosthesis)
Cervital TORP (Cervital total ossicular replacement prosthesis)
Cervital total ossicular replacement prosthesis (Cervital TORP)
CFE Taperloc hip prosthesis
Charcot prosthesis

prosthesis *continued*
Charnley cemented hip prosthesis
Charnley hip prosthesis
Charnley knee prosthesis
Charnley prosthesis
Charnley-cobra total hip prosthesis
Charnley-Moore hip prosthesis
Charnley-Mueller cemented hip prosthesis
chessboard prosthesis
chin prosthesis
Cintor knee prosthesis
cleft palate prosthesis
Cloutier knee prosthesis
$CO_2$ muscle prosthesis
cochlear prosthesis
collagen prosthesis
collagen tape prosthesis
compartmental total knee prosthesis
computerized assisted design prosthesis
condylar prosthesis
Conley prosthesis
constrained hinged knee prosthesis
constrained knee prosthesis
constrained nonhinged knee prosthesis
constrained total knee prosthesis
contoured Dow Corning Silastic prosthesis
convexoconcave valve prosthesis
Cooley-Bloodwell mitral valve prosthesis
Cooley-Bloodwell-Cutter prosthesis
Cooley-Cutter prosthesis
Coonrad prosthesis
Coonrad wrist prosthesis

prosthesis *continued*

Cox-Uphoff double-lumen breast prosthesis

Cox-Uphoff prosthesis

Creench insertion of vascular prosthesis

crimped Dacron prosthesis

crimped woven prosthesis

Cronin Silastic mammary prosthesis

crook measuring prosthesis

CROS hearing aid prosthesis

Cross-Jones disk valve prosthesis

Cross-Jones valve prosthesis

Crutchfield tongs prosthesis

cup hip prosthesis

Cutter aortic valve prosthesis

Cutter SCDK prosthesis

Cutter-Smeloff aortic valve prosthesis

Cutter-Smeloff cardiac valve prosthesis

Dacomed Omni Phase penile prosthesis

Dacron arterial prosthesis

Dacron bifurcation prosthesis

Dacron prosthesis

Dacron valve prosthesis

Dacron vascular prosthesis

Dacron vessel prosthesis

Dardik umbilical prosthesis

d'Aubigne prosthesis

Davis prosthesis

de la Caffiniere trapezio-metacarpal prosthesis

prosthesis *continued*

De Paco prosthesis

DeBakey ball-valve prosthesis

DeBakey prosthesis

DeBakey valve prosthesis

DeBakey vascular prosthesis

DeBakey Vasculour-II vascular prosthesis

Dee elbow prosthesis

Delrin frame of valve prosthesis

dental prosthesis

DePalma hip prosthesis

DePuy dual-lock hip prosthesis

DePuy prosthesis

DeVega prosthesis

Dilamezinsert penile prosthesis

discoid valve prosthesis

disk valve prosthesis

Doherty prosthesis

double-lumen endo-prosthesis

double-pigtail endo-prosthesis

double-rod penile prosthesis

Dow Corning mammary prosthesis

Dow Corning Silastic prosthesis

Dragstedt prosthesis

dual-lock DePuy hip prosthesis

dual-lock hip prosthesis

dual-lock prosthesis

Dubinet prosthesis

Duocondylar knee prosthesis

Duo-Lock hip prosthesis

Duo-Patella knee prosthesis

prosthesis *continued*
DuraPhase semirigid penile prosthesis
dynamic penile prosthesis
ear pinna prosthesis
ear piston prosthesis
Eaton prosthesis
Eaton upper limb prosthesis
Edwards prosthesis
Edwards seamless prosthesis
Edwards Teflon intracardiac patch prosthesis
Edwards Teflon intracardiac prosthesis
Efteklar-Charnley hip prosthesis
Ehmke ear prosthesis
Ehmke platinum Teflon prosthesis
Eicher hip prosthesis
Eicher prosthesis
elbow prosthesis
ELP femoral prosthesis
endoesophageal prosthesis
endoprosthesis
endoskeletal prosthesis
Engh porous metal hip prosthesis
Englehardt femoral prosthesis
English-McNab shoulder prosthesis
ESKA Jonas silicone-silver semirigid penile prosthesis
esophageal prosthesis
Esser prosthesis
Estecar prosthesis
Ethrone prosthesis
Ewald elbow prosthesis
Ewald prosthesis
external prosthesis

prosthesis *continued*
fallopian tube repair prosthesis
fascia lata prosthesis
femoral head prosthesis
femoral prosthesis
femorofemoral crossover prosthesis
fenestra prosthesis
finger prosthesis
Finney penile prosthesis
Finney prosthesis
Finney-flexirod penile prosthesis
Flatt prosthesis
Flatt thumb prosthesis
flexible penile prosthesis
Flexi-Flate inflatable penile prosthesis
Flexi-rod penile prosthesis
Flexi-rod semirigid penile prosthesis
Fox prosthesis
Fox-Blazina prosthesis
F.R. Thompson hip prosthesis
Fredricks mammary prosthesis
free prosthesis
Freeman-Samuelson knee prosthesis
Freeman-Swanson knee prosthesis
full-thickness prosthesis
Galante hip prosthesis
gel-filled prosthesis
gel-saline Surgitek prosthesis
Geomedic femoral condyle prosthesis
Geomedic knee prosthesis
Geomedic prosthesis
Geomedic total knee prosthesis

prosthesis *continued*

Geometric knee prosthesis
Georgiade breast prosthesis
Gilbert prosthesis
Giliberty prosthesis
Giliberty cup hip prosthesis
Giliberty total hip prosthesis
Gillies prosthesis
Girard keratoprosthesis
gliding prosthesis
golf tee-shaped polyvinyl prosthesis
Goodhill prosthesis
Gore-Tex prosthesis
Gore-Tex vascular prosthesis
Gott low-profile prosthesis
Gott mitral valve prosthesis
Gott prosthesis
Gott-Daggett heart valve prosthesis
Gruppe wire prosthesis
GSB knee prosthesis
Guepar hinge-knee prosthesis
Guepar knee prosthesis
Guepar prosthesis
Guepar total knee prosthesis
Gunston knee prosthesis
Gustilo knee prosthesis
Hall-Kaster mitral valve prosthesis
Hall-Kaster tilting-disk valve prosthesis
Hamas upper limb prosthesis
Hammersmith mitral prosthesis
Hammersmith prosthesis

prosthesis *continued*

Hancock aortic valve prosthesis
Hancock mitral valve prosthesis
Hancock porcine valve prosthesis
Hanger prosthesis
Hanslik patellar prosthesis
Harken prosthesis
Harris hip prosthesis
Harris precoat cemented hip prosthesis
Harris prosthesis
Harris total hip prosthesis
Harris-Galante hip prosthesis
Harris-Galante porous metal hip prosthesis
Harrison interlocked mesh prosthesis
Harrison prosthesis
Hartley mammary prosthesis
HD2 prosthesis
HD2 total hip prosthesis
heart prosthesis
heart valve prosthesis
Helanca prosthesis
Helanca seamless tube prosthesis
Henschke-Mauch SNS lower limb prosthesis
Herbert knee prosthesis
Herbert prosthesis
heterograft prosthesis
Hexcel total condylar knee system prosthesis
Heyer-Schulte breast prosthesis
Heyer-Schulte chin prosthesis
Heyer-Schulte malar prosthesis
Heyer-Schulte prosthesis

prosthesis *continued*

Heyer-Schulte testicular prosthesis
Hinderer malar prosthesis
Hinderer prosthesis
hinged constrained knee prosthesis
hinged total knee prosthesis
hinged-leaflet vascular prosthesis
hinge-knee prosthesis
hingeless heart valve prosthesis
hip cup prosthesis
hip prosthesis
HIP prosthesis (homograft incus prosthesis)
hollow sphere prosthesis
homograft prosthesis
Hosmer elbow prosthesis
House incus replacement prosthesis
House prosthesis
House stainless steel mesh prosthesis
House stapes wire prosthesis
House wire stapes prosthesis
House wire-fat prosthesis
Howmedica orthopedic prosthesis
Howmedica prosthesis
Howmedica Universal total knee prosthesis
Howorth prosthesis
Howse-Coventry prosthesis
HSS knee prosthesis
Hufnagel disk heart valve prosthesis
Hufnagel prosthesis
Hufnagel valve prosthesis
Hunter tendon prosthesis

prosthesis *continued*

hybrid prosthesis
hydraulic incontinent prosthesis
Hydroflex inflatable penile prosthesis
Hydroflex penile prosthesis
immediate fit prosthesis
immediate postoperative prosthesis (IPOP)
incontinence prosthesis
incus replacement prosthesis
Indong Oh prosthesis
inflatable mammary prosthesis
inflatable penile prosthesis with reservoir
inflatable prosthesis
inflatable urinary incontinence prosthesis
Insall-Burstein knee prosthesis
Insall-Burstein prosthesis
Insall-Burstein total knee prosthesis
interlocked mesh prosthesis
intracardiac patch prosthesis
intraluminal tube prosthesis
Ionescu-Shiley aortic valve prosthesis
Ionescu-Shiley prosthesis
Iowa total hip prosthesis
IPOP cast dressing (immediate postoperative prosthesis cast dressing)
iridium prosthesis
Ivalon prosthesis
Jenny mammary prosthesis
Jewett prosthesis

prosthesis *continued*

Jobst stocking prosthesis
Jonas penile prosthesis
Jonas silicone-silver penile prosthesis
Jonas silver penile prosthesis
Joplin toe prosthesis
Judet hip prosthesis
Judet press-fit hip prosthesis
Judet prosthesis
Kastec mitral valve prosthesis
Kaufman incontinence prosthesis
Kaufman penile prosthesis
Kaufman prosthesis
Kaufman urinary incontinence prosthesis
Kay-Shiley disk valve prosthesis
Kay-Shiley valve prosthesis
Kay-Suzuki disk prosthesis
Kay-Suzuki disk valve prosthesis
Kay-Suzuki valve prosthesis
Keeler cryoprosthesis
keratoprosthesis
Kessler prosthesis
Kessler upper limb prosthesis
Kinematic II total knee prosthesis
Kinematic prosthesis
Kinematic rotating-hinge knee prosthesis
Kirschner total shoulder prosthesis
knee prosthesis
knitted Teflon prosthesis
knitted vascular prosthesis

prosthesis *continued*

Krause-Wolfe prosthesis
L-type nose-bridge prosthesis
Lacey prosthesis
Lagrange-Letoumel hip socket prosthesis
LAI knee prosthesis
Lanceford porous metal hip prosthesis
large-bore bile duct endoprosthesis
laryngeal prosthesis
Lash-Masler penile prosthesis
Lash-Moser prosthesis
latex prosthesis
Leadbetter-Politano ureteral implant prosthesis
Leinbach prosthesis
Lillehei valve prosthesis
Lillehei-Cruz-Kaster prosthesis
Lillehei-Kaster aortic valve prosthesis
Lillehei-Kaster mitral valve prosthesis
Lillehei-Kaster prosthesis
Lippman hip prosthesis
Lippy incus prosthesis
Liverpool knee prosthesis
locking prosthesis
London prosthesis
Longhem prosthesis
Lo-Por arterial prosthesis
Lord press-fit hip prosthesis
Lorenzo SMO prosthesis
low-profile prosthesis
low-profile valve prosthesis
MacIntosh knee prosthesis
MacIntosh prosthesis
MacIntosh tibial plateau prosthesis

prosthesis *continued*

MacIntosh tibial prosthesis

Mackler intraluminal tube prosthesis

Mackler tube prosthesis

Macrofit hip prosthesis

Magnuson valve prosthesis

Magnuson-Cromie prosthesis

Magnuson-Cromie valve prosthesis

Magovern ball-valve prosthesis

Magovern-Cromie prosthesis

Magovern-Cromie valve prosthesis

malar prosthesis

Mallory-Head hip prosthesis

mammary prosthesis

mandibular prosthesis

Marlex mesh prosthesis

Marlex prosthesis

Marmor knee prosthesis

Marmor prosthesis

Marmor tibial prosthesis

Marmor total knee prosthesis

Matchett prosthesis

Matchett-Brown hip prosthesis

Mathys cementless prosthesis

maxillary dental prosthesis

maxillofacial prosthesis

Mayo elbow prosthesis

McBride prosthesis

McBride-Moore prosthesis

McGhan breast prosthesis

McKee prosthesis

prosthesis *continued*

McKee-Farrar hip prosthesis

McKee-Farrar total hip prosthesis

McKeever knee prosthesis

McKeever patella cap prosthesis

McKeever patella prosthesis

McKeever prosthesis

McKeever Vitallium cap prosthesis

McNaught keel laryngeal prosthesis

McNaught prosthesis

Meadox woven velour prosthesis

Meadox-Cooley woven low-porosity vascular prosthesis

Medi-graft vascular prosthesis

Medoc-Celestin endoprosthesis

Medtronic INTACT porcine bioprosthesis valve

Medtronic-Hall tilting-disk valve prosthesis

Mega prosthesis

Meme breast prosthesis

Mentor inflatable penile prosthesis

Mentor penile prosthesis with rear-tip extender

Mentor Resi prosthesis

Mentor Self-Cath penile prosthesis

Mersilene prosthesis

mesh prosthesis

metal prosthesis

Meyerding prosthesis

MGH knee prosthesis

Michael Reese prosthesis

microcrimped prosthesis

prosthesis *continued*

Microknit arterial prosthesis
Microvel prosthesis
Miller-Galante hip prosthesis
Milliknit arterial prosthesis
Milliknit vascular graft prosthesis
mitral valve prosthesis
Mittlemeir ceramic hip prosthesis
Mittlemeir femoral prosthesis
modified prosthesis
modular knee prosthesis
modular prosthesis
Monk prosthesis
Moore hip prosthesis
Moore hip-locking prosthesis
Moore prosthesis
Moore self-locking prosthesis
Moretz prosthesis
Mueller Duo-Lock hip prosthesis
Mueller hip prosthesis
Mueller micrograin prosthesis
Mueller prosthesis
Mueller-Charnley total hip prosthesis
Muhlberger orbital implant prosthesis
Mules prosthesis
Mulligan prosthesis
Mulligan Silastic prosthesis
Murray knee prosthesis
muscle prosthesis
myoelectric control prosthesis
Naden-Rieth prosthesis
Natural-Loc acetabular cup prosthesis

prosthesis *continued*

Natural-Y breast prosthesis
Neer prosthesis
Neer shoulder prosthesis
Neer shoulder replacement prosthesis
Neer I shoulder joint prosthesis
Neer II proximal humerus prosthesis
Neer II shoulder joint prosthesis
Neer II shoulder prosthesis
Neibauer hand prosthesis
Neibauer prosthesis
neural prosthesis
Neville tracheal prosthesis
Neville tracheobronchial prosthesis
Noiles prosthesis
noncemented prosthesis
nonconstrained knee prosthesis
nonhinged constrained knee prosthesis
nose-bridge prosthesis
nylon vascular prosthesis
ocular prosthesis
Odland ankle prosthesis
OEC hip prosthesis
offset hinge prosthesis
Ollier-Thiersch prosthesis
Ommaya reservoir prosthesis
OmniPhase semirigid penile prosthesis
onlay Dacron prosthesis
orbital floor prosthesis
orbital prosthesis
Oregon prosthesis
Orlon vascular prosthesis
Ortholoc prosthesis
ossicular chain replacement prosthesis

prosthesis *continued*

ossicular replacement prosthesis
Osteonics hip prosthesis
Osteonics prosthesis
Osteo-Stim prosthesis
Ottoback knee prosthesis
Oxford total knee prosthesis
Padgett prosthesis
Paladon prosthesis
Panje prosthesis
Panje voice button laryngeal prosthesis
paraffin prosthesis
partial ossicular reconstructive/replacement prosthesis (PORP)
patch prosthesis
patella cap prosthesis
patellar prosthesis
patellofemoral prosthesis
PCA knee prosthesis
Pearman penile Silastic prosthesis
pedicle prosthesis
peg-top prosthesis
Pemco valve prosthesis
penile prosthesis
peroral esophageal prosthesis
Perras mammary prosthesis
Phoenix total hip prosthesis
piggyback mammary prosthesis
Pillet hand prosthesis
piston prosthesis
piston-type prosthesis
plaster pants prosthesis
Plasticor torque-type prosthesis
Plasti-Pore ossicular replacement prosthesis

prosthesis *continued*

Plasti-Pore total ossicular replacement prosthesis (Plasti-Pore TORP)
Plasti-Pore TORP (Plasti-Pore total ossicular replacement prosthesis)
Plexiglas prosthesis
Plystan prosthesis
polycentric knee prosthesis
polycentric prosthesis
polyether prosthesis
polyethylene prosthesis
polyethylene talar prosthesis
polyurethane prosthesis
polyvinyl prosthesis
porcine heterograft prosthesis
porous coated anatomic knee prosthesis (PCA knee prosthesis)
PORP (partial ossicular reconstructive/replacement prosthesis)
press-fit prosthesis
Procter-Livingston endoprosthesis
Proplast prosthesis
Protasul femoral prosthesis
Protek hip prosthesis
Protek Protasul vanadium-free titanium alloy prosthesis
Rastelli prosthesis
replacement prosthesis
Reverdin prosthesis
Revive system penile prosthesis
Richards maximum contact total knee prosthesis (RMC total knee prosthesis)

prosthesis *continued*

Richards prosthesis
Ring hip prosthesis
Ring knee prosthesis
Ring total hip prosthesis
RMC total knee prosthesis (Richards maximum contact total knee prosthesis)
Robert Bent Brigham total knee prosthesis
Robert Brigham knee prosthesis
Robert Brigham prosthesis
Robinson prosthesis
Rock-Mulligan prosthesis
Rose L-type nose bridge prosthesis
Rosen prosthesis
Rosen urinary prosthesis
Rosenfeld hip prosthesis
Rosi bridge prosthesis
rotating-hinge knee prosthesis
S-ROM hip prosthesis
S-ROM system prosthesis
SACH prosthesis
Sampson prosthesis
Sauerbruch limb prosthesis
Sauerbruch prosthesis
Sauvage Bionit femoral prosthesis
Sauvage prosthesis
Savastano total knee prosthesis
Sbarbaro tibial prosthesis
SCDT heart valve prosthesis
Scheer Teflon prosthesis
Schlein total elbow prosthesis
Schuknecht piston prosthesis
Schuknecht stapes prosthesis

prosthesis *continued*

Schuknecht Teflon wire piston prosthesis
Schurring ossicle cup prosthesis
Scott inflatable penile prosthesis
scrotal-perineal incontinence prosthesis
Scuderi prosthesis
seamless prosthesis
seamless tube prosthesis
self-locking prosthesis
semiconstrained prosthesis
semirigid penile prosthesis
Servital prosthesis
Sevastano knee prosthesis
Shea bail-hook prosthesis
Shea malleus gripper prosthesis
Shea prosthesis
Shea Teflon piston prosthesis
Sheehan knee prosthesis
Sheehan total knee prosthesis
Sheehy incus replacement prosthesis
Sheehy-House incus replacement prosthesis
Sheehy-House prosthesis
shell prosthesis
Shier knee prosthesis
Shier prosthesis
shoulder prosthesis
Silastic mammary prosthesis
Silastic penile prosthesis
Silastic prosthesis
Silastic testicular prosthesis
silicone doughnut prosthesis

prosthesis *continued*

silicone prosthesis
Siloxane prosthesis
Singer-Blom electro-
larynx prosthesis
single-rod penile
prosthesis
Sivash hip prosthesis
Sivash prosthesis
Small-Carrion penile
prosthesis
Small-Carrion semirigid
penile prosthesis
Smeloff-Cutter aortic
valve prosthesis
Smeloff-Cutter ball-valve
prosthesis
Smeloff-Cutter heart
valve prosthesis
Smith prosthesis
Smith Silastic prosthesis
Smith-Petersen hip cup
prosthesis
Smith-Petersen prosthe-
sis
SMo prosthesis
solid silicone orbital
prosthesis
Spectron cemented hip
prosthesis
Spectron hip prosthesis
Spectron metal-backed
cup for Richards hip
prosthesis
Speed prosthesis
Speed radial cap
prosthesis
sphere prosthesis
split-thickness prosthesis
St. George total hip
prosthesis
St. George total knee
prosthesis
St. Jude Medical aortic
valve prosthesis
St. Jude Medical valve
prosthesis

prosthesis *continued*

St. Jude mitral valve
prosthesis
St. Jude valve prosthesis
stabilocondylar knee
prosthesis
stainless steel mesh
prosthesis
stainless steel prosthesis
stainless steel wire
prosthesis
Stanmore shoulder
prosthesis
stapedectomy prosthesis
stapes prosthesis
Starr ball heart prosthe-
sis
Starr-Edwards aortic
valve prosthesis
Starr-Edwards prosthesis
Starr-Edwards valve
prosthesis
steel wire prosthesis
Steffee prosthesis
stem prosthesis
Stenzel rod prosthesis
STH-2 total hip prosthe-
sis
straight-stem prosthesis
subdermal prosthesis
Supramid prosthesis
surgical prosthesis
Surgitek Flexi-Flate II
penile prosthesis
Surgitek Flexi-rod penile
prosthesis
Surgitek inflatable penile
prosthesis
Surgitek mammary
prosthesis
Surgitek penile prosthe-
sis
Sutter-Smeloff heart
valve prosthesis
sutureless valve prosthe-
sis
Swanson prosthesis

prosthesis *continued*

Swanson Silastic prosthesis
Syme prosthesis
Synatomic knee prosthesis
Synergist Erection penile prosthesis
tantalum mesh prosthesis
tantalum prosthesis
tantalum stapes prosthesis
TARA prosthesis
Teflon intracardiac patch prosthesis
Teflon mesh prosthesis
Teflon prosthesis
Teflon sheeting prosthesis
Teflon trileaflet prosthesis
Teflon wire piston prosthesis
tendon prosthesis
testicular prosthesis
Tevdek prosthesis
Tharies prosthesis
Thiersch prosthesis
Thompson femoral head prosthesis
Thompson prosthesis
threaded titanium acetabular prosthesis (TTAP)
Thrust femoral prosthesis
tibial prosthesis
tibiofemoral prosthesis
Ti/CoCr hip prosthesis
tilting-disk aortic valve prosthesis
titanium ball prosthesis
titanium prosthesis
Tivanium hip prosthesis
toe prosthesis
toe-to-thumb prosthesis

prosthesis *continued*

TORP (total ossicular reconstructive/replacement prosthesis)
torque-type prosthesis
total condylar knee prosthesis
total hip prosthesis
total knee prosthesis
total ossicular reconstructive/replacement prosthesis (TORP)
Townley knee prosthesis
Townley prosthesis
Townley TARA prosthesis
TR-28 hip prosthesis
Trapezoidal-28 total hip prosthesis
Trautman Locktite prosthesis
Triad prosthesis
trial prosthesis
triaxial elbow prosthesis
Tricon-M total knee prosthesis
trileaflet aortic prosthesis
trileaflet prosthesis
TTAP (threaded titanium acetabular prosthesis)
tube prosthesis
Turner prosthesis
two-prong stem finger prosthesis
Tygon esophageal prosthesis
UCI knee prosthesis
UCI prosthesis
UHI Universal head system hip prosthesis
umbrella-type prosthesis
unconstrained knee prosthesis
unconstrained prosthesis
undersized prosthesis
unicondylar prosthesis

prosthesis *continued*
- Universal femoral head prosthesis
- Universal proximal femur prosthesis (UPF prosthesis)
- UPF prosthesis (Universal proximal femur prosthesis)
- urinary incontinence prosthesis
- USCI Sauvage Bionit bifurcated vascular prosthesis
- USCI Sauvage EXS side-limb prosthesis
- Usher Marlex mesh prosthesis
- Valls prosthesis
- valve prosthesis
- Vanghetti limb prosthesis
- Vanghetti prosthesis
- vascular prosthesis
- Vascutek vascular prosthesis
- vessel prosthesis
- Vitallium hip prosthesis
- Vitallium Moore prosthesis
- Vitallium Moore self-locking prosthesis
- Vitallium prosthesis
- Vivosil prosthesis
- voice prosthesis
- Voltz wrist joint prosthesis
- Wada hingeless heart valve prosthesis
- Wada valve prosthesis
- Walldius knee prosthesis
- Walldius prosthesis
- Walldius total knee prosthesis
- Walldius Vitallium mechanical knee prosthesis
- Waugh ankle prosthesis
- Waugh knee prosthesis

prosthesis *continued*
- Weavenit prosthesis
- Weavenit valve prosthesis
- Weavenit vascular prosthesis
- Weck-cel prosthesis
- Wesolowski prosthesis
- Wesolowski Weavenit vascular prosthesis
- Wheeler prosthesis
- Whiteside prosthesis
- Whiteside total hip prosthesis
- Wilke boot prosthesis
- Wilson-Cook endo-prosthesis
- wire mesh prosthesis
- wire stapes prosthesis
- wire-fat ear prosthesis
- Wolfe prosthesis
- woven-tube vascular prosthesis
- Wright knee prosthesis
- Xenophor femoral prosthesis
- Zimaloy femoral head prosthesis
- Zimaloy hip prosthesis
- Zimaloy knee prosthesis
- Zimaloy prosthesis
- Zimmer prosthesis
- Zimmer shoulder prosthesis
- Zimmer tibial prosthesis
- Zimmer total hip prosthesis
- Zweymuller hip prosthesis

prosthesis extractor with hand grip
prosthesis fixation
prosthesis sizing set
prosthetic, prosthetics
prosthetic appliance
prosthetic ball valve
prosthetic device
prosthetic graft

prosthetic heart
prosthetic heart valve
prosthetic lens
prosthetic loop
prosthetic patch graft
prosthetic replacement arthro-
    plasty
prosthetic ring annuloplasty
prostheitic sizer
prosthetic system
prosthetic valve
prosthetic valve holder
prosthetic valve poppet
prosthetic valve sewing ring
prosthetic valve suture ring
prosthetist
Prosthex sponge
protamine sulfate
Protasul femoral prosthesis
Protasul prosthetic hip
protected bronchoscopic brush
protection
protective bandage
protective dressing
protective eye pad
protective eye shield
protective goggles
Protecto splint
protector
Protek hip prosthesis
Protek Protasul vanadium-free
    titanium alloy prosthesis
prothrombin time
Protouch synthetic orthopedic
    padding
Protozyme
protracted labor
protracted treatment
protraction
protractor
        Zimmer protractor
protruding
protruding fat
protrusio acetabulum
protrusio shill
protrusion
protrusive excursion

protrusive occlusion
protuberance
protuberant abdomen
proud flesh
provide
Providence Hospital artery
    forceps
Providence Hospital clamp
Providence Hospital classic
    forceps
Providence Hospital forceps
Providence Hospital hemostat
Providence Hospital hemostatic
    forceps
provisional canthoplasty
provisional ligature
provoked response
proximal
proximal articular set angle
    (PASA)
proximal colon
proximal electrode
proximal focal femoral defi-
    ciency (PFFD)
proximal gastrectomy
proximal incision
proximal interphalangeal
    joint
proximal jejunum
proximal ligatures
proximal row carpectomy
proximal shaft
proximal space
proximal splenorenal shunt
proximal third
proximal tibia
proximal to
proximal ureter
proximally retracted
proximate cause
Proximate flexible linear stapler
Proximate intraluminal stapler
Proximate linear stapler
Proximate skin staples
Proximate stapler
proximity
Proxi-Strip wound closures

PRP (proliferative retinopathy photocoagulation)
Pruitt anoscope
Pruitt irrigation catheter
Pruitt occlusion catheter
Pruitt proctoscope
Pruitt rectal speculum
Pruitt-Inahara autoperfusion shunt
Pruitt-Inahara carotid shunt
Pruitt-Inahara vascular shunt
pruned-tree appearance
pruned-tree arteriogram
prune-juice peritoneal fluid
Prussak fibers
Prussak pouch
Prussak space
Pryor-Péan retractor
PSA-1 monitor
psammoma bodies
PSC (posterior subcapsular cataract)
PSCE (presurgical clotting evaluation)
pseudarthrosis
pseudocapsule
pseudochylous ascites
pseudocyst
pseudocyst formation
pseudofollicular salpingitis
pseudohernia
pseudohypoparathyroidism
pseudojoint formation
pseudoligamentous
pseudomelia
pseudomembrane
pseudomembranous
pseudomotor cerebri
pseudo-obstruction
pseudoparalysis
pseudophake
pseudophakia
pseudophakos
pseudopolypoid changes
pseudotabes
PSIS (posterosuperior iliac spine)

PSKA antibiotic Hank solution
psoas abscess
psoas bladder hitch
psoas hitch procedure
psoas major, musculus
psoas margin
psoas minor, musculus
psoas muscle
psoas retractor
psoas sign
psoas test
PSVT (paroxysmal supraventricular tachycardia)
psychocardiac reflex
psychomotor
PTA (percutaneous transluminal angioplasty)
PTB (patellar tendon-bearing)
PTB brace
PTB cast
PTB walker
PTBD catheter (percutaneous transhepatic biliary drainage catheter)
PTC (percutaneous transhepatic cholangiography)
PTCA (percutaneous transluminal coronary angioplasty)
PTCA catheter
PTD (percutaneous transhepatic decompression/drainage)
pterygium
pterygium keratome
pterygium knife
pterygium operation
pterygium transplant
pterygoid canal
pterygoid muscle
pterygoid nerve
pterygoid notch
pterygoid plate
pterygoid process
pterygoideus lateralis, musculus
pterygoideus lateralis, nervus
pterygoideus medialis, musculus
pterygoideus medialis, nervus

pterygomandibular raphe
pterygomaxillary notch
pterygomaxillary region
pterygopalatine canal
pterygopalatine fossa
pterygopalatine ganglion
pterygopalatine nerves
pterygopalatini, nervi
PTFE (polytetrafluoroethylene;
    Teflon)
PTFE Gore-Tex graft
PTFE graft
PTLA (percutaneous translumi-
    nal angioplasty)
ptosis
ptosis clamp
ptosis correction
ptosis forceps
ptosis knife
ptosis sling
ptosis surgery
ptotic
ptotic breast
ptotic kidney
PTRA (percutaneous translumi-
    nal renal angioplasty)
ptyalectasis
ptyalolithiasis
ptyalolithotomy
pubarche
puberty
pubescent uterus
pubic arch
pubic bone
pubic crest
pubic hair
pubic hair line
pubic ramus
pubic region
pubic symphysis
pubic tubercle
pubioplasty
pubiotomy
pubis (pl. pubes)
pubocapsular ligament
pubocervical fascia
pubocervical ligament

pubococcygeal line
pubococcygeal muscle
pubococcygeoplasty
pubococcygeus, musculus
pubofemoral ligament
puboprostatic ligament
puboprostatic muscle
puboprostaticus, musculus
puborectal muscle
puborectalis loop
puborectalis, musculus
pubosacral diameter
pubotuberous diameter
pubovaginal muscle
pubovaginalis, musculus
pubovesical ligament
pubovesical muscle
pubovesicalis, musculus
pubovesicocervical fascia
puboxyphoid incision
PUD (peptic ulcer disease)
puddler's cataract
Puddu reconstruction
pudenda
pudenda interna, arteria
pudenda interna, vena
pudendae externae, arteriae
pudendae externae, venae
pudendal anesthesia
pudendal arteriography
pudendal artery
pudendal artery angiography
pudendal block
pudendal block anesthesia
pudendal canal
pudendal hernia
pudendal needle
pudendal nerve
pudendal vein
pudendal vessels
pudendum femininum
pudendum muliebre
pudendus, nervus
Pudenz reservoir
Pudenz shunt
Pudenz tube
Pudenz valve

Pudenz ventriculoatrial shunt
Pudenz-Heyer clamp
Pudenz-Heyer shunt
Pudenz-Heyer vascular catheter
Pudenz-Heyer-Schulte valve
pudic
pudic vessel
puerile respiration
puerperal eclampsia
puerperal sterilization
Puestow anastomosis
Puestow biliary tract procedure
Puestow dilator
Puestow guide wire
Puestow operation
Puestow pancreaticojejunos-
    tomy
Puestow pancreatojejunostomy
Puestow wires
Puestow-Gillesby operation
Puestow-Olander GI tube
PUF (pure ultrafiltration)
puffy gums
puffy tumor
Pugh driver
Pugh hip pin
Pugh nail
Pugh plate
Pugh tractor
Puig Massana-Shiley
    annuloplasty valve
puka chisel
pull knife
pull screw
pullback
pulled muscle
pulled taut
pulled tendon
pulley sutures
pulley tendon
pulleys
pull-out suture
pull-out wire
pull-out wire sutures
pull-through abdominoperineal
    resection
pull-through operation

pull-through procedure
pull-through proctectomy
pulmonalis dextra, arteria
pulmonalis inferior dextra, vena
pulmonalis inferior sinistra,
    vena
pulmonalis sinistra, arteria
pulmonalis superior dextra,
    vena
pulmonalis superior sinistra,
    vena
pulmonary abscess
pulmonary aneurysm
pulmonary angiogram
pulmonary aortic anastomosis
pulmonary apex
pulmonary arterial vent
pulmonary arteriography
pulmonary arteriole
pulmonary artery (PA)
pulmonary artery arteriogram
pulmonary artery balloon pump
    (PABP)
pulmonary artery banding
pulmonary artery catheter
pulmonary artery clamp
pulmonary artery forceps
pulmonary artery sling
pulmonary artery wedge
    angiogram
pulmonary balloon
pulmonary balloon
    valvuloplasty
pulmonary bed
pulmonary bypass
pulmonary capillary wedge
    (PCW)
pulmonary capillary wedge
    pressure
pulmonary circulation
pulmonary clamp
pulmonary conduit outflow tract
pulmonary disease
pulmonary edema
pulmonary embolism
pulmonary embolism clamp
pulmonary embolus

pulmonary fibrosis
pulmonary fields
pulmonary flotation catheter
pulmonary flow
pulmonary function
pulmonary function studies
pulmonary hemorrhage
pulmonary hilus
pulmonary hypertension
pulmonary infiltration
pulmonary innominate anasto-
    mosis
pulmonary lesion
pulmonary ligament
pulmonary lobule
pulmonary metastasis
pulmonary nodules
pulmonary outflow tract
pulmonary perfusion scanning
pulmonary pressure
pulmonary prominence
pulmonary pulse
pulmonary resection
pulmonary resistance
pulmonary retractor
pulmonary segment
pulmonary subclavian anasto-
    mosis
pulmonary surgery
pulmonary toilet
pulmonary triple-lumen catheter
pulmonary trunk
pulmonary trunk orifice
pulmonary valve
pulmonary valve knife
pulmonary valvotomy
pulmonary valvuloplasty
pulmonary valvulotome
pulmonary valvulotomy
pulmonary vascular markings
pulmonary vasculature
pulmonary vein
pulmonary venous congestion
pulmonary ventilation
pulmonary vesicles
pulmonary vessel clamp
pulmonary vessel forceps

pulmonary vessels
pulmonary wedge
pulmonary wedge pressure
pulmonic clamp
pulmonic closure
pulmonic insufficiency
pulmonic stenosis
pulmonic stenosis clamp
pulmonic valve
pulmonocoronary reflex
Pulmopak pump for arterial
    perfusion
pulp
pulp amputation
pulp canal
pulpa dentis
pulpa lienis
pulpal devitalization
pulpal excavations
pulpar cells
pulpectomy
pulped muscle dressing
pulpless tooth
pulposus
pulpotomy
pulpy testis
Pulsair system
Pulsar NI pacemaker
pulsatile
pulsatile assist device
pulsatile cardiopulmonary
    bypass
pulsatile hematoma
pulsatile mass
pulsatile perfusion
pulsating aneurysm
pulsating aorta
pulsating mass
pulsating pain
pulsation
pulsator
Pulsavac lavage debridement
    system
pulse
pulse generator
pulse monitor
pulse oximeter

pulse width
pulsed angiolaser
pulsed Doppler images
pulsed Doppler spectral
    analysis
pulsed echo methods
pulsed sonogram
pulsed-wave ultrasound
pulse-wave configurations
pulsion
pulsion hernia
pulsus alternans
pulsus tardus
pulverize
Pulvertaft fashion
Pulvertaft interweaving method
    for hand surgery
Pulvertaft sutures
pump
   Abbott PCA pump
   AccuPressure infusion
    pump
   Alvegniat pump
   angle port pump
   aortic balloon pump
   Argyle-Salem sump
    pump
   Arndorfer pneumocapil-
    lary infusion pump
   Autosyringe insulin
    pump
   Axiom double sump
    pump
   balloon pump
   Bard PCA pump
   Barron pump
   Bio-Medicus pump
   Bio-Pump for bypass
    surgery
   blood pump
   breast pump
   bubble trap oxygenator
    pump
   calcium pump
   Camel-Lindbergh pump
   cardiac balloon pump
   Carmody pump

pump *continued*
   Cobe double blood
    pump
   continuous suction
    pump
   Cordis Hakim pump
   Cormed infusion pump
   Crafon-Oretorp arthro-
    scopy pump
   Datascope intra-aortic
    balloon pump
   DeBakey heart pump
    oxygenator
   DeWall bubbler-type
    pump
   Dia pump
   disk oxygenator pump
   drainage pump
   drug-infusion pump
   Emerson pump
   extracorporeal pump
   Felig insulin pump
   fuser pump
   gastrostomy pump
   Gomco pump
   Gomco thermotic pump
   Gomco thoracic drainage
    pump
   Graseby pump
   Grieshaber air pump
   Hakim-Cordis pump
   hand pump
   Harvard PCA pump
   Harvard pump
   Hemopump
   Holter pump
   IABP (intra-aortic
    balloon pump)
   IMED infusion pump
   IMED pump
   implantable drug
    infusion pump
   implanted pump
   Infusaid chemotherapy
    pump
   Infusaid hepatic pump
   Infusaid infusion pump

pump *continued*
    Infusaid pump
    infusion pump
    infusion-withdrawal
      pump
    insulin pen pump
    interaortic balloon pump
    intra-aortic balloon
      pump (IABP)
    ion pump
    IVAC infusion pump
    IVAC pump
    IVAC volumetric infusion
      pump
    Jarvik-7 mechanical
      pump
    Jobst extremity pump
    kidney perfusion pump
    Life Care Pump
    Lindbergh pump
    Luer-Lok pump
    McGaw volumetric pump
    mechanical insulin pump
    Micro-Temp pump
    Novacor pump
    oxygenator pump
    PABP (pulmonary artery
      balloon pump)
    Pemco pump
    pressure pump
    pulmonary artery balloon
      pump (PABP)
    Pulmopak pump for
      arterial perfusion
    Razel pump
    Resipump pump-
      reservoir
    retroperfusion pump
    Salem sump pump
    Servo pump
    sodium pump
    Sorenson-Yankauer
      combination pump
    Stedman pump
    Stedman suction pump
    strap-on pump

pump *continued*
    suction pressure pump
    suction pump
    sump pump
    surgically implanted
      pump
    syringe pump
    thermotic pump
    Thoratec pump
    Travenol infusion pump
    vacuum hand pump
    VIP chemotherapy pump
    volumetric infusion
      pump
    volumetric pump
    Woodyatt pump
pump bump
pump failure
pump oxygenator
pump primed
pumper
pumping heart
punch
    Abrams biopsy punch
    Abrams pleural biopsy
      punch
    Abrams punch
    Accuflex punch
    Acufex duckbill punch
    Acufex linear punch
    Acufex rotary punch
    adenoid punch
    Adler attic ear punch
    Adler punch
    Ainsworth punch
    Alexander antrostomy
      punch
    Alexander biopsy punch
    Alexander punch
    Anderson antrum punch
    angular oval punch
    antral punch
    antrostomy punch
    aorta punch
    aortic punch
    attic ear punch

punch *continued*
- atticus punch
- Bailey punch
- Baumgartner punch
- Berens corneoscleral punch
- Berens punch
- Beyer atticus punch
- Beyer punch
- biopsy punch
- biting punch
- Braasch-Bumpus prostatic punch
- Brewster sinus punch
- Brock infundibular punch
- Brock punch
- Brooks adenoid punch
- Brooks punch
- Bruening punch
- canaliculus punch
- cartilage punch
- Castroviejo corneoscleral punch
- Castroviejo punch
- cervical foraminal punch
- cervical laminectomy punch
- cervical punch
- chalazion punch
- circular punch
- Citelli laminectomy punch
- Citelli punch
- Citelli-Meltzer atticus punch
- Citelli-Meltzer punch
- Cloward intervertebral punch
- Cloward punch
- Cloward-Dowel punch
- Cloward-English punch
- Cloward-Harper punch
- Cone bone punch
- Cone punch
- Cone skull punch
- Cordes punch

punch *continued*
- Cordes sphenoid punch
- Cordes-New laryngeal punch
- Cordes-New punch
- Corgill punch
- corneoscleral punch
- cup-biting punch
- cutaneous punch
- Davol punch
- Derlacki punch
- dermal punch
- Deyerle punch
- Dorsey cervical foraminal punch
- Dorsey punch
- DyoVac suction punch
- ear punch
- endocervical biopsy punch
- Eppendorfer biopsy punch
- Eppendorfer punch
- ethmoidal punch
- Faraci punch
- Faraci-Skillern punch
- Ferris Smith punch
- Ferris Smith-Gruenwald punch
- Ferris Smith-Gruenwald sphenoid punch
- foraminal punch
- Gass cervical punch
- Gass corneoscleral punch
- Gass punch
- Gass scleral punch
- Gaylor punch
- Gaylor-Alexander punch
- Gellhorn punch
- Gellhorn uterine biopsy punch
- Gendelach sphenoid punch
- glenoid punch
- Goldman cartilage punch
- Goldman punch

punch *continued*

Gossen vascular punch
Graham-Kerrison punch
grasping punch
Gruenwald nasal punch
Gruenwald punch
Gundelach punch
Gusberg endocervical
    biopsy punch
Gusberg punch
Haitz canaliculus punch
Hajek antral punch
Hajek-Koffler bone
    punch
Hajek-Koffler punch
Hajek-Koffler sphenoidal
    punch
Hajek-Skillern punch
Hancock aortic punch
Hardy sellar punch
Harper cervical laminec-
    tomy punch
Harris punch
Hartmann punch
Hartmann tonsillar
    punch
Hartmann-Citelli ear
    punch
Hartmann-Citelli punch
Hayek punch
Hoffmann biopsy punch
Hoffmann ear punch
Hoffmann punch
hole punch set
Holth corneoscleral
    punch
Holth punch
Holth sclerectomy punch
Holth-Rubin punch
Holtz corneoscleral
    punch
infundibular punch
Ingraham infant skull
    punch
Ingraham skull punch
intervertebral punch
intranasal punch

punch *continued*

Jackson punch
Jacobson punch
Jacobson vessel punch
Johnson tonsillar punch
Johnson-Kerrison punch
Joseph punch
Karp aortic punch
Kelly punch
Kelly-Descemet mem-
    brane punch
Kelly-Descemet punch
Kennan cervical punch
Kerrison punch
Kerrison-Rhoton punch
Kerrison-Rhoton sella
    punch
Kevorkian biopsy punch
Keyes cutaneous punch
Keyes dermal punch
Keyes punch
Keyes skin punch
kidney punch
King punch
Klause antrum punch
Klause-Carmody antrum
    punch
Klein punch
Knighton-Kerrison punch
Krause punch
laminectomy punch
Lange antrum punch
Lange punch
laryngeal punch
Lebsche punch
Leksell punch
Lempert malleus punch
Lempert punch
Lermoyez nasal punch
Lermoyez punch
MacKenty punch
MacKenty sphenoid
    punch
malleus punch
McElveney punch
McKenzie sphenoid
    punch

punch *continued*

Medtronic aortic punch
Medtronic Hancock
aortic punch
Meltzer adenoid punch
Meltzer punch
Mendez-Schubert aorta
punch
MGH glenoid punch
Miles nasal punch
Mixter punch
Mosher ethmoid punch
Mosher punch
Mulligan cervical biopsy
punch
Murphy kidney punch
Murphy punch
Myers punch
Myerson punch
Myles nasal punch
Myles punch
nasal punch
Noyes punch
Ostrom antral punch
Ostrom nose punch
Ostrom punch
Pfau atticus punch
Pfau punch
Phemister punch
pleural biopsy punch
Pollock punch
Pritikin punch
Pritikin scleral punch
prostatic punch
Raney punch
Reaves antral punch
Reaves punch
Rhoton punch
Richter laminectomy
punch
ring punch
Ronis adenoid punch
Rowe punch
Rubin-Holth corneo-
scleral punch
Rubin-Holth punch
Sachs cervical punch

punch *continued*

Sachs punch
Scheicker laminectomy
punch
Scheinmann biting
punch
Schlesinger cervical
punch
Schlesinger punch
Schmeden nasal punch
Schmeden punch
Schmeden tonsillar
punch
Schmithhuisen ethmoid
punch
Schmithhuisen sphenoid
punch
Schnaudigel sclerotomy
punch
Schubert biopsy punch
scleral punch
Seiffert punch
Seletz punch
Seletz Universal Kerrison
punch
semicircular punch
septal punch
Shastid punch
Shutt hook punch
Shutt punch
sinus punch
Skillern punch
skull cone punch
Smillie nail punch
Smithuysen ethmoidal
punch
Smithuysen sphenoidal
punch
Sokolowski punch
Spencer oval punch
Spencer punch
sphenoidal punch
Spies ethmoidal punch
Spies punch
Spurling-Kerrison
punch
square punch

punch *continued*
- Stammberger antral punch
- sternal punch
- Stevenson capsule punch
- Stevenson punch
- Storz antrum punch
- Storz punch
- Struempel ear punch
- Struyken punch
- suction punch
- Swan punch
- Sweet punch
- Sweet sternal punch
- Takahashi ethmoid punch
- Takahashi nasal punch
- Takahashi punch
- Thompson adenoid punch
- Thompson punch
- Thoms-Gaylor biopsy punch
- Tischler cervical biopsy punch
- Tischler punch
- tonsillar punch
- Troutman corneal punch
- Turkel punch
- Turrell angular rotating punch
- Turrell biopsy punch
- Universal antral punch
- Universal punch
- upbiting punch
- uterine biopsy punch
- Van Struyken nasal punch
- Van Struyken punch
- Veenema-Gusberg prostatic punch
- Veenema-Gusberg punch
- vessel punch
- Wagner antrum punch
- Wagner punch
- Walton punch

punch *continued*
- Walton-Schubert punch
- Watson-Williams ethmoidal punch
- Watson-Williams nasal punch
- Watson-Williams punch
- Whitcomb-Kerrison laminectomy punch
- Whitcomb-Kerrison punch
- Wilde nasal punch
- Wilde punch
- Wittner biopsy punch
- Wittner cervical punch
- Yankauer antral punch
- Yankauer punch
- Yeomans biopsy punch
- Yeomans punch

punch biopsy
punch forceps
punch forceps tip
punch resection of vocal cords
punch tip
punched-out
punched-out lesions
punched-out ulcer
puncta calcific stone
puncta vasculosa
punctate
punctate cataract
punctate electrode
punctate electrotome
punctate hemorrhage
punctate lesion
punctate ulcer
punctate wound
punctation
punctiform lesion
punctum
punctum dilator
punctum snip
puncture
puncture incision
puncture needle
puncture site
puncture wound

punctured lung
puncturing of skin
pungent odor
punktal lens
Puntenney forceps
Puntenney operation
Puntenney tying forceps
pupil
pupillary aperture
pupillary block
pupillary border
pupillary change
pupillary membrane
pupillary reflex
pupillotomy
pupils equal
pupils equal, round, react to light and accommodation (PERRLA)
pupils react to light and accommodation
pupils round and regular
pupils unequal
pupil-to-root iridectomy
Purcell retractor
Purcell self-retaining abdominal retractor
Purdue Pegs
pure ultrafiltration (PUF)
purification system
purified
purified cotton
purine-free diet
Puritan mask
Puritan-Bennett ventilator
Purkinje cells
Purkinje fibers
Purkinje images
Purlon sutures
puromucous
pursestring cervical closure
pursestring ligature
pursestring of black silk
pursestring sutures
pursue
pursuit
purulence
purulent

purulent discharge
purulent drainage
purulent material
purulent sputum
pus
pus accumulation
pus at incision site
pus basin
pus cells
pus tube
push fluids
push-back palatoplasty
push-back procedure
pusher
     Aker pusher
     chorda tympani pusher
     component pusher
     femoral component pusher
     femoral prosthetic pusher
     femoral pusher
     Geomedic femoral pusher
     Jacobson suture pusher
     palate pusher hook
     suture pusher
pusher catheter
pushing
push-pull ankle stress
push-up
Pusto dilatation
pustular lesion
pustular pharyngitis
pustular tonsillitis
pustule
putrefaction
putrid bronchitis
putrid empyema
Putti approach
Putti arthrodesis
Putti arthroplasty gouge
Putti bone rasp
Putti bone raspatory
Putti frame
Putti gouge
Putti knee arthrodesis
Putti operation

Putti rasp
Putti raspatory
Putti shoulder arthrodesis
Putti splint
Putti technique
Putti-Abbott approach
Putti-Platt arthroplasty
Putti-Platt director
Putti-Platt operation
Putti-Platt shoulder dislocation
    operation
Putti-Scaglietti procedure
putty
putty kidney
Puusepp operation
Puusepp reflex
PV (pressure velocity)
PVB sutures
PVC (premature ventricular
    contraction)
PVR (postvoiding residual)
PWB (partial weightbearing)
pyelectasia
pyelectasis
pyelitic
pyelocaliectasis
pyelocaliyceal system
pyelogram
pyelographic study
pyelography
pyeloileocutaneous
pyeloileocutaneous anastomosis
pyeloileostomy
pyelolithotomy
pyelolymphatic
pyeloplasty
pyelorrhaphy
pyeloscopy
pyelostomy
pyelotomy
pyelotomy incision
pyelotomy wound
pyeloureterogram
pyeloureterography
pyeloureterolysis
pyeloureteroplasty
pyelovenous backflow

Pyle-Greulich bone age scale
pylon
pylon fracture
pylorectomy
pyloric
pyloric antrum
pyloric cap
pyloric channel ulcer
pyloric gland
pyloric lymph node
pyloric mucosa
pyloric obstruction
pyloric occlusion operation
pyloric orifice
pyloric outlet obstruction
pyloric region
pyloric ring
pyloric sphincter
pyloric stenosis
pyloric stenosis dilator
pyloric stricture
pyloric string sign
pyloric vein
pyloric vein of Mayo
pyloric vestibule
pyloristenosis
pylorodilator
pyloroduodenal junction
pyloroduodenal obstruction
pyloroduodenal perforation
pyloroduodenotomy
pylorogastrectomy
pyloromyotomy
pyloroplasty
pyloroptosis
pyloroscopy
pylorospasm
pylorostenosis
pylorostomy
pylorotomy
pylorus
pylorus clamp
pylorus of stomach
pylorus separator
Pynchon applicator
Pynchon cannula
Pynchon decompressor

Pynchon mouth gag
Pynchon nasal speculum
Pynchon speculum
Pynchon suction tube
Pynchon tongue depressor
Pynchon tube
Pynchon-Lillie tongue depressor
pyocele
pyogenic
pyogenic abscess
pyoktanin catgut sutures
pyoktanin sutures
pyosalpinx
pyoureter
PYP scan (pyrophosphate scan)
pyramid of kidney
pyramid of thyroid
pyramidal
pyramidal cataract
pyramidal electrode
pyramidal eminence
pyramidal eye implant

pyramidal fracture
pyramidal function
pyramidal lobe
pyramidal lobe of thyroid
pyramidal muscle
pyramidal tract
pyramidal trocar
pyramidal tube
pyramidialis auriculae, musculus
pyramidialis, musculus
pyramidotomy
pyretic
Pyrex tube
pyrexia
Pyridium
pyriform (see *piriform*)
Pyrolite
Pyrolite carbon
Pyrolite heart valve
pyrolitic carbon
pyrophosphate scan (PYP scan)

# q

Q-angle
Q-band
Q-disk
Q-switched YAG laser system
Q-tip
QCT (quantitative computed tomography)
Quad-Lumen drain
quadrangular
quadrangular lobule of cerebellum
quadrangular space
quadrant
quadrant field
quadrantectomy, axillary dissection, radiotherapy (QUART)
quadrate gyrus
quadrate lobe
quadrate muscle
quadratus femoris, musculus
quadratus lumborum
quadratus, musculus
quadratus plantae, musculus
quadriceps
quadriceps atrophy
quadriceps femoris, musculus
quadriceps jerk
quadriceps muscle
quadriceps reflex
quadriceps tendon
quadricepsplasty
quadricuspid pulmonary valve
quadrilateral
quadrilateral brim
quadrilateral cartilage
quadrilateral septum
quadriplegia
quadriplegic

quadripolar catheter
Quadro dressing
quadruple amputation
Quaglino operation
Quantico needle
Quanticor catheter
quantitative
quantitative computed tomography (QCT)
quantitative hepatobiliary scintigraphy
quantitatively
Quantum pacemaker
QUART (quadrantectomy, axillary dissection, radiotherapy)
quartz lamp
quartz mercury ultraviolet lamp
quartz needle
quartz rod
quaternary ammonium chloride skin cleanser
Queckenstedt maneuver
Queckenstedt sign
Queckenstedt test
Queen Anne collar
Queen Anne dressing
Quelicin
quelling reaction
Quénu-Mayo operation
Quénu-Muret sign
quenuthoracoplasty
Quervain (also de Quervain)
Quervain abdominal retractor
Quervain cranial forceps
Quervain cranial rongeur forceps
Quervain elevator
Quervain forceps

Quervain fracture
Quervain incision
Quervain release
Quervain rongeur
Quervain tenolysis
Quervain-Sauerbruch retractor
questionable mass
questionable node
questionable sign
questionable significance
Quevedo forceps
quick pulse
Quick-cath
quickening
Quickert grooved director and
    tongue tie
Quickert probe
Quickert suture
Quickert tube
Quickert-Dryden probe
Quickert-Dryden tube
QuickFurl double-lumen
    balloon
QuickFurl single-lumen balloon
quiescence
quiescent
quiet

quiet bowel sounds
quietly
quilt sutures
quilted sutures
Quimby gum scissors
Quincke puncture
Quincke sign
Quinn holder
Quinn needle holder
quinsy tonsillectomy
Quinton biopsy catheter
Quinton catheter
Quinton Mahurkar double-
    lumen catheter
Quinton Mahurkar dual-lumen
    peritoneal catheter
Quinton Q-Port catheter
Quinton Q-Port vascular access
    port
Quinton suction biopsy
    instrument
Quinton tube
Quire finger forceps
Quire forceps
Quire mechanical finger forceps
Quisling hammer
Qwik-Clean dressing

R&R (recess-resect)
R-L shunt
R-synchronous VVT pacemaker
Raaf Cath vascular catheter
Raaf catheter
Raaf double-lumen catheter
Raaf dual-lumen catheter
Raaf flexible lighted spatula
Raaf forceps
Raaf rongeur
Raaf spatula
Raaf-Oldberg intervertebral disk
    forceps
Raaf-Oldberg rongeur
RAB (remote afterloading
    brachytherapy)
rabbit-ear sign
Rabiner neurological hammer
raccoon eyes
rachicentesis
rachigraph
rachilysis
rachiocentesis
rachiometer
rachiotome
rachiotomy
rachischisis
rachitic beads
rachitic pelvis
rachitic scoliosis
rachitome
rachitomy
rack
racket, racquet
racket amputation
racket incision
raclage
rad (radiation absorbed dose)
Radcliff retractor

radial
radial artery
radial artery catheter
radial artery of index finger
radial aspect
radial bone
radial bursa
radial collateral artery
radial collateral ligament
radial depression
radial deviation
radial drift
radial drift of metacarpal
radial extensor muscle
radial flexor muscle
radial fossa
radial foveola
radial fracture site
radial groove
radial head
radial incision
radial iridotomy
radial keratotomy (RK)
radial neck
radial nerve
radial nerve splint
radial notch
radial pulse
radial recurrent artery
radial reflex
radial shaft
radial shortening
radial styloid
radial styloid process
radial sutures
radial tuberosity
radial tunnel
radial tunnel syndrome
radial veins

radiales, venae
radialis, arteria
radialis indicis, arteria
radialis, nervus
radialis sign
radiate arteries of kidney
radiating chest pain
radiating pain
radiation
radiation absorbed dose (rad)
radiation and chemotherapy
radiation burn
radiation of pain
radiation surgery
radiation therapy
radiation treatment
radiational effect
radiation-induced carcinogenesis
radiation-induced ulceration
radical
radical abdominal hysterectomy
radical antrum operation
radical cure
radical excision
radical operation
radical operation for hernia
radical procedure
radical surgery
radical surgical procedure
radicle
radicotomy
radicular
radicular artery
radicular cyst
radicular pain
radiculectomy
radioactive
radioactive applicator
radioactive cobalt
radioactive iodine
radioactive rod
radioactive seeds
radioactive tag
radioactive tracer
radioactive uptake

radioactivity
radiocarpal articulation
radiocarpal disarticulation
radiocarpal implant
radiocarpal ligament
radiocurable tumor
radiodensity
radioencephalogram study
Radiofocus Glidewire angiography catheter
radiofrequency coil
radiofrequency pacemaker
radiogram
radiograph
radiographic density
radiographic effect
radiographic evidence
radiographic lesion
radiographic studies
radiography
radiohumeral joint
radioimmunoassay (RIA)
radioimmunoglobulin therapy
radioiodinated
radioisotope
radioisotope applicator
radioisotope scanning
radioisotope scintigraphy
radiologic, radiological
radiologic anatomy
radiologic diagnosis
radiologic examination
radiologic magnification study
radiologic procedure
radiologic studies
radiology
radiolucent
radiolucent calculus
radiolucent density
radiolucent gallstone
radiolucent splint
radiolucent stone
radiolus
Radiometer probe
Radionics lesion generator
radiononopaque stone
radionuclear dynamics

radionuclide
radionuclide angiogram
radionuclide cineangiogram
radionuclide imaging
radionuclide scanning
radiopaque
radiopaque bone cement
radiopaque bougie
radiopaque catheter
radiopaque contrast medium
radiopaque density
radiopaque dye
radiopaque intestinal tube
radiopaque lesion
radiopaque medium
radiopaque substance
radiopaque table
radiopharmaceutical
radioresistant
radioresistant tumor
radiosensitive
radiosensitivity
radiotherapy
radioulnar articulation
radioulnar joint
radioulnar subluxation
radioulnar synostosis
radium
radium application
radium applicator
radium capsule
radium implant
radium insertion
radium necrosis
radium needle
radium seeds
radium therapy
radius
radix arcus vertebrae
radix dentis
radix Raney jacket
Radley-Liebig-Brown technique
radon contamination
Radovan breast implant
Radovan subcutaneous tissue
    expander
Radovan tissue expander

RAE endotracheal tube
Ragnault incision
Ragnell double-ended retractor
Ragnell drain
Ragnell operation
Ragnell retractor
Ragnell scissors
Ragnell-Kilner scissors
railway catheter
Raimondi catheter
Raimondi forceps
Raimondi hemostat
Raimondi scalp hemostatic
    forceps
Raimondi shunt
Raimondi spring peritoneal
    catheter
Raimondi spring peritoneal
    valve
Raimondi tube
Raimondi ventricular catheter
Rainbow cast shoe
Rainbow envelope arm sling
Rainbow fracture frame
raised edge
raised skin flap
raised-arm method to reduce
    dislocated shoulder
raising
rake (see also *rake retractor*)
        amputation rake
        Blake rake
        Volkmann rake
rake retractor
        2-prong rake retractor
        4-prong rake retractor
        6-prong rake retractor
        arch rake retractor
        blunt rake retractor
        deep rake retractor
        finger rake retractor
        four-prong rake retractor
        Israel blunt rake retractor
        Israel rake retractor
        Murphy rake retractor
        Rollet rake retractor
        six-prong rake retractor

rake retractor *continued*
- Small rake retractor
- Tiko rake retractor
- two-prong rake retractor
- Volkmann rake retractor

rake teeth
rake ulcer
rales
Ralks applicator
Ralks bone drill
Ralks clamp
Ralks drill
Ralks ear forceps
Ralks ear knife
Ralks ear retractor
Ralks elevator
Ralks eye magnet
Ralks fingernail drill
Ralks forceps
Ralks hammer
Ralks knife
Ralks magnet
Ralks mallet
Ralks rachiotome
Ralks retractor
Ralks splinter forceps
Ralks stitch scissors
Ralks suction pressure anesthesia unit
Ralks tuning fork
Ralks wire-cutting forceps
Ralks-Davis mouth gag
RAM flap (rectus abdominis myocutaneous flap)
Ramadier operation
Rambo endaural incision
Ramdohr sutures
rami (*sing.* ramus)
ramicotomy
ramification
Ramirez arteriovenous shunt
Ramirez shunt
Ramirez straight Silastic tube
Ramirez tube
Ramirez winged catheter
ramisection
ramisectomy

Ramond point
Ramond sign
ramp
rampant
Rampley forceps
ram's horn toenail
Ramsbotham hook
Ramsbotham knife
Ramsbotham sickle
Ramsden eyepiece
Ramses diaphragm
Ramsey County pyoktanin catgut sutures
Ramstedt clamp
Ramstedt dilator
Ramstedt operation
Ramstedt pyloric stenosis dilator
Ramstedt pyloromyotomy
Ramstedt pyloroplasty
Ramstedt-Fredet pyloro-myotomy
ramus (*pl.* rami)
ramus bone
Ranawat-Defiore-Straub technique
Rand forceps
Rand Neuropledgets retractor for brain surgery
Randall biopsy curet
Randall curet
Randall endometrial biopsy curet
Randall forceps
Randall kidney stone forceps
Randall lip adhesion
Randall operation
Randall plaque
Randall sign
Randall stone forceps
Randall triangular flap repair
Randall-Brown needle holder
Rand-House suction tube
Randolph cannula
random access
random movement
randomized study

Rand-Wells pallidothalamec-
    tomy guide
Raney bone drill
Raney clip
Raney clip forceps
Raney cranial drill
Raney curet
Raney dissector
Raney drill
Raney flexion jacket brace
Raney forceps
Raney Gigli-saw guide
Raney jacket
Raney periosteal elevator
Raney punch
Raney retractor
Raney rongeur
Raney scalp clip
Raney scalp clip-applying
    forceps
Raney spinal fusion curet
Raney stainless steel scalp clip
Raney tube
Raney-Crutchfield skull traction
    tongs
Raney-Crutchfield tongs
range
range of motion (ROM)
ranine artery
ranine vein
Ranke complex
Ranke space
Rankin clamp
Rankin forceps
Rankin hemostat
Rankin hemostatic forceps
Rankin intestinal clamp
Rankin operation
Rankin prostatic retractor
Rankin retractor
Rankin suture
Rankin tractor
Rankin-Crile forceps
Rankin-Crile hemostat
Rankin-Crile hemostatic forceps
Rankin-Kelly hemostat
Rankin-Kelly hemostatic forceps

ranula
Ranvier membrane
Ranvier nodes
Ranvier segments
Ranvier tactile disk
Ranzewski clamp
RAO ventriculogram
raphe
rapid alternating movements
rapid emptying of dye
rapid exchange balloon catheter
rapid eye movements (REM)
rapid filling
rapid pull-through (RPT)
rapid pull-through esophageal
    manometry technique
rapid pull-through operation
rapid sequence filming
rapid Y descent
rapidly
Rapp forceps
Rapp technique
rarefaction
rarefaction click
rarefied area
Rasch sign
rash
Rashkind balloon
Rashkind balloon atrial sep-
    tostomy
Rashkind balloon catheter
Rashkind balloon septostomy
Rashkind cardiac procedure
Rashkind catheter
Rashkind procedure
Rashkind septostomy balloon
    catheter
Rashkind-Miller atrial sep-
    tostomy
Rasmussen aneurysm
rasp (see also *raspatory*)
    Alexander rib rasp
    Alexander-Farabeuf rib
        rasp
    AMS rasp
    antral rasp
    antrum rasp

rasp *continued*

Aufricht glabellar rasp
Aufricht nasal rasp
Aufricht rasp
Aufricht-Lipsett nasal rasp
Aufricht-Lipsett rasp
Austin Moore prosthesis rasp
Austin Moore rasp
Barsky rasp
Beck rasp
Berne nasal rasp
Berne rasp
Black bone and skin rasp
bone rasp
Bowen AMS rasp
Brawley antrum rasp
Brawley frontal sinus rasp
Brawley rasp
Brown rasp
Charnley-Mueller rasp
Christmas-tree rasp
circular rasp
Cohen rasp
Converse rasp
corneal rasp
Coryllos rasp
Cottle rasp
Cottle-MacKenty elevator rasp
Davidson-Mathieu-Alexander elevator rasp
Davidson-Sauerbruch rasp
Dean antral rasp
Dean rasp
diamond nasal rasp
diamond rasp
Doyen rib rasp
Eicher rasp
Epstein bone rasp
Epstein rasp
facet rasp
Farabeuf rasp

rasp *continued*

Farabeuf-Collen rasp
femoral shaft rasp
Filtzer interbody rasp
Fisher rasp
Fomon nasal rasp
Fomon rasp
F.R. Thompson rasp
frontal sinus rasp
Gallagher rasp
glabellar rasp
Gleason rasp
Good rasp
interbody circular rasp
interbody fusion rasp
interbody rasp
Israel nasal rasp
Israel rasp
Joseph nasal rasp
Joseph rasp
Lamont nasal rasp
Lamont rasp
Lewis rasp
Lorenz-Rees nasal rasp
Lundsgaard rasp
Lundsgaard-Burch rasp
Maliniac rasp
Maltz rasp
Maltz-Anderson nasal rasp
Maltz-Lipsett nasal rasp
Maltz-Lipsett rasp
McCabe rasp
McIndoe rasp
McKee-Farrar rasp
McKinty rasp
microbayonet rasp
Mitner rotary bone rasp
Moore prosthesis rasp
Moore rasp
nasal rasp
Parkes rasp
Peet nasal rasp
Phemister rasp
Plenk-Matson rasp
polyp grasper
Putti bone rasp

rasp *continued*
   Putti rasp
   rat-tail rasp
   Riordan rasp
   Ritter rasp
   Robb-Roberts rotary rasp
   Rubin rasp
   Saunders-Paparella rasp
   Saunders-Paparella
      window rasp
   Schantz sinus rasp
   Scheer rasp
   Schmidt rasp
   sinus rasp
   Spratt rasp
   stem rasp
   Stille-Doyen rasp
   Stille-Edwards rasp
   Sullivan sinus rasp
   Thompson antral rasp
   Thompson rasp
   Thompson sinus rasp
   trochanteric rasp
   Watson-Williams frontal
      sinus rasp
   Watson-Williams rasp
   Watson-Williams sinus
      rasp
   Wiener antral rasp
   Wiener rasp
   Wiener-Pierce antral rasp
   Wiener-Pierce rasp
   window rasp
   Woodward rasp
raspatory (see also *rasp*)
   Alexander raspatory
   Alexander rib raspatory
   Artmann raspatory
   Aufricht raspatory
   Aufricht-Lipsett raspa-
      tory
   Babcock raspatory
   Bacon periosteal
      raspatory
   Bacon raspatory
   Ballenger raspatory
   Barsky raspatory

raspatory *continued*
   Bastow laminectomy
      raspatory
   Bastow raspatory
   Beck raspatory
   Berne nasal raspatory
   Berry raspatory
   Berry rib raspatory
   Brawley antrum raspa-
      tory
   Brown raspatory
   Brunner raspatory
   Cohen sinus raspatory
   Converse raspatory
   Coryllos raspatory
   Coryllos rib raspatory
   Cottle raspatory
   Davidson-Mathieu
      raspatory
   Davidson-Sauerbruch rib
      raspatory
   Davis raspatory
   Dean raspatory
   Doyen raspatory
   Doyen rib raspatory
   Edwards raspatory
   Eicher raspatory
   facet raspatory
   Farabeuf raspatory
   Farrior raspatory
   fishtail raspatory
   Fomon raspatory
   French-pattern raspatory
   Friedrich raspatory
   Gallagher antral frontal
      raspatory
   Gleason raspatory
   Good frontal raspatory
   Hedblom raspatory
   Hein raspatory
   Herczel raspatory
   Herczel raspatory
      elevator
   Herczel rib raspatory
   Hill raspatory
   Hoen periosteal raspa-
      tory

raspatory *continued*

Hoen raspatory
Hopkins periosteal raspatory
Hopkins raspatory
Israel raspatory
Jansen mastoid raspatory
Jansen raspatory
Joseph nasal raspatory
Joseph raspatory
Kirmisson raspatory
Kleesattel raspatory
Kocher raspatory
Koenig raspatory
Kokowicz raspatory
Ladd raspatory
Lambert-Berry raspatory
Lambert-Berry rib raspatory
Lambotte raspatory
laminectomy raspatory
Lamont nasal raspatory
Lane periosteal raspatory
Lane raspatory
Langenbeck periosteal raspatory
Langenbeck raspatory
Langenbeck-O'Brien raspatory
Lebsche raspatory
Lewis nasal raspatory
Lewis raspatory
Lundsgaard-Burch corneal raspatory
Maliniac nasal raspatory
Maltz raspatory
Maltz-Lipsett raspatory
mastoid raspatory
Mathieu raspatory
Matson raspatory
microraspatory
Miller raspatory
Moore raspatory
Nelson first-rib raspatory
Nicola raspatory
Ollier raspatory
Overholt raspatory

raspatory *continued*

Parkes nasal raspatory
pericardial raspatory
periosteal raspatory
Phemister raspatory
Pierce raspatory
Plenk-Matson raspatory
Putti bone raspatory
Putti raspatory
rib raspatory
Ritter raspatory
Sauerbruch raspatory
Sauerbruch-Frey raspatory
Sayre periosteal raspatory
Sayre raspatory
Schantz sinus raspatory
Schmidt raspatory
Schneider raspatory
Sédillot elevator-raspatory
Sédillot raspatory
Semb raspatory
Sewall raspatory
Shuletz raspatory
Spratt raspatory
Sullivan raspatory
Thompson frontal sinus raspatory
Thompson raspatory
Trélat raspatory
Watson-Williams sinus raspatory
Wiberg raspatory
Wiener antral raspatory
Wiener Universal frontal sinus raspatory
Willauer raspatory
Williger raspatory
Woodward antral raspatory
xyster raspatory
Yasargil microraspatory
Yasargil raspatory
Zenker raspatory
Zoellner raspatory

raspberry mark
raspberry tongue
rasping pain
Rastelli graft
Rastelli implant
Rastelli operation
Rastelli prosthesis
ratchet
ratchet applicator
ratchet-type brace
rate of cerebral blood flow
    (rCBF)
rate-responsive pacemaker
Rathke folds
Rathke pocket
Rathke pouch
Rathke tumor
ratio
rational
Ratliff-Blake forceps
Ratliff-Blake gallstone forceps
Ratliff-Mayo forceps
Ratliff-Mayo gallstone forceps
rat-tail catheter
rat-tail rasp
rat-tail sign
rat-tooth forceps
rat-tooth rongeur
Rauchfuss sling
Rauchfuss sling splint
raucous murmur
Raven matrix
Raverdino operation
Ravich bougie
Ravich clamp
Ravich convertible cystoscope
Ravich cystoscope
Ravich dilator
Ravich lithotriptoscope
Ravich lithotriptoscope with
    Luer lock
Ravich lithotrite
Ravich needle holder
Ravich ureteral dilator
raw area
raw surface
rawhide bone hammer

ray amputation
Ray brain spatula
Ray brain spoon
Ray curet
Ray forceps
Ray nasal speculum
Ray pituitary curet
ray resection
Ray rhizotomy electrode
Ray screw
Ray speculum
Ray spoon
Ray tube
Rayner-Choyce eye implant
rayon gauze
rayon strip
Ray-Parsons-Sunday elevator
Ray-Parsons-Sunday staphylor-
    rhaphy elevator
Rayport dural dissector
Rayport dural knife
Rayport knife
Rayport muscle clamp
rays
Ray-Tec dressing
Ray-Tec gauze
Ray-Tec sponge
Ray-Tec surgical sponges
Ray-Tec x-ray detectable
    surgical sponge
Raz procedure for stress
    incontinence
Raz urethropexy
Razel pump
razor
      Castroviejo razor
razor blade
razor scalpel
rCBF (rate of cerebral blood
    flow)
RD (retinal detachment)
reabsorption
reaccumulation of fluid
reach-and-pin forceps
react
reacting
reaction

reactive
reactivity
reactor
Read chisel
Read facial curet
Read forceps
Read gouge
Read oral curet
Read osteotome
Read periosteal elevator
readable image
readjustment
Read-McIndoe operation
readmitted
readout
reagent
Real coronary artery scissors
real time
realigned fracture
realignment of fracture frag-
    ments
reality
real-time imaging
real-time ultrasonography
real-time ultrasound
ream
reamer
        acetabular reamer
        adjustable cup reamer
        Aufranc finishing ball
            reamer
        Aufranc finishing cup
            reamer
        Aufranc offset reamer
        Aufranc reamer
        Austin Moore bone
            reamer
        Austin Moore reamer
        ball reamer
        ball-tip reamer
        burred Wright reamer
        CAD reamer
        cannulated reamer
        Chamfer reamer
        Charnley reamer
        cylindrical reamer
        deepening reamer

Cloward

reamer *continued*
        DePuy reamer
        drill reamer
        engine reamer
        expanding reamer
        femoral head reamer
        femoral neck reamer
        finishing ball reamer
        finishing cup reamer
        Green-Armytage reamer
        grooving reamer
        Gruca hip reamer
        Harris reamer
        Harris-Norton hip reamer
        Henderson reamer
        Hewson-Richards reamer
        Indiana reamer
        Jergesen reamer
        Jewett reamer
        Küntscher reamer
        Küntscher shaft reamer
        Lorenzo reamer
        Lottes reamer
        MacAusland reamer
        Marin reamer
        medullary canal reamer
        Mira reamer
        Mira-Charnley reamer
        Moore bone reamer
        Moore reamer
        Murphy ball reamer
        Murphy reamer
        Norton adjustable cup
            reamer
        Norton ball reamer
        offset reamer
        Phemister reamer
        Reiswig reamer
        Richards barrel reamer
        Richards calibrated
            reamer
        Rowe reamer
        Rush reamer
        Schneider nail shaft
            reamer
        shaft reamer
        shelf reamer

reamer *continued*
    Smith-Petersen hip
      reamer
    Smith-Petersen reamer
    Sovak reamer
    spherical reamer
    spiral reamer
    spiral trochanteric
      reamer
    step-cut reamer
    Sturmdorf cervical
      reamer
    Sturmdorf reamer
    T-handle reamer
    trochanteric reamer
reamer awl
reamputation
reanastomosis
reapplication of cast
reapproximate
reapproximate skin edges
reapproximated
reassessment
reattached extremity
reattached surgically
reattachment
Reaumer temperature scale
Reaves antral punch
Reaves punch
REB rubber-reinforced bandage
rebleeding risk
rebound
rebound tenderness
rebreathing anesthesia
rebreathing bag
rebreathing mask
Rebuck skin window technique
Rebuck window
recalcitrant
recall
Récamier curet
Récamier operation
recanalization
recanalization of artery
recanalize
recanalizing thrombosis
recannulization

receding lower jaw
receiver coil
recent
receptacle
reception
receptive
receptivity
receptor
recess
recessed balloon septostomy
    catheter
recessed-head screw
recessing of tendon
recession
recession forceps
recessive
recess-resect procedure
rechecked
recipient
recipient of organ transplant
reciprocal rhythm
reciprocal transfusion
reciprocating saw
recirculation
Recklinghausen tonometer
reclamped
reclosure
recognition
recoil wave
recommend
recommended
recondition exercises
reconnected tissue
reconstruction
reconstruction operation
reconstructive microsurgery
reconstructive operation
reconstructive plastic procedure
reconstructive procedure
reconstructive surgery
reconstructive sutures
reconstructive technique
recontour
recontouring alveolectomy
record syringe
recorded measurements
recorded pattern

recorder
    Angus-Esterlie recorder
    Avionics two-channel
      Holter recorder
    Vas recorder
recording
recording cystometer
records
recovered
recovering
recovery
recovery room (RR)
recovery technique
rectal
rectal abscess
rectal ampulla
rectal anesthesia
rectal artery
rectal balloon
rectal biopsy forceps
rectal bleeding
rectal bougie
rectal canal
rectal catheter
rectal column
rectal crypt hook
rectal curet
rectal cutter
rectal dilator
rectal director
rectal distention
rectal enema
rectal examination
rectal finger cot
rectal fistula
rectal fistulectomy
rectal fold
rectal forceps
rectal gargle
rectal hemorrhoid
rectal hernia
rectal hook
rectal incontinence
rectal injection cannula
rectal injection needle
rectal irrigator
rectal lesion

rectal lithotomy
rectal mass
rectal mucosa
rectal muscle cuff
rectal needle
rectal nerves
rectal plexus
rectal polyp
rectal pouch
rectal pressure
rectal probe
rectal prolapse
rectal pull-through operation
rectal reflex
rectal retinaculum
rectal retractor
rectal scissors
rectal shelf
rectal sinuses
rectal site
rectal skin tag
rectal snare
rectal speculum
rectal sphincter
rectal stalks
rectal stenosis
rectal stricture
rectal stump
rectal suppository
rectal surgery
rectal swab
rectal tags
rectal tear
rectal temperature
rectal tenesmus
rectal trauma
rectal trocar
rectal tube
rectal valve
rectal vein
rectal verge
rectal warts
rectales inferiores, nervi
rectales inferiores, venae
rectales mediae, venae
rectalis inferior, arteria
rectalis media, arteria

rectalis superior, arteria
rectalis superior, vena
rectally
rectangular
rectangular amputation
rectangular flap
rectectomy
rectified microscope
rectified polarizing microscope
rectilinear
rectilinear scan
rectilinear scanner
rectoanal inhibitory reflex
rectocele
rectocele repair
rectoclysis
rectococcygeal muscle
rectococcygeus, musculus
rectococcypexy
rectocutaneous fistula
rectocystotomy
rectolabial fistula
rectoperineorrhaphy
rectopexy
rectoplasty
rectorectostomy
rectoromanoscope
rectoromanoscopy
rectorrhaphy
rectoscope
rectoscopy
rectosigmoid
rectosigmoid junction
rectosigmoid manometry
rectosigmoidectomy
rectosigmoidoscope
rectosigmoidoscopy
rectosigmoidostomy
rectostomy
rectotome
rectotomy
rectourethral muscle
rectourethralis, musculus
rectouterine fold
rectouterine ligament
rectouterine muscle
rectouterine pouch

rectouterinus, musculus
rectovaginal
rectovaginal dose
rectovaginal examination
rectovaginal fascia
rectovaginal fistula
rectovaginal fold
rectovaginal pouch
rectovaginal septum
rectovaginal space
rectovesical
rectovesical center
rectovesical fascia
rectovesical fistula
rectovesical fold
rectovesical lithotomy
rectovesical muscle
rectovesical pouch
rectovesical septum
rectovesical space
rectovesicalis, musculus
rectum
rectus
rectus abdominis, musculus
rectus abdominis myocutaneous
    flap (RAM)
rectus abdominis sheath
rectus capitis anterior, musculus
rectus capitis lateralis, musculus
rectus capitis posterior major,
    musculus
rectus capitis posterior minor,
    musculus
rectus fascia
rectus femoris, musculus
rectus incision
rectus inferior bulbi, musculus
rectus inferior, musculus
rectus lateralis bulbi, musculus
rectus lateralis, musculus
rectus medialis bulbi, musculus
rectus medialis, musculus
rectus muscle
rectus muscle hook
rectus muscle-splitting incision
rectus sheath
rectus sheath hematoma

rectus superior bulbi, musculus
rectus superior, musculus
rectus traction suture
recumbency cramps
recumbent film
recumbent incision
recumbent lateral projection
recumbent position
recuperation
recurrence
recurrens radialis, arteria
recurrens tibialis anterior, arteria
recurrens tibialis posterior,
    arteria
recurrens ulnaris, arteria
recurrent
recurrent artery
recurrent bandage
recurrent carcinoma
recurrent disease
recurrent dislocation
recurrent episode
recurrent hemorrhage
recurrent hernia
recurrent infection
recurrent interosseous artery
recurrent laryngeal nerves
recurrent lesion
recurrent nerve
recurrent stricture
recurrent tumor
recurrent ulcer
recurrent vaginal bleeding
recurrent vomiting
recurring hemorrhage
recurvatum
Red Cross adhesive dressing
red laser
red pessary
red reflex
red Robinson catheter
red rubber arch
red rubber catheter
reddened area
reddish macule
Redifocus guide wire
RediFurl catheter

RediFurl double-lumen balloon
RediFurl single-lumen balloon
redirection
Redi-Spec disposable vaginal
    speculum
redistribution
Redivac drain
Redivac drainage
Redivac tube
Redler nail
Redlich-Fisher miliary plaque
Redmond Smith operation
redness along incision site
Redo intestinal clamp
Redon drain
redressed wound
redressement
redressing
red-tip aspirator
red-top tube
reduce size of tumor
reduce tension
reduced
reduced fracture
reducible
reducible hernia
reducing fracture frame
reducing technique
reducing valve
reduction
reduction and internal fixation
reduction division
reduction en masse
reduction mammaplasty
reduction of fracture
reduction of hernia
reduction of intussusception
reduction of rectal prolapse
reduction of torsion
reduction of volvulus
reduction technique
reductive mammaplasty
redundancy
redundant
redundant foreskin
redundant pelvis
redundant prepuce

redundant prolapsed rectum
redundant tissue
reduplication
Redy hemodialysis system
Redy hemodialyzer
Reed ventriculorrhaphy
reef
reef knot
reef knot sutures
reefed vaginal cuff
reefing
reefing of joint capsule
reefing of vastus medialis
re-entrant loop
re-entry operation
Rees lighted retractor
Rees scissors
Reese advancement forceps
Reese dermatome
Reese forceps
Reese knife
Reese muscle forceps
Reese operation
Reese ptosis knife
Reese ptosis operation
Reese saw
Reese stimulator
Reese-Cleasby operation
Reese-Jones-Cooper operation
re-establishment
re-evaluate
re-excision
re-expansion of lung
reference
reference electrode
referential
referral
referred
referred pain
referred sensation
refill
refined
reflect
reflected
reflected from insertion
reflected laterally
reflected medially

reflected skin flap
reflected upward
reflecting microscope
reflecting ophthalmoscope
reflection
reflection of scalp
reflection of sternum
reflection site
reflector
reflex
reflex hammer
reflex ileus
reflex response
reflex stimulation
reflexes absent
reflexes equal
reflexive ileus
reflexively
reflex-like reaction
reflex-type ileus
reflux
reflux esophagitis
reflux filling
reflux from stomach
reflux of barium
reflux of gastric contents
reflux symptoms
reform eye
reform eye implant
reform implant
reformation of chamber
refracted x-ray
refractibility
refracting media
refraction
refraction of eye
refraction of lens
refraction test
refractive error
refractory ascites
refractory period
refracture
refracture following fracture
refracture of bone
refractured bone
refresh
refrigeration anesthesia

refusal
refused permission
refusion
refusion of blood
regained consciousness
Regen flexion exercises
regenerated
regeneration
regenerative activity
regimen
region
regional adenopathy
regional anesthesia
regional block
regional block anesthesia
regional cerebral blood flow
regional excision
regional ileitis
regional involvement
regional node
regional node involvement
regional perfusion
regional recurrence
regional spread
regional vasodilation
Register needle holder
regloving
regloving and regowning
Regnoli operation
regowning
regressed
regression
regression of symptoms
regrowth
regular contractions
regular eye spatula
regular rate and rhythm
regular sinus rhythm
regularity
regularly
regulate
regulation
regulator
regurgitant
regurgitated
regurgitation
rehabilitation

Rehbein rib spreader
Rehfuss tube
Rehne abdominal retractor
Rehne skin graft knife
Rehne-Delorme operation
Rehne-Delorme plication
rehospitalized
rehydrated
Reich curet
Reichel chondromatosis
Reichel cloacal duct
Reichenheim operation
Reichenheim-King operation
Reichenheim-King syndrome
Reichert antroscope
Reichert camera
Reichert fiberoptic sigmoido-
    scope
Reichert flexible sigmoidoscope
Reichert Ful-Vue ophthalmo-
    scope
Reichert Ful-Vue spot retino-
    scope
Reichert membrane
Reichert ophthalmodyna-
    mometer
Reichert radius gauge
Reichert refractor
Reichert retinoscope
Reichert scar
Reichert sigmoidoscope
Reichert slit lamp
Reichert tonometer
Reichling corneal scissors
Reichmann ivory rod
Reichmann rod
Reich-Nechtow cervical biopsy
    curet
Reich-Nechtow clamp
Reich-Nechtow curet
Reich-Nechtow dilator
Reich-Nechtow forceps
Reich-Nechtow hysterectomy
    forceps
Reich-Nechtow plug
Reicker pillow
Reid retinoscope

Reid-Baker procedure
Reif catheter
Reil island
Reilly granulations
reimplant
reimplantation
reimplantation of extremity
reimplantation of fingertip
reimplantation of ureter
reimplanted electrode
Reiner bone rongeur
Reiner curet
Reiner ear knife
Reiner ear syringe
Reiner knife
Reiner repair
Reiner rongeur
Reiner-Alexander syringe
Reiner-Beck tonsil snare
Reiner-Knight ethmoid-cutting
    forceps
reinforcement
reinforcing
reinforcing sutures
reinfusate
reinfusion
Reinke crystals
Reinke space
reinnervation
reinsertion
reintubation
Reisinger forceps
Reisinger lens-extracting forceps
Reisseisen muscle
Reissner canal
Reissner membrane
Reis-Wertheim operation
Reiswig reamer
Reiter syndrome
rejected graft
rejected organ
rejected transplant
rejection of graft
rejection of organ
rejection of transplant
related disorders
related injury

relation
relational coil
relationship
relatively
relax reflex
relaxant
relaxant effect
relaxation
relaxation sutures
relaxed
relaxed anterior wall
relaxed introitus
relaxed pelvic floor
relaxed perineal body
relaxed skin tension lines
relaxed vaginal outlet
relaxing incision
relaxing of muscles
release
release of carpal tunnel
release of patella
release of plantar fascia
release of pus
release of tendo Achillis
release of trigger finger
released
releasing
releasing incision
relevant
Reliavac drain
relief incision
relief of symptoms
relieve pressure
relieving
relining
Reliquet lithotrite
Relton-Hall frame
reluxation
REM (rapid eye movements)
Remak band
Remak fibers
Remak ganglion
Remak reflex
Remak sign
remarkable
remarkably
remineralization

remission
remission of disease
remission of symptoms
remittent fever
remnant
remnants
remobilization
remodeling
remodeling phase of wound
    healing
remote
remote afterloading brachy-
    therapy (RAB)
remote metastases
remottling fracture site
removable appliance
removable implant
removal
removal of calculus
removal of drain
removal of dressing
removal of emboli
removal of embryo
removal of fetal structure
removal of foreign body
removal of life support
removal of organ
removal of pack
removal of packing
removal of pin
removal of placenta
removal of placental frag-
    ments
removal of screw
removal of sutures
removed in part
removed in toto
removed manually
Remy separator
renal
renal angiography
renal arteriogram
renal arteriography
renal artery
renal artery clamp
renal artery forceps
renal artery-reverse saphenous

vein bypass
renal ballottement
renal biopsy
renal brush border membrane
renal calculi
renal capsulectomy
renal capsulotomy
renal clamp
renal colic
renal cyst
renal decortication
renal disease
renal failure
renal fascia
renal fossa
renal function
renal ganglia
renal infarction
renal injury
renal needle
renal obstruction
renal papillae
renal parenchyma
renal pedicle
renal pedicle clamp
renal pelvis
renal plexus
renal plication
renal pouch
renal ptosis
renal pyramid
renal scan
renal shadow
renal sinus
renal sinus retractor
renal transplant
renal transplantation
renal tubule
renal tumor
renal ultrasound
renal veins
renal venography
renales, venae
renalis, arteria
renewal
renewed tumor activity
renin

renis, arteriae
renogram study
renointestinal reflex
renorenal reflex
renovascular hypertension
rent
rent in uterus
rent of intestine
Rentrop catheter
Rentrop infusion catheter
Reo Macrodex sutures
reopen
reopened
reopening
reorientation
reoxygenation
repacking
repair
repair of defect
reparative closure
repeat chest x-ray
repeat study
repeated
reperfusion
reperitonealization
reperitonealize
repetition
repetitious
repetitive
replaced in cast
replacement
replacement fibrosis
replacement graft
replacement of joint
replacement of prosthesis
replacement prosthesis
replacement surgery
replacement therapy
replacement transfusion
replacer
replant
replantation
replantation of amputated digit
replica
replication
Replogle catheter
Replogle tube

repolarization
report
reposited
reposited iris
reposition
repositioned
repositioning
re-prepped
re-prepped and re-draped
reproduction
reproductive organs
required
requirement
Resano dissecting scissors
Resano scissors
rescreening
rescue
rescuer
rescuing pacemaker
research
resectable
resectable lesion
resectable tumor
resected aneurysm
resected tonsil
resecting fracture
resecting sheath
resection
resection clamp
resection of colon
resection-arthrodesis
resection-recession of eye
    muscles
resective colostomy
resector
    distal femoral resector
    femoral resector
    full-radius synovial
        resector
resectoscope
    ACMI pediatric resecto-
        scope
    ACMI resectoscope
    Bard resectoscope
    Baumrucker resecto-
        scope
    Bumpus resectoscope

resectoscope *continued*
    cold-punch resectoscope
    continuous irrigation-
      suction resectoscope
    continuous-flow resecto-
      scope
    Foroblique resectoscope
    French-Iglesias resecto-
      scope
    Gray resectoscope
    Green resectoscope
    Iglesias continuous-flow
      resectoscope
    Iglesias fiberoptic
      resectoscope
    Iglesias resectoscope
    Kaplan cold-punch
      resectoscope
    Kaplan resectoscope
    McCarthy miniature
      resectoscope
    McCarthy resectoscope
    multiple resectoscope
    obturator deflecting
      resectoscope
    obturator resectoscope
    rotating resectoscope
    Scott resectoscope
    Stern-McCarthy electro-
      tome resectoscope
    Stern-McCarthy resecto-
      scope
    Storz cold-punch
      resectoscope
    Storz continuous
      irrigation-suction
      resectoscope
    Storz resectoscope
    Storz-Iglesias resecto-
      scope
    Thompson direct full
      vision resectoscope
    Thompson resectoscope
    Timberlake resectoscope
    Wid-Med resectoscope
    Winter-Eber resecto-
      scope

resectoscope *continued*
    working element
      resectoscope
resectoscope adapter
resectoscope cable
resectoscope curet
resectoscope cutting loop
resectoscope sheath
resectoscopy
resemblance
reserve
reserve cell
reservoir
residual
residual air
residual barium
residual contrast material
residual deformity
residual disease
residual dye
residual node
residual pain
residual paralysis
residual scarring
residual stone
residual stool
residual tissue
residual tumor
residual urine
residual volume
residual weakness
residue
Resifilm
resin uptake
resin-uptake ratio
Resipump pump-reservoir
resistance
resistant
resistive
Resnick Button bipolar
    coagulator
resolution
resolving
resonance
resonant on percussion
resonant to percussion
resorb

resorption
resorption atelectasis
resorption of bone
resource
respect
respective
respiration
respiration assisted anesthesia
respiration bronchoscope
respiration pyelogram
respiration pyelography
respiration unassisted anesthesia
respirator
    Ambu respirator
    BABYbird respirator
    Bath respirator
    Bear respirator
    Bennett respirator
    Bird respirator
    Bourns infant respirator
    Bourns respirator
    Bragg-Paul respirator
    Clevedan positive
      pressure respirator
    cuirass respirator
    Dann respirator
    Drinker respirator
    Emerson respirator
    Emerson cuirass respirator
    Engstrom respirator
    Gill respirator
    Huxley respirator
    Kirmisson respirator
    mechanical respirator
    Med-Neb respirator
    Merck respirator
    Monaghan respirator
    Morch respirator
    Morsch-Retec respirator
    Moynihan respirator
    portable respirator
    Sanders jet ventilation
      device respirator
respiratory
respiratory activity

respiratory arrest
respiratory assistance
respiratory collapse
respiratory distress syndrome
respiratory effort
respiratory exchange
respiratory failure
respiratory function
respiratory murmur
respiratory paralysis
respiratory rales
respiratory secretions
respiratory therapy
respiratory tract
respiratory tube
respiratory wave
respiratory-dependent pacemaker
respiratory-esophageal fistula
respite
respondent
responding
response
Response external suction
    device for impotence
responsibility
responsive
rest and exercise gated nuclear
    angiogram
rest and recuperation
rest cyst
rest position
rest tissue
rested state contraction
resting
resting pan splint
Reston dressing
Reston foam
Reston foam dressing
Reston foam rubber padding
restoration
restorative dentistry
restrained
restraining tape
restraint
restraint belt
restricted

restriction
restrictive airway defect
restrictive heart disease
restrictive membrane
restrictor
result
resulting defect
resume
resumed
resumption
resurfacing procedure
resuscitate
resuscitated
resuscitation
resuscitative efforts
resuscitator
    Ambu resuscitator
    cardiopulmonary
      resuscitator
    heart-lung resuscitator
    Hope resuscitator
    infant Ambu resuscitator
    Kreiselman resuscitator
    Laerdal resuscitator
    Ohio Hope resuscitator
    pneuPAC resuscitator
    Robertshaw bag resusci-
      tator
re-suture
retained barium
retained contents
retained gallstone
retained placenta
retained placenta and membranes
retained root
retained stool
retained sutures
retained urine
retainer
    HygiNet elastic dressing
      retainer
    series II cup retainer
retainer arch bar
retaining
retaining device
retaining retractor

Retan treatment
retardant
retardation
retarded
rete pegs
rete plexus
rete ridges
rete testis
Retec machine
retention
retention catheter
retention cyst
retention polyp
retention sutures
retentive stabilization
Rethi incision
reticular cells
reticulated tissue
reticulocyte
reticuloendothelial cells
reticulohistiocytic granuloma
reticulopathy
reticulosis
reticulum cell
reticulum cell sarcoma
retina
retinacular release of patella
retinaculotomy
retinaculum (*pl.* retinacula)
retinal artery
retinal cones
retinal cryopexy
retinal detachment (RD)
retinal detachment repair
retinal diathermy electrode
retinal puncture cautery
retinal reattachment
retinal rods
retinal tear
retinal thinning
retinal vein
retinogram
retinoic acid
retinopathy
retinoscope
    Boilo retinoscope
    Copeland retinoscope

retinoscope *continued*
- electric retinoscope
- Ful-Vue spot retinoscope
- Ful-Vue streak retino-
  scope
- macula retinoscope
- Propper retinoscope
- Reichert Ful-Vue spot
  retinoscope
- Reichert retinoscope
- Reid retinoscope
- spot retinoscope
- streak retinoscope
- Welch Allyn retinoscope

retinoscopy
retract
retract proximally
retractable fiberoptic tube
retracted
retracted stoma
retraction
retractor (see also *rake retrac-
    tor*)
- 2-prong rake retractor
- 3-prong retractor
- 4-prong rake retractor
- 6-prong rake retractor
- Abadie self-retaining
  retractor
- abdominal retractor
- abdominal ring retractor
- abdominal-vascular
  retractor
- Ablaza retractor
- Ablaza-Blanco retractor
- Adams retractor
- Adson brain retractor
- Adson cerebellar
  retractor
- Adson retractor
- Adson splanchnic
  retractor
- Adson-Beckman retractor
- Agrikola lacrimal sac
  retractor
- Agrikola retractor
- Aim retractor

retractor *continued*
- alar retractor
- Alden retractor
- Alexander retractor
- Alexander-Ballen orbital
  retractor
- Alexander-Matson
  retractor
- Alexian Hospital model
  retractor
- Alfreck retractor
- Allen retractor
- Allis retractor
- Allison lung retractor
- Allport retractor
- Allport-Babcock retractor
- Allport-Gifford retractor
- Alm minor surgery
  retractor
- Alm retractor
- Alm self-retaining
  retractor
- Alter lip retractor
- aluminum cortex
  retractor
- Amenabar retractor
- Amoils iris retractor
- Amoils retractor
- amputation retractor
- anal retractor
- Anderson-Adson
  retractor
- Andrews retractor
- Andrews tracheal
  retractor
- Ankeney retractor
- Ankeney sternal retractor
- Ann Arbor phrenic
  retractor
- Ann Arbor retractor
- anterior retractor
- Anthony pillar retractor
- Anthony retractor
- antral retractor
- AOR collateral ligament
  retractor
- aorta retractor

retractor *continued*

aorta valve retractor
aortic retractor
aortic valve retractor
apicolysis retractor
appendectomy retractor
arch rake retractor
Arem-Madden retractor
Aren retractor
Army-Navy retractor
Aronson esophageal
    retractor
Aronson lateral sterno-
    mastoid retractor
Aronson medial eso-
    phageal retractor
Arruga eye retractor
Arruga globe retractor
Arruga retractor
Ashley retractor
atrial retractor
Aufranc cobra retractor
Aufranc femoral neck
    retractor
Aufranc hip retractor
Aufranc psoas retractor
Aufranc push retractor
Aufranc retractor
Aufricht nasal retractor
Aufricht retractor
Aufricht-Britetrac nasal
    retractor
Austin dental retractor
Austin retractor
automatic skin retractor
Babcock retractor
baby Adson brain
    retractor
baby Balfour retractor
baby retractor
baby Weitlaner retractor
Bacon cranial retractor
Bacon retractor
Badgley laminectomy
    retractor
Badgley retractor
Bahnson retractor

retractor *continued*

Bahnson sternal retractor
Bakelite retractor
Balfour abdominal
    retractor
Balfour pediatric
    retractor
Balfour retractor
Balfour self-retaining
    retractor
Ballantine hemilaminec-
    tomy retractor
Ballen-Alexander orbital
    retractor
Ballen-Alexander
    retractor
ball-type retractor
Bankart retractor
Bankart shoulder
    retractor
Baron retractor
Barr rectal retractor
Barr retractor
Barr self-retaining
    retractor
Barraquer lid retractor
Barrett-Adson cerebellum
    retractor
Barrett-Adson retractor
Barsky retractor
B.E. glass abdominal
    retractor
Beardsley esophageal
    retractor
Beatty pillar retractor
Beaver retractor
Becker retractor
Beckman laminectomy
    retractor
Beckman retractor
Beckman self-retaining
    retractor
Beckman-Adson
    laminectomy retractor
Beckman-Adson retractor
Beckman-Eaton laminec-
    tomy retractor

retractor *continued*

Beckman-Eaton retractor
Beckman-Weitlaner
    laminectomy retractor
Beckman-Weitlaner
    retractor
Bellfield wire retractor
Bellman retractor
Beneventi retractor
Beneventi self-retaining
    retractor
Bennett bone retractor
Bennett retractor
Bennett tibia retractor
Berens esophageal
    retractor
Berens eye retractor
Berens mastectomy
    retractor
Berens mastectomy skin
    flap retractor
Berens retractor
Berens skin flap retractor
Berens thyroid retractor
Bergen retractor
Berkeley retractor
Berlind-Auvard retractor
Berna infant abdominal
    retractor
Berna retractor
Bernay retractor
Bernay tracheal retractor
Bernstein retractor
Bethune phrenic
    retractor
Bethune retractor
Bicek retractor
Bicek vaginal retractor
bident retractor
bifid retractor
bifurcated retractor
Biggs mammaplasty
    retractor
biliary retractor
Billroth retractor
bivalved retractor
Black retractor

retractor *continued*

bladder retractor
blade retractor
Blair retractor
Blair-Brown retractor
Blair-Brown vacuum
    retractor
Blakesley retractor
Blakesley uvula retractor
Blanco retractor
Bland perineal retractor
Blount bone retractor
Blount hip retractor
Blount knee retractor
Blount retractor
blunt rake retractor
blunt retractor
boardlike retractor
Bodnar knee retractor
Boley retractor
Bookwalter retractor
Bose retractor
Bosworth retractor
bowel retractor
Boyd retractor
Boyes-Goodfellow hook
    retractor
Braastad costal arch
    retractor
Braastad retractor
brain retractor
brain silicone-coated
    retractor
Brantley-Turner retrac-
    tor
Brantley-Turner vaginal
    retractor
Brawley retractor
Brawley scleral wound
    retractor
Breen retractor
Brewster phrenic
    retractor
Brewster retractor
Briggs retractor
Brompton Hospital
    retractor

retractor *continued*

Bronson-Turtz iris retractor
Brophy tenaculum retractor
Brown retractor
Brown uvula retractor
Browne retractor set
Bruch mastoid retractor
Bruening retractor
Brunner retractor
Brunschwig retractor
Brunschwig visceral retractor
Buchwalter retractor
Bucy retractor
Buie retractor
Buie-Smith anal retractor
Buie-Smith retractor
bulb retractor
Burford retractor
Burford rib retractor
Burford-Finochietto retractor
Butler dental retractor
Butler retractor
buttonhook nerve retractor
buttonhook retractor
Byford retractor
Cairns retractor
Callahan retractor
Campbell lacrimal sac retractor
Campbell nerve root retractor
Campbell retractor
Campbell self-retaining retractor
Campbell suprapubic retractor
Cardillo retractor
Carlens retractor
Carroll offset hand retractor
Carroll retractor

retractor *continued*

Carten mitral valve retractor
Carter retractor
Castallo eyelid retractor
Castallo lid retractor
Castallo retractor
Castroviejo adjustable retractor
Castroviejo retractor
cat's paw retractor
Cave knee retractor
Cave retractor
cecostomy retractor
cerebellum retractor *Chevalier*
cerebral retractor
cervical retractor
chalazion retractor
Chandler laminectomy retractor
Chandler retractor
channel retractor
Charnley knee retractor
Charnley retractor
cheek retractor
Cherry laminectomy self-retaining retractor
Cherry retractor
Cherry S-shaped brain retractor
Cheyne retractor
Chitten-Hill retractor
Christie gallbladder retractor
claw retractor
Clevedent retractor
Cloward retractor
Cloward self-retaining retractor
Cloward-Cushing vein retractor
Cloward-Hoen laminectomy retractor
Cloward-Hoen retractor
Cobb retractor
cobra retractor
Cohen retractor

retractor *continued*

Cole duodenal retractor
Cole retractor
Coleman retractor
Collin abdominal
retractor
Collin sternal self-
retaining retractor
Collins-Mayo mastoid
retractor
Colonial retractor
Colver examining
retractor hook
Colver retractor
Colver tonsil retractor
Cone retractor
Cone scalp retractor
Cone self-retaining
retractor
contour retractor
contour scalp retractor
Converse alar retractor
Converse blade retractor
Converse double-ended
retractor
Converse nasal retractor
Converse retractor
Conway eye retractor
Conway lid retractor
Cook rectal retractor
Cook retractor
Cooley aorta retractor
Cooley atrial retractor
Cooley neonatal retractor
Cooley retractor
Cooley rib retractor
Cooley sternotomy
retractor
Cooley-Merz sternum
retractor
Cope double-ended
retractor
corner retractor
cortex retractor
Coryllos retractor
costal arch retractor
Cottle alar retractor

retractor *continued*

Cottle four-prong
retractor
Cottle pillar retractor
Cottle pronged retractor
Cottle retractor
Cottle sharp prong
retractor
Cottle single-blade
retractor
Cottle soft palate
retractor
Cottle upper lateral
retractor
Cottle weighted retractor
Cottle-Joseph retractor
Cottle-Neivert retractor
Crafoord retractor
Craig-Sheehan retractor
cranial retractor
Crawford aortic retractor
Crawford retractor
Crego retractor
Crile retractor
Crile thyroid double-
ended retractor
Crotti retractor
Crotti thyroid retractor
Cushing aluminum
retractor
Cushing angled retractor
Cushing brain retractor
Cushing decompression
retractor
Cushing nerve retractor
Cushing retractor
Cushing S-retractor
Cushing self-retaining
retractor
Cushing straight retractor
Cushing vein retractor
Cushing-Kocher retrac-
tor
dacryocystorhinostomy
retractor
Dallas retractor
Danis retractor

retractor *continued*

Darling popliteal
retractor
Darrach retractor
Dautrey retractor
Davidoff retractor
Davidson retractor
Davidson scapular
retractor
Davis brain retractor
Davis double-ended
retractor
Davis pillar retractor
Davis retractor
Davis self-retaining scalp
retractor
Deaver retractor
DeBakey chest retractor
DeBakey retractor
DeBakey-Balfour
retractor
DeBakey-Cooley
retractor
DeBakey-Cooley-Deaver
retractor
Decker retractor
decompressive retractor
deep rake retractor
deep retractor
DeLaginiere abdominal
retractor
Delaney phrenic
retractor
Delaney retractor
DeLee corner retractor
DeLee retractor
DeLee Universal retrac-
tor
DeLee vaginal retractor
DeLee vesical retractor
DeMartel retractor
Denis Browne adult
retractor set
Denis Browne adult
retractor set
Denis Browne pediatric
retractor set

retractor *continued*

Denis Browne pediatric
retractor set
Denis Browne ring
retractor
Denis Browne Universal
retractor set
Denis Browne Universal
retractor set
Dennis-Brown abdomi-
nal retractor
dental retractor
DePuy retractor
D'Errico nerve retractor
D'Errico retractor
D'Errico-Adson retractor
Desmarres lid retractor
Desmarres retractor
Deucher abdominal
retractor
Devine-Millard-Aufricht
retractor
Dingman flexible
retractor
Dingman Flexsteel
retractor
Dingman retractor
Dingman-Senn retractor
disposable iris retractor
disposable retractor
Doane knee retractor
Dohn-Carton brain
retractor
Dorsey retractor
Dott retractor
double-angled retractor
double-crank retractor
double-ended retractor
Downing retractor
Doyen abdominal
retractor
Doyen retractor
Doyen vaginal retractor
Drews iris retractor
Drews-Rosenbaum
retractor
dull retractor

retractor *continued*

dull-pronged retractor
Dumont retractor
duodenal retractor
dural retractor
Duryea retractor
Eastman retractor
Eastman vaginal retractor
East-West retractor
easy-out retractor
Echols retractor
Edinburgh retractor
Effenberger retractor
Elschnig lid retractor
Elschnig retractor
Emmet retractor
endaural retractor
Enker brain retractor
Enker self-retaining brain
    retractor
epicardial retractor
epiglottis retractor
erector spinae retractor
esophageal retractor
examination retractor
externofrontal retractor
eye retractor
eyelid retractor
Falk retractor
Falk vaginal retractor
Farabeuf double-ended
    retractor
Farabeuf retractor
Farr retractor
Farr self-retaining
    retractor
Farr spring retractor
Fasanella iris retractor
Fasanella retractor
fat-pad retractor
Favoloro atrial retractor
Favoloro retractor
Favoloro self-retaining
    sternal retractor set
Favoloro sternal retractor
Federspiel cheek
    retractor

retractor *continued*

Feldman lip retractor
Feldman retractor
femoral neck retractor
Ferguson retractor
Ferguson-Moon rectal
    retractor
Ferguson-Moon retractor
Ferris Smith retractor
Ferris Smith-Sewall
    orbital retractor
Ferris Smith-Sewall
    retractor
finger rake retractor
finger retractor
Fink lacrimal retractor
Fink retractor
Finochietto laminectomy
    retractor
Finochietto retractor
Finochietto rib retractor
Finochietto-Geissendor-
    fer rib retractor
Finsen retractor
Fisher retractor
Fisher tonsil retractor
Fisher-Nugent retractor
flexible retractor
flexible shaft retractor
Flexsteel retractor
Flexsteel ribbon retractor
Foerster abdominal
    retractor
Foerster abdominal ring
    retractor
Fomon nostril retractor
Fomon retractor
Ford-Deaver retractor
Foss bifid gallbladder
    retractor
Foss bifid retractor
Foss biliary retractor
Foss gallbladder retractor
Foss retractor
four-prong retractor
Fowler self-retaining
    retractor

retractor *continued*

Franklin malleable retractor
Franklin retractor
Franz abdominal retractor
Franz retractor
Frater intracardiac retractor
Frater retractor
Frazier laminectomy retractor
Frazier retractor
Frazier-Fay retractor
Freeman face-lift retractor
Freeman retractor
Freer retractor
Freer submucous retractor
Freiberg hip retractor
Freiberg retractor
Freidrich-Ferguson retractor
French brain retractor
French retractor
French S-shaped brain retractor
French S-shaped retractor
French-Stern-McCarthy retractor
Friedman perineal retractor
Friedman retractor
Fritsch retractor
Fulton retractor
Gabarro retractor
gallbladder retractor
gallows-type retractor
Gant gallbladder retractor
Garrett retractor
Garrigue vaginal retractor
gastric resection retractor
Gauthier retractor

retractor *continued*

Geissendorfer rib retractor
Gelpi perineal retractor
Gelpi retractor
Gelpi self-retaining retractor
Gerbode sternal retractor
Ghazi rib retractor
Gibson-Balfour abdominal retractor
Gibson-Balfour retractor
Gifford mastoid retractor
Gifford retractor
Gifford scalp retractor
Gifford-Jansen mastoid retractor
Gil-Vernet lumbotomy retractor
Gil-Vernet renal sinus retractor
Gil-Vernet retractor
Givner eye retractor
Glaser laminectomy retractor
Glaser retractor
Glass abdominal retractor
Glass retractor
Glenner retractor
Glenner vaginal retractor
Goelet double-ended retractor
Goelet retractor
goiter retractor
Goldstein lacrimal sac retractor
Goldstein retractor
Goligher retractor
Gomez retractor
Gooch mastoid retractor
Gooch retractor
Good retractor
Goodhill retractor
Goodyear retractor
Goodyear tonsillar retractor

retractor *continued*

Goodyear uvula retractor
Gosset abdominal retractor
Gosset appendectomy retractor
Gosset retractor
Gosset self-retaining retractor
Goulet retractor
Gradle eyelid retractor
Gradle retractor
Graether retractor
Grant gallbladder retractor
Grant retractor
Green goiter retractor
Green retractor
Greenberg Universal retractor
Greene retractor
Grieshaber Balfour retractor
Grieshaber retractor
Grieshaber wire retractor
Groenholm lid retractor
Groenholm retractor
Gross patent ductus retractor
Gross retractor
Gross-Pomeranz-Watkins atrial retractor
Gross-Pomeranz-Watkins retractor
Gruenwald retractor
Guttmann obstetrical retractor
Guttmann retractor
Guzman-Blanco epiglottis retractor
Haight baby retractor
Haight retractor
Haight-Finochietto retractor
Haight-Finochietto rib retractor
Hajek antral retractor

retractor *continued*

Hajek lip retractor
Hajek retractor
half-moon retractor
Hamby retractor
Hamby-Hibbs retractor
hand retractor
hand-held retractor
Hardy retractor
Hardy-Duddy vaginal retractor
Harken retractor
Harrington retractor
Harrington splanchnic retractor
Harrington-Pemberton retractor
Harrington-Pemberton sympathectomy retractor
Harrison chalazion retractor
Harrison retractor
Hartstein iris cryoretractor
Hartstein retractor
Hartzler rib retractor
Haslinger palate retractor
Haslinger retractor
Haslinger uvula retractor
Hasson retractor
Haverfield hemilaminectomy retractor
Haverfield retractor
Haverfield-Scoville hemilaminectomy retractor
Haverfield-Scoville retractor
Hayes retractor
Hays hand retractor
Heaney hysterectomy retractor
Heaney retractor
Heaney-Simon hysterectomy retractor
Heaney-Simon retractor

*Hasson retractor*

retractor *continued*

Hedblom retractor
Hedblom rib retractor
Heifitz retractor
Heiss mastoid retractor
Heiss retractor
Heiss soft tissue retractor
Helfrick anal retractor
Helfrick anal ring
    retractor
Helfrick retractor
hemilaminectomy
    retractor
Henderson retractor
Henley retractor
Henner endaural
    retractor
Henner retractor
Henner T-model
    endaural retractor
Henrotin retractor
hernia retractor
Hertzler baby retractor
Hertzler rib retractor
Heyer-Schulte brain
    retractor
Heyer-Schulte retractor
Hibbs laminectomy
    retractor
Hibbs retractor
Hibbs self-retaining
    retractor
Hill rectal retractor
Hill retractor
Hill-Ferguson rectal
    retractor
Hill-Ferguson retractor
Hillis eyelid retractor
Hillis lid retractor
Hillis retractor
Himmelstein retractor
Himmelstein sternal
    retractor
hip retractor
Hirschman retractor
Hoen hemilaminectomy
    retractor

retractor *continued*

Hoen retractor
Hoen scalp retractor
Hohmann retractor
Holman lung retractor
Holman retractor
Holscher nerve root
    retractor
Holscher root retractor
Holzbach retractor
Holzheimer mastoid
    retractor
Holzheimer retractor
Holzheimer skin retractor
horizontal retractor
House hand-held
    retractor
House retractor
House-Urban middle
    fossa retractor
House-Urban retractor
Howorth retractor
Howorth toothed
    retractor
Hudson bone retractor
Hudson retractor
Hunt bladder retractor
Hunt retractor
Hupp retractor
Hupp tracheal retractor
Hurd pillar retractor
Hurd retractor
Hutchinson iris retractor
hysterectomy retractor
incision retractor
infant abdominal
    retractor
infant eyelid retractor
infant rib retractor
Inge laminectomy
    retractor
Inge retractor
intestinal occlusion
    retractor
intracardiac retractor
iris disposable retractor
iris retractor

retractor *continued*

Iron interne retractor
irrigating mushroom
retractor
Israel blunt rake retractor
Israel rake retractor
Israel retractor
Jackson double-ended
retractor
Jackson goiter retractor
Jackson retractor
Jackson self-retaining
goiter retractor
Jackson tracheal retractor
Jackson vaginal retractor
Jacobson goiter retractor
Jacobson retractor
Jaeger lid plate retractor
Jaeger lid retractor
Jaeger retractor
Jaffe lid retractor
Jaffe wire lid retractor
Jannetta posterior fossa
retractor
Jannetta retractor
Jansen mastoid retractor
Jansen retractor
Jansen scalp retractor
Jansen-Gifford mastoid
retractor
Jansen-Gifford retractor
Jansen-Wagner mastoid
retractor
Jansen-Wagner retractor
Jefferson retractor
Johns Hopkins gallbladder retractor
Johns Hopkins retractor
Johnson retractor
Johnson ventriculogram
retractor
Jones retractor
Jorgenson retractor
Judd-Mason bladder
retractor
Judd-Mason retractor

retractor *continued*

Kalamarides dural
retractor
Kaufer type II retractor
Keizer eye retractor
Keizer lid retractor
Kel retractor
Kelly abdominal retractor
Kelly retractor
Kelly-Sims retractor
Kelly-Sims vaginal
retractor
Kelman retractor
Kennerdell-Maroon
orbital retractor set
Kerrison retractor
kidney retractor
Killian-King goiter
retractor
Killian-King retractor
Kilner retractor
King goiter retractor
King goiter self-retaining
retractor
King retractor
King-Hurd retractor
Kirby lid retractor
Kirby retractor
Kirchner retractor
Kirkland retractor
Kirklin atrial retractor
Kirschner abdominal
retractor
Kitner retractor
Kleinert-Ragdell retractor
Klemme appendectomy
retractor
Klemme gasserian
ganglion retractor
Klemme laminectomy
retractor
Klemme retractor
Knapp lacrimal sac
retractor
Knapp retractor
knee retractor

retractor *continued*

Knighton hemilaminec-
tomy self-retaining
retractor
Kocher bladder retractor
Kocher gallbladder
retractor
Kocher goiter self-
retaining retractor
Kocher retractor
Kocher-Crotti goiter
retractor
Kocher-Crotti goiter self-
retaining retractor
Kocher-Crotti retractor
Koerte retractor
Koneg retractor
Kozlinski retractor
Krasky retractor
Kretschmer retractor
Kristeller retractor
Kronfeld eyelid retrac-
tor
Kronfeld retractor
Krönlein-Berke retractor
Kuglen retractor
lacrimal retractor
lacrimal sac retractor
Lahey Clinic retractor
Lahey goiter retractor
Lahey retractor
Lahey thyroid retractor
laminectomy retractor
laminectomy self-
retaining retractor
Lane retractor
Lange retractor
Langenbeck retractor
Langenbeck-Cushing
vein retractor
Laplace liver retractor
Laplace retractor
laryngeal retractor
laryngofissure retractor
lateral retractor
Latrobe retractor
Laufe retractor

retractor *continued*

Lawton-Balfour self-
retaining retractor
leaflet retractor
Leasure tracheal retractor
Leatherman trochanteric
retractor
Lee double-ended
retractor
Legen self-retaining
retractor
Legueu kidney retractor
Legueu retractor
Lemmon self-retaining
sternal retractor
Lemmon sternal retractor
Lemole atrial valve self-
retaining retractor
Lempert retractor
Lempert-Colver retractor
Levy perineal retractor
Lewis retractor
Lewis uvula retractor
Leyla retractor
Leyla-Yasargil retractor
lid retractor
lighted retractor
Lilienthal-Sauerbruch
retractor
Lillehei retractor
Lillie retractor
Linton retractor
Linton splanchnic
retractor
lip retractor
Little retractor
liver retractor
Logan lacrimal sac self-
retaining retractor
Logan retractor
London retractor
loop retractor
Lorie retractor
Lothrop retractor
Lothrop uvula retractor
Love nerve retractor
Love retractor

retractor *continued*

Love uvula retractor
Lowman hand retractor
Lowsley prostate
   retractor
Lowsley retractor
Luer retractor
Luer tracheal double-
   ended retractor
Lukens retractor
Lukens thymus retractor
Lukens tracheal double-
   ended retractor
lumbotomy retractor
lung retractor
Luongo hand retractor
Luongo retractor
Luther-Peter retractor
MacAusland muscle
   retractor
MacAusland retractor
MacAusland-Kelly
   retractor
MacKay contour retractor
MacKay contour self-
   retaining retractor
MacKay retractor
Mahorner retractor
Mahorner thyroid
   retractor
Maison retractor
Maliniac nasal retractor
Maliniac retractor
Malis retractor
malleable blade retractor
malleable copper
   retractor
malleable retractor
malleable stainless steel
   retractor
Maltz retractor
Manning retractor
Markham-Meyerding
   retractor
Markley retractor
Martin abdominal
   retractor

retractor *continued*

Martin lip retractor
Martin palate retractor
Martin retractor
Mason-Judd retractor
Mason-Judd self-retaining
   retractor
mastoid retractor
mastoid self-retaining
   retractor
mastoid-retaining
   retractor
Mathieu double-ended
   retractor
Mathieu retractor
Matson-Mead apicolysis
   retractor
Mattison-Upshaw
   retractor
Mayfield retractor
Mayo abdominal
   retractor
Mayo retractor
Mayo-Adams appendec-
   tomy retractor
Mayo-Adams retractor
Mayo-Adams self-
   retaining retractor
Mayo-Adson self-
   retaining retractor
Mayo-Collins double-
   ended retractor
Mayo-Collins retractor
Mayo-Lovelace retrac-
   tor
Mayo-Simpson retractor
McBurney fenestrated
   retractor
McBurney retractor
McCullough externofron-
   tal retractor
McCullough retractor
McGannon eye retractor
McGannon iris retractor
McGannon retractor
McGill retractor
McIndoe retractor

retractor *continued*
McNealey visceral
retractor
Medicon rib retractor
Meigs retractor
Meller lacrimal sac
retractor
Meller retractor
meniscal retractor
Merrill-Levassier retractor
metacarpal double-ended
retractor
Meyerding double-ended
retractor with skin
hook
Meyerding finger
retractor
Meyerding laminectomy
self-retaining retractor
Meyerding retractor
Meyerding-Deaver
retractor
microsurgery retractor
Mikulicz retractor
Miles retractor
Milex retractor
Miller retractor
Miller-Senn double-
ended retractor
Miller-Senn retractor
Milligan self-retaining
retractor
Millin bladder retractor
Millin retractor
Millin retropubic bladder
retractor
Millin self-retaining
retractor
Millin-Bacon bladder
self-retaining retractor
Millin-Bacon retractor
Miltex retractor
Minnesota retractor
Miskimon cerebellar self-
retaining retractor
mitral valve retractor
Moberg retractor

retractor *continued*
Mollison retractor
Mollison self-retaining
retractor
Moon rectal retractor
Moore bone retractor
Moore retractor
Moorehead cheek
retractor
Moorehead dental
retractor
Moorehead retractor
Morris retractor
Morrison-Hurd pillar
retractor
Morrison-Hurd retractor
Morse retractor
Mosher retractor
Mott double-ended
retractor
Mott retractor
Mueller lacrimal sac
retractor
Mueller retractor
Mueller-Balfour retractor
Mueller-Balfour self-
retaining retractor
Muldoon lid retractor
Munro retractor
Munro self-retaining
retractor
Murphy gallbladder
retractor
Murphy rake retractor
Murphy retractor
Murphy-Balfour retractor
Murtagh self-retaining
infant scalp retractor
Myers knee retractor
Myers retractor
Naclerio diaphragm
retractor
narrow retractor
nasal retractor
nasopharyngeal retractor
Neivert double-ended
retractor

retractor *continued*

- Neivert retractor
- Nelson retractor
- Nelson rib self-retaining retractor
- nerve retractor
- Nevyas drape retractor
- New tracheal retractor
- New York Hospital retractor
- newborn eyelid retractor
- Newell lid retractor
- Noblock retractor
- North-South retractor
- Nuttall retractor
- Oberhill retractor
- Oberhill self-retaining retractor
- O'Brien rib retractor
- obstetrical retractor
- Obwegeser channel retractor
- Obwegeser periosteal retractor
- Obwegeser retractor
- Ochsner malleable retractor
- Ochsner retractor
- Ochsner-Favoloro self-retaining retractor
- O'Connor retractor
- O'Connor-O'Sullivan retractor
- O'Connor-O'Sullivan self-retaining retractor
- Oertli lid retractor
- Oettingen abdominal retractor
- Oettingen abdominal self-retaining retractor
- offset hand retractor
- Oldberg brain retractor
- Oldberg retractor
- Oliver retractor
- Oliver scalp retractor
- Ollier retractor
- Omni retractor

retractor *continued*

- orbital retractor
- Osher lid retractor
- O'Sullivan retractor
- O'Sullivan-O'Connor abdominal retractor
- O'Sullivan-O'Connor retractor
- O'Sullivan-O'Connor self-retaining retractor
- O'Sullivan-O'Connor vaginal retractor
- Otto Barkan Bident retractor
- Overholt retractor
- palate retractor
- Paparella retractor
- Paparella self-retaining retractor
- Parker double-ended retractor
- Parker retractor
- Parker-Mott double-ended retractor
- Parker-Mott retractor
- Parkes nasal retractor
- Parks retractor
- patent ductus retractor
- Paul lacrimal sac retractor
- Paul retractor
- Paulson knee retractor
- Payr retractor
- pediatric self-retaining retractor
- Peet lighted splanchnic retractor
- Pemberton retractor
- Penfield retractor
- Percy retractor
- Percy-Wolfson gallbladder retractor
- Percy-Wolfson retractor
- perineal prostatectomy retractor
- perineal retractor

retractor *continued*

perineal self-retaining retractor
Perkins retractor
Pheifer-Young retractor
Phoropter retractor
phrenic retractor
Picot retractor
Pierce cheek retractor
Pierce retractor
pillar retractor
Pilling-Favoloro retractor
Piper lateral wall retractor
Poliak eye retractor
Polytrac Gomez retractor
Polytrac retractor
Pomeranz retractor
Poppen-Gelpi laminectomy self-retaining retractor
Portmann retractor
posterior fossa retractor
Pratt bivalve retractor
Proctor cheek retractor
Proctor retractor
pronged retractor
prostatic retractor
Pryor-Péan retractor
psoas retractor
pulmonary retractor
Purcell retractor
Purcell self-retaining abdominal retractor
Quervain abdominal retractor
Quervain-Sauerbruch retractor
Radcliff retractor
Ragnell double-ended retractor
Ragnell retractor
rake retractor
Ralks ear retractor
Ralks retractor

retractor *continued*

Rand Neuropledgets retractor for brain surgery
Raney retractor
Rankin prostatic retractor
Rankin retractor
rectal retractor
Rees lighted retractor
Rehne abdominal retractor
renal sinus retractor
retaining retractor
retropubic retractor
rib retractor
ribbon retractor
Richards abdominal retractor
Richardson appendectomy retractor
Richardson retractor
Richardson-Eastman double-ended retractor
Richter retractor
Richter vaginal retractor
Rigby appendectomy retractor
Rigby bivalve retractor
Rigby rectal retractor
Rigby retractor
Rigby vaginal retractor
right-angle retractor
ring abdominal retractor
Rizzo retractor
Rizzuti retractor
Robin-Masse abdominal retractor
Robinson lung retractor
Robinson retractor
Rochester atrial retractor
Rochester atrial septal defect retractor
Rochester retractor
Rochester-Ferguson double-ended retractor
Rochester-Ferguson retractor

retractor *continued*

Rollet rake retractor
Rollet retractor
Roos retractor
Rose double-ended
   retractor
Rose tracheal retractor
Rosenbaum iris retractor
Rosenbaum-Drews
   retractor
Rosenberg full-radius
   blade synovial
   retractor
Rosenberg retractor
Ross aortic retractor
Ross retractor
Roux double-ended
   retractor
Roux retractor
Rowe retractor
Rowe scapular neck
   retractor
Rumel retractor
Ryerson bone retractor
Ryerson retractor
S-shaped retractor
Sachs retractor
Sachs vein retractor
Sachs-Cushing retractor
Sanchez-Bulnes lacrimal
   sac self-retaining
   retractor
Sanchez-Bulnes retractor
Sato lid retractor
Sauerbruch retractor
Sauerbruch-Zukschwerdt
   retractor
Sauerbruch-Zukschwerdt
   rib retractor
Sawyer rectal retractor
Sawyer retractor
Sayre retractor
scalp retractor
scalp self-retaining
   retractor
scapular retractor
Schepens eye retractor

retractor *continued*

Schepens orbital retractor
Schepens retractor
Schindler retractor
Schnitker scalp retractor
Schoenborn retractor
Schuknecht postauricu-
   lar self-retaining
   retractor
Schuknecht retractor
Schuknecht-Wullstein
   retractor
Schultz irrigating iris
   retractor
Schultz retractor
Schwartz laminectomy
   retractor
Schwartz laminectomy
   self-retaining retractor
Schwartz retractor
Scoville cervical disk
   self-retaining retractor
Scoville hemilaminec-
   tomy retractor
Scoville hemilaminec-
   tomy self-retaining
   retractor
Scoville nerve retractor
Scoville nerve root
   retractor
Scoville psoas muscle
   retractor
Scoville retractor
Scoville self-retaining
   retractor
Scoville-Richter self-
   retaining retractor
Seen retractor
Segond retractor
Seletz-Gelpi retractor
Seletz-Gelpi self-retaining
   retractor
self-retaining abdominal
   retractor
self-retaining retractor
self-retaining spring
   retractor

retractor *continued*
Semb lung retractor
Semb retractor
Senn double-ended retractor
Senn mastoid retractor
Senn retractor
Senn self-retaining retractor
Senn-Dingman double-ended retractor
Senn-Dingman retractor
Senn-Green retractor
Senn-Kanavel double-ended retractor
Senn-Kanavel retractor
Senturia retractor
serrated retractor
serrefine retractor
Sewall orbital retractor
Sewall retractor
Shambaugh endaural retractor
Shambaugh endaural self-retaining retractor
Shambaugh retractor
sharp-pronged retractor
Shearer lip retractor
Shearer retractor
Sheehan retractor
Sheldon hemilaminec-tomy retractor
Sheldon hemilaminec-tomy self-retaining retractor
Sheldon retractor
Sheldon-Gosset self-retaining retractor
Sherwin self-retaining retractor
Sherwood retractor
short Heaney retractor
Shriners Hospital interlocking retractor
Shriners Hospital retractor
Shurly retractor

retractor *continued*
Simon retractor
Sims double-ended retractor
Sims rectal retractor
Sims retractor
Sims vaginal retractor
Sims-Kelly retractor
Sims-Kelly vaginal retractor
Sisson-Love retractor
Sistrunk band retractor
Sistrunk double-ended retractor
Sistrunk retractor
six-prong rake retractor
skin flap retractor
skin retractor
skin self-retaining retractor
Sloan goiter retractor
Sloan goiter self-retaining retractor
Sloan retractor
Sluder palate retractor
Sluder retractor
Small rake retractor
Small tissue retractor
Smillie knee joint retractor
Smillie retractor
Smith rectal retractor
Smith rectal self-retaining retractor
Smith retractor
Smith vaginal self-retaining retractor
Smith-Buie anal retractor
Smith-Buie rectal retractor
Smith-Buie rectal self-retaining retractor
Smith-Buie retractor
Smith-Petersen capsule retractor
Smith-Petersen retrac-tor

retractor *continued*

Smithwick retractor
Snitman endaural retractor
Snitman endaural self-retaining retractor
Snitman retractor
Sofield retractor
soft palate retractor
spike retractor
spinal cord retractor
spinal retractor
Spivey iris retractor
splanchnic retractor
spoon retractor
spring retractor
spring-wire retractor
Spurling retractor
St. Luke retractor
Stack retractor
sternal retractor
Stevenson lacrimal retractor
Stevenson lacrimal sac retractor
Stevenson retractor
Stookey retractor
Storer retractor
Storz retractor
Strully retractor
Stuck laminectomy self-retaining retractor
submucous retractor
suprapubic retractor
suprapubic self-retaining retractor
Sweeney posterior vaginal retractor
Sweeney retractor
Sweet amputation retractor
Sweet retractor
sweetheart retractor
sympathectomy retractor
T-malleable retractor
Tara retropubic retractor
Taylor retractor

retractor *continued*

Temple-Fay laminectomy retractor
Temple-Fay retractor
Theis retractor
Theis self-retaining retractor
Thoma tissue retractor
three-prong retractor
Thurmond retractor
thymus retractor
thyroid retractor
tibial retractor
Tiko rake retractor
Tillary double-ended retractor
Tillary retractor
tissue retractor
tonsillar pillar retractor
tonsillar retractor
toothed retractor
Tower retractor
Tower rib retractor
Tower spinal retractor
tracheal retractor
Trent eye retractor
trigeminal retractor
trigeminal self-retaining retractor
Tubinger self-retaining retractor
Tuffier abdominal retractor
Tuffier retractor
Tuffier-Raney laminectomy retractor
Turner-Doyen retractor
Turner-Warwick retractor
two-prong rake retractor
U-shaped retractor
Ullrich laminectomy retractor
Ullrich retractor
Ullrich self-retaining retractor
Ullrich-St. Gallen self-retaining retractor

retractor *continued*
- Universal retractor
- Urban retractor
- U.S. Army double-ended retractor
- U.S. Army retractor
- U.S. Army-pattern retractor
- uvula retractor
- Vacher retractor
- Vacher self-retaining retractor
- vacuum retractor
- vaginal retractor
- vagotomy retractor
- Vail lid retractor
- Vaiser-Dibis muscle retractor
- Valin hemilaminectomy self-retaining retractor
- Vasco-Posada orbital retractor
- vascular retractor
- Veenema retractor
- Veenema retropubic retractor
- Veenema retropubic self-retaining retractor
- vein retractor
- ventriculogram retractor
- Verbrugge retractor
- vertical bone self-retaining retractor
- vertical retractor
- vesical retractor
- Viboch graft retractor
- Vinke retractor
- Volkmann rake retractor
- Volkmann retractor
- Walker gallbladder retractor
- Walker lid retractor
- Walker retractor
- Walter-Deaver retractor
- Wangensteen retractor
- Weary nerve root retractor

retractor *continued*
- Webb retractor
- Webb-Balfour abdominal retractor
- Webb-Balfour retractor
- Webb-Balfour self-retaining retractor
- Weber retractor
- Webster abdominal retractor
- Webster retractor
- Weder retractor
- Weder-Solenberger pillar retractor
- Weder-Solenberger retractor
- Weder-Solenberger tonsil pillar retractor
- weighted posterior retractor
- weighted retractor
- Weinberg "Joe's hoe" double-ended retractor
- Weinberg retractor
- Weinberg vagotomy retractor
- Weinstein intestinal retractor
- Weitlaner brain retractor
- Weitlaner retractor
- Weitlaner self-retaining retractor
- Wesson perineal retractor
- Wesson perineal self-retaining retractor
- Wesson retractor
- Wexler Bantam self-retaining retractor
- Wexler retractor
- Wexler self-retaining retractor
- Wexler-Balfour retractor
- White-Proud retractor
- Wiet retractor
- Wigderson ribbon retractor

retractor *continued*

Wilder retractor
Wilder scleral self-retaining retractor
Wilkes self-retaining retractor
Wilkinson abdominal retractor
Wilkinson abdominal self-retaining retractor
Wilkinson retractor
Willauer-Deaver retractor
Wills eye lacrimal retractor
Wilmer iris retractor
Wilmer retractor
Wilmer-Bagley retractor
Wilson retractor
Wiltse iliac retractor
Wiltse-Bankart retractor
Wiltse-Gelpi self-retaining retractor
Winsburg-White retractor
Wise retractor
Wolf meniscal retractor
Wolfson retractor
Woodward retractor
Worrall deep retractor
Worrall retractor
Wort antral retractor
Wullstein ear self-retaining retractor
Wullstein retractor
Wullstein-Weitlaner retractor
Wullstein-Weitlaner self-retaining retractor
Wylie retractor
Wylie splanchnic retractor
Yasargil retractor
Young lateral retractor
Young prostatic retractor
Young retractor
Zalkind lung retractor
Zalkind-Balfour self-retaining retractor

retractor *continued*

Zimberg esophageal hiatal retractor
retractor blade
retraining
retrenchment
retrieval
retroauricular incision
retroauricular sulcus
retrobulbar anesthesia
retrobulbar block
retrobulbar injection
retrobulbar neuralgia
retrobulbar prosthesis needle
retrobulbar pupillary reflex
retrocalcaneal
retrocardiac region
retrocardiac space
retrocaval ureter
retrocecal appendix
retrocecal hernia
retrocentral sulcus
retrocession
retroclusion
retrococcygeal air study
retrocochlear
retrocolic anastomosis
retrocolic choledochojejunostomy
retrodisplaced pessary
retrodisplacement
retroesophageal aorta
retroflexed
retroflexed uterus
retroflexion
retrogasserian neurotomy
retrogasserian rhizotomy
retroglandular sulcus
retrognathia
retrognathic profile
retrograde
retrograde aortogram
retrograde arteriogram
retrograde atherectomy
retrograde Beaver blade
retrograde bougie
retrograde cannulation

retrograde cardiac perfusion
retrograde cholangiogram
retrograde cystogram
retrograde electrode
retrograde fashion
retrograde filling
retrograde flow
retrograde hernia
retrograde injection
retrograde intussusception
retrograde knife
retrograde peristalsis
retrograde pyelogram
retrograde ureterogram
retrograde urogram
retrograde valvuloplasty
Retrografin dye
retroiliac ureter
retrojection
retrolental
retrolental space
retrolenticular
retrolisthesis
retromammary
retromandibular fossa
retromandibular vein
retromandibularis, vena
retromanubrial
retromolar
retromolar mucosa
retromolar triangle
retromolar trigone
retroparotid space
retropatellar fat pad
retroperfusion
retroperfusion catheter
retroperfusion pump
retroperitoneal
retroperitoneal abscess
retroperitoneal adenopathy
retroperitoneal anastomosis
retroperitoneal cavity
retroperitoneal fistula
retroperitoneal hernia
retroperitoneal injection of air
retroperitoneal lymph node
retroperitoneal space

retroperitoneal tumor
retroperitoneal-iliopsoas
    abscess
retroperitoneum
retropharyngeal abscess
retropharyngeal space
retroplacental lucencies
retropubic placement
retropubic prevesical prostatec-
    tomy
retropubic prostatectomy
retropubic retractor
retropubic space
retropulsion
retropulsion of nail
retrorectal lymph node
retroscopic lens
retrospective study
retrosternal abnormality
retrosternal fat pad
retrosternal hernia
retrosternal nodule
retrosternal pain
retrosternal thyroid
retrotarsal fold
retrotuberous mucosa
retrourethral catheterization
retrouterine hematocele
retrouterine hematoma
retrovaginal hernia
retrovaginal septum
retroversion
retroversion pessary
retroverted
retroverted uterus
retrusive excursion
retrusive occlusion
Retter needle
return flow
return-flow cannula
return-flow catheter
return-flow hemostatic catheter
returning cartilage
Retzius space
Retzius veins
Reuben insufflator
Reusner sign

Reuter bobbin stainless steel
    drain tube
Reuter bobbin tube
Reuter bobbin
Reuter button
Reuter stainless steel bobbin
Reuter tube
Reuter-Wolfe trocar
revascularization
revascularize
revealed
Reverdin abdominal spatula
Reverdin bunionectomy
Reverdin graft
Reverdin holder
Reverdin implant
Reverdin needle
Reverdin operation
Reverdin osteotomy
Reverdin prosthesis
Reverdin skin graft
Reverdin suturing needle
Reverdin-Green bunion
    procedure
reversal of cervical curve
reversal of lumbar curve
reverse
reverse bandage
reverse Cole arthrodesis
reverse flow
reverse gastrectomy
reverse Kingsley splint
reverse knuckle-bender splint
reverse sphincterotome
reverse Trendelenburg position
reverse Waters x-ray position
reverse-angle skid curet
reverse-bevel laryngoscope
reverse-curve clamp
reverse-cutting needle
reverse-cutting sutures
reversed bandage
reversed bypass
reversed peristalsis
reversed rhythm
reversed shunt (right-to-left)
reversed-three sign

reverse-shape eye implant
reverse-shape implant
reverse-threaded screw
reversible ischemic defect
reversible ischemic neurological
    defect (RIND)
reversible knife
reversible perfusion defect
reversible reaction
reversion pacemaker
reverted to normal position
reverting scope
review
revised wound margins
revision
revision and closure
revision and debridement
revision of amputation stump
revision of graft
revision of scar
revival techniques
Revive system penile prosthesis
revivification
revolutions per minute (rpm)
revulsant
revulsion
revulsive
Rex-Cantli-Serege line
Reynolds clamp
Reynolds infusion catheter
Reynolds resection clamp
Reynolds scissors
Reynolds tongs
Reynolds tube
Reynolds vascular clamp
Rezek forceps
Rezifilm dressing
Reziplast spray-on dressing
RF balloon catheter
rhabdoid suture
rhabdomyoma
rhabdomyosarcoma
rhabdosarcoma
rhegmatogenous retinal
    detachment
Rhein pick
Rheinberg microscope

Rheinstaedter curet
Rheinstaedter uterine curet
rheumatic mitral valve
rheumatic nodule
rheumatic scoliosis
rheumatic valvular disease
rheumatoid pannus
rhexis
Rhinelander clamp
Rhinelander guide
Rhinelander pin
Rhinelander plate
Rhino Rocket injector
rhinocheiloplasty
rhinokyphectomy
rhinolaryngoscope
rhinolith
rhinomanometer
rhinomanometry
rhinommectomy
rhinoplastic
rhinoplastic correction
rhinoplasty
rhinoplasty and submucous
    resection
rhinoplasty implant
rhinoplasty saw
rhinoplasty scissors
rhinorrhaphy
rhinoscopic mirror
rhinoscopy
rhinoseptoplasty
rhinostomy
rhinotomy
rhizodontropy
rhizolysis
rhizotomy
Rhode Island dissector
RhoGam
rhomboid fossa
rhomboid ligament
rhomboid muscle
rhomboid of Michaelis
rhomboideus major, musculus
rhomboideus minor, musculus
rhonchi (*sing.* rhonchus)
rhonchi and rales
Rhoton forceps

Rhoton neurodissector
Rhoton punch
Rhoton ring tumor forceps
Rhoton titanium microscissors
rhythm
rhythm strip
rhythmic, rhythmical
rhythmic activity
rhythmic breathing
rhythmic wave
rhythmic waxing and waning
rhytidectomy
rhytidoplasty
RIA (radioimmunoassay)
rib
rib belt
rib cage
rib contractor (see also *contractor*)
    Adams rib contractor
    baby rib contractor
    Bailey baby rib contractor
    Bailey rib contractor
    Bailey-Gibbon rib
        contractor
    Cooley rib contractor
    Graham rib contractor
    Rienhoff-Finochietto rib
        contractor
    Sellor rib contractor
    Waterman rib contractor
rib cutter
rib drill
rib elevator
rib elevator and raspatory
rib elevator and stripper
rib field treatment
rib graft
rib guillotine
rib involvement
rib lesion
rib needle
rib notches
rib raspatory
rib retractor
rib rongeur

rib rongeur forceps
rib shears (see also *shears*)
    Bacon rib shears
    Baer rib shears
    Bethune rib shears
    Bethune-Coryllos rib
      shears
    Brunner rib shears
    Collin rib shears
    Cooley first rib shears
    Coryllos rib shears
    Coryllos-Bethune rib
      shears
    Coryllos-Moure rib
      shears
    Coryllos-Shoemaker rib
      shears
    Doyen rib shears
    Duval-Coryllos rib shears
    Eccentric locked rib
      shears
    Exner rib shears
    Frey-Sauerbruch rib
      shears
    Giertz rib shears
    Giertz-Shoemaker rib
      shears
    Gluck rib shears
    Harrington-Mayo rib
      shears
    Horgan-Coryllos-Moure
      rib shears
    Horgan-Wells rib shears
    Horsley-Stille rib shears
    infant rib shears
    Liston-Key Horsley rib
      shears
    Moure-Coryllos rib
      shears
    Nelson-Bethune rib
      shears
    Potts infant rib shears
    Potts rib shears
    Roberts-Nelson rib shears
    Roos first-rib shears
    Roos rib shears
    Sauerbruch rib shears

rib shears *continued*
    Sauerbruch-Britsch rib
      shears
    Sauerbruch-Coryllos rib
      shears
    Sauerbruch-Frey rib
      shears
    Sauerbruch-Lebsche rib
      shears
    Schuchart pediatric rib
      shears
    Schumacher rib shears
    Semb rib shears
    Shallcross rib shears
    Shoemaker rib shears
    Stille rib shears
    Stille-Giertz rib shears
    Stille-Horsley rib shears
    Stille-pattern rib shears
    Thompson rib shears
    Tudor-Edwards rib
      shears
    Walton rib shears
rib spreader (see also *spreader)*
    Bailey rib spreader
    Burford rib spreader
    Burford-Finochietto rib
      spreader
    child's rib spreader
    Davis rib spreader
    DeBakey rib spreader
    Finochietto rib
      spreader
    Gerbode rib spreader
    Haight rib spreader
    Harken rib spreader
    Hertzler baby rib
      spreader
    Hertzler rib spreader
    infant rib spreader
    Lemmon rib spreader
    Lilienthal rib spreader
    Lilienthal-Sauerbruch rib
      spreader
    Matson rib spreader
    McGuire rib spreader
    Miltex rib spreader

rib spreader *continued*
    Nelson rib spreader
    Nissen rib spreader
    Overholt-Finochietto rib
      spreader
    Rehbein rib spreader
    Rienhoff rib spreader
    Rienhoff-Finochietto rib
      spreader
    Sauerbruch-Lilienthal rib
      spreader
    Sweet rib spreader
    Sweet-Burford rib
      spreader
    Sweet-Finochietto rib
      spreader
    Theis rib spreader
    Tuffier rib spreader
    Weinberg pediatric rib
      spreader
    Weinberg rib spreader
    Wilson rib spreader
rib stripper (see also *stripper)*
    Alexander rib stripper
    Dorian rib stripper
    Matson rib stripper
    Matson-Alexander rib
      stripper
    Nelson rib stripper
    Price-Thomas rib stripper
    Roberts-Nelson rib
      stripper
Riba electric ureteral meatotome
Riba electrourethrotome
    electrode
Riba urethrotome
Ribble bandage
Ribble dressing
ribbon gut
ribbon gut needle
ribbon gut sutures
ribbon muscles
ribbon retractor
ribbon stools
ribbonlike keratitis
ribbon-shaped stools

rib-edge stripper
Ribes ganglion
rib-vertebral angle
Ricard amputation
rice bodies
Richards abdominal retractor
Richards adjustable-angle guide
Richards adjustable hip screw
Richards barrel guide
Richards barrel reamer
Richards bone clamp
Richards bone curet
Richards calibrated reamer
Richards calibrated-tip threaded
    guide
Richards chisel
Richards clamp
Richards combination mallet
Richards compression device
Richards compression screw
Richards curet
Richards external fixation
    device for fractures
Richards forceps
Richards headrest
Richards hip screw plate
Richards lag screw
Richards mastoid curet
Richards mastoid ethmoid curet
Richards maximum contact total
    knee prosthesis (RMC total
    knee prosthesis)
Richards nail
Richards Phillips screwdriver
Richards probe
Richards prosthesis
Richards screw
Richards side plate
Richards stationary-angle guide
Richards tonsil-grasping forceps
Richards tonsil-seizing forceps
Richards-Moeller pneumatic air-
    filled dilator
Richardson angle suture
Richardson appendectomy
    retractor

Richardson hemostat
Richardson operation
Richardson retractor
Richardson right-angle ear knife
Richardson right-angle knife
Richardson sutures
Richardson technique
Richardson-Eastman double-
    ended retractor
Richards-Saltzman-Flynn
    technique
Richards-Schaefer gonioscope
Riche-Cannieu anastomosis
Richet aneurysm
Richet bandage
Richet dressing
Richet operation
Richmond bolt
Richmond forceps
Richmond screw
Richter bone drill
Richter episiotomy scissors
Richter forceps
Richter laminectomy punch
Richter retractor
Richter screwdriver
Richter suture clip-removing
    forceps
Richter sutures
Richter vaginal retractor
Richter-Heath clip-removing
    forceps
Richter-Heath forceps
Richter-Monro line
Rickham cup
Rickham intraventricular
    reservoir system
Rickham reservoir
Ridell operation
Rider-Moeller needle
Rider-Moeller pneumatic dilator
rider's bone
rider's muscle
rider's sprain
rider's tendon
ridge
ridge extension

ridge forceps
ridged-convoluted villi
ridging
riding embolus
riding-pants deformity
Ridley anterior chamber implant
Ridley forceps
Ridley implant cataract lens
Ridley lens
Ridley Mark II lens implant
Ridley operation
Ridley sinus
Ridlon hip dislocation
Ridlon knife
Ridlon operation
Ridlon plaster knife
Ridpath curet
Ridpath ethmoid curet
Riechert-Mundiger stereotaxic
    system
Riecker bronchoscope
Riecker respiration broncho-
    scope
Riedel lobe
Riedel lobe of liver
Riedel needle
Riedel struma
Rieger stethoscope
Rienhoff arterial clamp
Rienhoff arterial forceps
Rienhoff clamp
Rienhoff dissector
Rienhoff forceps
Rienhoff general operating
    scissors
Rienhoff needle holder
Rienhoff rib spreader
Rienhoff thoracic scissors
Rienhoff-Finochietto rib
    contractor
Rienhoff-Finochietto rib
    spreader
Rienhoff-Tanner operation
Rienke space
Riepe gastric bubble
Riepe-Bard gastric balloon
Ries-Wertheim hysterectomy

Rieux hernia
Rifkind sign
Rigal sutures
Rigaud operation
Rigby appendectomy retractor
Rigby bivalve retractor
Rigby rectal retractor
Rigby retractor
Rigby vaginal retractor
Rigg cannula
right antero-oblique position
right aortic arch
right atrial cuff
right bronchus
right colic artery
right colic vein
right colon
right colonic flexure
right coronary artery
right coronary catheter
right decubitus position
right ear (AD)
right gastric artery
right gastric vein
right gastroepiploic artery
right gastroepiploic vein
right gutter
right heart bypass
right hemicolectomy
right hepatic duct
right hilum
right hypogastric nerve
right inferior pulmonary vein
right lateral position
right lobe
right lower lobe (RLL)
right lower quadrant (RLQ)
right mentoanterior position
    (RMA position)
right mentoposterior position
    (RMP position)
right mentotransverse position
    (RMT position)
right occipitoanterior position
    (ROA position)
right occipitoposterior position
    (ROP position)

right occipitotransverse position
    (ROT position)
right ovarian vein
right pulmonary artery
right rectus incision
right sacroanterior position (RSA
    position)
right sacroposterior position
    (RSP position)
right scapuloanterior position
    (RScA position)
right scapuloposterior position
    (RScP position)
right superior pulmonary vein
right suprarenal vein
right temporoparietal craniot-
    omy
right testicular vein
right upper lobe (RUL)
right upper paramedian incision
right upper quadrant (RUQ)
right venous angle
right ventricle
right ventricular assist device
right ventricular inflow tract
right ventricular outflow tract
right-angle chest catheter
right-angle chest tube
right-angle clamp
right-angle curet
right-angle examining telescope
right-angle forceps
right-angle lens
right-angle mattress sutures
right-angle pick
right-angle retractor
right-angle scissors
right-angle telescope
right-angled bone cutter
right-angled erysiphake
right-curved scissors
right-handed
righting reflex
right-sided
right-to-left shunt
rigid abdomen
rigid biopsy forceps

rigid endoscope
rigid fixation
rigid hymen
rigid kidney stone forceps
rigid orthosis
rigid posture
rigid scoop
rigid sigmoidoscope
rigid sigmoidoscopy
rigidity
rigidly extended
Rigiflex balloon
Rigiflex balloon dilator
Rigiflex dilator
Rigiscan
Rigler sign
rigor nervorum
rigor tremens
Riley needle
rim incision
rim sign
rima (*pl.* rimae)
RIND (reversible ischemic
    neurological deficit)
Rindfleisch folds
ring
> Abbé ring
> abdominal ring
> Airy ring
> anorectal ring
> aortic ring
> atrioventricular ring
> Bandl obstetric ring
> Bickel ring
> Bonaccolto scleral ring
> Bonaccolto-Flieringa
>     scleral ring
> Bores twist fixation ring
> Cannon ring
> Carpentier ring
> cartilage ring
> cartilaginous ring
> Coats ring
> common tendinous ring
> constrictive ring
> contact ring
> Crawford suture ring

ring *continued*
> deep inguinal ring
> distal esophageal ring
> double-flanged valve-
>     sewing ring
> drop-lock ring
> Duran annuloplasty ring
> esophageal A-ring
> esophageal B-ring
> esophageal contractile
>     ring
> esophageal mucosal ring
> esophageal muscular
>     ring
> external inguinal ring
> external ring
> Falope ring
> Falope tubal sterilization
>     ring
> finger ring
> fixation ring
> Fleischer corneal ring
> Fleischer ring
> Flieringa fixation ring
> Flieringa scleral ring
> Graefenberg ring (also
>     Gräfenberg)
> half-ring
> halo ring
> hymenal ring
> inguinal ring
> internal abdominal ring
> internal inguinal ring
> intrahaustral contraction
>     ring
> Klein-Tolentino ring
> Landers vitrectomy ring
> Landolt ring
> Loomis ring
> Lowe ring
> McKinney fixation ring
> McNeill-Goldmann
>     blepharostat ring
> McNeill-Goldmann ring
> McNeill-Goldmann
>     scleral ring
> mitral valve ring

ring *continued*
    Ochsner ring
    O'Harris-Petruso ring
    olive ring
    orbicular ring
    pyloric ring
    Schatzki esophageal ring
    Schatzki ring
    scleral ring
    semicircular ring
    sewing ring
    Silastic ring
    silicone ring
    Soemmering ring
    sphincter contraction
      ring
    superficial inguinal ring
    supra-annular suture ring
    suture ring
    tantalum ring
    tendinous ring
    Thiersch ring
    third cartilaginous ring
    Thomas ring
    titanium ring
    Tolentino ring
    tracheal rings
    Tru-Arc blood vessel ring
    tubal ring
    Universal valve prosthe-
      sis sewing ring
    valve ring
    vascular ring
    Vossius lenticular ring
    Waldeyer ring
    Waldeyer tonsillar ring
ring abdominal retractor
ring avulsion injury
Ring biliary drainage catheter
Ring cataract mask
Ring catheter
ring curet
ring epiphyses
ring finger
ring forceps
ring fracture
ring graft

Ring hip prosthesis
Ring knee prosthesis
ring man shoulder
ring of bone
ring pessary
ring punch
Ring ribbon scissors
Ring total hip prosthesis
ring ulcer of cornea
ring-enhancing lesion
Ringer lactate solution
Ringer solution
ringing in ears
Ring-McLean catheter
Ring-Moore total hip
ring-rotation forceps
ring-toothed tenaculum
ring-wall lesion
Rinman sign
Rinne sign
rinse
Riolan arc
Riolan arch
Riolan muscle
Riordan flexible silver cannula
Riordan osteostat
Riordan pin
Riordan procedure
Riordan rasp
Riordan repair of muscle
ripe cataract
ripe cervix
ripple voltage
Ripstein anterior sling recto-
    pexy
Ripstein arterial forceps
Ripstein forceps
Ripstein operation for rectal
    prolapse
Ripstein presacral rectopexy
Ripstein proctopexy
Ripstein rectopexy
Ripstein tissue forceps
RISA cisternography
Risdon approach
Risdon extraoral incision
Risdon wire

Riseborough-Radin classification of humeral fractures
Rish chisel
Rish knife
Rish osteotome
rising pulse
rising sun appearance of olecranon on x-ray
risk category
risk potential
risk/benefit ratio
risks and benefits
Risley pliers
risorius muscle
risorius, musculus
Risser cast
Risser cast table
Risser jacket
Ritch lens
Ritchie articular pain scale
Ritchie tenaculum
Ritisch sutures
Ritter bougie
Ritter Bovie
Ritter coagulator
Ritter dilator
Ritter double-orifice tip
Ritter drain
Ritter fibers
Ritter forceps
Ritter meatal dilator
Ritter rasp
Ritter raspatory
Ritter single-orifice tip
Ritter sound
Ritter suprapubic suction drain
Ritter suprapubic suction tube
Ritter table
Ritter-Oleson technique
ritual circumcision
Riva-Rocci manometer
Riva-Rocci sphygmomano-meter
Rivero-Carvallo maneuver
Rivero-Carvallo sign
Rives operation
Rives splenectomy

Riviere sign
rivinian foramen
rivinian notch
rivinian segment
Rivinus duct
Rivinus gland
Rivinus membrane
Rivinus notch
Rivinus segment
rivus lacrimalis
Rizzo retractor
Rizzoli operation
Rizzoli osteoclast
Rizzuti eye expressor
Rizzuti forceps
Rizzuti iris expressor
Rizzuti lens hook
Rizzuti retractor
Rizzuti scleral knife
Rizzuti scissors
Rizzuti-Furness cornea-holding forceps
Rizzuti-McGuire corneal-section scissors
Rizzuti-McGuire scissors
Rizzuti-Spizziri knife
Rizzuti-Verhoeff forceps
RK (radial keratotomy)
RLL (right lower lobe)
RLQ (right lower quadrant)
RMA position (right mento-anterior position)
RMC total knee prosthesis (Richards maximum contact total knee prosthesis)
RMP position (right menoto-posterior position)
RMT position (right mentotrans-verse position)
r/o (rule out)
ROA position (right occipito-anterior position)
Roaf approach
Robb cannula
Robb forceps
Robb knife

Robb needle
Robb syringe
Robb tonsillar forceps
Robb tonsillar knife
Robb tonsillar sponge forceps
Robb-Roberts rotary rasp
Robert Bent Brigham total knee
    prosthesis
Robert Brigham knee prosthesis
Robert Brigham prosthesis
Robert Jones bandage
Robert Jones compressive
    dressing
Robert Jones dressing
Robert Jones splint
Robert ligament
Robert pelvis
Roberts bronchial forceps
Roberts chisel
Roberts episiotomy scissors
Roberts esophagoscope
Roberts forceps
Roberts laryngoscope
Roberts nasal snare
Roberts needle
Roberts self-retaining laryngo-
    scope
Roberts shears
Roberts snare
Roberts speculum
Roberts trocar
Roberts-Gill periosteal elevator
Robertshaw bag resuscitator
Robertshaw double-lumen
    endotracheal tube
Roberts-Nelson rib shears
Roberts-Nelson rib stripper
Roberts-Nelson tourniquet
Robertson forceps
Robertson knife
Robertson sign
Robertson suprapubic drain
Robertson suprapubic trocar
Robertson tonsillar forceps
Robertson tonsillar knife
Robertson tonsil-seizing
    forceps

Robicheck wire
Robin-Masse abdominal
    retractor
Robinson artificial apparatus
Robinson bag
Robinson belt
Robinson catheter
Robinson dislodger
Robinson equalizing tube
Robinson flap knife
Robinson hook
Robinson lung retractor
Robinson pocket arthrometer
Robinson procedure
Robinson prosthesis
Robinson retractor
Robinson stone basket
Robinson stone dislodger
Robinson strut
Robinson tonsillar suction
Robinson urethral catheter
Robinson-Brauer trocar
Robinson-Riley cervical
    arthrodesis
Robinson-Smith procedure
Robinson-Southwick spinal
    fusion
Robson intestinal forceps
Robson line
Robson point
Robson position
Robson staging of renal cancer
    (I–IV)
Rochester atrial retractor
Rochester atrial septal defect
    retractor
Rochester awl
Rochester clamp
Rochester dissector
Rochester dressing
Rochester elevator
Rochester forceps
Rochester gallstone forceps
Rochester knife
Rochester laminar dissector
Rochester laminar elevator
Rochester mitral stenosis knife

rhytid

Rochester needle
Rochester needle holder
Rochester retractor
Rochester syringe
Rochester tube
Rochester-Carmalt forceps
Rochester-Carmalt hemostat
Rochester-Carmalt hemostatic
    forceps
Rochester-Davis forceps
Rochester-Ewald tissue forceps
Rochester-Ferguson double-
    ended retractor
Rochester-Ferguson retractor
Rochester-Ferguson scissors
Rochester-Harrington forceps
Rochester-Mixter artery forceps
Rochester-Mixter forceps
Rochester-Ochsner forceps
Rochester-Ochsner hemostat
    forceps
Rochester-Péan clamp
Rochester-Péan forceps
Rochester-Péan hemostat
Rochester-Rankin forceps
Rochester-Rankin hemostatic
    forceps
Rochester-Russian forceps
Rochet procedure
Rock endometrial suction curet
rock-candy lesion
rocker-bottom foot
Rockey cannula
Rockey clamp
Rockey dilating probe
Rockey endoscope
Rockey forceps
Rockey probe
Rockey scoop
Rockey trachea cannula
Rockey-Davis appendectomy
    incision
Rockey-Davis incision
rocking motion
rocking-leg splint
Rock-Mulligan hood
Rock-Mulligan prosthesis

Rockwood classification
Rockwood shoulder procedure
Rockwood-Green technique
rod
    Auer rod
    Baden Silastic rod
    Bailey rod
    Biethium ostomy rod
    Bobechko rod
    cloverleaf rod
    colostomy rod
    compression rod
    Corti rod
    Cotrel-Dubousset rod
    distraction rod
    Dwyer rod
    enamel rod
    flexible round silicone
        rod
    germinal rod
    glass rod
    Hansen-Street intra-
        medullary rod
    Harrington rod
    Heidenhain rod
    House measuring rod
    House rod
    Hunter rod
    Hunter Silastic rod
    Hydroflex penile implant
        rod
    intramedullary rod
    Knodt distraction rod
    Knodt rod fusion of
        spine
    knurled CD rod (knurled
        Cotrel-Dubousset rod)
    knurled Cotrel-
        Dubousset rod
        (knurled CD rod)
    Koenig rod
    Küntscher rod
    Lottes rod
    Luque rod
    Maddox rod
    malleable rod
    Marafioti-Westin rod

rod *continued*
- measuring rod
- Meckel rod
- metal rod
- Moore measuring rod
- Moore rod
- quartz rod
- radioactive rod
- Reichmann ivory rod
- Reichmann rod
- retinal rod
- Rush rod
- Sage forearm rod
- Sage intramedullary rod
- Sage rod
- Samson rod
- Schneider rod
- short rod
- silicone rod
- Sofield rod
- Stenzel rod
- Street rod
- telescoping medullary rod
- Veirs canaliculus rod
- Veirs malleable rod
- Veirs rod
- Y-glass rod
- Zickel rod
- Zielke rod

rod electrode
rod fixation
Rodenstock lens
Rodin implant
Rodin orbital implant
rodlike structure
Rodman mastectomy incision
Rodney Smith biliary stricture operation
Rodney Smith drainage
Rodney Smith operation
Rodriguez aneurysm
Rodriguez catheter
Rodriguez-Alvarez catheter
rods and cones
Roe aortic clamp
Roe solution

Roeder clamp
Roeder forceps
Roeder towel clamp
Roeder towel forceps
roentgen
roentgen dosage
roentgen equivalent
roentgen ray
roentgen therapy
roentgenogram
roentgenography
Roger amputation
Roger Anderson apparatus
Roger Anderson external fixator
Roger Anderson external skeletal fixation device
Roger Anderson fixation bar
Roger Anderson operation
Roger Anderson pin
Roger Anderson splint
Roger Anderson table
Roger Anderson well-leg splint
Roger cervical spine fusion
Roger dissector
Roger forceps
Roger needle holder
Roger scissors
Roger septal elevator
Roger sign
Roger spinal fusion
Roger submucous dissector
Roger vascular-toothed hysterectomy forceps
Roger wire-cutting scissors
Rogers sphygmomanometer
Rogge sterilizing forceps
ROHO cushion
Rokitansky diverticulum
Rokitansky hernia
Rokitansky kidney
Rokitansky tumor
Rokitansky-Aschoff sinus
Rokitansky-Cushing ulcer
Roland dilator
rolandic cortex
rolandic region

Rolando fracture
role
Rolf dilator
Rolf forceps
Rolf jeweler's forceps
Rolf lacrimal probe
Rolf lance
Rolf muscle hook
Rolf punctum dilator
Rolf-Jackson cannula
roll stitch
roll tube
rolled back
rolled Colles splint
rolled sheet
rolled tendon anchovy
    procedure
roller
        Devonshire roller
        hand tubing roller
        intravenous tubing roller
        Spence cranioplastic
          roller
        Unger adenoid pressure
          roller
roller bandage
roller dressing
roller electrode
roller forceps
roller knife
Rollet incision
Rollet irrigator
Rollet rake retractor
Rollet retractor
rollflap operation
rolling hernia
rolling hiatal hernia
rolling motion
rolling movement
rolling of conjunctiva
Rolnel catheter
Rolyan brace
Rolyan tibial fracture brace
ROM (range of motion)
ROM exercises (range-of-motion
    exercises)
romanoscope

Romberg facial deformity
Romberg sign
Romberg test
ROMI (rule out myocardial
    infarction)
Rommel cautery
Rommel-Hildreth cautery
Rondic sponge dressing
rongeur
        Adson bone rongeur
        Adson cranial rongeur
        Adson rongeur
        Andrews-Hartmann ear
          rongeur
        Andrews-Hartmann
          rongeur
        angular rongeur
        antral rongeur
        aortic valve rongeur
        Bacon bone rongeur
        Bacon cranial rongeur
        Bacon rongeur
        Bailey aortic valve
          rongeur
        Bailey rongeur
        Bane bone rongeur
        Bane rongeur
        Bane-Hartmann bone
          rongeur
        bayonet rongeur
        Belz lacrimal sac ron-
          geur
        Bethune rib rongeur
        Bethune rongeur
        Beyer bone rongeur
        Beyer endaural rongeur
        Beyer rongeur
        Beyer-Stille bone
          rongeur
        Blumenthal rongeur
        Böhler bone rongeur
        bone rongeur
        bone-cutting rongeur
        bony rongeur
        Brock cardiac dilator
          rongeur
        Bruening-Citelli rongeur

rongeur *continued*
    Bucy laminectomy
      rongeur
    Cairns rongeur
    Campbell laminectomy
      rongeur
    Campbell rongeur
    Carroll rongeur
    cervical rongeur
    Cherry-Kerrison laminec-
      tomy rongeur
    chicken-bill rongeur
    Cicherelli bone rongeur
    Cicherelli rongeur
    Citelli rongeur
    Cleveland bone rongeur
    Cloward rongeur
    Cloward-English
      laminectomy rongeur
    Cloward-Harper laminec-
      tomy rongeur
    Codman-Kerrison
      laminectomy rongeur
    Codman-Leksell laminec-
      tomy rongeur
    Codman-Schlesinger
      cervical rongeur
    Colclough rongeur
    Converse nasal rongeur
    Converse rongeur
    Costen-Kerrison rongeur
    Cottle nasal-biting
      rongeur
    Cottle-Jansen bone
      rongeur
    Cottle-Jansen rongeur
    Cottle-Kazanjian bone
      rongeur
    cranial bone rongeur
    cranial rongeur
    Cushing bone rongeur
    Cushing rongeur
    cystoscopic rongeur
    Dahlgren rongeur
    Dale first rib rongeur
    Davol rongeur
    Dean bone rongeur

rongeur *continued*
    Dean mastoid rongeur
    Dean rongeur
    Decker microrongeur
    Decker pituitary rongeur
    Defourmental bone
      rongeur
    Defourmental rongeur
    Dench rongeur
    DePuy rongeur
    DeVilbiss cranial rongeur
    DeVilbiss rongeur
    double-action rongeur
    double-biting rongeur
    duckbill rongeur
    ear rongeur
    Echlin bone rongeur
    Echlin duckbill rongeur
    Echlin-Luer rongeur
    endaural rongeur
    Ferris Smith interverte-
      bral disk rongeur
    Ferris Smith pituitary
      rongeur
    Ferris Smith rongeur
    Ferris Smith-Gruenwald
      rongeur
    Ferris Smith-Kerrison
      rongeur
    Ferris Smith-Spurling
      rongeur
    Ferris Smith-Takahashi
      rongeur
    Friedman bone rongeur
    Frykholm bone rongeur
    Frykholm rongeur
    Fulton laminectomy
      rongeur
    Fulton rongeur
    Garrison rongeur
    Giertz rongeur
    Glover rongeur
    gooseneck rongeur
    Gruenwald neurosurgical
      rongeur
    Gruenwald rongeur
    Guleke bone rongeur

rongeur *continued*

Hajek antral rongeur
Hajek rongeur
Hakansson bone rongeur
Hakansson-Olivecrona
  rongeur
Harper rongeur
Hartmann bone rongeur
Hartmann ear rongeur
Hartmann mastoid
  rongeur
Hartmann rongeur
Hartmann-Herzfeld ear
  rongeur
Hartmann-Herzfeld
  rongeur
Hein rongeur
Henny rongeur
Heyman septum-cutting
  rongeur
Hoen intervertebral disk
  rongeur
Hoen laminectomy
  rongeur
Hoen rongeur
Hoffmann ear rongeur
Horsley bone rongeur
Horsley cranial rongeur
Houghton rongeur
Hudson cranial rongeur
Hudson rongeur
Husks bone rongeur
Husks mastoid rongeur
Husks rongeur
infundibular rongeur
infundibulectomy
  rongeur
intervertebral disk
  rongeur
IV disk rongeur
Ivy mastoid rongeur
Ivy rongeur
Jackson intervertebral
  disk rongeur
Jansen bayonet rongeur
Jansen mastoid rongeur
Jansen rongeur

rongeur *continued*

Jansen-Cottle rongeur
Jansen-Middleton
  rongeur
Jansen-Zaufel bone
  rongeur
Jansen-Zaufel rongeur
Jarit-Kerrison laminec-
  tomy rongeur
Jarit-Ruskin bone
  rongeur
Juers-Lempert endaural
  rongeur
Juers-Lempert rongeur
Kerr rongeur
Kerrison laminectomy
  rongeur
Kerrison mastoid rongeur
Kerrison rongeur
Kerrison-Costen ear
  rongeur
Kerrison-Ferris Smith
  rongeur
Kerrison-Spurling
  rongeur
Killian rongeur
Kleinert-Kutz bone
  rongeur
laminectomy rongeur
Lane rongeur
Lange-Converse rongeur
Lebsche rongeur
Leksell bone rongeur
Leksell cardiovascular
  rongeur
Leksell rongeur
Leksell-Stille thoracic-
  cardiovascular rongeur
Lempert bone rongeur
Lempert endaural
  rongeur
Lempert rongeur
Lillie rongeur
Lillie sinus bone-nibbling
  rongeur
Liston rongeur
Littauer rongeur

rongeur *continued*
- Lombard mastoid rongeur
- Lombard rongeur
- Lombard-Beyer rongeur
- Lombard-Boies rongeur
- Love-Gruenwald cranial rongeur
- Love-Gruenwald pituitary rongeur
- Love-Gruenwald rongeur
- Love-Kerrison rongeur
- Lowman rongeur
- Luer bone rongeur
- Luer rongeur
- Luer-Friedman bone rongeur
- Luer-Hartmann rongeur
- Luer-Liston-Wheeling rongeur
- Luer-Whiting mastoid rongeur
- Markwalder bone rongeur
- Marquardt bone rongeur
- mastoid rongeur
- Mayfield bone rongeur
- Mead bone rongeur
- Mead mastoid rongeur
- Mead rongeur
- microrongeur
- Mollison mastoid rongeur
- monster rongeur
- Montenovesi rongeur
- Mount laminectomy rongeur
- multiple-action rongeur
- nasal rongeur
- Nichol rongeur
- Nicola pituitary rongeur
- Noyes rongeur
- O'Brien rongeur
- Oldberg pituitary rongeur
- Oldberg rongeur

rongeur *continued*
- Oldberg intervertebral disk rongeur
- Olivecrona endaural rongeur
- Olivecrona mastoid rongeur
- Olivecrona rongeur
- oral surgery rongeur
- Parham-Martin rongeur
- peapod intervertebral disk rongeur
- peapod rongeur
- pediatric bone rongeur
- Peiper-Beyer bone rongeur
- Peiper-Beyer laminectomy rongeur
- Pierce mastoid rongeur
- Pilling-Ruskin rongeur
- pituitary rongeur
- Poppen pituitary rongeur
- Poppen rongeur
- Quervain rongeur
- Raaf rongeur
- Raaf-Oldberg rongeur
- Raney rongeur
- rat-tooth rongeur
- Reiner bone rongeur
- Reiner rongeur
- rib rongeur
- Röttgen-Ruskin bone rongeur
- Rowland nasal rongeur
- Rowland rongeur
- Ruskin bone rongeur
- Ruskin cranial rongeur
- Ruskin duckbill rongeur
- Ruskin mastoid rongeur
- Ruskin multiple-action rongeur
- Ruskin rongeur
- Ruskin-Jansen bone rongeur
- Ruskin-Jay heavy-duty rongeur

rongeur *continued*

Ruskin-Liston bone-cutting rongeur
Ruskin-Rowland bone rongeur
Sauerbruch rib rongeur
Sauerbruch-Coryllos bone rongeur
Sauerbruch-Coryllos rib rongeur
Sauerbruch-Lebsche rongeur
Sauerbruch-Stille bone rongeur
Sauer-Lebsche rongeur
Schlesinger cervical rongeur
Schlesinger intervertebral disk rongeur
Schlesinger rongeur
Schwartz-Kerrison rongeur
Selverstone intervertebral disk rongeur
Selverstone rongeur
Semb gouging rongeur
Semb rongeur
Semb-Sauerbruch rongeur
Semb-Stille bone rongeur
Shearer bone rongeur
Shearer chicken-bill rongeur
Shearer rongeur
Shoemaker rongeur
side-curved rongeur
Simplex mastoid rongeur
skinny-nose rongeur
slender-nose rongeur
Smith-Petersen laminectomy rongeur
Smith-Petersen rongeur
Spence intervertebral disk rongeur
Spurling laminectomy rongeur

rongeur *continued*

Spurling pituitary rongeur
Spurling rongeur
Spurling-Kerrison down-biting rongeur
Spurling-Kerrison laminectomy rongeur
Spurling-Kerrison rongeur
Spurling-Kerrison up-biting rongeur
Spurling-Love-Gruen-wald-Cushing rongeur
St. Luke rongeur
Stille bone rongeur
Stille rongeur
Stille-Lauer bone rongeur
Stille-Leksell rongeur
Stille-Liston double-action rongeur
Stille-Liston rongeur
Stille-Luer bone rongeur
Stille-Luer multiple-action rongeur
Stille-Luer rongeur
Stille-Luer-Echlin bone rongeur
Stookey cranial rongeur
Stookey rongeur
Storz cystoscopic rongeur
Storz rongeur
straight rongeur
Struempell rongeur
Strully-Kerrison rongeur
Takahashi rongeur
taper-jaw rongeur
Tobey rongeur
Urschel first-rib rongeur
Urschel-Leksell rongeur
von Seemen rongeur
Voris IV disk rongeur
Walton rongeur
Walton-Liston bone rongeur

rongeur *continued*
  Walton-Ruskin bone
    rongeur
  Watson-Williams
    intervertebral disk
    rongeur
  Watson-Williams rongeur
  Weil pituitary rongeur
  Weil rongeur
  Weil-Blakesley in-
    tervertebral disk
    rongeur
  Weingartner rongeur
  Whitcomb-Kerrison
    laminectomy rongeur
  Whitcomb-Kerrison
    rongeur
  White mastoid rongeur
  Wilde intervertebral disk
    rongeur
  Yasargil pituitary ron-
    geur
  Young rongeur
  Zaufel bone rongeur
  Zaufel-Jansen rongeur
rongeur forceps (see also
    *forceps, rongeur*)
  Adson cranial rongeur
    forceps
  Bacon cranial rongeur
    forceps
  Bane rongeur forceps
  Cherry-Kerrison rongeur
    forceps
  chicken-bill rongeur
    forceps
  Cicherelli rongeur
    forceps
  Cottle-Jansen rongeur
    forceps
  cranial rongeur forceps
  Cushing cranial rongeur
    forceps
  Defourmental rongeur
    forceps
  DeVilbiss rongeur
    forceps

rongeur forceps *continued*
  double-action rongeur
    forceps
  Echlin rongeur forceps
  Ferris Smith cup rongeur
    forceps
  Ferris Smith-Kerrison
    rongeur forceps
  Friedman rongeur
    forceps
  Glover infundibular
    rongeur forceps
  Glover rongeur forceps
  Hudson cranial rongeur
    forceps
  Hudson rongeur forceps
  infundibular rongeur
    forceps
  intervertebral disk
    rongeur forceps
  Juers-Lempert rongeur
    forceps
  Lempert rongeur forceps
  Lombard-Beyer rongeur
    forceps
  Lowis IV disk rongeur
    forceps
  mastoid rongeur forceps
  Montenovesi cranial
    rongeur forceps
  Mount intervertebral disk
    rongeur forceps
  oral rongeur forceps
  pituitary rongeur forceps
  Quervain cranial rongeur
    forceps
  rib rongeur forceps
  spinal rongeur forceps
Ronis adenoid punch
Ronis cutting forceps
Rönne nasal step
roof disk
roof of mouth
roofing
rooming-in patient
Roos first-rib shears
Roos hip flexor release

Roos osteotome
Roos procedure for thoracic
    outlet syndrome
Roos retractor
Roos rib cutter
Roos rib shears
Roos test for thoracic outlet
Roos transaxillary approach
Roosevelt clamp
Roosevelt gastroenterostomy
    clamp
Roosevelt gastrointestinal
    clamp
root amputation
root canal
root cap
root dehiscence
root elevator
root needle
root of lung
root of tongue
root perforation
root pliers
root sheath
root sleeve
root-canal broach
root-canal filling
root-canal spreader
Rooter splint
rooting reflex
rooting response
rootlet
ROP position (right occipito-
    posterior position)
rope flap
rope graft
Roper cannula
Roper scissors
Roper-Hall localizer
Roper-Rumel tourniquet
ropy mass
ropy saliva
ropy tumor
Rosa-Berens implant
Rosa-Berens orbital implant
rosary bougie
rosary-bead esophagus

Rosch-Thurmond fallopian tube
    catheterization set
Roscoe-Graham anterior
    gastrojejunostomy
Roscoe-Graham jejunostomy
Rose bed dressing
rose bengal scan
rose bengal sodium I-131 biliary
    scan
Rose cleft lip repair
Rose disimpaction forceps
Rose double-ended retractor
Rose head-extension position
Rose L-type nose bridge
    prosthesis
Rose operation
Rose position
Rose tamponade
Rose tracheal retractor
Rose-Bradford kidney
rosebud stoma
Rosen curet
Rosen dissector
Rosen ear probe
Rosen elevator
Rosen endaural probe
Rosen fenestrator
Rosen guide wire
Rosen incision
Rosen incision knife
Rosen knife
Rosen needle
Rosen pick
Rosen probe
Rosen prosthesis
Rosen separator
Rosen suction tube
Rosen tube
Rosen urinary prosthesis
Rosen wire
Rosenbach sign
Rosenbaum iris retractor
Rosenbaum-Drews retractor
Rosenberg full-radius blade
    synovial retractor
Rosenberg retractor
Rosenburg drill guide

Rosenburg operation
Rosenfeld hip prosthesis
Rosenfeld total hip prosthesis
Rosengren operation
Rosenmueller (also
    Rosenmüller)
Rosenmueller body
Rosenmueller curet
Rosenmueller fossa
Rosenmueller gland
Rosenmüller (see *Rosenmueller*)
Rosenthal ascending vein
Rosenthal fibers
Rosenthal needle
Rosenthal speculum
Rosenthal vein
Roser mouth gag
Roser needle
Roser-Braun sign
Rose-Thompson cleft lip repair
Rose-Thompson operation
rose-thorn ulcer
rosette
rosette cataract
Rosi bridge prosthesis
Rosomoff cordotomy
Rosomoff percutaneous
    cordotomy
Ross aortic retractor
Ross catheter
Ross needle
Ross procedure
Ross retractor
Rosser crypt hook
Rosser hook
Rossetti modification of Nissen
    fundoplication
Rostan shunt
rostral aspect
rostral pole
rostrally
rostrate pelvis
rostrum of sinus
rostrum of sphenoid
ROT position (right occipi-
    totransverse position)
Rotablator

Rotalink flexible shaft
Rotalok cup
Rotalok cup cementless
    acetabular component
rotary cutting tip
rotary dissector
rotary hub saw
rotary joint
rotary microtome
rotary subluxation
rotate scope
rotated down
rotated kidney
rotated to left
rotated to right
rotated upward
rotating anoscope
rotating disk oxygenator
rotating forceps
rotating hinge
rotating laryngoscope
rotating resectoscope
rotating speculum anoscope
rotating speculum proctoscope
rotating sphincterotome
rotating tourniquet
rotating transilluminator
rotating-hinge knee prosthesis
rotation
rotation advancement flap
rotation flap
rotation forceps
rotation of colon
rotation of flap
rotation of pelvis
rotation operative delivery
rotation osteotomy
rotation skin flap
rotation skin flap technique
rotation therapy
rotational atherectomy device
rotational flap graft
rotational instability
rotational irradiation therapy
rotational x-ray beam dosimetry
rotator cuff
rotator cuff injury

rotator cuff tear
rotator cuff tendinitis
rotator muscles
rotatores, musculi
rotatory
rotatory hammer
rotatory instability
rotatory motion
rotatory spasm
Rotch sign
Rotex II biopsy needle
Rotex needle
Roth urethral suture guide
Rothene catheter
Roticulator clamp stapler
Roto Kinetic bed
rotoextraction
Roto-Rest bed
rotoscoliosis
rotosteotome
Rotozyme diagnostic procedure
Rotter interpectoral nodes
Rotter node
Röttgen-Ruskin bone rongeur
Rouge operation
Rouget muscle
rouleaux formation
round bur
round cell
round counterbore
round ligament of femur
round ligament of liver
round ligament of uterus
round ligament
round needle
round nucleus
round pronator muscle
round punch forceps
round ulcer
round window
round-blade scissors
rounded edge
round-loop electrode
round-tip catheter
round-wire electrode
roused
route

Routier operation
routine manner
routine procedure
routine urinalysis (RUA)
routine workup
Routte operation
Roux double-ended retractor
Roux gastroenterostomy
Roux operation
Roux retractor
Roux sign
Roux spatula
Roux-en-Y (also Roux-Y)
Roux-en-Y anastomosis
Roux-en-Y esophagojejunos-
    tomy
Roux-en-Y gastrectomy
Roux-en-Y gastric bypass
Roux-en-Y gastrojejunostomy
Roux-en-Y hepaticojejunostomy
Roux-en-Y incision
Roux-en-Y jejunal limb
Roux-en-Y jejunal loop incision
Roux-en-Y jejunoileostomy
Roux-en-Y operation
Roux-en-Y pancreaticojejunos-
    tomy
Roux-Goldthwait operation
Roux-Goldthwait patella repair
Roux-Goldthwait patellar
    tendon transfer
Roveda technique
Rovenstine catheter-introducing
    forceps
Rovighi sign
Rovsing operation
Rovsing sign
Rovsing-Blumberg sign
row of sutures
Rowbotham operation
Rowe approach
Rowe disimpaction forceps
Rowe elevator
Rowe forceps
Rowe posterior approach
Rowe punch
Rowe reamer

Rowe retractor
Rowe scapular neck retractor
Rowe-Killey forceps
Rowen spinal fusion gouge
Rowinski operation
Rowland double-action hump
    forceps
Rowland eye knife
Rowland forceps
Rowland keratome
Rowland nasal hump forceps
Rowland nasal rongeur
Rowland osteotome
Rowland rongeur
Rowsey cannula
Royal Flush angiographic flush
    catheter
Royal Hospital dilator
Royal Moore opponens pollicis
    transfer
Royal spoon
Royalite body jacket
Royalite splint
Royce ear knife
Royce forceps
Royce knife
Royce perforator
Royle operation
Royle-Thompson FDS transfer
Royle-Thompson opponens-
    plasty
rpm (revolutions per minute)
RPT (rapid pull-through)
RPT operation
RR (recovery room)
RS4 pacemaker
RScA position (right scapu-
    loanterior position)
RScP position (right scapulopos-
    terior position)
RSP position (right sacropos-
    terior position)
RUA (routine urinalysis)
rub
rubber acorn
rubber airway
rubber arch
rubber bolster

rubber catheter
rubber dam
rubber drain
rubber endoscopic tube
rubber glove
rubber padding
rubber pegs
rubber Scan spray dressing
rubber sponge
rubber sutures
rubber tip
rubber tissue
rubber tube
rubber vessel loop
rubber-band hemorrhoid
    ligation
rubber-band ligation
rubber-bulb syringe
rubber-dam clamp
rubber-dam clamp forceps
rubber-dam drain
rubber-shod catheter
rubber-shod clamp
rubber-shod forceps
rubber-shod hook
rubber-tip, rubber-tipped
Rubbrecht operation
Rubin Brandborg biopsy tube
Rubin bronchus clamp
Rubin cannula
Rubin cartilage planer
Rubin clamp
Rubin gouge
Rubin hydraulic biopsy tube
Rubin needle
Rubin operation
Rubin osteotome
Rubin rasp
Rubin septal morselizer
Rubin tube
Rubin-Holth corneoscleral
    punch
Rubin-Holth punch
Rubin-Quinton small-bowel
    biopsy tube
Rubinstein cryoprobe
Rubovits clamp
rubs or murmurs

ruby knife
ruby laser
ruby laser operation for retinal
    detachment
Rudd Clinic forceps
Rudd Clinic hemorrhoidal
    forceps
Rudd Clinic hemorrhoidal
    ligator
Rudd Clinic ligator
Ruddy dissector
Rudich treatment unit
rudimentary
rudimentary bone
rudimentary disk space
rudimentary eye
rudimentary ribs
rudimentary uterus
rudimentary vagina
Ruedemann eye evisceration
Ruedemann eye implant
Ruedemann operation
Ruedemann-Todd tendon
    tucker
Ruel aorta clamp
Ruel forceps
ruffed canal
ruga (*pl.* rugae)
rugae gastricae
rugae of stomach
rugae of vagina
rugae vaginales
rugal coarsening
rugal folds
rugal pattern
rugal pattern of stomach
Rugby deep-surgery forceps
Rugby forceps
rugby knee
rugger jersey spine
rugine
Ruiz plano fundus lens implant
Ruiz-Mora operation for claw
    toe
Ruiz-Morgan procedure
RUL (right upper lobe)
rule

rule of nines formula for
    percentage of body surface
    burned
rule out myocardial infarction
    (ROMI)
rule out (r/o)
ruled out
ruler
    Berndt hip ruler
    Chernov notched ruler
    hip ruler
    Joseph ruler
    metal ruler
    millimeter ruler
    notched ruler
    Pischel scleral ruler
    scleral ruler
    Scott ruler
    Tabb ruler
    V.M. & Co. ruler calipers
    Walker scleral ruler
rumble
rumbling bowel sounds
Rumel bronchial hemostat
Rumel cardiac tourniquet
Rumel cardiovascular tourniquet
Rumel catheter
Rumel clamp
Rumel forceps
Rumel lobectomy forceps
Rumel myocardial clamp
Rumel myocardial tourniquet
Rumel retractor
Rumel rubber clamp
Rumel rubber forceps
Rumel splint
Rumel technique
Rumel thoracic clamp
Rumel thoracic forceps
Rumel thoracic-dissecting
    forceps
Rumel tourniquet
Rumel tourniquet eyed
    obturator
Rumel-Belmont tourniquet
Rumpel-Leede sign
Rumpuffet vessel tourniquet

runner
running chromic sutures
running continuous sutures
running imbricating sutures
running subcuticular sutures
running sutures
running technique
running-locked stitch
running-locked sutures
run-off
rupture
ruptured
ruptured aneurysm
ruptured appendix
ruptured bag of waters
ruptured bladder
ruptured diaphragm
ruptured disk
ruptured disk curet
ruptured ligament
ruptured membranes
ruptured spleen
ruptured uterus
RUQ (right upper quadrant)
Rusch catheter
Rusch laryngoscope
Rusch nephrostomy instrument
Rusch tube
Ruschelit bougie
Ruschelit catheter
Ruschelit urethral bougie
Rusch-Foley catheter
Rush bone clamp
Rush clamp
Rush driver
Rush driver-bender-extractor
Rush extractor
Rush hammer
Rush incision
Rush intramedullary nail
Rush intramedullary pin
Rush nail
Rush pin
Rush pin bender
Rush pin driver-bender
    extractor
Rush pin instrument

Rush pin lead-filled head mallet
    with extractor
Rush pin prosthesis extractor
    with hand grip
Rush pin reamer awl
Rush pin round bevel-point pin
    set
Rush reamer
Rush rod
Rush rod insertion
Rush rod instrument
Rush safety pin
Rushkin balloon
Ruskin antral needle
Ruskin antral trocar
Ruskin bone rongeur
Ruskin bone-cutting forceps
Ruskin bone-splitting forceps
Ruskin cranial rongeur
Ruskin duckbill rongeur
Ruskin forceps
Ruskin mastoid rongeur
Ruskin multiple-action rongeur
Ruskin needle
Ruskin rongeur
Ruskin trocar
Ruskin-Jansen bone rongeur
Ruskin-Jay heavy-duty rongeur
Ruskin-Liston bone-cutting
    rongeur
Ruskin-Liston forceps
Ruskin-Rowland bone rongeur
Ruskin-Rowland forceps
Russe bone graft
Russe incision
Russe inlay bone graft
Russe operation
Russell dilator
Russell forceps
Russell frame
Russell gastrostomy
Russell hysterectomy forceps
Russell percutaneous endo-
    scopic gastrostomy
Russell pin traction
Russell suction tube
Russell traction

Russell tractor
Russell-Buck extension tractor
Russell-Buck tractor
Russell-Davis forceps
Russell-Taylor interlocking nail
Russell-Taylor nail
Russell-Taylor tibial interlocking
    nail
Russian bath
Russian fixation hook
Russian forceps
Russian thumb forceps
Russian tissue forceps
Russian-Péan forceps
Rust amputation saw
rusty sputum
Rutner catheter

Rutner stone basket
Rutner wedge catheter
Ruuska meniscotome
Ruysch muscle
Ruysch tube
Ruysch veins
Ruysch-Armor tube
Rx (take, therapy, treatment)
Rycroft cannula
Ryder needle holder
Ryerson bone retractor
Ryerson operation
Ryerson retractor
Ryerson tenotome
Ryerson triple arthrodesis
Ryle duodenal tube
Ryle tube

**S**

6-prong rake retractor
S&C (sclerae and conjunctivae)
S-A node (sinoatrial node)
S-B tube (Sengstaken-Blake-
    more tube)
S-cannula
S-flap incision
S-L dissociation (scapholunate
    dissociation)
S-O (salpingo-oophorectomy)
S-plasty
S-ROM gripper
S-ROM hip prosthesis
S-ROM modular total hip system
S-ROM system prosthesis
S-shaped anal anastomosis
S-shaped ileal pouch
S-shaped incision
S-shaped pouch
S-shaped reservoir
S-shaped retractor
S-shaped scar
S-shaped scoliosis
SA position (sacroanterior
    position)
Saalfeld comedo extractor
SAB (spontaneous abortion;
    subarachnoid block)
SAB anesthesia (subarachnoid
    block anesthesia)
Saba classification of shoulder
    muscles
saber incision
saber saw
saber tibia
saber-back scissors
saber-cut approach
saber-cut incision
saber-slash incision

sable brush
sabot heart
Sabreloc needle
Sabreloc spatula needle
Sabreloc sutures
sac
SAC (short-arm cast)
sac cushion
sacciform kidney
saccular
saccular aneurysm
saccular bronchiectasis
saccular colon
saccular nerve
saccularis, nervus
sacculated
sacculation
saccule
sacculus (*pl.* sacculi)
saccus operation
SACH (solid ankle cushioned
    heel)
SACH heel
SACH implant
SACH prosthesis
Sachs brain suction tube
Sachs brain-exploring cannula
Sachs bur
Sachs cannula
Sachs cervical punch
Sachs dural hook
Sachs dural separator
Sachs elevator
Sachs forceps
Sachs hook
Sachs needle
Sachs nerve separator
Sachs nerve spatula
Sachs punch

963

Sachs retractor
Sachs separator
Sachs skull bur
Sachs spatula
Sachs suction tube
Sachs tissue forceps
Sachs tube
Sachs urethrotome
Sachs vein retractor
Sachs-Cushing retractor
Sachs-Freer dissector
Sacks biliary drain
Sacks-Vine feeding gastrostomy
Sacks-Vine feeding gastrostomy
    tube
Sacks-Vine gastrostomy kit
Sacks-Vine PEG tube (percuta-
    neous endoscopic gastros-
    tomy tube)
Sacks-Vine percutaneous
    endoscopic gastrostomy
    tube (PEG tube)
sacral ala
sacral anesthesia
sacral arteries
sacral block anesthesia
sacral bone
sacral canal
sacral cul-de-sac
sacral flexure
sacral ganglia
sacral nerves
sacral plexus
sacral prominence
sacral reflexes
sacral region
sacral spine
sacral splanchnic nerves
sacral tuberosity
sacral veins
sacral vertebrae
sacrales laterales, arteriae
sacrales laterales, venae
sacrales, nervi
sacralis mediana, arteria
sacralis mediana, vena
sacralization

sacrectomy
sacroabdominoperineal pull-
    through operation
sacroanterior position (SA
    position)
sacrococcygeal
sacrococcygeal articulation
sacrococcygeal cyst
sacrococcygeal joint
sacrococcygeal muscle
sacrococcygeal region
sacrococcygeal sinus
sacrococcygeus dorsalis,
    musculus
sacrococcygeus ventralis,
    musculus
sacrodextra anterior position
sacrodextra posterior position
sacrofetal pregnancy
sacrofixation
sacrogenital ligament
sacrohorizontal angle
sacrohysteric pregnancy
sacroiliac
sacroiliac articulation
sacroiliac belt
sacroiliac joint
sacroiliac notch
sacroiliac strain
sacroperineal
sacroposterior position (SP
    position)
sacropubic diameter
sacrosciatic notch
sacrospinal muscle
sacrospinous ligament
sacrotomy
sacrotransverse position
sacrotuberous ligament
sacrouterine ligament
sacrum
saddle area
saddle block anesthesia
saddle block spinal anesthesia
saddle coil
saddle deformity
saddle deformity of nose

saddle embolism
saddle joint
saddle nose
saddle-back nose
saddlebag hernia
Sade modification of Norwood
    operation
Sadler bone hook
Sadler cartilage scissors
Sadler tissue scissors
Saemisch operation
Saemisch ulcer
Saenger macula
Saenger operation
Saenger ovum forceps
Saenger reflex
Saenger sign
Saenger sutures
SAF hip replacement (self-
    articulating femoral hip
    replacement)
Safar bronchoscope
Safar operation
Safar tube
Safar ventilation bronchoscope
Safar-S airway
safety belt
safety goggles
safety pessary
safety pin
safety pin closer
safety pin finger orthosis
safety pin orthosis
safety pin splint
safety strap
safety technique
safety tube
safety-bolt sutures
safety-sterility disk
Saf-T-Cath
Saf-T-Coil intrauterine device
sag foot
Sage forearm rod
Sage intramedullary rod
Sage pin
Sage rod
Sage snare

Sage technique
Sage tonsil snare
Sage-Clark cheilectomy
Sage-Salvatore classification of
    A-C joint injuries
sagittal area
sagittal diameter
sagittal fontanelle
sagittal linear transducer
sagittal orientation
sagittal plane
sagittal rotation
sagittal sector transducer
sagittal sinus
sagittal suture
sagittal suture line
sagittal suture synostosis
sagittalis inferior, sinus
sagittalis superior, sinus
sagittal-split osteotomy
Saha shoulder procedure
Sahli whistle
Sahlin restrictor
sail of cartilage
sail of pin
sailor's knot
Saint (see St.)
Saint triad
Sajou laryngeal forceps
Sakellarides technique for
    forearm contracture
Sakler erysiphake
SAL (suction-assisted lipectomy)
Salah needle
Salah sternal needle
Salem duodenal sump tube
Salem nasogastric tube
Salem sump
Salem sump drain
Salem sump pump
Salem sump tube
Salenius meniscus knife
Salibi carotid artery clamp
Salibi carotid clamp
Salibi clamp
salicylated cotton
salient symptom

saline
saline compress
saline dressing
saline infusion
saline irrigation
saline solution
saline-moistened sponge
Salinger nasal reducer
Salinger reducer
saliva
salivary
salivary duct
salivary gland
salivary tube
salmon backcut incision
Salmon catheter
Salmon sign
salmon-patch hemorrhage
Salmon-Rickham reservoir
Salonpas plaster
salpingeal curet
salpingeal probe
salpingectomy
salpingitis
salpingography
salpingo-oophorectomy (S-O)
salpingo-oophoroplasty
salpingo-oophorostomy
salpingo-oophorotomy
salpingo-oophorrhaphy
salpingo-ovarian salpingolysis
salpingo-ovariolysis
salpingopalatine fold
salpingopexy
salpingopharyngeal fold
salpingopharyngeal muscle
salpingopharyngeus, musculus
salpingoplasty
salpingorrhaphy
salpingoscopy
salpingostomy
salpingotomy
salpingo-ureteroscopy
salt and pepper duodenal
    erosion
Salter fracture (I–VI)
Salter incremental lines

Salter innominate osteotomy
Salter operation
Salter osteotomy
Salter-Harris fracture (I–IV)
Saltzman-Flynn-Richards
    technique
Salus arch
Salus incision
salvage technique
salvage therapy
salvarsan throat irrigation tube
salvarsan tube
salvatella vein
Salvatore ligator
Salvatore-Maloney tracheotome
salve
Salyer modification of Obweg-
    eser mandibular osteotomy
Sam Roberts bronchial biopsy
    forceps
Sam Roberts esophagoscope
Sam Roberts forceps
Sam Roberts headrest
Sam Roberts laryngoscope
Sam Roberts self-retaining
    laryngoscope
same-day surgery
Samilson calcaneal osteotomy
Samonara palatoplasty
sample
sampling
Sampson cyst
Sampson nail
Sampson prosthesis
Samson rod
Samuel position
Samuels forceps
Samuels hemoclip-applying
    forceps
Samuels vein stripper
Samuelson total knee
Samway tourniquet
Sana-Lok syringe
Sanborn metabolator
Sanborn oscilloscope
Sanchez-Bulnes lacrimal sac
    self-retaining retractor

Sanchez-Bulnes retractor
sanctuary disease
sanctuary site
sandbag
sandbag placed for support
Sanders bed
Sanders forceps
Sanders incision
Sanders intubation laryngo-
    scope
Sanders jet ventilation device
    respirator
Sanders laryngoscope
Sanders operation
Sanders valve
Sanders vasectomy forceps
Sanders-Brown needle
Sanders-Brown-Shaw needle
Sanders-Castroviejo forceps
Sandhill probe
Sandor foam bath
sandpaper dermabrader
sandpaper disk
sandpapering
Sandt utility forceps
sandwich flap
sandwich patch closure
Sanfilippo syndrome
sanguineous (also sanguinous)
sanguineous cataract
sanguineous drainage
sanguineous fluid
sanguineous material
sanguinous (see *sanguineous*)
Sani-dril sutures
Santorini cartilage
Santorini concha
Santorini duct
Santorini muscle
Santorini parietal vein
Santorini plexus
Santulli clamp
Santy dissecting forceps
Santy forceps
saphena accessoria, vena
saphena magna, vena
saphena parva, vena

saphenectomy
saphenofemoral
saphenofemoral juncture
saphenous
saphenous artery
saphenous graft
saphenous hiatus
saphenous nerve
saphenous pulse
saphenous system
saphenous vein
saphenous vein bypass graft
    (SVBG)
saphenous vein ligation and
    stripping
Sappey fibers
Sappey vein
sapphire knife
saprophyte
Saraf toenail operation
Saratoga sump
Saratoga sump catheter
sarcogenic cells
sarcoid
sarcoidosis
sarcoma (*pl.* sarcomas, sarco-
    mata)
sarcoplasmic reticulum
Sargis uterine manipulator
Sarmiento brace
Sarmiento cast
Sarmiento osteotomy for
    intertrochanteric fracture
Sarmiento osteotomy of hip
Sarnoff aortic clamp
Sarnoff clamp
Sarns aortic arch cannula
Sarns cannula
Sarns electric saw
Sarns intracardiac suction tube
Sarns safety loop
Sarns saw
Sarns temperature probe
Sarns two-stage cannula
Sarns venous drainage cannula
Sarns vent
Sarot artery clamp

Sarot artery forceps
Sarot bold sutures
Sarot bronchial clamp
Sarot cardiovascular needle
    holder
Sarot clamp
Sarot forceps
Sarot needle
Sarot needle holder
Sarot petit point needle holder
Sarot pleurectomy forceps
Sarot thoracic needle holder
Sarot thoracoscope
sartorius muscle
sartorius, musculus
SASMAS (skin-adipose superfi-
    cial musculoaponeurotic
    system)
SASMAS face-lift
satellite
satellite cells
satellite lesion
satellite nodule
Saticon vacuum chamber
    pickup tube
Saticon vacuum tube
Satinsky aortic clamp
Satinsky cardiac scissors
Satinsky clamp
Satinsky double-curve scissors
Satinsky forceps
Satinsky scissors
Satinsky thoracic scissors
Satinsky tourniquet
Satinsky vascular clamp
Satinsky vena cava clamp
satisfactorily
satisfactory general anesthesia
satisfactory recovery
Sato corneal knife
Sato eye knife
Sato knife
Sato lid retractor
Sato operation
Sato speculum
Satterlee advancement forceps
Satterlee amputating saw

Satterlee amputation saw
Satterlee aseptic saw
Satterlee bone saw
Satterlee capital saw
Satterlee muscle forceps
Satterlee saw
Sattler layer
Sattler veil
saturate
saturated solution
saturation
saturation index
saturnine nephritis
saucer
saucerization
saucerize
saucerizing a cyst
Sauer debrider
Sauer eye speculum
Sauer forceps
Sauer guillotine
Sauer speculum
Sauer tonometer
Sauer tonsillectome
Sauer-Bacon operation
Sauerbruch elevator for first rib
Sauerbruch forceps
Sauerbruch implant
Sauerbruch limb prosthesis
Sauerbruch pickup forceps
Sauerbruch prosthesis
Sauerbruch raspatory
Sauerbruch retractor
Sauerbruch rib guillotine
Sauerbruch rib rongeur
Sauerbruch rib shears
Sauerbruch rongeur
Sauerbruch-Britsch rib shears
Sauerbruch-Coryllos bone
    rongeur
Sauerbruch-Coryllos rib rongeur
Sauerbruch-Coryllos rib shears
Sauerbruch-Frey raspatory
Sauerbruch-Frey rib elevator
Sauerbruch-Frey rib shears
Sauerbruch-Lebsche rib shears
Sauerbruch-Lebsche rongeur

Sauerbruch-Lilienthal rib spreader
Sauerbruch-Stille bone rongeur
Sauerbruch-Zukschwerdt retractor
Sauerbruch-Zukschwerdt rib retractor
Sauer-Lebsche rongeur
Sauer-Sluder tonsillectome
Sauer-Storz tonometer
Sauer-Wiener intranasal instruments
Sauflon contact lens
Saunders needle
Saunders-Paparella hook
Saunders-Paparella needle
Saunders-Paparella pick
Saunders-Paparella rasp
Saunders-Paparella stapes hook
Saunders-Paparella window rasp
sausaging of vein
Sauvage arterial graft
Sauvage Bionit femoral prosthesis
Sauvage Bionit graft
Sauvage Dacron graft
Sauvage graft
Sauvage prosthesis
Sauvage vein graft
Savage intestinal decompressor
Savary bougie
Savary dilator
Savary esophageal dilator
Savary gastrointestinal endoscopy
Savary tapered thermoplastic dilator
Savary-Gilliard dilator
Savary-Gilliard esophageal dilator
Savastano total knee prosthesis
Savin operation
saw
    Adams saw
    Aesculap saw

saw *continued*
    Albee bone saw
    Albee saw
    amputating saw
    amputation saw
    angular saw
    antral saw
    Arbuckle antral saw
    Arruga saw
    bayonet saw
    Beaver finger ring saw
    Beaver saw
    Becker-Joseph saw
    Bier amputation saw
    Bishop oscillatory electric bone saw
    Bishop saw
    bone saw
    Bosworth nasal saw
    Bosworth saw
    Brown saw
    bur saw
    Butcher saw
    Cayo saw
    chain saw
    Chamfer saw
    Charrière bone saw
    Charrière saw
    circular saw
    circular twin saw
    Clerf laryngeal saw
    Clerf saw
    Converse nasal saw
    Converse saw
    Cottle nasal saw
    Cottle saw
    Cottle Universal nasal saw
    Cottle-Joseph saw
    counterrotating saw
    Crego Gigli saw
    crosscut saw
    crown saw
    crurotomy saw
    double-concave rotating saw
    Farabeuf saw

saw *continued*
Hey saw
intranasal saw
Jesse-Stryker saw
Joseph nasal saw
Joseph saw
Joseph-Maltz nasal saw
Joseph-Maltz saw
Lamont nasal saw
Lamont saw
Langenbeck metacarpal saw
Langenbeck saw
laryngeal saw
laryngectomy saw
laryngofissure saw
Lell laryngofissure saw
Lell saw
Luck bone saw
Luck saw
Luck-Bishop saw
Macewen saw
Magnuson circular twin saw
Magnuson saw
Magnuson single circular saw
Maltz bayonet saw
Maltz nasal saw
Maltz saw
McCabe crurotomy saw
metacarpal saw
Micro-Aire bone saw
Mueller round Gigli saw
Mueller saw
Myerson saw
nasal saw
Ogura saw
Olivecrona saw
Orthair oscillating saw
oscillating saw
oscillating sternotomy saw
oscillatory saw
Paparella-McCabe crurotomy saw
plaster saw

saw *continued*
reciprocating saw
Reese saw
rhinoplasty saw
rotary hub saw
Rust amputation saw
saber saw
Sarns electric saw
Sarns saw
Satterlee amputation saw
Satterlee aseptic saw
Satterlee bone saw
Satterlee capital saw
Satterlee saw
Schwartz saw
Seltzer saw
Shrady saw
silver saw
single circular saw
Skil Saw
skull saw
Slaughter nasal saw
Slaughter saw
sternotomy saw
Stille Gigli saw
Stille saw
Stille-Joseph saw
Stryker oscillating saw
Stryker saw
subcutaneous saw
transverse saw
Tuke saw
Tyler Gigli saw
Universal saw
V.M. & Co. amputating saw
Wigmore saw
Williams microsurgery saw
Woakes saw
saw guide (see also *guide*)
Adson Gigli-saw guide
Adson saw guide
Bailey Gigli-saw guide
Blair Gigli-saw guide
Blair saw guide
Cushing Gigli-saw guide

saw guide *continued*
    Davis saw guide
    Joseph saw guide
    Kendrick Gigli-saw guide
    Lebsche wire saw guide
    Mumford Gigli-saw guide
    Poppen Gigli-saw guide
    Raney Gigli-saw guide
    Schlesinger Gigli-saw
      guide
    Stille Gigli-saw guide
saw incision
Sawar ptosis operation
sawdust bed
Sawtell applicator
Sawtell forceps
Sawtell gallbladder forceps
Sawtell hemostat
Sawtell hemostatic forceps
Sawtell nasal applicator
Sawtell tonsillar forceps
Sawtell-Davis forceps
Sawtell-Davis hemostat
Sawtell-Davis tonsillar hemostat
    forceps
saw-tooth appearance sign
saw-toothed curet
Sawyer rectal retractor
Sawyer rectal speculum
Sawyer retractor
Saxtorph maneuver
Sayoc operation
Sayre apparatus
Sayre bandage
Sayre cast application
Sayre double-ended elevator
Sayre dressing
Sayre elevator
Sayre head sling
Sayre jacket
Sayre operation
Sayre periosteal elevator
Sayre periosteal raspatory
Sayre raspatory
Sayre retractor
Sayre splint
Sayre traction

Sbarbaro operation
Sbarbaro tibial prosthesis
SBE (subacute bacterial
    endocarditis)
SBO (small-bowel obstruction)
SBRN (sensory branch of radial
    nerve)
SC (supracondylar)
SC-5A fiberscope
scab
scabbard trachea
scabiform
Scaeffer orthosis
Scaglietti procedure
scalar time
scald
scale
scalene
scalene adenopathy
scalene biopsy
scalene elevator
scalene lesion
scalene lymph node
scalene maneuver
scalene muscle
scalene node
scalene node biopsy
scalenectomy
scalenotomy
scalenovertebral triangle
scalenus
scalenus anterior, musculus
scalenus anterior syndrome
scalenus anticus, musculus
scalenus anticus syndrome
scalenus medius, musculus
scalenus minimus, musculus
scalenus, musculus
scalenus posterior, musculus
scaler
scaling
scallop sign
scalloping
scalloping of vertebrae
scalp
scalp clip
scalp clip forceps

scalp clip-applying forceps
scalp electrode
scalp forceps
scalp hemostasis clip
scalp hemostat
scalp incision
scalp retractor
scalp self-retaining retractor
scalp sutures
scalp tourniquet
scalpel (see also *knife*)
    ASR scalpel
    Bard-Parker disposable
       scalpel
    Cavitron scalpel
    disposable scalpel
    disposable sterile scalpel
    Green pendulum scalpel
    Jackson scalpel
    John Green pendulum
       scalpel
    LaserSonics Nd:YAG
       LaserBlade scalpel
    lid scalpel
    pendulum scalpel
    plasma scalpel
    razor scalpel
    Shaw scalpel
scalpel blade
scalpel vulvectomy
scalpene needle
scan
Scan spray dressing
scan-directed biopsy
Scanmate stethoscope
scanner
scanning
scanning electron microscope
scanography
Scanpore hypoallergenic tape
Scanzoni forceps
Scanzoni maneuver
Scanzoni operation
scaphoconchal angle
scaphoid
scaphoid abdomen
scaphoid bone

scaphoid fossa
scaphoid fracture
scaphoid gouge
scaphoid projection
scaphoid scapula
scaphoid screw guide
scaphoid spatula
scapholunate
scapholunate advanced collapse
    (SLAC)
scapholunate dissociation (S-L
    dissociation)
scaphotrapeziotrapezoid joint
    (STT joint)
scapula
scapular area
scapular artery
scapular notch
scapular reflex
scapular region
scapular retractor
scapulary
scapulectomy
scapuloanterior position
scapuloclavicular articulation
scapuloclavicular joint
scapulohumeral reflex
scapulohumeral type
scapulopexy
scapuloposterior position
scapulothoracic
scapulothoracic bursa
scapulothoracic motion
scar
scar contracture
scar formation
scar tissue
Scardino pyeloplasty
Scardino ureteropelvioplasty
scarf bandage
scarf sign
scarification
scarified duodenum
scarifier
scarifying curet
scarlet red gauze dressing
Scarpa fascia

Scarpa ganglion
Scarpa ligament
Scarpa membrane
Scarpa nerve
Scarpa operation
Scarpa sheath
Scarpa shoe
Scarpa triangle
scarred
scarring
scatoma
scatter
scattered
scattering
scavenger cell
SCDK heart valve prosthesis
SCDK-Cutter valve
Schaaf foreign body forceps
Schachar implant cataract lens
Schachar lens
Schachar-Gills microsponge
Schachowa tube
Schaedel clip
Schaedel towel forceps
Schaeffer curet
Schaeffer ethmoid curet
Schaeffer mastoid curet
Schaldach electrode pacemaker
Schall tube
Schamberg extractor
Schantz sinus rasp
Schantz sinus raspatory
Schanz brace
Schanz collar brace
Schanz operation
Schanz osteotomy
Schanz screw
Schanzioni craniotomy forceps
Scharf implant cataract lens
Scharf lens
Schatten mammaplasty
Schatz laser technique
Schatz maneuver
Schatzki esophageal ring
Schatzki ring
Schaudinn fluid
Schauffler operation

Schauta operation
Schauta radical vaginal hyster-
    ectomy
Schauta vaginal operation
Schauta-Amreich operation
Schauta-Amreich vaginal
    operation
Schauta-Wertheim operation
Schauwecker compression
    wiring
Scheck-Mensor hanging hip
    operation
Schede curet
Schede operation
Schede osteotomy
Schede rotation osteotomy
Schede sequestrectomy
Schede thoracoplasty
Scheer crimper forceps
Scheer elevator
Scheer hook
Scheer knife
Scheer needle
Scheer pick
Scheer rasp
Scheer Teflon prosthesis
Scheer-Wullstein cutting bur
Scheicker laminectomy punch
Scheie anterior chamber
    cannula
Scheie cannula
Scheie cataract aspiration
Scheie cataract needle
Scheie cataract-aspirating
    needle
Scheie cautery
Scheie electrocautery
Scheie goniopuncture knife
Scheie goniotomy knife
Scheie knife
Scheie needle
Scheie operation
Scheie ophthalmic cautery
Scheie syndrome
Scheie-Graefe fixation forceps
Scheier hinge
Scheie-Westcott eye scissors

Scheinmann biting punch
Scheinmann biting tip
Scheinmann forceps
Scheinmann laryngeal forceps
schematic eye
schematic representation
scheme
Schepens binocular indirect
    camera
Schepens binocular indirect
    ophthalmoscope
Schepens clip
Schepens depressor
Schepens electrode
Schepens eye decompressor
Schepens eye retractor
Schepens forceps
Schepens hollow hemisphere
    implant
Schepens indirect ophthal-
    moscope
Schepens operation
Schepens ophthalmoscope
Schepens orbital retractor
Schepens retractor
Schepens-Okamura-Brockhurst
    retinal detachment repair
Scherback speculum
Scherback-Porges vaginal
    speculum
Scheuermann kyphosis
Schick forceps
Schick sign
Schiller D&C technique
Schiller iodine
Schiller test
Schimek operation
Schimelbush ether inhaler
Schindler esophagoscope
Schindler gastroscope
Schindler peritoneal forceps
Schindler retractor
Schindler syndrome
Schiøtz tonometer
Schiøtz tonometry
Schirmer test
Schlange sign

Schlatter disease
Schlatter operation
Schlein arthroplasty
Schlein clamp
Schlein total elbow prosthesis
Schlemm canal
Schlesinger cervical punch
Schlesinger cervical rongeur
Schlesinger clamp
Schlesinger forceps
Schlesinger Gigli-saw guide
Schlesinger instrument
Schlesinger intervertebral disk
    forceps
Schlesinger intervertebral disk
    rongeur
Schlesinger punch
Schlesinger rongeur
Schlesinger sign
schlieren microscope
Schlösser treatment
Schmalz operation
Schmeden dural scissors
Schmeden nasal punch
Schmeden punch
Schmeden scissors
Schmeden tonsillar punch
Schmidt rasp
Schmidt raspatory
Schmidt rod holder
Schmiedel ganglion
Schmieden-Taylor neurodissec-
    tor
Schmieden-Taylor scissors
Schmithhuisen ethmoid punch
Schmithhuisen sphenoid punch
Schmorl body
Schmorl furrow
Schmorl groove
Schmorl node
Schmorl nodule
Schnaudigel sclerotomy
    punch
Schneider arthrodesis
Schneider catheter
Schneider driver-extractor
Schneider hip fusion

Schneider intramedullary
    fixation of femur
Schneider intramedullary nail
Schneider medullary nail
Schneider nail
Schneider nail driver
Schneider nail extractor
Schneider nail shaft reamer
Schneider pelvimeter
Schneider pin
Schneider raspatory
Schneider rod
Schneider self-broaching pin
Schneider technique
schneiderian carcinoma
Schneider-Shiley catheter
Schneider-Shiley dilatation
    catheter
Schnidt clamp
Schnidt forceps
Schnidt gall duct forceps
Schnidt hemostat
Schnidt passer
Schnidt thoracic forceps
Schnidt tonsillar forceps
Schnidt tonsillar hemostat
Schnidt tonsillar hemostatic
    forceps
Schnidt-Rumpler forceps
Schnitker scalp retractor
Schnitman skin hook
Schnute wedge resection
Schobinger incision
Schocket depressor
Schoemaker (see also *Schuma-
    cher, Schumaker, Shoe-
    maker*)
Schoemaker anastomosis
Schoemaker gastrectomy
Schoemaker gastroenterostomy
Schoemaker goiter scissors
Schoemaker line
Schoemaker thyroid scissors
Schoemaker-Billroth I anasto-
    mosis
Schoemaker-Billroth II gastrec-
    tomy

Schoemaker-Billroth II intestinal
    anastomosis
Schoemaker-Loth ligature
    scissors
Schoemaker-Wangensteen
    operation
Schoenberg forceps
Schoenberg intestinal forceps
Schoenberg uterine forceps
Schoenberg uterine-elevating
    forceps
Schoenborn retractor
Scholl knife
Scholl meniscus knife
Scholl solution
Schonander technique
Schönbein operation
Schoonmaker catheter
Schoonmaker femoral catheter
Schoonmaker multipurpose
    catheter
Schott bath
Schott Fiber Optics
Schreger striae
Schröder (see *Schroeder*)
Schroeder curet
Schroeder episiotomy scissors
Schroeder forceps
Schroeder forceps tenaculum
Schroeder interlocking sound
Schroeder operating scissors
Schroeder operation
Schroeder scissors
Schroeder tenaculum
Schroeder uterine curet
Schroeder uterine tenaculum
    forceps
Schroeder vulsellum forceps
Schroeder-Braun forceps
Schroeder-Braun uterine
    tenaculum forceps
Schroeder-Van Doren tenacu-
    lum forceps
Schrotter catheter
Schubert biopsy punch
Schubert forceps
Schubert uterine biopsy forceps

Schubert uterine biopsy punch forceps
Schubert uterine tenaculum forceps
Schuchardt incision
Schuchardt operation
Schuchardt-Pfeifer operation
Schuchart pediatric rib shears
Schuknecht chisel
Schuknecht crimper
Schuknecht cutter
Schuknecht elevator
Schuknecht excavator
Schuknecht footplate hook
Schuknecht gouge
Schuknecht hook
Schuknecht knife
Schuknecht needle
Schuknecht operation
Schuknecht pick
Schuknecht piston prosthesis
Schuknecht postauricular self-retaining retractor
Schuknecht retractor
Schuknecht roller knife
Schuknecht scissors
Schuknecht spatula
Schuknecht speculum
Schuknecht stapedectomy
Schuknecht stapes hook
Schuknecht stapes prosthesis
Schuknecht suction tube
Schuknecht Teflon crimper
Schuknecht Teflon piston
Schuknecht Teflon wire piston prosthesis
Schuknecht temporal trephine
Schuknecht trephine
Schuknecht wire
Schuknecht wire crimper
Schuknecht wire-cutting scissors
Schuknecht-Wullstein retractor
Schuletz pacemaker
Schuller position
Schulte valve
Schultz irrigating iris retractor
Schultz retractor

Schultze bundle
Schultze embryotomy knife
Schultze fold
Schultze knife
Schultze method
Schultze placenta
Schumacher (see also *Schoemaker, Schumaker, Shoemaker*)
Schumacher aorta clamp
Schumacher biopsy forceps
Schumaker (see also *Shoemaker, Schumacher, Shoemaker*)
Schumaker gynecologic scissors
Schumaker umbilical cord scissors
Schurring ossicle cup prosthesis
Schutz clamp
Schutz clip
Schutz forceps
Schwalbe fissure
Schwalbe foramen
Schwalbe line
Schwalbe membrane
Schwalbe sheath
Schwalbe spaces
Schwann cell
Schwann sheath
Schwann tumor
schwannoma
Schwarten balloon dilatation catheter
Schwarten guide wire
Schwartz arterial aneurysm clamp
Schwartz bulldog clamp
Schwartz clamp
Schwartz clip
Schwartz clip-applying forceps
Schwartz cordotomy knife
Schwartz curet
Schwartz endocervical curet
Schwartz expression hook
Schwartz forceps
Schwartz hook

Schwartz intracranial clamp
Schwartz knife
Schwartz laminectomy retractor
Schwartz laminectomy self-retaining retractor
Schwartz obstetrical forceps
Schwartz retractor
Schwartz saw
Schwartz tenaculum
Schwartz trephine
Schwartz trocar
Schwartz-Baumgard technique
Schwartze operation
Schwartze-Stacke operation
Schwartz-Kerrison rongeur
Schweigger capsular forceps
Schweigger capsule
Schweigger extracapsular forceps
Schweigger forceps
Schweigger hand perimeter
Schweigger perimeter
Schweitzer pin
Schweitzer spring plate
Schweizer cervix-holding forceps
Schweizer forceps
sciatic
sciatic artery
sciatic foramen
sciatic hernia
sciatic nerve
sciatic notch
sciatic pain
sciatic scoliosis
sciatica
Science-Med balloon catheter
Sci-Med oxygenator
Sci-Med skinny catheter
scimitar blade
scimitar-blade knife
scintigram
scintigraphic balloon
scintigraphic perfusion defect
scintigraphic study
scintigraphy

scintillating sesamoids sign
scintillation camera
scintillation counter
scintillation scanner
scintiphoto
scintiphotography
scintiscan
scirrhous (adj.)
scirrhous adenocarcinoma
scirrhous cancer
scirrhous carcinoma
scirrhous lesion
scirrhus (noun)
scissor dissection
scissors
    abdominal scissors
    Acufex scissors
    Ada dissecting scissors
    Ada scissors
    Adson dural scissors
    Adson ganglion scissors
    Adson scissors
    Aebli corneal scissors
    Aebli corneal section scissors
    Aebli scissors
    Aebli-Manson scissors
    alligator scissors
    aloe stitch scissors
    American umbilical scissors
    American-pattern scissors
    American-pattern umbilical scissors
    angled scissors
    angular scissors
    aortic scissors
    arterial scissors
    arteriotomy scissors
    Asta ligature scissors
    Atkinson-Walker scissors
    Aufricht scissors
    automated intravitreal scissors
    baby Metzenbaum scissors
    backward-cutting scissors

scissors *continued*

Bakst scissors
ballpoint scissors
ball-tipped scissors
Baltimore nasal scissors
bandage scissors
Bantam wire scissors
Bantam wire-cutting
scissors
Bard-Parker scissors
Barkan scissors
Barnes scissors
Barraquer corneal
section scissors
Barraquer iris scissors
Barraquer scissors
Barraquer section
scissors
Barraquer-DeWecker iris
scissors
Barraquer-DeWecker
scissors
Barsky scissors
Baruch circumcision
scissors
Baruch scissors
Baum scissors
bayonet microscissors
bayonet scissors
beaded-tip scissors
Beall circumflex artery
scissors
Bechert intraocular
scissors
Becker corneal suture
scissors
Becker scissors
Becker septum scissors
Beckman nasal scissors
Beebe collar scissors
Beebe scissors
Bell scissors
Bellucci alligator scissors
Bellucci ear scissors
Bellucci otolaryngology
scissors
Bellucci scissors

scissors *continued*

Bellucci-Paparella
scissors
Berbridge scissors
Berens corneal transplant
scissors
Berens iridocapsulotomy
scissors
Berens scissors
Bergman bandage
scissors
Bergman plaster scis-
sors
Berridge gauze scissors
Blanco scissors
Blot scissors
Blum arterial scissors
blunt scissors
Bodian scissors
Boettcher scissors
Boettcher tonsil scissors
Boochai scissors
Bowman iris scissors
Bowman scissors
Bowman strabismus
scissors
Boyd dissecting scissors
Boyd scissors
brain scissors
Braun episiotomy
scissors
Braun scissors
Braun-Stadler bandage
scissors
Brook wire-stitch scissors
Brooks gallbladder
scissors
Brooks scissors
Brophy plastic surgery
scissors
Brophy scissors
Brown scissors
Bruns plastic surgery
scissors
Bruns scissors
Bruns-Stadler episiotomy
scissors

scissors *continued*

Buerger-McCarthy scissors
Buie operating scissors
Buie rectal scissors
Buie scissors
bulldog nasal scissors
bulldog scissors
Bunge scissors
Burnham bandage scissors
Burnham finger bandage scissors
Burnham scissors
Busch scissors
Busch umbilical scissors
calcified tissue scissors
canalicular scissors
cannula scissors
Caplan double-action scissors
Caplan nasal scissors
capsulotomy scissors
carbide-jaw scissors
cardiac scissors
cardiovascular scissors
cartilage scissors
Castanares face-lift scissors
Castanares scissors
Castroviejo corneal microscissors
Castroviejo corneal scissors
Castroviejo microscissors
Castroviejo scissors
Castroviejo section scissors
Castroviejo-Troutman scissors
Castroviejo-Vannas capsulotomy scissors
cataract scissors
Caylor scissors
Chadwick scissors
chemopallidectomy scissors

scissors *continued*

Cherry S-shape scissors
Cherry scissors
Chevalier Jackson scissors
Church cardiovascular scissors
Church deep-surgery scissors
Church pediatric scissors
Church scissors
Cinelli scissors
Cinelli-Fomon scissors
circumcisional scissors
circumflex artery scissors
circumflex scissors
Classon deep-surgery scissors
Classon pediatric scissors
Classon scissors
cloth scissors
Cohan-Vannas scissors
Cohan-Westcott scissors
Collis scissors
combined needle holder and scissors
Converse nasal tip scissors
Converse plastic surgery scissors
Converse scissors
Cooley arteriotomy scissors
Cooley cardiovascular scissors
Cooley probe-point scissors
Cooley reverse-cut scissors
Cooley scissors
Cooper scissors
cornea scissors
corneal scissors
corneal section scissors
corneal transplant scissors
corneoscleral scissors

scissors *continued*

- coronary artery scissors
- coronary scissors
- Cottle angular scissors
- Cottle bulldog scissors
- Cottle dorsal scissors
- Cottle dressing scissors
- Cottle heavy septum scissors
- Cottle nasal scissors
- Cottle scissors
- Cottle spring scissors
- Cottle stent scissors
- Cottle Vital dorsal angled scissors
- Crafoord lobectomy scissors
- Crafoord scissors
- Crafoord thoracic scissors
- Craig angular scissors
- Craig scissors
- craniotomy scissors
- crown and bridge scissors
- crown-collar scissors
- curved Mayo scissors
- curved scissors
- curved-on-flat scissors
- cuticle scissors
- cystoscopic scissors
- Dahlgren scissors
- Dandy neurosurgical scissors
- Dandy scissors
- Dandy trigeminal scissors
- Davis scissors
- Dean scissors
- Dean tonsillar scissors
- Dean-Trusler scissors
- Deaver operating scissors
- Deaver scissors
- DeBakey endarterectomy scissors
- DeBakey scissors
- DeBakey stitch scissors
- DeBakey valve scissors

scissors *continued*

- DeBakey vascular scissors
- DeBakey-Metzenbaum dissecting scissors
- DeBakey-Metzenbaum scissors
- DeBakey-Potts scissors
- decapitation scissors
- Decker scissors
- deep-surgery scissors
- delicate scissors
- DeMartel neurosurgical scissors
- DeMartel scissors
- DeMartel vascular scissors
- DeWecker eye scissors
- DeWecker iridectomy scissors
- DeWecker iris scissors
- DeWecker scissors
- DeWecker-Pritikin scissors
- diamond-edge scissors
- diathermic scissors
- Diethrich coronary scissors
- Diethrich scissors
- Diethrich valve scissors
- dissecting scissors
- dissecting tonsillar scissors
- dissecting Vital scissors
- dorsal scissors
- dorsal-angled scissors
- Douglas nasal scissors
- Doyen abdominal scissors
- Doyen scissors
- Dubois decapitation scissors
- Dubois scissors
- Duffield cardiovascular scissors
- Duffield scissors
- Dumont angular scissors

scissors *continued*
- Dumont scissors
- Dumont thoracic scissors
- dural scissors
- ear scissors
- Eiselberg uterine scissors
- Emmet scissors
- Emmet uterine scissors
- endarterectomy scissors
- enterotomy scissors
- enucleation scissors
- episiotomy scissors
- Esmarch plaster scissors
- Esmarch scissors
- esophageal scissors
- Essrig dissecting scissors
- Essrig scissors
- eye scissors
- face-lift scissors
- Favoloro scissors
- Federspiel scissors
- Ferguson abdominal scissors
- Ferguson scissors
- Ferguson-Metzenbaum scissors
- Fine scissors
- fine-dissecting scissors
- fine-stitch scissors
- fine-suture scissors
- Finochietto scissors
- Finochietto thoracic scissors
- flap scissors
- Fomon angular scissors
- Fomon dorsal scissors
- Fomon lower lateral scissors
- Fomon scissors
- Fomon upper lateral scissors
- Fomon Vital dorsal scissors
- Foster scissors
- Fox scissors
- Frahur scissors
- Frazier dural scissors

scissors *continued*
- Frazier scissors
- Freeman rhytidectomy scissors
- Freeman scissors
- Fulton deep-surgery scissors
- Fulton scissors
- gallbladder scissors
- gauze scissors
- general operating scissors
- Gill scissors
- Gillies scissors
- Gillies suture scissors
- Glassman scissors
- goiter scissors
- Goldman scissors
- gold-plated bandage scissors
- Gonin-Amsler sclera marker scissors
- Good scissors
- Good tonsillar scissors
- Good-Reiner scissors
- Good-Reiner tonsillar scissors
- Gorney face-lift scissors
- Gorney rhytidectomy scissors
- Gorney scissors
- Gorney septal scissors
- Gorney turbinate scissors
- Graham cardiovascular scissors
- Graham pediatric scissors
- Graham scissors
- Griffon tonsil scissors
- Guggenheim scissors
- Guilford ear scissors
- Guilford-Schuknecht scissors
- Guilford-Schuknecht wire-cutting scissors
- guillotine scissors
- Guist enucleation scissors

scissors *continued*

Guist scissors
gum scissors
Guyton scissors
Habaley-Stille Super Cut scissors
Haenig irrigating scissors
Haenig scissors
Haglund scissors
Haimovici arteriotomy scissors
Halsey nail scissors
Harrington deep surgical scissors
Harrington scissors
Harrington-Mayo scissors
Harrington-Mayo thoracic scissors
Harrison scissors
Harrison suture-removing scissors
Harvey wire-cutting scissors
Heath scissors
Heath suture scissors
Heath suture-cutting scissors
heavy-angled scissors
Hegemann scissors
Hercules scissors
Heyman nasal scissors
Heyman-Paparella angular scissors
Heyman-Paparella scissors
Hi-level bandage scissors
Hill stitch scissors
Hoen laminectomy scissors
Hoen scissors
Holinger scissors
hook scissors
Hooper deep-surgery scissors
Hooper pediatric scissors
Hooper scissors
Hough scissors
House alligator scissors

scissors *continued*

House dissecting scissors
House Metzenbaum scissors
House scissors
House-Bellucci alligator scissors
House-Bellucci scissors
House-Bellucci-Shambaugh alligator scissors
House-Bellucci-Shambaugh scissors
Howell coronary scissors
Huey scissors
Huey suture scissors
hysterectomy scissors
incision scissors
intestinal scissors
intraocular scissors
iridectomy scissors
iridocapsulotomy scissors
iris microscissors
iris miniature scissors
iris scissors
Irvine corneal scissors
Irvine probe-point scissors
Irvine scissors
Jabaley-Stille Supercut scissors
Jackson scissors
Jackson turbinate scissors
Jacobson microscissors
Jacobson scissors
Jacobson spring-handled scissors
Jaffe scissors
Jako laryngeal microscissors
Jameson dissecting scissors
Jameson-Metzenbaum scissors
Jannetta bayonet scissors
Jannetta scissors
Jannetta-Kurze dissecting scissors
Jannetta-Kurze scissors

scissors *continued*

- Jansen scissors
- Jarit flat-top scissors
- Jolly prostatic scissors
- Jones dissecting scissors
- Jones scissors
- Jorgenson dissecting scissors
- Jorgenson scissors
- Jorgenson thoracic scissors
- Joseph nasal scissors
- Joseph scissors
- Joseph serrated scissors
- Joseph-Maltz scissors
- Kahn dissecting scissors
- Kahn scissors
- Kantrowitz vascular dissecting scissors
- Kantrowitz vascular scissors
- Karmody venous scissors
- Katena Vannas scissors
- Katzeff cartilage scissors
- Katzin corneal scissors
- Katzin corneal transplant scissors
- Katzin scissors
- Katzin transplant scissors
- Kaye scissors
- Kayess bandage scissors
- Kazanjian scissors
- Keith scissors
- Kelly fistula scissors
- Kelly scissors
- Kelly uterine scissors
- Kelly-Littauer stitch scissors
- keratoplasty scissors
- Kilner scissors
- Kirby scissors
- Kleinsasser laryngeal microscissors
- Klinkenberg-Loth scissors
- Knapp iris scissors
- Knapp scissors
- Knapt scissors

scissors *continued*

- Knight nasal scissors
- Knight scissors
- Knowles bandage scissors
- Knowles scissors
- Kocher scissors
- Koenig nail-splitting scissors
- Kreuscher scissors
- Kurze dissecting scissors
- Kurze microscissors
- Kurze scissors
- Lagrange scissors
- Lahey dissecting scissors
- Lahey scissors
- Lahey thyroid scissors
- Lahey-Metzenbaum dissecting scissors
- Lakeside scissors
- laminectomy scissors
- Landolt enucleation scissors
- laryngeal scissors
- laryngofissure scissors
- Lawton scissors
- Leather-Carmody scissors
- left-curved scissors
- Lejeune scissors
- Lexer dissecting scissors
- Lexer scissors
- Lillie alligator scissors
- Lillie scissors
- Lillie tonsillar scissors
- Lincoln cardiovascular scissors
- Lincoln deep scissors
- Lincoln pediatric scissors
- Lincoln scissors
- Lincoln-Metzenbaum scissors
- Lipsett scissors
- Lister bandage scissors
- Lister scissors
- Liston scissors
- Littauer scissors
- Littauer stitch scissors

scissors *continued*

Littauer suture scissors
Littler carrying scissors
Littler scissors
Litwak mitral valve scissors
Litwak scissors
Litwak utility scissors
Litwin dissecting scissors
Litwin scissors
lobectomy scissors
Locklin stitch scissors
long scissors
Long stitch scissors
Lorenz bandage scissors
Lower lateral scissors
lung scissors
Lynch scissors
MacKenty scissors
Maclay scissors
Maclay tonsillar scissors
Malis neurological scissors
Malis scissors
Manson-Aebli scissors
Martin cartilage scissors
Martin scissors
Martin throat scissors
Mattis corneal scissors
Mattis scissors
Maunoir iris scissors
Maunoir scissors
Mayo dissecting scissors
Mayo scissors
Mayo uterine scissors
Mayo-Harrington dissecting scissors
Mayo-Harrington scissors
Mayo-New scissors
Mayo-Noble dissecting scissors
Mayo-Noble scissors
Mayo-Potts dissecting scissors
Mayo-Potts scissors
Mayo-Sims dissecting scissors

scissors *continued*

Mayo-Sims scissors
Mayo-Stille dissecting scissors
Mayo-Stille scissors
McAllister scissors
McClure eye scissors
McClure iris scissors
McClure scissors
McGuire corneal scissors
McGuire scissors
McHenry scissors
McIndoe cartilage scissors
McIndoe scissors
McLean capsulotomy scissors
McLean scissors
McPherson scissors
McPherson-Castroviejo corneal microscissors
McPherson-Castroviejo scissors
McPherson-Vannas iris microscissors
McPherson-Vannas iris scissors
McPherson-Vannas scissors
McPherson-Westcott conjunctival scissors
McPherson-Westcott stitch scissors
McReynolds pterygium scissors
McReynolds scissors
Medi bandage scissors
meniscectomy scissors
Metzenbaum baby tonsillar scissors
Metzenbaum dissecting scissors
Metzenbaum dressing scissors
Metzenbaum scissors
Metzenbaum tonsillar scissors

scissors *continued*
 Metzenbaum-Lipsett
  plastic scissors
 Metzenbaum-Lipsett
  scissors
 microscissors
 microscopic scissors
 microsurgical scissors
 microvascular scissors
 microvit scissors
 Microwec scissors
 Miller dissecting scissors
 Miller rectal scissors
 Miller scissors
 Mills arteriotomy scissors
 miniature scissors
 minor surgery scissors
 Mira scissors
 Mixter general operating
  scissors
 Mixter scissors
 Moehle scissors
 moleskin and felt
  scissors
 Morse aortic scissors
 Morse scissors
 MPC scissors
 Mueller scissors
 Munro brain scissors
 Munro scissors
 Murphy scissors
 Nagel scissors
 nasal dorsal-angled
  scissors
 nasal scissors
 Nelson general operating
  scissors
 Nelson scissors
 Nelson thoracic scissors
 Nelson uterine scissors
 Nelson-Metzenbaum
  scissors
 Neubauer scissors
 Neumann scissors
 neurological scissors
 New scissors
 Noble scissors

scissors *continued*
 Northbent scissors
 Northbent suture scissors
 Noyes iridectomy
  scissors
 Noyes iris scissors
 Noyes scissors
 Noyes-Shambaugh
  alligator scissors
 Noyes-Shambaugh
  scissors
 Nugent-Gradle stitch
  scissors
 O'Brien suture scissors
 Ochsner scissors
 O'Connor hook scissors
 Olivecrona dura scissors
 Olivecrona guillotine
  scissors
 Olivecrona scissors
 O'Neill scissors
 operating scissors
 Panzer gallbladder
  scissors
 Panzer scissors
 Paparella scissors
 Paparella wire-cutting
  scissors
 Pardos scissors
 Péan scissors
 Peck scissors
 pediatric scissors
 Penn scissors
 Penn umbilical scis-
  sors
 plaster-of-Paris scissors
 plastic scissors
 plastic surgery scissors
 PMH scissors
 pointed scissors
 Poppen scissors
 Potts 60-degree angled
  scissors
 Potts scissors
 Potts tenotomy scissors
 Potts vascular scissors
 Potts-DeMartel scissors

scissors *continued*
  Potts-Smith cardiovascu-
    lar scissors
  Potts-Smith scissors
  Potts-Smith vascular
    scissors
  Potts-Yasargil scissors
  Pratt rectal scissors
  Pratt scissors
  Prince scissors
  Prince tonsillar scissors
  Prince-Potts scissors
  Prince-Potts tonsillar
    scissors
  probe-point scissors
  prostatic scissors
  Quimby gum scissors
  Ragnell scissors
  Ragnell-Kilner scissors
  Ralks stitch scissors
  Real coronary artery
    scissors
  rectal scissors
  Rees scissors
  Reichling corneal scis-
    sors
  Resano dissecting
    scissors
  Resano scissors
  Reynolds scissors
  rhinoplasty scissors
  Rhoton titanium micro-
    scissors
  Richter episiotomy
    scissors
  Rienhoff general
    operating scissors
  Rienhoff thoracic
    scissors
  right-angle scissors
  right-curved scissors
  Ring ribbon scissors
  Rizzuti scissors
  Rizzuti-McGuire corneal
    section scissors
  Rizzuti-McGuire scissors
  Roberts episiotomy
    scissors

scissors *continued*
  Rochester-Ferguson
    scissors
  Roger scissors
  Roger wire-cutting
    scissors
  Roper scissors
  round-blade scissors
  saber-back scissors
  Sadler cartilage scissors
  Sadler tissue scissors
  Satinsky cardiac scissors
  Satinsky double-curve
    scissors
  Satinsky scissors
  Satinsky thoracic scissors
  Scheie-Westcott eye
    scissors
  Schmeden dural scissors
  Schmeden scissors
  Schmieden-Taylor
    scissors
  Schoemaker goiter
    scissors
  Schoemaker thyroid
    scissors
  Schoemaker-Loth ligature
    scissors
  Schroeder episiotomy
    scissors
  Schroeder operating
    scissors
  Schroeder scissors
  Schuknecht scissors
  Schuknecht wire-cutting
    scissors
  Schumaker gynecologic
    scissors
  Schumaker gynecologic
    umbilical cord scissors
  sclerectomy scissors
  Sealy dissecting scissors
  Seiler scissors
  Seiler turbinate scissors
  semilunar cartilage
    scissors
  septal scissors
  serrated scissors

scissors *continued*

Serratex scissors
Serratex-Mayo dissecting
scissors
Seutin plaster scissors
Shea vein graft scissors
Shea-Bellucci scissors
Shepard scissors
Shortbent scissors
Shortbent stitch scissors
Shutt scissors
Siebold uterine scissors
Sims general operating
scissors
Sims scissors
Sims uterine scissors
Sims-Siebold uterine
scissors
Sistrunk dissecting
scissors
Sistrunk scissors
slender-tip scissors
small spring scissors
Smart enucleation
scissors
Smart scissors
Smellie obstetrical
scissors
Smellie scissors
Smith scissors
Smith wire-cutting
scissors
Smith-Potts scissors
Snowden-Pencer
scissors
Southbent scissors
Spencer scissors
Spencer stitch scissors
spring-handled scissors
Stevens scissors
Stevens tenotomy
scissors
Stevenson scissors
Stille dissecting scissors
Stille scissors
Stille Super Cut scissors
Stille-Mayo scissors
stitch scissors

scissors *continued*

Storz cystoscopic scissors
Storz delicate iris scissors
Storz intraocular scissors
Storz-Westcott conjuncti-
val scissors
strabismus scissors
straight scissors
Strully dissecting scissors
Strully neurological
scissors
Strully scissors
surgical scissors
Sutherland scissors
Sutherland-Grieshaber
scissors
suture scissors
suture-removing scissors
Sweet esophageal
scissors
Sweet scissors
sympathectomy scissors
Taylor craniotomy
scissors
Taylor neurosurgical
scissors
Taylor scissors
tenotomy scissors
Thompson-Walker
scissors
thoracic scissors
Thorek gallbladder
scissors
Thorek scissors
Thorek-Feldman
gallbladder scissors
Thorek-Feldman scissors
Thorpe pupillary
membrane scissors
Thorpe scissors
Thorpe-Castroviejo
cataract scissors
Thorpe-Castroviejo
scissors
Thorpe-Westcott scissors
throat scissors
Toennis anastomosis
scissors

scissors *continued*

Toennis dissecting scissors
Toennis scissors
Toennis-Adson scissors
Toennis-Adson utility scissors
tonsil-dissecting scissors
tonsillar scissors
tracheal scissors
tracheostomy scissors
trigeminus scissors
Troutman conjunctival scissors
Troutman corneal scissors
Troutman corneal section scissors
Troutman scissors
Troutman-Castroviejo scissors
Troutman-Katzin corneal transplant scissors
Trusler-Dean scissors
turbinate scissors
Twisk scissors
umbilical scissors
U.S. Army-pattern gauze scissors
uterine scissors
utility scissors
valve scissors
Vannas capsulotomy scissors
Vannas corneal scissors
Vannas microcapsu-lotomy scissors
Vannas scissors
vascular scissors
vena caval scissors
Verdi scissors
Verhoeff dissecting scissors
Verhoeff scissors
Vernon scissors
Vezien scissors
Vital iris scissors
Vital scissors

scissors *continued*

von Graefe scissors
Wadsworth scissors
Walker scissors
Walker-Apple corneal scissors
Walker-Apple scissors
Walker-Atkinson corneal scissors
Walker-Atkinson scissors
Walkmann episiotomy scissors
Walton scissors
Watzke scissors
Weber scissors
Weber tissue scissors
Webster meniscectomy scissors
Weck suture-removal scissors
Weller dissecting scissors
Wells enucleation scissors
Werb rhinostomy scissors
Werb scissors
Wertheim deep-surgery scissors
Westcott microscissors
Westcott scissors
Westcott tenotomy scissors
Westcott-Scheie scissors
Wester scissors
Wexteel scissors
White scissors
Wiechel scissors
Willauer scissors
Willauer thoracic scissors
Wilmer iris scissors
Wilmer scissors
Wilmer-Converse conjunctival scissors
Wincor enucleation scissors
Wincor scissors
wire carbide-jaw suture scissors

scissors *continued*
  wire-cutting scissors
  Wolf curved scissors
  Wolf scissors
  Woods tonsillar scissors
  Wullstein ear scissors
  Wullstein scissors
  Wutzler circumcision
   scissors
  Wutzler scissors
  Yankauer scissors
  Yankauer tonsillar
   scissors
  Yasargil bayonet scissors
  Yasargil microscissors
  Yasargil microvascular
   bayonet scissors
  Yasargil scissors
  Zoellner scissors
scissors dissection
scissors forceps
scissors probe
sclera (*pl.* sclerae)
sclerae and conjunctivae (S&C)
scleral bed
scleral buckle eye implant
scleral buckle procedure for
 retinal detachment
scleral buckler implant
scleral buckling
scleral buckling operation
scleral canal
scleral cauterization
scleral depressor
scleral ectasia
scleral eye implant
scleral fistula
scleral fistula operation
scleral flap
scleral hook
scleral implant
scleral marker (see also *marker*)
  Amsler scleral marker
  Gass scleral marker
  Gonin-Amsler scleral
   marker
scleral punch
scleral rim

scleral ring
scleral ruler
scleral shortening
scleral shortening operation
scleral spatula needle
scleral spur
scleral trephine
sclerectoiridectomy
sclerectoiridodialysis
sclerectomy
sclerectomy by punch
sclerectomy by scissors
sclerectomy by trephining
sclerectomy punch
sclerectomy punch forceps
sclerectomy scissors
sclerectomy with punch
sclerectomy with scissors
sclerectomy with trephine
scleriritomy
sclerocorneal junction
scleroderma
sclerolimbal junction
scleronyxis
scleroplasty
sclerosed
sclerosed lens
sclerosing
sclerosing injection
sclerosing therapy
sclerosis
sclerostomy
sclerotherapy
sclerotherapy needle
sclerotic rind
sclerotic thickening
scleroticectomy
scleroticochoroidal canal
scleroticonyxis
scleroticopuncture
sclerotome (see also *knife*)
  Alvis-Lancaster scle-
   rotome
  Atkinson sclerotome
  Castroviejo sclerotome
  Curdy sclerotome
  Guyton-Lundsgaard
   sclerotome

sclerotome *continued*
    Lancaster sclerotome
    Lundsgaard sclerotome
    Lundsgaard-Burch
       sclerotome
    Walker-Lee sclerotome
sclerotomy
sclerotomy knife
sclerotomy with drainage
sclerotomy with exploration
sclerotomy with removal of
    foreign body
sclerous tissues
Scobee hook
Scobee muscle hook
Scobee oblique muscle hook
Scobee-Allis forceps
scoliosis
scoliosis brace
scoliosis osteotome
Scolitron screw
Scomac outrigger system
scoop
    Abbott scoop
    abdominal scoop
    Arlt fenestrated lens
       scoop
    Arlt lens scoop
    Arlt scoop
    Beck abdominal scoop
    Beck gastrostomy scoop
    Beck scoop
    Berens lens scoop
    Berens scoop
    common duct scoop
    Councill stone scoop
    cystic duct scoop
    Daviel scoop
    Desjardins gall duct
       scoop
    Desjardins gallbladder
       scoop
    Desjardins gallstone
       scoop
    Desjardins scoop
    Elschnig lens scoop
    Elschnig scoop

scoop *continued*
    enucleation scoop
    fenestrated lens scoop
    Ferguson gallstone scoop
    Ferguson scoop
    Ferris common duct
       scoop
    Ferris scoop
    gall duct scoop
    gallbladder scoop
    gallstone scoop
    gastrostomy scoop
    Green lens scoop
    Green scoop
    Hess lens scoop
    Hess scoop
    Kirby intracapsular scoop
    Klebanoff gallstone
       scoop
    Klebanoff scoop
    Knapp lens scoop
    Knapp scoop
    Lang scoop
    lens scoop
    Lewis lens scoop
    Lewis scoop
    Luer gallstone scoop
    Luer scoop
    Luer-Koerte scoop
    malleable scoop
    Mayo common duct
       scoop
    Mayo cystic duct scoop
    Mayo gallstone scoop
    Mayo scoop
    Mayo-Robson gallstone
       scoop
    Mayo-Robson scoop
    microbayonet scoop
    Moore gallstone scoop
    Moore scoop
    Moynihan gallstone
       scoop
    Moynihan scoop
    Mules scoop
    Pagenstecher scoop
    rigid scoop

scoop *continued*
  Rockey scoop
  Sellet common duct
    scoop
  Wells enucleation scoop
  Wells scoop
  Wilder lens scoop
  Wilder scoop
  Yasargil scoop
Scoop transtracheal catheter
scoops and loops
scooter
scope
scope-straightening twists and
  fold-gathering (on colon-
  oscopy)
Scopinaro pancreaticobiliary
  bypass
scopolamine
score
Scotch douche
Scotchcast casting tape
Scotchcast Plus
Scotchflex casting tape
scotoma
scotometer
scotometry
scotopic vision
Scott attic cannula
Scott cannula
Scott humerus splint
Scott inflatable penile prosthesis
Scott jejunoileal bypass
Scott operation
Scott resectoscope
Scott rubber ventricular cannula
Scott ruler
Scott speculum
Scott splint
Scott suction tube
Scott ventricular cannula
Scott-Harden tube
Scottish Rite brace
Scottish Rite hip orthosis
Scottish Rite orthosis
Scottish Rite procedure
Scottish Rite splint

Scott-McCracken elevator
Scott-McCracken periosteal
  elevator
scout film
scout negative
scout positive
Scoville brain forceps
Scoville brain spatula
Scoville brain spatula forceps
Scoville cervical disk self-
  retaining retractor
Scoville clip
Scoville clip applier
Scoville curet
Scoville curved hook
Scoville curved nerve hook
Scoville flat brain spatula
Scoville forceps
Scoville hemilaminectomy
Scoville hemilaminectomy
  retractor
Scoville hemilaminectomy self-
  retaining retractor
Scoville hook
Scoville needle
Scoville nerve hook
Scoville nerve retractor
Scoville nerve root retractor
Scoville psoas muscle retractor
Scoville retractor
Scoville ruptured disk curet
Scoville self-retaining retractor
Scoville skull trephine
Scoville spatula
Scoville trephine
Scoville ventricular needle
Scoville-Greenwood forceps
Scoville-Lewis clamp
Scoville-Lewis clip
Scoville-Richter self-retaining
  retractor
scraped
scraping
scrapings
scratch
scratch incision
scratch-type incision

scratcher
screen
screen oxygenator
screen pneumotach
screening
screw
    A-O screw
    Ace cannulated
      cancellous hip screw
    Ace cannulated
      cancellous screw
    Ace captured hip screw
    Ace cortical bone screw
    Ace hip screw
    Ace screw
    afterloading screw
    Allen screw
    Ambi compression hip
      screw
    Ambi hip screw
    arthrodesis screw
    ASIF screw
    Asner screw
    Asnis cannulated screw
    Asnis screw
    Basile hip screw
    Basile screw
    Bechtol screw
    bone screw
    Bosworth coracoclavicu-
      lar screw
    Bosworth screw
    Bristow screw
    buttress thread screw
    cancellous bone screw
    cancellous screw
    carpal scaphoid screw
    Carroll-Girard screw
    Collison screw
    compression hip screw
      (CHS)
    compression screw
    Concept screw
    coracoclavicular screw
    corkscrew
    cortex screw
    cortical screw

screw *continued*
    cotton screw
    crown drill screw
    cruciate head screw
    cruciate screw
    cruciform head-bone
      screw
    cruciform screw
    Cubbins screw
    Deyerle screw
    double-threaded Herbert
      screw
    Doyen screw
    Doyen tumor screw
    Druck-Schrauben screw
    Duo-Drive cortical bone
      screw
    Dwyer cancellous screw
    Dwyer screw
    dynamic condylar screw
      (DCS)
    ECT internal fracture
      fixation and bone
      screw
    Eggers screw
    eyelet lag screw
    Filtzer corkscrew
    fixing screw
    foreign body screw
    German A-O hip
      compression screw
    Harris hip screw
    Henderson lag screw
    Herbert bone screw
    Herbert scaphoid bone
      screw
    Herbert screw
    hex screw (hexagon
      screw)
    hexagon screw
    hexhead screw
    hip screw
    Hi-Torque screw
    Hoffmann screw
    Howmedica lag screw
    Howmedica screw
    Howmedica Luer screw

screw *continued*
- Howse-Coventry screw
- Jewett pickup screw
- Jewett screw
- Johannsen lag screw
- key-free compression screw
- Kristiansen screw
- Kurosaka bone screw
- Kurosaka cannulated screw
- Kurosaka extremity screw
- Kurosaka interference fixation screw
- lag screw
- Leinbach olecranon screw
- Leinbach screw
- Lewin tonsil screw
- Lorenzo bone fixation screw
- Lorenzo screw
- malleable screw
- Marion screw
- Martin screw
- McAtee screw
- McLaughlin screw
- Mecron cannulated cancellous screw
- metal screw
- Morris biphase screw
- Neufeld screw
- Omega screw
- Phillips recessed-head screw
- Phillips screw
- pickup screw
- plates and screws
- pull screw
- Ray screw
- recessed-head screw
- removal of screw
- reverse-threaded screw
- Richards adjustable hip screw

screw *continued*
- Richards compression screw
- Richards lag screw
- Richards screw
- Richmond screw
- Schanz screw
- Scolitron screw
- Scuderi screw
- self-tapping bone screw
- Sherman bone screw
- Sherman molybdenum screw
- Sherman plate and screws
- Sherman screw
- Sherman Vitallium screw
- Simmons screw
- Simmons-Martin screw
- slotted screw
- spongiosa screw
- stainless steel screw
- Steffee screw
- Stryker screw
- syndesmosis screw
- syndesmotic screw
- Syntex screw
- Synthes compression hip screw
- Synthes screw
- Thatcher screw
- Thornton screw
- titanium mesh screw
- titanium screw
- tonsillar screw
- Townley screw
- transfixion screw
- transsyndesmotic screw
- Tronzo screw
- tumor screw
- Venable hip screw
- Venable screw
- Vitallium screw
- Wood screw
- Woodruff screw
- Y-screw
- Z-screw

screw *continued*
    Zielke screw
    Zimmer compression hip
        screw
    Zimmer screw
screw compressor
screw elevator
screw home mechanism
screw plate
screw tenaculum
screwdriver
    Allen-headed screw-
        driver
    automatic screwdriver
    Becker screwdriver
    Children's Hospital
        screwdriver
    Collison screwdriver
    cross-slot screwdriver
    cruciform screwdriver
    Cubbins screwdriver
    DePuy screwdriver
    Dorsey screwdriver
    heavy cross-slot screw-
        driver
    hexhead screwdriver
    Johnson screwdriver
    Ken screwdriver
    Lane screwdriver
    lever-type screwdriver
    light cross-slot screw-
        driver
    Lok-it screwdriver
    Lok-screw double-slot
        screwdriver
    Lok-screw screwdriver
    Massie screwdriver
    Master screwdriver
    medium screwdriver
    Moore-Blount screw-
        driver
    Phillips screwdriver
    plain screwdriver
    Richards Phillips
        screwdriver
    Richter screwdriver
    Sherman screwdriver

screwdriver *continued*
    Sherman-Pierce screw-
        driver
    single cross-slot screw-
        driver
    Stryker screwdriver
    Trenkle screwdriver
    V.M. & Co. screwdriver
    White screwdriver
    Williams screwdriver
    Woodruff screwdriver
    Zimmer screwdriver
screwdriver teeth
screw-in lead
screw-in lead pacemaker
Scribner arteriovenous shunt
Scribner shunt
scrotal
scrotal area
scrotal compartment
scrotal dressing
scrotal hernia
scrotal hydrocele
scrotal incision
scrotal mass
scrotal nerves
scrotal sac
scrotal septum
scrotal suspensory support
scrotal swelling
scrotal veins
scrotales anteriores, nervi
scrotales anteriores, venae
scrotales posteriores, nervi
scrotales posteriores, venae
scrotal-perineal incontinence
        prosthesis
scrotectomy
scrotocele
scrotoplasty
scrotum
scrub
scrub person
scrub prep
scrub preparation
scrub sink
scrub suit

Tisseel fibrin sealant

scrubbed, prepped, and draped
Scudder clamp
Scudder forceps
Scudder intestinal clamp
Scudder intestinal forceps
Scudder skid
Scudder stomach clamp
Scuderi forceps
Scuderi prosthesis
Scuderi screw
Scuderi tendon repair
Scuderi-Callahan flange
SCUF therapy (slow continuous
    ultrafiltration therapy)
scultetus
scultetus bandage
scultetus binder
scultetus binder band
scultetus binder dressing
scultetus dressing
scultetus position
scutum
scybalous
scybalous feces
scybalous stool
scybalum (pl. scybala)
SDC anesthesia
sea anemone ulcer
sea fronds
seal
SealEasy resuscitation mask
sealed applicator
sealed vacuum bottle
sealing
Sealy dissecting scissors
seam
seamless arterial graft
seamless prosthesis
seamless tube prosthesis
searcher (see also bougie,
    sound)
        Allport mastoid searcher
        Allport searcher
        Allport-Babcock mastoid
            searcher
        Allport-Babcock searcher
        mastoid searcher

searcher continued
        Shea searcher
        stone searcher
Searcy capsule forceps
Searcy chalazion trephine
Searcy erysiphake
Searcy fixation hook
Searcy forceps
Searcy hook
Searcy tonsillectome
Searcy trephine
searing pain
seat belt
seat belt injury
seated securely
seating
sebaceous
sebaceous cyst
sebaceous glands
sebaceous material
Sebileau elevator
Sechrist infant ventilator
Sechrist neonatal ventilator
secobarbital anesthetic agent
Seconal anesthetic agent
secondary
secondary amputation
secondary branch
secondary carcinoma
secondary cataract
secondary cause
secondary closure of wound
secondary condition
secondary constriction
secondary fracture
secondary hemorrhage
secondary infection
secondary process
secondary repair
secondary site
secondary stage
secondary sutures
secondary to
second-degree burn (2nd-
    degree burn)
second-degree sprain
second-look laparotomy

second-look operation
second-look procedure
Secretan disease
secrete
secreting
secretion
secretory
secretory activity
secretory nerve
secretory otitis media (SOM)
section
sectional
sectioned
sector iridectomy
sector scan echocardiography
Secu clip
Secund fracture
secundigravida
secundum
secundum atrial septal defect
secundum foramen
secured
secured hemostasis
secured with tape
secured with ties
security
sedated
sedation
sedative
Seddon arthrodesis
Seddon costotransversectomy
Seddon nerve graft
Seddon operation
Seddon wrist arthrodesis
Sédillot elevator
Sédillot elevator-raspatory
Sédillot operation
Sédillot periosteal elevator
Sédillot raspatory
sediment
sedimentary cataract
sedimentation
sedimentation rate (SR)
sedimented red cells
Seecor pacemaker
seed graft

seed implant
seeding
seeker
Seen retractor
seesaw murmur
segment
segmental
segmental arteries
segmental atelectasis
segmental bronchus
segmental buckle
segmental colon resection
segmental fracture
segmental graft
segmental innervation
segmental lung resection
segmental orifices
segmental pulmonary resection
segmental resection
segmental resection of lung
segmental stripping
segmental washings
segmentation
segmentectomy
segmented forms
segmented fracture
Segond forceps
Segond fracture
Segond retractor
Segond spatula
Segond tumor forceps
Segond vaginal spatula
Segond-Landau hysterectomy
    forceps
segregator
        Cathelin segregator
        Harris segregator
        Luys segregator
Segura procedure
Segura stone basket
Segura surgery for esophageal
    varices
Sehrt clamp
Sehrt compressor
Seidel bone-holding clamp
Seidel plug

Seidel sign
Seidel test for aqueous fluid
    leak
Seiffert forceps
Seiffert punch
Seiffert tip
Seiler conization knife
Seiler knife
Seiler scissors
Seiler tonsillar knife
Seiler turbinate scissors
Seinsheimer classification of
    subtrochanteric fractures
seize
seizure
Seldinger cardiac catheterization
Seldinger catheter
Seldinger cystic duct catheteri-
    zation
Seldinger needle
Seldinger percutaneous
    technique
Seldinger technique
Seldinger wire
Seldinger-Desilet technique
selected
selection
selective cannulation
selective catheterization
selective coronary arteriogram
selective coronary cineangi-
    ogram
selective injection
selective studies
selective subendocardial
    resection
selective vagolysis
selective vagotomy
Selective-HI catheter
Seletz cannula
Seletz catheter
Seletz foramen-plugging forceps
Seletz forceps
Seletz punch
Seletz Universal Kerrison punch
Seletz ventricular cannula
Seletz-Gelpi retractor

Seletz-Gelpi self-retaining
    retractor
self-adjusting nail
self-administered
self-articulating femoral hip
    replacement (SAF hip
    replacement)
self-broaching nail
self-broaching pin
self-compressing plate
self-induced
self-induced injury
self-limited
self-locking prosthesis
self-locking stitch
self-retaining abdominal
    retractor
self-retaining catheter
self-retaining laryngoscope
self-retaining retractor
self-retaining retractor blade
self-retaining speculum
self-retaining spring retractor
self-sealing
self-suspension
self-tapering pin
self-tapping bone screw
self-treatment
Selig intrapelvic obturator
    neurectomy
Selinger operation
Selker reservoir
Selkin speculum
sella turcica
Sellet common duct scoop
Sellheim uterine catheter
Sellick maneuver
Sellor clamp
Sellor contractor
Sellor knife
Sellor rib contractor
Sellor valvulotome
Selman clamp
Selman clip
Selman forceps
Selman nonslip tissue
    forceps

Selman peripheral blood vessel
    forceps
Selman tissue forceps
Selman vessel forceps
Selofix dressing
Selopor dressing
Selsi sport telescope
Seltzer saw
Selverstone carotid artery clamp
Selverstone carotid clamp
Selverstone clamp
Selverstone cordotomy hook
Selverstone forceps
Selverstone hook
Selverstone intervertebral disk
    rongeur
Selverstone rongeur
SEM (systolic ejection murmur)
Semb bone-cutting forceps
Semb dissecting forceps
Semb forceps
Semb gouging rongeur
Semb ligature forceps
Semb lung retractor
Semb operation
Semb raspatory
Semb retractor
Semb rib shears
Semb rongeur
Semb shears
Semb-Ghazi dissecting forceps
Semb-Sauerbruch rongeur
Semb-Stille bone rongeur
SEMI (subendocardial myocar-
    dial infarction)
semiambulatory
semiaxial anteroposterior
    projection
semiaxial projection
semiaxial transcranial projection
semibarber position
semicanal for tensor tympani
semicanal of auditory tube
semicircular canals
semicircular ducts
semicircular incision
semicircular punch

semicircular rings
semicircular trochlear notch
semiclosed anesthesia
semiclosed endotracheal
    anesthesia
semicomatose
semicompressive dressing
semiconscious
semiconstrained prosthesis
semierect position
semiflat tip electrode
semiflexed incision
semiflexible endoscope
semiflexible intraocular lens
semi-Fowler position
semi-invasive electrical stimula-
    tion system
semilunar bone
semilunar cartilage
semilunar cartilage knife
semilunar cartilage scissors
semilunar fibrocartilage
semilunar fold
semilunar ganglion
semilunar hiatus
semilunar incision
semilunar line
semilunar lobule
semilunar notch
semilunar valve
semimembranosus, musculus
semimembranous
semimembranous muscle
seminal ducts
seminal fluid
seminal sutures
seminal vesicles
seminiferous tubules
seminoma
semiopen anesthesia
semiopen endotracheal
    inhalation anesthesia
semioval center
semipermeable membrane
semipermeable membrane
    dressing
semipressure dressing

semiprone position
semireclining position
semirecumbent position
semirigid
semirigid catheter
semirigid endoscope
semirigid penile prosthesis
semirigid sigmoidoscope
semishell eye implant
semishell implant
semishelving incision
semisolid material
semispinal muscle
semispinalis capitis, musculus
semispinalis cervicis, musculus
semispinalis thoracis, musculus
semistuporous patient
semitendinosus, musculus
semitendinous muscle
semitubular plate
semiupright film
semiupright position
Semken forceps
Semken infant forceps
Semken tissue forceps
Semm cannula
Semm uterine catheter
Semmes dural forceps
Semmes spinal fusion curet
Semon triangle
senescent changes
Sengstaken balloon
Sengstaken nasogastric tube
Sengstaken tube
Sengstaken-Blakemore balloon
Sengstaken-Blakemore device
Sengstaken-Blakemore tube
senile atrophy
senile cataract
Senn bone plate
Senn double-ended retractor
Senn forceps
Senn mastoid retractor
Senn operation
Senn retractor
Senn self-retaining retractor
Senn speculum

Senn-Dingman double-ended
    retractor
Senn-Dingman retractor
Senn-Green retractor
Senning atrial baffle repair
Senning baffle
Senning bulldog clamp
Senning clamp
Senning correction of transposi-
    tion of great vessels
Senning forceps
Senning intra-arterial baffle
Senning operation
Senning suction tube
Senning transposition operation
Senning-Stille clamp
Senn-Kanavel double-ended
    retractor
Senn-Kanavel retractor
Sens dissector
sensation
sense
sensibility
sensing catheter
sensitive to pain
sensitivity
Sensolog pacemaker
sensor
Sensor Kelvin pacemaker
Sensor Pad
sensor-based single-chamber
    pacemaker
sensorimotor
sensorimotor cortex
sensorimotor neuropathy
sensorimotor rhythm
sensorimuscular
sensorineural
sensorineural deafness
sensorineural hearing loss
sensorium
sensory branch of radial nerve
    (SBRN)
sensory deficit
sensory functions
sensory hyperesthesia
sensory loss

sensory nerve
sensory pathway
sensory tract
sentinel blood clot
sentinel cells
sentinel fold
sentinel gland
sentinel loop
sentinel node
sentinel pile
sentinel polyp
sentinel tag
Senturia forceps
Senturia pharyngeal speculum
Senturia retractor
Senturia speculum
SEP (somatosensory evoked
   potential)
separate stab wound
separated
separating wire
separation
separation anxiety
separator
   bayonet separator
   Benson pylorus separa-
      tor
   Benson separator
   curved zonule separator
   cylindrical zonule
      separator
   Davis nerve separator
   Davis separator
   Dorsey dural separator
   Dorsey separator
   double-ball separator
   dural separator
   flat zonule separator
   Frazier dural separator
   Frazier separator
   Grant separator
   Harris separator
   Hoen dural separator
   Hoen separator
   Horsley dural separator
   Horsley separator
   House separator

separator *continued*
   Hunter dural separator
   Hunter separator
   Kirby flat zonule
      separator
   Kirby intracapsular lens
      separator
   Kirby separator
   Luys separator
   posterior canal separator
   pylorus separator
   Remy separator
   Rosen separator
   Sachs dural separator
   Sachs nerve separator
   Sachs separator
   tonsillar separator
   Williger separator
   Woodson dural separator
      and packer
   zonule separator
sepsis
septa (*sing.* septum)
septal annuloplasty
septal bone forceps
septal branch
septal cartilage
septal chisel
septal clamp
septal compression forceps
septal defect
septal deviation
septal elevator
septal forceps
septal fracture
septal gouge
septal knife
septal lines
septal needle
septal posterior nasal arteries
septal punch
septal raphe
septal ridge forceps
septal scissors
septal separation
septal speculum
septal splint

septal straightener
septal trephine
septate hymen
septate uterus
septectomy
septi pellucidi, venae
septic
septic abortion
septic joint
septic process
septic shock
septic wound
septicemia
Septisol prep
Septisol soap dressing
septoplasty
septorhinoplasty
septostomy
septostomy balloon catheter
Septotome septum trimmer
septotomy
septum (*pl.* septa)
septum femorale
septum-cutting forceps
septum-straightening forceps
sequela (*pl.* sequelae)
sequence
sequential
sequential graft
sequestration
sequestrectomy
sequestrotomy
sequestrum (*pl.* sequestra)
sequestrum forceps
sequestrum formation
Sequicor II pacemaker
Sequicor III pacemaker
Sequicor pacemaker
SER fracture (supination, external rotation fracture)
SER-IV fracture
Serafini hernia
Seraflo A-V fistula needle sets
Seraphim clip
Serature clip
Serature spur clip
serial angiogram

serial chest x-rays
serial cholangiograms
serial EKGs
serial examinations
serial films
serial injection
serial sonography
serial studies
serial wedged cast
serially clamped
serially clamped, cut, and ligated
serially dilated
series
series II acetabular cup positioner
series II cup retainer
series II femoral broach
seriscission
serocystadenoma
serofibrinous
seromucous glands
seromuscular
seromuscular coat
seromuscular layer
seromuscular stitch
seromuscular sutures
seromuscular-to-edge sutures
seropurulent
seropurulent discharge
seropurulent sputum
serosa
serosal fibroids
serosal fold
serosal layer
serosal reflection
serosal surface
serosanguineous (also serosanguinous)
serosanguineous drainage
serosanguineous fluid
serosanguinous (see *serosanguineous*)
seroserosal
seroserosal silk
seroserosal silk sutures
seroserosal sutures

serous
serous fluid
serous glands
serous membrane
serous otitis media (SOM)
serous tumor
serpentine aneurysm
serpentine bone plate
serpentine incision
serpentine plate
serpiginous
serpiginous chancroid
serpiginous ulcer
serpiginous ulceration
serrate
serrated curet
serrated forceps
serrated grasping tip
serrated knife
serrated retractor
serrated scissors
serrated sutures
serrated T-spatula
Serratex scissors
Serratex-Mayo dissecting
    scissors
serratus anterior, musculus
serratus muscle
serratus, musculus
serratus posterior inferior,
    musculus
serratus posterior superior,
    musculus
Serre operation
serrefine (see also *forceps*)
serrefine clamp
serrefine forceps
serrefine implant
serrefine retractor
Sertoli cells
serum
serum transfusion
Servital prosthesis
Servo pump
Servo ventilator
Servox speech aid (post-
    laryngectomy)

sesamoid
sesamoid bones
sesamoid cartilages
sesamoidectomy dissector
sesamoiditis
sessile
sessile adenoma
sessile hydatid
sessile lesion
sessile polyp
setback
seton
seton drain
seton hip brace
seton needle
seton operation
seton sutures
seton tube
seton wound
Settegast position
setting
setup
Seutin bandage
Seutin plaster scissors
Seutin plaster shears
Sevastano knee prosthesis
seventh cranial nerve (VII)
sever
Sever operation
severance
severance transurethral bag
severe
severed
severed digit
severed limb
severed surface
severed tendon
severely
Severin intraocular lens
Severin lens
severing
severity of injury
Sever-L'Episcopo operation
Sever-L'Episcopo shoulder
    repair
Sewall antral cannula
Sewall antral trocar

Sewall brain clip-applying
   forceps
Sewall cannula
Sewall chisel
Sewall elevator
Sewall ethmoidal chisel
Sewall ethmoidal elevator
Sewall forceps
Sewall mucoperiosteal elevator
Sewall orbital retractor
Sewall raspatory
Sewall retractor
Sewall trocar
Sewell internal mammary
   implantation
Sewell-Boyden flap
Sewell-Boyden operation
SEWHO (shoulder-elbow-wrist-
   hand orthosis)
sewing ring
sewing-machine stitch sutures
sewn-in waterproof drape
SEX fracture (supination,
   external rotation fracture)
Sexton bayonet ear knife
Sexton ear knife
Sexton knife
Seyfert forceps
Seyfert speculum
SGA (small for gestational age)
SGIA stapler
SGIA staples
SGIA stapling device
Shaaf eye forceps
Shaaf forceps
Shaaf foreign body forceps
shadow
shadow cath
shadow-free laryngoscope
Shadow-Stripe catheter
Shaffer eye knife
shaft
shaft of bone
shaft of femur
shaft of fibula
shaft of humerus
shaft of phalanx

shaft reamer
shaggy pericardium
shagreen lesions of lens
shagreen patch
shagreen skin
Shahan ophthalmic lamp
Shahan thermophore
shaking
shaking sound
Shaldach pacemaker
Shaldon tube
Shallcross bone shears
Shallcross forceps
Shallcross gallbladder forceps
Shallcross hemostat
Shallcross hemostatic forceps
Shallcross nasal forceps
Shallcross nasal-packing forceps
Shallcross plaster shears
Shallcross rib shears
Shallcross screwdriver
Shallcross tonsillar hemostat
shallow breathing
shallow chamber
Shambaugh adenotome
Shambaugh elevator
Shambaugh endaural elevator
Shambaugh endaural hook
Shambaugh endaural incision
Shambaugh endaural retractor
Shambaugh  endaural self-
   retaining retractor
Shambaugh fistula hook
Shambaugh hook
Shambaugh incision
Shambaugh irrigator
Shambaugh knife
Shambaugh needle
Shambaugh operating micro-
   scope
Shambaugh retractor
Shambaugh technique
Shambaugh-Derlacki chisel
Shambaugh-Derlacki elevator
Shambaugh-Derlacki endaural
   elevator
Shambaugh-Derlacki knife

Shambaugh-Derlacki microhook
Shambaugh-Derlacki micro-
    scope
Shambaugh-Lempert knife
Shantz dressing
Shantz osteotomy
Shantz pin
shape
shaped
shaping
Shapiro internal fixation system
Shapiro sign
Shapleigh curet
Shapleigh ear curet
Sharley tracheostomy tube
sharp blow
sharp curet
Sharp derma curet
sharp disk
sharp dissection
sharp elevator
sharp hook
sharp incision
sharp pain
sharp spoon
sharp-and-slow wave
Sharpey fibers
Sharplan CO2 laser
Sharplan laser
Sharplav laparoscope
sharply demarcated
Sharpoint knife
Sharpoint microsurgical knife
Sharpoint slit knife
Sharpoint V-lance blade
sharp-pointed forceps
sharp-pronged retractor
sharps
sharp-toothed tenaculum
Sharpy fibers
Sharrard iliopsoas transfer
Sharrard kyphectomy
Sharrard operation
Sharrard transfer
Shastid punch
shatter hammer
shattering needle

shave biopsy
shaver catheter
Shaver sign
shaving
Shaw carotid artery clot
    stripper
Shaw carotid clot stripper
Shaw clot stripper
Shaw knife
Shaw operation
Shaw scalpel
Shaw tube
shawl scrotum
Shea bail-hook prosthesis
Shea bur
Shea curet
Shea drill
Shea ear drill
Shea elevator
Shea footplate hook
Shea headrest
Shea hook
Shea incision
Shea irrigator
Shea knife
Shea malleus gripper prosthesis
Shea pick
Shea polyethylene drainage
    tube
Shea prosthesis
Shea speculum holder
Shea stapedectomy
Shea Teflon piston prosthesis
Shea tube
Shea vein graft scissors
Shea-Anthony bag
Shea-Anthony balloon
Shea-Bellucci scissors
Shea-Hough incision
Shealy facet rhizotomy elec-
    trode
shear force
shear fracture
shear strain
shear stress
Shearer bone rongeur
Shearer chicken-bill forceps

Shearer chicken-bill rongeur
Shearer external fixation
  system
Shearer forceps
Shearer lip retractor
Shearer retractor
Shearer rongeur
Shearing intraocular implant
  lens
Shearing lens
shears (see also *rib shears*)
  Bacon rib shears
  Bacon thoracic shears
  Baer rib shears
  Bethune rib shears
  Bethune shears
  Bethune-Coryllos rib
    shears
  bone shears
  Brun plaster shears
  Brun plastic shears
  Brunner rib shears
  Clayton laminectomy
    shears
  Clayton shears
  Collin rib shears
  Cooley first-rib shears
  Cooley-Pontius shears
  Cooley-Pontius sternum
    shears
  Coryllos rib shears
  Coryllos-Bethune rib
    shears
  Coryllos-Moure rib
    shears
  Coryllos-Shoemaker rib
    shears
  Diertz shears
  Doyen rib shears
  Dubois shears
  Duval-Coryllos rib shears
  Eccentric locked rib
    shears
  Esmarch plaster shears
  Esmarch shears
  esophageal shears
  Exner rib shears

shears *continued*
  Frey-Sauerbruch rib
    shears
  Giertz rib shears
  Giertz-Shoemaker rib
    shears
  Giertz-Shoemaker
    shears
  Gluck rib shears
  Gluck shears
  Harrington-Mayo rib
    shears
  Horgan-Coryllos-Moure
    rib shears
  Horgan-Wells rib shears
  Horsley-Stille rib shears
  infant rib shears
  Jackson shears
  Jackson-Moore shears
  Kazanjian shears
  laminectomy shears
  laryngofissure shears
  Lebsche shears
  Liston shears
  Liston-Key Horsley rib
    shears
  Liston-Ruskin shears
  Moure-Coryllos rib
    shears
  Nelson-Bethune rib
    shears
  Pilling shears
  plaster shears
  Potts infant rib shears
  Potts rib shears
  Potts shears
  rib shears (see separate
    listing)
  Roberts shears
  Roberts-Nelson rib shears
  Roos first-rib shears
  Roos rib shears
  Sauerbruch rib shears
  Sauerbruch-Britsch rib
    shears
  Sauerbruch-Coryllos rib
    shears

shears *continued*

Sauerbruch-Frey rib
shears
Sauerbruch-Lebsche rib
shears
Schuchart pediatric rib
shears
Semb rib shears
Semb shears
Seutin plaster shears
Shallcross bone shears
Shallcross plaster shears
Shallcross rib shears
Shoemaker rib shears
Shoemaker shears
sternal shears
Stille plaster shears
Stille rib shears
Stille shears
Stille-Giertz rib shears
Stille-Horsley rib shears
Stille-pattern rib shears
Thompson rib shears
Thomson rib shears
Tudor-Edwards rib
shears
Walton rib shears
Weck shears

sheath

adventitial sheath
angioplasty sheath
anterior rectus sheath
arterial sheath
Bakelite resectoscope
sheath
beaked sheath
Berry rotating sheath
biceps tendon sheath
carotid sheath
catheter sheath
check-valve sheath
concave sheath and
obturator
connective tissue sheath
convex sheath and
obturator
Cook transseptal sheath

sheath *continued*

Cordis sheath
cystoscope sheath
dilator-sheath
documentation sheath
enamel rod sheath
external rectus sheath
fascial sheath
femoral artery sheath
femoral sheath
fiberoptic photographic
sheath
fiberoptic sheath
fibrous sheath
glial sheath
guiding sheath
Hemaquet sheath
hysteroscope sheath
incandescent sheath
integral fiberoptic sheath
introducer sheath
Mecron titanium
Voorhoeve sheath
medullated fibers and
sheaths
meniscotome sheath
Mullins sheath
Mullins transseptal
sheath
myelin sheath
O'Connor sheath
peel-away sheath
penile sheath
periosteum sheath
peroneal sheath
peroneal tendon sheath
posterior rectus sheath
rectus abdominis sheath
rectus sheath
resecting sheath
resectoscope sheath
root sheath
Scarpa sheath
Schwalbe sheath
Schwann sheath
sigmoidoscope docu-
mentation sheath

sheath *continued*
    split-sheath catheter
    Storz sheath
    subclavian peel-away
      sheath
    synovial sheath
    tearaway sheath
    Teflon sheath
    tendinous sheath
    tendon sheath
    transseptal sheath
    trocar sheath
    USCI angioplasty guiding
      sheath
    vascular sheath
    venous sheath
sheath and side-arm
sheath cystoscope
sheath of rectus abdominis
    muscle
sheath of rectus muscle
sheath with side-arm adapter
sheath-dilator
sheathed flexible gastric
    forceps
sheathed flexible gastroscopic
    forceps
Shea-TORP shunt
shedding
Sheehan chisel
Sheehan knee prosthesis
Sheehan nasal chisel
Sheehan osteotome
Sheehan retractor
Sheehan total knee prosthesis
Sheehy button
Sheehy canal knife
Sheehy collar-button tube
Sheehy forceps
Sheehy incus replacement
    prosthesis
Sheehy knife
Sheehy ossicle-holding clamp
Sheehy ossicle-holding forceps
Sheehy tube
Sheehy-House chisel
Sheehy-House incus replace-
    ment prosthesis

Sheehy-House knife
Sheehy-House prosthesis
sheen
Sheen airway reconstruction
Sheen tip graft
sheepskin dressing
Sheer probe
sheer spot Band-Aid dressing
sheet
sheet wadding
sheeting
Sheets cannula
Sheets cyclodialysis
Sheets glide
Sheets intraocular lens
Sheets irrigating vectis
Sheets lens
Sheets lens forceps
Sheets lens guide
Sheets intraocular lens
sheet-wadding dressing
Sheffield splint
Sheffield treadmill test
Sheinmann laryngeal forceps
Shekelton aneurysm
Sheldon catheter
Sheldon hemilaminectomy
    retractor
Sheldon hemilaminectomy self-
    retaining retractor
Sheldon retractor
Sheldon-Gosset self-retaining
    retractor
Sheldon-Pudenz dissector
Sheldon-Pudenz operation
Sheldon-Pudenz tube
Sheldon-Pudenz valve
Sheldon-Spatz needle
Sheldon-Swann needle
shelf hip procedure
shelf life
shelf operation
shelf osteotomy
shelf reamer
shelf reconstruction of acetabu-
    lum
shell eye implant
shell fragment

shell graft
shell implant
shell prosthesis
shellac-covered catheter
shelled out
shell-type eye implant
shell-type implant
Shelton plate
shelving edge
shelving edge of Poupart
    ligament
shelving incision
shelving operation
shelving portion of ligament
Shenstone tourniquet
Shenton arch
Shenton line
Shepard cannula
Shepard forceps
Shepard grommet tube
Shepard intraocular lens forceps
Shepard intraocular lens implant
Shepard intraocular lens-
    inserting forceps
Shepard lens
Shepard lens forceps
Shepard osteotome
Shepard scissors
Shepard Teflon tube
Shepard tube
Shepard ventilation tube
Shepard-Reinstein intraocular
    lens forceps
Shepherd fracture
Shepherd hook catheter
shepherd's crook deformity of
    proximal femur
Sheridan tube
Sherk-Probst technique
Sherman bone plates
Sherman bone screw
Sherman knife
Sherman molybdenum screw
Sherman plate
Sherman plate and screws
Sherman screw
Sherman screwdriver

Sherman suction tube
Sherman Vitallium screw
Sherman-Pierce screwdriver
Sherman-Stille drill
Sherwin self-retaining retractor
Sherwood retractor
shield (see also *eye shield*)
    aluminum eye shield
    AME PinSite shield
    Barraquer eye shield
    binocular shield
    bronchoscopic face
        shield
    Buller eye shield
    Carapace disposable face
        shield
    circumcisional shield
    Dacron shield
    eye shield
    face shield
    Faraday shield
    Fox aluminum eye shield
    Fox eye shield
    Fuller shield
    gonad shield
    Green shield
    lead shield
    Mueller shield
    protective eye shield
    Storz face shield
    Universal eye shield
shield incision
shielding
Shier knee prosthesis
Shier prosthesis
Shiffrin bone wire
Shiffrin wire crimper
shift
shift to the left
shift to the right
shifting
shifting border
shifting dullness
shifting dullness on percussion
shifting pacemaker
Shiley cardioplegia system
Shiley catheter

Shiley endotracheal tube
Shiley French sump tube
Shiley guiding catheter
Shiley heart valve
Shiley JL-4 guiding catheter
Shiley JR-4 guiding catheter
Shiley MultiPro catheter
Shiley oxygenator
Shiley shunt
Shiley soft-tip guiding catheter
Shiley sump tube
Shiley tracheostomy tube
Shiley tube
Shiley valve
Shiley-Björk tube
Shiley-Ionescu catheter
Shiller solution
shin bone
Shiner tube
Shin-Pak
shiny material
Shipps cholangiographic tunnel
Shirodkar cerclage
Shirodkar needle
Shirodkar operation
Shirodkar probe
Shirodkar sutures
Shirodkar-Barter cervical
    cerclage
Shirodkar-Barter operation
Shirodkar-McDonald cervical
    repair
Shirodkar-Page cerclage
SHJR4s catheter (side-hole
    Judkins right, curve 4, short
    catheter)
Shober index for spondylitis
shock
shock liver
shock position
shocky
shoe-and-stocking position
shoehorn speculum
shoelace-type repair
Shoemaker (see also *Schoe-
    maker, Schumacher,
    Schumaker*)

Shoemaker intestinal clamp
Shoemaker rib shears
Shoemaker rongeur
Shoemaker shears
Shoepinger incision
shooting pains
short abductor muscle
short adductor muscle
short anconeus muscle
short arc exercises
short axis
short bundle colonoscope
short bursts
short calcaneocuboid ligament
short ciliary arteries
short ciliary nerves
short course
short crus of incus
short extensor muscle
short fibular muscle
short flexor muscle
short gastric arteries
short gastric branch of lienal
    artery
short gastric veins
short Heaney retractor
short increment sensitivity index
    (SISI)
short levator muscles
short needle
short of breath (SOB)
short palmar muscle
short peroneal muscle
short plantar ligament
short posterior ciliary artery
short posterior ciliary axis
short pulse
short QRS complex
short radial extensor muscle
short rectangular flap
short rod
short rotator muscles
short-acting barbiturate
short-arm cast (SAC)
Shortbent scissors
Shortbent stitch scissors
short-bowel syndrome

shortening
shortening of bone
shortening of eyeball
shortening of ocular muscle
shortening of round ligament
shortening of sacrouterine
    ligament
shortening of tendon
short-gut syndrome
shorthand vertical mattress
    stitch suture technique
short-leg brace
short-leg cast (SLC)
short-leg walking cast (SLWC)
short-length tracheal tube
short-lived
shortness of breath (SOB)
short-term
short-tip bag
short-tip hemostatic bag
short-tooth forceps
short-wave diathermy
short-winded
shot compressor
shot-gun approach
shot-perforated
shot-silk retina
shotted sutures
shotty lymph node
shotty node
shoulder
shoulder arthrodesis
shoulder blade
shoulder brace
shoulder drop
shoulder girdle
shoulder impingement syn-
    drome
shoulder joint
shoulder pointer
shoulder prosthesis
shoulder subluxation inhibitor
    (SSI) brace
shoulder-elbow-wrist-hand
    orthosis (SEWHO)
shoulder-strap incision
Shouldice hernia repair

Shouldice herniorrhaphy
Shouldice inguinal hernia repair
Shouldice inguinal hernior-
    rhaphy
shoveller's fracture
shovel-shaped incisor
ShowerSafe cast and bandage
    protector
Shrady saw
shrapnel fragment
shred
Shriners Hospital instruments
Shriners Hospital interlocking
    retractor
Shriners Hospital retractor
Shriners pin
shrinking
shriveled
shrunken
shrunken liver
Shug device for male contracep-
    tion
Shugrue operation
Shuletz raspatory
Shunn gun
Shunn gun transilluminator
shunt
    Allen-Brown shunt
    Ames shunt
    Ames ventriculoperi-
        toneal shunt
    aorta to pulmonary
        artery shunt
    aorticopulmonary shunt
    aortopulmonary shunt
    arteriovenous shunt
    ascending aorta to
        pulmonary artery
        shunt
    ascites shunt
    Assal-Javid cerebrospinal
        shunt
    AV shunt
    balloon shunt
    Beck shunt
    bidirectional shunt
    biliopancreatic shunt

shunt *continued*
Blalock shunt
Blalock-Taussig shunt
Brenner carotid bypass
shunt
Buselmeier shunt
cardiac shunt
cardiovascular shunt
carotid bypass shunt
carotid endarterectomy
shunt
carotid shunt
cavamesenteric shunt
Cavin shunt
central nervous system
shunt
cerebrospinal fluid shunt
Cimino arteriovenous
shunt
Codman shunt
conventional shunt
Cordis Hakim shunt
CSF shunt system
Denver hydrocephalus
shunt
Denver peritoneal-
venous shunt
descending thoracic
aorta to pulmonary
artery shunt
dialysis shunt
distal splenorenal shunt
Dow Corning shunt
Drapanas mesocaval
shunt
Drapanas shunt
endolymphatic subarach-
noid shunt
end-to-side portacaval
shunt
esophageal shunt
extracardiac shunt
Fischer shunt
Foltz shunt
Foltz-Overton shunt
function shunt
Garner balloon shunt

shunt *continued*
gastric vena caval shunt
Glenn shunt
Gore-Tex shunt
Gott shunt
Gott-Daggett shunt
Groshong shunt
H-H neonatal shunt for
hydrocephalus
Hakim shunt
Hepacon shunt
Heyer-Schulte shunt
instruments
Heyer-Schulte shunt
system
Holter shunt
House shunt
Hyde shunt
hydrocephalus shunt
Inahara shunt
Inahara-Pruitt vascular
shunt
initial venous shunt
input shunt
interposition mesocaval
H-graft shunt
intracardiac shunt
intrapericardial aortico-
pulmonary shunt
intrapulmonary shunt
Javid bypass shunt
Javid endarterectomy
shunt
Javid internal carotid
shunt
Javid shunt
L-R shunt (left-to-right
shunt)
left-to-right shunt (L-R
shunt)
LeVeen dialysis shunt
LeVeen peritoneal shunt
LeVeen peritoneovenous
shunt
Levine shunt
Linton shunt
lumboperitoneal shunt

shunt *continued*

magnitude shunt
mesobi-ileal shunt
mesocaval H-graft shunt
mesocaval interposition
   shunt
mesocaval shunt
Mischler shunt
Mischler-Pudenz shunt
modified shunt
net shunt
obstructed shunt
Ommaya shunt
otic shunt
Overton shunt
parietal shunt
peritoneal shunt
peritoneal-atrial shunt
peritoneal-venous shunt
peritoneocaval shunt
peritoneovenous shunt
PFTE shunt (polyfluoro-
   tetraethylene shunt)
Polystan shunt
portacaval shunt
portal shunt
portal to systemic venous
   shunt
portal-systemic shunt
Portnoy ventricular-end
   shunt
portopulmonary shunt
portorenal shunt
portosystemic shunt
portosystemic vascular
   shunt
postcaval shunt
Potts shunt
proximal splenorenal
   shunt
Pruitt-Inahara autoperfu-
   sion shunt
Pruitt-Inahara carotid
   shunt
Pruitt-Inahara vascular
   shunt
Pudenz shunt

shunt *continued*

Pudenz ventriculoatrial
   shunt
Pudenz-Heyer shunt
R-L shunt (right-to-left
   shunt)
Raimondi shunt
Ramirez arteriovenous
   shunt
Ramirez shunt
reversed shunt (right-to-
   left)
right-to-left shunt (R-L
   shunt)
Rostan shunt
Scribner arteriovenous
   shunt
Scribner shunt
selective distal spleno-
   renal shunt
Shea-TORP shunt
Shiley shunt
side-to-side portacaval
   shunt
Silastic shunt
Silastic ventriculoperi-
   toneal shunt
small-bowel shunt
Spetzler lumboperitoneal
   shunt
Spetzler shunt
Spitz-Holter VA shunt
splenorenal shunt
spongiosa shunt
subarachnoid shunt
systemic-pulmonary
   artery shunt
temporary aortic shunt
Torkildsen shunt
Uresil Vascu-Flo carotid
   shunt
Vascu-Flo carotid shunt
Vascushunt
vena cava to pulmonary
   artery shunt
venous shunt
ventriculoatrial shunt

shunt *continued*
    ventriculocaval shunt
    ventriculocisternal shunt
    ventriculoperitoneal shunt
    Vitagraft arteriovenous shunt
    VP shunt (ventriculoperitoneal shunt)
    Warren shunt
    Warren splenorenal shunt
    Waterston shunt
    Waterston-Cooley shunt
    winged shunt
    Winters shunt
shunt cyanosis
shunt for aortic aneurysm
shunt function
shunt infection
shunt obstruction
shunt operation
shunt site
shunt system
shunt tube
shunt-site drainage
shunt-site leaking
shunt-site oozing
shunt-tube introducer
Shuppe biting forceps
Shur-Clens
Shurly retractor
Shur-Strip tape
Shur-Strip wound closure tape
Shuster forceps
Shuster suture forceps
Shuster tonsillar forceps
shutoff clamp
Shutt forceps
Shutt grasper
Shutt grasping forceps
Shutt hook
Shutt minibasket
Shutt punch
Shutt scissors
shuttle forceps
sialadenectomy

sialadenotomy
sialoadenectomy
sialoadenolithotomy
sialoadenotomy
sialodochoplasty
sialogram
sialography
sialolithotomy
sialosyrinx
sibilant rale
Sibson fascia
Sibson notch
Sibson vestibule
Sichel implant
Sichel iris knife
Sichel knife
Sichel movable implant
Sichel orbital implant
sick sinus syndrome
sickle
sickle cell anemia
sickle knife
sickle middle-ear knife
sickle tonsillar knife
sickle-shaped Beaver blade
sickle-shaped blade
sickle-shaped House knife
sickle-shaped knife
SICOR cardiac catheterization system
side channel of scope
side effect
side mouth gag
side plate
side view
side-arm adapter
side-biting clamp
side-curved forceps
side-curved rongeur
side-cutting spatulated needle
side-flattened needle
side-grasping forceps
side-hole catheter
side-hole pigtail catheter
sideline examination
sideswipe fracture
side-to-end anastomosis

side-to-side anastomosis
side-to-side jejunal pouch
side-to-side portacaval shunt
side-to-side vein bypass
side-viewing endoscope
side-viewing fiberscope
side-viewing scope
sidewall infusion cannula
sidewinder catheter
Siebold pubiotomy
Siebold uterine scissors
Siegel otoscope
Siegel technique
Siegle otoscope
Siegle speculum
Siegler-Hellman clamp
Siemens cyclographic tomogram
Siemens Lithostar
Siemens Orbix head unit
Siemens Orbix image intensifier
Siemens PTCA open-heart
    sutures
Siemens Servo ventilator
Siemens-Elema AB pulse
    transducer
Siemens-Elema multiprogram-
    mable pacemaker
Siemens-Elema pacemaker
Siemens-Pacesetter pacemaker
Sierra-Sheldon trabeculotome
Sierra-Sheldon tracheotome
sieve
sieve graft
sievelike pores
Siffert-Forster-Nachamie
    clubfoot procedure
sigmoid
sigmoid anastomosis
sigmoid arteries
sigmoid bladder
sigmoid clamp
sigmoid colon
sigmoid colostomy
sigmoid flexure
sigmoid folds
sigmoid loop
sigmoid loop colostomy

sigmoid mesocolon
sigmoid notch
sigmoid sinus
sigmoid speculum
sigmoid veins
sigmoid volvulus
sigmoidal branch of inferior
    mesenteric artery
sigmoideae, arteriae
sigmoideae, venae
sigmoidectomy
sigmoid-end colostomy
sigmoid-loop rod colostomy
sigmoidocutaneous fistula
sigmoidopexy
sigmoidoproctectomy
sigmoidoproctostomy
sigmoidorectostomy
sigmoidorrhaphy
sigmoidoscope
    ACMI fiberoptic procto-
        sigmoidoscope
    ACMI flexible sigmoido-
        scope
    ACMI proctosigmoido-
        scope
    adult sigmoidoscope
    anosigmoidoscope
    Boehm sigmoidoscope
    Buie sigmoidoscope
    disposable sigmoido-
        scope
    Eder sigmoidoscope
    ESI sigmoidoscope
    fiberoptic procto-
        sigmoidoscope
    fiberoptic sigmoido-
        scope
    flexible sigmoidoscope
    Frankfeldt sigmoido-
        scope
    Fujinon flexible
        sigmoidoscope
    Gorsch sigmoidoscope
    Heinkel sigmoidoscope
    Hopkins sigmoidoscope
    Kelly sigmoidoscope

sigmoidoscope *continued*
    KleenSpec disposable
       sigmoidoscope
    KleenSpec sigmoido-
       scope
    Lieberman sigmoido-
       scope
    Lloyd-Davis sigmoido-
       scope
    Montague sigmoido-
       scope
    Olympus fiberoptic
       sigmoidoscope
    Olympus flexible
       sigmoidoscope
    Olympus sigmoidoscope
    Pentax fiberoptic
       sigmoidoscope
    Pentax flexible sigmoido-
       scope
    proctosigmoidoscope
    rectosigmoidoscope
    Reichert fiberoptic
       sigmoidoscope
    Reichert flexible
       sigmoidoscope
    Reichert sigmoidoscope
    rigid sigmoidoscope
    Solow sigmoidoscope
    Strauss sigmoidoscope
    Turrell sigmoidoscope
    Tuttle sigmoidoscope
    Welch Allyn flexible
       sigmoidoscope
    Welch Allyn sigmoido-
       scope
    Yeomans sigmoidoscope
sigmoidoscope biopsy forceps
sigmoidoscope documentation
    sheath
sigmoidoscope inflation bulb
sigmoidoscope insulated
    suction tube
sigmoidoscope suction tube
sigmoidoscope with swinging
    window
sigmoidoscopy

sigmoidoscopy table
sigmoidoscopy with rectal
    polypectomy
sigmoidosigmoidostomy
sigmoidostomy
sigmoidotomy
sigmoidovesical
sign mechanism for ventilator
    breathing
sign of clearing
signal
signet-ring carcinoma
signet-ring cell carcinoma
signet-ring pattern
significance
significant
significant abnormality
significant pathology
signs and symptoms
Sigualt symphysiotomy
Sigvaris compression
    stockings
Sigvaris stockings
Sigvaris support stockings
Siker laryngoscope
Silastic
Silastic adhesive
Silastic bead embolization
Silastic cannula
Silastic catheter
Silastic collar-reinforced stoma
Silastic corneal implant
Silastic coronary artery cannula
Silastic Cronin implant
Silastic Cronin medical adhesive
    silicone
Silastic Cystocath
Silastic disk heart valve
Silastic drain
Silastic dressing
Silastic eye implant
Silastic graft
Silastic grommet
Silastic HP 100 Swanson flexible
    toe hinge
Silastic HP tissue expander
Silastic implant

Silastic injection
Silastic keel of vomer
Silastic loop
Silastic mammary prosthesis
Silastic material
Silastic mushroom catheter
Silastic obstetrical vacuum cup
Silastic patch
Silastic penile prosthesis
Silastic plate
Silastic prosthesis
Silastic prosthetic sizer
Silastic ring
Silastic scleral buckler implant
Silastic sheet
Silastic shunt
Silastic silicone rubber implants
Silastic silo
Silastic silo reduction of
   gastroschisis
Silastic sphere
Silastic sponge
Silastic stent
Silastic subdermal implant
Silastic tape
Silastic testicular prosthesis
Silastic thyroid drain
Silastic tube
Silastic ventriculoperitoneal
   shunt
silent abdomen
silent area
silent attack
silent chest
silent gallstone
silent infection
Silesian bandage
Silesian belt
Silesian belt suspension
Silfverskiold knee procedure
silhouette
silhouette sign
silicate filling
silicon ion therapy
silicon nitride
silicone
silicone ball heart valve

silicone cannula
silicone copolymer
silicone doughnut prosthesis
silicone drain
silicone dressing
silicone elastomer band
silicone elastomer catheter
silicone elastomer infusion
   catheter
silicone eye implant
silicone implant
silicone prosthesis
silicone ring
silicone rod implant
silicone rods
silicone rubber
silicone rubber Dacron-cuffed
   catheter
silicone rubber joint
silicone sleeve
silicone sponge
silicone sponge implant
silicone sump drain
silicone thoracic drain
silicone tube
silicone-filled breast implant
silicone-treated surgical silk
   sutures
silicone-treated sutures
Silicore catheter
Silitek catheter
Silitek ureteral stent
silk glove sign
silk implantation
silk interrupted mattress sutures
silk pop-off sutures
silk seton
silk sign
silk stay sutures
silk sutures
silk ties
silk traction suture
silk-and-wax catheter
silk-braided sutures
silkworm gut
silkworm gut sutures
Silon pouch chimney

Silon tent
Silovi incision
Silovi procedure
Silovi saphenous vein bypass
	graft
Siloxane graft
Siloxane implant
Siloxane prosthesis
Silva-Costa operation
Silvadene
Silver bunionectomy
Silver cannula
Silver chisel
silver clip
Silver forceps
Silver knife
silver material
silver nitrate cautery
silver nitrate cautery stick
Silver osteotome
silver probe
Silver procedure
silver saw
silver suture wire
silver sutures
silver-fork deformity
silver-fork fracture
Silver-Hildreth eyelid operation
silverized catgut sutures
Silverman biopsy needle
Silverman needle
Silverman-Boeker needle
Silver-Skin bunionectomy
Silverstein dressing
Silverstein malleus clip wire
Silverstein tube
silver-wire appearance of retinal
	arteries
silver-wiring of retinal arteries
SIMA reconstruction (single
	internal mammary artery
	reconstruction)
Simcoe anterior chamber lens
Simcoe eye implant
Simcoe handpiece
Simcoe I&A unit
Simcoe implant

Simcoe intraocular implant lens
Simcoe intraocular lens implant
Simcoe lens
Simcoe needle
Simcoe posterior chamber lens
Simcoe-Amo eye implant
Simmons catheter
Simmons chisel
Simmons osteotome
Simmons screw
Simmons technique
Simmons-Martin screw
Simon bone curet
Simon cheiloplasty
Simon colpocleisis
Simon dermatome
Simon fistula hook
Simon incision
Simon operation
Simon perineorrhaphy
Simon position
Simon retractor
Simon sign
Simon speculum
Simon spinal curet
Simon sutures
Simon vaginal speculum
Simonart band
Simons stone-removing forceps
simple comminuted fracture
simple dislocation
simple excision
simple fracture
simple ganglion
simple interrupted fashion
simple iridectomy
simple joint
simple mastectomy
simple mastoidectomy
simple mechanical obstruction
simple microscope
simple operation
simple reflex
simple sinusotomy
simple skull fracture
simple sutures
Simplex adhesive

Simplex cement
Simplex mastoid rongeur
Simplex P&C cement
Simplex P cement
Simplus catheter
Simplus dilatation catheter
Simpson antral curet
Simpson atherectomy
Simpson AtheroCath catheter
Simpson atherectomy catheter
Simpson curet
Simpson forceps
Simpson hysteropexy
Simpson lacrimal dilator
Simpson lacrimal probe
Simpson light
Simpson obstetrical forceps
Simpson operation
Simpson PET balloon atherec-
    tomy device
Simpson sound
Simpson splint
Simpson sugar-tong splint
Simpson tampon
Simpson Ultra Lo-Profile II
    balloon catheter
Simpson uterine dilator
Simpson uterine sound
Simpson-Luikart forceps
Simpson-Luikart obstetrical
    forceps
Simpson-Robert ACS dilatation
    catheter
Simpson-Robert ACS guide wire
Simpson-Robert catheter
Simpulse irrigating system
Simpulse lavage system
Simpulse pulsed lavage
Simrock speculum
Sims anoscope
Sims cannula
Sims curet
Sims dilator
Sims double-ended retractor
Sims double-ended speculum
Sims general operating scissors
Sims knife

Sims needle
Sims plug
Sims position
Sims probe
Sims proctoscope
Sims rectal retractor
Sims rectal speculum
Sims retractor
Sims scissors
Sims sound
Sims speculum
Sims suction tip
Sims sutures
Sims tenaculum
Sims uterine curet
Sims uterine dilator
Sims uterine probe
Sims uterine scissors
Sims uterine sound
Sims vaginal decompressor
Sims vaginal retractor
Sims-Kelly retractor
Sims-Kelly vaginal retractor
Sims-Maier sponge and dressing
    forceps
Sims-Siebold uterine scissors
simulate
simulation
simulator
simultaneous
sine qua non
Sinexon dilator
Singer needle
Singer portable apparatus
Singer-Blom electrolarynx
    prosthesis
Singer-Blom tube
Singer-Blom valve
singer's node
singer's nodule
single circular saw
single cross-slot screwdriver
single injection anesthesia
single need catheter
single onlay cortical bone graft
single-armed sutures
single-balloon valvotomy

single-balloon valvuloplasty
single-chamber pacemaker
single-contrast study
single-fiber EMG electrode
single-guarded osteotome
single-handed knot sutures
single-J urinary diversion stent
single-pass pacemaker
single-phase current
single-plane angiogram
single-puncture laparoscopy
single-rod penile prosthesis
single-stage catheter
single-stage omphalocele repair
Singleton incision
Singleton trocar
single-tooth tenaculum
single-toothed tenaculum
single-use dermatome
single-wire electrode
Singley clamp
Singley forceps
Singley intestinal clamp
Singley intestinal forceps
Singley intestinal tissue forceps
Singley tissue forceps
Singley-Tuttle dressing forceps
Singley-Tuttle tissue forceps
singultus gastricus nervosus
sinoatrial
sinoauricular
sinodural angle
sinogram
sinography
sinospiral muscle bundle
sinotubular junction
sinoventricular
Sinskey blue loop intraocular
   lenses
Sinskey forceps
Sinskey hook
Sinskey intraocular lens
Sinskey intraocular lens forceps
Sinskey lens
Sinskey lens implant
Sinskey posterior chamber
   intraocular lens

Sinskey posterior chamber lens
Sinskey-McPherson forceps
Sinskey-Wilson forceps
Sinskey-Wilson foreign body
   forceps
SinStat preformed skin staple
sinuous incision
sinus (pl. sinuses)
sinus antral cannula
sinus arrest
sinus arrhythmia
sinus balloon
sinus biopsy forceps
sinus block
sinus bradycardia
sinus bur
sinus cannula
sinus chisel
sinus curet
sinus defect
sinus dilator
sinus drainage
sinus groove
sinus in the tentorium
sinus nerve
sinus node
sinus node pacemaker
sinus operation
sinus pacemaker
sinus probe
sinus punch
sinus rasp
sinus rhythm
sinus suction syringe
sinus tachycardia
sinus tract
sinus tympani excavator
sinus wash bottle
sinus wash tube
sinusectomy
sinus-irrigating cannula
sinusography
sinusoid
sinusoidal circulation
sinusoidal spaces
sinusotomy
sinu-vertebral nerve

siphon
siphon suction tube
siphonage
Sippy dilating olives
Sippy dilator
Sippy esophageal dilator
Sippy point
sireniform fetus
sirenomelia
Sisson forceps
Sisson fracture-reducing
    elevator
Sisson hook
Sisson-Cottle septal speculum
Sisson-Love retractor
Sisson-Vienna nasal speculum
Sister Mary Joseph lymph node
Sister Mary Joseph node
Sistrunk band retractor
Sistrunk dissecting scissors
Sistrunk double-ended retractor
Sistrunk operation
Sistrunk retractor
Sistrunk scissors
site
SITE argon laser
SITE aspiration machine
SITE irrigation machine
SITE laser
SITE microsurgical instrument
sitting position
sitting-up view angiogram
situation
situational
situs
situs inversus
situs inversus viscerum
situs perversus
situs solitus
situs transversus
Sivash hip prosthesis
Sivash hip replacement
Sivash prosthesis
six-eye catheter
six-hole stainless steel plate
six-prong rake retractor
sixth cranial nerve (VI)

size and condition normal
sizer
Sjöqvist operation
skate flap
Skeele chalazion curet
Skeele corneal curet
Skeele curet
Skeele eye curet
Skeggs-Leonard dialyzer
skeletal abnormalities
skeletal deformity
skeletal maturation
skeletal muscle
skeletal pin
skeletal series
skeletal structure
skeletal tissue
skeletal traction
skeletalization
skeleton
skeleton hand
skeletonize
skeletonized
Skene catheter
Skene duct
Skene forceps
Skene glands
Skene spoon
Skene tenaculum
Skene uterine curet
Skene uterine forceps
Skene uterine spoon
Skene uterine spoon curet
Skene uterine tenaculum
Skene uterine vulsellum
Skene vulsellum forceps
skenoscope
skewfoot
ski needle
ski position
skiagram study
skiametry
skid
    Austin Moore-Murphy
        bone skid
    bone skid
    Davis bone skid

skid *continued*
    Davis skid
    hip skid
    MacAusland skid
    Meyerding bone skid
    Meyerding skid
    Murphy bone skid
    Murphy-Lane bone skid
    Murphy-Lane skid
    Scudder skid
Skil Saw
skill
skilled movements
skilled nursing facility
Skillern cannula
Skillern curet
Skillern forceps
Skillern fracture
Skillern phimosis forceps
Skillern probe
Skillern punch
Skillern sinus curet
Skillern sinus probe
Skillern sphenoid cannula
Skillern sphenoid probe
Skillman forceps
Skillman hemostatic forceps
Skillman prepuce forceps
skin barrier
skin biopsy
skin breakdown
skin cancer
skin clip
skin closed
skin closure strips
skin crease
skin dry and itchy
skin edges approximated
skin elevator
skin exfoliation
skin flap
skin flap retractor
skin flap rotation
skin forceps
skin graft
skin graft hook
skin graft knife

skin grafting
skin gun
skin hook
skin incision
skin integrity
skin knife
skin layers
skin lesion
skin lines
skin loss
skin maceration
skin margins
skin markings
skin mesh
skin moist
skin numbness
skin pale
skin pallor
skin pencil
skin planing
skin preparation
skin rash
skin reaction
skin relaxation
skin response
skin retractor
skin self-retaining retractor
Skin Skribe pen
skin splint
skin spots
skin staples
skin stitch
skin surface
skin sutures
skin sutures intact
skin tag
skin test
skin towels
skin traction
skin turgor
skin window
skin-adipose superficial
    musculoaponeurotic system
    (SASMAS)
skin-adipose unit (SA unit)
Skin-Cottle hook
skin-equivalent tissue

skinfold
skinfold calipers
skinfold incision
skinline incision
skinned
skinning colpectomy
skinning vaginectomy
skinning vulvectomy
skinning vulvovaginectomy
skinny Chiba needle
skinny needle
skinny needle cholangiography
skinny-nose rongeur
skip lesion
skipped beat
skive
skiving knife
Sklar anoscope
Sklar bone pin cutter
Sklar cutter
Sklar evacuator
Sklar proctoscope
Sklar tonometer
Sklar-Junior Tompkins aspirator
Sklar-Kleen
Sklar-Schiøtz jewel tonometer
Sklar-Schiøtz tonometer
Skoda rale
Skoda sign
Skoda tympany
skodaic resonance
skodaic tympany
Skoog cleft lip repair
Skoog fasciectomy
Skoog incision in palmar
   fasciectomy
Skoog mammaplasty
Skoog method
Skoog nasal chisel
Skoog operation
Skoog procedure for Dupuytren
   contracture
Skoog release of Dupuytren
   contracture
Skoog technique
skull
skull base

skull bur
skull clamp
skull closure
skull cone punch
skull film
skull fracture
skull plate
skull radiography
skull saw
skull survey
skull tantalum
skull tongs
skull traction
skull traction drill
skull tractor
skull trephine
skyline projection
skyline view
skyline view of patella
Skytron air-fluidized bed
Skytron operating table
SLAC (scapholunate advanced
   collapse)
SLAC wrist
slant
slant muscle operation
Slatis frame
Slaughter nasal saw
Slaughter saw
SLC (short-leg cast)
Sled implant
sleeper sutures
sleeve
> Dent sleeve
> Dunlop sleeve
> Hemmer connection
>    sleeve
> Keene self-sealing sleeve
>    and obturator
> laparoscopic trocar
>    sleeve
> Lidge reducer sleeve
> Malleotrain ankle sleeve
> mucosal sleeve resection
> neoprene sleeve
> Palumbo sleeve
> root sleeve

sleeve *continued*
    silicone sleeve
    Supramid ptosis sleeve
    Watzke silicone sleeve
    Watzke sleeve
    Williams overtube sleeve
sleeve adapter
sleeve clot
sleeve graft
sleeve lobectomy
sleeve-resection circumcision
sleeve-spreading dilating
    forceps
slender-nose rongeur
slender-tip scissors
slice graft
slide plate
slide specimen
sliding capsule forceps
sliding esophageal hiatal hernia
sliding flap
sliding hernia
sliding hiatal hernia
sliding inguinal hernia
sliding inlay bone graft
sliding laryngoscope
sliding microtome
sliding nail
sliding skin flap technique
sliding technique
sliding-type hiatal hernia
slight deformity
slightly curved ear pick
slightly curved pick
slightly displaced
sling
    acromioclavicular
      dislocation harness
      sling
    adjustable strap arm
      sling
    Bobath sling
    CircOlectric sling
    clavicle strap sling
    Colles sling
    cradle arm sling
    fascial sling

sling *continued*
    Freidenwald-Guyton
      sling
    frontalis sling
    Glisson sling
    Goebel-Stoeckel sling
    hand cock-up sling
    Harris sling
    Hoyer lift sling
    levator sling
    Marlex mesh sling
    Mason-Allen Universal
      sling
    Meek clavicle sling
    pelvic sling
    pericardial sling
    Posey sling
    ptosis sling
    pulmonary artery sling
    Rainbow envelope arm
      sling
    Rauchfuss sling
    Sayre head sling
    Snoopy arm sling
    strap sling
    Supramid ptosis sling
    suspension sling
    Teare arm sling
    Teare sling
    Veeder tip sling
    Velpeau sling
    Weil pelvic sling
    Weil sling
    Zimmer arm sling
    Zimmer clavicular cross
      sling
    Zimmer sling
sling dressing
sling operation
sling sutures
sling-and-swathe bandage
slip hernia
slip-joint pliers
slip-knot ties
slipped capital femoral epiphy-
    sis
slipped disk

slipped epiphysis
slipped hernia
slipped meniscus
slipped Nissen fundoplication
slipper cast
slipping epiphysis
slipping patella
slipping ribs
slit
slit illuminator
slit lamp (see also *light*)
    binocular slit lamp
    Gullstrand slit lamp
    Haag slit lamp
    Haag-Streit slit lamp
    Kowa hand-held slit
      lamp
    Kowa slit lamp
    Reichert slit lamp
    Thorpe slit lamp
    Zeiss slit lamp
slit scanography
slit-lamp camera attachment
slit-lamp examination
slit-lamp instrument table
slit-lamp microscope
slitting
slitting of canaliculus
sliver
sliver bone graft
Sloan abdominal incision
Sloan dissector
Sloan goiter flap dissector
Sloan goiter retractor
Sloan goiter self-retaining
    retractor
Sloan incision
Sloan retractor
Slocum amputation tech-
    nique
Slocum anterior rotary drawer
    test
Slocum elevator
Slocum knee repair
Slocum meniscal clamp
Slocum operation
Slocum pes transfer

Slocum splint
Slocum test
Slocum-Smith-Petersen nail
slope
sloping surface
slot incision
slotted bronchoscope
slotted handle
slotted laryngoscope
slotted needle vent
slotted plate
slotted screw
slotted speculum
slotted sutures
slotted wrench
slotting bur
slotting-bur osteotome
slot-type rim incision
slough
sloughed area
sloughing
sloughing of skin
slough off
slow continuous ultrafiltration
    therapy (SCUF therapy)
slow infusion IV drip
slow phleboclysis
slow spike and wave
slow wave
slowly developing
slowly growing
slowness
slow-twitch fibers
SLR test (straight leg-raising test)
Sluder adenotome
Sluder cautery electrode
Sluder guillotine
Sluder headband
Sluder hook
Sluder knife
Sluder mouth gag
Sluder needle
Sluder palate retractor
Sluder retractor
Sluder speculum
Sluder sphenoidal hook
Sluder sphenoidal speculum

Sluder tonometer
Sluder tonsillar guillotine
Sluder tonsillar knife
Sluder tonsillectome
Sluder tonsillectomy
Sluder Universal handle
Sluder-Ballenger tonsillectome
Sluder-Demarest tonometer
Sluder-Ferguson mouth gag
Sluder-Jansen mouth gag
Sluder-Mehta electrode
Sluder-Sauer guillotine
Sluder-Sauer tonometer
Sluder-Sauer tonsil guillotine
Sluder-Sauer tonsillectome
sludged blood
sluggish reaction
sluggishly
sluggishness
Slumber mask
slush
SLWC (short-leg walking cast)
SMA (superior mesenteric artery)
smacking
small blood vessel
small bone chisel
small bone-cutting forceps
small bowel
small brass mallet
small caliber
small cardiac vein
small cell carcinoma
small circumflex system
small for gestational age (SGA)
small head mallet
small intestine
small loop electrode
small pelvis
small pick
Small rake retractor
small saphenous vein
small sciatic nerve
small spring scissors
small square-groove silicone
Small tissue retractor
small uterus

small-bowel enema
small-bowel follow-through
small-bowel meal
small-bowel obstruction (SBO)
small-bowel resection
small-bowel series
small-bowel shunt
small-bowel tube
Small-Carrion penile prosthesis
Small-Carrion semirigid penile prosthesis
Small-Carrion Silastic rod for penile implant
small-cell carcinoma
small-cell tumor
small-droplet fatty liver
smaller pectoral muscle
smaller psoas muscle
smallest adductor muscle
smallest cardiac veins
smallest scalene muscle
small-loop electrode
Smart chalazion forceps
Smart enucleation scissors
Smart forceps
smart laser
Smart nonslipping chalazion forceps
Smart scissors
SMAS (superficial musculo-aponeurotic system)
SMAS face-lift technique
SMAS fascia
SMAS layer
SMAS level
Smead closure
Smead-Jones closure
Smead-Jones stitches
Smead-Jones sutures
smear
smear and culture
smear culture
smear slides
Smedberg brace
Smedberg dilator
Smedberg drill
Smedberg hemostat

smegma
Smellie crochet hook
Smellie hook
Smellie maneuver
Smellie method
Smellie obstetrical forceps
Smellie obstetrical hook
Smellie obstetrical perforator
Smellie obstetrical scissors
Smellie perforator
Smellie scissors
Smellie-Veit method
Smeloff prosthetic valve
Smeloff-Cutter aortic valve
    prosthesis
Smeloff-Cutter ball-valve
    prosthesis
Smeloff-Cutter ball-cage
    prosthetic valve
Smeloff-Cutter heart valve
    prosthesis
SMI cannula
SMI Surgi-Med arthroscopy
    instruments
SMI Surgi-Med CPM device
smile incision
Smiley-Williams needle
smiling incision
Smillie cartilage chisel
Smillie cartilage knife
Smillie chisel
Smillie knee joint retractor
Smillie knife
Smillie meniscotome
Smillie meniscus knife
Smillie nail
Smillie nail punch
Smillie pin
Smillie retractor
Smith aneurysmal clip
Smith anoscope
Smith bone clamp
Smith cartilage stripper
Smith cataract extraction
Smith cataract knife
Smith clamp
Smith clip

Smith cordotomy clamp
Smith cordotomy knife
Smith dislocation
Smith dissector
Smith drill
Smith electrode
Smith expressor
Smith expressor hook
Smith eye speculum
Smith eyelid operation
Smith forceps
Smith fracture
Smith grasping forceps
Smith head lamp
Smith hook
Smith intraocular implant
    lens
Smith knife
Smith lens
Smith lens expressor
Smith lid expressor
Smith lid hook
Smith lid-retracting hook
Smith marginal clamp
Smith operation
Smith orbital floor implant
Smith perforator
Smith pessary
Smith posterior cartilage
    stripper
Smith prosthesis
Smith rectal retractor
Smith rectal self-retaining
    retractor
Smith retractor
Smith scissors
Smith Silastic prosthesis
Smith speculum
Smith technique
Smith tonsillar dissector
Smith trabeculotomy
Smith vaginal self-retaining
    retractor
Smith wire-cutting scissors
Smith-Boyce operation
Smith-Buie anal retractor
Smith-Buie rectal retractor

Smith-Buie rectal self-retaining
    retractor
Smith-Buie retractor
Smith-Fisher cataract knife
Smith-Fisher cataract lamp
Smith-Fisher iris replacer
Smith-Fisher knife
Smith-Fisher spatula
Smith-Green cataract knife
Smith-Green double-end spatula
Smith-Green knife
Smith-Green spatula
Smith-Hodge pessary
Smith-Indian operation
Smith-Kuhnt-Szymanowski
    operation
Smith-Petersen acromioplasty
Smith-Petersen approach
Smith-Petersen arthrodesis
Smith-Petersen arthroplasty
    gouge
Smith-Petersen cannulated nail
Smith-Petersen capsule retractor
Smith-Petersen chisel
Smith-Petersen cup
Smith-Petersen cup arthroplasty
Smith-Petersen curet
Smith-Petersen elevator
Smith-Petersen extractor
Smith-Petersen forceps
Smith-Petersen fracture pin
Smith-Petersen gouge
Smith-Petersen hammer
Smith-Petersen hip cup prosthe-
    sis
Smith-Petersen hip reamer
Smith-Petersen incision
Smith-Petersen laminectomy
    rongeur
Smith-Petersen mallet
Smith-Petersen nail
Smith-Petersen nail extractor
Smith-Petersen nailing
Smith-Petersen operation
Smith-Petersen osteotome
Smith-Petersen osteotomy
Smith-Petersen pin

Smith-Petersen plate
Smith-Petersen prosthesis
Smith-Petersen reamer
Smith-Petersen retractor
Smith-Petersen rongeur
Smith-Petersen spatula
Smith-Petersen tucker
Smith-Petersen wrist arthrodesis
Smith-Potts scissors
Smith-Robinson anterior
    approach
Smith-Robinson cervical fusion
Smith-Robinson operation
Smithuysen ethmoidal punch
Smithuysen sphenoidal punch
Smithwick anastomotic clamp
Smithwick blunt nerve hook
Smithwick buttonhook
Smithwick clamp
Smithwick clip
Smithwick clip-applying forceps
Smithwick dissector
Smithwick dissector hook
Smithwick forceps
Smithwick hook
Smithwick nerve hook
Smithwick operation
Smithwick retractor
Smithwick silk buttonhook
Smithwick silver clip
Smithwick sympathectomy
Smithwick sympathectomy
    hook
Smithwick-Hartmann forceps
SMo (stainless steel with
    molybdenum)
SMo Moore pin
SMo plate
SMo prosthesis
smoker's heart
smoker's palate
smoker's patches
smoker's tongue
smooth broach
smooth liver edge
smooth margin
smooth muscle

smooth tissue forceps
smooth-tooth forceps
smooth-walled uterus
smothering sensation
SMR (submucous resection)
SMR speculum
Smuckler tucker
snaggle tooth
snake graft
snakebite
SNAP (sensory nerve action
   potential)
snap gauge band
snap-lock brace
snapping
snapping finger
snapping hip
snapping tendon
snare
   Alfred snare
   Banner enucleation snare
   Banner snare
   Beck-Schenck tonsil
    snare
   Beck-Storz tonsil snare
   Boettcher-Farlow snare
   Bosworth nasal snare
   Bosworth snare
   Brown snare
   Brown tonsil snare
   Bruening ear snare
   Bruening nasal snare
   Bruening snare
   Buerger snare
   Castroviejo enucleation
    snare
   Castroviejo snare
   cautery snare
   caval snare
   cold snare
   Crapeau nasal snare
   Crapeau snare
   cut snare wire
   cystoscopic snare
   Dean ear snare
   dissection and snare
   Douglas mucosal snare

snare *continued*
   Douglas rectal snare
   Douglas snare
   Douglas-Roberts snare
   ear snare
   electrosurgical snare
   endoscopic snare
   enucleation snare
   Eves snare
   Eves tonsillar snare
   Eves-Neivert tonsillar
    snare
   eye enucleation snare
   Farlow snare
   Farlow tonsil snare
   Farlow-Boettcher snare
   Farlow-Boettcher tonsil
    snare
   Foerster snare
   Frankfeldt rectal snare
   Frankfeldt snare
   galvanocaustic snare
   hot snare
   Jarvis snare
   Krause ear snare
   Krause nasal snare
   Krause snare
   Lange-Wilde snare
   laryngeal snare
   Layman-Storz snare
   Lewis snare
   Lewis tonsillar snare
   long-nose retriever
    snare
   Martin snare
   Myles snare
   Myles tonsillectome
    snare
   nasal snare
   Neivert snare
   Neivert tonsillar snare
   Neivert-Eves snare
   Nesbit snare
   Norwood rectal snare
   Norwood snare
   polyethylene snare
   polyp snare

snare *continued*
    rectal snare
    Reiner-Beck snare
    Reiner-Beck tonsil snare
    Roberts nasal snare
    Roberts snare
    Sage snare
    Sage tonsil snare
    Storz snare
    Storz-Beck snare
    Storz-Beck-Schenck snare
    Stutsman nasal snare
    Stutsman snare
    tonsillar snare
    Tydings snare
    Tydings tonsil snare
    Weston rectal snare
    Wilde nasal snare
    Wilde-Bruening snare
    Wright nasal snare
    Wright snare
snare cautery
snare loop
snare loop biopsy
snare technique
snare tonsillectomy
snare wire
Snellen entropion forceps
Snellen entropion operation
Snellen eye chart
Snellen eye implant
Snellen forceps
Snellen operation
Snellen ptosis operation
Snellen reform eye
Snellen sutures
Snellen vectis
Snitman endaural retractor
Snitman endaural self-retaining retractor
Snitman retractor
Snoopy arm sling
Snowden-Pencer forceps
Snowden-Pencer scissors
snowflake cataract
snowstorm cataract

snuffbox
snugness
Snyder deep-surgery forceps
Snyder forceps
Snyder hemostat
Snyder Hemovac
Snyder Hemovac drain
Snyder Hemovac evacuator
Snyder Hemovac suction tube
Snyder Hemovac tube
Snyder mini-Hemovac drain
Snyder Surgivac drainage
Snyder trocar
Snyder tube
soaked cotton
SOA-MCA (superficial occipital artery–middle cerebral artery)
soaks
soap-bubble pattern
soapsuds enema
Soave abdominal pull-through procedure
Soave endorectal pull-through procedure
Soave operation
Soave procedure for mega-colon
Soave pull-through procedure
SOB (short of breath, shortness of breath)
Sober ureterostomy
soccer-style kicker
Socin operation
socket
socks
soda-lime mechanism
sodium pentothal anesthetic agent
sodium pump
Soemmering area
Soemmering arterial vein
Soemmering external radial vein
Soemmering foramen
Soemmering ring
Soemmering ring cataract
Soemmering spot

Sofield operation
Sofield osteotomy
Sofield pseudarthrosis of tibia
Sofield retractor
Sofield rod
Soflens contact lens
Sof-Rol cast padding
Sof-Rol dressing
SOF-T guide wire
SOF-T guiding catheter
soft abdomen
soft cartilage
soft cataract aspirator
soft catheter
soft disk
soft fold
soft lens
soft palate
soft palate retractor
soft rubber curet
soft rubber drain
soft structure injury
soft tissue
soft tissue elevator
soft tissue mass
soft tissue stranding
soft tissue windowing
Softcon contact lens
Softcon lens
softener
softening
Softgut chromic suture
Softgut sutures
Softies wrist and forearm splint
Softip arteriography catheter
Softip catheter
Softip diagnostic catheter
Softjaw clamp
Softjaw handless clamp
Softouch guiding catheter
soft-tipped guide wire
Sof-Wick drain
Sof-Wick drain sponges
Sof-Wick dressing
Sof-Wick sponge
Soilleau tube
Sokolec elevator

Sokolowski punch
solar cautery
Solcotrans autotransfusion unit
Solcotrans orthopedic drainage
    system
Solcotrans orthopedic reinfusion
    system
soldier's heart
sole of foot
sole reflex
sole wedge
solenoid coil
soleus muscle
soleus, musculus
solid ankle cushioned heel
    (SACH)
solid organ
solid silicone orbital prosthesis
solid silicone with Supramid
    mesh implant
solid stool
solid tumor
solid waste
solid-appearing mass
solid-state esophageal manom-
    etry catheter
solid-state silk sutures
solid-tip catheter
solitary
solitary lesion
solitary nodule
Solo cast sole
Sol-O-Pake barium
Solow sigmoidoscope
solubility
soluble bougie
soluble ligature
Soluset device
solution
solution basin
solution bowl
Solvang graft
solving
SOM (serous otitis media;
    secretory otitis media)
Somagyi reflex
somatic death

somatic muscles
somatic nerves
somatic sarcoma
somatization reactions
somatointestinal reflex
somatosensory area
somatosensory evoked potential (SEP)
Somers clamp
Somers forceps
Somers tonsillar knife
Somers uterine clamp
Somers uterine elevator
Somers uterine forceps
Somers uterine-elevating forceps
Somerset bur
Somerset-Mack hand operation
Somerville open reduction
SOMI (skull, occiput, mandibular immobilization)
SOMI brace
SOMI orthosis
Sommers compression dressing
SON anesthetic agent
sonde coudé
Sondergaard cleft
Sondergaard groove
Sondergaard operation
Sondermann canal
Sondermann suction tip
Sones arteriography
Sones brachial cutdown technique
Sones cardiac catheterization
Sones Cardio-Marker catheter
Sones catheter
Sones cineangiography technique
Sones coronary arteriography
Sones coronary catheter
Sones guide wire
Sones hemostatic bag
Sones Hi-Flow catheter
Sones Positrol catheter
Sones selective coronary arteriogram

Sones vent catheter
sonic applicator
sonic curet
sonic surgery
sonic wave
Sonneberg operation
Sonnenschein nasal speculum
Sonnenschein speculum
sonoencephalographic study
sonography
sonolucent
sonolucent area
sonolucent mass
Sonop ultrasonic aspiration system
Soonawalla uterine elevator
Soonawalla vasectomy forceps
Soper cone hard contact lens
Sophy pressure valve
Sophy valve
sorbose cushion
Sorbothane orthotic device
Sorbsan dressing
SorbSystem
Sordille operation
Sorenson catheter for CVP line
Sorenson sinus cleanser
Sorenson-Yankauer combination pump
Soresi cannula
Soria operation
Sorin cardiac prosthetic valve
Sorin pacemaker
Sorin prosthetic valve
Sorondo hindquarter amputation
Sorondo-Ferre amputation
SOS guide wire
Soto-Hall bone graft technique
Soto-Hall patellectomy
Soto-Hall sign
Soto-Hall-West patellectomy
Sotteau operation
Souligoux-Morestin lavage
sound (see also *bougie, searcher*)
    Allport mastoid sound

sound *continued*
    Allport-Babcock sound
    Bellocq sound
    Bellows sound
    Béniqué sound
    Campbell miniature
      sound
    Campbell sound
    Campbell urethral sound
    Collin sound
    common duct sound
    Davis sound
    Dittel sound
    Ellik sound
    Fowler sound
    Fowler urethral sound
    French sound
    French-following metal
      sound
    Gouley sound
    Gouley tunneled urethral
      sound
    Gouley urethral sound
    graduated sound
    Greenwald sound
    Guyon sound
    Guyon urethral sound
    Guyon-Béniqué sound
    Hunt metal sound
    Hunt sound
    infant sound
    infant urethral sound
    interlocking sound
    Jewett urethral sound
    Klebanoff common duct
      sound
    Kocher bronchocele
      sound
    Kocher sound
    Korotkoff sound
    lacrimal sound
    LeFort sound
    LeFort urethral sound
    McCrea infant sound
    McCrea sound
    meatal sound
    Mercier sound

sound *continued*
    metal sound
    miniature sound
    Otis prostatic urethral
      sound
    Otis urethral sound
    Pratt sound
    Ritter sound
    Schroeder interlocking
      sound
    shaking sound
    Simpson sound
    Simpson uterine sound
    Sims sound
    Sims uterine sound
    urethral sound
    uterine sound
    uterus sound
    van Buren sound
    van Buren urethral
      sound
    Walther sound
    Walther urethral sound
    Winternitz sound
    Woodward sound
sounded
sounding
sounds and bougies
soupy material
source
Sourdille keratoplasty
Sourdille operation
Sourdille ptosis operation
Souter hinge
Southbent scissors
Southey anasarca trocar
Southey cannula
Southey capillary drainage tube
Southey trocar
Southey tube
Southey-Leech trocar
Southey-Leech tube
Southwick clamp
Southwick osteotomy
Southwick procedure
Southwick screw extractor
Southwick-Robinson approach

Souttar cautery
Souttar craniotomy incision
Souttar iliac crest fasciotomy
Souttar incision
Souttar operation
Souttar skin incision
Souttar tube
Souttar-Campbell slide
Sovak reamer
Sovally suprapubic suction cup
    drain
SP (status post; suprapatellar;
    sacroposterior)
SP position (sacroposterior
    position)
space of Fontana
space of Forel
space of Retzius
space of Tenon
space of Traube
space shoes
space-occupying lesion
spacer
spacing
spade hand
Spaeth cystic bleb operation
Spaeth facial nerve block
Spaeth operation
Spaeth ptosis operation
spaghetti drain
Spalding-Richardson hysterec-
    tomy
Spalding-Richardson operation
span
Span-aid abduction pillow
Span-aid bed supports
Spanish blue virgin silk sutures
Spanish tourniquet
sparsity of bone formation
Sparta micro iris forceps
spasm
spasmodic
spasmodic entropion operation
spasmodic stricture
spasmoid talipes
spastic
spastic stricture

spasticity
spatial resolution
spatial vectorcardiogram
spatially separated foci
spatula
    Bakelite spatula
    Bangerter spatula
    Barraquer cyclodialysis
        spatula
    Barraquer iris spatula
    Barraquer spatula
    Bechert irrigating spatula
    Berens plastic spatula
    Berens spatula
    brain spatula
    Castroviejo cyclodialysis
        spatula
    Castroviejo spatula
    Cave scaphoid spatula
    Cave spatula
    Children's Hospital brain
        spatula
    Children's Hospital
        spatula
    Cleasby iris spatula
    Crile spatula
    Culler iris spatula
    Culler spatula
    Cushing brain spatula
    Cushing S-shaped brain
        spatula
    Cushing spatula
    cyclodialysis spatula
    Davis brain spatula
    Davis spatula
    D'Errico brain spatula
    D'Errico spatula
    DeWecker iris spatula
    Dorsey spatula
    double spatula
    double-ended spatula
    Drews suture pickup
        spatula
    Elschnig cyclodialysis
        spatula
    Elschnig spatula
    endarterectomy spatula

spatula *continued*

Fisher-Smith spatula
fishtail spatula
flat spatula
Freer spatula
French-pattern eye
   spatula
French-pattern spatula
Garron spatula
Gass endarterectomy
   spatula
Green eye spatula
Green spatula
Gross spatula
Haberer abdominal
   spatula
Halle vascular spatula
Hirschman lens spatula
Hirschman spatula
hook with spatula
Hough spatula
iris spatula
irrigating eye spatula
Jacobson endarterectomy
   spatula
Jacobson spatula
Katena iris spatula
Kellman-Elschnig
   cyclodialysis spatula
Kimura platinum spatula
Kimura spatula
Kirby iris spatula
Kirby spatula
Knapp iris spatula
Knapp spatula
Laird cyclodialysis
   spatula
Laird spatula
lens spatula
Lindner cyclodialysis
   spatula
Lindner spatula
lingual spatula
Lynch spatula
malleable spatula
Maumenee-Barraquer
   vitreous sweep spatula

spatula *continued*

Mayfield brain spatula
Mayfield spatula
McPherson iris spatula
McPherson spatula
McReynolds eye spatula
McReynolds spatula
Meller spatula
microsurgical spatula
Milex spatula
O'Brien spatula
Olivecrona brain spatula
Olivecrona spatula
Paton spatula
Paton transplant spatula
Peyton brain spatula
phakodialysis spatula
platinum conjunctival
   smear spatula
platinum spatula
Raaf flexible lighted
   spatula
Raaf spatula
Ray brain spatula
regular eye spatula
Reverdin abdominal
   spatula
Roux spatula
Sabreloc spatula needle
Sachs nerve spatula
Sachs spatula
scaphoid spatula
Schuknecht spatula
scleral spatula needle
Scoville brain spatula
Scoville brain spatula
   forceps
Scoville flat brain spatula
Scoville spatula
Segond spatula
Segond vaginal spatula
serrated T-spatula
side-cutting spatulated
   needle
Smith-Fisher spatula
Smith-Green double-end
   spatula

spatula *continued*
   Smith-Green spatula
   Smith-Petersen spatula
   spoon and spatula
   stainless spatula
   Suker cyclodialysis spatula
   Tan spatula
   Tauber spatula
   Tennant eye spatula
   Thomas spatula
   Tooke spatula
   transplant spatula
   Troutman iris spatula
   Tuffier abdominal spatula
   ultrasound spatula
   University of Kansas eye spatula
   University of Kansas spatula
   Weary brain spatula
   Weary spatula
   Wecker iris spatula
   Wecker silver spatula
   Wecker spatula
   Wheeler spatula
   Wills eye spatula
   Woodruff spatula knife
   Woodson spatula
   Wullstein spatula
   Wullstein transplant spatula
   Wurmuth spatula
   Wylie endarterectomy spatula
spatula and spoon
spatula needle sutures
spatula-split needle
Spaulding-Richardson hysterectomy
speaking tube
Speare dural hook
spearing
Speas operation
Speas strabismus operation
special wound care

specialized equipment
specialty care
specific
specifications
specimen
specimen container
specimen forceps
specimen jar
specimen sent to lab
speckled pattern
speckled pattern of myocardium
Speclite
SPECT (single photon emission computed tomography)
SPECT imaging
SPECT scan
SPECT-Bullseye scans
Spectraflex pacemaker
spectral analysis
Spectra-Physics argon laser
Spectra-Physics microsurgical laser
Spectraprobe-PLS laser angioplasty catheter
Spectrax bipolar pacemaker
Spectrax pacemaker
Spectrax programmable Medtronic pacemaker
spectrometer
spectrometry
Spectron cemented hip prosthesis
Spectron femoral component
Spectron hip prosthesis
Spectron metal-backed cup for Richards hip prosthesis
Spectron total hip
Spectron total hip stem
spectrophotometer
spectrophotometry
spectrum
specular microscope
specular microscopy
speculum
   Adson speculum
   Alfonso speculum

speculum *continued*

Allen-Heffernan nasal speculum
Allingham rectal speculum
Allingham speculum
Amko vaginal speculum
anal speculum
anoscope speculum
Arruga eye speculum
Arruga speculum
Aufricht retractor-speculum
Aufricht septum speculum
Aufricht speculum
Aumence eyelid speculum
aural speculum
Auvard speculum
Auvard weighted vaginal speculum
Auvard-Remine speculum
Auvard-Remine vaginal speculum
Auvard-Remine weighted speculum
Azar lid speculum
Barnes speculum
Barr anal speculum
Barr rectal speculum
Barr speculum
Barraquer eye speculum
Barraquer speculum
Barraquer wire lid speculum
Barraquer wire speculum
Barraquer-Colibri eye speculum
Barraquer-Kratz speculum
Barr-Shuford rectal speculum
Beard eye speculum
Beard speculum

speculum *continued*

Becker-Park eye speculum
Beckman nasal speculum
Beckman speculum
Beckman-Colver nasal speculum
Beckman-Colver speculum
Bedrossian eye speculum
Berens eye speculum
Berens speculum
Berlind-Auvard speculum
beveled speculum
bivalved ear speculum
bivalved speculum
Bodenheimer rectal speculum
Bodenheimer speculum
Bosworth nasal speculum
Bosworth speculum
Boucheron speculum
Bozeman speculum
brain speculum
Breisky vaginal speculum
Breisky-Navratil vaginal speculum
Brescio-Breisky-Navratil speculum
Brewer speculum
Brewer vaginal speculum
Brinkerhoff rectal speculum
Brinkerhoff speculum
Bronson speculum
Bronson-Park speculum
Brown ear speculum
Bruening speculum
Bruner vaginal speculum
Buie-Hirschman speculum
Buie-Smith speculum
Carter speculum
Castallo speculum
Castroviejo eye speculum

speculum *continued*

Castroviejo speculum
Castroviejo-Barraquer speculum
Chelsea-Eaton anal speculum
Chelsea-Eaton speculum
Chevalier Jackson laryngeal speculum
Chevalier Jackson speculum
child-size eye speculum
Clark eye speculum
Clark speculum
Coakley nasal speculum
Coakley speculum
Coldlite speculum
Coldlite vaginal speculum
Coldlite-Graves vaginal speculum
Colibri speculum
Collin speculum
Collin vaginal speculum
Converse nasal speculum
Converse speculum
Cook eye speculum
Cook rectal speculum
Cook speculum
Cottle nasal speculum
Cottle septum speculum
Cottle speculum
Cusco speculum
Cusco vaginal speculum
Cushing-Landolt transsphenoidal speculum
Czerny rectal speculum
David rectal speculum
Davy speculum
DeLee speculum
DeRoaldes nasal speculum
DeVilbiss speculum
DeVilbiss vaginal speculum

speculum *continued*

DeVilbiss-Stacey speculum
disposable speculum
disposable vaginal speculum
Douglas mucosal speculum
Douglas speculum
Douvas-Barraquer speculum
Doyen speculum
duckbill speculum
Dudley-Smith rectal speculum
Dudley-Smith speculum
Duplay nasal speculum
Duplay-Lynch nasal speculum
Duplay-Lynch speculum
ear speculum
Eaton nasal speculum
Eaton speculum
endaural speculum
endospeculum
Erhardt ear speculum
Erhardt speculum
esophageal speculum
eye speculum
eyelid speculum
Fansler rectal speculum
Fansler speculum
Fanta eye speculum
Farkas urethral speculum
Farrior ear speculum
Farrior oval ear speculum
Farrior oval speculum
Farrior speculum
Fergusson speculum
Fergusson tubular vaginal speculum
Flannery ear speculum
Flannery speculum
Floyd-Barraquer speculum
Forbes speculum

speculum *continued*

Foster-Ballenger nasal speculum
Foster-Ballenger speculum
Fox eye speculum
Fox speculum
Fraenkel speculum
Freeway speculum
Freeway-Graves speculum
Gaffee speculum
Garrigue speculum
Garrigue vaginal speculum
Gerzog nasal speculum
Gerzog speculum
Gilbert-Graves speculum
Gleason speculum
Goldbacher anoscope speculum
Goldbacher speculum
Goldstein mucosa speculum
Goldstein speculum
Goligher speculum
Good speculum
Graefe eye speculum
Graefe speculum
Graves Britetrac vaginal speculum
Graves speculum
Graves vaginal speculum
Green eye speculum
Gruber ear speculum
Gruber speculum
Guild-Pratt rectal speculum
Guild-Pratt speculum
Guist eye speculum
Guist speculum
Guist-Black eye speculum
Guist-Black speculum
Guttmann speculum
Guttmann vaginal speculum

speculum *continued*

Guyton-Maumenee speculum
Guyton-Park eye speculum
Guyton-Park lid speculum
Guyton-Park speculum
Gyn-A-Lite speculum illuminator
Haglund speculum
Hajek-Tieck nasal speculum
Halle infant speculum
Halle nasal speculum
Halle speculum
Halle-Tieck nasal speculum
Halle-Tieck speculum
Hardy bivalve speculum
Hardy speculum
Hardy-Cushing speculum
Hardy-Duddy weighted vaginal speculum
Harrison speculum
Hartmann nasal speculum
Hartmann speculum
Hartmann-Dewaxer speculum
heavy weighted speculum
Heffernan speculum
Henrotin speculum
Henrotin vaginal speculum
Hertel nephrostomy speculum
Hertel speculum
Higbee speculum
Higbee vaginal speculum
Hinkle-James rectal speculum
Hinkle-James speculum
Hirschman speculum

speculum *continued*

Holinger speculum
Hood-Graves speculum
Hood-Graves vaginal
speculum
House speculum
House stapes speculum
Huffman speculum
Huffman-Graves
speculum
Huffman-Graves vaginal
speculum
Iliff-Park speculum
illuminated nasal
speculum
Imperatori laryngeal
speculum
infant eye speculum
infant vaginal speculum
Ingals speculum
intranasal antral specu-
lum
Ives speculum
Jackson speculum
Jackson vaginal specu-
lum
Jaffe speculum
Jonas-Graves speculum
Jonas-Graves vaginal
speculum
Kahn-Graves speculum
Kahn-Graves vaginal
speculum
Kaiser speculum
Keizer-Lancaster
speculum
Kelly rectal speculum
Kelly speculum
Kelman speculum
Killian nasal speculum
Killian rectal speculum
Killian septal speculum
Killian speculum
Klaff septal speculum
Klaff speculum
KleenSpec disposable
speculum

speculum *continued*

KleenSpec speculum
KleenSpec vaginal
speculum
Knapp eye speculum
Knapp speculum
Knolle lens speculum
Kogan endospeculum
Kogan speculum
Kramer bivalve ear
speculum
Kramer ear speculum
Kramer speculum
Kristeller speculum
Kristeller vaginal
speculum
Kyle nasal speculum
Kyle speculum
Lancaster eye speculum
Lancaster lid speculum
Lancaster speculum
Lancaster-O'Connor
speculum
Landolt pituitary
speculum
Lang speculum
Lange eye speculum
Lange speculum
laryngeal speculum
Lawford speculum
LeFort urethral speculum
Lempert-Colver specu-
lum
Lester-Burch eye
speculum
lid speculum
Lillie nasal speculum
Lillie speculum
Lister-Burch eye specu-
lum
Lister-Burch speculum
Lucae ear speculum
Luer speculum
Macon Hospital specu-
lum
Mahoney intranasal
antral speculum

speculum *continued*

Mahoney speculum
Martin rectal speculum
Martin speculum
Martin-Davy rectal
    speculum
Martin-Davy speculum
Mason-Auvard speculum
Mason-Auvard weighted
    vaginal speculum
Mathews rectal speculum
Mathews speculum
Matzenauer speculum
Maumenee-Park eye
    speculum
Maumenee-Park lid
    speculum
Mayer speculum
Mayer vaginal speculum
McHugh speculum
McKinney eye speculum
McKinney speculum
McLaughlin speculum
McPherson eye specu-
    lum
McPherson speculum
Meller speculum
Mellinger eye speculum
Mellinger speculum
Metcher eye speculum
Metcher speculum
Miller speculum
Miller vaginal speculum
Milligan speculum
Monosmith nasal
    speculum
Montgomery speculum
Montgomery vaginal
    speculum
Montgomery-Bernstine
    speculum
Mosher speculum
Moynihan-Navratil
    speculum
mucosa speculum
Mueller speculum
Murdock eye speculum

speculum *continued*

Murdock speculum
Murdock-Wiener eye
    speculum
Murdock-Wiener
    speculum
Myles nasal speculum
Myles speculum
Myles-Ray speculum
nasal speculum
nasopharyngeal specu-
    lum
National speculum
nephrostomy speculum
New York speculum
Nichol speculum
Nott speculum
Nott-Guttmann specu-
    lum
Nott-Guttmann vaginal
    speculum
Noyes speculum
Omni-Park eyelid
    speculum
oral speculum mouth
    gag
O'Sullivan-O'Connor
    speculum
O'Sullivan-O'Connor
    vaginal speculum
oval speculum
Park eye speculum
Park-Guyton eye
    speculum
Park-Guyton-Callahan
    eye speculum
Park-Maumenee eye
    speculum
Park-Maumenee lid
    speculum
Patton nasal speculum
Patton speculum
Peck-Vienna nasal
    speculum
Pederson speculum
Pederson vaginal
    speculum

speculum *continued*
Pennington rectal
speculum
Pennington speculum
pharyngeal speculum
Picot speculum
Picot vaginal speculum
Picot weighted speculum
plain wire speculum
Politzer ear speculum
Politzer speculum
Portmann speculum
Pratt rectal speculum
Pratt sigmoid speculum
Pratt speculum
Preefer eye speculum
Pritchard speculum
proctoscopic speculum
Pruitt rectal speculum
Pynchon nasal speculum
Pynchon speculum
Ray nasal speculum
Ray speculum
rectal speculum
Redi-Spec disposable
vaginal speculum
Roberts speculum
Rosenthal speculum
rotating speculum
anoscope
rotating speculum
proctoscope
Sato speculum
Sauer eye speculum
Sauer speculum
Sawyer rectal speculum
Scherback speculum
Scherback-Porges vaginal
speculum
Schuknecht speculum
Scott speculum
self-retaining speculum
Selkin speculum
Senn speculum
Senturia pharyngeal
speculum
Senturia speculum

speculum *continued*
septal speculum
Seyfert speculum
shoehorn speculum
Siegle speculum
sigmoid speculum
Simon speculum
Simon vaginal speculum
Simrock speculum
Sims double-ended
speculum
Sims rectal speculum
Sims speculum
Sisson-Cottle septal
speculum
Sisson-Vienna nasal
speculum
slotted speculum
Sluder speculum
Sluder sphenoidal
speculum
Smith eye speculum
Smith speculum
SMR speculum
Sonnenschein nasal
speculum
Sonnenschein speculum
SRT vaginal speculum
stapes speculum
Stearns speculum
Steiner-Auvard speculum
Steiner-Auvard vaginal
speculum
Stevenson eye speculum
stop eye speculum
Storz ear speculum
Storz nasal speculum
Storz speculum
Storz-Vienna speculum
Subramanian valve
speculum
Sweeney speculum
Tauber speculum
Taylor speculum
Taylor vaginal speculum
Terson speculum
Tieck nasal speculum

speculum *continued*
- Tieck speculum
- Tieck-Halle speculum
- Toynbee ear speculum
- Toynbee speculum
- Trélat speculum
- Trélat vaginal speculum
- Troeltsch ear speculum
- Troeltsch speculum
- tubular vaginal speculum
- urethral speculum
- vaginal speculum
- Vernon-David speculum
- Vienna nasal speculum
- Vienna speculum
- Vilbiss-Miller speculum
- Voltolini septum speculum
- Voltolini speculum
- von Graefe speculum
- Walton speculum
- Walton-Pederson speculum
- Walton-Vienna speculum
- Watson speculum
- Weeks eye speculum
- Weeks speculum
- weighted obstetrical speculum
- weighted speculum
- weighted vaginal speculum
- Weisman-Graves speculum
- Weisman-Graves vaginal speculum
- Weiss speculum
- Welch Allyn speculum
- Wiener eye speculum
- Wiener speculum
- Wilde ear speculum
- Williams eye speculum
- Williams speculum
- winged speculum
- wire bivalve obstetrical speculum

speculum *continued*
- wire bivalve vaginal speculum
- wire eye speculum
- wire lid speculum
- wire speculum
- wire-winged lid speculum
- Worcester City Hospital vaginal speculum
- Yankauer nasopharyngeal speculum
- Yankauer pharyngeal speculum
- Yankauer speculum
- Ziegler eye speculum
- Ziegler speculum
- Zower speculum

speculum anoscope
speculum forceps
speculum holder
speculum illuminator
speculum transilluminator
Speed hand splint
speed lock clamp
Speed operation
Speed osteotomy
Speed osteotomy and bone graft
Speed prosthesis
Speed radial cap prosthesis
Speed sternoclavicular procedure
Speed-Boyd fracture reduction
Speed-Boyd open reduction
Speed-Boyd reduction technique
Speed-Sprague knife
Speer periosteotome
Spence cranioplastic roller
Spence forceps
Spence gel flotation
Spence gel mattress pad
Spence intervertebral disk rongeur
Spence urethral meatotomy

Spence-Adson clip-introducing
    forceps
Spence-Adson forceps
Spence-Allen hypospadias
    repair
Spencer cannula
Spencer chalazion forceps
Spencer forceps
Spencer labyrinth exploration
    probe
Spencer oval punch
Spencer oval tip
Spencer probe
Spencer punch
Spencer scissors
Spencer stitch scissors
Spencer-Wells chalazion forceps
Spencer-Wells forceps
Spencer-Wells hemostatic
    forceps
Spencer-Watson operation
Spencer-Watson Z-plasty
Spenco neoprene foam rubber
Spenco orthotic device
spermatic artery
spermatic calculus
spermatic cord
spermatic fascia
spermatic nerve
spermatic veins
spermatic vesicle
spermatic vessel
spermatica externa, arteria
spermatica, vena
spermatocele
spermatocele implant
spermatocelectomy
spermatocystectomy
spermatocystotomy
spermatogenic cells
spermatozoon (*pl.* spermatozoa)
spermectomy
Spero forceps
Spero meibomian expressor
    forceps
Spero meibomian forceps
Spetzler catheter

Spetzler lumboperitoneal shunt
Spetzler MacroVac surgical
    suction device
Spetzler shunt
Spetzler subarachnoid catheter
Spetzler technique for shunt
    placement
sphenoethmoidal recess
sphenoethmoidal suture
sphenofrontal suture
sphenofrontal suture line
sphenoid
sphenoid bone
sphenoid sinusotomy
sphenoidal bur
sphenoidal cannula
sphenoidal concha
sphenoidal fontanelle
sphenoidal knife
sphenoidal paranasal sinus
sphenoidal probe
sphenoidal process
sphenoidal punch
sphenoidal punch forceps
sphenoidal ridge
sphenoidal sinus
sphenoidal turbinate
sphenoidal wing
sphenoidectomy
sphenoidostomy
sphenoidotomy
sphenomalar suture
sphenomaxillary fissure
sphenomaxillary ganglion
sphenomaxillary suture
spheno-occipital suture
spheno-orbital suture
sphenopalatina, arteria
sphenopalatine artery
sphenopalatine branch of
    internal maxillary artery
sphenopalatine ganglion
sphenopalatine ganglionectomy
sphenopalatine needle
sphenopalatine nerves
sphenopalatine notch of
    palatine bone

sphenopalatini, nervi
sphenoparietal sinus
sphenoparietal suture
sphenoparietal suture line
sphenopetrosal suture
sphenosquamous suture
sphenotemporal suture
sphenozygomatic suture
sphere
sphere eye implant
sphere implant
sphere introducer (see also
   *introducer*)
      Carter sphere introducer
      eye sphere introducer
      metallic sphere intro-
        ducer
sphere prosthesis
spherical
spherical eye implant
spherical implant
spherical mass
spherical reamer
spherical shape
spherical-shaped form
spheroid joint
sphincter
sphincter ampullae hepatopan-
   creaticae, musculus
sphincter ani
sphincter ani externus, musculus
sphincter ani internus, musculus
sphincter atony
sphincter contraction ring
sphincter dilator
sphincter ductus choledochi,
   musculus
sphincter iridis
sphincter muscle
sphincter oculi
sphincter of Oddi
sphincter of pupil
sphincter pupillae, musculus
sphincter pylori, musculus
sphincter tone
sphincter urethrae, musculus

sphincter vaginae
sphincter vesicae
sphincter vesicae urinariae,
   musculus
sphincter-saving operation
sphincteral
sphincteral achalasia
sphincteralgia
sphincterectomy
sphincterismus
sphincterolysis
sphincteroplasty
sphincterorrhaphy
sphincteroscope
     Kelly sphincteroscope
sphincteroscopy
sphincterotome
     Demling-Classen
      sphincterotome
     Doubilet sphincterotome
     Erlangen endoscopic
      sphincterotome
     needle-knife
      sphincterotome
     Olympus sphinctero-
      tome
     precut sphincterotome
     reverse sphincterotome
     rotating sphincterotome
sphincterotomy
sphincterotomy basket
sphygmograph
sphygmomanometer
     Faught sphygmo-
      manometer
     Freemont spinal sphyg-
      momanometer
     Janeway sphygmo-
      manometer
     Kompak sphygmo-
      manometer
     Monoject sphygmo-
      manometer
     Riva-Rocci sphygmo-
      manometer
     Rogers sphygmo-
      manometer

sphygmomanometer *continued*
    Staunton sphygmoma-
       nometer
sphygmomanometer cuffs
sphygmometry
sphygmoscope
sphygmoscopy
spica bandage
spica cast
spica dressing
spica splint
spicular
spiculated
spiculated calcification
spicule
spicule forceps
spiculum (*pl.* spicula)
spider angiomata
spider cell
spider nevus
spider projection
Spieghel line
Spielberg dilator
Spielberg sinus cannula
Spies ethmoidal punch
Spies punch
Spiesman fistula probe
spigelian hernia
Spigelman baseball finger splint
spike
spike discharges
spike focus
spike pattern
spike retractor
spike rhythm
spike waves
spike-and-dome complex
spike-and-sharp waves
spike-and-slow wave
spike-and-wave
spikelike emanation
spikelike formation
spikey activity
spiking
spin technique
spina bifida
spinal accessory nerve

spinal anesthesia
spinal arachnoid
spinal artery
spinal block
spinal canal
spinal cord
spinal cord abscess
spinal cord compression
spinal cord retractor
spinal cord stimulator
spinal cordotomy
spinal curet
spinal elevator
spinal epidural space
spinal fluid
spinal fluid tap
spinal fracture
spinal fusion
spinal fusion chisel
spinal fusion curet
spinal fusion elevator
spinal fusion gouge
spinal fusion instrument set
spinal fusion osteotome
spinal fusion plate
spinal ganglion
spinal gouge
spinal graft tamp
spinal impactor
spinal manometer
spinal marrow
spinal meningitis
spinal muscle
spinal needle
spinal nerves
spinal neurectomy
spinal paralysis
spinal perforating forceps
spinal puncture
spinal reflex
spinal retractor
spinal retractor blade
spinal rongeur forceps
spinal stenosis
spinal subarachnoid block
spinal tap
spinal thrust

spinal trephine
spinal veins
spinales, nervi
spinales, venae
spinalis anterior, arteria
spinalis capitis, musculus
spinalis posterior, arteria
spinalis thoracis, musculus
Spinal-Stim bone growth
    stimulator
spindle cataract
spindle cell
spindle colonic groove
spindle-shaped
spindle-shaped cataract
spindling patterns
spine
spine board
spine of Henle
spin-echo MRI
spin-echo scanning technique
Spinelli biopsy needle
Spinelli operation
Spinhaler
spinoneural artery
spinothalamic
spinothalamic tract
spinothalamic tract cauterized
spinous process
spinous process of vertebra
spinous process spreader
spiny projection
Spira procedure
spiral
spiral arterioles
spiral bandage
spiral drill
spiral elevator
spiral flap
spiral fold
spiral forceps
spiral fracture
spiral ganglion
spiral groove
spiral incision
spiral joint
spiral probe

spiral reamer
spiral reverse bandage
spiral stone dislodger
spiral sutures
spiral trochanteric reamer
spiral valve
spiral vein
spiral vein of modiolus
spiral vein stripper
spiral wound
spiralis modioli, vena
spiral-tipped bougie
spiral-tipped catheter
Spirec drill
spirogram
spirometer
        Calculair spirometer
        Collis spirometer
        DeVilbiss spirometer
        Eagle spirometer
spirometry
spit cyst
Spittle biceps muscle cineplasty
Spitz nevus
Spitz-Holter flushing device
Spitz-Holter VA shunt
Spitz-Holter valve
Spivack cystostomy
Spivack gastrostomy
Spivack operation
Spivack valve
Spivack valve technique
Spivey iris retractor
Spizziri knife
splanchnic anesthesia
splanchnic AV fistula
splanchnic block
splanchnic circulation
splanchnic ganglion
splanchnic nerve
splanchnic neurectomy
splanchnic retractor
splanchnicectomy
splanchnici lumbales, nervi
splanchnici pelvini, nervi
splanchnici sacrales, nervi
splanchnicotomy

splanchnicus imus, nervus
splanchnicus major, nervus
splanchnicus minor, nervus
splanchnoscopy
splanchnotribe
splayfoot
spleen
splenectomize
splenectomy
splenectopia
splenic
splenic abscess
splenic artery
splenic AV fistula
splenic capsule
splenic dullness
splenic flexure
splenic flexure of colon
splenic hilum
splenic portogram
splenic portography
splenic pulp
splenic puncture
splenic recess of omental bursa
splenic rupture
splenic shadow
splenic souffle
splenic system angiogram
splenic tissue
splenic vein
splenic vein thrombosis
splenic venogram
splenic-renal angle
splenium
splenius capitis, musculus
splenius cervicis, musculus
splenius muscle
splenocele
splenocleisis
splenocolic
splenocolic ligament
splenogastric omentum
splenogram
splenography
splenolaparotomy
splenolymph glands
splenolysis

splenomegaly
splenoncus
splenopexy
splenoplasty
splenoportal venography
splenoportogram
splenoportography
splenoptosis
splenorenal
splenorenal anastomosis
splenorenal angle
splenorenal ligament
splenorenal shunt
splenorenal venous operation
splenorrhagia
splenorrhaphy
splenosis
splenotomy
splenulus
spline
    dorsal plaster spline
    os pubis spline
    plaster spline
    stapes spline
splint
    abduction finger splint
    abduction splint
    abduction thumb splint
    acrylic cap splint
    acrylic splint
    acrylic surgical splint
    Adam and Eve rib belt
      splint
    adhesive aluminum
      splint
    adjustable cross splint
    adjustable splint
    Agnew splint
    airfoam splint
    airplane splint
    airsplint
    Alumafoam splint
    aluminum bridge splint
    aluminum fence splint
    aluminum finger-cot
      splint
    aluminum foam splint

splint *continued*

aluminum splint
anchor splint
Anderson splint
Angle splint
anterior acute-flexion elbow splint
anterior splint
any-angle splint
application of splint
Aquaplast splint
arch bar splint
arm splint
Asch nasal splint
Asch splint
Ashhurst splint
bail-lock splint
Balkan splint
banjo splint
banjo traction splint
baseball finger splint
baseball splint
basswood splint
Bavarian splint
Baylor adjustable cross splint
Baylor splint
Beatty aluminum finger splint
bite splint
Böhler splint
Böhler wire splint
Böhler-Braun splint
Bond splint
Bowlby splint
bracketed splint
Brady suspension splint
Brant aluminum splint
Brant splint
Bremmer-Breeze splint
Browne splint
Buck extension splint
Buck splint
buddy splint
Bunnell active hand splint
Bunnell finger splint

splint *continued*

Bunnell modified safety-pin splint
Bunnell outrigger splint
Bunnell splint
C-splint
Cabot leg splint
Cabot splint
calibrated clubfoot splint
Campbell airplane splint
Campbell splint
canine-to-canine lingual splint
cap splint
Capner splint
Capner boutonnière splint
cardboard splint
Carl P. Jones traction splint
Carter splint
cast cap splint
cast lingual splint
Chandler splint
Chatfield-Girdlestone splint
clavicle splint
clavicular cross splint
Clayton splint
clean acrylic template splint
clubfoot splint
coaptation splint
cock-up arm splint
cock-up hand splint
Colles splint
compression splint
contact splint
Converse splint
countertraction splint
Craig abduction splint
Craig splint
Cramer splint
Cramer wire splint
Cullen abduction splint
Culley splint
Curry splint

splint *continued*

Curry walking splint
Darco medical-surgical shoe and toe alignment splint
Darco toe alignment splint
Davis metacarpal splint
Davis splint
Delbet splint
Denis Browne splint
Denis Browne talipes hobble splint
dental splint
denture splint
Denver nasal splint
Denver splint
DePuy open-thimble splint
DePuy rocking-leg splint
DePuy splint
DePuy-Potts splint
double-J silicone splint
double-occlusal splint
Doyle nasal splint
drop-foot splint
Dupuytren splint
Duran-Houser wire splint
dynamic splint
dynamic splinting
Easton cock-up splint
Eggers contact splint
Eggers splint
elephant-ear clavicle splint
Engelmann splint
Erich maxillary splint
Erich nasal splint
Erich splint
Essig splint
Essig wire acrylic splint
extension splint
external nasal splint
external splint
felt-collar splint
femoral splint
fence splint

splint *continued*

Ferciot splint
Fillauer night splint
Fillauer splint
finger splint
finger-cot splint
Flexisplint flexed-arm board
fore-and-aft splint
forearm and metacarpal splint
forearm splint
Forrester splint
Fosler splint
Fox clavicle splint
Fractomed splint
fracture splint
Frejka pillow splint
frog splint
frog-leg splint
Fruehevald splint
full occlusal splint
functional splint
Funsten supination splint
Futura splint
Galveston splint
gauntlet splint
Gilmer splint
Gilmer tooth splint
Glisson sling splint
gnathological splint
Goode nasal splint
Goode-Magne nasal airway splint
Gordon arm splint
Gordon splint
greenstick fracture splint
Guerrant-Cochran splint
Gunning jaw splint
Gunning splint
gutter finger splint
gutter splint
half-ring leg splint
half-ring Thomas splint
Hammond splint
hand cock-up splint
hand splint

splint *continued*

Hanna splint
Hare traction splint
Hart extension finger
    splint
Hart splint
Haynes-Griffin mandible
    splint
Haynes-Griffin splint
Hilgenreiner splint
hinged Thomas splint
Hirschtick splint
Hirschtick utility
    shoulder splint
Hodgen splint
humerus splint
Ilfeld splint
Ilfeld-Gustafson splint
infant abduction splint
inflatable splint
INRO surgical nail splint
interdental splint
intranasal splint
jaw splint
Jelenko splint
Jobe-Patt splint
Johnson splint
Jonell countertraction
    metacarpal splint
Jonell finger splint
Jonell splint
Jones forearm splint
Jones metacarpal splint
Jones splint
Joseph splint
Kanavel cock-up splint
Kanavel splint
Kazanjian splint
Keller-Blake half-ring leg
    splint
Keller-Blake splint
Kenny-Howard splint
Kerr abduction splint
Kerr splint
Kingsley splint
Kinney-Brown AC splint
Kirschner-wire splint

splint *continued*

Kleinert rubber-band
    splint
Kleinert volar pedicle
    splint
Klenzak splint
knee splint
knuckle-binder splint
labial splint
Lambrinudi splint
leg extension splint
leg splint
Levis splint
Lewin baseball finger
    splint
Lewin splint
Lewin-Stern finger splint
Lewin-Stern thumb splint
limb splint
lingual splint
Link boutonnière finger
    splint
Liston splint
live splint
Lively splint
Love nasal splint
Love splint
lumiform splint
Lynch splint
Lytle metacarpal splint
Lytle splint
Magnuson abduction
    humerus splint
Magnuson splint
mandible splint
Mason splint
Mason-Allen splint
Mason-Allen Universal
    hand splint
Mayer nasal splint
Mayer splint
McGee splint
McIntire splint
McKibbin splint
metacarpal splint
metal splint
metatarsal splint

splint *continued*

Middeldorpf splint
Mohr splint
molded splint
Morris splint
Murray-Thomas arm
    splint
nasal splint
neoprene splint
Neubeiser splint
night splint
O'Donaghue knee splint
O'Donaghue splint
O'Donaghue stirrup
    splint
OEC forearm splint
Olliger splint
Omnivac splint
open thimble splint
Oppenheimer splint
opponens splint
Ortho Tech cock-up
    wrist splint
Ortho-last splint
orthopedic strap clavicle
    splint
outrigger splint
outrigger wrist splint
padded splint
Pallab finger splint
palmar splint
pan splint
Parke-Davis splint
Peabody splint
Pearson clavicle attach-
    ment splint
Pehr abduction splint
pelvic splint
Phelps splint
Pier abduction splint
pillow splint
plastic splint
Plexiglas splint
pneumatic splint
polyvinyl alcohol splint
Pond splint
Ponseti splint

splint *continued*

poroplastic splint
Porzett splint
posterior splint
Pott splint
Protecto splint
Putti splint
radial nerve splint
radiolucent splint
Rauchfuss sling splint
resting pan splint
reverse Kingsley splint
reverse knuckle-bender
    splint
Robert Jones splint
rocking-leg splint
Roger Anderson splint
Roger Anderson well-leg
    splint
rolled Colles splint
Rooter splint
Royalite splint
Rumel splint
safety pin splint
Sayre splint
Scott humerus splint
Scott splint
Scottish Rite splint
septal splint
Sheffield splint
Simpson splint
Simpson sugar-tong
    splint
skin splint
Slocum splint
Softies wrist and forearm
    splint
Speed hand splint
spica splint
Spigelman baseball
    finger splint
spreading hand splint
spring cock-up splint
spring-wire safety-pin
    splint
Stack splint
Stader splint

splint *continued*

Stax splint
stirrup splint
Strampelli eye splint
strap clavicle splint
Stromeyer splint
sugar-tong plaster splint
sugar-tong splint
supination splint
surgical splint
T-finger splint
T-splint
talipes hobble splint
Taylor splint
Teare arm sling splint
Teflon splint
template splint
therapeutic splint
thigh splint
Thomas full-ring leg splint
Thomas leg splint
Thomas splint
Thompson modification of Denis Browne splint
thumb splint
Ticonium splint
Titus forearm splint
Titus wrist splint
Tobruk splint
tong splint
Toronto splint
torsion bar splint
U-splint
ulnar splint
Universal gutter splint
Universal splint
Universal support splint
utility shoulder splint
Valentine splint
Valpo splint
Van Rosen splint
Velcro splint
volar splint
Volkmann splint
von Rosen hip splint
von Rosen splint

splint *continued*

Wamarline wrist splint
Warm "N" Form splint
Weil splint
well-leg splint
Wertheim splint
Wilson splint
Winter splint
Wirefoam splint
wraparound splint
Xomed Silastic splint
Xomed-Doyle nasal airway splint
Zimfoam finger splint
Zimfoam splint
Zimmer airplane splint
Zimmer clavicular cross splint
Zimmer splint
Zim-Trac traction splint
Zim-Zip rib belt splint
Zollinger splint
Zucker splint

splinted
splinter forceps
splinter hemorrhage
splintered fracture
splintered to pieces
splinting
splinting material
splinting tube
split
split drape
split graft
split hand
split ileostomy
split incision
split Russell traction
split sheet
split shot
split skin graft
split-course treatment
split-heel incision
split-sheath catheter
splitter

beam splitter
Zeiss beam splitter

splitter *continued*
    Zeiss small-beam splitter
split-thickness graft
split-thickness implant
split-thickness prosthesis
split-thickness skin graft
splitting
splitting chisel
splitting forceps
splitting of heart sounds
spondylolisthesis
spondylolysis
spondylopathy
spondylosis
spondylosyndesis
sponge
    absorbable gelatin
      sponge
    absorbable sponge
    Alcon microsponge
    blue sponge
    bronchoscopy sponge
    C-sponge
    cherry sponge
    Codman sponge
    Collostat hemostatic
      sponge
    Collostat sponge
    Custodis sponge
    4 x 4 sponge
    fibrin sponge
    free sponge
    gauze sponge
    gelatinous sponge
    Gelfoam sponge
    Helistat sponge
    Hibbs sponge
    Ivalon sponge
    Kitner sponge
    lap sponge
    laparotomy sponge
    Lapwall laparotomy
      sponge
    Lapwall sponge
    latex sponge
    Lincoff Silastic sponge
    Marlex sponge

sponge *continued*
    Medistat hemostatic
      sponge
    Merocel sponge
    microsponge
    nasopharyngeal sponge
    Nu-Gauze sponge
    peanut sponge
    pledget sponge
    polyvinyl alcohol sponge
    polyvinyl sponge
    Prosthex sponge
    Ray-Tec sponge
    Ray-Tec surgical sponge
    Ray-Tec x-ray detectable
      surgical sponge
    Rondic sponge
    rubber sponge
    saline-moistened sponge
    Schachar-Gills micro-
      sponge
    Silastic sponge
    silicone sponge
    Sof-Wick drain sponge
    Sof-Wick sponge
    stainless sponge
    stick sponge
    surgical sponge
    Surgtex x-ray detectable
      sponge
    tonsil sponge
    tonsillar sponges
    Topper dressing sponges
    Topper sponge
    vaginal sponge
    Vaiser eye sponge
    Vistec sponge
    Vistec x-ray detectable
      sponge
    Weck-cel sponge
    Weck-sorb airwick
      sponge
    wet lap sponge
    Zobec sponge
sponge and lap count
sponge and needle count
sponge basin

sponge biopsy
sponge carrier (see also *carrier*)
    bronchoscopic sponge
      carrier
    Jackson sponge carrier
sponge clamp
sponge count
sponge dissector
sponge forceps
sponge graft
sponge implant
sponge kidney
sponge patties
sponge test
sponge-and-dressing forceps
sponge-holding forceps
sponging forceps
spongiosa bone graft
spongiosa graft
spongiosa screw
spongiosa shunt
spongiosaplasty
Spongostan hemostat
spongy bone
spongy tissue
Sponsel osteotomy
spontaneous
spontaneous abortion (SAB)
spontaneous amputation
spontaneous breech delivery
spontaneous delivery
spontaneous fracture
spontaneous labor
spontaneous miscarriage
spontaneous pneumothorax
spontaneous respiration
spontaneous rupture
spontaneous vaginal delivery
spontaneous version
spontaneous voiding
spontaneously
spool
spoon
    appendectomy spoon
    Ballance mastoid spoon
    brain spatula spoon
    brain spoon

spoon *continued*
    Bunge exenteration
      spoon
    Bunge spoon
    Castroviejo spoon
    cataract spoon
    Culler lens spoon
    Cushing brain spatula
      spoon
    Cushing pituitary spoon
    Cushing spatula spoon
    Cushing spoon
    Daviel lens spoon
    Daviel spoon
    ear spoon
    Elschnig eye spoon
    Elschnig lens spoon
    Elschnig spoon
    enucleation spoon
    evisceration spoon
    exenteration spoon
    eye evisceration spoon
    eye spoon
    Falk appendectomy
      spoon
    Falk spoon
    Fisher spoon
    gall duct spoon
    gallbladder spoon
    Gross ear spoon
    Gross spoon
    Hardy pituitary spoon
    Hatt spoon
    Hess lens spoon
    Hess spoon
    Hiebert esophageal
      suture spoon
    Hoke spoon
    Hoke-Roberts spoon
    intracapsular lens spoon
    Kalt eye spoon
    Kalt spoon
    Kirby intracapsular lens
      spoon
    Kirby lens spoon
    Kirby spoon
    Knapp spoon

spoon *continued*
    Kocher brain spoon
    Kocher spoon
    lens spoon
    Lindner cyclodialysis
      spoon
    marrow spoon
    Mayo common duct
      spoon
    Moore gallbladder spoon
    Moore spoon
    obstetrical spoon
    Ray brain spoon
    Ray spoon
    Royal spoon
    sharp spoon
    Skene spoon
    Skene uterine spoon
    Troutman lens spoon
    uterine spoon
    Volkmann pancreatic
      calculus spoon
    Volkmann spoon
    Weber-Elschnig lens
      spoon
    Wells enucleation spoon
    Wells spoon
    Wills eye spoon
    Woodson spoon
spoon anastomosis clamp
spoon and spatula
spoon clamp
spoon retractor
spoon-shaped forceps
sporadic
sporadically occurring
spore
spore formation
spot cautery
spot film
spot retinoscope
spot view
Spot-quartz light
spotting and cramping
Sprague-Rappaport stethoscope
sprain
sprain fracture

sprain of joint
sprain of ligament
Spratt bone curet
Spratt curet
Spratt ear curet
Spratt mastoid curet
Spratt rasp
Spratt raspatory
spray
Spray Band dressing
spray bandage
spray bottle
Spray N Stretch
spread
spread pattern
spreader (see also *rib spreader*)
    Bailey rib spreader
    Bailey spreader
    Beeson plaster spreader
    bladder neck spreader
    Blanco valve spreader
    Blount bone spreader
    Burford rib spreader
    Burford spreader
    Burford-Finochietto rib
      spreader
    Burford-Finochietto
      spreader
    chest spreader
    child's rib spreader
    Cloward vertebral
      spreader
    Davis rib spreader
    DeBakey rib spreader
    deep spreader blade
    ductus spreader
    Favoloro-Morse sternal
      spreader
    Finochietto rib
      spreader
    Finochietto spreader
    Gerbode rib spreader
    Gross ductus spreader
    Gross spreader
    Haglund spreader
    Haight rib spreader
    Haight spreader

spreader *continued*

Haight-Finochietto spreader
Harken rib spreader
Harken spreader
Henning cast spreader
Henning plaster spreader
Hertzler baby rib spreader
Hertzler rib spreader
infant rib spreader
Inge lamina spreader
Inge spreader
Kimpton spreader
Kimpton vein spreader
Kirschner wire spreader
lamina spreader
Leksell sternal spreader
Lemmon rib spreader
Lemmon sternal spreader
Lilienthal rib spreader
Lilienthal spreader
Lilienthal-Sauerbruch rib spreader
Matson rib spreader
McGuire rib spreader
Medicon spreader
Millin-Bacon spreader
Miltex rib spreader
mitral valve spreader
Morse sternal spreader
Nelson rib spreader
Nissen rib spreader
Overholt spreader
Overholt-Finochietto rib spreader
Rehbein rib spreader
Rienhoff-Finochietto rib spreader
Rienhoff rib spreader
root-canal spreader
Sauerbruch-Lilienthal rib spreader
spinous process spreader
sternal spreader
Stille plaster spreader
Stille-Quervain spreader

spreader *continued*

Suarez spreader
Sweet rib spreader
Sweet-Burford rib spreader
Sweet-Finochietto rib spreader
Theis rib spreader
toe spreader
tonsillar spreader
Tudor-Edwards spreader
Tuffier rib spreader
Tuffier spreader
Turek spinous process spreader
Turek spreader
vertebral spreader
Weinberg pediatric rib spreader
Weinberg rib spreader
Weinberg spreader
Welsh pupil spreader-retractor forceps
Wilson rib spreader
Wilson spreader
Wiltberger spreader

spreader bar
spreading hand splint
Sprengel deformity
spring

Weiss spring

spring clip
spring cock-up splint
spring finger
spring holder
spring hook
spring lancet
spring ligament
spring pin
spring plate
spring retractor
spring swivel thumb
spring-eye needle
spring-handled forceps
spring-handled needle holder
spring-handled scissors
spring-holder instrument tray

spring-hook wire needle
spring-loaded vascular stent
spring-wire retractor
spring-wire safety-pin splint
sprinter's fracture
Sprong sutures
sprung knee
SPT technique (station pull-
    through technique)
spud
    Alvis spud
    Bahn spud
    Bennett foreign body
      spud
    Bennett spud
    Corbett foreign body
      spud
    Corbett spud
    curved needle eye spud
    curved needle spud
    Davis foreign body
      spud
    Davis spud
    Dix foreign body spud
    Dix spud
    Ellis foreign body spud
    Ellis spud
    eye spud
    Fisher spud
    flat eye spud
    foreign body eye spud
    foreign body spud
    Francis knife spud
    Francis spud
    golf-club eye spud
    golf-club spud
    Gross ear spud
    Gross spud
    Hosford foreign body
      spud
    Hosford spud
    LaForce knife spud
    LaForce spud
    Levine foreign body
      spud
    O'Brien foreign body
      spud
    Plange spud

spud *continued*
    Storz folding handle eye
      spud
    Walter corneal spud
    Walter spud
    Walton round gouge
      spud
    Whittle spud
spud dissector
spur
spur crusher
    baby spur crusher
    Garlock spur crusher
    Gross spur crusher
    Mayo-Lovelace spur
      crusher
    Ochsner-DeBakey spur
      crusher
    Pemberton spur crusher
    Stetten spur crusher
    Warthen spur crusher
    Wolfson spur crusher
    Wurth spur crusher
spur formation
spur-crushing clamp
spurious aneurysm
spurious pregnancy
Spurling forceps
Spurling IV disk forceps
Spurling laminectomy rongeur
Spurling maneuver
Spurling periosteal elevator
Spurling pituitary rongeur
Spurling retractor
Spurling rongeur
Spurling sign
Spurling tissue forceps
Spurling-Kerrison down-biting
    rongeur
Spurling-Kerrison forceps
Spurling-Kerrison laminectomy
    rongeur
Spurling-Kerrison punch
Spurling-Kerrison rongeur
Spurling-Kerrison up-biting
    rongeur
Spurling-Love-Gruenwald-
    Cushing rongeur

spurring
spurter
Sputnik-Federov lens
sputum
sputum collection
sputum culture
sputum production
sputum studies
sputum tube
squama
squama alveolaris
squamocolumnar junction
squamosal suture
squamosomastoid suture
squamosoparietal suture
squamososphenoid suture
squamous bone
squamous cell carcinoma
squamous epithelium
squamous suture lines
squamous suture of cranium
square
square knot
square punch
square specimen forceps
squared
square-off sign of shoulder
squares of dressing
square-tipped artery dissector
squatting
squatting maneuver
squeeze dynamometer
squeeze-handle forceps
Squibb Sur-Fit ostomy pouch
squint
squint hook
squinting eye
squinting patella
Squire catheter
SRH (stigmata of recent hemorrhage)
SRP (synchronized retroperfusion)
SRT vaginal speculum
SRVG (silicone elastomer ring vertical gastroplasty)
SS (stainless steel)

SS staple
SS sutures
SSA total hip system
Ssabanejew-Frank gastrostomy
Ssabanejew-Frank operation
SSI brace (shoulder subluxation inhibitor brace)
SST deformity
SSW forceps
St. Clair forceps
St. Clair-Thompson abscess forceps
St. Clair-Thompson adenoid curet
St. Clair-Thompson adenotome
St. Clair-Thompson curet
St. Clair-Thompson forceps
St. Clair-Thompson peritonsillar abscess forceps
St. George total hip prosthesis
St. George total knee prosthesis
St. Jude bileaflet prosthetic valve
St. Jude composite valve graft
St. Jude Medical aortic valve prosthesis
St. Jude Medical bileaflet heart valve
St. Jude Medical prosthetic heart valve
St. Jude Medical valve prosthesis
St. Jude mitral valve prosthesis
St. Jude valve
St. Jude valve prosthesis
St. Luke retractor
St. Luke rongeur
St. Mark clamp
St. Mark excision
St. Mark hemorrhoidectomy
St. Mark incision
St. Martin eye forceps
St. Martin forceps
St. Martin suturing forceps
St. Martin-Franceschetti secondary cataract hook

St. Urban Berlin hip joint
    surface replacement
St. Vincent forceps
St. Vincent tube clamp
St. Vincent tube-clamping
    forceps
stab drain
stab form
stab incision
stab needle
stab wound
stabbing pain
stability
stabilization
stabilization of joint
stabilized condition
stabilized course
stabilizing
stabilocondylar knee pros-
    thesis
stable condition
stable fracture
stable sprain
stable vital sign
Stableflex lens
stab-wound drain
stab-wound incision
Stack perfusion coronary
    dilatation catheter
Stack retractor
Stack splint
Stacke chisel guard
Stacke gouge
Stacke mastoidectomy
Stacke operation
Stader pin
Stader splint
Stader wrench
Stadie-Riggs microtome
stadium-type of ureteral orifice
Staecker nerve protector
stage of labor
staghorn calculus
staghorn stone
staging laparotomy
staging lymphadenectomy
staging operation

staging process and imaging
staging system
staging systems in radiation
    therapy
Stagnera procedure
Staheli shelf operation
Stahl calipers
Stahl ear
Stähli line
stain
stained smear
staining
stainless
stainless irrigator
stainless spatula
stainless sponge
stainless steel
stainless steel bobbin
stainless steel clamp
stainless steel cup
stainless steel graft
stainless steel implant
stainless steel mesh
stainless steel mesh prosthesis
stainless steel piston
stainless steel prosthesis
stainless steel screw
stainless steel strut
stainless steel stud
stainless steel sutures
stainless steel wire
stainless steel wire prosthesis
stainless steel wire sutures
stainless steel with molybde-
    num
stalagmometer
stalk
stalk of polyp
stalked hydatid
stall bars
Stallard  dissector
Stallard flap operation
Stallard operation
Stallard scleral hook
Stallard sutures
Stallard-Liegard suture
Stallworthy placenta

STA-MCA (superficial temporary artery-middle cerebral artery)
STA-MCA bypass procedure
Stamey bladder neck suspension
Stamey catheter
Stamey needle
Stamey paraurethral suspension
Stamey procedure
Stamey ureteral catheter
Stamey urethropexy
Stamey-Pereyra bladder neck suspension
Stamey-Pereyra urethropexy
Stamm arthrodesis
Stamm bunionectomy
Stamm gastroplasty
Stamm gastrostomy
Stamm hip fusion
Stamm operation
Stamm osteotomy
Stamm tube
Stammberger antral punch
stammering bladder
Stamm-Kader operation
Stamm-Senn gastroscopy
Stamm-Seu gastroscopy
stamp test
standard 6-lumen perfused catheter
standard artery forceps
standard arthroscope
standard bronchoscope
standard configuration
standard laryngoscope
standard neck Universal for Richards hip prosthesis
standard procedure
standard radical neck dissection
standard therapy
standard trocar
standard-pattern hammer
standard-pattern mallet
standby
standby assist
standby assistance

standby Baumanometer
standby pacemaker
standing ambulation
standing frame orthosis
standing orders
standpoint
standstill
Stanford chemotherapy protocol
Stanford end-hole pigtail catheter
Stanicor Gamma pacemaker
Stanicor Lambda demand pacemaker
Stanicor pacemaker
Stanischeff operation
Stanley-Kent bundle
Stanmore shoulder arthroplasty
Stanmore shoulder prosthesis
Stanmore total hip
Stanton cautery clamp
Stanton cautery with mousetrap clamp
Stanton clamp
stapedectomy
stapedectomy forceps
stapedectomy knife
stapedectomy prosthesis
stapedial crus
stapedial fold
stapedial footplate auger
stapedial nerve
stapedial tendon
stapedial tendon cut
stapediolysis
stapediotenotomy
stapedius muscle
stapedius, musculus
stapedius, nervus
stapedius tendon
stapedius tendon knife
stapes
stapes bone
stapes chisel
stapes curet
stapes dilator
stapes elevator

stapes excavator
stapes fixed
stapes footplate
stapes forceps
stapes hoe
stapes hook
stapes mobilization
stapes mobilization operation
stapes pick
stapes piston
stapes prosthesis
stapes speculum
stapes spline
stapes superstructure
stapes tapping hammer
stapes wire guide
staphylectomy
staphylopharyngorrhaphy
staphyloplasty
staphylorrhaphy
staphylorrhaphy elevator
staphylorrhaphy needle
staphylotome
staphylotomy
staple
    Accustaple
    barb staple
    Blount knee staple
    Blount staple
    Coventry staple
    duToit staple
    Dwyer staple
    Ellison fixation staple
    Ethicon staple
    GIA staple
    ICLH staple
    Mario-Stone staple
    Oswestry staple
    Proplast staple
    Proximate skin staple
    SGIA staple
    SinStat preformed skin
      staple
    skin staple
    SS staple
    step staple
    Stone staple

staple *continued*
    30-V staple
    titanium staple
    von Petz staple
    Zimaloy epiphyseal
      staple
    Zimaloy staple
staple forceps
staple gun (see also *stapler*)
    Auto-Suture TA-50 staple
      gun
    Cobe staple gun
staple line dehiscence
staple procedure
staple sutures
stapler (see also *staple gun*)
    American vascular
      stapler
    Appose disposable skin
      stapler
    Appose skin stapler
    Auto-Suture GIA stapler
    Auto-Suture stapler
    Auto-Suture surgical
      stapler
    Barstow stapler
    CEEA stapler (curved
      end-to-end anasto-
      mosis stapler)
    circular stapler
    Cobe stapler
    Davis-Geck surgical
      stapler
    double-headed P190
      stapler
    EEA Auto-Suture stapler
    EEA circular stapler
    EEA stapler
    GIA circular stapler
    GIA stapler
    ILA surgical stapler
    ILS (intraluminal stapler)
    LDA stapler
    LDF stapler
    LDS stapler
    linear stapler
    One Time skin stapler

stapler *continued*
   PI surgical stapler
   Precise disposable skin
     stapler
   Proximate flexible linear
     stapler
   Proximate intraluminal
     stapler
   Proximate linear stapler
   Proximate stapler
   Roticulator clamp stapler
   SGIA stapler
   Staplizer powered
     metaphyseal stapler
   Surgeon's Choice stapler
   TA-30 stapler
   TA-50 stapler
   TA-55 stapler
   TA-60 stapler
   TA-90 stapler
   TA-90-BN stapler
   Uhlrich stapler
   Watt skin closure stapler
   Weck stapler
   Wiberg fracture stapler
Staples elbow arthrodesis
Staples osteotomy nail
Staples-Black-Brostrom ankle
   procedure
stapling
stapling device
stapling instruments
stapling procedure
stapling technique
Staplizer powered metaphyseal
   stapler
starch bandage
Starck cardiodilator
Starck dilator
Starlinger dilator
Starlinger uterine dilator
Starr ball heart prosthesis
Starr ball heart valve
Starr fixation forceps
Starr forceps
Starr-Bloodwell low-profile
   valve

Starr-Edwards aortic valve
   prosthesis
Starr-Edwards heart valve
Starr-Edwards hermetically
   sealed pacemaker
Starr-Edwards pacemaker
Starr-Edwards prosthesis
Starr-Edwards prosthetic aortic
   valve
Starr-Edwards prosthetic ball
   valve
Starr-Edwards prosthetic mitral
   valve
Starr-Edwards prosthetic valve
Starr-Edwards Silastic valve
Starr-Edwards silicone rubber
   ball valve
Starr-Edwards valve
Starr-Edwards valve prosthesis
starting and stopping of urinary
   stream
stasis (*pl.* stases)
stasis changes
stasis edema
stasis gallbladder
stasis ulcer
stat (immediately)
Stat aspirating instrument
Stat cutting instrument
stat orders
Stat Scrub handwasher
   machine
state
State colorectal anastomosis
state of consciousness
State operation
state-of-the-art
Statham cautery
Statham flowmeter
Statham pressure transducer
Statham strain gauge
Statham transducer
Statham transensor
static disorder
static tendon transfer
station
station pull-through operation

station pull-through technique
(SPT technique)
stationary bridge
stationary cataract
Sta-Tite gauze dressing
Staude forceps
Staude tenaculum forceps
Staude uterine tenaculum
forceps
Staude-Jackson tenaculum
forceps
Staude-Moore forceps
Staude-Moore tenaculum
Staude-Moore uterine tenaculum forceps
Staunig position
Staunton sphygmomanometer
Stax splint
stay knot
stay sutures
steadily advancing
steadily deteriorating
steadiness
steady downhill course
steal procedure
steam cautery
steam sterilization
steam sterilizer
steam under pressure
Stearns speculum
steatorrhea
Stecher arachnoid knife
Stecher position
Stedman aspirator
Stedman pump
Stedman suction pump
Stedman suction pump aspirator
Stedman suction tube
steel mallet
steel mesh
steel mesh sutures
steel plate
steel sutures
steel wire prosthesis
Steele bronchial dilator
Steele dilator
Steele osteotomy

Steele periosteal elevator
Steele-Stewart operation
Steelquist amputation
steep Trendelenburg position
steeple sign
steerable catheter
steerable guide wire
steerable wire
steering-wheel injury
Steffanoff ear reconstruction
Steffee plate
Steffee prosthesis
Steffee screw
Steichen technique
Steide fracture of femur
Stein cheiloplasty
Stein intraocular implant lens
Stein lens
Stein membrane perforator
Stein operation
Stein perforator
Stein-Abbé lip flap
Steinach method
Steinach operation
Steinberg thumb sign
Steindler arthrodesis
Steindler flexorplasty
Steindler matricectomy
Steindler operation
Steindler stripping
Steindler technique
Steiner-Auvard speculum
Steiner-Auvard vaginal
speculum
Stein-Kazanjian flap
Stein-Leventhal syndrome
Steinmann calibrated pin
Steinmann extension
Steinmann holder
Steinmann intestinal forceps
Steinmann intestinal grasping
forceps
Steinmann nail
Steinmann pin
Steinmann pin chuck
Steinmann pin with Crowe pilot
point

Steinmann traction
Steinmann traction bow
Steinmann tractor
stellatae renis, venulae
stellate block
stellate block anesthesia
stellate cataract
stellate fracture
stellate ganglion
stellate ganglion block
stellate incision
stellate veins
stellate veins of kidney
stellectomy
Stellite ring material of
    prosthetic valve
stem
stem pessary
stem prosthesis
stem rasp
stem-cell marrow harvesting
Stemp compound
stencil wire
Stener lesion
Stener-Gunterberg sacrum
    resection
Stengstrom nerve cutter
stenopeic disk
stenopeic iridectomy
stenosed aortic valve
stenosing
stenosis (*pl.* stenoses)
stenosis clamp
stenotic
stenotic femoral artery
stenotic segment
stenotic valve
Stensen canal
Stensen duct
Stensen foramen
Stensen veins
Stenstrom foot flap
stent
        activated balloon
            expandable intravascu-
            lar stent
        adjustable vaginal stent

stent *continued*
    Amsterdam stent
    balloon expandable
        intravascular stent
    Bard coil stent
    Bard soft double-pigtail
        stent
    biliary stent
    Carpentier stent
    coil vascular stent
    Cook ureteral stent
    Cook Urosoft stent
    core mold stent
    Dacron stent
    double-J indwelling
        catheter stent
    double-J silicone internal
        ureteral catheter stent
    double-J ureteral stent
    double-pigtail stent
    endoluminal stent
    esophageal stent
    foam rubber stent
    foam rubber vaginal
        stent
    French stent
    gauze stent
    Gianturco stent
    Gibbon indwelling
        ureteral stent
    Gibbon stent
    Gibbon ureteral stent
    indwelling stent
    indwelling ureteral stent
    intraoral stent
    iridium-192 loaded stent
    J-stent
    keel stent
    Medinvent vascular stent
    Ossof-Sisson surgical
        stent
    Palmaz stent
    Palmaz vascular stent
    pancreatic duct stent
    percutaneous stent
    pigtail stent
    polyethylene stent

stent *continued*

- Silastic stent
- Silitek ureteral stent
- single-J urinary diversion stent
- spring-loaded vascular stent
- straight stent
- Surgitek double-J ureteral stent
- Surgitek Tractfinder ureteral stent
- Surgitek Uropass stent
- T-tube stent
- ties-over-stent
- transhepatic biliary stent
- U-tube stent
- ureteral stent
- Urosoft stent
- vaginal stent
- Wilson-Cook French stent

stent dressing
stent graft
Stent mass
stent placement
stent plugging
stent skin graft technique
stent tube
stent tube with pigtail curl
Stenver position
Stenver view
Stenver x-ray view
Stenzel rod
Stenzel rod prosthesis
step graft
step staples
step-cut lengthening
step-cut osteotomy
step-cut reamer
step-down drill
step-down osteotomy
step-down transformer
Stephee joint replacement
Stephenson corneal trephine
Stephenson holder
Stephenson-Donovan transfer

Stepita clamp
Stepita meatus clamp
stepladder incision
step-off fracture
step-osteotomy
step-up
step-up transformer
stepwise sutures
stercoraceous
stercoral appendicitis
stercoral ulcer
stereo views
stereo x-ray views
stereoarthrolysis
stereoencephalotome
stereoencephalotomy
stereoroentgenography
stereoscopic
stereotactic laser
stereotactic surgery
stereotaxic
stereotaxic device
stereotaxic hypophysectomy
stereotaxic neuroradiography
stereotaxic neurosurgery
stereotaxic procedure
stereotaxic surgery
stereotaxy
Steri-Drape
sterile
sterile absorbent gauze
sterile adhesive plaster
sterile adhesive tape
sterile bone wax
sterile compression dressing
sterile connecting tube
sterile drape
sterile dressing
sterile examination
sterile field
sterile fluffs
sterile fluid
sterile procedure
sterile saline
sterile site
sterile specimen
sterile tape

sterile technique
sterile towels
sterile vacuum collection tube
sterilely
sterilely draped
sterilely prepared and draped
sterilely prepped and draped
sterility
sterilization
sterilized instruments
sterilizer
sterilizer forceps
Steri-pads dressing
Sterisol
steri-stripped incision
Steri-Strips
Steritapes
Sterivac drain
Sterles sign
Stern position
sternal approximator (see also
    *approximator*)
        Leksell sternal approxi-
            mator
        Lemmon sternal approxi-
            mator
        Nunez sternal approxi-
            mator
        Pilling Wolvek sternal
            approximator
        Wolvek sternal approxi-
            mator
sternal biopsy
sternal blade
sternal border
sternal depression
sternal fissure
sternal infection
sternal instruments
sternal knife
sternal lead
sternal muscle
sternal needle
sternal notch
sternal perforating awl
sternal punch
sternal puncture

sternal puncture by aspiration
sternal puncture by curettage
sternal puncture needle
sternal retractor
sternal retractor blade
sternal shears
sternal spreader
sternal trephine
sternal wire
sternal wire sutures
sternal-splitting incision
sternalis, musculus
Sternberg sign
Stern-Castroviejo forceps
Stern-McCarthy electrode
Stern-McCarthy electrotome
Stern-McCarthy electrotome
    resectoscope
Stern-McCarthy knife
Stern-McCarthy resectoscope
sternoclavicular
sternoclavicular angle
sternoclavicular articulation
sternoclavicular joint
sternoclavicular junction
sternoclavicular ligament
sternoclavicular notch
sternocleidomastoid artery
sternocleidomastoid hemor-
    rhage
sternocleidomastoid muscle
sternocleidomastoid region
sternocleidomastoid vein
sternocleidomastoidea, arteria
sternocleidomastoidea, vena
sternocleidomastoideus,
    musculus
sternocostal articulation
sternocostal ligament
sternocostal muscle
sternocostal surface of heart
sternohyoid muscle
sternohyoideus, musculus
sternomastoid muscle
sternothyroid muscle
sternothyroideus, musculus
sternotomy

sternotomy saw
sternotracheal
sternotrypesis
sternum
sternum depressed
sternum-splitting procedure
steroids
Stertzer brachial guiding
   catheter
Stertzer catheter
Stertzer-Myler extension wire
stethoscope
   Albion-Ford stetho-
      scope
   Allen fetal stethoscope
   binaural stethoscope
   Bowles stethoscope
   Cammann stethoscope
   combination stethoscope
   DeLee-Hillis obstetrical
      head stethoscope
   DeLee-Hillis obstetrical
      stethoscope
   DeLee-Hillis stethoscope
   diaphragm stethoscope
   Doppler stethoscope
   Doptone fetal stetho-
      scope
   Duo-Sonic stethoscope
   electronic stethoscope
   esophageal stethoscope
   fetal stethoscope
   Ford stethoscope
   Gordon stethoscope
   Howell tunable dia-
      phragm stethoscope
   Leff stethoscope
   Littman Class II pediatric
      stethoscope
   micromembranous
      stethoscope
   Pilling stethoscope
   Rieger stethoscope
   Scanmate stethoscope
   Sprague-Rappaport
      stethoscope
   Tiemann stethoscope

stethoscope *continued*
   tunable diaphragm
      stethoscope
   Wechsler obstetrical
      stethoscope
Stetten colostomy crusher
Stetten intestinal clamp
Stetten spur crusher
Stevens elevator
Stevens eye knife
Stevens fixation forceps
Stevens forceps
Stevens hook
Stevens iris forceps
Stevens needle holder
Stevens scissors
Stevens tenotomy hook
Stevens tenotomy scissors
Stevens tissue knife
Stevens traction hook
Stevenson capsule punch
Stevenson clamp
Stevenson eye speculum
Stevenson forceps
Stevenson grasping forceps
Stevenson lacrimal retractor
Stevenson lacrimal sac retractor
Stevenson LaForce adenotome
Stevenson needle holder
Stevenson operation
Stevenson punch
Stevenson retractor
Stevenson scissors
Stewart cartilage knife
Stewart crypt hook
Stewart guide
Stewart hook
Stewart incision
Stewart knife
Stewart ligament guide
Stewart sutures
Stewart technique
Stewart-Hamilton cardiac output
   technique
Stewart-Harley ankle procedure
Stewart-Treves syndrome
STH-2 total hip prosthesis

stick
stick sponge
stick ties
stick-on electrode
stick-tie sutures
Stieda disease
Stieda fracture
Stieglitz splinter forceps
stiff neck
stiff pupil
stiff ray
stiffening of joint
stiff-heart syndrome
stiffness
stiffness and pain
stiffness of joints
stiffness of neck
stifle joint
Stifneck immobilizing collar
stigma (*pl.* stigmata)
stigmata of recent hemorrhage
   (SRH)
Stiles-Bunnell transfer
stilet (see *stylet*)
stilette (see *stylet*)
stiletto
stiletto knife
stillbirth
stillborn infant
Stille bone rongeur
Stille chisel
Stille clamp
Stille cranial drill
Stille dissecting scissors
Stille drill
Stille forceps
Stille gallstone forceps
Stille Gigli saw
Stille Gigli-saw guide
Stille Gigli-saw wire
Stille gouge
Stille kidney clamp
Stille mallet
Stille osteotome
Stille periosteal elevator
Stille plaster shears
Stille plaster spreader

Stille rib shears
Stille rongeur
Stille saw
Stille scissors
Stille shears
Stille Super Cut scissors
Stille tissue forceps
Stille trephine
Stille uterine dilator
Stille vessel clamp
Stille-Adson forceps
Stille-Barraya intestinal forceps
Stille-Barraya intestinal-grasping
   forceps
Stille-Björk forceps
Stille-Crawford clamp
Stille-Crawford coarctation
   clamp
Stille-Crile forceps
Stille-Doyen rasp
Stille-Edwards rasp
Stille-French needle holder
Stille-Giertz rib shears
Stille-Halsted forceps
Stille-Horsley bone-cutting
   forceps
Stille-Horsley forceps
Stille-Horsley rib shears
Stille-Joseph saw
Stille-Langenbeck elevator
Stille-Lauer bone rongeur
Stille-Leksell rongeur
Stille-Liston bone forceps
Stille-Liston bone-cutting
   forceps
Stille-Liston double-action
   rongeur
Stille-Liston forceps
Stille-Liston rib-cutting forceps
Stille-Liston rongeur
Stille-Luer bone rongeur
Stille-Luer forceps
Stille-Luer multiple-action
   rongeur
Stille-Luer rongeur
Stille-Luer-Echlin bone rongeur
Stille-Mathieu needle holder

Stille-Mayo scissors
Stille-Mayo-Hegar needle
Stille-Metzenbaum needle
  holder
Stille-pattern bone chisel
Stille-pattern bone drill
Stille-pattern bone gouge
Stille-pattern osteotome
Stille-pattern rib shears
Stille-Quervain spreader
Stiller sign
Stille-Russian forceps
Stille-Seldinger needle
Stillette catheter
Stilli knife
Stimson maneuver
stimulant
stimulate
stimulating catheter
stimulation
stimulation of peripheral nerves
stimulator (see also *bone growth stimulator, nerve stimulator*)
  ACUTENS transcutaneous nerve stimulator
  AME bone growth stimulator
  Burdick muscle stimulator
  Concept nerve stimulator
  cutaneous stimulator
  DCS (dorsal column stimulator/stimulation)
  dorsal column stimulator (DCS)
  implantable bone growth stimulator
  nerve stimulator
  Orgen SpF spinal bone growth stimulator
  Orthofuse implantable growth stimulator
  OrthoGen bone growth stimulator
  OrthoPak bone growth stimulator

stimulator *continued*
  OsteoGen bone growth stimulator
  Osteo-Stim electrical bone growth stimulator
  percutaneous dorsal column stimulator
  spinal cord stimulator
  Spinal-Stim bone growth stimulator
  TCNS (transcutaneous nerve stimulator)
  TENS (terminal electrode nerve stimulator)
  TENS (transcutaneous electrical nerve stimulation/stimulator)
  terminal electrode nerve stimulator (TENS)
  TNS (transcutaneous nerve stimulator)
  transcutaneous electrical nerve stimulation/stimulator (TENS)
  transcutaneous nerve stimulator (TCNS, TNS)
  transcutaneous stimulator
stimulus
stimulus response
stipple cell
stippled epiphysis
stippled tongue
stippling
stirrup anastomosis
stirrup bone
stirrup brace
stirrup splint
stirrup-loop curet
stirrups
stitch
stitch abscess
stitch scissors
stitched together
Stitt catheter
Stock eye trephine
Stock operation

Stocker cyclodiathermy
    puncture needle
Stocker needle
Stocker operation
stockinette
stockinette amputation bandage
stockinette bandage
stockinette cap
stockinette dressing
stocking-and-glove-type
    hypesthesia
stocking-glove distribution
stocking-seam incision
Stockman clamp
Stockman penis clamp
Stoerck loop
Stoffel operation
Stokes amputation
Stokes lens
Stokes operation
Stokes sign
Stokes-Adams seizures
Stokes-Adams syndrome
Stokes-Gritti amputation
Stolte dissector
Stoltz laparoscope
Stoltz pubiotomy
stoma (*pl.* stomas, stomata)
stoma irrigated
stoma site
stomach
stomach acid
stomach brush
stomach bubble
stomach calculus
stomach cancer
stomach capacity
stomach clamp
stomach contents
stomach distention
stomach irrigation tube
stomach lining
stomach magnet
stomach rugae
stomach spasms
stomach stapling
stomach tube

stomach ulcer
stomach wall
Stomahesive
stomal
stomal bag
stomal stenosis
stomal ulcer
stomatoplasty
stomatorrhagia gingivarum
stomatorrhaphy
stone
stone basket (see also *basket*)
    Barnes-Dormia stone
        basket
    biliary stone basket
    Browne stone basket
    Councill stone basket
    disposable stone basket
    Dormia biliary stone
        basket
    Dormia stone basket
    Ellik kidney stone basket
    Ellik stone basket
    Ferguson stone basket
    Howard stone basket
    Johns Hopkins stone
        basket
    Johnson stone basket
    Johnson ureteral stone
        basket
    Mitchell stone basket
    Pfister stone basket
    Pfister-Schwartz stone
        basket
    Robinson stone basket
    Rutner stone basket
    Segura stone basket
    ureteral stone basket
Stone bunionectomy
Stone clamp
stone cutter's phthisis
stone dislodger (see also
    *dislodger*)
    Cook helical stone
        dislodger
    Councill stone dislodger
    Creevy stone dislodger

stone dislodger *continued*
    Davis loop stone dislodger
    Davis stone dislodger
    Dormia stone dislodger
    Dormia ureteral stone dislodger
    Ellik loop stone dislodger
    filiform stone dislodger
    Howard stone dislodger
    Johnson stone dislodger
    Levant stone dislodger
    Morton stone dislodger
    Porges stone dislodger
    Robinson stone dislodger
    spiral stone dislodger
    Storz stone dislodger
    ureteral basket stone dislodger
    ureteral stone dislodger
    woven-loop stone dislodger
    Wullen stone dislodger
    Zeiss stone dislodger
stone dislodger filiform
stone extractor
Stone eye implant
Stone forceps
Stone hip arthrodesis
stone impaction
Stone implant
stone locking device
stone placenta
Stone procedure for hallux rigidus
stone removal
Stone staple
Stone tissue forceps
stone-crushing forceps
stone-extraction forceps
stone-grasping forceps
Stone-Holcombe anastomosis clamp
Stone-Holcombe clamp
Stone-Holcombe intestinal clamp

stone-holding basket
Stoneman forceps
stony hard
Stony splenorenal shunt clamp
Stookey cranial rongeur
Stookey reflex
Stookey retractor
Stookey rongeur
Stookey-Scarff operation
stool
stooping
stop eye speculum
stop needle
stopcock
stoppage
storage
stored fat
Storer retractor
Storey forceps
Storey gall duct forceps
Storey-Hillar dissecting forceps
Stork arthroscope
Stormer viscosimeter
Storz adjustable headrest
Storz adjustable magnifier
Storz anterior commissure laryngoscope
Storz anti-fog solution
Storz anti-fog tube
Storz antrum punch
Storz applicator
Storz arthroscope
Storz arthroscopy operating instruments
Storz aspiration biopsy needle
Storz atomizer
Storz atraumatic distending obturator
Storz attachment
Storz binocular loupe
Storz binocular prism
Storz binocular prism loupe
Storz biopsy forceps
Storz biopsy thoracoscope
Storz bladder evacuator
Storz bougie-urethrotome
Storz bronchial catheter

Storz bronchoscope
Storz bronchoscopic forceps
Storz bronchoscopic specimen
    collector
Storz bronchoscopic suction
    tube
Storz bronchoscopic telescope
Storz cable
Storz camera equipment
Storz catheter adapter
Storz catheter connector
Storz choledochoscope
Storz cleaning accessories
Storz cleaning brush
Storz cold-light fountain
Storz cold-punch resectoscope
Storz conductor
Storz continuous irrigation-
    suction resectoscope
Storz corneal bur
Storz cotton carrier
Storz cystoscope
Storz cystoscope tip
Storz cystoscope-urethroscope
Storz cystoscopic accessories
Storz cystoscopic electrode
Storz cystoscopic forceps
Storz cystoscopic rongeur
Storz cystoscopic scissors
Storz deflecting obturator
Storz delicate iris scissors
Storz direct-vision cystoscope
Storz disposable trephine
Storz ear speculum
Storz emergency ventilation
    bronchoscope
Storz endocamera
Storz endomagnifier
Storz esophageal conductor
Storz esophagoscope
Storz esophagoscopic forceps
Storz evacuator
Storz examination insert tube
Storz examining arthroscope
Storz eyepiece
Storz eyepiece attachment
Storz face shield

Storz face-shield headband
Storz fiberoptic cable
Storz fiberoptic cable adapter
Storz fiberoptic light cable
Storz fiberoptic light source
Storz flash generator
Storz flash tube
Storz flexible biopsy instru-
    ments
Storz flexible esophageal
    conductor
Storz flexible injection needle
Storz folding emergency
    ventilation bronchoscope
Storz folding-handle ear knife
Storz folding-handle eye spud
Storz forceps
Storz grasping biopsy forceps
Storz guillotine
Storz gynecological instruments
Storz headlight
Storz high-frequency cord
Storz hysteroscope
Storz infant bronchoscope
Storz infection ventilation
    laryngoscope
Storz Injecttimer
Storz insert tube
Storz intraocular scissors
Storz intratracheal tube
Storz kidney stone forceps
Storz knife
Storz laparoscope
Storz laryngopharyngoscope
Storz magnet
Storz meatus clamp
Storz meniscotome
Storz miniature forceps
Storz nasal speculum
Storz nasopharyngeal biopsy
    forceps
Storz needle cannula
Storz nephroscope
Storz operating esophago-
    scope
Storz optical biopsy forceps
Storz optical esophagoscope

Storz otolaryngological instru-
ments
Storz pediatric esophagoscope
Storz peritoneoscope
Storz proctoscopic instruments
Storz punch
Storz resectoscope
Storz resectoscope cable
Storz resectoscope curet
Storz resectoscope electrode
Storz retractor
Storz rongeur
Storz safety-sterility disk
Storz scope
Storz sheath
Storz sinus biopsy forceps
Storz snare
Storz speculum
Storz sterilizing case
Storz stone dislodger
Storz stone-crushing forceps
Storz stone-extraction forceps
Storz suprapubic cystoscope
Storz synchronizing cords
Storz teaching attachment
Storz telescope
Storz tube
Storz urological instrument
Storz-Beck snare
Storz-Beck-Schenck snare
Storz-Bell erysiphake
Storz-Bonn forceps
Storz-Bonn suturing forceps
Storz-Bowman lacrimal probe
Storz-Bruenings diagnostic head
Storz-Bruenings ear magnifier
Storz-Castroviejo needle holder
Storz-DeKock two-way bron-
chial catheter
Storz-Denecke headlight
Storz-Doesel-Huzly broncho-
scope tube
Storz-Duredge cataract knife
Storz-Ellik evacuator
Storz-Hopkins laryngoscope
Storz-Hopkins telescope
Storz-Hopkins telescopic optics

Storz-Iglesias resectoscope
Storz-Kirkheim urethrotome
Storz-LaForce adenotome
Storz-LaForce-Stevenson
adenotome
Storz-Moltz tonometer
Storz-Urban surgical microscope
Storz-Vienna speculum
Storz-Westcott conjunctival
scissors
Stout continuous loop wire
Stout wire
Stout wiring
Straatsma intraocular implant
lens
Straatsma lens
strabismus
strabismus correction
strabismus forceps
strabismus hook
strabismus needle
strabismus operation
strabismus scissors
strabismus tucker
straddle fracture
straddling aorta
straddling embolus
straight AP pelvic injection
straight arterioles of kidney
straight catheter
straight cautery
straight chest tube
straight clamp
straight connector
straight Crile clamp
straight cutting knife
straight dural hook
straight elevator
straight flush percutaneous
catheter
straight forceps
straight graft
straight guide wire
straight hemostat
straight incision
straight lacrimal cannula
straight last shoes

straight leg raising
straight leg-raising test (SLR test)
straight line
straight needle
straight nerve hook
straight rongeur
straight scissors
straight single tenaculum
    forceps
straight sinus
straight stem femoral compo-
    nent
straight stent
straight stylet
straight suture needle
straight tenaculum
straight tubular graft
straight-blade electrode
straight-blade laryngoscope
straight-end cup forceps
straightener
        Asch septal straightener
        Asch straightener
        Cottle-Walsham septal
            straightener
        Cottle-Walsham straight-
            ener
        Walsham straightener
straight-pin teeth
straight-point electrode
straight-stem prosthesis
straight-stemmed
straight-tipped electrode
strain
strain film
strain fracture
strain gauge
strain pattern
strain x-rays
strain-gauge manometer
strain-gauge transducer
straining
strait
Straith operation
Straith otoplasty
Straith profilometer
Strampelli eye splint

Strampelli implant
Strampelli implant cataract lens
Strampelli lens
strandy infiltrate
strangulated
strangulated bowel
strangulated bowel obstruction
strangulated hemorrhoid
strangulated hernia
strangulated inguinal hernia
strangulated viscus
strangulation
strangulation obstruction
stranguria
strangury
strap clavicle splint
strap muscles
Strap operation
strap sling
strap-on pump
strapping
Strassman metroplasty
Strassman operation
Strassman-Jones operation
Strassmann uterine-elevating
    forceps
strata (*sing.* stratum)
strategy procedure
stratification
stratified squamous epithelium
Stratte clamp
Stratte forceps
Stratte needle holder
stratum (*pl.* strata)
stratum corneum
stratum granulosum
Strauss cannula
Strauss clamp
Strauss meatus clamp
Strauss needle
Strauss proctoscope
Strauss sigmoidoscope
Strauss sign
strawberry cervix
strawberry gallbladder
strawberry hemangioma
strawberry mark

strawberry tongue
straw-colored ascites
straw-colored fluid
straw-colored urine
Strayer knife
Strayer operation to lengthen
    heel cord
streak culture
streak retinoscope
streaked ovaries
streaked with blood
streaking
streaks
stream
stream of urine
Street diamond-shaped nail
Street medullary pin
Street nail
Street pin
Street rod
Street tonsillar syringe
Street-Stevens humeral replace-
    ment
Strelinger catheter-introducing
    forceps
Strelinger colon clamp
Strelinger right-angle colon
    clamp
strength
strength and mobility
stress action
Stress Cath catheter
stress fracture
stress incontinence
stress on cannula
stress on needle
stress responses
stress roentgenogram
stress skin lines
stress test
stress ulcer
stress ulceration
stressful
stress-induced condition
stressor
stress-related condition
stress-strain curve

stretch
stretch marks
stretch reflex
stretch stricture
stretcher
stretching of iris
stretching of muscle
stretching of nerve
Stretzer bent-tip USCI catheter
stria (*pl.* striae)
striae of abdomen
striae of breasts
striae of pregnancy
striae of thighs
striata, vena
striate vein
striated
striated muscle
striated reticulum
striation
Strickland tendon repair
stricture
        annular stricture
        bridle stricture
        cicatricial stricture
        contractile stricture
        false stricture
        functional stricture
        impassable stricture
        impermeable stricture
        irritable stricture
        organic stricture
        permanent stricture
        recurrent stricture
        spasmodic stricture
        spastic stricture
        temporary stricture
stricture formation
stricture scope
stricturoplasty
stricturotome
stricturotomy
stride length
stridor
string bladder
string carcinoma
string operation

string test for peptic ulcer
stringent
Stringer catheter-introducing
    forceps
Stringer forceps
Stringer newborn throat forceps
string-of-beads appearance
stringy infiltration
stringy opacification
stringy vitreous floaters
striocerebellar tremor
strip of gauze
stripe
striped muscle
stripped and ligated
stripper (see also *rib stripper,
    tendon stripper, vein
    stripper*)
    Alexander rib stripper
    Babcock jointed vein
        stripper
    Babcock vein stripper
    Bartlett fascia stripper
    Bartlett stripper
    Brand tendon stripper
    Bunnell tendon stripper
    Callahan zonule lens
        stripper
    Cannon stripper
    Cannon vein stripper
    Carroll forearm tendon
        stripper
    cartilage stripper
    Clark vein stripper
    clot stripper
    Codman vein stripper
    Cole polyethylene vein
        stripper
    Cole vein stripper
    Crawford fascial stripper
    Crile stripper
    Crile vagotomy stripper
    DeBakey intraluminal
        stripper
    DeBakey stripper
    disposable stripper
    Dorian rib stripper

stripper *continued*
    Doyle vein stripper
    Dunlop stripper
    Dunlop thrombus
        stripper
    elevator and stripper
    Emerson stripper
    Emerson vein stripper
    endarterectomy stripper
    endotracheal stripper
    external stripper
    external vein stripper
    extraluminal stripper
    fascia stripper
    Friedman vein stripper
    Holley vascular stripper
    hydraulic vein stripper
    improved Webb strip-
        per
    internal vein stripper
    intraluminal stripper
    J-stripper
    jointed vein stripper
    Joplin stripper
    Keeley stripper
    Keeley vein stripper
    Kurten stripper
    Kurten vein stripper
    Leigh zonule lens
        stripper
    Lempka stripper
    Lempka vein stripper
    Linton vein stripper
    Martin stripper
    Masson fascial stripper
    Matson rib stripper
    Matson stripper
    Matson-Alexander rib
        stripper
    Matson-Mead periosteal
        stripper
    Matson-Mead stripper
    Mayo stripper
    Mayo vein stripper
    Mayo-Myers external
        vein stripper
    Mayo-Myers stripper

stripper *continued*
- Myers intraluminal stripper
- Myers stripper
- Myers vein stripper
- Nabatoff stripper
- Nabatoff vein stripper
- Nelson rib stripper
- Nelson-Roberts stripper
- New Orleans endarterectomy stripper
- New Orleans stripper
- Obwegeser stripper
- olive-tipped stripper
- periosteum stripper
- polyethylene vein stripper
- Price-Thomas rib stripper
- rib elevator and stripper
- rib-edge stripper
- Roberts-Nelson rib stripper
- Samuels vein stripper
- Shaw carotid artery clot stripper
- Shaw carotid clot stripper
- Shaw clot stripper
- Smith cartilage stripper
- Smith posterior cartilage stripper
- spiral vein stripper
- thrombus stripper
- Trace stripper
- Trace vein stripper
- vagotomy stripper
- vein stripper
- Webb stripper
- Webb vein stripper
- Wilson stripper
- Wilson vein stripper
- Wurth vein stripper
- Wylie endarterectomy stripper
- Wylie stripper

stripper *continued*
- Zollinger-Gilmore intraluminal vein stripper
- Zollinger-Gilmore vein stripper

stripper and elevator
stripper with bullet end
stripping
stripping and dissection
stripping and ligation
stripping of cord
stripping of kidney capsule
stripping of vocal cord
stroboscopic microscope
stroke
stroke index
stroke risk
stroke victim
stroking
stroma (*pl.* stromata)
stromal hyperplasia
stromal tissue
Strömbeck breast reduction
Strömbeck incision
Strömbeck mammaplasty
Strömbeck mammaplasty incision
Strömbeck operation
Strömbeck template
Stromeyer cephalhematocele
Stromeyer splint
Stromeyer-Little operation
strong and equal pulses
strong and regular pulses
strong pulse
Struble everter
structural abnormality
structural anomaly
structural change
structural damage
structural lesion
structural pathology
structural surgery
structure
structured
Struempel (also Strümpel)

Struempel ear alligator forceps
Struempel ear punch
Struempel ear punch forceps
Struempel forceps
Struempel rongeur
Struempel-Voss ethmoidal
    forceps
Strully curet
Strully dissecting scissors
Strully dressing forceps
Strully dural twist hook
Strully Gigli-saw handle
Strully hook
Strully neurological scissors
Strully retractor
Strully ruptured disk curet
Strully scissors
Strully tissue forceps
Strully-Kerrison rongeur
struma
strumectomy
Strümpel (see *Struempel*)
strung-out
Strunsky sign
strut
        Adkins strut
        Anderson nasal strut
        calipers strut
        dorsal strut
        Harrington strut
        House calipers strut
        Magnuson strut
        nasal strut
        pinch nose strut
        piston strut
        Plasti-Pore strut
        polyethylene strut
        Robinson strut
        stainless steel strut
        Teflon strut
        TORP strut
        tricuspid valve strut
        valve outflow strut
        wire-loop strut
strut bar
strut bar hook
strut calipers

strut forceps
strut graft
strut guide
strut hook
strut pick
strut rhinoplasty
Struthers ligament
strut-measuring instrument
strut-type pin
struvite calculus
struvite urinary tract stones
Struyken forceps
Struyken nasal forceps
Struyken nasal-cutting forceps
Struyken punch
Struyken turbinate forceps
Stryker blade
Stryker cast cutter
Stryker chip camera
Stryker chondrotome
Stryker CircOlectric fracture
    frame
Stryker Dacron prosthetic
    ligament
Stryker dermabrader
Stryker dermatome
Stryker drill
Stryker equipment
Stryker fracture frame
Stryker fracture table
Stryker frame
Stryker impact osteotome
Stryker knee arthrometer
Stryker oscillating saw
Stryker perforator
Stryker Rolo-dermatome
Stryker saw
Stryker saw trephine
Stryker screw
Stryker screwdriver
Stryker Surgilav machine
Stryker turning frame
STSG (split-thickness skin graft)
STT joint (scaphotrapeziotrape-
    zoid joint)
Stubbs adenoid curet
Stubbs curet

Stuck laminectomy self-retaining
    retractor
Stucker bile duct dilator
stump
stump hallucination
stump inverted
stump ligation
stump of appendix
stump of bronchus
stump of esophagus
stump of pedicle
stump pressure
stump shrinker
stump shrinking
stump sock
stunted
Sturgis tenaculum
Sturmdorf amputation of cervix
Sturmdorf cervical needle
Sturmdorf cervical reamer
Sturmdorf colporrhaphy
Sturmdorf needle
Sturmdorf obstetrical sutures
Sturmdorf operation
Sturmdorf pedicle needle
Sturmdorf reamer
Sturmdorf sutures
Stutsman nasal snare
Stutsman snare
stuttering urinary stream
stye
stylet (also stilet, stilette)
styletted catheter
styletted tracheobronchial
    catheter
Stylex syringe
styloglossus, muscle
styloglossus, musculus
stylohyoid muscle
stylohyoid nerve
stylohyoideus, musculus
styloid
styloid bone
styloid process
stylomandibular ligament
stylomastoid artery
stylomastoid foramen

stylomastoid vein
stylomastoidea, arteria
stylomastoidea, vena
stylopharyngeal muscle
stylopharyngeal nerve
stylopharyngeus, musculus
stylus
styptic
styptic cotton
styptic wool
Styrofoam dressing
Suarez spreader
Suarez-Villafranca operation
subacromial bursa
subacute condition
subaortic stenosis
subapical osteotomy
subaponeurotic fascial cleft
subarachnoid
subarachnoid anesthesia
subarachnoid bleeding
subarachnoid block
subarachnoid block anesthesia
    (SAB anesthesia)
subarachnoid cavity
subarachnoid cisterna
subarachnoid hemorrhage
subarachnoid pathways
subarachnoid sac
subarachnoid septum
subarachnoid shunt
subarachnoid space
subarachnoid ureterostomy
subarachnoidal cisterns
subarachnoidal sinus
subarcuate fossa
subareolar
subareolar region
subastragalar amputation
subastragalar dislocation
subauricular region
subcallosal gyrus
subcapital fracture
subcapsular cataract
subcapsular cortex
subcapsular nephrectomy
subcapsular opacity

subcardinal veins
subcarinal angle
subcarinal lymphadenopathy
subchondral bone
subchondral bony resorption
subchondral cyst
subclavia, arteria
subclavia, vena
subclavian
subclavian aortic anastomosis
subclavian arteriogram
subclavian artery
subclavian catheter
subclavian dialysis catheter
subclavian endarterectomy
subclavian flap technique
subclavian introducer
subclavian line
subclavian loop
subclavian nerve
subclavian peel-away sheath
subclavian steal syndrome
subclavian sulcus of lung
subclavian Tegaderm dressing
subclavian triangle
subclavian vein
subclavian-carotid bypass
subclavian-subclavian bypass
subclavicular murmur
subclavius muscle
subclavius, musculus
subclavius, nervus
subclinical disease
subclinical infection
subcollateral gyrus
subcondylar osteotomy
subconjunctival hemorrhage
subconjunctival injection
subconscious
subcoracoid dislocation
subcortical encephalopathy
subcortical structures
subcostal
subcostal area
subcostal artery
subcostal flank incision
subcostal incision

subcostal muscles
subcostal nerve
subcostal retractions
subcostal vein
subcostales, musculi
subcostalis, arteria
subcostalis, nervus
subcostalis, vena
subcrepitant rales
subcutaneae abdominis, venae
subcutaneous
subcutaneous adipose tissue
subcutaneous bleeders
subcutaneous connective tissues
subcutaneous fascia
subcutaneous fat
subcutaneous fracture
subcutaneous injection
subcutaneous intraocular node
subcutaneous mass
subcutaneous mastectomy
subcutaneous metastasis
subcutaneous nodule
subcutaneous operation
subcutaneous perineal mass
subcutaneous plane
subcutaneous saw
subcutaneous swelling
subcutaneous temporal nerves
subcutaneous tenotomy
subcutaneous tissue
subcutaneous tissue expander
subcutaneous tissues approxi-
    mated
subcutaneous tissues reapproxi-
    mated
subcutaneous tumor
subcutaneous tunnels
subcutaneous veins of abdomen
subcutaneous venous arch at
    root of fingers
subcutaneous wound
subcutaneously
subcuticular
subcuticular fat
subcuticular level
subcuticular stitch

subcuticular sutures
subcuticular wire
subdeltoid bursa
subdermal graft
subdermal implant
subdermal layer
subdermal prosthesis
subdiaphragmatic abscess
subdiaphragmatic fields
subdiaphragmatic hernia
subdiaphragmatic involvement
subdiaphragmatic radiation
    therapy
subdiaphragmatic sympathec-
    tomy
subdigastric lymph nodes
subdural abscess
subdural fluid
subdural hematoma
subdural hygroma
subdural puncture
subdural space
subendocardial infarction
subendocardial injury
subendocardial ischemia
subendocardial myocardial
    infarction (SEMI)
subepicardial fat
subepicardial injury
subepithelial plexus
subfascial
subgaleal space
subgingival curettage
subglenoid dislocation
subglottic area
subglottic forceps
subglottic stenosis
subhepatic abscess
subhyaloid hemorrhage
subhyoid laryngotomy
subhyoid region
subinguinal incision
subintimal structure
subinvolution of uterus
subjacent
subject
subjective

subjective change
subjective improvement
sublabial
sublabial adhesion
Sublimaze anesthesia
sublimis tendon
sublingual
sublingual artery
sublingual caruncle
sublingual ducts
sublingual fold
sublingual glands
sublingual hematoma
sublingual nerve
sublingual saliva
sublingual tablet
sublingual vein
sublingualis, arteria
sublingualis, nervus
sublingualis, vena
sublobular veins
subluxated
subluxation
subluxed radial head
subluxed shoulder
submammary
submammary incision
submandibular
submandibular duct
submandibular ganglion
submandibular gland
submandibular lymph nodes
submandibular salivary gland
submandibular triangle
submaxillary
submaxillary duct
submaxillary ganglion
submaxillary gland
submaxillary nerves
submaxillary region
submaxillary triangle
submental artery
submental glands
submental hematoma
submental lymph nodes
submental region
submental vein

submental vertex roent-
genogram
submentalis, arteria
submentalis, vena
submentovertical axial projection
submerged tonsil
submerged tooth
submitral area
submitral calcification
submitted for biopsy
submitted for frozen section
submitted for microsection
submitted to pathologist
submucosa
submucosal connective tissue
submucosal dissection
submucosal hemorrhage
submucosal implant
submucosal vascular pattern
submucosal venous plexus
submucosal vessels
submucous chisel
submucous curet
submucous dissection
submucous dissector
submucous elevator
submucous knife
submucous leiomyoma
submucous myomata
submucous resection (SMR)
submucous resection and
rhinoplasty
submucous retractor
suboccipital craniectomy
suboccipital decompression
suboccipital incision
suboccipital nerve
suboccipital puncture
suboccipital triangle
suboccipital trigeminal
rhizotomy
suboccipitalis, nervus
suboccipitobregmatic diameter
suboccluding ligature
suboptimal
subpapillary zone

subperiosteal abscess of frontal
sinus
subperiosteal amputation
subperiosteal bone
subperiosteal calcification
subperiosteal dissection
subperiosteal fracture
subperiosteal implant
subperiosteally
subperiosteally resected
subperitoneal appendicitis
subperitoneal Baldy-Webster
hysteropexy
subperitoneal space
subphrenic
subphrenic abscess
subphrenic collection
subpleural mass
subpleural mediastinal plexus
subpubic angle
subpubic hernia
subpyramidal fossa
Subramanian aortic clamp
Subramanian clamp
Subramanian miniature aortic
clamp
Subramanian valve speculum
subretinal fluid
subscapular
subscapular angle
subscapular artery
subscapular bursa
subscapular muscle
subscapular nerves
subscapular splenectomy
subscapularis, arteria
subscapularis, musculus
subscapularis, nervus
subscapularis tendon
subsegmental area
subsegmental resection
subsequent treatment
subserosa
subserous
subserous fascia
subsiding
subsigmoid fossa

subspinous dislocation
substance
substernal
substernal goiter
substernal thyroid
substitute
substitution
substitution transfusion
substrate
substrate phase of wound
    healing
subsynaptic web
subtalar arthrodesis
subtalar articulation
subtalar joint
subtalar motion
subtemporal decompression
subtend
subtended
subtendinous bursa
subtentorial structures
subtentorial tumor
subthalamus
subtle difficulties
subtotal cataract extraction
subtotal colectomy
subtotal cystectomy
subtotal excision
subtotal gastrectomy
subtotal hysterectomy
subtotal laminectomy
subtotal orbital exenteration
subtotal pancreatectomy
subtotal removal of tumor
subtotal resection
subtotal thyroidectomy
subtraction films
subtraction scintigraphy
subtrigonal spheroids
subtrochanteric fracture
subtrochanteric incision
subtrochanteric osteotomy
subumbilical incision
subumbilical space
subungual hematoma
subungual melanoma
subunit

suburethral melanoma
suburethral sling procedure
subvalvular aortic stenosis
subvertebral muscles
subvesical duct
subvesical fascia
subvolution
subxiphoid
succedaneous teeth
succenturiate lobe
succenturiate placenta
successful passage of instru-
    ment
successional teeth
successive responses
successive stages
succinylcholine anesthetic
    agent
succinylcholine drip
succulent nodes
succus
succussion
succussion sounds
succussion splash
sucker
sucking and swallowing
    difficulties
sucking wound
Sucquet-Hoyer anastomosis
suction
suction abortion
suction adapter
suction airway
suction and intubation
suction apparatus
suction aspirator
suction biopsy
suction biopsy instrument
suction biopsy needle
suction bulb
suction cannula
suction catheter
suction connector
suction cup
suction curet
suction curettage
suction cutter

suction D&C
suction device
suction dilatation and curettage
suction dissector
suction drain
suction drain system
suction drainage
suction elevator
suction evacuator
suction forceps
suction hemostatic agent
suction knife
suction lipectomy
suction machine
suction ophthalmodynamometer
suction plate
suction pressure pump
suction probe
suction pump
suction pump aspirator
suction punch
suction reservoir
suction stomach
suction tip (see also *tip*)
    Adson brain suction tip
    Andrews suction tip
    aortographic suction tip
    Blue rectal suction tip
    brain suction tip
    Brawley nasal suction tip
    Brawley suction tip
    Buie rectal suction tip
    exploratory suction tip
    Frazier nasal suction tip
    Frazier suction tip
    glass nasal suction tip
    glass suction tip
    Sims suction tip
    Sondermann suction tip
    T&A suction tip
    tonsil suction tip
    Yankauer suction tip
suction tip curet
suction tonsillar dissector
suction tube (see also *tube*)
    Adson brain suction
        tube

suction tube *continued*
    Adson straight suction
        tube
    Adson suction tube
    Anderson flexible suction
        tube
    Anderson suction tube
    Andrews suction tube
    Andrews-Pynchon
        suction tube
    Andrews-Yankauer
        suction tube
    angled suction tube
    Anthony mastoid suction
        tube
    Anthony suction tube
    ascites suction tube
    Asepto suction tube
    Barnes nasal suction
        tube
    Barnes suction tube
    Baron suction tube
    bedside suction tube
    Bellucci nasal suction
        tube
    Bellucci suction tube
    brain suction tube
    Bron suction tube
    bronchoscopic suction
        tube
    Bucy-Frazier suction tube
    Buie rectal suction tube
    Buie suction tube
    Butler tonsil suction tube
    Buyes air-vent suction
        tube
    C-P suction tube
    Chaffin suction tube
    Chaffin-Pratt suction
        tube
    closed suction tube
    closed water-seal suction
        tube
    Cone suction tube
    continuous suction tube
    Cook County suction
        tube

suction tube *continued*

Cook County tracheal
suction tube
Cooley cardiovascular
suction tube
Cooley suction tube
coronary sinus suction
tube
Cottle suction tube
Coupland nasal suction
tube
Coupland suction tube
Dandy suction tube
Davol suction tube
DeBakey suction tube
DeVilbiss suction tube
Devine-Millard-Frazier
suction tube
ear suction tube
Emerson suction tube
Fay suction tube
Ferguson brain suction
tube
Ferguson-Frazier suction
tube
Finsterer suction tube
Fitzpatrick suction tube
flexible suction tube
Frazier brain suction
tube
Frazier insulated suction
tube
Frazier modified suction
tube
Frazier nasal suction
tube
Frazier straight suction
tube
Frazier suction tube
Frazier-Paparella suction
tube
Glover suction tube
Gomco suction tube
Gwathmey suction
tube
Hemovac suction tube
House suction tube

suction tube *continued*

Humphrey coronary
sinus suction tube
Immergut suction tube
insulated suction tube
irrigator-suction tube
Jako suction tube
Jarit-Pol suction tube
Jarit-Yankauer suction
tube
Killian suction tube
Lennarson suction tube
lifesaving suction tube
Lukens suction tube
Madoff suction tubes
Mason suction tube
mastoid suction tube
Methodist suction tube
Millin suction tube
Monoject suction tube
Morse-Andrews suction
tube
Morse-Ferguson suction
tube
Mosher suction tube
Mueller suction tube
Mueller-Frazier suction
tube
Mueller-Poole suction
tube
Mueller-Pynchon suction
tube
Mueller-Yankauer
suction tube
nasal suction tube
New York Hospital
suction tube
pleural suction tube
Pleur-Evac suction tube
Poole abdominal suction
tube
Poole suction tube
Poppen suction tube
Porto-vac suction tube
Pribram suction tube
Proctor suction tube
Pynchon suction tube

suction tube *continued*

Rand-House suction tube
Ritter suprapubic suction tube
Rosen suction tube
Russell suction tube
Sachs brain suction tube
Sachs suction tube
Sarns intracardiac suction tube
Schuknecht suction tube
Scott suction tube
Senning suction tube
Sherman suction tube
sigmoidoscope insulated suction tube
sigmoidoscope suction tube
siphon suction tube
Snyder Hemovac suction tube
Stedman suction tube
Storz bronchoscopic suction tube
sump suction tube
Supramid suction tube
three-bottle tidal suction tube
tonsil suction tube
Toomey suction tube
tracheal suction tube
tracheobronchial suction tube
Tucker suction tube
Tufts suction tube
underwater-seal suction tube
Walter-Poole suction tube
Walter-Yankauer suction tube
Wangensteen suction tube
Waring tonsil suction tube
Watkins suction tube
Weck suction tube

suction tube *continued*

Welch Allyn suction tube
Yankauer suction tube
Yasargil suction tube
Zollner suction tube
suction unit
suction-assisted lipectomy (SAL)
suction-coagulation tube
suctioned
suction-electrocoagulator
suctioning
suction-irrigator
sudden body jerk
sudden death
sudden movement
sudden pain
sudden paralysis
sudden trauma
suddenly
sudomotor nerves
sudoriferous cyst
sudoriferous glands
sudorific
sudorific centers
sudoriparous glands
sufficient quantity
suffocative goiter
Sugar aneurysm clip
Sugar clip
Sugarbaker operation
Sugarbaker retrocolic clamp
sugar-tong cast
sugar-tong plaster splint
sugar-tong splint
suggestion
Suggs catheter
Sugioki osteotomy of hip
Sugita aneurysm clip
Sugita catheter
Sugita clip
Sugiura abdominal pull-through operation
Sugiura devascularization of esophagus and stomach
Sugiura esophageal varices
Sugiura procedure for esophageal varices

suitable beam film localization
suitcase kidney
Suker cyclodialysis spatula
Suker iris forceps
Suker knife
sulcated tongue
sulci (*sing.* sulcus)
sulci in brain
sulciolar gastric mucosa
sulcus (*pl.* sulci)
sulcus angle
sulcus blunting
sulcus of heart
sulcus of lung
sulcus of subclavian artery
sulcus tumor
sulfa film
sulfa level
sulfate
sulfur colloid liver scan
sulfur colloid nuclear medicine
sulfur colloid scan
Sullivan raspatory
Sullivan sinus rasp
SULP II catheter
Sultrin cream
Sultrin impregnated vaginal
    pack
summary
summit
summit of nose
Sumner clamp
Sumner elevator
Sumner sign
sump catheter
sump drain
sump drainage
sump nasogastric tube
sump Penrose drain
sump pump
sump pump catheter
sump suction tube
sump thoracic drainage
    system
sump tube
sun cautery
Sunday elevator

Sunday staphylorrhaphy
    elevator
Sundt clip
Sundt encircling clip
Sundt-Kees aneurysmal clip
Sundt-Kees clip
sunflower cataract
sunken acetabulum
sunrise projection
sunrise view
sunrise view of patella on x-ray
sunscreen
sunset view
sunset view of patella on x-ray
sunset x-ray view
Super Pinky
Superblade
superciliary depressor muscle
superficial
superficial abdominal fascia
superficial abrasion
superficial bleeders
superficial blood vessels
superficial brachial artery
superficial bullae
superficial circumflex iliac artery
superficial circumflex iliac vein
superficial dorsal veins
superficial epigastric artery
superficial epigastric vein
superficial erosion
superficial fascia
superficial femoral arch
superficial fibular nerve
superficial flexor muscle
superficial implant
superficial infection
superficial inguinal ring
superficial laceration
superficial layers
superficial middle cerebral vein
superficial middle petrosal
    nerve
superficial musculoaponeurotic
    system (SMAS)
superficial nerve
superficial nodes

superficial palmar arch
superficial perineal artery
superficial perineal fascia
superficial perineal space
superficial peroneal nerve
superficial radial nerve
superficial reflex
superficial sclera
superficial structures
superficial sutures
superficial temporal branch of
    external carotid artery
superficial temporal vein
superficial transverse fibers
superficial transverse muscle of
    perineum
superficial ulceration
superficial varicosities
superficial vein
superficial venous markings
superficial vertebral veins
superficial wound
superficially explored
Superflex elastic dressing
Superglue adhesive
superimposed bowel gas
superimposed depression
superimposition
superior
superior alveolar nerve
superior ampullar nerve
superior anastomotic vein
superior annulus
superior articular facet
superior articulating process
superior aspect
superior astragalonavicular
    ligament
superior auricular muscle
superior azygos vein
superior border
superior bulb of internal jugular
    vein
superior cardiac cervical nerve
superior carotid ganglion
superior carotid triangle
superior cerebellar artery

superior cerebellar peduncle
superior cerebellar vein
superior cerebral veins
superior cervical cardiac nerve
superior cervical chain
superior cervical ganglion
superior clunial nerves
superior colliculus
superior commissure
superior constrictor pharyngeal
    muscle
superior corner
superior crus
superior cul-de-sac
superior duodenal fold
superior duodenal recess
superior epigastric artery
superior epigastric veins
superior fascia of urogenital
    diaphragm
superior flexure of duodenum
superior fornix
superior fovea
superior frontal gyrus
superior ganglion
superior gemellus muscle
superior gluteal artery
superior gluteal nerve
superior gluteal veins
superior hemorrhoidal artery
superior hemorrhoidal branch
    of inferior mesenteric artery
superior hemorrhoidal vein
superior iliac spine
superior intercostal vein
superior iridotomy
superior labial artery
superior labial region
superior labial veins
superior lacrimal gland
superior laryngeal artery
superior laryngeal nerve
superior laryngeal vein
superior lateral cutaneous nerve
    of arm
superior ligament of incus
superior lip

superior lobe
superior longitudinal muscle of
    tongue
superior longitudinal sinus
superior lumbar hernia
superior maxilla
superior meatus
superior mediastinum
superior mesenteric angiogram
superior mesenteric artery
superior mesenteric ganglion
superior mesenteric lymph
    nodes
superior mesenteric vein
superior mesenteric-caval
    anastomosis
superior muscle
superior nasal venule of retina
superior oblique muscle
superior oblique tendon
superior occipital gyrus
superior omental recess
superior ophthalmic vein
superior orbital fissure
superior ossicular chain
superior palpebral region
superior palpebral vein
superior pancreaticoduodenal
    artery
superior parathyroid gland
superior parietal lobule
superior pelvic strait
superior perihilar mass
superior petrosal sinus
superior phrenic vein
superior pole of calyx
superior pole of thyroid
superior portion of
    mesencephalon
superior posterior serratus
    muscle
superior pulmonary vein
superior ramus
superior rectal artery
superior rectal veins
superior rectus
superior rectus bridle sutures

superior rectus forceps
superior rectus muscle
superior rectus traction
    sutures
superior root ansa cervicalis
superior sagittal sinus
superior segment of lung
superior semilunar lobule
superior spine
superior suprarenal artery
superior tarsal muscle
superior temporal gyrus
superior temporal sulcus
superior temporal venule of
    retina
superior thoracic aperture
superior thyroid artery
superior thyroid gland
superior thyroid notch
superior thyroid vein
superior tracheobronchial
    lymph nodes
superior tracheotomy
superior turbinate
superior tympanic artery
superior ulnar collateral artery
superior vagal ganglion
superior vena cava
superior vena cavography
superior venula nasalis retinae
superior vesical artery
superiorly
superiorly milked
supernatant
supernumerary
supernumerary bone
supernumerary digits
supernumerary organ
superoinferior projection
superoinferior tangential
    projection
superolateral
superolateral aspect
superomedial
supersede
supersonic frequency
superstructure

Super-Trac adhesive traction
    dressing
supervision
supinate
supination
supination splint
supination, external rotation
    fracture (SER fracture, SEX
    fracture)
supinator
supinator longus reflex
supinator muscle
supinator, musculus
supine film
supine mediolateral view
supine position
Suppan procedure for nail
    deformity
supple neck
supplement
supplemental
supplies
support
    Abée support
    advanced cardiac life
        support (ACLS)
    Andrews rigid chest
        support
    arch support
    Bard cardiopulmonary
        support
    Biomet Velcro wrist
        support
    cardiovascular support
    cervical support
    Dale abdominal support
    Dale ankle support
    Dale knee support
    Dale pelvic support
    Dale rib support
    Dale tennis elbow
        support
    Dale wrist support
    Dobutrex support
    Epitrain active elbow
        support
    Epitrain-N elbow support

Fredricks mammary
    support
Genutrain knee support
Glattelast elastic knee
    support
hemodynamic support
Houston halo cervical
    support
Jahnke-Barron heart
    support
Jobst mammary support
Kamp support
knee support
laryngoscope chest
    support
Logan bow support
longitudinal arch
    support
lumbosacral support
Lynco arch support
Malleotrain active ankle
    support
mammary support
mastectomy support
Morgan pelvic support
neoprene support
padded knee support
pelvic muscular support
pelvic support
perineal support
Philadelphia collar
    cervical support
Posey support
scrotal suspensory
    support
Span-aid bed supports
therapeutic support
support measures
support stockings
    Jobst-Stride support
        stockings
    Jobst-Stridette support
        stockings
    Sigvaris support stock-
        ings
    True Form support
        stockings

support stockings *continued*
  venous pressure gradient
    support stockings
    (VPGSS)
  VPGSS (venous pressure
    gradient support
    stockings)
  Zimmer antiembolism
    support stockings
support sutures
supported
supported angioplasty
supporting stitches
supporting structures
supporting tissue
supportive halo cast
supportive intervention
supportive measures
supportive therapy
supportive tissue
supportive treatment
suppress
suppressant
suppressing
suppression
suppurate
suppuration
suppurative
suppurative appendicitis
suppurative infection
suppurative otitis media (SOM)
suppurative tonsillitis
supra-annular suture ring
supra-aortic angiography
supracallosal gyrus
supracardiac silhouette
supracardinal veins
supracervical amputation
supracervical hysterectomy
supracervical incision
suprachoroid lamina
supraciliary canal
supraclavicular
supraclavicular adenopathy
supraclavicular area
supraclavicular bruit
supraclavicular fossa

supraclavicular lymph nodes
supraclavicular nerves
supraclavicular node
supraclavicular port
supraclavicular region
supraclavicular triangle
supraclaviculares intermedii,
  nervi
supraclaviculares laterales, nervi
supraclaviculares mediales,
  nervi
supracolliculus
supracondylar
supracondylar fracture
supracondylar plate
supradiaphragmatic diverticulum
supradiaphragmatic sympathectomy
supraduction
supraglenoid
supraglenoid tubercle
supraglottic larynx
supraglottic structures
suprahepatic caval cuff
suprahepatic venous obstruction
suprahilar mass
suprahyoid muscles
suprahyoidei, musculi
supralevator abscess
supralevator space
supramalleolar
supramarginal gyrus
suprameatal spine
supramediastinal mantle
Supramid Extra sutures
Supramid graft
Supramid implant
Supramid mesh implant
Supramid prosthesis
Supramid ptosis sleeve
Supramid ptosis sling
Supramid suction tube
Supramid sutures
supramohyoid neck dissection
supraoptic canal

supraoptic commissure
supraoptico-hypophyseal axis
supraorbital area
supraorbital artery
supraorbital canal
supraorbital foramen
supraorbital nerve
supraorbital notch
supraorbital region
supraorbital vein
supraorbitalis, arteria
supraorbitalis, nervus
supraorbitalis, vena
suprapatellar effusion
suprapatellar plica
suprapatellar pouch
suprapatellar reflex
suprapiriform foramen
suprapubic
suprapubic appendectomy
    incision
suprapubic aspiration
suprapubic bag
suprapubic cannula
suprapubic catheter
suprapubic cystoscope
suprapubic cystostomy
suprapubic cystotomy
suprapubic drain
suprapubic excision of prostate
suprapubic hemostatic bag
suprapubic incision
suprapubic lithotomy
suprapubic prostatectomy
suprapubic rami
suprapubic reflex
suprapubic region
suprapubic retractor
suprapubic self-retaining
    retractor
suprapubic sinus
suprapubic suction drain
suprapubic tenderness
suprapubic transvesical
    prostatectomy
suprapubic trocar
suprapubic tube

suprapubic urethroplasty
suprarenal area
suprarenal arteries
suprarenal capsule
suprarenal epithelioma
suprarenal ganglion
suprarenal glands
suprarenal medulla
suprarenal plexus
suprarenal vein
suprarenales superiores,
    arteriae suprarenalis dextra,
    vena
suprarenalis inferior, arteria
suprarenalis media, arteria
suprarenalis sinistra, vena
suprascapular artery
suprascapular nerve
suprascapular notch
suprascapular vein
suprascapularis, arteria
suprascapularis, nervus
suprascapularis, vena
suprasellar
suprasellar aneurysm
suprasellar cisterna
suprasellar tumor
suprasphincteric fistula
supraspinatus fossa
supraspinatus, musculus
supraspinatus tendon
supraspinous muscle
suprasternal
suprasternal fossa
suprasternal notch
suprasternal pulsation
suprasternal region
suprasternal retraction
supratentorial parts of central
    nervous system
supratrochlear artery
supratrochlear depression
supratrochlear nerve
supratrochlear veins
supratrochleares, venae
supratrochlearis, arteria
supratrochlearis, nervus

supraumbilical incision
supraumbilical reflex
supravaginal hysterectomy
supravaginal septum
supravalvular aortic stenosis
supravalvular aortogram
supravesical fossa
supravesical hernia
supreme cardiac nerves
sural arteries
sural nerve
surales, arteriae
suralis, nervus
Surcan knee holder
Surcan leg holder
surcingle
Surefit anterior chamber
    intraocular lens
Sure-Fit surgical garments
Sureflow catheter
Surfacaine anesthetic agent
surface analgesia
surface anatomy
surface anesthesia
surface antibody
surface area
surface biopsy
surface coil
surface cooling hypothermia
surface electrode
surface eye implant
surface implant
surface tension
surface trauma
surface vessels
surface wrinkling retinopathy
surfactant test
Surfasoft dressing
surfer's nodules
Sur-Fit adhesive
Sur-Fit colostomy bag
Sur-Fit Mini pouch
Surgairtome
Surgaloy metallic sutures
Surgaloy sutures
Surgaloy wire
surgeon

Surgeon's Choice stapler
surgeon's footstool
surgeon's headlight
surgeon's knot
surgeon's knot sutures
surgeon's regular needle
surgery
Surg-E-Trol
surgibone
surgibone implant
surgical
surgical abdomen
surgical abscess
surgical absence of (breast,
    limb, uterus, etc.)
surgical amputation
surgical anastomosis
surgical anatomy
surgical anesthesia
surgical ankylosis
surgical approach
surgical assistant
surgical biopsy
surgical blade
surgical chromic sutures
surgical closure
surgical complications
surgical consultation
surgical contraception
surgical correction
surgical corset
surgical course
surgical current
surgical debridement
surgical decompression
surgical defect
surgical disease
surgical dome
surgical drapes
surgical dressing
surgical electrode
surgical emphysema
surgical engine
surgical evaluative staging
surgical excision
surgical exploration
surgical field

surgical film
surgical fixation
surgical flap
surgical gauze
surgical grade stainless steel
    wire
surgical gut sutures
surgical hand scrubs
surgical hazard
surgical history
surgical immobilization of joint
surgical implantation
surgical incision
surgical infection
surgical intervention
surgical iridectomy
surgical isolator
surgical knife handle
surgical knot
surgical laser
surgical lesion
surgical limbus
surgical linen sutures
Surgical Lint Pic-Ups
surgical loupe
surgical management
surgical menopause
surgical microscope
surgical neck
surgical neck fracture
surgical neck of humerus
surgical neck of tooth
surgical needle
Surgical Nu-Knit
surgical nurse
surgical option
surgical pathogens
surgical pathology
surgical permit
surgical pharmacology
surgical prep
surgical procedure
surgical prosthesis
surgical recovery
surgical removal (of organ,
    tissue, etc.)
surgical resection

surgical resident
surgical risk
surgical scar
surgical scissors
surgical shock
surgical shoe
surgical silk sutures
Surgical Simplex cement
Surgical Simplex P radiopaque
    bone cement
surgical site
surgical soft diet
surgical splint
surgical sponge
surgical staging
surgical steel sutures
surgical stockinette
surgical suite
surgical supplies
surgical sutures
surgical swelling
surgical team
surgical technique
surgical technologist
surgical technology
surgical template
surgical therapy
surgical trauma
surgical treatment
surgical triangle
surgical urachus
surgical vagolysis
surgical vagotomy
surgical wound
surgical wound classification
surgical wound infection
surgical wound surveillance
surgical-assist leg holder
surgically absent
surgically implanted pump
surgically implanted tube
surgically severed limb
Surgicel dressing
Surgicel gauze
Surgicel gauze dressing
Surgicel implant placement
Surgicel implantation

Surgiclip
Surgidev intraocular lens
Surgidev iris clip
Surgidev lens
Surgifix dressing
Surgifix outer expandable
    netting
Surgiflex bandage
Surgilar suture
Surgilav drain
Surgilav machine
Surgilene sutures
Surgilift
Surgiloid sutures
Surgilon braided nylon sutures
Surgilon sutures
Surgilone monofilament
    polypropylene sutures
Surgilone sutures
Surgilope sutures
Surgi-Med clamp
Surgi-Pad combined dressing
Surgi-Prep
Surgiset sutures
Surgitek catheter
Surgitek double-J ureteral
    catheter
Surgitek double-J ureteral stent
Surgitek expander
Surgitek Flexi-Flate II penile
    implant
Surgitek Flexi-Flate II penile
    prosthesis
Surgitek Flexi-rod penile
    prosthesis
Surgitek implant
Surgitek inflatable penile
    prosthesis
Surgitek mammary implant
Surgitek mammary prosthesis
Surgitek penile prosthesis
Surgitek T-Span tissue expander
Surgitek Tractfinder ureteral
    stent
Surgitek Uropass stent
Surgitome bur
Surgitool prosthetic valve
Surgitron

Surgitube dressing
Surgivac drainage
Surgtex x-ray detectable sponge
Surital anesthesia
surrounding graft material
surrounding structures
surrounding tissues
surveillance
surveillance procedure
survey
survival
survival rate
survivor
susceptibility
susceptible
suspected transfusion reaction
suspended in saline solution
suspension
suspension apparatus (see also
    *apparatus*)
        Killian suspension
            apparatus
        Lewy suspension
            apparatus
        Lynch suspension
            apparatus
suspension laryngoscope
suspension of kidney
suspension of uterus
suspension sling
suspension traction
suspensorius, musculus
suspensory
suspensory bandage
suspensory dressing
suspensory ligament
suspensory muscle
suspicious
suspicious area
sustaining
sustentacular tissue
Sutherland hamstring transfer
Sutherland hip procedure
Sutherland scissors
Sutherland thigh procedure
Sutherland-Greenfield osteot-
    omy
Sutherland-Grieshaber scissors

Sutro procedure
Sutter-Smeloff heart valve
    prosthesis
Sutton needle
Sutupak sutures
sutural cataract
sutural ligament
suturation
suture (see also *ligature*)
    absorbable surgical
        sutures
    absorbable sutures
    Acutrol sutures
    Albert sutures
    Alcon sutures
    Allgower sutures
    Allison sutures
    already-threaded sutures
    alternating sutures
    aluminum wire sutures
    aluminum-bronze wire
        sutures
    Ancap braided silk
        sutures
    Ancap silk sutures
    anchoring sutures
    angle sutures
    anterior palatine suture
    Appolito sutures
    apposition sutures
    approximation sutures
    arcuate sutures
    Argyll Robertson sutures
    Arlt sutures
    Arruga encircling suture
    arterial silk sutures
    AS (Auto-Suture)
    Atraloc sutures
    Atraloc-Ethilon sutures
    atraumatic braided silk
        sutures
    atraumatic chromic
        sutures
    atraumatic sutures
    Aureomycin sutures
    Auto-Suture (AS)
    Axenfeld sutures

suture *continued*
    B&S gauge sutures
        (Brown-Sharp gauge
        sutures)
    Babcock wire sutures
    back-and-forth sutures
    Barraquer silk sutures
    Barraquer sutures
    barrel knot sutures
    baseball sutures
    basilar sutures
    bastard sutures
    Bauer-Black sutures
    Béclard sutures
    Bell sutures
    Bertrandi sutures
    Bigelow sutures
    biparietal suture
    black braided sutures
    black silk sutures
    black twisted sutures
    Blalock sutures
    blanket sutures
    blue cotton sutures
    blue twisted cotton
        sutures
    bolster sutures
    bone wax sutures
    Bonney sutures
    bony sutures
    Bozeman sutures
    braided Ethibond
        sutures
    braided Mersilene
        sutures
    braided Nurolon sutures
    braided nylon sutures
    braided polyamide
        sutures
    braided silk sutures
    braided sutures
    braided wire sutures
    bregmatomastoid suture
    bridle sutures
    bronchial sutures
    bronze sutures
    bronze wire sutures

suture *continued*
 Brown-Sharp gauge
  sutures (B&S gauge
  sutures)
 Buckston sutures
 bulb sutures
 bunching sutures
 Bunnell sutures
 buried sutures
 button sutures
 cable wire sutures
 Callaghan sutures
 capitonnage sutures
 cardinal sutures
 cardiovascular sutures
 Cargile sutures
 Carrel sutures
 catgut sutures (CGS)
 celluloid linen sutures
 celluloid sutures
 cervical sutures
 CGS (catgut sutures)
 chain sutures
 Champion sutures
 Cherney sutures
 Chinese twisted silk
  sutures
 chloramine catgut
  sutures
 chromated catgut sutures
 chromic blue dyed
  sutures
 chromic catgut mattress
  sutures
 chromic catgut sutures
 chromic collagen sutures
 chromic gut sutures
 chromic sutures
 chromicized catgut
  sutures
 circular sutures
 circumcisional sutures
 clavate clove-hitch
  sutures
 clavate sutures
 clove-hitch sutures
 Cloward stitch sutures

suture *continued*
 Coakley sutures
 coaptation sutures
 coated polyester sutures
 coated sutures
 coated Vicryl sutures
 cobbler's sutures
 cocoon thread sutures
 collagen sutures
 compound sutures
 Connell inverting sutures
 Connell sutures
 continuous catgut
  sutures
 continuous circular
  inverting sutures
 continuous cuticular
  sutures
 continuous hemostatic
  sutures
 continuous interlocking
  sutures
 continuous inverting
  sutures
 continuous key-pattern
  sutures
 continuous Lembert
  sutures
 continuous locked
  sutures
 continuous mattress
  sutures
 continuous over-and-
  over sutures
 continuous running
  locked sutures
 continuous running
  sutures
 continuous silk sutures
 continuous sutures
 continuous U-shaped
  sutures
 Cooley U-sutures
 corneal sutures
 corneoscleral sutures
 corneoscleroconjunctival
  sutures

suture *continued*

>coronal suture
cotton Deknatel sutures
cotton sutures
cranial sutures
crown sutures
Cushing sutures
cushioning sutures
Custodis sutures
cutaneous suture of
   palate
cutaneous sutures
cuticular sutures
Czerny sutures
Czerny-Lembert sutures
D&G sutures
Dacron bolstered sutures
Dacron sutures
Dacron traction sutures
Daily sutures
Davis-Geck eye sutures
Davis-Geck sutures
Degnon sutures
dekalon sutures
Deklene sutures
Deknatel silk sutures
Deknatel sutures
delayed sutures
DeMartel sutures
dentate sutures
dermal sutures
dermal tension nonab-
   sorbing sutures
Dermalene sutures
Dermalon cuticular
   sutures
Dermalon sutures
Dexon Plus sutures
Dexon subcuticular
   sutures
Dexon sutures
DG Softgut sutures
direct radial sutures
Docktor suture
Donnati sutures
double-armed mattress
   sutures

suture *continued*

>double-armed retention
   sutures
double-armed sutures
double-button sutures
doubled black silk
   sutures
doubled chromic catgut
   sutures
doubled pursestring
   sutures
doubled sutures
double-stop sutures
doubly armed sutures
doubly ligated sutures
Douglas sutures
Drews suture
Dulox sutures
Dupuytren sutures
dural tenting sutures
Duvergier sutures
echelon sutures
edge-to-edge sutures
Edinburgh sutures
EEA Auto-Sutures
elastic sutures
Emmet sutures
end-on mattress sutures
end-over-end running
   sutures
EPTFE vascular sutures
   (expanded
   polytetrafluoroeth-
   ylene vascular sutures)
Equisetene sutures
Ethibond polyester
   sutures
Ethibond sutures
Ethicon silk sutures
Ethicon sutures
Ethicon-Atraloc sutures
Ethiflex retention sutures
Ethiflex sutures
Ethilon nylon sutures
Ethilon sutures
Ethi-pack sutures
ethmoidomaxillary suture

suture *continued*
 everting interrupted
  sutures
 everting sutures
 extrachromic sutures
 eye sutures
 40-day chromic catgut
  sutures
 Faden sutures
 false sutures
 far sutures
 far-and-near sutures
 far-near sutures
 figure-of-eight sutures
 filament sutures
 fine chromic sutures
 fine silk sutures
 fine sutures
 Finsterer sutures
 fish-mouth sutures
 fixation sutures
 flat sutures
 Flaxedil sutures
 Flexitone sutures
 Flexon steel sutures
 Flexon sutures
 formaldehyde catgut
  sutures
 forty-day chromic catgut
  sutures
 Fothergill sutures
 free ligature sutures
 free-tie sutures
 French sutures
 Friedmann sutures
 frontal suture
 frontal zygomatic suture
 frontoethmoidal suture
 frontolacrimal suture
 frontomalar suture
 frontonasal suture
 frontoparietal suture
 frontosphenoid suture
 frontozygomatic suture
 Frost sutures
 funicular sutures
 Furniss sutures

suture *continued*
 furrier's sutures
 Gaillard-Arlt sutures
 Gambee sutures
 Gamophen suture
 gastrointestinal surgical
  gut sutures
 gastrointestinal surgical
  linen sutures
 gastrointestinal surgical
  silk sutures
 Gély sutures
 general closure sutures
 general eye surgery
  sutures
 GI pop-off silk sutures
 GI silk sutures
 Gianturco sutures
 Gibson sutures
 Gillies horizontal dermal
  sutures
 glover's sutures
 glue-in sutures
 Goethe sutures
 gossamer silk sutures
 Gould sutures
 granny knot sutures
 green braided sutures
 green monofilament
  polyglyconate sutures
 Gregory stay sutures
 groove sutures
 Gudebrod sutures
 guide sutures
 Gussenbauer sutures
 gut chromic sutures
 gut plain sutures
 gut sutures
 guy steadying sutures
 guy sutures
 Guyton sutures
 Guyton-Friedenwald
  sutures
 half-hitch sutures
 Halsted interrupted
  mattress sutures
 Halsted mattress sutures

suture *continued*

Halsted sutures
Hamis suture
harelip sutures
harmonic sutures
Harrington sutures
Harris sutures
Heaney sutures
heavy gauge sutures
heavy retention
    sutures
heavy silk retention
    sutures
heavy silk sutures
heavy wire sutures
helical sutures
hemostatic sutures
Herculon sutures
Hill sutures
horizontal mattress
    sutures
horizontal sutures
horseshoe sutures
Horsley sutures
IKI catgut sutures
imbricated sutures
imbricating sutures
implanted sutures
incisive sutures
India rubber sutures
infraorbital sutures
insert mattress sutures
intact skin sutures
interdermal buried
    sutures
interlocking sutures
intermaxillary sutures
intermittent sutures
internasal suture
interpalpebral suture
interrupted black silk
    sutures
interrupted chromic
    catgut sutures
interrupted chromic
    sutures
interrupted cotton
    sutures

suture *continued*

interrupted far-near
    sutures
interrupted fine silk
    sutures
interrupted Lembert
    sutures
interrupted mattress
    sutures
interrupted near-far
    sutures
interrupted plain catgut
    sutures
interrupted silk
    sutures
interrupted sutures
interrupted vertical
    mattress sutures
intestinal sutures
intracuticular nylon
    sutures
intracuticular sutures
intradermal mattress
    sutures
intradermal sutures
inverted knot sutures
inverted sutures
inverting sutures
iodine catgut sutures
iodized surgical gut
    sutures
iodochromic catgut
    sutures
Ivalon sutures
Jobert de Lamballe
    sutures
Jobert sutures
Jones sutures
jugal sutures
Kal-Dermic sutures
Kalt sutures
kangaroo tendon
    sutures
Keisley sutures
Kelly plication
    sutures
Kelly sutures
Kelly-Kennedy sutures

suture *continued*

Kessler sutures
Kirby sutures
Kirschner sutures
Kleinert sutures
Krause transverse sutures
Küstner sutures
Kypher sutures
lace sutures
lacidem sutures
lacrimoconchal suture
lacrimoethmoidal suture
lacrimomaxillary suture
lacrimoturbinal suture
Lahey sutures
lambdoid suture
Lang sutures
LaRoque sutures
lead-shot tie sutures
LeDentu sutures
LeDran sutures
LeFort sutures
Lembert sutures
Lespinasse sutures
Ligapak sutures
ligation sutures
ligature sutures
limbal sutures
limbic sutures
Lindner corneoscleral sutures
linear polyethylene sutures
linen sutures
linen thread sutures
lip sutures
Littre sutures
living sutures
lock sutures
locked sutures
locking running sutures
locking sutures
lock-stitch sutures
Loeffler sutures
longitudinal sutures
loop sutures
Lukens catgut sutures

suture *continued*

lumbar sutures
Lytle sutures
malomaxillary suture
mamillary suture
Marlex sutures
Marshall V-sutures
mastoid sutures
mattress sutures
Maunsell sutures
Maxam sutures
Maxon absorbable sutures
Maxon sutures
Mayo linen sutures
Mayo sutures
McCannel sutures
McGraw sutures
McKissock sutures
McLean corneoscleral sutures
Measuroll sutures
median palatine suture
medium chromic sutures
Medrafil sutures
Medrafil wire sutures
Meigs sutures
Mers sutures
Mersilene sutures
mesh sutures
metal band sutures
metopic suture
middle palatine suture
mild chromic sutures
Millipore sutures
monofilament clear sutures
monofilament green sutures
monofilament nylon sutures
monofilament sutures
monofilament wire sutures
multifilament sutures
multistrand sutures
Mustardé sutures

suture *continued*

nasal suture
nasofrontal suture
nasomaxillary suture
natural sutures
near-and-far sutures
near-far sutures
nerve sutures
Nesta stitch sutures
neurological sutures
neurosutures
Nissen sutures
nonabsorbable surgical
    sutures
nonabsorbable sutures
noneverting sutures
noose sutures
Novofil sutures
Nurulon sutures
nylon monofilament
    sutures
nylon retention sutures
nylon sutures
obstetrical double-armed
    sutures
occipital suture
occipitomastoid suture
occipitoparietal suture
occipitosphenoidal
    suture
O'Connell sutures
Oertli sutures
oiled silk sutures
on-edge mattress sutures
osteosutures
outer interrupted silk
    sutures
over-and-over sutures
over-and-over whip
    sutures
overlapping sutures
Owen sutures
Oyloidin sutures
Pagenstecher linen
    thread sutures
Pagenstecher sutures
palatine suture

suture *continued*

palatoethmoid suture
palatoethmoidal suture
palatomaxillary suture
Palfyn sutures
Pancoast sutures
pants-over-vest sutures
Paré sutures
parietal suture
parietomastoid suture
parieto-occipital suture
Parker-Kerr sutures
patch-reinforced mattress
    sutures
PDS (polydioxanone
    sutures)
PDS Vicryl sutures
Pearsall Chinese twisted
    sutures
Pearsall silk sutures
pericostal suture
perineal support sutures
Perlon sutures
Perma-Hand braided silk
    sutures
Perma-Hand silk sutures
Perma-Hand sutures
Petit sutures
petrobasilar suture
petrosphenobasilar
    suture
petrospheno-occipital
    suture of Gruber
petrosquamous suture
Pilling sutures
pin sutures
pink twisted cotton
    sutures
plain catgut sutures
plain gut sutures
plain interrupted sutures
plain sutures
plastic sutures
pledget sutures
pledgeted Ethibond
    sutures
pledgeted sutures

suture *continued*
plicating sutures
plication sutures
polyamide sutures
Polydek sutures
polydioxanone sutures
(PDS)
polyester fiber sutures
polyester sutures
polyethylene sutures
polyfilament sutures
polyglycolic sutures
polypropylene button
sutures
polypropylene sutures
pop-off sutures
posterior palatine suture
postplaced sutures
Potts tie sutures
precut sutures
premaxillary suture
preplaced sutures
presection sutures
primary sutures
Prolene sutures
pulley sutures
pull-out sutures
pull-out wire sutures
Pulvertaft sutures
Purlon sutures
pursestring sutures
PVB sutures
pyoktanin catgut sutures
pyoktanin sutures
Quickert sutures
quilt sutures
quilted sutures
radial sutures
Ramdohr sutures
Ramsey County
pyoktanin catgut
sutures
Rankin sutures
reconstructive sutures
rectus traction sutures
reef knot sutures
reinforcing sutures

suture *continued*
relaxation sutures
Reo Macrodex sutures
retained sutures
retention sutures
reverse-cutting sutures
rhabdoid suture
ribbon gut sutures
Richardson angle sutures
Richardson sutures
Richter sutures
Rigal sutures
right-angle mattress
sutures
Ritisch sutures
rubber sutures
running chromic sutures
running continuous
sutures
running imbricating
sutures
running subcuticular
sutures
running sutures
running-locked sutures
Sabreloc sutures
Saenger sutures
safety-bolt sutures
sagittal suture
Sani-dril sutures
Sarot bold sutures
scalp sutures
secondary sutures
seminal sutures
seromuscular sutures
seromuscular-to-edge
sutures
seroserosal silk sutures
seroserosal sutures
seroserous sutures
serrated sutures
seton sutures
sewing-machine stitch
sutures
Shirodkar sutures
shorthand vertical
mattress stitch sutures

suture *continued*

shotted sutures
Siemens PTCA open-heart sutures
silicone-treated surgical silk sutures
silicone-treated sutures
silk braided sutures
silk interrupted mattress sutures
silk pop-off sutures
silk stay sutures
silk sutures
silk traction sutures
silkworm gut sutures
silver suture wire
silver sutures
silverized catgut sutures
Simon sutures
simple sutures
Sims sutures
single-armed sutures
single-handed knot sutures
skin sutures
sleeper sutures
sling sutures
slotted sutures
Smead-Jones sutures
Snellen sutures
Softgut chromic sutures
Softgut sutures
solid-state silk sutures
Spanish blue virgin silk sutures
spatula needle sutures
sphenoethmoidal suture
sphenofrontal suture
sphenomalar suture
sphenomaxillary suture
spheno-occipital suture
spheno-orbital suture
sphenoparietal suture
sphenopetrosal suture
sphenosquamous suture
sphenotemporal suture
sphenozygomatic suture

suture *continued*

spiral sutures
Sprong sutures
squamosal suture
squamosomastoid suture
squamosoparietal suture
squamososphenoid suture
squamous suture
squamous suture of cranium
SS sutures (stainless steel sutures)
stainless steel sutures (SS sutures)
stainless steel wire sutures
Stallard sutures
Stallard-Liegard sutures
staple sutures
stay sutures
steel mesh sutures
steel sutures
stepwise sutures
sternal wire sutures
Stewart sutures
stick-tie sutures
Sturmdorf obstetrical sutures
Sturmdorf sutures
subcuticular sutures
superficial sutures
superior rectus bridle sutures
superior rectus traction sutures
support sutures
Supramid Extra sutures
Supramid sutures
Surgaloy metallic sutures
Surgaloy sutures
surgeon's knot sutures
surgical chromic sutures
surgical gut sutures
surgical linen sutures
surgical silk sutures
surgical steel sutures
surgical sutures

suture *continued*

Surgilar suture
Surgilene sutures
Surgiloid sutures
Surgilon braided nylon
   sutures
Surgilon sutures
Surgilone sutures
Surgilone monofilament
   polypropylene sutures
Surgilope sutures
Surgiset sutures
Sutupak sutures
swaged sutures
swaged-on sutures
Swedgeon sutures
Swiss blue virgin silk
   sutures
synthetic absorbable
   sutures
synthetic sutures
20-day gut sutures
tacking sutures
Tagima sutures
tantalum wire monofil-
   ament sutures
tantalum wire sutures
Tapercut sutures
Taylor sutures
Teflon-coated Dacron
   sutures
Teflon-pledgeted sutures
temporal suture
temporomalar suture
temporozygomatic suture
tendinosutures
tendon sutures
tenosutures
tension sutures
tenting sutures
Tevdek pledgeted
   sutures
Tevdek sutures
thermo-flex sutures
Thiersch sutures
thoracic sutures
thread sutures

suture *continued*

through-and-through
   continuous sutures
through-and-through
   sutures
Ti-Cron sutures (also
   Tycron)
tie sutures
tiger gut sutures
Tinel sutures
Tom Jones sutures
tongue sutures
tongue-and-groove
   sutures
tongue-in-groove sutures
tonsillar sutures
track sutures
traction sutures
transfixing sutures
transfixion sutures
transition sutures
transverse suture
transverse suture of
   Krause
traumatic sutures
true sutures
Trumbull sutures
twenty-day gut sutures
twisted cotton sutures
twisted dermal sutures
twisted linen sutures
twisted silk sutures
twisted sutures
Tycron sutures (also Ti-
   Cron)
Tyrrell-Gray sutures
U-double-barrel suture
U-shaped continuous
   sutures
U-sutures
umbilical tape sutures
unabsorbable sutures
undyed sutures
uninterrupted sutures
uteroparietal suture
Van Hillman suture
vascular silk sutures

suture *continued*
    venesuture
    venisuture
    Verhoeff sutures
    vertical mattress sutures
    vertical sutures
    VEST traction sutures
    Vicryl pop-off sutures
    Vicryl SH sutures
    Vicryl sutures
    Vienna wire sutures
    virgin silk sutures
    Viro-Tec sutures
    visceroparietal suture
    von Pirquet sutures
    Werner suture
    whipstitch sutures
    white braided sutures
    white nylon sutures
    white silk sutures
    white sutures
    white twisted sutures
    wing sutures
    wire sutures
    wire Zytor sutures
    Wölfler sutures
    Woodbridge sutures
    Worst medallion sutures
    Wysler sutures
    Y-sutures
    Z-sutures
    zygomatic suture
    zygomaticofrontal
      suture
    zygomaticomaxillary
      suture
    zygomaticotemporal
      suture
    Zytor sutures
suture and tying forceps
suture carrier
suture clip
suture clip applier
suture forceps
suture hole drill
suture hook
suture ligated
suture ligation

suture ligature
suture line
suture line of skull
suture material
suture needle (see also *needle*)
    Adson suture needle
    atraumatic suture needle
    Bonney suture needle
    cervix suture needle
    corneal suture needle
    curved suture needle
    Dees suture needle
    diamond-point suture
      needle
    Douglas suture needle
    eyed suture needle
    eyeless atraumatic suture
      needle
    eyeless suture needle
    Ferguson suture needle
    Gardner suture needle
    Hagedorn suture needle
    Henton suture needle
    Henton tonsillar suture
      needle
    Hurd suture needle
    kidney suture needle
    King suture needle
    Lane suture needle
    nasal suture needle
    noncutting suture needle
    straight suture needle
    taper-point suture needle
    tonsillar suture needle
    Yankauer suture needle
suture needle holder
suture plication
suture pusher
suture repair
suture ring
suture scissors
suture sizes (1-0, 2-0, 3-0, 4-0
    [or 0, 00, 000, 0000], 5-0,
    etc.)
suture sizing
Suture Strip Plus wound closure
    strip
suture wire

suture-carrying forceps
sutured in place
sutured parallel with wound
    edges
suture-holding forceps
sutureless pacemaker electrode
sutureless valve prosthesis
suture-line dehiscence
suture-pulling forceps
suture-release needle
suture-removing scissors
sutures attached to arterial wall
sutures tied
sutures tied down over cotton
sutures tied over rubber shoes
suture-tying forceps
suture-tying platform forceps
suturing forceps
suturing instruments
suturing needle
suturing
suturing of cyst inside out
suturing silks
SVBG (saphenous vein bypass
    grafting)
swab
swab stick
swabbed
swabbing
swaged needle
swaged sutures
swaged-on needle
swaged-on sutures
swallow
swallower
swallowing center
swallowing mechanism
Swan aortic clamp
Swan clamp
Swan gouge
Swan incision
Swan knife-needle
Swan eye needle holder
Swan operation
Swan punch
Swan-Ganz catheter
Swan-Ganz catheterization

Swan-Ganz guide wire TD
    catheter
Swan-Ganz pulmonary artery
    catheter
Swan-Ganz pulmonary
    catheterization
Swan-Ganz thermodilution
    catheter
Swan-Ganz tube
Swan-Jacob goniotomy pliers
swan-neck clamp
swan-neck deformity
swan-neck gouge
Swann-Morton blade
Swann-Morton surgical blade
Swann-Sheldon needle
Swanson arthroplasty
Swanson carpal lunate im-
    plant
Swanson carpal scaphoid
    implant
Swanson classification of
    congenital skeletal limb
    deficiency
Swanson finger joint implant
Swanson great toe implant
Swanson hemi-implant
Swanson implant
Swanson knife
Swanson operation
Swanson prosthesis
Swanson radial head implant
Swanson radiocarpal implant
Swanson Silastic prosthesis
Swanson trapezium implant
Swanson ulnar head implant
Swanson wrist joint implant
swayback
swayback deformity
swayback nose
swaying of body
sweat glands
Swede-O brace
Swedgeon already-threaded
    needle
Swedgeon sutures
Swedish knee cage

Sweeney posterior vaginal
    retractor
Sweeney retractor
Sweeney speculum
Sweet amputation retractor
Sweet antral trocar
Sweet clip-applying forceps
Sweet dissecting forceps
Sweet electric magnet
Sweet esophageal scissors
Sweet eye magnet
Sweet forceps
Sweet ligature forceps
Sweet magnet
Sweet punch
Sweet retractor
Sweet rib spreader
Sweet scissors
Sweet sternal punch
Sweet trocar
Sweet-Burford rib spreader
Sweet-Finochietto rib spreader
sweetheart retractor
swelling
swelling and pain
Swenko bag
Swenko gastric-cooling appara-
    tus
Swenson abdominal pull-
    through procedure
Swenson operation
Swenson pull-through proce-
    dure
swimmer's knee
swimmer's view of cervical
    spine on x-ray
swimmer's x-ray view
swimming injury
swim-up test
swine xenograft
swing phase
Swiss blade
Swiss blade breaker
Swiss blade holder
Swiss blue virgin silk sutures
Swiss bulldog clamp
Swiss MP joint implants
Swiss-cheese endometrium
Swiss-cheese hyperplasia
Swiss-pattern osteotome
switch
switch flap
Switzerland dilatation catheter
swivel connector tubing
swivel hook
swivel knife
swivel tracheostomy tube
swollen and painful joints
swollen and tender
swollen glands
swollen joints
swollen lymph nodes
swollen mucosa
sword knife
Syark vulsellum forceps
Sydenham mouth gag
Syed radium applicator
Syed template
Syed template flange
Syed template implant
Syed-Neblett implant
Syed-Neblett template
Sylva eye irrigator
Sylva irrigating cannula
Sylva irrigator
sylvian aqueduct
sylvian area
sylvian artery
sylvian fissure
sylvian fossa
sylvian line
sylvian point
sylvian waves
Symbion artificial heart
Symbion pneumatic assist
    device
Symbios dual-chamber pace-
    maker
Symbios pacemaker
symbiosis
symblepharon
symbol
Syme amputation
Syme amputation at ankle

Syme amputation of foot
Syme external urethrotomy
Syme operation
Syme prosthesis
Syme urethrotomy
symmetrical
symmetrical in contour
symmetrically
symmetry
Symmonds enterocele repair
Symmonds vaginal prolapse
    repair
sympathectomy
sympathectomy hook
sympathectomy retractor
sympathectomy scissors
sympathetic block
sympathetic block anesthesia
sympathetic carotid plexus
sympathetic chain
sympathetic ganglia
sympathetic nerve
sympathetic nerve block
sympathetic nerve fibers
sympathetic nervous system
sympathetic reaction
sympathetic trunk
sympathicectomy
sympathicodiaphtheresis
sympathicotripsy
symphysiorrhaphy
symphysiotomy
symphysis (*pl.* symphyses)
symphysis pubis
symphysis to umbilicus
symplastic tissue
symptom
symptomatic
symptomatic gallstone
symptomatically
symptomatology
Syms traction
Syms tractor
synapse
synaptic blocking agents
synaptic transmission
synarthrodial joint

Synatomic knee prosthesis
Synatomic total knee
Synatomic total knee system
    with Porocoat
synchondrectomy
synchondroseotomy
synchondrosis
synchondrotomy
synchronized retroperfusion
    (SRP)
synchronizing cords
synchronous amputation
synchronous bilateral breast
    cancer
synchronous burst pacemaker
synchronous mode pacemaker
synchronous pacemaker
synchronous with heart beat
synchronously
synchrony
Synchrony pacemaker
synchrotron-based transvenous
    angiography
synchysis of vitreous
synclitism
syncytial
syncytial cell
syncytial knots
syncytiovascular membrane
syndactylism release
syndactylization
syndactyly
syndectomy
syndesmectomy
syndesmochorial placenta
syndesmo-odontoid
syndesmopexy
syndesmophytes of spine
syndesmoplasty
syndesmorrhaphy
syndesmosis
syndesmosis screw
syndesmotic screw
syndesmotomy
syndrome
synechia (*pl.* synechiae)
synechialysis

synechotomy
synechtenterotomy
synergic muscles
synergism
synergist
Synergist Erection penile
    prosthesis
synergistic muscles
synergistic pressor effect
synergy
syngeneic graft
syngeneic transplantation
syngenesioplastic transplant
syngenesioplastic transplanta-
    tion
syngraft
synkinesis
synkinetic
Syn-optics camera
synoptoscopy
synosteotomy
synostosis (*pl.* synostoses)
synovectomy
synovia (*sing.* synovium)
synovial
synovial capsule
synovial cavity
synovial chondroma
synovial cyst
synovial flap
synovial fluid
synovial fold
synovial ganglion
synovial hernia
synovial joint
synovial membrane
synovial osteochondromatosis
synovial plica
synovial sac
synovial sheath
synovial villi
synoviochondromatosis
synovium (*sing.* synovia)
synovium biopsy forceps
Syntex screw
Synthaderm dressing
Synthes compression hip screw
Synthes external fixator

Synthes facial curet
Synthes facial drill
Synthes metallic plate
Synthes nail
Synthes plate
Synthes screw
synthesis
synthetic absorbable sutures
synthetic graft
synthetic human growth
    hormone
synthetic mesh
synthetic suture material
synthetic wool
synulosis
synulotic
syringe
    air syringe
    Alcock bladder syringe
    Alcock syringe
    Alexander syringe
    all-metal ear syringe
    Allegist syringe
    Anel lacrimal syringe
    Anel syringe
    antral syringe
    Asepto aspirating syringe
    Asepto bulb syringe
    Asepto irrigation syringe
    Asepto syringe
    aspiration syringe
    Autosyringe insulin
        pump
    B-D Luer-Lok syringe
    B-D Yale syringe
    bladder syringe
    bulb syringe
    Carpule syringe
    catheter-tip syringe
    chip syringe
    colonoscope syringe
    control syringe
    Davidson syringe
    dental syringe
    DeVilbiss irrigating
        syringe
    DeWecker syringe
        cannula

syringe *continued*
- displacement syringe
- disposable syringe
- Duval irrigating syringe
- ear syringe
- Eccentric syringe
- Fischer syringe
- fountain syringe
- Fuchs two-way eye syringe
- Gabriel syringe
- Goldstein eye syringe
- Goldstein syringe
- Green-Armytage syringe
- Heath anterior chamber syringe
- Higgenson syringe
- hypodermic syringe
- irrigation syringe
- Isaacs aspiration syringe
- Kaufman syringe
- Keyes-Ultzmann syringe tube
- Kramer syringe
- lacrimal syringe
- laryngeal syringe
- Lehman syringe
- Luer syringe
- Luer tip syringe
- Luer-Lok syringe
- metal syringe
- Nourse syringe
- Parker-Heath eye syringe
- Pierce syringe
- Pitkin syringe
- plastic syringe
- Pomeroy ear syringe
- Pomeroy syringe
- Pravay syringe
- Pritchard syringe
- Proetz displacement syringe
- record syringe
- Reiner ear syringe
- Reiner-Alexander syringe
- Robb syringe
- Rochester syringe
- rubber-bulb syringe

syringe *continued*
- Sana-Lok syringe
- sinus suction syringe
- Street tonsillar syringe
- Stylex syringe
- Thompson syringe
- tonsillar syringe
- Toomey syringe
- Tuber syringe
- van Buren cervix syringe
- Vim Gabriel aspirating syringe
- Vim tonsil syringe

syringe extension
syringe pump
syringe push
syringe suction
syringectomy
syringing
syringomyelia
syringomyelic
syringotome
syringotomy
system
systematic anatomy
systematic approach
systemic blood flow
systemic cancer
systemic circulation
systemic lesion
systemic pressure
systemic sepsis
systemic shock
systemic treatment
systemic-pulmonary artery shunt
systemic-to-pulmonary artery anastomosis
systole
systolic
systolic murmur
systolic pressure
Szilagyi approach
Sztehlo clamp
Sztehlo umbilical clamp
Szuler forceps
Szymanowski operation
Szymanowski-Kuhnt operation

10-20 electrode system
10-20 system
2D echo (two-dimensional echo)
20-day gut sutures
3-point chuck
3-way Foley catheter
30-V staples
3D CT (three-dimensional computed tomography)
3D knee system
3D PTB walker
3D short-leg walker
3M bone mill
3M drape
3M dressing
3M mammary implant
3M Vi-Drape
T&A (tonsillectomy and adenoidectomy)
T&A suction tip
T&C (type and crossmatch)
T-bandage
T-bandage dressing
T-bar elevator
T-binder
T-binder pressure dressing
T-condylar fracture
T-contact lens
T-drain
T-finger splint
T-handle
T-handle elevator
T-handle reamer
T-handle wrench
T-incision
T-lens
T-loop
T-malleable retractor

T-piece
T-plate
T-shaped forceps
T-shaped fracture
T-shaped incision
T-shaped scar
T-Span tissue expander
T-spine
T-splint
T-tube
T-tube catheter
T-tube cholangiogram (TTC)
T-tube cholangiography
T-tube drain
T-tube drainage
T-tube incision
T-tube stent
T-tube technique
T-type ileocystoplasty
T-vent connector
T-wave
Ta-182 (tantalum-182)
TA-30 stapler
TA-50 stapler
TA-55 stapler
TA-60 stapler
TA-90 stapler
TA-90-BN stapler
Taarnhøj operation
TAB (therapeutic abortion)
Tabb curet
Tabb ear elevator
Tabb ear knife
Tabb elevator
Tabb knife
Tabb myringoplasty knife
Tabb ruler
tabes
tabes dorsalis

tabescent
tabetic foot
table
    Abbott table
    Albee fracture table
    Albee table
    Albee-Compere fracture
        table
    Allen arm surgery table
    Allen hand surgery table
    Andrews spinal table
    anesthetist's table
    anterior table
    back table
    Bell fracture table
    Bird table
    bony table
    Boren-Mayo table
    Boyd table
    Burgess table
    Castle laminectomy table
    chair-table
    Chick fracture table
    Chick operating table
    Chick-Hyde fracture
        table
    Chick-Langren table
    conversion table
    Dextra surgical table
    DMI ambulatory surgery
        table
    Elgin table
    external table
    fracture table
    hand table
    Hayley table
    Heidelberg-R surgical
        table
    Holley table
    hydraulic chair-table
    hydraulic table
    inner table
    inner table bones of
        skull
    inner table frontal bone
    inner table of skull
    instrument table

table *continued*
    internal table
    Karlin spinal table
    LeBerne treatment table
    Maquet endoscopy table
    Maquet table
    Mayfield overhead table
    Mayfield table
    Mayo instrument table
    McKee table
    McPheeters table
    Mimer table
    operating table
    orthopedic table
    outer table bones of
        skull
    outer table of frontal
        bone
    outer table of skull
    posterior table
    radiopaque table
    Risser cast table
    Ritter table
    Roger Anderson table
    sigmoidoscopy table
    Skytron operating table
    slit-lamp instrument
        table
    Stryker fracture table
    tilt table
    Tower fracture table
    Tower table
table band
table bones of skull
table of skull
tabs
Tab-Strap knee immobilizer
TAC (total abdominal colec-
    tomy)
TAC atherectomy catheter
Tachdjian hamstring technique
tachography study
tachyarrhythmia
tachycardia
tachycardia-terminating
    pacemaker
Tachylog pacemaker

tachypacing
tachypnea
tachysystole
tack
    Cody sacculotomy tack
    Cody tack
    Cody tack inserter
    Cody tack procedure
    Effler tack
    inserter tack
tack hammer
tack inserter
tack operation
tack-and-pin forceps
tacking
tacking sutures
tackler's arm
tactics
tactile disk
tactile fremitus
tactile probe
tactile sensation
tactile stimulation
tactile tension
TAD guide wire
taenia organism
tagged muscles
Tagima sutures
tagliacotian operation
tagliacotian rhinoplasty
Tagliacozzi flap
Tagliacozzi nasal reconstruction
tags
TAH (total abdominal hysterectomy)
tail fold
tail of pancreas
tail of Spence
tail sign
tailbone
tailbone area
tailgut
tailoring of flap
tailor's ankle
tailor's bunion
Tait flap
Tait graft
Tait perineoplasty

Takahashi cutting forceps
Takahashi elevator
Takahashi ethmoid forceps
Takahashi ethmoid punch
Takahashi forceps
Takahashi nasal forceps
Takahashi nasal punch
Takahashi neurological forceps
Takahashi punch
Takahashi rongeur
takedown
takedown of adhesions
takedown of anastomosis
takeoff
takeoff of vessel
taking down of adhesions
TAL (tendon Achilles lengthening)
talar component
talar tendon
talar tilt
talar tilt test
talc
talc operation
talc plaque
talc poudrage
tali (*sing.* talus)
talipes
talipes calcaneovalgus
talipes calcaneovarus
talipes calcaneus
talipes cavovalgus
talipes cavus
talipes correction
talipes equinovalgus
talipes equinovarus
talipes equinus
talipes hobble splint
talipes planovalgus
talipes valgus
talipes varus
talipomanus
talking tracheostomy tube
Talma operation
talocalcaneal ligament
talocalcaneonavicular articulation
talocalcaneonavicular ligament

talofibular ligament
talonavicular articulation
talonavicular joint
talonavicular ligament
talus (*pl.* tali)
talus foot deformity
talus head
Tamai clamp approximator
Tamai stitch
Tamai technique
tamp
> graft tamp
> interbody graft tamp
> Kiene bone tamp
> spinal graft tamp

tamper
tampon
> Corner tampon
> Doyle nasal tampon
> Dührssen tampon
> Genupak tampon
> nasal tampon
> Simpson tampon
> tonsillar tampon
> tracheal tampon
> Trendelenburg tampon
> vaginal tampon

tampon applicator
tampon injury
tampon tube
tamponade
tamponade action
tamponing
tamponment
Tan spatula
Tanagho modification of Burch
> procedure

tandem
tandem insertion
tangential beam
tangential clamp
tangential cut
tangential field
tangential forceps
tangential occlusion clamp
tangential plane
tangential projection
tangential view

tangential view on x-ray
tangential wound
tangentially
tangles
tank
Tanner herniorrhaphy
Tanner mesher
Tanner method
Tanner operation
Tanner Rue-19 esophagogastro-
> jejunostomy

Tanner-19 anti-bile reflux
> operation

Tanner-Vandeput graft
Tanner-Vandeput mesh
> dermatome

Tansini breast amputation
Tansini gastric resection
Tansini operation
Tansini removal of liver cyst
Tansini sign
Tansley operation
tantalum
tantalum bronchogram
tantalum clip
tantalum eye implant
tantalum graft
tantalum hemostasis clip
tantalum implant
tantalum material
tantalum mesh
tantalum mesh graft
tantalum mesh implant
tantalum mesh prosthesis
tantalum plate
tantalum prosthesis
tantalum ring
tantalum sheet
tantalum stapes prosthesis
tantalum wire
tantalum wire fixation
tantalum wire monofilament
> sutures

tantalum wire sutures
tantalum-182 (Ta-182)
Tanzer operation
tap
> bloody tap

tap drill
tape
tape ligature
taper
taper needle
Tapercut needle
Tapercut sutures
tapered bougie
tapered needle
tapered rubber bougie
tapering
taper-jaw rongeur
taper-point needle
taper-point needle holder
taper-point suture needle
tapping hammer
tapping of chest for fluid
tar cancer
TARA (total articular replace-
    ment arthroplasty)
TARA prosthesis
Tara retropubic retractor
target
target cell
target lesion
target tissue
target volume
target-to-nontarget ratio
Tarlov cyst
Tarlov nerve elevator
Tarnier forceps
Tarnier obstetrical forceps
Tarrant position
tarsal arteries
tarsal bar
tarsal bone
tarsal canal
tarsal coalition
tarsal cyst
tarsal fold
tarsal gland
tarsal joint
tarsal muscle
tarsal plate
tarsal sinus
tarsal synostosis
tarsal tunnel
tarsal tunnel syndrome

tarsal wedge osteotomy
tarsalis inferior, musculus
tarsalis superior, musculus
tarsals
tarsea lateralis, arteria
tarseae mediales, arteriae
tarsectomy
tarsoclasis
tarsoepiphyseal aclasis
tarsometatarsal articulations
tarsometatarsal ligament
tarsophalangeal reflex
tarsoplasia
tarsoplasty
tarsorrhaphy
tarsotibial amputation
tarsotomy
tarsus (*pl.* tarsi)
tarsus inferior palpebrae
tarsus orbital septum
tarsus superior palpebrae
Tascon prosthetic valve
Tasia operation
task
Tassett vaginal cup bag
taste bud
taste cells
Tate flap
tattoo
tattoo injury
tattoo surgery
tattooing
tattooing instrument
tattooing needle
Tatum clamp
Tatum ureteral transilluminator
Tauber catheter
Tauber hook
Tauber ligature carrier
Tauber needle
Tauber spatula
Tauber speculum
Taucher tunneler
Taussig operation
Taussig-Bing anomaly
Taussig-Bing malformation
Taussig-Bing syndrome
Taussig-Morton operation

taut
taut foot
tautening
Tavernetti-Tennant-Cutter knee
Tawara node
taxis
Tay choroiditis
Tay spot
Taylor apparatus
Taylor aspirator
Taylor back brace
Taylor blade
Taylor brace
Taylor craniotomy scissors
Taylor curet
Taylor dissecting forceps
Taylor forceps
Taylor gastric balloon
Taylor knife
Taylor Merocel ear wick
Taylor neurosurgical scissors
Taylor position
Taylor retractor
Taylor scissors
Taylor speculum
Taylor sutures
Taylor technique
Taylor tissue forceps
Taylor vaginal speculum
Tay-Sachs disease
TC IV total knee
TC needle holder
Tc-99m phosphate bone
    imaging
TcHIDA scan
TCNS (transcutaneous nerve
    stimulator)
TCPM pneumatic tourniquet
    system
TCS knee immobilizer (tri-
    panel, convoluted, Y-strap
    knee immobilizer)
TDD (thoracic duct drainage)
TDI hip (three-dimensional
    interlocking hip)
TE fistula (tracheoesophageal
    fistula)
TEA (thromboendarterectomy)

teaching attachment
Teale amputation
Teale director
Teale forceps
Teale lithotomy gorget guide
Teale operation
Teale uterine vulsellum forceps
Teale vulsellum forceps
Teale-Knapp operation
team approach
tear at 1 (2, 3, etc.) o'clock
tear duct
tear duct tube
tear of capsule
tear of ligament
tear of meniscus
tear of mucosa
tear of muscle
tear sac
tearaway sheath
teardrop fracture
teardrop vertebral outgrowth
Teare arm sling
Teare arm sling splint
Teare sling
teased open
Teca therapeutic generator
Techmedica CAD/CAM custom
    implant system
Techmedica total hip
Techmedica total pelvis
technetium
technetium pertechnetate
    scan
technetium pyrophosphate
technetium scan
technetium-99m scan
technical precautions
technician
technique
Technomed Sonolith 3000
    lithotriptor
tectonic keratoplasty
tectorial membrane
tectum of brain stem
tectum of midbrain
TED (thromboembolic disease)
TED hose

TED pneumatic compression boots
TED socks
TED stockings
TEE (transesophageal echo-cardiography)
teeth
Teevan lithotrite
Teflon
Teflon Bardic plug
Teflon block
Teflon bolster
Teflon button
Teflon cannula
Teflon catheter
Teflon endolymphatic shunt tube
Teflon ERCP cannula
Teflon felt
Teflon felt bolster
Teflon felt patch
Teflon felt pledget
Teflon graft
Teflon implant
Teflon intracardiac patch
Teflon intracardiac patch prosthesis
Teflon mesh
Teflon mesh implant
Teflon mesh prosthesis
Teflon nasobiliary drain
Teflon needle
Teflon orbital floor implant
Teflon paste
Teflon paste injection for incontinence
Teflon patch
Teflon plate
Teflon pledget
Teflon probe
Teflon prosthesis
Teflon sheath
Teflon sheeting prosthesis
Teflon shunt tube
Teflon sling rectopexy
Teflon sling repair
Teflon splint

Teflon strut
Teflon strut-cutting block
Teflon tape
Teflon tip
Teflon trileaflet prosthesis
Teflon tube
Teflon wire piston prosthesis
Teflon-coated Dacron sutures
Teflon-coated guide wire
Teflon-covered needle
Teflon-Delrin cutting block
Teflon-pledgeted sutures
Teflon-tipped catheter
Teflon-wire piston
Tegaderm
Tegaderm dressing
Tegaderm occlusive dressing
Tegaderm transparent dressing
tegmental cells
tegmental region
tegmental wall
tegmentum of midbrain
Tehl clamp
Tek tube
telangiectasia
telangiectatic glioma
telangiectatic wart
Telectronics lithium pacer
Telectronics pacemaker
telecurietherapy
telemetric monitoring
telemetric pressure sensor
telemetric technique
telemetry
telemetry monitor
telephone probe
teleradiography
teleradiology
teleroentgenogram
telescope
    ACMI microlens Foroblique telescope
    ACMI microlens telescope
    ACMI telescope
    Atkins esophagoscopic telescope

telescope *continued*
  Best telescope
  biopsy telescope
  bioptic telescope
  Bridge telescope
  bronchoscopic telescope
  Broyles telescope
  Burns telescope
  clamp-on telescope
  convertible telescope
  direct forward-vision
    telescope
  direct-vision telescope
  double-catheterizing
    telescope
  endoscopic telescope
  examining telescope
  fiberoptic right-angle
    telescope
  fiberoptic telescope
  Foroblique telescope
  Holinger bronchoscopic
    telescope
  Holinger telescope
  Hopkins endoscopy
    telescope
  Hopkins nasal endos-
    copy telescope
  Hopkins pediatric
    telescope
  Hopkins rod lens
    telescope
  Hopkins telescope
  infant telescope
  Keeler panoramic
    surgical telescope
  Kramer telescope
  LUMINA-operating
    telescope
  LUMINA-SL telescope
  McCarthy miniature
    telescope
  McCarthy telescope
  nasal endoscopy
    telescope
  operating telescope
  pediatric telescope

telescope *continued*
  right-angle examining
    telescope
  right-angle telescope
  Selsi sport telescope
  Storz bronchoscopic
    telescope
  Storz telescope
  Storz-Hopkins telescope
  transilluminating
    telescope
  Tucker telescope
  Vest telescope
  Walden telescope
telescope adapting bridge
telescope bridge
telescope of cystoscope
telescoping guide
telescoping medullary rod
teletherapy
Teletrast gauze
television microscope
television microscopy
Telfa 4 x 4 bandage
Telfa dressing
Telfa gauze dressing
Telfa pad
Telfa plastic film
Telfa plastic film dressing
TeLinde hysterectomy
TeLinde operation
TeLinde-Everett operation
Telson hinged walking heel
Temens curet
Temp-Bond
temperature
temperature probe
template
  acetabular cup template
  McKissock keyhole
    areolar template
  Moore template
  Strömbeck template
  surgical template
  Syed template
  Syed-Neblett template
  Thompson template

template *continued*
    wire template
    x-ray template
template markings
template splint
Temple procedure
Temple University nail
Temple University plate
Temple-Fay laminectomy
    retractor
Temple-Fay retractor
Templeton-Zim carpal tunnel
    projection
temporal
temporal arcade
temporal area
temporal arteries
temporal arteriole of retina
temporal bone
temporal bone bank
temporal bone holder
temporal canthus
temporal diameter
temporal diploic vein
temporal electrode
temporal facial nerve
temporal field
temporal fossa
temporal gyrus
temporal horn of lateral
    ventricle
temporal incision
temporal line
temporal lobe
temporal muscle
temporal nerves
temporal region
temporal retina
temporal suture
temporal trephine
temporal vein
temporal venule
temporales profundae, arteriae
temporales profundae, venae
temporales profundi, nervi
temporales superficiales, venae
temporalis media, arteria

temporalis media, vena
temporalis, musculus
temporalis superficialis, arteria
temporally
temporary
temporary aortic shunt sub-
    clavian-subclavian bypass
temporary callus
temporary clip
temporary end colostomy
temporary loop ileostomy
temporary magnet
temporary pacemaker
temporary pacing catheter
temporary pacing wire
temporary stricture
temporary transvenous pace-
    maker
temporary vascular clip
temporary vessel clip
temporofacial graft
temporomalar suture
temporomandibular articulation
temporomandibular joint
temporomandibular joint
    dislocation
temporomaxillary articulation
temporomaxillary joint
temporoparietal muscle
temporoparietalis, musculus
temporozygomatic suture
tenacious mucoid secretion
tenaculum
    Adair breast tenaculum
    Adair tenaculum
    Adair uterine tenaculum
    Adair-Allis tenaculum
    atraumatic tenaculum
    Barrett tenaculum
    Barrett uterine tenaculum
    Bierer tenaculum
    Braun tenaculum
    Braun uterine tenaculum
    breast tenaculum
    Brophy tenaculum
    bullet tenaculum
    cervical tenaculum

tenaculum *continued*
- cleft palate tenaculum
- Corey tenaculum
- Cottle sharp tenaculum
- Cottle tenaculum
- Crossen puncturing tenaculum
- DeLee tenaculum
- double-hook skin tenaculum
- double-tooth tenaculum
- Dudley tenaculum
- Duplay tenaculum
- Duplay uterine tenaculum
- Emmet tenaculum
- Emmet uterine tenaculum
- Ferguson tenaculum
- Gaylor tenaculum
- goiter tenaculum
- Hulka tenaculum
- Hulka uterine tenaculum
- Jackson tenaculum
- Jackson tracheal tenaculum
- Jacob tenaculum
- Jacob uterine tenaculum
- Jarcho tenaculum
- Joseph tenaculum
- Kahn tenaculum
- Kahn traction tenaculum
- Kelly uterine tenaculum
- labiotenaculum
- Lahey goiter tenaculum
- Lahey tenaculum
- Lahey thyroid tenaculum
- Lillie-White tenaculum
- lion-jaw tenaculum
- Marlex atraumatic obstetrical tenaculum
- Marlex atraumatic tenaculum
- Marlex tenaculum
- nasal tenaculum
- Newman tenaculum

tenaculum *continued*
- Newman uterine tenaculum
- Potts tenaculum
- Potts-Smith tenaculum
- Pozzi tenaculum
- ring-toothed tenaculum
- Ritchie tenaculum
- Schroeder tenaculum
- Schwartz tenaculum
- screw tenaculum
- sharp-toothed tenaculum
- Sims tenaculum
- single-tooth tenaculum
- single-toothed tenaculum
- Skene tenaculum
- Skene uterine tenaculum
- Staude-Moore tenaculum
- straight tenaculum
- Sturgis tenaculum
- Tensor tenaculum
- Thoms tenaculum
- tonsillar screw tenaculum
- tonsillar tenaculum
- toothed tenaculum
- tracheal tenaculum
- uterine tenaculum
- Watts tenaculum
- Weisman tenaculum

tenaculum forceps
tenaculum hook
tenaculum traction
Tenckhoff catheter
Tenckhoff peritoneal catheter
Tenckhoff renal dialysis catheter
tendency
tender and swollen
tender mass
Tenderfoot incision-making device
tenderness
tenderness on palpation
tenderness on pressure
tenderness on rebound
tenderness to percussion
tenderness to touch
tendines (*sing.* tendo)

tendinoplasty
tendinosutures
tendinotrochanteric ligament
tendinous
tendinous arch of levator ani
tendinous center
tendinous chiasm
tendinous galea
tendinous ring
tendinous sheath
tendo (*pl.* tendines)
tendocalcaneus
tendolysis
tendon
tendon Achilles lengthening
    (TAL)
tendon advancement
tendon aspiration and injec-
    tion
tendon blockage
tendon calcaneus
tendon cartilage
tendon forceps
tendon graft
tendon implant
tendon injury
tendon insertion
tendon intact
tendon laceration
tendon lengthening
tendon passer (see also *passer*)
    Brand tendon passer
    Bunnell tendon passer
    Gallie tendon passer
    Joplin tendon passer
    Kleinert tendon passer
    Ober tendon passer
tendon prosthesis
tendon release
tendon rupture
tendon severed
tendon sheath
tendon shortening
tendon stripper (see also
    *stripper*)
    Brand tendon stripper
    Bunnell tendon stripper

tendon stripper *continued*
    Carroll forearm tendon
        stripper
tendon sutures
tendon transfer
tendon transplant
tendon transplantation
tendon tucker (see also *tucker*)
    Bishop tendon tucker
    Bishop-Black tendon
        tucker
    Bishop-DeWitt tendon
        tucker
    Bishop-Peter tendon
        tucker
    Burch-Greenwood
        tendon tucker
    Fink tendon tucker
    Ruedemann-Todd
        tendon tucker
tendon-holding forceps
tendon-tucking instruments
tendon-tunneling forceps
tendoplastic amputation
tendoplasty
tendosynovial tissue sarcoma
tendotome
tendotomy
tendovaginitis
tenectomy
tenia libera coli
tenia of thalamus
teniamyotomy
Tennant Anchorflex anterior
    chamber intraocular lens
Tennant Anchorflex lens
    implant
Tennant eye spatula
Tennant forceps
Tennant intraocular implant
    lens
Tennant intraocular lens forceps
Tennant iris hook
Tennant lens
Tennant needle holder
Tennant-Maumenee forceps
Tenner cannula

Tenner eye cannula
Tennessee polisher
tennis elbow
tennis leg
Tennis Racquet angiographic
    catheter
Tennis Racquet catheter
tennis thumb
tennis toe
Tennison cheiloplasty
Tennison operation
Tennison Z-plasty
Tennison-Randall cleft lip
    repair
Tennison-Randall operation
tennis-racket incision
tenodesis
tenography
tenolysis
tenomyoplasty
tenomyotomy
tenon
Tenon capsule
Tenon fascia
Tenon membrane
Tenon space
tenonectomy
tenonometer
tenontomyoplasty
tenontomyotomy
tenontoplasty
tenontotomy
tenoplastic
tenoplasty
tenorrhaphy
tenosuspension
tenosutures
tenosynovectomy
tenosynovial chondrometa-
    plasia
tenosynovitis
tenotome
tenotomy
tenotomy hook
tenotomy knife
tenotomy of ocular tendon
tenotomy scissors

TENS (transcutaneous electrical/
    electrode nerve stimula-
    tion/stimulator)
TENS unit
tense abdomen
tense ascites
tensile strength
Tensilon anesthetic agent
Tensilon implant
tensing
tensiometer
tension
tension band wiring
tension planes
tension skin lines
tension sutures
tension-free anastomosis
tensionless anastomosis
Tensoplast elastic adhesive
    dressing
tensor
Tensor elastic dressing
tensor fascia lata
tensor fasciae latae, musculus
tensor muscle
Tensor tenaculum
tensor tympani, musculus
tensor veli palatini, musculus
tensoris tympani, nervus
tensoris veli palatini, nervus
tent
tentative
tented
tenth cranial nerve (X)
tenting of diaphragm
tenting of hemidiaphragm
tenting sutures
tentorial herniation
tentorial line
tentorial nerve
tentorial notch
tentorium cerebelli
tentorium cyst
tentorium of cerebellum
tentorium of hypophysis
tenuous
Tenzel elevator

Tenzel periosteal elevator
Tenzel semicircular flap
tepee incision
tepid water
teratic implantation
teratocarcinoma
teratogenic
teratogenic potential
teratogenicity
teratoid tumor
teratoma
Terblanche decompression of
    common bile duct
terebration
teres major muscle
teres major, musculus
teres minor muscle
teres minor, musculus
teres muscle
term delivery
term pregnancy
terminal
terminal adapter electrode
terminal aorta
terminal bile duct
terminal cancer
terminal carcinoma
terminal care
terminal colostomy
terminal condition
terminal disease
terminal electrode
terminal electrode adapter
terminal electrode nerve
    stimulator (TENS)
terminal ganglion
terminal ileal loop
terminal ileal pouch
terminal ileal segment
terminal ileostomy
terminal ileum
terminal ligature
terminal line
terminal nerves
terminal occlusion
terminal phalanx
terminal sigmoid colostomy
terminal state

terminal sulcus
terminal tuft fracture
terminal vein
terminal ventricle
terminal web
terminate
termination of labor
termination of pregnancy
termination of procedure
terminoterminal anastomosis
Ter-Pogossian applicator
Terrien degeneration
Terrillon operation
Terry fingernail sign
Terry keratometer
Terry keratotomy
Terry nails
Terry skin lines
Terry-Mayo needle
Terson capsule forceps
Terson forceps
Terson operation
Terson speculum
tertiary amputation
tertiary carina
tertiary contractions
tertiary dehiscence
tertiary peristaltic activity
tertiary radicle
tertiary transmission
tertiary vitreous
Terumo dialyzer
Terwilliger excision
Tes Tape dressing
Tesberg esophagoscope
Tesla measurement
tessellated fundus
Tessier bone bender
Tessier craniofacial cleft
Tessier craniofacial operation
Tessier disimpaction device
    forceps
Tessier disimpaction elevator
Tessier dislodger
Tessier elevator
Tessier facial dysostosis
    operation
Tessier operation

Tessier rib morcellizer
test
test tube
testectomy
testes (*sing.* testis)
testes in scrotum
testicle
testicle transplant
testicular
testicular abscess
testicular appendage
testicular artery
testicular atrophy
testicular cancer
testicular choriocarcinoma
testicular implant
testicular lymphoma
testicular plexus
testicular prosthesis
testicular shock
testicular swelling
testicular torsion
testicular tubules
testicular vein
testicularis, arteria
testicularis dextra, vena
testicularis sinistra, vena
testing
testis (*pl.* testes)
testis tumor
tethered
tethered spinal cord
tethered-bowel sign
tethered-cord syndrome
tetracaine hydrochloride
    anesthetic agent
tetrad
tetralogy of Fallot
Teufel brace
Teuffer tendocalcaneus repair
Tevdek graft
Tevdek implant
Tevdek pledgeted sutures
Tevdek prosthesis
Tevdek sutures
Texas catheter
Textor operation
Textor vasectomy clamp

texture
TF-II total hip system
TFT cervix (tight fingertip
    dilated)
TGA (transposition of great
    arteries)
TGAR (total graft area rejected)
TGV (transposition of great
    vessels)
Thackston retropubic bag
Thal esophageal stricture repair
Thal esophagogastrostomy
Thal gastric patch
Thal hiatal hernia repair
thalamectomy
thalamic tumor
thalamomammillary bundle
thalamostriata vena
thalamotomy
thalamus
Tham flap
THARIES (total hip articular
    replacement by internal
    eccentric shells)
Tharies hip arthroplasty
Tharies prosthesis
Tharies surface hip replacement
Thatcher nail
Thatcher screw
THC (transhepatic cholangi-
    ogram)
thebesian valve
thebesian vein
theca (*pl.* thecae)
theca cordis
theca folliculi
theca lutein cells
theca vertebralis
thecal
thecal cell
thecal cell tumor
thecal puncture
thecal whitlow
Theden bandage
Theile glands
Theis retractor
Theis rib spreader
Theis self-retaining retractor

thelarche
theleplasty
thelerethism
thelorrhagia
thenar
thenar atrophy
thenar cleft
thenar compartment
thenar eminence
thenar fascia
thenar flap
thenar muscle
thenar space
thenar surface
thenar web
Theobald lacrimal dilator
Theobald probe
Theobald sinus probe
TheraBand
therapeutic
therapeutic abortion (TAB)
therapeutic approach
therapeutic D&C
therapeutic endoscopy
therapeutic intervention
therapeutic iridectomy
therapeutic measures
therapeutic splint
therapeutic support
therapeutic treatment
Thera-Putty
Therapybird
TheraSeed
thermal agents
thermal burn
thermal dilution technique
thermal dose
thermal effect
thermal imaging
thermal injury
thermistor catheter
thermistor probe
thermocauterectomy
thermocautery
thermocoagulation
thermodilution balloon catheter
thermodilution pacing catheter

thermodilution Swan-Ganz
    catheter
thermo-flex sutures
thermography
thermometer
Thermophore bandage
Thermophore hot pack
Thermophore moist heat pad
thermoplastic orthosis
thermoplastic polymer
Therm-O-Rite blanket
Thermos pacemaker
thermosetting polymer
thermotherapy
thermotic pump
Theurig sterilizer forceps
THI needle
thialbarbitone anesthetic agent
thiamylal sodium anesthetic
    agent
thick adhesions
thick elastic tissue
thick visceral peel
thickened
thickened folds
thickened musculature
thickened pleura
thickening
thick-layer autoradiography
thickness
thick-split graft
thick-walled
thick-walled gallbladder
Thiersch anal incontinence
    operation
Thiersch cerclage
Thiersch graft
Thiersch implant
Thiersch knife
Thiersch operation
Thiersch procedure for rectal
    prolapse
Thiersch prosthesis
Thiersch repair of rectal
    procidentia
Thiersch ring
Thiersch skin graft

Thiersch skin graft knife
Thiersch sutures
Thiersch wire
Thiersch-Duplay urethroplasty
thigh
thigh bone
thigh splint
Thillaye bandage
Thillaye dressing
thin adhesions
thin disk
thin edge
thin osteotome
thin plastic membrane
Thinlith II pacemaker
thin-needle percutaneous
    cholangiogram
thin-split graft
thin-walled
thin-walled needle
thiopental sodium anesthetic
    agent
third cartilaginous ring
third cranial nerve
third molar
third nerve
third occipital nerve
third peroneal muscle
third trimester
third ventricle of brain
third-degree (3rd-degree)
third-degree burn
third-degree sprain
third-spacing
Thiry fistula
Thiry-Vella fistula
Thole pelvimeter
Thom flap
Thom flap laryngeal reconstruc-
    tion
Thoma clamp
Thoma tissue retractor
Thomas Allis forceps
Thomas Allis tissue forceps
Thomas brace
Thomas cervical collar brace
Thomas collar

Thomas cryoextractor
Thomas cryopter
Thomas curet
Thomas fracture frame
Thomas full-ring leg splint
Thomas heel
Thomas hyperextension frame
Thomas knife
Thomas leg splint
Thomas leg splint with Pearson
    attachment
Thomas operation
Thomas pelvimeter
Thomas ring
Thomas shot compression
    forceps
Thomas spatula
Thomas splint
Thomas uterine curet
Thomas uterine tissue-grasping
    forceps
Thomas Waldon wrench
Thomas walking calipers brace
Thomas-Thompson-Straub
    gluteus medius procedure
Thomas-Thompson-Straub
    transfer
Thomas-Warren incision
Thomayer sign
Thombostat
Thompson adenoid punch
Thompson antral rasp
Thompson bronchial catheter
Thompson carotid artery clamp
Thompson carotid vascular
    clamp
Thompson catheter
Thompson clamp
Thompson curet
Thompson direct full-vision
    resectoscope
Thompson drape
Thompson evacuator
Thompson femoral head
Thompson femoral head
    prosthesis
Thompson fracture frame

Thompson frontal sinus
    raspatory
Thompson lithotrite
Thompson modification of
    Denis Browne splint
Thompson operation
Thompson prosthesis
Thompson punch
Thompson rasp
Thompson raspatory
Thompson reduction technique
Thompson resectoscope
Thompson rib shears
Thompson root extractor
Thompson sinus rasp
Thompson squeeze test of
    Achilles
Thompson squeeze test of
    gastrocnemius
Thompson syndrome
Thompson syringe
Thompson telescoping
    V-osteotomy
Thompson template
Thompson-Compere hip
    arthrodesis
Thompson-Epstein classification
    of hip dislocations
Thompson-Henry approach
Thompson-Walker scissors
Thoms cervical collar brace
Thoms forceps
Thoms method
Thoms pelvimeter
Thoms tenaculum
Thoms tissue-grasping forceps
Thoms-Allis forceps
Thoms-Allis tissue forceps
Thoms-Gaylor biopsy forceps
Thoms-Gaylor biopsy punch
Thoms-Gaylor forceps
Thoms-Gaylor uterine forceps
thoracectomy
thoracentesis
thoracic
thoracic aneurysm
thoracic aorta

thoracic aortography
thoracic arch aortogram
thoracic artery
thoracic artery forceps
thoracic cage
thoracic cardiac nerve
thoracic cavity
thoracic clamp
thoracic drain
thoracic drainage tube
thoracic duct
thoracic duct drainage (TDD)
thoracic empyema
thoracic esophagus
thoracic fascia
thoracic forceps
thoracic ganglia
thoracic hemostatic forceps
thoracic inferior vena cava
thoracic inlet
thoracic laminectomy
thoracic nerve
thoracic nerve block
thoracic outlet compression
thoracic outlet syndrome
thoracic region
thoracic roentgenogram
thoracic scissors
thoracic spinal cord
thoracic spine
thoracic surgery
thoracic sutures
thoracic sympathectomy
thoracic tissue forceps
thoracic vein
thoracic vertebrae
thoracic viscera
thoracic wall
thoracica interna, arteria
thoracica lateralis, arteria
thoracica lateralis, vena
thoracica suprema, arteria
thoracicae internae, venae
thoracici, nervi
thoracicoabdominal incision
thoracicoabdominal splenec-
    tomy

thoracicolumbar division
thoracicus longus, nervus
thoracoabdominal incision
thoracoacromial artery
thoracoacromial vein
thoracoacromialis, arteria
thoracoacromialis, vena
thoracobronchotomy
thoracocentesis
thoracodorsal
thoracodorsal artery
thoracodorsal nerve
thoracodorsalis, arteria
thoracodorsalis, nervus
thoracoepigastric veins
thoracoepigastricae, venae
thoracolaparotomy
thoracolumbar division
thoracolumbar fascia
thoracolumbar nerve block
thoracolumbar standing orthosis
    brace (TLSO brace)
thoracolysis
thoracoplasty
thoracoscope
        Coryllos thoracoscope
        Jacobaeus thoracoscope
        Jacobaeus-Unverricht
            thoracoscope
        Moore thoracoscope
        Sarot thoracoscope
        Storz biopsy thoraco-
            scope
thoracoscopy
Thoracoseal drainage
thoracostomy
thoracostomy tube
thoracotome
        Bettman-Forash thoraco-
            tome
thoracotomy
thoracotomy incision
thoracotomy tray
thoracotomy tube
thoracotomy wound
Thora-Drain chest drainage
    unit

Thora-Klex chest drainage
    system
Thora-Klex chest tube
Thoratec biventricular assist
    device
Thoratec pump
Thoratec right ventricular assist
    device
Thoratec ventricular assist
    device
thorax
Thorek aspirator
Thorek gallbladder aspirator
Thorek gallbladder forceps
Thorek gallbladder scissors
Thorek operation
Thorek scissors
Thorek-Feldman gallbladder
    scissors
Thorek-Feldman scissors
Thorek-Mixter forceps
Thorek-Mixter gall duct
    forceps
Thorek-Mixter gallbladder
    forceps
Thorel bundle
Thornell microlaryngoscopy
Thornell operation
Thornton nail
Thornton plate
Thornton screw
Thornton side plate
Thornwald antral drill
Thornwald antral trephine
Thornwald drill
Thornwald irrigator
Thornwald perforator
Thornwald trephine
Thorpe calipers
Thorpe corneal forceps
Thorpe curet
Thorpe fixation forceps
Thorpe forceps
Thorpe foreign body knife
Thorpe plastic lens
Thorpe pupillary membrane
    scissors

Thorpe scissors
Thorpe slit lamp
Thorpe-Castroviejo cataract
    scissors
Thorpe-Castroviejo scissors
Thorpe-Westcott scissors
Thow gastrostomy tube
Thow tube
THR (total hip replacement)
thread
thread sutures
threaded pin
threaded portion of nail
threaded titanium acetabular
    prosthesis (TTAP)
thready pulse
threat reflex
threatened abortion
threatened labor
threatened miscarriage
threatened premature delivery
threatened transplant rejection
threatening
three major leads
three-armed basket forceps
three-bladed clamp
three-bottle drainage
three-bottle drainage system
three-bottle system
three-bottle tidal suction tube
three-chambered heart
three-clamp technique
three-dimensional image
three-dimensional interlocking
    hip (TDI hip)
three-finger spica cast
three-flanged nail
three-flanged spike
three-legged cage heart valve
three-loop ileal pouch
three-mirror contact lens
three-pillow orthopnea
three-pronged forceps
three-pronged grasping forceps
three-pronged retractor
three-snip punctum operation
three-step tenotomy

three-vein graft
three-vessel umbilical cord
three-way bridge
three-way catheter
three-way Foley catheter
three-way irrigating catheter
three-way stopcock
threshold
thrill
throat
throat forceps
throat irrigation tube
throat mucosa
throat scissors
throat smear
throat swab
throat washings
throbbing
throbbing aorta
throbbing pain
Throckmorton reflex
thrombectomy
thrombectomy catheter
thrombi (*sing.* thrombus)
thrombin
thrombin clotting time
thrombin time
thromboembolic disease (TED)
thromboembolic disease hose
thromboembolic disease socks
thromboembolic disease
    stockings
thromboembolism
thromboendarterectomy (TEA)
thrombolysis
thrombolytic therapy
thrombopenia
thromboplastin
thrombosed hemorrhoid
thrombosed veins
thrombosis (*pl.* thromboses)
Thrombostat
thrombotic
thrombotic occlusion
thrombus (*pl.* thrombi)
thrombus formation
thrombus stripper

through drainage
through-and-through avulsion injury
through-and-through continuous sutures
through-and-through sutures
through-cutting forceps tip
through-the-scope dilator (TTS dilator)
thrower's elbow
Thruflex PTCA balloon catheter
thrust
Thrust femoral prosthesis
thumb abduction
thumb cushion
thumb finger
thumb forceps
thumb fracture
thumb pad
thumb sign
thumb spica cast
thumb splint
thumb tissue forceps
thumb-dressing forceps
thumb-in-palm deformity
Thunberg restrictor
Thunberg tube
Thurmond retractor
Thurston-Holland fragment forceps
thymectomize
thymectomy
thymic aplasia
thymic cyst
thymic nodule
thymic tumor
thymic vein
thymicae, venae
thymopexy
thymus
thymus gland
thymus retractor
thymusectomy
thyroarytenoid muscle
thyroarytenoideus, musculus
thyrocervical
thyrocervical trunk

thyrochondrotomy
thyrocricoidectomy
thyrocricotomy
thyroepiglottic ligament
thyroepiglottic muscle
thyroepiglotticus, musculus
thyroglossal
thyroglossal cyst
thyroglossal duct
thyroglossal duct cystectomy
thyroglossal sinus
thyrohyal
thyrohyoid
thyrohyoid laryngotomy
thyrohyoid ligament
thyrohyoid membrane
thyrohyoid muscle
thyrohyoideus, musculus
thyroid
thyroid abscess
thyroid artery
thyroid bruit
thyroid cancer
thyroid capsule
thyroid cartilage
thyroid collar
thyroid drain
thyroid forceps
thyroid gland
thyroid imaging
thyroid isthmectomy
thyroid isthmus
thyroid lobe
thyroid loop
thyroid notch
thyroid region
thyroid retractor
thyroid scan
thyroid sheet
thyroid tissue
thyroid traction forceps
thyroid tray
thyroid tumor
thyroid uptake
thyroid vein
thyroidal
thyroidea

thyroidea accessoria
thyroidea ima, arteria
thyroidea ima, vena
thyroidea inferior, arteria
thyroidea inferior, vena
thyroidea superior, arteria
thyroidea superior, vena
thyroideae mediae, venae
thyroidectomize
thyroidectomy
thyroidorrhaphy
thyroidotomy
thyrolaryngeal fascia
thyrolingual trunk
thyromegaly
thyroparathyroidectomy
thyropharyngeal muscle
thyrotome
thyrotomy
thyrotoxic goiter
thyrotoxicosis
thyroxine
Ti (titanium)
TI measurement (transischial
    measurement)
Ti-28 total hip replacement
TIA (transient ischemic attack)
Ti-BAC acetabular component
tibia
tibia valga
tibia vara
tibial
tibial artery
tibial calipers
tibial collateral ligament
tibial compartment
tibial condyle
tibial crest
tibial driver
tibial fixation plate
tibial fracture
tibial impactor
tibial insertion
tibial lymph node
tibial muscle
tibial nerve
tibial peg holes

tibial perforator
tibial pin
tibial plafond
tibial plateau
tibial plateau fracture
tibial plateau prosthesis
tibial prosthesis
tibial pulse
tibial relocation plate
tibial resection guide
tibial resection jig
tibial retractor
tibial shaft
tibial sign
tibial spine
tibial stress reaction
tibial torsion
tibial tray
tibial tubercle
tibial tuberosity
tibial vein
tibiales anteriores, venae
tibiales posteriores, venae
tibialis anterior, arteria
tibialis anterior, musculus
tibialis, musculus
tibialis, nervus
tibialis posterior, arteria
tibialis posterior, musculus
tibialis sign
tibioadductor reflex
tibiocollateral ligament
tibiofemoral fossa
tibiofemoral prosthesis
tibiofibular articulation
tibiofibular joint
tibiofibular ligament
tibiofibular mortise
tibiofibular syndesmosis
tibioperoneal trunk
tibiotalar joint
tibiotarsal articulation
Tickner forceps
Ticonium splint
Ti/CoCr hip prosthesis
Ti-Cron sutures (also Tycron)
tics and fasciculations

tidal air
tidal drainage
tidal thoracic drainage system
tidal volume
tidal wave
tie sutures
Tieck nasal speculum
Tieck speculum
Tieck-Halle speculum
tied down over cotton sutures
tied over rubber shoes
Tiedemann nerve
Tiemann bullet forceps
Tiemann catheter
Tiemann coudé catheter
Tiemann Foley catheter
Tiemann nail
Tiemann stethoscope
tie-over dressing
ties (see *sutures*)
ties-over-stent
tiger gut sutures
tight adhesions
tight fingertip dilated cervix
 . (TFT cervix)
tight seal
tightened
tightener (see also *wire
    tightener*)
    Kirschner wire tightener
tightly
tightness
Tikhoff-Lindberg operation
Tikhoff-Lindberg shoulder
    girdle resection
Tiko rake retractor
Tilastan femoral components
Tilderquist eye needle holder
Tilderquist needle holder
Tile-Pennal classification of
    pelvic ring fractures
Tillary double-ended retractor
Tillary retractor
Tillaux fracture of ankle
Tillett operation
Tilley dressing forceps
Tillman resurfacing technique

tilt table
tilting-disk aortic valve prosthe-
    sis
tilting-disk heart valve
tilting-disk valve
Timberlake electrode
Timberlake evacuator
Timberlake obturator
Timberlake resectoscope
Timbrall-Fisher incision
timed contractions
tin-bullet probe
tincture of benzoin
tincture of time
tincture of Zephiran
tined
tined lead
tined lead pacemaker
Tinel sign
Tinel sutures
tinge
tingling
tingling of fingertips
tingling sensation
tinkling bowel sounds
tip (see also *suction tip*)
    ACMI cystoscopic tip
    Adson brain suction tip
    Andrews suction tip
    aortographic suction tip
    Artus cutting tip
    aspirating tip
    B-D irrigating tip
    Bard cystoscope tip
    Bard tip
    Bishop-Harmon tip
    Blasucci tip
    Blue rectal suction tip
    Bovie coagulation tip
    brain suction tip
    Brawley nasal suction tip
    Brawley suction tip
    Buie rectal suction tip
    catheter tip
    Clerf aspirating tip
    Cordes punch forceps tip
    coronary perfusion tip

tip *continued*

- cystoscope tip
- diamond-dusted tip
- disposable ear tip
- disposable otoscopic ear tips
- double-articulated laryngeal forceps tip
- electrosurgical resec- toscope tip
- epsilon tip
- exploratory suction tip
- eye irrigating tip
- Fell sucker tip
- fingertip
- Flex-i-Tip
- forceps tip
- Frazier nasal suction tip
- Frazier suction tip
- Girard irrigating tip
- glass nasal suction tip
- glass nasal tip
- glass suction tip
- Grieshaber vitrectomy tip
- Hanafee catheter tip
- Henke forceps tip
- Henke punch forceps tip
- Hildreth tip
- House oiler tip
- House-Urban oiler tip
- House-Urban tip
- interchangeable forceps tips
- interchangeable laryn- geal forceps tips
- irrigating tip
- irrigating-aspirating tip
- Jackson square punch tip
- Kelman irrigation- aspiration tip
- Kidde Flex-i-Tip
- Killian cutting forceps tip
- Killian double-articulated forceps tip
- Killian forceps tip
- KleenSpec otoscope tip

tip *continued*

- Kleinert fingertip
- Krause forceps tip
- Krause punch forceps tip
- Krause through-cutting forceps tip
- Kutler fingertip
- laryngeal forceps tip
- laser tip
- leaflet tip
- nasal-cutting tip
- olive tip
- punch tip
- Q-tip
- Ritter double-orifice tip
- Ritter single-orifice tip
- rotary cutting tip
- rubber tip
- Scheinmann biting tip
- Seiffert tip
- serrated grasping tip
- Sims suction tip
- Sondermann suction tip
- Spencer oval tip
- Storz cystoscope tip
- suction tip (see separate listing)
- T&A suction tip
- Teflon tip
- through-cutting forceps tip
- tonsil-suction tip
- ultrasonic tip
- Universal Kerrison set and tips
- valve tip
- vitrectomy tip
- vitrector tip
- Wagener punch tip
- Watson-Williams punch tip
- whistle-tip
- Yankauer antral-punch tip
- Yankauer multi-orifice tip

Tisseel fibrin sealant

tip *continued*
　　　Yankauer single-orifice
　　　　tip
　　　Yankauer suction tip
tire eye implant
tire implant
tiredness
tire-grooved silicone
tire-iron maneuver
Tischler cervical biopsy forceps
Tischler cervical biopsy punch
Tischler cervical forceps
Tischler forceps
Tischler punch
tissue
tissue ablation
tissue attenuation
tissue band
tissue bank
tissue bed
tissue biopsy
tissue burn
tissue culture
tissue damage
tissue desiccation needle
tissue drain
tissue dressing forceps
tissue expander
tissue fluid
tissue forceps
tissue forceps with teeth
tissue forceps without teeth
tissue gouge
tissue graft
tissue homogeneity
tissue mass
tissue occlusion clamp
tissue perfusion
tissue process
tissue regeneration
tissue rejection
tissue repair
tissue retractor
tissue samples
tissue spaces
tissue transplant
tissue turgor

tissue typing
tissue wedge
tissue welding by laser
tissue-grasping forceps
tissue-holding forceps
Titan femoral component
Titan hip cup
Titan hip system
Titan total hip system
titanium (Ti)
titanium ball heart valve
titanium ball prosthesis
titanium cage heart valve
titanium mesh screw
titanium needle
titanium optimized design plate
　　　(TOD plate)
titanium prosthesis
titanium proximal-loading, 6-in.
　　　stem total hip system (TPL-
　　　6 total hip system)
titanium ring
titanium screw
titanium staple
Titus decompressor
Titus forearm splint
Titus needle
Titus tongue depressor
Titus wrist splint
Tivanium
Tivanium hip prosthesis
Tivnen forceps
Tivnen tonsil-seizing forceps
TJF endoscope
TKR (total knee replacement)
TLC Baxter balloon catheter
TLS drain
TLS suction drain
TLSO brace (thoracolumbar
　　　standing orthosis brace)
TMA (transmetatarsal amputa-
　　　tion)
TMP (transmembrane pressure)
TNB (Tru-Cut needle biopsy)
TNM (tumor, nodes, metastases)
TNM classification of malignant
　　　tumors

TNS (transcutaneous nerve
    stimulator)
to-and-fro anesthesia
to-and-fro friction sounds
to-and-fro murmur
Tobey forceps
Tobey rongeur
Tobey-Ayer maneuver
Tobold forceps
Tobold knife
Tobold laryngeal forceps
Tobold-Fauvel forceps
Tobold-Fauvel grasping forceps
Tobolsky elevator
tocolysis
tocolytic agent
TOD plate (titanium optimized
    design plate)
Todd bodies
Todd button
Todd cautery
Todd gouge
Todd needle
Todd-Heyer cannula guide
Todd-Wells guide
Todd-Wells stereotaxic appara-
    tus
Todd-Wells stereotaxic guide
Todd-Wells stereotaxic unit
toe bones
toe flexed
toe prosthesis
toe sign
toe spica cast
toe spread sign for Morton
    neuroma
toe spreader
toe tag
toedrop brace
toeing in
toeing out
toenail
Toennis anastomosis scissors
Toennis dissecting scissors
Toennis needle holder
Toennis scissors
Toennis tumor-grasping forceps

Toennis-Adson forceps
Toennis-Adson scissors
Toennis-Adson utility scissors
toe-to-thumb prosthesis
toggle
toggled
toggling
Tohen transfer
toilet
toilette
Toldt ligament
Toldt line
Tolentino cutter
Tolentino lens
Tolentino ring
Tolentino vitreous cutter
tolerable
tolerance
toluidine blue
Tom Jones closure
Tom Jones hysterectomy
    closure
Tom Jones sutures
Toma sign
Tomac catheter
Tomac clip
Tomac foam rubber traction
    dressing
Tomac forceps
Tomac goniometer
Tomac knitted rubber elastic
    dressing
Tomac sphygmomanometer
Tomac vest-style holder
Tomas iris hook
Tomas suture hook
Tomasini brace
Tomasini split
Tomkins anesthesia unit
Tommy hip bar
tomogram
tomograph
tomographic cut
tomographic examination
tomographic images
tomographic study
tomography

Tompkins operation
tone
tone and elasticity
tone burst
tone contraction
tone decay
tong splint
tongs (see also *traction tongs*)
    Ace Universal tongs
    Barton tongs
    Barton-Cone tongs
    biopsy tongs
    Böhler tongs
    cervical traction tongs
    Cherry tongs
    Cherry traction tongs
    Cohen-Eder tongs
    Crutchfield skull tongs
    Crutchfield tongs
    Crutchfield traction
      tongs
    Crutchfield-Raney tongs
    Crutchfield-Raney
      traction tongs
    Eder tongs
    Gardner tongs
    Gardner-Wells skull
      tongs
    Gardner-Wells tongs
    Gardner-Wells traction
      tongs
    Heifitz tongs
    Heifitz traction tongs
    Raney-Crutchfield skull
      traction tongs
    Raney-Crutchfield tongs
    Reynolds tongs
    skull tongs
    Trippi-Wells tongs
    Vinke tongs
    Wells-Gardner tongs
tongue
tongue blade
tongue depressor (see also
    *depressor*)
    Andrews tongue
      depressor

tongue depressor *continued*
    Andrews-Pynchon
      tongue depressor
    Blakesley tongue
      depressor
    Dorsey tongue depressor
    Dunn tongue depressor
    Farlow tongue depressor
    Hamilton tongue
      depressor
    Lewis tongue depressor
    oral screw tongue
      depressor
    Proetz tongue depressor
    Pynchon tongue
      depressor
    Pynchon-Lillie tongue
      depressor
    Titus tongue depressor
    Weder tongue depressor
tongue forceps
tongue plate electrode
tongue retractor blade
tongue sutures
tongue traction
tongue-in-groove advancement
tongue-in-groove sutures
tongue-seizing forceps
tongue-shaped villi
tongue-tie operation
tonic
tonic contraction
tonicity
Tonnis clip
Tonnis dura hook
Tonnis dura knife
Tonnis-Adson neurodissector
tonoclonic spasm
tonography
tonometer
    calibration tonometer
    Daniels tonometer
    Digilab pneumatonome-
      ter
    Draeger tonometer
    electronic tonometer
    Gärtner tonometer

tonometer *continued*
- Goldmann applanation tonometer
- Goldmann tonometer
- Gradle tonometer
- Harrington tonometer
- hemostatic tonometer
- impression tonometer
- LaForce tonometer
- Mack tonometer
- MacKay-Marg tonometer
- McLean tonometer
- Meding tonsil enucleator tonometer
- Mueller electronic tonometer
- Mueller tonometer
- Musken tonometer
- Non-Contact tonometer
- Pach-Pen tonometer
- Perkins tonometer
- pneumatic tonometer
- pneumatonometer
- Recklinghausen tonometer
- Reichert tonometer
- Sauer tonometer
- Sauer-Storz tonometer
- Schiøtz tonometer
- Sklar tonometer
- Sklar-Schiøtz jewel tonometer
- Sklar-Schiøtz tonometer
- Sluder tonometer
- Sluder-Demarest tonometer
- Sluder-Sauer tonometer
- Storz-Moltz tonometer

tonometry
tonsil
tonsil dissector
tonsil position
tonsil sponge
tonsil suction dissector
tonsil suction tip
tonsil suction tube

tonsil-dissecting scissors
tonsil-holding forceps
tonsillar abscess
tonsillar abscess forceps
tonsillar artery forceps
tonsillar calculus
tonsillar calipers
tonsillar clamp
tonsillar compressor
tonsillar crypts
tonsillar electrode
tonsillar elevator
tonsillar enucleator
tonsillar expressor
tonsillar exudate
tonsillar forceps
tonsillar fossa
tonsillar guillotine
tonsillar hemostat
tonsillar hemostatic forceps
tonsillar hernia
tonsillar hook
tonsillar knife
tonsillar needle
tonsillar needle holder
tonsillar needle holder forceps
tonsillar nerves
tonsillar pillar
tonsillar pillar retractor
tonsillar punch
tonsillar retractor
tonsillar scissors
tonsillar screw
tonsillar screw tenaculum
tonsillar separator
tonsillar slitter
tonsillar snare
tonsillar snare wire
tonsillar sponges
tonsillar spreader
tonsillar suture hook
tonsillar suture needle
tonsillar sutures
tonsillar syringe
tonsillar syringe extension
tonsillar tag

tonsillar tampon
tonsillar tenaculum
tonsillar tissue
tonsillectome
    Daniels hemostatic
        tonsillectome
    Daniels tonsillectome
    hemostatic tonsillectome
    LaForce hemostatic
        tonsillectome
    LaForce tonsillectome
    lingual tonsillectome
    Mack tonsillectome
    Meding tonsil enucleator
        tonsillectome
    Molt-Storz tonsillectome
    Myles tonsillectome
    Sauer tonsillectome
    Sauer-Sluder tonsillec-
        tome
    Searcy tonsillectome
    Sluder tonsillectome
    Sluder-Ballenger
        tonsillectome
    Sluder-Sauer tonsillec-
        tome
    Tydings tonsillectome
    Van Osdel tonsillar
        enucleator tonsillec-
        tome
    Van Osdel tonsillectome
tonsillectomy
tonsillectomy and adenoidec-
    tomy (T&A)
tonsil-ligating forceps
tonsilloadenoidectomy
tonsilloscope
tonsillotome
tonsillotomy
tonsils
tonsil-seizing forceps
tonsil-suturing forceps
tonsil-suturing instrument
tonus fracture
Tooke blade
Tooke corneal forceps
Tooke knife

Tooke spatula
Toomey adaptor
Toomey bladder evacuator
Toomey evacuator
Toomey forceps
Toomey suction tube
Toomey syringe
tooth band
tooth elevator
tooth extraction
tooth socket
toothed forceps
toothed retractor
toothed tenaculum
toothed thumb forceps
toothed tissue forceps
tooth-extracting forceps
tooth-like calcification
Topcon camera
Topcon refractor
tophaceous
tophus (*pl.* tophi)
topical
topical anesthetic spray
topical application
topical cocaine anesthetic agent
topical therapy
toposcopic catheter
Topper cannula
Topper dressing sponges
Topper sponge
top-valve airway obstruction
Torcon angiographic catheter
Torcon catheter
torcular tourniquet
Torek esophagectomy
Torek operation
Torek orchiopexy
Torek resection of thoracic
    esophagus
Torek-Bevan operation
toric lens
Torkildsen operation
Torkildsen shunt
Torkildsen shunt procedure
Torkildsen shunt ventriculo-
    cisternostomy

Torkildsen tube
Torkildsen ventriculocisternos-
    tomy
torn cartilage
torn knee cartilage
torn lateral meniscus
torn ligament
torn medial meniscus
torn muscle
Tornwaldt cyst
Toronto orthosis
Toronto splint
TORP (total ossicular recon-
    structive/replacement
    prosthesis)
TORP strut
Torpin operation
torque guide
torque heel
torque-type prosthesis
torr units of pressure
Torrence steel hook
torsion
torsion bar splint
torsion forceps
torsion fracture
torsional rigidity
torso crease
torso presentation
torticollis
tortuosity
tortuosity of glands
tortuosity of vessel
tortuous
tortuous aorta
tortuous esophagus
tortuous root canal
tortuous varicosities
tortuous vessels
torus
torus crush
Toshiba video endoscope
total abdominal colectomy
    (TAC)
total abdominal hysterectomy
    (TAH)
total anesthesia

total articular replacement
    arthroplasty (TARA)
total artificial heart
total biopsy
total bladder resection
total blood loss
total blood volume
total body
total breech delivery
total breech extraction
total capsulectomy
total cardiopulmonary bypass
total cataract
total cataract extraction
total condylar knee prosthesis
total enteral nutrition (TEN)
total gastrectomy
total gastric wrap
total graft area rejected (TGAR)
total hip arthroplasty
total hip prosthesis
total hip replacement (THR)
total hysterectomy
total joint replacement
total keratoplasty
total knee prosthesis
total knee replacement (TKR)
total laryngectomy
total laryngectomy with radical
    neck dissection
total mastectomy
total meniscectomy
total obstruction
total ossicular reconstruction/
    replacement prosthesis
    (TORP)
total pancreatectomy
total parenteral alimentation
total parenteral nutrition (TPN)
total pelvic exenteration
total penile reconstruction
total placenta previa
total pneumonectomy
total spinal anesthesia
Totco Autoclip
Totco clip
Toti operation

_Toupet proc.(?caps) fundoplication (as per Dr. Dietz_

Toti-Mosher operation
toughness
tourniquet
    Adams tourniquet
    automatic rotating
      tourniquet
    automatic tourniquet
    Bethune lobectomy
      tourniquet
    Bethune lung tourniquet
    Bethune tourniquet
    Campbell-Boyd tourni-
      quet
    cardiovascular tourniquet
    Carr lobectomy tourni-
      quet
    Carr tourniquet
    caval tourniquet
    Conn tourniquet
    Davol tourniquet
    deflated tourniquet
    Dupuytren tourniquet
    Esmarch tourniquet
    flexible tourniquet
    garrote tourniquet
    Gaylord pneumatic
      tourniquet
    horseshoe tourniquet
    Ideal automatic tourni-
      quet
    inflated tourniquet
    Kidde tourniquet
    Kidde-Robbins tourni-
      quet
    Linton tourniquet
    lobectomy tourniquet
    lung tourniquet
    Medi-quet surgical
      tourniquet
    Momberg tourniquet
    Penrose tourniquet
    pneumatic tourniquet
    Roberts-Nelson tourni-
      quet
    Roper-Rumel tourniquet
    rotating tourniquet
    Rumel cardiac tourniquet

tourniquet _continued_
    Rumel cardiovascular
      tourniquet
    Rumel myocardial
      tourniquet
    Rumel tourniquet
    Rumel-Belmont tourni-
      quet
    Rumpuffet vessel
      tourniquet
    Samway tourniquet
    Satinsky tourniquet
    scalp tourniquet
    Shenstone tourniquet
    Spanish tourniquet
    TCPM pneumatic
      tourniquet
    torcular tourniquet
    Trussdale tourniquet
    Universal tourniquet
    Velcro tourniquet
    Velket-Velcro tourniquet
    Weiner tourniquet
tourniquet control
tourniquet cuff
tourniquet inflation unit
tourniquet tightened
toward
towel clamp
towel clip
towel clip forceps
towel forceps
Tower forceps
Tower fracture table
Tower muscle forceps
Tower prong
Tower retractor
Tower rib retractor
Tower spinal retractor
Tower table
Towne position
Towne projection
Towne projection roent-
    genogram
Towne view of skull on
    x-ray
Towne x-ray view

Townley anatomic instruments
Townley anatomic knee
    replacement
Townley calipers
Townley femur calipers
Townley forceps
Townley implant
Townley inside-outside femur
    calipers
Townley knee prosthesis
Townley prosthesis
Townley screw
Townley TARA prosthesis
Townley tissue forceps
Townley-Paton operation
toxemia curet
toxic
toxic goiter
toxic megacolon
toxicity
Toynbee ear speculum
Toynbee maneuver
Toynbee speculum
TPL-6 total hip system (titanium
    proximal-loading, 6-in.
    stem total hip system)
TPN (total parenteral nutrition)
TPN catheter
TPN line
TR-28 hip prosthesis
trabecula (pl. trabeculae)
trabecular
trabecular bone
trabecular degeneration
trabecular meshwork
trabecular region
trabecular vein
trabeculated
trabeculation
trabeculectomy
trabeculodialysis
trabeculoplasty
trabeculotome
        Sierra-Sheldon trabeculo-
            tome
trabeculotomy
trace

Trace stripper
Trace vein stripper
tracer
tracer study
trachea
tracheal adenoma
tracheal biopsy
tracheal bistoury
tracheal bougie
tracheal bronchial knife
tracheal bronchus
tracheal calcification
tracheal cannula
tracheal cartilage
tracheal catheter
tracheal catheterization
tracheal compression
tracheal deviation
tracheal dilator
tracheal fistula
tracheal forceps
tracheal fracture
tracheal hemostat
tracheal hemostatic forceps
tracheal hook
tracheal incision
tracheal intubation
tracheal knife
tracheal lavage
tracheal mucosa
tracheal muscle
tracheal obstruction
tracheal papilloma
tracheal reflex
tracheal retractor
tracheal rings
tracheal scissors
tracheal secretions
tracheal stenosis
tracheal stump
tracheal suction tube
tracheal tampon
tracheal tenaculum
tracheal tree
tracheal tube
tracheal tube brush
tracheal tube cuff

tracheal tube with obturator
tracheal tug
tracheal ulceration
tracheal vein
tracheal wall
tracheales, venae
trachealis, musculus
trachelectomy
trachelomastoid muscle
trachelopexy
tracheloplasty
trachelorrhaphy
trachelotome
trachelotomy
tracheobronchial
tracheobronchial suction
    tube
tracheobronchial tree
tracheocele
tracheocricotomy
tracheoesophageal (TE)
tracheoesophageal fistula
tracheoesophageal fistula
    closure
tracheoesophageal junction
tracheofissure
tracheogram
tracheography
tracheolaryngotomy
tracheoplasty
tracheopulmonary secretions
tracheorrhaphy
tracheoscope
    Haslinger tracheo-
        scope
    Jackson tracheoscope
tracheoscopy
tracheostomy
tracheostomy button
tracheostomy cannula
tracheostomy care
tracheostomy hook
tracheostomy scissors
tracheostomy stoma
tracheostomy tray
tracheostomy trocar
tracheostomy tube

tracheotome
    Salvatore-Maloney
        tracheotome
    Sierra-Sheldon tracheo-
        tome
tracheotomic bistoury
tracheotomize
tracheotomy
tracheotomy cannula
tracheotomy hook
tracheotomy set
tracheotomy site
tracheotomy tube
Trach-Mist
trachoma
trachoma forceps
tracing
track
track sutures
track valve
Tracker knee brace
tract
traction
traction bar
traction diverticulum
traction forceps
traction halter collar
traction handle (see also
    *handle*)
    Barton traction handle
    Bill axis traction handle
    Bill traction handle
    Castroviejo-Kalt traction
        handle
    Luikart-Bill traction
        handle
    obstetrical traction
        handle
traction spur from disk degen-
    eration
traction sutures
traction tongs (see also *tongs*)
    cervical traction tongs
    Cherry traction tongs
    Crutchfield traction tongs
    Crutchfield-Raney
        traction tongs

traction tongs *continued*
Gardner-Wells traction tongs
Heifitz traction tongs
Raney-Crutchfield skull traction tongs
Tracto-Halter
tractor
Anderson tractor
axial tractor
banjo tractor
Blackburn tractor
Böhler tractor
Buck tractor
circumtractor
Conco tractor
curved tractor
extension tractor
Freiberg tractor
halo pelvic tractor
Lowsley prostatic tractor
Lowsley tractor
Naugh os calcis apparatus tractor
Neufeld tractor
Perkins tractor
prostatic tractor
Pugh tractor
Rankin tractor
Russell tractor
Russell-Buck extension tractor
Russell-Buck tractor
skull tractor
Steinmann tractor
Syms tractor
Vinke skull tractor
Vinke tractor
Watson-Jones tractor
Wells tractor
Young prostatic tractor
Young tractor
Zimcode traction frames tractor
Zim-Trac traction splint tractor
tractotomy

traditional
tragicus, musculus
tragus
tragus muscle
trailer gauze
training
Trainor operation
Trainor-Nida operation
trajector
TRAM procedure (transverse rectus abdominis myocutaneous procedure)
transabdominal
transabdominal cholangiography
transabdominal colonoscopy
transabdominal repair
transacromial incision
transanal puncture
transannular patch
transaxial tomography
transaxillary incision
transbasal
transbrachial arch aortogram
transcarpal
transcatheter
transcatheter closure of atrial septal defect
transcellular fluid
transcervical fracture
transcolonic endoscopy
transcondylar fracture
transcorneal transillumination
transcortical
transcranial Doppler
transcranial projection
transcutaneous electrical nerve stimulation (TENS)
transcutaneous electrical nerve stimulator (TENS)
transcutaneous nerve stimulator (TCNS, TNS)
transcutaneous pacemaker
transcutaneous stimulator
transcystoscopically
transdiaphragmatic sympathectomy

transducer
transducer-tipped catheter
transduction
transduodenal
transduodenal choledo-
    cholithotomy
transduodenal endoscopic
    decompression
transduodenal excision of
    common duct stone
transduodenal fiberscopic duct
    injection
transduodenal sphincterotomy
transdural approach
transect
transected
transection
transection incision
transection of artery
transection of nerve roots
transection of nerve tracts
transection of tube
transection of vein
Transelast surgical drape
transendoscopic electrocoagula-
    tion
transesophageal echocardiogra-
    phy
transesophageal ligation of
    varices
transesophageal probe
transethmoidal hypophysec-
    tomy
transethmoidal sphenoidotomy
transfer
transfer forceps
transfer of tendon
transference
transference of muscle
transferred
transfibular arthrodesis
transfixing sutures
transfixion
transfixion bolt
transfixion screw
transfixion sutures
transformation

transformer
transfused
transfusion
transgastric ligation
transgastric plication
transhepatic biliary stent
transhepatic cholangiogram
    (THC)
transhepatic cholangiography
transhepatic embolization
transhepatic portography
transient anesthesia
transilluminating telescope
transillumination
transilluminator (see also
    *illuminator*)
        all-purpose transillumina-
        tor
        Briggs transilluminator
        Coldlite transilluminator
        Finnoff transilluminator
        hooded transilluminator
        Lancaster transilluminator
        National transilluminator
        rotating transilluminator
        Shunn gun transillumina-
        tor
        speculum transillumina-
        tor
        Tatum ureteral transillu-
        minator
        Welch Allyn transillumi-
        nator
        Whitelite transilluminator
        Widner transilluminator
transischial measurement (TI
    measurement)
transit time
transition
transition sutures
transitional
transitional cell carcinoma
transitional development
transitional lumbosacral joint
transitional lumbosacral
    vertebra
transitional tumor

transitional vertebra
transjugular liver biopsy
translateral films
translatory movement
translumbar aortogram
transluminal angioplasty
transluminal balloon
transluminal balloon
    angioplasty
transluminal coronary
    angioplasty
transluminal coronary
    angioplasty guide wire
transluminal coronary artery
    angioplasty
transluminal extraction catheter
    (TEC)
transmeatal atticotomy
transmeatal incision
transmeatal labyrinthotomy
transmembrane pressure (TMP)
transmesenteric hernia
transmesenteric plication
transmetatarsal
transmetatarsal amputation
    (TMA)
transmission
transmitted
transmitter
transmural
transmural resection
transnasal bile duct catheteriza-
    tion
transnasal drain
transnasal sphenoidotomy
transoral projection
transorbital leukotomy
transorbital lobotomy
transosseous
transosseous holes
transpalatal
transpapillary biopsy
transpapillary drain
transparent drape
transparent dressing
transpedicular segmental
    fixation

transpericardial pacemaker
transperitoneal cesarean section
transperitoneal nephrectomy
transperitoneal technique
transplacental hemorrhage
transplant
transplant spatula
transplantation
transplantation metastasis
transplantation of cornea
transplantation of kidney
transplantation of muscle
transplantation of ocular muscle
transplantation of tendon
transplantation surgery
transplantation tissue
transplanted organ
transplant-grafting forceps
transpleural
transpleural approach
Transpore surgical tape
Transpore surgical tape dressing
transport
transport tube
transporter
transposition
transposition of colon
transposition of great arteries
    (TGA)
transposition of great vessels
    (TGV)
transposition of pulmonary
    veins
transposition of tendon
transposition operation
transpubic
transpyloric tube
transrectal perineal needle
    biopsy
transrectal transsphincteric
    approach
transrectal ultrasonography
    (TRUS)
transrectus incision
transsacral
transsacral anesthesia
transsacral block

transscrotal
transscrotal orchiopexy
transseptal
transseptal cannula
transseptal catheter
transseptal sheath
transseptal stylet
transsphenoidal
transsphenoidal forceps
transsphenoidal hypophysec-
    tomy
transsphenoidal resection
transsternal thyroidectomy
transsyndesmotic screw
transtentorial herniation
transthoracic approach
transthoracic biopsy
transthoracic catheter
transthoracic diameter
transthoracic hepatotomy
transthoracic pacemaker
transthoracic ultrasound
transthoracotomy
transtracheal anesthesia
transtrochanteric osteotomy
transudate
transudation of fluid
transudative ascites
transureteroureteral anasto-
    mosis
transureteroureterostomy
transurethral biopsy
transurethral perineal biopsy
transurethral prostatectomy
transurethral resection (TUR)
transurethral resection of
    bladder tumor (TURBT)
transurethral resection of
    prostate (TURP)
transvaginal cone
transvaginal puncture
transvenous
transvenous approach
transvenous catheter pacemaker
transvenous digital subtraction
    angiogram
transvenous electrodes

transvenous implantation of
    pacemaker leads
transvenous pacemaker
transvenous pacemaker catheter
transvenous pacer
transvenous packing
transvenous ventricular demand
    pacemaker
transventricular closed valvot-
    omy
transventricular dilator
transventricular valvotomy
transversa colli, arteria
transversa faciei, arteria
transversa faciei, vena
transversae colli, venae
transversal tomography
transversalis, fascia
transverse
transverse abdominal incision
transverse acetabular ligament
transverse amputation
transverse appendectomy
    incision
transverse arch
transverse arteriotomy
transverse artery of face
transverse artery of neck
transverse artery of scapula
transverse arytenoid muscle
transverse axis
transverse bipolar montage
transverse carpal ligament
transverse cervical artery
transverse cervical nerve
transverse cervical veins
transverse cesarean section
transverse circumflex vessels
transverse colectomy
transverse colon
transverse colostomy
transverse commissure
transverse diameter
transverse diameter of inlet
transverse diameter of pelvic
    outlet
transverse disk

transverse facial artery
transverse facial fracture
transverse facial vein
transverse fascia
transverse fibers
transverse folds of rectum
transverse fracture
transverse head
transverse humeral ligament
transverse incision
transverse lie presentation
transverse ligament
transverse maxillary fracture
transverse mesocolon
transverse metatarsal ligament
transverse mucosal rugae
transverse muscle
transverse nerve
transverse occipital protuberance
transverse occipital sulcus
transverse orientation
transverse osteotomy
transverse palatine folds
transverse pelvic inlet
transverse perineal muscle
transverse plane
transverse presentation
transverse process
transverse projection
transverse rectal folds
transverse rectus abdominis myocutaneous procedure (TRAM procedure)
transverse row of sutures
transverse saw
transverse scapular ligament
transverse section
transverse sheet
transverse sinus
transverse sulcus of heart
transverse suture
transverse suture of Krause
transverse tarsal joint
transverse temporal gyri
transverse tomography
transverse vein

transverse wave
transversectomy
transverse-loop rod colostomy
transversely
transversospinal muscle
transversospinalis, musculus
transversostomy
transversotomy
transversus abdominis, musculus
transversus auriculae, musculus
transversus colli, nervus
transversus linguae, musculus
transversus menti, musculus
transversus, musculus
transversus nuchae, musculus
transversus perinei profundus, musculus
transversus perinei superficialis, musculus
transversus situs
transversus thoracis, musculus
transvesical prostatectomy
Trantas operation
trap
trap bottle
trap incision
trapdoor incision
trapdoor scleral buckle operation
trapdoor technique for retinal detachment
trapeze bar
trapeziectomy
trapezii, musculi
trapezium
trapezium bone
trapezium implant
trapezius muscle
trapezius, musculus
trapezius ridge sign
trapezoid
trapezoid bone
trapezoid ligament
Trapezoidal-28 total hip prosthesis

trapped
trapping of air
Trattner catheter
Traube murmur
Traube semilunar space
Traube sign
Traube space
trauma
traumatherapy
traumatic
traumatic abscess
traumatic amputation
traumatic avulsion
traumatic brain death
traumatic capsule
traumatic cataract
traumatic dislocation
traumatic hemorrhage
traumatic injury
traumatic lacerations
traumatic occlusion
traumatic pain
traumatic perforation
traumatic rupture
traumatic shock
traumatic sutures
traumatic wound
traumatism
traumatize
traumatized
traumatogenic
traumatogenic occlusion
traumatogenic pulpal occlusion
traumatopnea
traumatopneic wound
traumatosis
traumatotherapy
Trauner operation
Trautman Locktite hook
Trautman Locktite prosthesis
Trautmann triangle
Travel jejunostomy
Travel operation
Travenol bag
Travenol biopsy needle
Travenol dialyzer
Travenol infusion pump

Travenol infusor device
Travenol needle
Travenol twin coil for hemo-
    dialysis
Travert needle
Treace drill
Treace microdrill
Treace stapes drill
Treacher Collins syndrome
treadmill electrocardiogram
treadmill exercise stress test
treatable
treated
treatment
treatment and observation
treatment as indicated
treatment sequelae
treatment-resistant
trefoil deformity
trefoil tendon
Treitz arch
Treitz fossa
Treitz hernia
Treitz ligament
Treitz muscle
Trélat raspatory
Trélat speculum
Trélat vaginal speculum
trembling
tremors
Trendelenburg cannula
Trendelenburg operation
Trendelenburg position
Trendelenburg pulmonary
    embolectomy
Trendelenburg synchondros-
    teotomy
Trendelenburg tampon
Trendelenburg vein ligation
Trendelenburg-Crafoord clamp
Trendelenburg-Craoord
    coarctation clamp
Trendelenburg-position
    lithotomy
Trenkle screwdriver
Trent eye pick
Trent eye retractor

trephination
trephine
    antral trephine
    Arruga eye trephine
    Arruga lacrimal trephine
    Arruga trephine
    automatic corneal
      trephine
    Barraquer corneal
      trephine
    Barraquer trephine
    Becker trephine
    Blakesley lacrimal
      trephine
    Blakesley trephine
    Boiler septal trephine
    Boiler trephine
    Boston model trephine
    Brown-Pusey corneal
      trephine
    Brown-Pusey trephine
    Cardona corneal
      prosthesis trephine
    Castroviejo corneal
      trephine
    Castroviejo transplant
      trephine
    Castroviejo trephine
    chalazion trephine
    Cloward trephine
    corneal trephine
    cranial trephine
    Cross scleral trephine
    dacryocystorhinostomy
      trephine
    dacryotrephine
    Damshek sternal
      trephine
    Damshek trephine
    D'Errico skull trephine
    D'Errico trephine
    DeVilbiss cranial
      trephine
    DeVilbiss skull trephine
    DeVilbiss trephine
    Dimitry dacryocysto-
      rhinostomy trephine

trephine *continued*
    Dimitry trephine
    electric trephine
    Elliot corneal trephine
    Elliot eye trephine
    Elliot trephine
    exploratory trephine
    Franceschetti trephine
    Galt skull trephine
    Galt trephine
    Gradle corneal trephine
    Gradle trephine
    Green automatic corneal
      trephine
    Green trephine
    Greenwood trephine
    Grieshaber corneal
      trephine
    Grieshaber trephine
    Guyton trephine
    hand trephine
    Harris trephine
    Hessburg trephine
    Hessburg-Barron
      trephine
    Hessburg-Barron vacuum
      trephine
    Hippel trephine
    Horsley trephine
    Iliff lacrimal trephine
    Iliff trephine
    Jentzer trephine
    Katena trephine
    Katzin trephine
    King trephine
    lacrimal trephine
    Lahey trephine
    Leksell trephine
    Lichtenberg trephine
    Lichtwicz antral trephine
    Londermann corneal
      trephine
    Lorie antral trephine
    Lorie trephine
    Maumenee trephine
    Michel trephine
    Mueller electric trephine

trephine *continued*
    Mueller trephine
    nasal trephine
    Paton corneal trephine
    Paton trephine
    Paufique corneal
      trephine
    Paufique trephine
    Polley-Bickel trephine
    Schuknecht temporal
      trephine
    Schuknecht trephine
    Schwartz trephine
    scleral trephine
    Scoville skull trephine
    Scoville trephine
    Searcy chalazion
      trephine
    Searcy trephine
    septal trephine
    skull trephine
    spinal trephine
    Stephenson corneal
      trephine
    sternal trephine
    Stille trephine
    Stock eye trephine
    Storz disposable trephine
    Stryker saw trephine
    temporal trephine
    Thornwald antral
      trephine
    Thornwald trephine
    Turkel trephine
    Walker trephine
    Weck trephine
    Wilder trephine
    Wilkins trephine
trephine blade
trephine drill
trephinement
trephiner
trephining
Trethawain bunionectomy
Treves fold
Treves operation
triad

triad hip system
triad knee repair
triad of symptoms
Triad prosthesis
triaditis
triage
trial acetabular cups
trial basis
trial cup
trial fracture frame
trial frame
trial of labor
trial prosthesis
trial reduction
trial results
trial visit
triangle
triangle of Calot
triangle of Farabeuf
triangle of Langenbeck
triangle of lingual artery
triangle of Livingston
triangle of Trautmann
triangle of Ward
triangular
triangular bandage
triangular bipolar montage
triangular bone
triangular defect
triangular dressing
triangular fold
triangular fossa
triangular ligament
triangular muscle
triangular punch forceps
triangular resection of leaflet
triangular space
triangulation technique
triatrial heart
triaxial elbow prosthesis
triaxial hinge
triazine polymer resin
tribasilar synostosis
tributaries and perforators
tributary
triceps brachii, musculus
triceps muscle

triceps reflex
triceps surae jerk
triceps surae, musculus
triceps surae reflex
tricepsplasty
trichiasis operation
trichloroethylene anesthetic
    agent
trick knee
tricompartmental knee replace-
    ment
Tricon-M total knee prosthesis
Tricon-P tibial component with
    Flex-Lok pegs
tricrotic pulse
tricrotic wave
tricuspid annuloplasty
tricuspid aortic valve
tricuspid atresia
tricuspid commissurotomy
tricuspid orifice
tricuspid stenosis
tricuspid valve
tricuspid valve annuloplasty
tricuspid valve strut
tricuspid valvotomy
tricuspid valvulotomy
trident hand
tri-fin chisel
triflange intramedullary nail
triflange nail
Tri-flow incentive spirometer
Tri-flow incentive spirometry
triflow oxygen
trifurcate incision
trigeminal ganglion
trigeminal gland
trigeminal nerve (cranial
    nerve V)
trigeminal nerve compression
trigeminal nerve sign
trigeminal neuralgia
trigeminal pulse
trigeminal retractor
trigeminal rhizotomy
trigeminal self-retaining
    retractor
trigeminus

trigeminus cannula
trigeminus nervus
trigeminus reflex
trigeminus scissors
trigeminy
trigger cannula
trigger digit
trigger finger
trigger finger release
trigger point
trigger reaction
trigger thumb
triggered
trigone
trigonectomy
trileaflet aortic prosthesis
trileaflet aortic valve
trileaflet prosthesis
Trilene anesthetic agent
Trillat patellar tendon
    transfer
Trillat procedure
Trillaux fracture
trilobar hyperplasia
trilobate placenta
Tri-lock total hip system with
    Porocoat
trilocular heart
trilogy of Fallot
trimalleolar fracture
Trimar anesthetic agent
trimester
Tri-Met apnea monitor
Trimline knee immobilizer
trimmed
trimming
Trinkle brace
Trinkle power drill
trinocular microscope
tripanel, convoluted 4-strap
    (TCS) knee immobilizer
Trios M pacemaker
tripartite
tripartite patella
tripartite placenta
triphalangeal thumb
trip-hammer pulse
Tripier amputation

Tripier operation
triplane arthrodesis
triplane fracture
triple amputation
triple arthrodesis
triple bypass heart surgery
triple innominate osteotomy
triple strength
triple thermistor coronary sinus
   catheter
triple vessel disease
triple voiding cystogram
triple-A repair (AAA; abdominal
   aortic aneurysm)
triple-angle
triple-lumen catheter
triple-lumen central catheter
triple-lumen central venous
   catheter
triple-lumen manometric
   catheter
triple-lumen needle
triple-lumen perfusion to
   measure jejunal absorption
triple-lumen Sengstaken-
   Blakemore tube
triple-lumen sump drain
triplets
triplication of ureter
tripod
tripod cane
tripod pin traction
tripolar catheter
Trippi-Wells tongs
tripronged loop
triquetral bone
triquetrum
triradial
triradiate cartilage
trivalve
trivascular umbilical cord
trocar
     Abelson cricothyrotomy
      trocar
     accessory trocar
     Allen cecostomy trocar
     Allen trocar
     amniotic trocar

trocar *continued*
     anasarca trocar
     antral trocar
     Arbuckle-Shea trocar
     aspirating trocar
     Axiom thoracic trocar
     B-D Potain thoracic
      trocar
     Babcock empyema trocar
     Babcock trocar
     Barnes internal decom-
      pression trocar
     Barnes trocar
     Beardsley cecostomy
      trocar
     Beardsley trocar
     Bernay hydrocele trocar
     Billroth ovarian trocar
     Birch trocar
     Bishop antrum trocar
     bladder trocar
     Boettcher trocar
     Boettcher-Schnidt antrum
      trocar
     bore trocar
     brain-exploring trocar
     Bueleau empyema trocar
     Campbell trocar
     Castens trocar
     cecostomy trocar
     Charlton trocar
     Coakley trocar
     conical trocar
     Corb biopsy trocar
     cricothyroid trocar
     cricothyrotomy trocar
     Cross needle trocar
     Curschmann trocar
     cystotrocar
     Davidson thoracic trocar
     Davidson trocar
     Dean antral trocar
     Dean trocar
     decompressive trocar
     Denker trocar
     Diederich empyema
      trocar
     Douglas antral trocar

trocar *continued*
Douglas trocar
Doyen trocar
Duchenne trocar
Duke trocar
Durham tracheotomy
    trocar
Durham trocar
Emmet ovarian trocar
Emmet trocar
empyema trocar
Faulkner trocar
Fein antrum trocar
Fein trocar
fiberglass sleeve trocar
Frazier brain-exploring
    trocar
Frazier trocar
Gallagher trocar
gallbladder trocar
Hargin antrum trocar
Hargin trocar
Havlicek trocar
Hunt trocar
Hurwitz thoracic trocar
Hurwitz trocar
hydrocele trocar
intercostal trocar
internal decompression
    trocar
intestinal decompression
    trocar
intestinal trocar
Judd trocar
Kemp trocar
Kidd trocar
Klima-Rosegger trocar
Kolb trocar
Krause trocar
Kreutzmann trocar
Landau pelvic access
    trocar
Landau trocar
laparoscopic trocar
Lichtwicz antral trocar
Lichtwicz trocar
Lillie antral trocar

trocar *continued*
Lillie trocar
Livermore trocar
Lovelace gallbladder
    trocar
Lower trocar
Mayo-Ochsner trocar
Myerson antrum trocar
Myerson trocar
Neal catheter trocar
Nelson thoracic trocar
Nelson trocar
nested trocar
Ochsner gallbladder
    trocar
Ochsner trocar
ovarian trocar
Patterson trocar
Penn trocar
Pierce antral trocar
Pierce trocar
piloting trocar
Poole trocar
Post trocar
Potain aspirating trocar
Potain trocar
prostatic trocar
pyramidal trocar
rectal trocar
Reuter-Wolfe trocar
Roberts trocar
Robertson suprapubic
    trocar
Robinson-Brauer trocar
Ruskin antral trocar
Ruskin trocar
Schwartz trocar
Sewall antral trocar
Sewall trocar
Singleton trocar
Snyder trocar
Southey anasarca trocar
Southey trocar
Southey-Leech trocar
standard trocar
suprapubic trocar
Sweet antral trocar

trocar *continued*
Sweet trocar
tracheostomy trocar
Ueckermann cricothyroid trocar
Ueckermann-Denker trocar
Universal trocar
Van Alyea antral trocar
Van Alyea trocar
Veirs trocar
Veress trocar
Walther trocar
Wangensteen trocar
Wiener-Pierce antral trocar
Wiener-Pierce trocar
Wilson trocar
Wolf needle trocar
Yankauer antral trocar
Yankauer trocar
trocar needle
trocar sheath
trocar tunneling instrument
trochanter
trochanter-holding clamp
trochanteric bursa(e) of gluteus maximus
trochanteric pin
trochanteric plate
trochanteric rasp
trochanteric reamer
trochanterplasty
trochlea
trochlear nerve (cranial nerve IV)
trochlear nerve sign
trochlear notch
trochlear process
trochlear ridge
trochlearis, nervus
trochoid joint
trochoidal articulation
Troeltsch (also Tröltsch)
Troeltsch ear forceps
Troeltsch ear speculum
Troeltsch forceps

Troeltsch speculum
Troisier ganglion
Troisier node
Trolard vein
Tröltsch (see *Troeltsch*)
Troncoso gonioscope
Troncoso implant
Tronothane hydrochloride anesthetic agent
Tronzo approach to hip
Tronzo classification of trochanteric fractures
Tronzo elevator
Tronzo hip surgery
Tronzo lateral approach to hip
Tronzo screw
Tronzo total hip
trophic cicatrix
trophic fracture
trophic lesion
trophic nerve
trophoblastic tumor
Trotter forceps
Trotter syndrome
trough
trough and peak levels
trough gouge
trough level
trousers
Trousseau bougie
Trousseau dilator
Trousseau forceps
Trousseau-Jackson dilator
Trousseau-Jackson esophageal dilator
Trousseau-Jackson tracheal dilator
Troutman alpha-chymotrypsin cannula
Troutman cannula
Troutman cataract extractor
Troutman chisel
Troutman conjunctival scissors
Troutman corneal dissector
Troutman corneal forceps
Troutman corneal knife
Troutman corneal punch

Troutman corneal scissors
Troutman corneal section
    scissors
Troutman eye dissector
Troutman eye implant
Troutman forceps
Troutman gouge
Troutman implant
Troutman iris spatula
Troutman lens loupe
Troutman lens spoon
Troutman magnetic implant
Troutman mastoid chisel
Troutman mastoid gouge
Troutman needle
Troutman needle holder
Troutman operation
Troutman rectal forceps
Troutman scissors
Troutman-Barraquer colibri
    forceps
Troutman-Barraquer iris forceps
Troutman-Barraquer needle
    holder
Troutman-Castroviejo scissors
Troutman-Katzin corneal
    transplant scissors
Troutman-Llobera fixation
    forceps
Troutman-Llobera Flieringa
    forceps
Tru-Arc blood vessel ring
Tru-Arc trachea tube
Truc flap
Truc operation
Tru-Clip
Tru-Cut biopsy needle
Tru-Cut liver biopsy needle
Tru-Cut needle
Tru-Cut needle biopsy (TNB)
true aneurysm
true cords
True Form support stockings
true labor
true lateral x-ray view
true pelvis
true ribs

true sutures
true vocal cords
Trueta method
Trueta technique
Trueta treatment
Trumble arthrodesis
Trumble hip arthrodesis
Trumbull sutures
trumpet needle guide
trumpeting on x-ray
truncal abrasions
truncal vagotomy
truncate
truncated cone
truncated osteotomy
truncus arteriosus
truncus brachiocephalicus
truncus celiacus
truncus clamp
truncus costocervicalis
truncus pulmonalis
truncus thyrocervicalis
trunk
trunk movement
trunk muscles
trunk valves
TRUS (transrectal ultrasonogra-
    phy)
Trusler aortic valve technique
Trusler clamp
Trusler-Dean scissors
truss
Trussdale tourniquet
TSH (thyroid stimulating
    hormone)
Tsuge technique to reconstruct
    hand tendons
Tsuge tendon repair
Tsuji laminaplasty
TTAP (threaded titanium
    acetabular prosthesis)
TTC (T-tube cholangiogram)
TTS dilator (through-the-scope
    dilator)
tub
tubal abortion
tubal block

tubal implantation into uterus
tubal inflation
tubal insufflation
tubal insufflation cannula
tubal insufflator
tubal ligation
tubal obstruction
tubal occlusion
tubal patency
tubal pregnancy
tubal ring
tubal sterilization
Tubbs dilator
Tubbs mitral valve dilator
Tubbs valvulotome
Tubby knife
Tubby-Steindler operation
tube (see also *suction tube*)
    Abbott tube
    Abbott-Miller tube
    Abbott-Rawson double-
      lumen gastrointestinal
      tube
    Abbott-Rawson tube
    Abramson tube
    ACMI Valentine tube
    Adson brain suction tube
    Adson straight suction
      tube
    Adson suction tube
    Adson tube
    AF tube (anti-fog tube)
    air inflatable tube
    air tube
    Air-Lon laryngectomy
      tube
    Air-Lon tracheal tube
    Air-Lon tube
    Alesen tube
    American tracheotomy
      tube
    Amsterdam tube
    anaerobic culture tube
    Anderson flexible suction
      tube
    Anderson suction tube
    Anderson tube

tube *continued*
    Andrews suction tube
    Andrews-Pynchon
      suction tube
    Andrews-Pynchon tube
    Andrews-Yankauer
      suction tube
    anesthetic tube
    angled suction tube
    anode tube
    Anthony mastoid suction
      tube
    Anthony mastoid tube
    Anthony suction tube
    Anthony tube
    anti-fog tube (AF tube)
    antral drainage tube
    antral wash tube
    antrum-irrigating tube
    Argyle chest tube
    Argyle Sentinel Seal
      chest tube
    Argyle tube
    Argyle-Salem sump tube
    Armour endotracheal
      tube
    Armour tube
    Armstrong tube
    Armstrong V-vent tube
    Arrow tube
    ascites drainage tube
    ascites suction tube
    Asepto suction tube
    aspirating tube
    Atkins-Cannard tube
    Atkinson silicone rubber
      tube
    Ayre tube
    Babcock tube
    Baker intestinal decom-
      pression tube
    Baker jejunostomy tube
    Baker tube
    Bard tube
    Bardic tube
    Barnes nasal suction
      tube

tube *continued*

Barnes suction tube
Baron ear tube
Baron suction tube
Bavrona tube
Baylor cardiovascular
    sump tube
Baylor sump tube
Beardsley empyema tube
Beardsley tube
Beck mouth tube airway
bedside suction tube
Bellini tube
Bellocq tube
Bellucci nasal suction
    tube
Bellucci suction tube
Bellucci tube
Bettman empyema tube
Bilboa-Dotter nasogastric
    tube
Billroth tube
binocular tube
bivalve tube
Bivona tracheostomy
    tube
bladder tube
Blake esophageal tube
Blakemore esophageal
    tube
Blakemore tube
Blakemore-Sengstaken
    tube
blue Shepard grommet
    tube
Bonina-Jacobson tube
Bonnano tube
Bouchut tube
Bowman tubes
Boyce tube
brain suction tube
Brawley tube
breathing tube
Bron suction tube
bronchial tube
Broncho-Cath endo-
    tracheal tube

tube *continued*

bronchoscopic aspirating
    tube
bronchoscopic suction
    tube
Broyles tube
buccal tube
Bucy tube
Bucy-Frazier suction tube
Buie rectal suction tube
Buie suction tube
Buie tube
Butler tonsil suction tube
Buyes air-vent suction
    tube
bypass tube
C-P suction tube
Camel tube
Cantor intestinal tube
Cantor tube
Carabelli tube
Carlens double-lumen
    endotracheal tube
Carlens tube
Carmalt tube
Carman rectal tube
Carman tube
Carrel tube
cartilaginous tube
Casselberry sphenoid
    washing tube
Casselberry tube
Castelli tube
Castelli-Paparella collar-
    button-tube
Castelli-Paparella
    myringotomy tube
Cattel tube
Cattell forked-type
    T-tube
Cattell T-tube
Causse-Shea tube
Celestin esophageal tube
Celestin latex rubber
    tube
Celestin tube
cerebromedullary tube

tube *continued*

cesium tube
Chaffin suction tube
Chaffin sump tube
Chaffin tube
Chaffin-Pratt suction tube
Chaffin-Pratt tube
Chaoul tube
Chassin tube
Chaussier tube
chest tube
Chevalier Jackson tracheal tube
Chevalier Jackson tube
cholangiography tube
Christopher-Williams overtube
Christopher-Williams tube
Cilastin tube
circle nephrostomy tube
Clerf tube
closed drainage tube
closed suction drainage tube
closed suction tube
closed water-seal suction tube
coagulation-aspiration tube
Coakley tube
Cole pediatric tube
Cole tube
collar-button tube
collecting tube
collection tube
Collin tube
colostomy tube
Colton empyema tube
Cone suction tube
Cone tube
Connell breathing tube
Connell ether vapor tube
continuous suction tube
Cook County suction tube

tube *continued*

Cook County tracheal suction tube
Cooley cardiovascular suction tube
Cooley suction tube
Cooley sump tube
Coolidge tube
Cope nephrostomy tube
corneal tube
coronary sinus suction tube
Corpak feeding tube
Costen tube
Cottle suction tube
Coupland nasal suction tube
Coupland suction tube
Crookes tube
cuffed endotracheal tube
cuffed tube
cuffless tube
culture tube
Cummings tube
cystostomy tube
Dakin tube
Dandy suction tube
Davol colon tube
Davol suction tube
Davol tube
Deane tube
Deaver T-tube
DeBakey suction tube
Debove tube
decompressive tube
DeLee tube
Denker tube
Dennis intestinal tube
Dennis tube
Depaul tube
DeVilbiss suction tube
Devine tube
Devine-Millard-Frazier suction tube
diagnostic tube
diagnostic ear tube
Diamond tube

tube *continued*

digestive tube
discharge tube
Dobbhoff feeding tube
Doesel-Huzly broncho-
    scopic tube
Dominici tube
Donaldson eustachian
    tube
Donaldson myringotomy
    tube
Donaldson Silastic ear
    tube
Donaldson Teflon tube
Donaldson tube
double-cuffed tube
double-lumen endo-
    bronchial tube
double-lumen tube
Dr. Twiss duodenal tube
drain tube
drainage tube
Dreiling tube
dressed tube
Dryden-Quickert tube
Duke tube
Dumon-Gilliard prosthe-
    sis-pushing tube
Dumon-Harrell tracheal
    tube
Dundas Grant tube
duodenal tube
Duplay tube
Durham tracheostomy
    tube
Durham tube
ear suction tube
Eastman tube
Edlich gastric lavage tube
Edlich lavage tube
Einhorn tube
Emerson suction tube
empyema tube
encircling silicone tube
encircling tube
end tube
endobronchial tube

tube *continued*

endolymphatic shunt
    tube
endolymphatic tube
endoscopic tube
endotracheal tube
Endotrol endotracheal
    tube
Endotrol tracheal tube
EntriFlex small-bowel
    feeding tube
Esmarch tube
esophageal tube
esophagonasogastric
    tube
esophagoscopic tube
Ethox lavage tube
eustachian tube
Ewald stomach tube
Ewald tube
examination insert tube
fallopian tubes
Faucher stomach tube
Fay suction tube
Fazio-Montgomery tube
feeding gastrostomy tube
feeding tube
fenestrated tracheostomy
    tube
fenestrated tube
Ferguson brain suction
    tube
Ferguson-Frazier suction
    tube
fermentation tube
Feuerstein ear tube
Feuerstein myringotomy
    drain tube
fiberoptic tube
fil d'Arion tube
Finsterer suction tube
Fitzpatrick suction tube
flash tube
flexible rubber endo-
    scopic tube
flexible rubber tube
flexible suction tube

tube *continued*

flush tube
Foregger tube
forked T-tube
four-lumen tube
Frazier brain suction tube
Frazier insulated suction tube
Frazier modified suction tube
Frazier nasal suction tube
Frazier straight suction tube
Frazier suction tube
Frazier tube
Frazier-Paparella mastoid tube
Frazier-Paparella suction tube
French chest tube
Friend aspirating tube
frontal sinus wash tube
Fuller bivalve trach tube
Fuller tube
fusion tube
Gabriel Tucker tube
gallbladder tube
gas tube
gastric aspiration tube
gastric lavage tube
gastric tube
gastroduodenal tube
gastroenterostomy tube
gastrointestinal tube
gastrostomy tube
gavage tube
Geissler tube
Geissler-Pluecker tube
Gilman-Abrams gastric tube
Gilman-Abrams tube
Glasser gastrostomy tube
Glover suction tube
glutaraldehyde-tanned bovine collagen tube

tube *continued*

Gomco suction tube
Goode T-tube
Goode tube
Goodhill-Pynchon tube
Gore-Tex tube
Gott tube
granulation tube
Great Ormand Street tube
Greiling gastroduodenal tube
Greiling tube
grommet drain tube
grommet tube
Guibor canalicular tube
Guibor eye tube
Guibor Silastic tube
Guibor tube
Guisez tube
Gwathmey suction tube
Hakim tube
Haldane tube
Harris tube
Heimlich tube
hemodialysis tube
Hemovac suction tube
Hemovac tube
heparin-bonded tube
Herring tube
Hilger tracheal tube
Hilger tube
Hi-Lo Jet tracheal tube
Hi-Lo tracheal tube
Hittorf tube
Hodge intestinal decompression tube
Holinger aspirating tube
Holinger tube
Hollister tube
Holter tube
Honore-Smathers tube
horizontal tube
hot cathode tube
House endolymphatic shunt tube

tube *continued*

House shunt tube
House suction tube
House suction-irrigator tube
House tube
Humphrey coronary sinus suction tube
Hurwitz gastrostomy tube
Hyst T-tube
Immergut suction tube
Immergut suction-coagulation tube
Immergut tube
implanted tube
infant feeding tube
infusion tube
ingress tube
insert tube
insulated suction tube
intercostal tube
intestinal tube
intraluminal tube
intranasal tube
intratracheal tube
intubation tube
irrigating tube
irrigator-suction tube
Israel tube
Jackson cane-shaped tube
Jackson laryngectomy tube
Jackson tracheal tube
Jackson tube
Jacques stomach tube
Jako suction tube
Jarit-Pol suction tube
Jarit-Yankauer suction tube
Javid bypass tube
Javid tube
jejunal feeding tube
jejunostomy tube
Jergesen tube
Jesberg aspirating tube

tube *continued*

Jesberg tube
Joel-Baker tube
Johns Hopkins tube
Johnson intestinal tube
Johnson tube
Jones Pyrex tube
Jones tear duct tube
Jones tube
Jutte tube
Kaslow intestinal tube
Kaslow irrigation tube
Kaslow stomach tube
Kaslow tube
Kehr T-tube
Kehr tube
Keidel tube
Kelly tube
Keofeed feeding tube
Keyes-Ultzmann syringe tube
Kidd tube
Killian suction tube
Killian tube
Killian washing tube
Kimpton-Brown tube
Kistner plastic tube
Kistner tracheostomy tube
Kistner tube
Kobelt tube
Kozlowski tube
Kuhn tube
Kurze suction-irrigator tube
lacrimal tube
Lahey tube
Lahey Y-tube
Lanz low-pressure cuff endotracheal tube
Lanz tracheostomy tube
Lanz tube
Lapides tube
large-bore gastric lavage tube
LaRocca lacrimal tube
LaRocca tube

tube *continued*

- laryngeal tube
- laryngectomy tube
- latex tube
- Leiter tube
- Lell tube
- Lennarson suction tube
- Lennarson tube
- Lentz tracheotomy tube
- Leonard tube
- Lepley-Ernst tube
- Levin duodenal tube
- Levin tube
- Levin-Davol tube
- Lewis tube
- lifesaving suction tube
- lifesaving tube
- Lindeman-Silverstein tube
- Lindholm anatomical tracheal tube
- Lindholm tracheal tube
- Linton tube
- Linton-Nachlas tube
- Lloyd tube
- Loening stomach tube
- long intestinal tube
- Lo-Pro tracheal tube
- Lord-Blakemore tube
- Lore tube
- Lore-Lawrence tube
- Lorenz tube
- Luer tracheal tube
- Luer tube
- Lukens suction tube
- Lyon tube
- Lyster tube
- M-A tube (Miller-Abbott tube)
- MacKenty antral tube
- MacKenty tube
- Mackler esophageal tube
- Mackler tube
- Madoff suction tubes
- Magill tube
- Malecot gastrostomy tube

tube *continued*

- Malecot tube
- Mark IV nasogastric tube
- Martin drainage tube
- Martin laryngectomy tube
- Martin tube
- Mason suction tube
- mastoid suction tube
- Matzner tube
- McCollum tube
- McGowan-Keeley tube
- McIver nephrostomy tube
- McKesson mouth tube
- Medina ileostomy catheter tube
- Medoc-Celestin pulsion tube
- medullary tube
- membranous tube
- mercury-weighted tube
- metal-weighted Silastic feeding tube
- Methodist suction tube
- Mett tube
- middle ear arrow-tube
- Miescher tube
- Miller tube
- Miller-Abbott double-channel intestinal tube
- Miller-Abbott intestinal tube
- Miller-Abbott tube (M-A tube)
- Millin suction tube
- Millin tube
- Minnesota tube
- Mixter tube
- MLT tube
- Momberg tube
- Monoject suction tube
- monomer suction biopsy tube
- Montefiore tracheal tube
- Montefiore tube

tube *continued*

Montgomery T-piece
tube
Montgomery T-tube
Moore tube
Morch swivel
tracheostomy tube
Morch tracheostomy tube
Morch tube
Morsch-Retec respirator
tube
Morse-Andrews suction
tube
Morse-Ferguson suction
tube
Mosher esophagoscope
tube
Mosher lifesaver tube
Mosher lifesaving tube
Mosher suction tube
Mosher tube
Moss gastrostomy tube
Moss Mark IV gastros-
tomy tube
Moss Mark IV nasal tube
Moss tube
Mousseau-Barbin
prosthetic tube
Mueller suction tube
Mueller-Frazier suction
tube
Mueller-Frazier tube
Mueller-Poole suction
tube
Mueller-Poole tube
Mueller-Pynchon suction
tube
Mueller-Pynchon tube
Mueller-Yankauer
suction tube
Mueller-Yankauer tube
Muldoon tube
multiholed tube
multiple-lumen tube
Murphy drip tube
Murphy endotracheal
tube

tube *continued*

Murphy tube
myringotomy drain tube
myringotomy tube
Nachlas tube
Nachlas-Linton tube
nasal suction tube
nasal tube
nasobiliary tube
nasoduodenal feeding
tube
nasoesophageal feeding
tube
nasogastric feeding tube
nasogastric tube
nasojejunal feeding tube
nasolacrimal tube
nasopharyngeal tube
nasotracheal tube
Natelson tube
nephrostomy tube
Neuber drainage tube
Neuber tube
neural tube
New tube
New York Hospital
suction tube
Newvicon vacuum tube
NG tube
Nunez tube
Nutraflex Poole tube
Nyhus-Nelson gastric
decompression tube
Nyhus-Nelson jejunal
feeding tube
O'Beirne tube
obstructed tube
Ochsner gallbladder tube
Ochsner tube
O'Dwyer intubation tube
O'Hanlon-Pool tube
Olschevksy tube
Ommaya tube
open-end aspirating tube
oral endotracheal tube
orogastric tube
orotracheal tube

tube *continued*

Oto-mid permanent
ventilation tube
otopharyngeal tube
ovarian tube
Oxford tube
Paparella polyethylene
tube
Paparella tube
parasol tube
patent fallopian tube
patent tube
Paul drainage tube
Paul-Mixter tube
PE tube (polyethylene
tube; pressure
equalization tube)
pediatric feeding tube
pediatric nasogastric tube
PEG tube (percutaneous
endoscopic gastros-
tomy tube)
Penrose tube
Per-Lee middle ear tubes
Per-Lee myringotomy
tube
Per-Lee ventilating tube
Pezzar tube
Pfluger tube
pharyngeal tube
pharyngotympanic tube
Pierce antral wash tube
Pierce tube
Pierce washing tube
Pilling duralite tracheal
tube
Pilling tracheostomy tube
Pilling tube
Pitot tube
Pitt tracheostomy tube
plastic tube
pleural suction tube
pleural tube
Pleur-Evac suction tube
Pleur-Evac tube
plugged tube
Polisar-Lyons tube

tube *continued*

polyethylene drainage
tube
polyethylene tube
polyvinyl tube
Ponsky-Gauderer PEG
tube
Poole abdominal suction
tube
Poole suction tube
Poole tube
Poppen suction tube
Portex speaking tube
Portex tracheostomy
tube
Portex tube
Porto-vac suction tube
postnasal tube
precipitin tube
pressure equalization
tube (PEG tube)
Pribram suction tube
Procter-Livingston tube
Proctor suction tube
Pudenz tube
Puestow-Olander GI
tube
pus tube
Pynchon suction tube
Pynchon tube
pyramidal tube
Pyrex tube
Quickert tube
Quickert-Dryden tube
Quinton tube
radiopaque intestinal
tube
RAE endotracheal tube
Raimondi tube
Rainey tube
Ramirez straight Silastic
tube
Ramirez tube
Rand-House suction tube
Ray tube
rectal tube
Redivac tube

tube *continued*

red-top tube
Rehfuss tube
Replogle tube
respiratory tube
retractable fiberoptic
tube
Reuter bobbin stainless
steel drain tube
Reuter bobbin tube
Reuter tube
Reynolds tube
right-angle chest tube
Ritter suprapubic suction
tube
Robertshaw double-
lumen endotracheal
tube
Robinson equalizing
tube
Rochester tube
roll tube
Rosen suction tube
Rosen tube
rubber endoscopic tube
rubber tube
Rubin Brandborg biopsy
tube
Rubin hydraulic biopsy
tube
Rubin tube
Rubin-Quinton small-
bowel biopsy tube
Rusch tube
Russell suction tube
Ruysch tube
Ruysch-Armor tube
Ryle duodenal tube
Ryle tube
S-B tube (Sengstaken-
Blakemore tube)
Sachs brain suction
tube
Sachs suction tube
Sachs tube
Sacks-Vine feeding
gastrostomy tube

tube *continued*

Sacks-Vine PEG tube
(percutaneous
endoscopic gastros-
tomy tube)
Sacks-Vine percutaneous
endoscopic gastros-
tomy tube (PEG tube)
Safar tube
safety tube
Salem duodenal sump
tube
Salem nasogastric tube
Salem sump tube
salivary tube
Salvarsan throat irrigation
tube
Salvarsan tube
Sarns intracardiac suction
tube
Saticon vacuum chamber
pickup tube
Saticon vacuum tube
Schachowa tube
Schall tube
Schuknecht suction tube
Scott suction tube
Scott-Harden tube
seamless tube
Sengstaken nasogastric
tube
Sengstaken tube
Sengstaken-Blakemore
tube (S-B tube)
Senning suction tube
seton tube
Shaldon tube
Sharley tracheostomy
tube
Shaw tube
Shea polyethylene
drainage tube
Shea tube
Sheehy collar-button
tube
Sheehy tube
Sheldon-Pudenz tube

tube *continued*

Shepard grommet tube
Shepard Teflon tube
Shepard tube
Shepard ventilation tube
Sheridan tube
Sherman suction tube
Shiley endotracheal tube
Shiley French sump tube
Shiley sump tube
Shiley tracheostomy tube
Shiley tube
Shiley-Björk tube
Shiner tube
short-length tracheal tube
shunt tube
sigmoidoscope insulated suction tube
sigmoidoscope suction tube
Silastic tube
silicone tube
Silverstein tube
Singer-Blom tube
sinus wash tube
siphon suction tube
small-bowel tube
Snyder Hemovac suction tube
Snyder Hemovac tube
Snyder tube
Soilleau tube
Southey capillary drainage tube
Southey tube
Southey-Leech tube
Souttar tube
speaking tube
splinting tube
sputum tube
Stamm tube
Stedman suction tube
stent tube
sterile connecting tube
sterile vacuum collection tube

tube *continued*

stomach irrigation tube
stomach tube
Storz anti-fog tube
Storz bronchoscopic suction tube
Storz examination insert tube
Storz flash tube
Storz insert tube
Storz intratracheal tube
Storz tube
Storz-Doesel-Huzly bronchoscope tube
straight chest tube
suction tube (see separate listing)
suction-coagulation tube
sump nasogastric tube
sump suction tube
sump tube
Supramid suction tube
suprapubic tube
surgically implanted tube
Surgitube dressing
Swan-Ganz tube
swivel tracheostomy tube
T-tube
talking tracheostomy tube
tampon tube
tear duct tube
Teflon endolymphatic shunt tube
Teflon shunt tube
Teflon tube
Tek tube
test tube
thoracic drainage tube
thoracostomy tube
thoracotomy tube
Thora-Klex chest tube
Thow gastrostomy tube
Thow tube
three-bottle tidal suction tube
throat irrigation tube

tube *continued*
Thunberg tube
tonsil-suction tube
Toomey suction tube
Torkildsen tube
tracheal suction tube
tracheal tube
tracheal tube with obturator
tracheobronchial suction tube
tracheostomy tube
tracheotomy tube
transport tube
transpyloric tube
triple-lumen Sengstaken-Blakemore tube
Tru-Arc trachea tube
Tucker suction tube
Tucker tube
Tufts suction tube
Turkel tube
Tygon tube
tympanostomy ventilation tube
U-tube
underwater-seal suction tube
underwater-seal tube
uterine tube
Vacutainer tube
vacuum tube
Valentine irrigation tube
Valentine tube
valve tube
Van Alyea tube
Veillon tube
velvet-eye tube
ventilation tube
ventricular ventilation tube
Ventrol Levin tube
Venturi tube
Vernon antral tube
Vernon tube
vertical tube

tube *continued*
Vidicon vacuum chamber pickup tube
Vidicon vacuum tube
Vivonex Moss tube
Voltolini ear tube
Voltolini tube
Von Eichen antral tube
Von Eichen antral wash tube
Von Eichen tube
Walter-Poole suction tube
Walter-Yankauer suction tube
Wangensteen duodenal tube
Wangensteen suction tube
Wangensteen tube
Waring tonsil suction tube
warning stop tube
wash tube
washing tube
water-seal chest tube
Watkins suction tube
Watzke tube
Webster infusion tube
Webster tube
Weck suction tube
Weck tube
Welch Allyn suction tube
Welch Allyn tube
Wesolowski Dacron tube
West tube
Whelan-Moss T-tube
Winsburg-White bladder tube
wire-wound endo-tracheal tube
Witzel tube
Wookey skin tube
Xomed endotracheal tube
Y-tube
Yankauer suction tube

tube *continued*
- Yankauer tube
- Yankauer washing tube
- Yasargil suction tube
- Yeder tube
- Ygon tube
- Zeiss binocular tube
- Zollner suction tube
- Zyler tube

tube carrier
tube cecostomy
tube decompression
tube flap
tube gauze
tube graft
tube inflation
tube inserted
tube insufflator
tube introducer
tube intubation
tube obstruction
tube pedicle graft
tube placement
tube prosthesis
tube stockinette
tubed pedicle flap
tubeless cystostomy
tube-occluding clamp
Tuber syringe
tubercle
tuberosity
Tubex injector
Tubi-Grip
Tubi-Grip elastic support
    bandages
tubing
tubing clamp
tubing clamp forceps
tubing compressor
Tubinger self-retaining
    retractor
Tubiton tubular bandage
tubo-insufflation
tuboligation
tubo-ovarian
tubo-ovarian abscess
tubo-ovarian cyst
tubo-ovarian pregnancy
tubo-ovarian varicocele
tuboplasty
tubouterine pregnancy
tubular
tubular adenoma
tubular aneurysm
tubular blade
tubular defect
tubular dressing
tubular ectasia
tubular forceps
tubular gouge
tubular graft
tubular necrosis
tubular polyp
tubular vaginal speculum
tubular vertical gastroplasty
tubule
tubulization
tubulovillous adenoma
tubulovillous polyp
tuck
tucker (see also *tendon tucker*)
- Bishop tendon tucker
- Bishop-Black tendon
    tucker
- Bishop-Black tucker
- Bishop-DeWitt tendon
    tucker
- Bishop-DeWitt tucker
- Bishop-Peter tendon
    tucker
- Burch-Greenwood
    tendon tucker
- Burch-Greenwood
    tucker
- Cooley cardiac tucker
- Crafoord-Cooley tucker
- DeBakey tucker
- Fink tendon tucker
- Fink tucker
- Green tucker
- Harrison tucker
- Kelly combined packer
    and tucker
- Kelly tucker

tucker *continued*
    Ruedemann-Todd
      tendon tucker
    Smith-Petersen tucker
    Smuckler tucker
    strabismus tucker
Tucker appendix clamp
Tucker bougie
Tucker bronchoscope
Tucker dilator
Tucker forceps
Tucker laryngoscope
Tucker suction tube
Tucker telescope
Tucker tube
Tucker-Jako laryngoscope
Tucker-Luikart blade
Tucker-McLean obstetrical
    forceps
tucking
Tudor operation
Tudor-Edwards costotome
Tudor-Edwards rib shears
Tudor-Edwards spreader
Tudor-Thomas graft
Tudor-Thomas operation
Tuffier abdominal retractor
Tuffier abdominal spatula
Tuffier bone bender
Tuffier forceps
Tuffier operation
Tuffier retractor
Tuffier rib spreader
Tuffier spreader
Tuffier-Raney laminectomy
    retractor
Tuffnell bandage
tuft fracture
tuft of bone
Tufts suction tube
Tuke saw
Tulevech lacrimal cannula
Tulip harvesting system for
    suction lipectomy
tulip probe
tulle gras
tulle gras dressing

tumble flap
tumble-flap hypospadias repair
tumbler graft
tumbler skin flap
tumbling fashion
tumbling procedure
tumbling technique
tumbling-technique cataract
    extraction
tumefaction
tummy tuck
tumor
tumor blush
tumor forceps
tumor plop
tumor screw
tumorous portion
tunable diaphragm stethoscope
tunable dye laser
tunable dye laser lithotripsy
tungsten arc lamp
tunic
tunica (*pl.* tunicae)
tunica abdominalis
tunica adventitia
tunica conjunctiva
tunica dartos
tunica fibrosa hepatis
tunica fibrosa lienis
tunica intima
tunica media
tunica mucosa ventriculi
tunica mucosa vesicae felleae
tunica muscularis coli
tunica muscularis intestini
    tenuis
tunica muscularis recti
tunica muscularis ventriculi
tunica propria
tunica serosa coli
tunica serosa hepatis
tunica serosa intestini tenuis
tunica serosa lienis
tunica serosa peritonei
tunica serosa ventriculi
tunica serosa vesicae felleae
tunica vaginalis

tunicary
tunicary hernia
tuning fork
tunnel
tunnel flap
tunnel graft
tunnel projection
tunnel view
tunnel view on x-ray
tunnel x-ray view
tunneled bougie
tunneled eye implant
tunneled implant
tunneler
> Crafoord-Cooley tunneler
> DeBakey tunneler
> Eidemiller tunneler
> Favoloro tunneler
> Oregon tunneler
> Taucher tunneler

tunneling
tunneling instrument
Tuohy aortography needle
Tuohy catheter
Tuohy needle
Tuohy spinal needle
Tuohy-Bost introducer
Tuohy-Bost micropuncture introducer
TUR (transurethral resection)
turbid
turbid fluid
turbid milky fluid
turbid peritoneal fluid
turbidity
turbinate bone
turbinate electrode
turbinate forceps
turbinate knife
turbinate scissors
turbinates
turbine pneumotach
turbinectomy
turbo-bit craniotome
turbo-tip of phacoemulsification unit

TURBT (transurethral resection of bladder tumor)
turbulence
Türck bundle
Turco clubfoot release
Turco operation for talipes equinovarus
Turek spinous process spreader
Turek spreader
turf toe
turgescence
turgescent
turgescent vessel
turgid
turgor
Turkel liver biopsy needle
Turkel needle
Turkel punch
Turkel trephine
Turkel tube
turkey gobbler neck
turkey-claw clamp
turmoil
turnbuckle
turnbuckle cast
Turnbull applicator
Turnbull cannula
Turnbull colostomy
Turnbull forceps
Turnbull multiple ostomy
Turnbull nail nipper
Turnbull nipper
Turnbull technique
Turner cystoscopic fulguration electrode
Turner dilator
Turner elevator
Turner gouge
Turner hip pin
Turner intraparietal sulcus
Turner operation
Turner periosteal elevator
Turner pin
Turner prosthesis
Turner sign
Turner spinal gouge
Turner tooth

Turner-Babcock tissue forceps
Turner-Doyen retractor
Turner-Warwick incision
Turner-Warwick needle
Turner-Warwick retractor
Turner-Warwick stone forceps
Turner-Warwick suction
Turner-Warwick urethroplasty
Turner-Warwick-Adson forceps
turning fracture frame
turnover
TURP (transurethral resection of prostate)
Turrell angular rotating punch
Turrell biopsy forceps
Turrell biopsy punch
Turrell forceps
Turrell proctoscope
Turrell sigmoidoscope
Turrell specimen forceps
Turrell-Wittner rectal biopsy forceps
Turrell-Wittner rectal forceps
turret exostosis
Tuttle forceps
Tuttle proctoscope
Tuttle sigmoidoscope
Tuttle test
Tuttle tissue forceps
tweezers
        Dumont tweezers
twelfth cranial nerve (XII)
twenty-day gut sutures
twilight anesthesia
twill dressing
twin knife
twinge
Twining position
twin-pattern chisel
Twisk forceps
Twisk needle holder
Twisk scissors
twist
twist drill
twist drill catheter
twist drill points
twist drill set

twisted cotton sutures
twisted dermal sutures
twisted linen sutures
twisted silk sutures
twisted sutures
twisted wire loop
twisting
twisting injury
twitch
twitching
two-bladed dilator
two-bottle drainage
two-bottle thoracic drainage system
two-clamp anastomosis
two-dimensional echocardiogram
two-dimensional echocardiography
two-layer anastomosis
two-loop ileal J-pouch
Twombly operation
Twombly-Ulfelder operation
two-piece ostomy pouch
two-pin technique
two-poster orthosis
two-prong dural hook
two-prong rake retractor
two-prong stem finger prosthesis
two-pronged retractor
two-stage operation
two-stage pancreatoduodenectomy
two-stage Sarns cannula
two-step corneal section
two-toothed forceps
two-way adapter for K-Temp thermometer
two-way bag
two-way catheter
two-way hemostatic bag
two-wing drain
two-wing Malecot drain
Tycos sphygmomanometer
Tycron sutures (also Ti-Cron)
Tydings forceps

Tydings knife
Tydings snare
Tydings tonsil clamp
Tydings tonsil forceps
Tydings tonsil knife
Tydings tonsil snare
Tydings tonsillectome
Tydings-Lakeside forceps
Tydings-Lakeside tonsil-seizing
   forceps
Tygon catheter
Tygon esophageal prosthesis
Tygon surgical tubing
Tygon tube
Tygon tubing
tying
tylectomy
Tyler Gigli saw
tylosis
tympanectomy
tympanic annulus
tympanic antrum
tympanic artery
tympanic bone
tympanic cavity
tympanic ganglion
tympanic membrane
tympanic nerve
tympanic notch
tympanic orifice
tympanic plexus
tympanic sinus
tympanic sulcus
tympanic vein
tympanica anterior, arteria
tympanica inferior, arteria
tympanica posterior, arteria
tympanica superior, arteria
tympanicae, venae
tympanicus, nervus
tympanites
tympanitis
tympanogram
tympanography
tympanomastoid abscess

tympanomastoid cavity
tympanomastoidectomy
tympanomeatal
tympanomeatal flap
tympanometry
tympanoplastic knife
tympanoplasty (type I, II, III,
   IV, V)
tympanoplasty knife
Tympan-O-Scope
tympanoscope
tympanostomy ventilation
   tube
tympanosympathectomy
tympanotomy
tympanotomy flap
tympanum
tympanum perforator
tympany
Tym-tap
Tyndall light
type and crossmatch (T&C)
type I imperforate anus
type I tympanoplasty
type II imperforate anus
type II tympanoplasty
type III imperforate anus
type IV imperforate anus
type IV tympanoplasty
type V tympanoplasty
typhlectomy
typhlopexy
typhlorrhaphy
typhlostomy
typhlotomy
typhloureterostomy
typical
Tyrrell clamp
Tyrrell foreign body forceps
Tyrrell hook
Tyrrell iris hook
Tyrrell skin hook
Tyrrell-Gray sutures
Tyson glands
Tzanck operation

**U**

U-clip
U-connector
U-double-barrel suture
U-shaped continuous sutures
U-shaped forceps
U-shaped incision
U-shaped retractor
U-shaped scar
U-splint
U-stitch
U-sutures
U-tube
U-tube stent
U-wave
UAC catheter (umbilical artery catheter)
UBC brace (University of British Columbia brace)
UCB orthosis (University of California, Berkeley, orthosis)
Uchida fimbriectomy
Uchida incision
Uchida operation
Uchida technique
Uchida tubal banding
Uchida tubal ligation
UCI knee prosthesis
UCI prosthesis
UCI total knee replacement
UCI-Barnard aortic valve
UCI-Barnard valve
UCLA functional long-leg brace
UCLA ureterosigmoidostomy
Uebe applicator
Ueckermann cricothyroid trocar
Ueckermann-Denker trocar
Uematsu shoulder arthrodesis

UES (upper esophageal sphincter)
UF (ultrafiltrate, ultrafiltration)
UGI (upper gastrointestinal) tract
UHI Universal head system hip prosthesis
Uhlrich stapler
ulcer
ulcer bed
ulcer disease
ulcerated area
ulcerated lesion
ulcerated nodule
ulcerated wound
ulcerating
ulcerating adenocarcinoma
ulcerating area
ulcerating granuloma
ulcerating lesion
ulceration
ulcerative lesion
ulcerogenic tumor
ulceromembranous
ulectomy
Ulloa operation
Ullrich drill guard
Ullrich forceps
Ullrich laminectomy retractor
Ullrich retractor
Ullrich self-retaining retractor
Ullrich tubing clamp
Ullrich uterine knife
Ullrich-St. Gallen self-retaining retractor
ulna
ulnar artery
ulnar aspect
ulnar bursa

Ultratome (sp.check)

ulnar collateral ligament
ulnar deviation
ulnar extensor muscle
ulnar flexor muscle
ulnar groove
ulnar ligament
ulnar nerve
ulnar notch
ulnar recurrent artery
ulnar reflex
ulnar resection
ulnar shaft
ulnar splint
ulnar styloid bone
ulnar tunnel
ulnar tunnel syndrome
ulnar variance
ulnar veins
ulnares, venae
ulnaris, arteria
ulnaris, nervus
ulnocarpal
ulnocarpal ligament
ulnoradial
ulotomy
ULP (ultra low profile)
Ultex bifocal lens
Ultex implant
Ultex lens
ultimate
ultimate load
ultimobranchial body
Ultra COM monitor
ultra low profile (ULP)
Ultra pacemaker
ultra x-ray
Ultracor prosthetic valve
Ultra-Cut surgical instruments
ultrafiltrate (UF)
ultrafiltration (UF)
ultraflow
Ultramark 8 transducer
Ultramer catheter
ultramicroscope
ultrasonic cleaner
ultrasonic diathermy

ultrasonic diathermy electrosurgical unit
ultrasonic dissector
ultrasonic electrode
ultrasonic fragmentation of urinary calculi
ultrasonic lithotripsy
ultrasonic lithotriptor
ultrasonic microscope
ultrasonic tip
ultrasonic wand
ultrasonogram
ultrasonographic
ultrasonography
ultrasound
ultrasound cardiogram
ultrasound scan
ultrasound spatula
Ultrastop anti-fogging solution
ultraviolet
ultraviolet microscope
Ultra-X external fixation system
Ultroid device for hemorrhoid treatment
Ultroid for nonsurgical hemorrhoidal management
umbilectomy
umbilical
umbilical artery
umbilical artery catheter (UAC)
umbilical catheter
umbilical circulation
umbilical clamp
umbilical clip
umbilical cord
umbilical cord clamp
umbilical fissure
umbilical fold
umbilical graft
umbilical hernia
umbilical hernia repair
umbilical hernia repair with omphalectomy
umbilical hernia repair with umbilectomy
umbilical herniorrhaphy
umbilical ligament

umbilical notch
umbilical region
umbilical scissors
umbilical stump
umbilical tape
umbilical tape drain
umbilical tape sutures
umbilical vein
umbilical vein catheter
umbilical vein graft
umbilicalis, arteria
umbilicalis sinistra, vena
umbilicalis, vena
umbilicated mass
umbiliclamp
umbiliclip
umbilicus
umbrella
umbrella filter
umbrella-type prosthesis
unabsorbable sutures
unassisted delivery
unassisted respiration
unavoidable
unbalanced
unbanded gastroplasty
unbridling
unciform bone
uncinate bone
uncinate gyrus
uncinate process
uncomplicated birth
uncomplicated delivery
uncomplicated postoperative
    course
unconditioned
unconscious
unconsciousness
unconstrained knee prosthesis
unconstrained prosthesis
uncontaminated
uncontrollable
uncontrollable bleeding
uncontrollable pain
uncotomy
uncovering
uncovertebral joint

underarm orthosis
undercut
underlay fascial graft
underlying
underlying chest muscles
underlying fascia
underlying skin
underlying structures
underlying tissue
undermine
underpad
underrunning
undersensing malfunction of
    pacemaker
underside
undersized
undersized prosthesis
understanding
undersurface
underwater drainage
underwater electrode
underwater seal
underwater suction
underwater-seal drainage
underwater-seal suction tube
underwater-seal thoracic
    drainage system
underwater-seal tube
undescended testicle
undescended testis
undetermined cause
undetermined etiology
undifferentiated
undifferentiated
    adenocarcinoma
undifferentiated carcinoma
undifferentiated lesion
undifferentiated lymphoma
undifferentiated type
undirected
undisplaced
undisplaced fracture
undyed sutures
unengaged
unenhanced study
unequal
unequivocal diagnosis

uneven contour
uneventful course
unexpected
unexpectedly
Unger adenoid pressure roller
ungual process
ungual tuft
unguis (*pl.* ungues)
unguis incarnatus
uniarticular
uniaxial joint
unicameral bone cyst
unicommissural aortic valve
unicompartmental knee implant
unicompartmental knee
    replacement
unicondylar prosthesis
Uniflex dressing
unifocal PVCs
uniform
uniformity
Unilab surgibone surgical
    implant
unilateral
unilateral aortofemoral graft
unilateral bar
unilateral facet subluxation
unilateral fracture
unilateral procedure
unilateral salpingo-oophorec-
    tomy
Unilink system for hand surgery
Unilith pacemaker
unilobar
unilocular joint
unimpaired function
unimpeded
unimproved
uninterrupted sutures
union
unipennate muscle
unipolar
unipolar atrial pacemaker
unipolar atrioventricular
    pacemaker
unipolar electrode
unipolar lead

unipolar limb leads
unipolar pacemaker
unipolar pacemaker lead
unipolar sequential pacemaker
unit
United Max-E pouch
United Surgical Bongort
    Lifestyle pouch
United Surgical Featherlite
    ileostomy pouch
United Surgical Shear Plus
    pouch
United Surgical Soft & Secure
    pouch
Univalve cast
Universal antral punch
Universal appliance
Universal aspirator
Universal condenser
Universal conformer
Universal cystoscope
Universal drill
Universal drill point
Universal esophagoscope
Universal eye shield
Universal femoral head
    prosthesis
Universal forceps
Universal gastroscope
Universal gutter splint
Universal hand drill with chuck
    key
Universal handle
Universal handle for punch tips
Universal handle with nasal-
    cutting tips
Universal joint cervix
Universal joint device
Universal Kerrison set and tips
Universal lamp
Universal malleable valvulo-
    tome
Universal mirror handle
Universal nerve hook
Universal proximal femur
    prosthesis (UPF prosthesis)
Universal punch

Universal retractor
Universal saw
Universal splint
Universal support splint
Universal T-adapter
Universal tourniquet
Universal trocar
Universal two-speed hand drill
Universal valve prosthesis
    sewing ring
University forceps
University of British Columbia
    brace (UBC brace)
University of California,
    Berkeley orthosis (UCB
    orthosis)
University of Illinois marrow
    needle
University of Illinois needle
University of Kansas eye spatula
University of Kansas forceps
University of Kansas hook
University of Kansas spatula
University of Michigan Mixter
    thoracic forceps
unknown
unlimited
unmanageable
unmyelinated
unmyelinated nerve fibers
Unna boot
Unna boot cast
Unna comedo extractor
Unna extractor
Unna paste
Unna paste boot
Unna wrap
unobstructed
unossified cartilage
unpigmented
unproductive
unremarkable
unresectable tumor
unresolved
unresponsive
unripe cataract
unroof

unroofing
unruptured ectopic pregnancy
unruptured vascular anomalies
Unschuld sign
unsealed
unsegmented bar
unstable
unstable joint
unstriated muscle
unsuspected
untimely
untoward reaction
untreatable
ununited fracture
unusual
up-and-down flap
up-biting biopsy forceps
up-biting cup forceps
up-biting forceps
up-biting punch
up-cutting rongeur
update
Updegraff cleft palate needle
Updegraff hook
Updegraff needle
updrawn pupil
UPF prosthesis (Universal
    proximal femur prosthesis)
upgated technique
upgoing
upgoing toes
UPJ (ureteropelvic junction)
UPJ stricture (ureteropelvic
    junction stricture)
UPP (urethral pressure profile)
upper abdomen
upper abdominal midline
    incision
upper abdominal organs
upper body dressing
upper cervical region
upper esophageal sphincter
    (UES)
upper esophagoscope
upper esophagus
upper extremity
upper eyelid

upper gastrointestinal (UGI) tract
upper GI series
upper jaw
upper jaw bone
upper lid
upper limb
upper lip
upper lobe of lung
upper mantle field
upper midline incision
upper panendoscopy
upper respiratory tract
uppermost
UPPP (uvulopalato-pharyngoplasty)
Uppsala gall duct forceps
upright film
upright position
upset
upsloping
uptake
uptake studies
upward and downward
upward movement
upward-gaze incision
urachal cyst
urachal fossa
urachal sinus of bladder
urachus (*pl.* urachi)
uraniscoplasty
uraniscorrhaphy
uranoplasty
uranorrhaphy
uranostaphyloplasty
uranostaphylorrhaphy
Urban mastectomy
Urban operation
Urban retractor
Urbaniak technique
Urbantschitsch bougie
Urbantschitsch forceps
uremia
uremic
Uresil Vascu-Flo carotid shunt
ureter
ureteral

ureteral basket stone dislodger
ureteral biopsy
ureteral bougie
ureteral catheter
ureteral catheter forceps
ureteral catheter obturator
ureteral catheterization
ureteral clamp
ureteral dilation
ureteral dilator
ureteral illuminator
ureteral implant
ureteral isolation forceps
ureteral meatotome
ureteral meatotomy
ureteral orifice
ureteral reflux
ureteral stent
ureteral stone
ureteral stone basket
ureteral stone dislodger
ureteral stone extractor
ureteral stone forceps
ureterectasis
ureterectomy
ureteric opening
ureteric plexus
ureteric ridge
ureteritis
ureterocecostomy
ureterocele
ureterocelectomy
ureterocentesis
ureterocolectomy
ureterocolostomy
ureterocutaneostomy
ureterocystanastomosis
ureterocystoneostomy
ureterocystoscope
ureterocystostomy
ureteroduodenal fistula
ureteroenteroanastomosis
ureteroenterostomy
ureterogram
ureteroileal loop
ureteroileobladder anasto-mosis

ureteroileocutaneous anasto-
    mosis
ureteroileostomy
ureterointestinal anastomosis
ureterolithiasis
ureterolithotomy
ureterolysis
ureteromeatotomy
ureteroneocystostomy
ureteroneopyelostomy
ureteronephrectomy
ureteropelvic junction (UPJ)
ureteropelvic junction stricture
ureteropelvioneostomy
ureteropelvioplast
ureteropelvioplasty
ureteropexy
ureteroplasty
ureteroplication
ureteroproctostomy
ureteropyelogram
ureteropyelography
ureteropyeloneostomy
ureteropyelonephrostomy
ureteropyeloplasty
ureteropyelostomy
ureterorectoneostomy
ureterorenoscope
ureterorenoscopy
ureterorrhaphy
ureteroscopy
ureterosigmoidostomy
ureterostomy
ureterotomy
ureterotrigonoenterostomy
ureterotrigonosigmoidostomy
ureterotubal anastomosis
ureteroureteral anastomosis
ureteroureterostomy
ureterovaginal fistula
ureterovesical implantation
ureterovesical junction (UVJ)
ureterovesicoplasty
ureterovesicostomy
urethra
urethral
urethral artery

urethral bougie
urethral bougienage
urethral catheter
urethral catheterization
urethral chill
urethral crest
urethral dilatation
urethral dilator
urethral filiforms
urethral forceps
urethral gland
urethral incompetence
urethral instillation cannula
urethral instrumentation
urethral meatotomy
urethral meatus dilator
urethral opening
urethral orifice
urethral pressure profile (UPP)
urethral sound
urethral speculum
urethral stricture
urethral suspension
urethral wall
urethral whip bougie
urethralis, arteria
urethrascope
urethrectomy
urethreurynter
urethroblennorrhea
urethrocele
urethrocystogram
urethrocystography
urethrocystopexy
urethrogram
urethrographic cannula
urethrographic cannula clamp
urethrographic catheter
urethrographic clamp
urethrography
urethrolithotomy
urethrometer
urethrometry
urethroperineal fistula
urethroperineoscrotal
urethropexy
urethrophyma

urethroplasty
urethrorectal fistula
urethrorrhaphy
urethroscope
    ACMI cystourethroscope
    ACMI microlens
        cystourethroscope
    ACMI urethroscope
    Albarran urethroscope
    Ballenger urethroscope
    cystourethroscope
    female urethroscope
    Foroblique cystourethro-
        scope
    Guiteras urethroscope
    Lowsley urethroscope
    obturator urethroscope
    posterior urethroscope
urethroscopic examination
urethroscopy
urethrostomy
urethrotome
    bougie-urethrotome
    Hertel bougie-
        urethrotome
    Hertel urethrotome
    Huffman-Huber infant
        urethrotome
    infant urethrotome
    Keitzer infant
        urethrotome
    Keitzer urethrotome
    Kirkheim-Storz
        urethrotome
    Maisonneuve
        urethrotome
    Otis urethrotome
    Riba electrourethrotome
    Riba urethrotome
    Sachs urethrotome
    Storz bougie-
        urethrotome
    Storz-Kirkheim
        urethrotome
urethrotomy
urethrovaginal fistula
urethrovaginal space

urethrovesical angle
urethrovesicular differential
    reflux
Uribe implant
Uribe orbital implant
uric acid
urinary bladder
urinary bladder hernia
urinary blockage
urinary calculus
urinary catheter
urinary diversion
urinary diversion procedure
urinary drainage
urinary hesitancy
urinary incontinence
urinary incontinence clamp
urinary incontinence prosthesis
urinary infection
urinary opening
urinary output
urinary reflux
urinary reservoir
urinary retention
urinary sphincter
urinary stasis
urinary stone
urinary stream
urinary stress incontinence
    (USI)
urinary symptoms
urinary tract
urinary tract infection
urinary urgency
urinary volume
urinary washings
urination
urine
urine culture
Urist-Matchett-Brown total hip
uroflow study
uroflowmeter
uroflowmetry
urogenital
urogenital diaphragm
urogenital fold
urogenital region

urogenital surgery
urogenital tract
urogenital trigone
urogenital vestibule
urogram
urography
urologic catheter
urologic surgery instrument set
urologic ultrasonography
Uro-San Plus external catheter
Uroscan Uroflow system
Urosoft stent
urostomy pouch
urothelial tumor
urothelioma
urothelium
Urschel first rib rongeur
Urschel-Leksell rongeur
U.S. Army chisel
U.S. Army double-ended
    retractor
U.S. Army gouge
U.S. Army osteotome
U.S. Army retractor
U.S. Army-pattern gauze
    scissors
U.S. Army-pattern knife
U.S. Army-pattern osteotome
U.S. Army-pattern retractor
USCI angioplasty guiding sheath
USCI Bard catheter
USCI cannula
USCI catheter
USCI Finesse guiding catheter
USCI guide wire
USCI guiding catheter
USCI Mini-Profile balloon
    dilatation catheter
USCI nonsteerable system
USCI pacing electrode
USCI Positrol coronary catheter
USCI Sauvage Bionit bifurcated
    vascular prosthesis
USCI Sauvage EXS side-limb
    prosthesis
USCI Sauvage graft
USCI steerable system

USCI Vario permanent pace-
    maker
Usher Marlex mesh
Usher Marlex mesh dressing
Usher Marlex mesh graft
Usher Marlex mesh implant
Usher Marlex mesh prosthesis
Usher-Bellis hernia repair
USI (urinary stress inconti-
    nence)
Uskow pillar
usual anatomic position
Utah artificial arm
uterina, arteria
uterinae, venae
uterine appendage
uterine artery
uterine artery forceps
uterine aspiration
uterine aspirator
uterine atony
uterine biopsy forceps
uterine biopsy punch
uterine bleeding
uterine canal
uterine cannula
uterine cavity
uterine cervix
uterine configuration
uterine corpus
uterine cramping
uterine cuff
uterine curet
uterine curettage
uterine curettement
uterine curettings
uterine cycle
uterine descensus
uterine didelphys
uterine dilatation
uterine dilator
uterine elevator
uterine enlargement
uterine evacuation
uterine fibroid
uterine fibroidectomy
uterine fibroma

uterine forceps
uterine fundus
uterine hemorrhage
uterine hernia
uterine incision
uterine knife
uterine leiomyosarcoma
uterine lining
uterine manipulating forceps
uterine manipulator
uterine mucus
uterine muscle
uterine myoma
uterine myomata
uterine myomectomy
uterine needle
uterine nerve
uterine orifice
uterine placenta
uterine plexus
uterine polyp forceps
uterine pregnancy
uterine probe
uterine procidentia
uterine prolapse
uterine prolapse repair
uterine radium insertion
uterine reflection
uterine sarcoma
uterine scissors
uterine scrapings
uterine secundines
uterine segment
uterine shadow
uterine sound
uterine specimen forceps
uterine spoon
uterine suction curet
uterine suspension
uterine suspension operation
uterine tenaculum
uterine tenaculum forceps
uterine tenaculum hook
uterine tissue
uterine trigger cannula
uterine tube
uterine tube fimbria

uterine vacuum cannula
uterine veins
uterine vessels
uterine vulsellum forceps
uterine wall
uterine-dressing forceps
uterine-elevating forceps
uterine-holding forceps
uterine-irrigating curet
uterine-packing forceps
uteroabdominal pregnancy
uterocentesis
uterofixation
utero-ovarian pregnancy
uteroparietal suture
uteropelvic ligaments
uteropexy
uteroplacental apoplexy
uteroplacental insufficiency
uteroplasty
uterorectal fistula
uterosacral
uterosacral ligament
uterosalpingography
uterotubal pregnancy
uterovaginal fistula
uterovaginal plexus
uterovesical fold
uterovesical junction (UVJ)
uterus
uterus arcuatus
uterus didelphys
uterus massaged
uterus mobilized
uterus normal in length
uterus normal in size and shape
uterus packed
uterus packed with gauze
uterus septus
uterus simplex
uterus sounded
uterus unicornis
utility forceps
utility scissors
utility shoulder splint
utility-type incision
utilization

Utrata capsulorrhexis forceps
utricle
utricular nerve
utricularis, nervus
utriculoampullar nerve
utriculoampullaris, nervus
uvea
uveal melanoma
uveal staphyloma
uveomeningeal syndrome
uviol light

UVJ (ureterovesical junction)
uvula
uvula retractor
uvula vesicae
uvulae, musculus
uvulectomy
uvulitis
uvulopalatine musculature
uvulopalatopharyngoplasty
uvulotome
uvulotomy

V-blade plate
V-clip
V-fib (ventricular fibrillation)
V-medullary nail
V-osteotomy
V-shaped incision
V-shaped scar
V-shaped ulcer
V-tach (ventricular tachycardia)
V-type intertrochanteric plate
V-wave
V-Y advancement flap
V-Y flap
V-Y muscle-plasty
V-Y operation
V-Y palatoplasty
V-Y plasty
V-Y plasty of bladder neck
V-Y procedure
V-Y push back
V-Y push-back cleft palate
    repair
V-Y repair of cheek defect
V-Y retroposition cleft palate
    repair
V-Z advancement in buccal
    sulcus
V1, V2, V3, V4, V5, V6 EKG
    leads
VA (visual acuity)
VA magnetic implant
VA magnetic orbital implant
Vabra aspirator
Vabra aspirator disposable
    system
Vabra cannula
Vabra catheter
Vabra cervical aspirator
Vabra curettage

Vabra endometrial biopsy
Vabra endometrial study
Vabra uterine aspiration
    curettage
Vacher retractor
Vacher self-retaining retractor
Vac-Pac positioner
Vacurette
Vacurette catheter
Vacurette suction curet
Vacutainer drain
Vacutainer holder
Vacutainer needle
Vacutainer tube
Vacu-tome knife
vacuum
vacuum abortion
vacuum aspiration
vacuum aspiration apparatus
vacuum aspirator
vacuum curet
vacuum curettage
vacuum drain
vacuum drainage
vacuum drainage system
vacuum erection device (VED)
vacuum extraction
vacuum extraction operation
vacuum hand pump
vacuum intrauterine cannula
vacuum intrauterine probe
vacuum retractor
vacuum thoracic drainage
    system
vacuum tube
vacuum tumescence-constrictor
    device
vacuum tumescence-enhance-
    ment therapy

vacuum vaginal delivery
vacuuming needle
VAD (ventricular assist device; vascular/venous access device)
vagal
vagal accessory nerve
vagal ganglion
vagal nerve
vagal trunk
vagina
vagina bulbi
vaginal
vaginal artery
vaginal atrophy
vaginal bag
vaginal birth
vaginal birth after cesarean section (VBAC)
vaginal bleeding
vaginal candle
vaginal celiotomy
vaginal cervix
vaginal cesarean section
vaginal construction
vaginal cuff
vaginal cuff clamp
vaginal delivery
vaginal dilator
vaginal flow
vaginal folds
vaginal fornix
vaginal graft
vaginal hernia
vaginal hysterectomy
vaginal hysterectomy forceps
vaginal ligaments
vaginal lithotomy
vaginal lubrication
vaginal lumen
vaginal mucosa
vaginal muscles
vaginal nerves
vaginal orifice
vaginal outlet
vaginal pack
vaginal packing

vaginal pad
vaginal plexus
vaginal prolapse
vaginal radium insertion
vaginal reconstruction
vaginal repair
vaginal retractor
vaginal speculum
vaginal sponge
vaginal stent
vaginal suppository
vaginal suspension procedure
vaginal swab
vaginal tampon
vaginal tissue
vaginal varicose vein
vaginal vault
vaginal vault repair
vaginal vertex delivery
vaginal wall
vaginal, cervical, endocervical smears (VCE smears)
vaginalectomy
vaginales, nervi
vaginalis, arteria
vaginectomy
vaginismus
vaginocutaneous fistula
vaginofixation
vaginolabial
vaginolabial hernia
vaginoperineal fistula
vaginoperineotomy
vaginoplasty
vaginorectal examination
vaginorrhaphy
vaginoscope
    Huffman infant vaginoscope
    Huffman vaginoscope
    Huffman-Huber infant vaginoscope
    Huffman-Huber vaginoscope
    infant vaginoscope
vaginoscopy
vaginotomy

vagolysis
vagotomy
vagotomy and pyloroplasty
vagotomy retractor
vagotomy stripper
Vag-Pack
vagus nerve (cranial nerve X)
vagus, nervus
Vail everter
Vail lid retractor
Vainio arthroplasty
Vairox high compression
    vascular stockings
Vairox vascular stockings
Vaiser eye sponge
Vaiser-Dibis muscle retractor
Valdoni clamp
Valentine irrigation tube
Valentine irrigator
Valentine position
Valentine splint
Valentine tube
valgus
valgus deformity
valid
Valin hemilaminectomy self-
    retaining retractor
valise handle graft
vallecula (*pl.* valleculae)
vallecular
vallecular pouch
Valley Lab cautery
Vallis instrument for hair
    transplant
Valls needle biopsy
Valls prosthesis
Valpo splint
Valsalva maneuver
Valsalva sinus
Valtchev uterine manipulator
Valtchev uterine mobilizer
valvanocautery
valve (see also *prosthesis*)
    4-A Magovern heart
      valve
    Abrams-Lucas flap heart
      valve

valve *continued*
    ACMI irrigating valve
    ACMI valve
    Angell-Shiley bio-
      prosthetic valve
    Angell-Shiley xenograft
      prosthetic valve
    Angiocor prosthetic valve
    annuloplasty valve
    aortic valve
    Arenberg-Denver valve
    artificial valve
    atrioventricular valve
    auriculoventricular valve
    ball heart valve
    ball valve
    ball-and-cage prosthetic
      valve
    ball-cage valve
    ball-type valve
    Bard-Apter valve
    Bauer air valve
    Bauhin valve
    Beall heart valve
    Beall prosthetic valve
    Beall valve
    Beall-Surgitool ball-cage
      prosthetic valve
    Beall-Surgitool disk
      prosthetic valve
    Beall-Surgitool prosthetic
      valve
    Bennett valve
    Bicer-val prosthetic valve
    bicuspid aortic valve
    bicuspid valve
    bileaflet heart valve
    bileaflet tilting-disk
      prosthetic valve
    Biocor heart valve
    Biocor prosthetic valve
    bioprosthetic heart
      valve
    bioprosthetic valve
    Bio-Vascular prosthetic
      valve
    Björk-Shiley heart valve

valve *continued*

Björk-Shiley prosthetic aortic valve
Björk-Shiley prosthetic mitral valve
Blom-Singer post-laryngectomy valve
Blom-Singer voice valve
Bochdalek valve
bovine heart valve
Braunwald valve
Braunwald-Cutter caged-ball heart valve
Brauwald-Cutter prosthetic valve
bronchial check-valve
butterfly heart valve
C-C heart valve (convexoconcave heart valve)
caged-ball heart valve
caged-disk heart valve
Capetown aortic prosthetic valve
cardiac valve
Carpentier valve
Carpentier-Edwards bioprosthetic valve
Carpentier-Edwards mitral annuloplasty valve
Carpentier-Edwards pericardial valve
Carpentier-Edwards porcine prosthetic valve
Carpentier-Edwards valve
caval valve
colic valve
commissural pulmonary valve
convexoconcave disk prosthetic valve
Cooley-Bloodwell low profile valve
Cooley-Bloodwell-Cutter valve

valve *continued*

Cooley-Cutter disk prosthetic valve
Coratomic prosthetic valve
Cross-Jones mitral valve
CSF flushing valve
Cutter mitral valve
Cutter-Smeloff disk valve
Cutter-Smeloff heart valve
Cutter-Smeloff mitral valve
DeBakey heart valve
DeBakey-Surgitool prosthetic valve
Delrin heart valve
Denver-Krupin valve
disk valve
double-angled valve
dysplastic valve
eccentric monocuspid tilting-disk prosthetic valve
echo-dense valve
ectatic aortic valve
Edmark mitral valve
Edwards heart valve
Edwards-Carpentier aortic valve brush
Edwards-Duromedics bileaflet valve heart valve
Edwards-Duromedics prosthetic valve
Edwards-Duromedics valve
Elgiloy frame of prosthetic valve
esophagogastric flap valve
eustachian valve
fenestrated valve
fibrotic mitral valve
flail mitral valve
floating disk heart valve
floppy mitral valve
flushing valve

valve *continued*

Foltz valve
free-hand allograft valve
glutaraldehyde-tanned
    bovine heart valve
glutaraldehyde-tanned
    porcine heart valve
Gott butterfly heart
    valve
Gott valve
Guangzhou GD-1
    prosthetic valve
Hakim valve
Hall prosthetic heart
    valve
Hall-Kaster disk pros-
    thetic valve
Hall-Kaster heart valve
Hancock aortic 242
    prosthetic valve
Hancock bioprosthetic
    valve
Hancock pericardial
    prosthetic valve
Hancock porcine
    heterograft heart valve
Hancock porcine
    heterograft valve
Hancock valve
Harken prosthetic valve
Harken valve
Hasner valve
heart valve
Heimlich valve
Heister valve
Hemex prosthetic valve
heterograft valve
Heyer valve
Heyer-Pudenz valve
hinged-leaflet aortic
    valve
hockey-stick tricuspid
    valve
Holter valve
homograft valve
Houston valve
Hufnagel disk heart
    valve

valve *continued*

Hufnagel caged-ball
    heart valve
Hufnagel prosthetic
    valve
Hufnagel valve
Huschke valve
hypoplastic valve
ileocecal valve
Ionescu valve
Ionescu-Shiley bio-
    prosthetic valve
Ionescu-Shiley bovine
    pericardial valve
Ionescu-Shiley heart
    valve
Ionescu-Shiley pericar-
    dial valve graft
Ionescu-Shiley porcine
    heterograft heart
    valve
Ionescu-Shiley standard
    pericardial prosthetic
    valve
Ionescu-Shiley valve
irrigating valve
Jatene-Macchi prosthetic
    valve
Kay-Shiley disk pros-
    thetic valve
Kay-Shiley mitral valve
Kerckring valve
Krupin glaucoma valve
Krupin valve
Krupin-Denver eye valve
LeVeen valve
Lillehei-Kaster pivoting-
    disk prosthetic valve
Liotta-BioImplant
    prosthetic valve
lipomatous ileocecal
    valve
Magnuson valve
Magovern-Cromie ball-
    cage prosthetic valve
Medtronic Hancock valve
Medtronic prosthetic
    valve

valve *continued*

- Medtronic-Hall heart valve
- Medtronic-Hall monocuspid tilting-disk valve
- Mischler valve
- mitral valve
- Mitroflow pericardial prosthetic valve
- monocuspid tilting-disk heart valve
- monostrut valve
- native valve
- nipple valve
- nonrebreathing valve
- Omnicarbon prosthetic valve
- Omniscience heart valve
- Omniscience prosthetic valve
- Omniscience tilting-disk valve
- Panje voice valve
- parachute mitral valve
- parachute valve
- Pemco prosthetic valve
- peristaltic valve
- pivotal disk heart valve
- poppet valve
- porcine heart valve
- porcine valve
- prosthetic ball valve
- prosthetic heart valve
- prosthetic valve
- Pudenz valve
- Pudenz-Heyer-Schulte valve
- Puig Massana-Shiley annuloplasty valve
- pulmonary valve
- pulmonic valve
- Pyrolite heart valve
- quadricuspid pulmonary valve
- Raimondi spring peritoneal valve

valve *continued*

- rectal valve
- reducing valve
- rheumatic mitral valve
- Rigby bivalve retractor
- Sanders valve
- SCDK-Cutter valve
- Schulte valve
- semilunar valve
- Sheldon-Pudenz valve
- Shiley heart valve
- Shiley valve
- Silastic disk heart valve
- silicone ball heart valve
- Singer-Blom valve
- Smeloff prosthetic valve
- Smeloff-Cutter ball-cage prosthetic valve
- Sophy pressure valve
- Sophy valve
- Sorin cardiac prosthetic valve
- Sorin prosthetic valve
- spiral valve
- Spitz-Holter valve
- Spivack valve
- St. Jude bileaflet prosthetic valve
- St. Jude Medical bileaflet heart valve
- St. Jude Medical prosthetic heart valve
- St. Jude valve
- Starr ball heart valve
- Starr-Bloodwell low profile valve
- Starr-Edwards heart valve
- Starr-Edwards prosthetic aortic valve
- Starr-Edwards prosthetic ball valve
- Starr-Edwards prosthetic mitral valve
- Starr-Edwards prosthetic valve
- Starr-Edwards Silastic valve

valve *continued*

Starr-Edwards silicone
    rubber ball valve
Starr-Edwards valve
Surgitool prosthetic valve
Tascon prosthetic valve
thebesian valve
three-legged cage heart
    valve
tilting-disk heart valve
tilting-disk valve
titanium ball heart valve
titanium cage heart valve
track valve
tricuspid aortic valve
tricuspid valve
trivalve
trunk valve
UCI-Barnard aortic valve
UCI-Barnard valve
Ultracor prosthetic valve
unicommissural aortic
    valve
Vascor porcine prosthetic
    valve
VentEasy II isolation
    valve
ventricular valve
Wada-Cutter disk
    prosthetic valve
Wessex prosthetic valve
xenograft heart valve
Xenomedica prosthetic
    valve
valve dilator
valve formation
valve holder
valve hook
valve of Bauhin
valve of Heister
valve of Houston
valve of Kerckring
valve outflow strut
valve prosthesis
valve replacement
valve ring
valve scissors

valve structure
valve tip
valve tube
valved graft
valvotome
valvotomy
valvotomy knife
valvula (*pl.* valvulae)
valvula ileocolica
valvula pylori
valvular defect
valvular disease
valvular insufficiency
valvular sclerosis
valvular stenosis
valvulectomy
valvuloplasty
valvuloplasty balloon
    catheter
valvulotome

Bailey-Glover-O'Neill
    valvulotome
Bakst valvulotome
bread-knife valvulotome
Brock valvulotome
cardiovalvulotome
Carmody valvulotome
curved valvulotome
Derra valvulotome
Dogliotti valvulotome
expansile valvulotome
Gerbode mitral valvulo-
    tome
Gohrbrand valvulotome
Harken valvulotome
Himmelstein pulmonary
    valvulotome
Himmelstein valvulotome
Leather venous valvulo-
    tome
LeMaitre valvulotome
Longmire valvulotome
Longmire-Mueller curved
    valvulotome
Malm-Himmelstein
    pulmonary valvulo-
    tome

valvulotome *continued*
  Malm-Himmelstein valvulotome
  Mills valvulotome
  Niedner valvulotome
  Potts expansile valvulotome
  Potts valvulotome
  Potts-Riker valvulotome
  pulmonary valvulotome
  Sellor valvulotome
  Tubbs valvulotome
  Universal malleable valvulotome
valvulotomy
Van Alyea antral cannula
Van Alyea antral trocar
Van Alyea cannula
Van Alyea trocar
Van Alyea tube
van Buren cervix syringe
van Buren dilator
van Buren forceps
van Buren operation
van Buren sequestrum forceps
van Buren sound
van Buren urethral sound
Van de Graaf generator
Van Doren forceps
Van Doren uterine biopsy punch forceps
Van Doren uterine forceps
Van Gorder approach
Van Gorder arthrodesis
Van Gorder operation
Van Hillman suture
van Hook operation
van Hook ureteroureterostomy
van Hoorn maneuver
Van Hove bag
Van Lint akinesia
Van Lint block
Van Lint conjunctival flap
Van Lint injection
Van Lint technique
Van Lint-Atkinson akinesia
Van Lint-Atkinson block

Van Lint-Atkinson lid akinetic block
Van Lint-O'Brien akinesia
van Loonen operating keratoscope
Van Mandach capsule fragment and clot forceps
Van Millingen eyelid repair technique
Van Millingen graft
Van Millingen operation
van Ness rotation
Van Osdel antral wash bottle
Van Osdel guillotine
Van Osdel irrigating cannula
Van Osdel tonsillar enucleator
Van Osdel tonsillar enucleator tonsillectome
Van Osdel tonsillar knife
Van Osdel tonsillectome
Van Rosen splint
Van Slyke analysis
van Sonnenberg catheter
van Sonnenberg sump
van Sonnenberg sump catheter
van Sonnenberg sump drain
Van Struyken forceps
Van Struyken nasal forceps
Van Struyken nasal punch
Van Struyken punch
Van Tassel angled pigtail catheter
Van Tassel pigtail catheter
Vander Pool sterilizer forceps
Vanderbilt clamp
Vanderbilt deep vessel forceps
Vanderbilt forceps
Vanderbilt University hemostatic forceps
Vanderbilt University vessel clamp
Vanderbilt vessel clamp
Vanghetti cineplasty
Vanghetti limb prosthesis
Vanghetti prosthesis
Vannas abscess knife
Vannas capsulotomy scissors

Vannas corneal scissors
Vannas fixation forceps
Vannas knife
Vannas microcapsulotomy
    scissors
Vannas scissors
Vantage tube-occluding forceps
Vantec dilator
Vantos vacuum
Vantos vacuum extraction
vapor
vaporization
vaporizer
vaporizing diseased tissue
Varco dissecting clamp
Varco forceps
Varco gallbladder forceps
Varco thoracic forceps
variability
variable findings
variable rate pacemaker
variable resistance exercise
variance
vari-angle clip applier
variant
variation
variceal bleed
variceal decompression
variceal wall
varices (*sing.* varix)
Varick elastic dressing
varicocele
varicocele ligation
varicocelectomy
varicose
varicose aneurysm
varicose ulceration
varicose ulcers
varicose veins
varicosity
varicotomy
variegated lesions
Variflex catheter
Varigray implant
Varigray lens implant
Varilux implant
varix (*pl.* varices)

varus
varus knee
varus osteotomy
varying
vas (*pl.* vasa)
vas aberrans
vas clamp
vas deferens (*pl.* vasa deferen-
    tia)
vas efferens
vas hook
vas isolation forceps
Vas projectors
Vas recorder
vasa (*sing.* vas)
vasa brevia
vasa deferentia
vasa nervorum
Vas-Cath
Vasconcelos amputation
Vasconcelos-Barretto clamp
Vasconez tensor fascia lata flap
Vasco-Posada orbital retractor
Vascor porcine prosthetic valve
Vascu-Flo carotid shunt
vascular
vascular anastomosis
vascular angiography
vascular bed
vascular catheter
vascular channel
vascular circle of optic nerve
vascular clamp
vascular clip
vascular collapse
vascular compromise
vascular congestion
vascular dilator
vascular dissector
vascular engorgement
vascular epiploic arch
vascular extravasation
vascular forceps
vascular graft
vascular graft clamp
vascular loop
vascular malformation

vascular needle holder
vascular nerve
vascular nevus
vascular obstruction
vascular occlusion
vascular pattern
vascular pedicle
vascular permeability
vascular prosthesis
vascular reconstruction
vascular redistribution
vascular reflex
vascular resistance
vascular retractor
vascular ring
vascular scissors
vascular sheath
vascular silk sutures
vascular spasm
vascular structure
vascular system
vascular tape
vascular tissue
vascular tissue forceps
vascular tunic
vascularis, nervus
vascularity
vascularization
vascularize
vascular/venous assist device
   (VAD)
vasculature
vasculitic lesion
Vasculour II DeBakey graft
Vascushunt
vascustat
Vascutech circular blade
Vascutek vascular prosthesis
vasectomized
vasectomy
vasectomy forceps
vasectomy reversal
Vaseline dressing
Vaseline gauze
Vaseline gauze dressing
Vaseline petrolatum gauze
   dressing

Vaseline petrolatum packing
Vaseline wick dressing
Vasocillator fracture appliance
vasoconstriction
vasoconstrictor nerve
vasodepression
vasodepressor material
vasodilatation
vasodilation
vasodilator
vasoepididymectomy
vasoepididymostomy
vasogram
vasography
vasoligation
vasomotor
vasomotor activity
vasomotor center
vaso-orchidostomy
vasopressor
vasopressor agent
vasopressor reflex
vasopuncture
vasoresection
vasorrhaphy
vasosection
vasosensory nerve
vasospasm
vasospastic angina
vasostomy
vasotomy
vasotribe
vasotripsy
vasovagal attack
vasovasostomy
vasovasostomy clamp
vasovesiculectomy
vastus intermedius, musculus
vastus lateralis, musculus
vastus medialis, musculus
vastus medialis obliquus,
   musculus (VMO)
VAT pacemaker
Vater ampulla
Vater papilla
VATER syndrome
Vaughan abscess knife

Vasoseal (Dr. Dash) per

Vaughan periosteotome
Vaughn sterilizer forceps
vault
Vaumgartner Vital needle
    holder
VBAC (vaginal birth after
    cesarean section)
VBG (vertical-banded gastro-
    plasty)
VCE smears (vaginal, cervical,
    endocervical smears)
VCUG (voiding cystourethro-
    gram; vesicoureterogram)
VDD pacemaker
Veau cleft lip repair
Veau elevator
Veau operation
Veau palatoplasty
Veau straight-line closure
Veau-Axhausen operation
Veau-Wardill palatal push-back
Veau-Wardill palatoplasty
Veau-Wardill-Kilner cleft palate
    repair
vectis
vectis blade
vectis cesarean section forceps
vectis forceps
vector
vector guide to knee system
    from Dyonics
vector loop
vector lunate joint
vectorcardiogram
vectorcardiography
VED (vacuum erection device)
Veeder tip sling
Veenema retractor
Veenema retropubic retractor
Veenema retropubic self-
    retaining retractor
Veenema-Gusberg needle
Veenema-Gusberg prostatic
    biopsy punch
Veenema-Gusberg prostatic
    punch
Veenema-Gusberg punch

vegetation growth
vegetations
vegetative lesions
Veidenheimer clamp
Veillon tube
vein
vein dilator
vein graft
vein of Galen
vein of Labbé
vein of Thebesius
vein patch graft
vein retractor
vein sign
vein stripper (see also *stripper*)
    Babcock jointed vein
      stripper
    Babcock vein stripper
    Cannon vein stripper
    Clark vein stripper
    Codman vein stripper
    Cole polyethylene vein
      stripper
    Cole vein stripper
    Doyle vein stripper
    Emerson vein stripper
    external vein stripper
    Friedman vein stripper
    hydraulic vein stripper
    internal vein stripper
    jointed vein stripper
    Keeley vein stripper
    Kurten vein stripper
    Lempka vein stripper
    Linton vein stripper
    Mayo vein stripper
    Mayo-Myers external
      vein stripper
    Myers vein stripper
    Nabatoff vein stripper
    polyethylene vein
      stripper
    Samuels vein stripper
    spiral vein stripper
    Trace vein stripper
    vein stripper
    Webb vein stripper

vein stripper *continued*
    Wilson vein stripper
    Wurth vein stripper
    Zollinger-Gilmore
        intraluminal vein
        stripper
    Zollinger-Gilmore vein
        stripper
vein stripping
Veirs canaliculus rod
Veirs cannula
Veirs malleable rod
Veirs needle
Veirs operation
Veirs rod
Veirs trocar
velamenta cerebri
velamentum (*pl.* velamenta)
Velcro belt
Velcro binder
Velcro crackles
Velcro dressing
Velcro fastener dressing
Velcro rales
Velcro rales in lungs
Velcro splint
Velcro tapes
Velcro tourniquet
Veleanu-Rosianu-Ionescu
    procedure
Veley head holder
Veley headrest
Velket-Velcro tourniquet
Vella fistula
velocimetry
velocity
velopharyngeal portal
velopharynx
velour graft
velour patch
Velpeau axillary view
Velpeau bandage
Velpeau cast
Velpeau deformity
Velpeau dressing
Velpeau hernia
Velpeau sling

Velpeau sling-dressing
Velpeau stockinette dressing
Velpeau tendon transfer
Velroc dressing
velvet-eye tube
vena (*pl.* venae) (see specific
    venae)
vena azygos
vena cava
vena cava to pulmonary artery
    shunt
vena cava-gallbladder line
vena caval cannula
vena caval clamp
vena caval clip
vena caval forceps
vena caval obstruction
vena caval scissors
vena caval umbrella
vena caval umbrella filter
vena comitans of hypoglossal
    nerve
Venable bone plate
Venable hip screw
Venable plate
Venable screw
Venable-Stuck fracture pin
Venable-Stuck nail
Venable-Stuck pin
venacavogram
venacavography
venectomy
venereal
venereal wart
VenES antiembolism stockings
VenES II Medical stockings
VenES vascular stocking
venesection
venesuture
Venflon cannula
venipuncture
venipuncture needle
venipuncture side
venisection
venisuture
venocapillary congestion
Venocath

venoclysis
venoclysis cannula
Venodyne pneumatic inflation device
venogram
venography
veno-occlusive disease
venoperitoneostomy
venorrhaphy
venotomy
venotripsy
venous
venous access
venous anastomosis
venous aneurysm
venous angiocardiography
venous angle
venous aortography
venous bifurcation
venous bleeding
venous cannula
venous cannulation
venous capacitance bed
venous catheter
venous claudication
venous congestion
venous cutdown
venous distention
venous drainage
venous embolism
venous engorgement
venous flow
venous graft
venous hemorrhage
venous insufficiency
venous intravasation
venous lakes
venous needle
venous obstruction
venous plexus
venous pressure
venous pressure gradient support stockings (VPGSS)
venous pulse
venous puncture
venous reflux
venous return

venous sheath
venous shunt
venous sinus of dura mater
venous spread
venous stasis
venous thrombectomy catheter
venous thromboembolism
venous thrombosis
venous ulcer
venous vertebral plexus
venous wave
venous web  *Ventak PRX III*
venovenostomy
venovenous bypass
Ventak AICD (automatic implantable cardioverter-defibrillator)
Ventak AICD pacemaker
VentEasy II isolation valve
Ventfoam traction dressing
Venti mask
ventilation
ventilation bronchoscope
ventilation perfusion scan
ventilation tube
ventilation-perfusion defect
ventilation-perfusion lung scan (V/Q lung scan)
ventilator
   Bear adult-volume ventilator
   Bear Cub infant ventilator
   Bear ventilator
   Bennett pressure-cycled ventilator
   Bennett ventilator
   Bio-Med MVP-10 pediatric ventilator
   Bird pressure-cycled ventilator
   blow-by ventilator
   Bourns infant ventilator
   Bourns-Bear ventilator
   Carass ventilator
   IVAC ventilator
   mechanical ventilator

ventilator *continued*
    Monaghan ventilator
    Morch ventilator
    Ohio critical care
      ventilator
    pneuPAC ventilator
    Puritan-Bennett ventila-
      tor
    Sechrist infant ventilator
    Sechrist neonatal
      ventilator
    Servo ventilator
    Siemens Servo ventilator
    Venturi ventilator
    Vix infant ventilator
ventilatory assistance
ventilatory capacity
ventilatory equivalent
venting aortic Bengash needle
venting catheter
ventral
ventral aorta
ventral aspect
ventral celiotomy
ventral cleft of thyroid cartilage
ventral column
ventral hernia
ventral hernia repair
ventral herniorrhaphy
ventral nerve root
ventral nerve root rhizotomy
ventral root
ventral sacrococcygeal muscle
ventral septal defect
ventral surface
ventricle
Ventricor pacemaker
ventricular aneurysm
ventricular angiogram
ventricular aqueduct
ventricular assist device (VAD)
ventricular band
ventricular bigeminy
ventricular block
ventricular cannula
ventricular capture
ventricular catheter

ventricular catheter introducer
ventricular contraction
ventricular defect
ventricular demand pacemaker
ventricular ejection
ventricular end-diastolic
    pressure
ventricular enlargement
ventricular exclusion
ventricular failure
ventricular fibrillation (V-fib)
ventricular flow tract
ventricular fluid
ventricular flutter
ventricular fold
ventricular ganglion
ventricular heart failure
ventricular hypertrophy
ventricular laryngocele
ventricular lead
ventricular ligament
ventricular loop
ventricular needle
ventricular outflow tract
ventricular pacemaker
ventricular pressure
ventricular puncture
ventricular rate
ventricular response
ventricular sacculation
ventricular septal defect (VSD)
ventricular system
ventricular tachycardia
ventricular tap
ventricular trigeminy
ventricular valve
ventricular ventilation tube
ventricular wall
ventricular-suppressed
    pacemaker
ventricular-triggered pacemaker
ventriculoarterial graft
ventriculoatrial shunt
ventriculoatriostomy
ventriculocaval shunt
ventriculocholecystostomy
ventriculocisternal shunt

ventriculocisternostomy
ventriculocordectomy
ventriculogram
ventriculogram retractor
ventriculography
ventriculography catheter
ventriculomyocardiotomy
ventriculomyotomy
ventriculoperitoneal shunt (VP shunt)
ventriculoperitoneostomy
ventriculopuncture
ventriculorrhaphy
ventriculoscope
ventriculoscopy
ventriculoseptal defect
ventriculoseptopexy
ventriculoseptoplasty
ventriculostomy
ventriculotomy
ventriculovenostomy
ventrigulography
ventrocystorrhaphy
ventrofixation of uterus
ventrohysteropexy
Ventrol Levin tube
ventrolateral mass
ventroposterolateral (VPL)
ventroposterolateral thalamic electrode (VPL thalamic electrode)
ventrorostral
ventroscopy
ventrosuspension of uterus
ventrotomy
Venturi apparatus
Venturi insufflator
Venturi mask
Venturi spirometer
Venturi tube
Venturi ventilation adapter
Venturi ventilator
venule engorgement
VEP (visual evoked potential)
VER (visual evoked response)
Veraguth fold
Verbrugge bone clamp

Verbrugge bone-holding forceps
Verbrugge clamp
Verbrugge forceps
Verbrugge retractor
Verbrugge-Souttar craniotome
Verdan graft
Verdan hand procedure
Verdan tendon repair
Verdi scissors
Veress cannula
Veress laparoscopic cannula
Veress needle
Veress spring-loaded laparoscopy needle
Veress trocar
Veress-Frangenheim needle
Verga lacrimal groove
verge
Verhoeff advancement
Verhoeff capsule forceps
Verhoeff cataract forceps
Verhoeff dissecting scissors
Verhoeff expressor
Verhoeff forceps
Verhoeff operation
Verhoeff scissors
Verhoeff sclerotomy
Verhoeff sutures
Verhoeff-Chandler operation
verification
verified
VeriFlex guide wire
Veri-Soft graft
Verlow brace
Vermale amputation
Vermale operation
vermicular
vermicular appendage
vermiculation
vermiculous
vermiform
vermiform appendix
vermiform process
vermifugal
vermilion
vermilion border

vermilion laceration
vermilion margin
vermilion surface of lip
vermilionectomy
verminous aneurysm
vermis
vermis incision
vermis of cerebellum
Verner operation for talipes
    equinovarus
Verneuil operation
Vernier calipers
Vernon antral tube
Vernon scissors
Vernon tube
Vernon-David operation
Vernon-David proctoscope
Vernon-David speculum
verruca (*pl.* verrucae)
verruca acuminata
verruca digitata
verruca filiformis
verruca plana
verruca plantaris
verruca vulgaris
verrucae (*sing.* verruca)
verrucous carcinoma
verrucous lesion
Versadopp Doppler probe
Versafil tissue expander
Versaflex steerable catheter
Versatrax cardiac pacemaker
Versatrax II pacemaker
Versatrax pacemaker
Versed anesthesia
versicolor
version
versus
vertebra (*pl.* vertebrae)
vertebrae cervicales
vertebrae coccygeae
vertebrae lumbales
vertebrae sacrales
vertebrae thoracicae
vertebral angiography
vertebral arch
vertebral arch fusion defect

vertebral arteriogram
vertebral arteriography
vertebral artery
vertebral body
vertebral body biopsy instru-
    ments
vertebral body impactor
vertebral canal
vertebral column
vertebral disk
vertebral endplate
vertebral epiphysitis
vertebral foramen
vertebral ganglion
vertebral interspace
vertebral nerve
vertebral notch
vertebral outgrowth
vertebral plexus
vertebral prominence
vertebral region
vertebral ribs
vertebral spine
vertebral spreader
vertebral surface
vertebral vein
vertebralis, arteria
vertebralis, nervus
vertebralis, vena
vertebrated catheter
vertebrated probe
vertebrectomy
vertebrocostal
vertebrocostal ribs
vertebromammary diameter
vertebrosacral
vertebrosternal ribs
vertex
vertex presentation
vertical
vertical axis
vertical bone self-retaining
    retractor
vertical bur-hole incision
vertical elliptical incision
vertical flap pyeloplasty
vertical groove

vertical incision
vertical lateral parapatellar
    incision
vertical mattress sutures
vertical midline incision
vertical muscle
vertical overlap
vertical plane
vertical retractor
vertical ring curet
vertical ring gastroplasty (VRG)
vertical Silastic ring gastroplasty
vertical sternotomy
vertical sutures
vertical talus
vertical tract
vertical tube
vertical-banded gastroplasty
    (VBG)
verticalis linguae, musculus
verticality
verticosubmental projection
verumontanum
Verwey eyelid operation
Verwey operation
vesalian bone
vesalian vein
Vesely nail
Vesely-Street nail
vesical
vesical artery
vesical fascia
vesical fistula
vesical hernia
vesical orifice
vesical retinaculum
vesical retractor
vesicales superiores, arteriae
vesicalis inferior, arteria
vesicle
vesicoabdominal fistula
vesicocervical fistula
vesicoclysis
vesicocutaneous fistula
vesicoenteric fistula
vesicofixation
vesicointestinal

vesicointestinal reflex
vesicolithotomy
vesicoperineal fistula
vesicoprostatic calculus
vesicoprostatic plexus
vesicosigmoidostomy
vesicospinal center
vesicostomy
vesicotomy
vesicoureteral fistula
vesicoureteral reflux
vesicoureterogram (VCUG)
vesicourethral orifice
vesicourethral suspension
vesicourethroplasty
vesicouterine deflection
vesicouterine excavation
vesicouterine fistula
vesicouterine ligament
vesicouterine peritoneum
vesicouterine pouch
vesicovaginal fascia
vesicovaginal fistula
vesicovaginal lithotomy
vesicular
vesicular appendages
vesiculation
vesiculectomy
vesiculography
vesiculotomy
Vesi-loop
vessel
vessel band
vessel clamp
vessel clip
vessel clip-applying forceps
vessel forceps
vessel knife
vessel loop
vessel pediatric forceps
vessel peripheral clamp
vessel peripheral forceps
vessel prosthesis
vessel punch
vessel-occluding clamp
Vest lens
vest restraint

Vest technique
Vest telescope
VEST traction sutures
vestibular canal
vestibular clamp
vestibular disease
vestibular dysfunction
vestibular fold
vestibular function
vestibular ganglion
vestibular gland
vestibular ligament
vestibular nerve
vestibular osteotomy
vestibular region
vestibular saccule
vestibular trough
vestibular veins
vestibular window
vestibulares, venae
vestibule
vestibule of inner ear
vestibule of vagina
vestibulocochlear nerve (cranial
    nerve VIII)
vestibulocochlearis, nervus
vestibuloplasty
vestibulotomy
vestige
vestigial
vestigial muscle
vestigial nodule
vest-over-pants hernia repair
vest-over-pants herniorrhaphy
vest-over-pants inguinal
    herniorrhaphy
vest-over-pants technique
Vezien scissors
viability
viable
Viamonte-Hobbs dye injector
Viamonte-Hobbs electrosurgical
    unit
Viamonte-Hobbs injector
    hydrotherapy
Viamonte-Jutzy electrosurgical
    unit

Viboch graft retractor
vibrametry
vibratory hammer
vibratory massage
vibrocardiography study
Vibrodilator
Vibrodilator probe
Vicat needle
vice-grip pliers
Vick-Blanchard forceps
Vick-Blanchard hemorrhoidal
    forceps
Vickers microsurgical instru-
    ment
Vickers Venti-mask
Vicor pacemaker
Vicq d'Azyr bundle
Vicq d'Azyr operation of larynx
Vicryl pop-off sutures
Vicryl SH sutures
Vicryl sutures
Victor blood lancet knife
Victor-Gomel microsurgical
    tubal reconstruction
Victorian collar dressing
Victorian collar-type dressing
Vidal device
Vidal operation
Vidal operation for varicocele
Vidal-Ardrey modified Hoffman
    device
Vidal-Hoffman fixator frame
video endoscope
video endoscope system
video image
video image colonoscope
video image gastrointestinal
    scope
videolaseroscopy
video-stroboscopy
vidian canal
vidian nerve
vidianectomy
Vidicon vacuum chamber
    pickup tube
Vidicon vacuum tube
Vi-Drape dressing

Vi-Drape surgical film
Vienna nasal speculum
Vienna speculum
Vienna wire sutures
Viers erysiphake
Viers rod
Vieussens annulus
Vieussens loop
Vieussens veins
Vieussens ventricle
view
viewing instrument
Vigger-5 eye forceps
Vigilon drain
Vigilon dressing
vigorous
Vilbiss-Miller speculum
Villard button
villi (*sing.* villus)
villoglandular
villoglandular polyp
villoma
villous adenoma
villous polyp
villus (*pl.* villi)
villusectomy
Vim Gabriel aspirating syringe
Vim needle
Vim tonsil syringe
Vim-Silverman needle
Vim-Silverman technique for
    liver biopsy
VIN (vulvar intraepithelial
    neoplasia)
Vineberg cardiac revasculariza-
    tion
Vineberg operation
Vinethene and ether
Vinke retractor
Vinke skull tractor
Vinke tong skull traction
Vinke tong traction
Vinke tongs
Vinke tractor
vinyl ether anesthetic agent
vinyl ethyl ether anesthetic
    agent

Vioform dressing
Vioform gauze dressing
violaceous
violin-string adhesions
VIP chemotherapy pump
Virchow brain knife
Virchow chisel
Virchow knife
Virchow node
Virchow sentinel node
Virchow skin graft knife
Virchow space
Virchow-Troisier node
Virden catheter
virgin silk sutures
virginal abdomen
virginal introitus
Viro-Tec sutures
virtual cautery
Virtus forceps
Virtus splinter forceps
virulent
virulent appendix
virulent cancer
Visatec cystotome
VISC (vitreous infusion suction
    cutter)
viscera (*sing.* viscus)
viscera-holding forceps
visceral angiography
visceral aortography
visceral arteriography
visceral forceps
visceral lamina
visceral muscle
visceral pain
visceral peritoneum
visceral pleura
visceral surface
viscerocardiac reflex
visceromotor manifestations
visceromotor reflex
visceroparietal
visceroparietal suture
visceroperitoneal
visceropleural
visceroptosis

viscerosensory
viscerosensory reflex
viscerotrophic reflex
Vischer incision
Vischer lumboiliac incision
viscid
viscidity
Visco surgery
Viscoat
viscoelastic
viscoelastic agents
viscosity
viscous bile
viscus (*pl.* viscera)
viscus perforation
vise forceps
VISI (volar intercalated segmental instability)
Visi-Black needle
Visi-Black surgical needle
Visitec anterior chamber cannula
Visitec cannula
Visitec cystotome
Visitec needle
Visitec retrobulbar needle
visor flap operation
Vi-Spray
Vista pacemaker
Vista T pacemaker generator
Vistaril
Vistec sponge
Vistec x-ray detectable sponge
visual evoked potential (VEP)
visual evoked response (VER)
visual hemostatic forceps
visual inspection
visual line
visualization
visualized
visualizing
Visulas Nd:YAG laser
visuscope
Vitacuff
Vitagraft arteriovenous shunt
Vitagraft vascular graft
vital capacity

Vital Cooley microvascular needle holder
Vital forceps
Vital intestinal forceps
Vital intracardiac needle holder
Vital iris scissors
Vital lung-grasping forceps
Vital needle holder
Vital needle holder forceps
vital organs
Vital Ryder microvascular needle holder
Vital scissors
vital sign
vital sign check
Vital tissue forceps
Vitalcor cardioplegia infusion cannula
Vitalcor catheter
Vitalcor venous catheter
Vitalcor venous return catheter
Vitallium cap
Vitallium clip
Vitallium cup
Vitallium drill
Vitallium eye implant
Vitallium graft
Vitallium hip prosthesis
Vitallium implant
Vitallium mesh
Vitallium Moore prosthesis
Vitallium Moore self-locking prosthesis
Vitallium nail
Vitallium plate
Vitallium prosthesis
Vitallium screw
Vitatrax II pacemaker
Vitatron pacemaker
Vitax female catheter
vitelline circulation
vitelline duct
vitelline vein
vitellointestinal cyst
vitrectomy
vitrectomy tip

vitrector
    Kaufman vitrector
    ocutome vitrector
    Peyman vitrector
vitrector tip
vitreolenticular
vitreous abscess
vitreous base
vitreous body
vitreous cavity
vitreous chamber
vitreous detachment
vitreous floater
vitreous fluff
vitreous fluid
vitreous hemorrhage
vitreous herniation
vitreous humor
vitreous infusion suction cutter
    (VISC)
vitreous knife
vitreous membrane
vitreous opacity
vitreous ossification
vitreous space
vitreous-grasping forceps
Vitrophage Peyman system
Vivalith-10 pacemaker
Vivatron pacemaker
Vivonex jejunostomy catheter
Vivonex Moss tube
Vivonex TEN system
Vivosil graft
Vivosil implant
Vivosil prosthesis
Vix infant ventilator
Vladimiroff (also Wladimiroff)
Vladimiroff operation
Vladimiroff tarsectomy
Vladimiroff-Mikulicz amputation
V.M. & Co. amputating saw
V.M. & Co. mastoid curet
V.M. & Co. ruler calipers
V.M. & Co. screwdriver
VMO (vastus medialis obliquus)
vocal cordectomy
vocal cordotomy
vocal cords

vocal ligament
vocal muscle
vocal process
vocalis, musculus
Vogel adenoid curet
Vogel curet
Vogel infant adenoid curet
Vogel nephropexy
Vogel operation
Vogel otoplasty
Vogt cataract
Vogt forceps
Vogt operation
Vogt point
Vogt-Barraquer eye needle
Vogt-Hueter point
voice box
voice button
voice prosthesis
voice restoration
voiding cystogram
voiding cystourethrogram
    (VCUG)
voiding difficulty
volar artery
volar aspect
volar carpal ligament
volar flap
volar intercalated segmental
    instability (VISI)
volar interosseous fascia
volar ligament
volar pad
volar plate
volar plate injury
volar radiocarpal ligament
volar region
volar shelf arthroplasty
volar splint
volar surface
volatile
Volk conoid implant
Volk conoid ophthalmic lens
Volk Pan retinal lens
Volkmann bone curet
Volkmann bone hook
Volkmann canal
Volkmann contracture

Volkmann curet
Volkmann membrane
Volkmann operation for
    hydrocele
Volkmann oval curet
Volkmann pancreatic calculus
    spoon
Volkmann rake
Volkmann rake retractor
Volkmann retractor
Volkmann splint
Volkmann spoon
Volkmann subluxation
Voller curet
volsella (see *vulsella*)
volsellum (see *vulsellum*)
volt
voltage
voltage clamp
Voltolini ear tube
Voltolini septum speculum
Voltolini speculum
Voltolini tube
Voltz wrist joint prosthesis
volume
volumetric infusion pump
volumetric pump
volumetric solution
voluminous hernia
voluntary activity
voluntary control
voluntary guarding
voluntary movement
voluntary muscle
voluntary voiding
Volutrol
Volutrol apparatus for IV
volvulus
Volz elbow hinge
Volz total elbow
vomer
vomer bone
vomer forceps
vomer osteotome
vomer septal forceps
vomerine groove
vomerine ridge

vomerine spur
vomeronasal cartilage
Von Ammon operation
Von Andel catheter
Von Andel dilation catheter
von Bergmann hernia
von Bergmann operation
von Blaskovics-Doyen opera-
    tion
Von Brunn nests in bladder
    carcinoma
von Burow operation
Von Eichen antral tube
Von Eichen antral wash tube
Von Eichen cannula
Von Eichen tube
von Gies joint
von Graefe (see *Graefe*)
von Haberer gastrectomy
von Haberer gastroenterostomy
von Haberer-Aquirre gastrec-
    tomy
von Haberer-Finney anasto-
    mosis
von Haberer-Finney gastrec-
    tomy
von Haberer-Finney gastro-
    enterostomy
von Hackler operation
von Hippel (see *Hippel*)
von Kraske operation
Von Lackum surcingle
Von Lackum transection shift
    jacket brace
von Langenbeck bipedicle
    mucoperiosteal flap
von Langenbeck cleft lip repair
von Langenbeck flap
von Langenbeck incision
von Langenbeck operation
von Langenbeck periosteal
    elevator
von Mondak forceps
Von Noorden flap
Von Noorden incision
von Petz clamp
von Petz clip

von Petz forceps
von Petz intestinal clamp
von Petz  staple
von Petz stomach clamp
von Petz suturing apparatus
von Pirquet sutures
von Recklinghausen disease
von Rosen hip splint
von Rosen splint
von Rosen view
von Rosen view for determining
    hip dislocation
von Saal medullary pin
von Saal pin
von Seemen rongeur
von Willebrandt knee
Voohr needle holder
Voorhees bag
Voorhees needle
Voris IV disk rongeur
Voris-Oldberg IV disk rongeur
    forceps
Voris-Wester forceps
Voronoff operation
Vorse occluding clamp
Vorse-Webster clamp
Vorse-Webster tube-occluding
    clamp
vortex
vortex vein
Voshell bursa
Voss hanging-hip operation
Vossius lenticular ring
VP shunt (ventriculoperitoneal
    shunt)
VPGSS (venous pressure
    gradient support stockings)
VPI nonadhesive pouch
VPL (ventroposterolateral)
VPL thalamic electrode (ventro-
    posterolateral thalamic
    electrode)
V/Q lung scan (ventilation-
    perfusion lung scan)

VRG (vertical ring gastroplasty)
VSD (ventricular septal defect)
VSP plates
vulcanite bur
vulcanite dental plate
vulnerable
Vulpius operation
Vulpius-Compere operation
Vulpius-Compere procedure for
    tight heel cords
vulsella (*sing.* vulsellum)
vulsella forceps
vulsellum (*pl.* vulsella) (see also
    *forceps*)
    Bland cervical traction
        vulsellum
    Donald vulsellum
    Skene uterine vulsel-
        lum
vulsellum forceps
vulva
vulvar biopsy
vulvar carcinoma
vulvar condylomata
vulvar intraepithelial neoplasia
    (VIN)
vulvar lesions
vulvar neoplasia
vulvectomy
vulvorectal fistula
vulvovaginal
vulvovaginal cyst
vulvovaginal glands
vulvovaginectomy
VVI bipolar Programalith
    pacemaker
VVI pacemaker
VVI single-chamber pace-
    maker
VVI/AAI pacemaker
VVIR single-chamber rate-
    adaptive pacemaker
VVT pacemaker
Vygon Nutricath S catheter

W-hernia
W-plasty
W-plasty in scar revision
W-plasty revision
W-shaped anal anastomosis
W-shaped ileal pouch
W-shaped incision
W-shaped pouch
W-V palatal repositioning
W-Y operation
W-Y palatoplasty
Wachenheim-Reder sign
Wachsberger bur
Wachtenfeldt butterfly clip
Wachtenfeldt clip
Wachtenfeldt clip-applying
    forceps
Wachtenfeldt clip-removing
    forceps
Wachtenfeldt forceps
Wachtenfeldt wound clip
Wada hingeless heart valve
    prosthesis
Wada monocuspid tilting-disk
    heart valve
Wada valve prosthesis
Wada-Cutter disk prosthetic
    valve
wadding
Wadsworth approach
Wadsworth hinge
Wadsworth lid clamp
Wadsworth lid forceps
Wadsworth scissors
Wadsworth-Todd eye cautery
Wagener ear hook
Wagener punch tip
Wagner advancement
Wagner antrum punch

Wagner apparatus
Wagner external fixator
Wagner fracture reduction
Wagner hammer
Wagner hand operation
Wagner laryngeal brush
Wagner leg-lengthening device
Wagner limb-lengthening
    technique
Wagner needle holder
Wagner operation
Wagner procedure to correct
    leg length discrepancy
Wagner punch
Wagner reduction technique
Wagner resurfacing technique
Wagner skull resection
Wagner tibial lengthening
    procedure
wagon wheel fracture
Wagoner approach
Wagoner operation
Wagoner osteotomy
Wagstaffe fracture
Wahl sign
Wainwright osteotomy plate
waisting of nerve contour
waiver and consent
WAK (wearable artificial
    kidney)
Walcher position
Waldeau fixation forceps
Waldeau forceps
Walden telescope
Waldenberg apparatus
Waldeyer colon
Waldeyer fascia
Waldeyer fluid
Waldeyer forceps

Waldeyer glands
Waldeyer ring
Waldeyer sulcus
Waldeyer tonsillar ring
Waldhauer operation
Waldhausen subclavian flap
    repair of coarctation of
    aorta
Wales bougie
Wales dilator
Wales rectal bougie
Walker cautery
Walker curet
Walker dissector
Walker electrode
Walker elevator
Walker everter
Walker forceps
Walker gallbladder retractor
Walker lid everter
Walker lid retractor
Walker needle
Walker pin
Walker retractor
Walker ruptured disk curet
Walker scissors
Walker scleral ruler
Walker tonsil dissector
Walker tonsil suction dissector
Walker trephine
Walker ureteral meatotomy
    electrode
Walker-Apple corneal scissors
Walker-Apple scissors
Walker-Atkinson corneal
    scissors
Walker-Atkinson scissors
Walker-Lee eye knife
Walker-Lee sclerotome
Walker-Murdock wrist sign
walking aids
walking boot
walking brace
walking calipers
walking cast
walking heel
Walkmann episiotomy scissors

wall
wall bracket
Wallace cesarean forceps
Wallach colposcope
Wallach Colpostar-V6
Wallach freezer cryosurgical
    device
Wallach pencil
Wallach pencil cryosurgical
    device
Wallach surgical devices
Wallach ZoomScope
Walldius knee arthroplasty
Walldius knee prosthesis
Walldius prosthesis
Walldius total knee prosthesis
Walldius Vitallium mechanical
    knee prosthesis
wallerian degeneration
Wallich curet
Walsh chisel
Walsh curet
Walsh dermal curet
Walsh forceps
Walsh hook
Walsh hook-type dermal curet
Walsh procedure
Walsham forceps
Walsham nasal forceps
Walsham septal forceps
Walsham septum-straightening
    forceps
Walsham straightener
Walsh-Ogura orbital decom-
    pression
Walter corneal spud
Walter forceps
Walter Reed implant
Walter splinter forceps
Walter spud
Walter-Deaver retractor
Walter-Poole suction tube
Walter-Yankauer suction tube
Walthardt operation
Walther canal
Walther catheter
Walther clamp

*Wall stent (urethral)
? caps - spelling per
Dr. Coles*

Walther dilator
Walther duct
Walther female catheter
Walther forceps
Walther ganglion
Walther kidney pedicle clamp
Walther pedicle clamp
Walther sound
Walther tissue forceps
Walther trocar
Walther urethral dilator
Walther urethral sound
Walther-Crenshaw clamp
Walther-Crenshaw meatus
    clamp
Walton clamp
Walton curet
Walton ear knife
Walton extractor
Walton forceps
Walton foreign body gouge
Walton gouge
Walton knife
Walton meniscus clamp
Walton punch
Walton rib shears
Walton rongeur
Walton round gouge spud
Walton scissors
Walton speculum
Walton-Allis tissue forceps
Walton-Liston bone rongeur
Walton-Pederson speculum
Walton-Ruskin bone rongeur
Walton-Schubert forceps
Walton-Schubert punch
Walton-Schubert uterine biopsy
    forceps
Walton-Vienna speculum
waltzed skin flap
Walzl hysterectomy forceps
Wamarline wrist splint
wandering atrial pacemaker
    (WAP)
wandering gallbladder
wandering heart
wandering kidney

wandering liver
wandering ovary
wandering pacemaker
Wang needle
Wangensteen anastomosis
    clamp
Wangensteen apparatus
Wangensteen awl
Wangensteen carrier
Wangensteen clamp
Wangensteen colostomy
Wangensteen dissector
Wangensteen drain
Wangensteen drainage
Wangensteen dressing
Wangensteen duodenal tube
Wangensteen forceps
Wangensteen gastric-crushing
    anastomotic clamp
Wangensteen herniorrhaphy
Wangensteen ligature carrier
Wangensteen needle
Wangensteen needle holder
Wangensteen operation
Wangensteen retractor
Wangensteen suction
Wangensteen suction tube
Wangensteen tissue forceps
Wangensteen tissue inverter
Wangensteen trocar
Wangensteen tube
waning chest pain
WAP (wandering atrial pace-
    maker)
Wappler cautery
Wappler cold cautery
Wappler cystoscope
Wappler electrode
Ward elevator
Ward triangle
Ward triangle on pelvic x-ray
Ward-French needle
Ward-Hendrick incision
Wardill palatoplasty
Wardill-Kilner cleft palate repair
Wardill-Kilner operation
Ward-Lempert lens

Ward-Mayo operation
Ward-Mayo vaginal hysterectomy
Waring tonsil suction tube
Warm "N" Form cast
Warm "N" Form corset
Warm "N" Form splint
warm moist heat
Warm Springs brace
warmer
warmth and redness
warm-up
Warner-Farber operation
warning sign
warning stop tube
Warren incision
Warren operation
Warren shunt
Warren splenorenal shunt
Warren-Mack drill
wart
Wartenberg sign
Warthen clamp
Warthen crusher
Warthen forceps
Warthen spur crusher
Warthen spur-crushing clamp
Warthin sign
Warthin tumor
warty cicatricial tumor
wash catheter
wash tube
washer-sterilizer
washing catheter
washing tube
washings
Washio skin flap
washout
washout cannula
washout pyelography
Wasko common duct probe
Wasko probe
wasp-waist effect
wasp-waist laryngoscope
Wassel classification of thumb polydactyly
wastage

waste products
wasting of muscle
Watanabe arthroscope
Watanabe arthroscopic system
Watanabe arthroscopy
Watanabe catheter
Watanabe pin remover
Water cesarean section
water cystometer
water dressing
water fissures in lens
water probe
Waterhouse urethroplasty
water-infusion esophageal manometry catheter
watering-can scrotum
Waterman bronchoscope
Waterman folding bronchoscope
Waterman rib contractor
Waterman sump drain
waterproof
Waters operation
Waters position
Waters view of sinuses
Waters x-ray position
water-seal chest tube
water-seal drain
water-seal drainage
water-seal drainage bottle
water-seal drainage system
Waterston extrapericardial anastomosis
Waterston groove
Waterston operation
Waterston pacing wire
Waterston shunt
Waterston-Cooley shunt
Waters-Waldron position
watertight
watertight seal
watery discharge
Watkins operation
Watkins spinal fusion
Watkins suction tube
Watkins transposition operation for uterine prolapse

Watkins-Wertheim operation
Watson forceps
Watson operation
Watson skin-grafting knife
Watson speculum
Watson tonsil-seizing forceps
Watson-Cheyne dissector
Watson-Cheyne dry dissector
Watson-Cheyne wedge resection
Watson-Jones ankle procedure
Watson-Jones approach
Watson-Jones arthrodesis
Watson-Jones bone gouge
Watson-Jones dressing
Watson-Jones elevator
Watson-Jones gouge
Watson-Jones guide pin
Watson-Jones incision
Watson-Jones ligament reconstruction
Watson-Jones nail
Watson-Jones operation
Watson-Jones repair of ankle fracture
Watson-Jones tractor
Watson-Williams ethmoid-biting forceps
Watson-Williams ethmoidal punch
Watson-Williams forceps
Watson-Williams frontal sinus rasp
Watson-Williams intervertebral disk rongeur
Watson-Williams nasal forceps
Watson-Williams nasal polypus
Watson-Williams nasal punch
Watson-Williams needle
Watson-Williams polyp forceps
Watson-Williams punch
Watson-Williams punch tip
Watson-Williams rasp
Watson-Williams rongeur
Watson-Williams sinus rasp
Watson-Williams sinus raspatory

Watt skin closure stapler
Watts clamp
Watts locking clamp
Watts tenaculum
watt-second
Watzke operation
Watzke scissors
Watzke self-holding sleeve operation
Watzke Silicone sleeve
Watzke sleeve
Watzke tube
Waugh ankle prosthesis
Waugh dissection forceps
Waugh knee prosthesis
Waugh operation
Waugh tissue forceps
Waugh-Clagett pancreatico-duodenostomy
wave
wave guide catheter
wavelength
wax (see also *bone wax*)
    bone wax
    casting bone wax
    Horsley bone wax
    Horsley wax
    Mosetig-Moorhof bone wax
    sterile bone wax
wax and wane
wax bougie
waxing and waning
waxlike rigidity
waxlike secretion
wax-tipped bougie
waxy cast
waxy kidney
Wayne laminectomy seat
weak
weakened
weakening
weakly positive
weakly reactive
weakness
wean off ventilator
weaned off bypass

wearable artificial kidney (WAK)
Weary brain spatula
Weary hook
Weary nerve hook
Weary nerve root retractor
Weary spatula
Weavenit graft
Weavenit implant
Weavenit patch graft
Weavenit prosthesis
Weavenit valve prosthesis
Weavenit vascular prosthesis
Weaver chalazion clamp
Weaver chalazion curet
Weaver chalazion forceps
Weaver clamp
Weaver forceps
Weaver sinus probe
Weaver-Dunn repair of acromioclavicular separation
Weaver-Dunn technique
weaver's bottom
web
web ligament
web of fingers
web of larynx
web space
Webb bolt
Webb cannula
Webb nail
Webb pin
Webb retractor
Webb stove bolt
Webb stove nail
Webb stripper
Webb vein stripper
Webb-Balfour abdominal retractor
Webb-Balfour retractor
Webb-Balfour self-retaining retractor
webbed
webbed fingers
webbed toes
webbing

Weber aortic clamp
Weber canaliculus knife
Weber catheter
Weber classification of fractures
Weber colonic insufflator
Weber douche
Weber eye knife
Weber gland
Weber hip implant
Weber implant
Weber insufflator
Weber knife
Weber nasal douche
Weber retractor
Weber scissors
Weber sign
Weber tissue scissors
Weber-Elschnig lens loupe
Weber-Elschnig lens spoon
Weber-Elschnig loupe
Weber-Fergusson incision
Weber-Fergusson-Longmire incision
Weber-Vasey technique
Webril bandage
Webril dressing
Webster abdominal retractor
Webster cheiloplasty
Webster coronary sinus catheter
Webster infusion cannula
Webster infusion tube
Webster knife
Webster meniscectomy scissors
Webster needle holder
Webster operation
Webster retractor
Webster skin graft knife
Webster skin lines
Webster tube
Wechsler obstetrical stethoscope
Weck ceiling-mount operating microscope
Weck clamp
Weck clip
Weck dermatome
Weck electrosurgery pencil

Weck forceps
Weck hemoclip
Weck instrument holder
Weck knife
Weck operating microscope
Weck shears
Weck stapler
Weck suction tube
Weck suture-removal scissors
Weck towel forceps
Weck trephine
Weck tube
Weck-Baggish hysteroscopy
    system
Weck-blade knife
Weck-cel dressing
Weck-cel graft
Weck-cel implant
Weck-cel operating microscope
Weck-cel prosthesis
Weck-cel sponge
Wecker iris spatula
Wecker silver spatula
Wecker spatula
Weck-Harms forceps
Weck-sorb airwick sponge
Weder retractor
Weder tongue depressor
Weder-Solenberger pillar
    retractor
Weder-Solenberger retractor
Weder-Solenberger tonsil pillar
    retractor
wedge arteriogram
wedge biopsy
wedge catheter
wedge colon resection
Wedge Cook catheter
wedge elevator
wedge excisional biopsy
wedge fracture
wedge heel
wedge hepatic biopsy
wedge incision
wedge liver biopsy
wedge of skin

wedge of tissue
wedge ostectomy
wedge osteotomy
wedge pressure
wedge resection
wedge resection clamp
wedge-line needle
wedge-shaped
wedge-shaped sleeve aneurys-
    mal resection
wedging of olisthetic vertebra
wedging of vertebra
Weeks eye forceps
Weeks eye speculum
Weeks needle
Weeks operation
Weeks speculum
weeping
Wegener granulomatosis
Wehmerlite IV-A headlight
Wehrbein hypospadias repair
Wehrbein urethroplasty
Wehrbein-Smith hypospadias
    repair
Weiger-Zollner forceps
weight
weightbearing
weightbearing brace
weighted obstetrical speculum
weighted posterior retractor
weighted radiograph
weighted retractor
weighted speculum
weighted vaginal speculum
weightlifter's headache
weight-reduction operation
Weil cannula
Weil ear forceps
Weil ethmoidal forceps
Weil forceps
Weil lacrimal cannula
Weil pelvic sling
Weil pituitary rongeur
Weil rongeur
Weil sling
Weil splint

Weil-Blakesley intervertebral
disk rongeur
Weinberg blade
Weinberg Joe's hoe double-
ended retractor
Weinberg modification of
pyloroplasty
Weinberg operation
Weinberg pediatric rib spreader
Weinberg pyloroplasty
Weinberg retractor
Weinberg rib spreader
Weinberg spreader
Weinberg vagotomy retractor
Weiner cannula
Weiner operation
Weiner tourniquet
Weingartner ear forceps
Weingartner forceps
Weingartner rongeur
Weinstein intestinal retractor
Weir appendectomy
Weir excision
Weir incision
Weir operation
Weir wedge
Weir-pattern skin flap technique
Weis operation
Weisenbach forceps
Weise-pattern markings
Weisinger operation
Weisman curet
Weisman ear curet
Weisman forceps
Weisman infant ear curet
Weisman tenaculum
Weisman uterine tenaculum
forceps
Weisman-Graves speculum
Weisman-Graves vaginal
speculum
Weiss eye knife
Weiss hook
Weiss needle
Weiss procedure
Weiss speculum

Weiss spring
Weiss-pattern knife
Weitbrecht ligament
Weitlaner brain retractor
Weitlaner hemostat
Weitlaner retractor
Weitlaner self-retaining retractor
Weitter plaster knife
Welch Allyn anal biopsy forceps
Welch Allyn battery handle
Welch Allyn cord handle
Welch Allyn flexible sigmoido-
scope
Welch Allyn forceps
Welch Allyn hook
Welch Allyn instrument
Welch Allyn Kleenspec laryngo-
scope
Welch Allyn laryngoscope
Welch Allyn ophthalmoscope
Welch Allyn otoscope
Welch Allyn probe
Welch Allyn proctoscope
Welch Allyn retinoscope
Welch Allyn sigmoidoscope
Welch Allyn speculum
Welch Allyn suction tube
Welch Allyn transilluminator
Welch Allyn tube
well-aerated lungs
Wellaminski antral perforator
Wellaminski perforator
well-being
well-compensated
well-controlled
well-defined
well-demarcated margin
well-demarcated scar
well-developed
well-differentiated
well-differentiated adenoma
well-epithelialized
Weller cartilage forceps
Weller dissecting scissors
well-healed scar
well-leg cast

well-leg holder
well-leg raising test
well-leg splint
well-leg traction
wellness
well-nourished
well-outlined
Wells cannula
Wells clamp
Wells enucleation scissors
Wells enucleation scoop
Wells enucleation spoon
Wells eye spatula
Wells eye spoon
Wells forceps
Wells irrigator
Wells Johnson cannula
Wells pedicle clamp
Wells pick
Wells posterior rectopexy
Wells rectopexy
Wells scleral suture pick
Wells scoop
Wells spoon
Wells tractor
Wells-Gardner tongs
Welsh erysiphake
Welsh olive-tipped needles
Welsh ophthalmological
    forceps
Welsh pupil spreader-retractor
    forceps
Welt bronchoscopic treatment
    unit
Welt bronchoscopic unit
wen
Wenckebach block
Wenckebach disease
Wenger slotted plate
Werb operation
Werb rhinostomy scissors
Werb scissors
Wermer syndrome
Werner suture
Wernicke area of brain
Wernicke disease
Wernicke sign

Wertheim clamp
Wertheim deep-surgery scissors
Wertheim forceps
Wertheim hysterectomy
Wertheim hysterectomy forceps
Wertheim needle holder
Wertheim operation
Wertheim splint
Wertheim vaginal forceps
Wertheim-Cullen clamp
Wertheim-Cullen forceps
Wertheim-Cullen pedicle clamp
Wertheim-Cullen pedicle
    forceps
Wertheim-Navratil needle
Wertheim-Reverdin clamp
Wertheim-Reverdin pedicle
    clamp
Wertheim-Schauta operation
Wertheim-Taussig operation
Wesley Jessen lens
Wesolowski bifurcation
    replacement
Wesolowski bypass graft
Wesolowski Dacron tube
Wesolowski prosthesis
Wesolowski Teflon graft
Wesolowski Weavenit vascular
    prosthesis
Wess vectis
Wessex prosthetic valve
Wesson mouth gag
Wesson perineal retractor
Wesson perineal self-retaining
    retractor
Wesson retractor
West blunt elevator
West bone chisel
West bone gouge
West cannula
West chisel
West gouge
West hand dissector
West lacrimal cannula
West nasal-dressing forceps
West operation
West osteotome

West patellectomy
West plastic dissector
West Point view of shoulder on x-ray
West tube
West-Beck periosteotome
West-Beck spoon curet
Westcott microscissors
Westcott scissors
Westcott tenotomy scissors
Westcott-Scheie scissors
Wester clamp
Wester scissors
Westerman-Jansen needle
Westlake bull's eye bulb
Westmacott dressing forceps
Westmacott forceps
Weston rectal snare
Westphal forceps
Westphal gall duct forceps
Westphal hemostat
Westphal sign
West-Soto-Hall knee procedure
wet bandage
wet colostomy
wet cup
wet dressing
wet lap sponge
wet lung
wet pack
wet reading of x-ray
wet smear
wet swallows
wet voice
wet-field cautery
wet-field coagulator
wet-field eraser cautery
wet-sheet pack
wetting
wet-to-dry dressing
Wetzel grid
Weve operation
Wexler Bantam self-retaining retractor
Wexler retractor
Wexler self-retaining retractor
Wexler-Balfour retractor

Wexteel scissors
whalebone eustachian bougie
whalebone eustachian probe
whalebone filiform bougie
whalebone filiform catheter
Wharton construction of artificial vagina
Wharton duct
Wharton operation
Wharton tumor
Wharton-Jones V-Y operation
Wheeler cystoscope
Wheeler cystotome
Wheeler discission knife
Wheeler eye implant
Wheeler eye sphere
Wheeler graft material
Wheeler halving procedure
Wheeler implant
Wheeler incision
Wheeler knife
Wheeler malleable-shape knife
Wheeler operation
Wheeler prosthesis
Wheeler spatula
Wheeler sphere eye implant
Wheeler vessel forceps
Wheeler-Reese operation
Wheelhouse operation
wheezing
Whelan-Moss T-tube
whenever necessary (p.r.n., prn, PRN)
whip
whip bougie
whiplash injury
whiplash pain
Whipple incision
Whipple operation
Whipple pancreatectomy
Whipple pancreaticoduodenec-tomy
Whipple pancreaticoduodenos-tomy
Whipple pancreatoduodenec-tomy
Whipple procedure

Whipple triad
whipstitch sutures
whipstitched
whirlpool
whirlybird excavator
whirlybird knife
whirlybird needle
whirlybird probe
whirlybird stapes excavator
whisk-packets dressing
whistle
Bárány noise apparatus whistle
Edelmann-Galton whistle
Galton ear whistle
Galton whistle
hearing whistle
Sahli whistle
whistle bougie
whistle-tip catheter
whistle-tip drain
whistle-tip Foley catheter
whistle-tip ureteral catheter
whistling rales
Whitacre operation
Whitaker malar sizer
Whitcomb-Kerrison laminectomy punch
Whitcomb-Kerrison laminectomy rongeur
Whitcomb-Kerrison punch
Whitcomb-Kerrison rongeur
White bone chisel
white braided sutures
White chisel
White foam pessary
White forceps
white graft
White hammer
white line of Toldt
White mallet
White mastoid rongeur
white matter
white nylon sutures
White operation
white patch

White procedure to shorten femur
white roll border
White scissors
White screwdriver
white silk sutures
white sutures
White tonsil forceps
White tonsil hemostat forceps
White tonsil-seizing forceps
white twisted sutures
Whitehead deformity
Whitehead mouth gag
Whitehead operation
White-Lillie forceps
White-Lillie tonsil forceps
Whitelite transilluminator
White-Oslay forceps
White-Oslay prostatic lobe-holding forceps
White-Proud retractor
Whiteside Ortholoc total knee system
Whiteside prosthesis
Whiteside total hip prosthesis
White-Smith forceps
Whitman arthroplasty
Whitman astragalectomy
Whitman fracture appliance
Whitman fracture frame
Whitman frame
Whitman operation
Whitman osteotomy
Whitman plate
Whitman procedure for long thoracic nerve palsy
Whitman technique
Whitman-Thompson procedure
Whitmore bag
Whitnall ligament
Whittle spud
Whitver clamp
Whitzel tunnel
WHO (wrist-hand orthosis)
whole body irradiation
whole bone transplant graft
whole brain irradiation

whole pelvis radiation
Wholey guide wire
Wholey Hi-Torque floppy guide
    wire
Wholey Hi-Torque modified J-
    guide wire
Wholey Hi-Torque standard
    guide wire
Wholey wire
Wholey-Edwards catheter
whorled cells
whorling
whorls
Wiberg fracture stapler
Wiberg raspatory
Wiberg shelf procedure
Wicherkiewicz eyelid repair
Wicherkiewicz operation
wick
Wick catheter
wick dressing
Wickham-Miller triradiate
    optical kidney stone
    grasper
Wickman uterine forceps
Wickstrom arthrodesis
Wickstrom wrist arthrodesis
Wickwitz esophageal stricture
wide excision
wide local excision
wide skin incision
wide-angle glaucoma
wide-angle system
wide-field eyepiece
widely patent orifice
wide-mouth sac
widened
widening
widening of abdominal aorta
widening of suture lines
widespread
Widia needle holder
Wid-Med resectoscope
Widner transilluminator
Wiechel scissors
Wieder decompressor
Wieder dissector

Wieder retractor
Wieger ligament
Wiener antral rasp
Wiener antral raspatory
Wiener breast reduction
Wiener corneal hook
Wiener eye knife
Wiener eye needle
Wiener eye speculum
Wiener eyelid repair
Wiener gold plate
Wiener hook
Wiener hysterectomy forceps
Wiener keratome
Wiener operation
Wiener rasp
Wiener scleral hook
Wiener speculum
Wiener suture hook
Wiener Universal frontal sinus
    raspatory
Wiener-Pierce antral rasp
Wiener-Pierce antral trocar
Wiener-Pierce rasp
Wiener-Pierce trocar
Wiener-Sauer intranasal tear-sac
    operation instruments
Wies chalazion forceps
Wies entropion excision
Wies entropion incision
Wies forceps
Wies operation
Wiet retractor
Wigand maneuver
Wigand version
Wigby-Taylor position
Wigderson ribbon retractor
Wigmore saw
Wikstroem artery forceps
Wild operating microscope
Wild surgical microscope
Wilde ear forceps
Wilde ear speculum
Wilde ethmoidal exenteration
    forceps
Wilde ethmoidal forceps
Wilde forceps

Wilde incision
Wilde intervertebral disk
    rongeur
Wilde laminectomy forceps
Wilde nasal punch
Wilde nasal snare
Wilde punch
Wilde septal forceps
Wilde-Blakesley ethmoidal
    forceps
Wilde-Bruening snare
Wilder cystoscope
Wilder cystotome
Wilder dilating forceps
Wilder dilator
Wilder eye knife
Wilder hook
Wilder lens hook
Wilder lens loop
Wilder lens scoop
Wilder loupe
Wilder retractor
Wilder scleral depressor
Wilder scleral self-retaining
    retractor
Wilder scoop
Wilder sign
Wilder trephine
Wilde-Troeltsch forceps
Wildgen-Reck localizer
Wildgen-Reck magnet
Wilhelm cystoscope
Wilke boot
Wilke boot brace
Wilke boot prosthesis
Wilke brace
Wilkerson bur
Wilkes self-retaining retractor
Wilkin classification of radial
    neck fractures
Wilkins trephine
Wilkinson abdominal retractor
Wilkinson abdominal self-
    retaining retractor
Wilkinson operation
Wilkinson retractor
Willauer raspatory

Willauer scissors
Willauer thoracic scissors
Willauer-Allis forceps
Willauer-Allis thoracic forceps
Willauer-Allis thoracic tissue
    forceps
Willauer-Allis tissue forceps
Willauer-Deaver retractor
Willauer-Gibbon periosteal
    elevator
Willett clamp
Willett forceps
Willett placental forceps
Williams brace
Williams clamp
Williams colpopoiesis
Williams craniotome
Williams dilator
Williams ear perforator
Williams eye speculum
Williams flexion exercises
Williams forceps
Williams gastrointestinal forceps
Williams intestinal forceps
Williams L-R guiding catheter
Williams lacrimal dilator
Williams lacrimal probe
Williams lumbosacral orthosis
Williams microsurgery saw
Williams nail system
Williams operation
Williams orthosis
Williams overtube sleeve
Williams pelvimeter
Williams perforator
Williams position
Williams probe
Williams screwdriver
Williams sign
Williams speculum
Williams tonsil electrode
Williams tracheal tone
Williams uterine forceps
Williams vessel-holding forceps
Williams-Haddad procedure
Williams-Richardson operation
Williger bone curet

Williger elevator
Williger raspatory
Williger separator
Willis antrum
Willis circle
Willis pancreas
Willis pouch
Willock jacket
Willock respiratory jacket
willow fracture
Wills eye lacrimal retractor
Wills eye spatula and spoon
Wills Hospital eye cautery
Wills Hospital forceps
Wills Hospital ophthalmology
   forceps
Wills Hospital utility forceps
Willy Meyer incision
Willy Meyer radical mastectomy
Wilman clamp
Wilmer chisel
Wilmer iris forceps
Wilmer iris retractor
Wilmer iris scissors
Wilmer operation
Wilmer retractor
Wilmer scissors
Wilmer wedge chisel
Wilmer-Bagley expressor
Wilmer-Bagley retractor
Wilmer-Converse conjunctival
   scissors
Wilmington jacket
Wilms operation
Wilms tumor
Wilson amniotic perforator
Wilson approach
Wilson arthrodesis
Wilson awl
Wilson bolt
Wilson chamber
Wilson clamp
Wilson fracture appliance
Wilson frame
Wilson graft
Wilson knee test
Wilson leads

Wilson muscle
Wilson operation
Wilson plate
Wilson retractor
Wilson rib spreader
Wilson right-angled awl
Wilson spinal frame
Wilson splint
Wilson spreader
Wilson stripper
Wilson technique
Wilson trocar
Wilson vein stripper
Wilson vitreous foreign body
   forceps
Wilson wrench
Wilson-Cook biopsy forceps
Wilson-Cook catheter
Wilson-Cook endoprosthesis
Wilson-Cook French stent
Wilson-Cook gastric balloon
Wilson-Cook mechanical
   lithotriptor
Wilson-Jacobs procedure
Wilson-Jones patellar operation
Wilson-Jones procedure
Wilson-McKeever procedure
Wilson-McKeever shoulder
   procedure
Wiltberger spreader
Wilton-Webster coronary sinus
   catheter
Wiltse iliac retractor
Wiltse-Bankart retractor
Wiltse-Gelpi self-retaining
   retractor
Winberger line
Winberger line on x-ray
Wincor enucleation scissors
Wincor scissors
wind sock sign
window
window operation
window rasp
windowing of cortex
windpipe
windshield wiper sign

Winer catheter
wing clip
wing of scapula
wing sutures
winged catheter
winged retractor blade
winged scapula
winged shunt
winged speculum
winged V-flap operation
Wingfield frame
Winiwarter cholecystoenteros-
    tomy
Winiwarter operation
Winkelman hydrocele repair
winking patella
winking spasm
Winograd ingrown nail proce-
    dure
Winquist-Hansen classification
    of femoral fractures
Winsburg-White bladder tube
Winsburg-White retractor
Winslow foramen
Winslow ligament
Winslow pancreas
Winter anterior osteotomy
Winter arch bar
Winter elevation torque
    technique
Winter elevator
Winter splint
Winter syndrome
Winter-Eber resectoscope
Winternitz sound
Winters shunt
wire (see also *guide wire*)
        ACS exchange guide
            wire
        ACS exchange wire
        ACS floppy-tip guide
            wire
        ACS gold-standard guide
            wire
        ACS gold-standard wire
        ACS guide wire
        ACS SOF-T guide wire

wire *continued*
        Amplatz Super Stiff guide
            wire
        Amplatz torque wire
        angiographic guide wire
        arch wire
        atrial pacing wire
        Babcock stainless suture
            wire
        Babcock suture wire
        Bentson floppy-tip guide
            wire
        Bentson guide wire
        Bentson wire
        Bunnell pull-out wire
        catheter forming wires
        cerclage wire
        circumcoronal wire
        closer wire
        Cole pull-out wire
        Compere fixation wire
        continuous loop wire
        coronary wire
        crimped wire
        crimper wire
        cut snare wire
        dock wire
        docking wire
        double-woven wire
        ear cut snare wire
        Eder-Puestow wire
        epicardial pacing wire
        Fegerstra wire
        Flex guide wire
        flexible guide wire
        flexible steerable wire
        flexible-J guide wire
        floppy guide wire
        floppy-tipped guide
            wire
        forming wires
        Gigli-saw wire
        guide wire (see separate
            listing)
        high-torque guide wire
        hinged-loop snare wire
        Hi-Per Flex guide wire

wire *continued*
    Hi-Torque Flex-T guide
      wire
    Hi-Torque floppy guide
      wire
    Hi-Torque intermediate
      guide wire
    Hi-Torque standard
      guide wire
    House wire
    Hyams wire
    Hyams-Timberlake wire
      loop for electrode
    Hyperflex guide wire
    Ideal arch wire
    interdental wire
    intramedullary wire
    intraoral wire
    Ivy wire
    J-guide wire
    J-tip guide wire
    J-tip wire
    J-tipped exchange guide
      wire
    J-tipped wire
    J-wire
    K-wire (Kirschner wire)
    Kazanjian wire
    Killip wire
    Kirschner wire (K-wire)
    Lassoe wire
    ligature wire
    Linx exchange guide
      wire
    Lunderquist guide wire
    Lunderquist wire
    Lunderquist working
      wire
    Lundquist nephrostomy
      wire
    Luque wire
    Meditech guide wire
    Micro-Glide exchange
      wire
    monofilament stainless
      steel wire
    monofilament wire

wire *continued*
    multifilament wire
    olive wire
    pacing electrode wire
    pacing wire
    PDT guide wire
    Puestow guide wire
    Puestow wires
    pull-out wire
    TAD guide wire
    tantalum wire
    Teflon-coated guide
      wire
    Teflon-wire piston
    temporary pacing wire
    Thiersch wire
    tonsillar snare wire
    transluminal coronary
      angioplasty guide wire
    USCI guide wire
    VeriFlex guide wire
    Waterston pacing wire
    Wholey guide wire
    Wholey Hi-Torque
      floppy guide wire
    Wholey Hi-Torque
      modified J-guide wire
    Wholey Hi-Torque
      standard guide wire
    Wholey wire
wire appliance
wire bivalve obstetrical specu-
    lum
wire bivalve vaginal speculum
wire carbide-jaw suture scissors
wire crimper (see also *crimper*)
    Caparosa wire crimper
    Francis-Gray wire
      crimper
    Gruppe wire crimper
    McGee-Caparosa wire
      crimper
    Schuknecht wire crimper
    Shiffrin wire crimper
wire cutter (see also *cutter*)
    Berbecker wire cutter
    Martin wire cutter

wire eye speculum
wire lid speculum
wire ligature
wire loop dilator
wire loop stapes dilator
wire mandrin
wire mesh eye implant
wire mesh graft
wire mesh implant
wire mesh prosthesis
wire needle holder
wire osteotomy plane
wire pass bur
wire probe
wire speculum
wire stapes prosthesis
wire stylet catheter
wire sutures
wire template
wire tightener (see also *tight-ener*)
    Kirschner wire tightener
wire Zytor suture
wire-bending die
wire-closure forceps
wire-crimper forceps
wire-cutting scissors
wired jaw
wire-fat ear prosthesis
Wirefoam splint
wire-loop lesion
wire-loop strut
wire-pulling forceps
wire-tightening clamp
wire-twister needle holder
wire-twisting forceps
wire-winged lid speculum
wire-wound cannula
wire-wound endotracheal tube
wiring
wiring of jaw
Wirsung duct
Wirsung pancreatic duct
Wirth-Jager posterior cruciate reconstruction

Wirthlin splenorenal clamp
Wirthlin splenorenal shunt clamp
wiry pulse
wisdom tooth
Wise breast incision
Wise dilator
Wise operation
Wise pattern in breast reduction
Wise retractor
Wis-Foregger laryngoscope
Wishard catheter
Wishard tip catheter
Wishard ureteral catheter
Wis-Hipple laryngoscope
Wister clamp
Wister nipper
Wister wire-and-pin cutter
withdrawal
withdrawn
Wittner biopsy punch
Wittner cervical punch
Wittner forceps
Wittner uterine biopsy forceps
Witzel duodenostomy
Witzel enterostomy
Witzel enterostomy catheter
Witzel gastrostomy
Witzel jejunostomy
Witzel operation
Witzel tube
Witzel tunnel for feeding jejunostomy
Wizard disposable inflation device
Wladimiroff (see *Vladimiroff*)
Woakes saw
Wobig entropion repair
Woelfe-Boehler cast breaker
Woelfe-Boehler cutter
Wolf antral needle
Wolf arthrosocpe
Wolf biopsy forceps
Wolf biting basket forceps
Wolf cannula

Wolf catheter
Wolf chisel knife
Wolf curved basket forceps
Wolf curved scissors
Wolf drainage cannula
Wolf draw knife
Wolf fiberoptic cord
Wolf laparoscope
Wolf Loktite gag
Wolf meniscal knife
Wolf meniscal retractor
Wolf mouth gag
Wolf needle trocar
Wolf nephrostomy bag catheter
Wolf panendoscope
Wolf procedure
Wolf procedure for plantar
    callosity
Wolf scissors
Wolfe breast dysplasia
Wolfe cheiloplasty
Wolfe classification of breast
    dysplasia
Wolfe eye forceps
Wolfe graft
Wolfe implant
Wolfe mammographic par-
    enchymal patterns
Wolfe operation
Wolfe prosthesis
Wolfe ptosis operation
Wolfe uterine cuff forceps
Wolfe-Kawamoto iliac graft
Wolfe-Krause graft
Wolfe-Krause implant
Wolfenden position
Wolferman drill
Wolff dermal curet
Wolff drain
wolffian body
wolffian cyst
wolffian drain
wolffian duct
Wölfler gastroenterostomy
Wölfler operation
Wölfler sign
Wölfler sutures

Wolf-Schindler gastroscope
Wolfson clamp
Wolfson forceps
Wolfson retractor
Wolfson spur crusher
Wolf-Veress needle
Wolkowitsch sign
Wolvek approximator
Wolvek fixation device
Wolvek sternal approximator
Wood applicator
Wood black light
Wood bulldog clamp
Wood lamp
Wood light
Wood needle
Wood operation
Wood osteotome
Wood screw
wood tongue blade
Woodbridge sutures
Wood-Doig vacuum biopsy
    instrument
Woodman operation
Woodruff catheter
Woodruff nasopalatine plexus
Woodruff screw
Woodruff screwdriver
Woodruff spatula knife
Woodruff ureteropyelographic
    catheter
Woods maneuver
Woods tonsillar scissors
Woodson double-ended
    dissector
Woodson dural separator and
    packer
Woodson elevator
Woodson spatula
Woodson spoon
Woodward antral raspatory
Woodward elevation of scapula
Woodward forceps
Woodward hemostat
Woodward hemostatic forceps
Woodward operation
Woodward rasp

Woodward retractor
Woodward scapula procedure
Woodward sound
Woodward thoracic hemostatic
    forceps
Woodyatt pump
Wookey neck flap
Wookey radical neck dissection
Wookey skin tube
wool roll dressing
Wooler mitral anuloplasty
Wooten eye needle
Worcester City Hospital vaginal
    speculum
Worcester instrument holder
Word catheter
work up (verb)
worked up
working diagnosis
working element resectoscope
workup (adj., noun)
wormian bone
wormy veins
Worrall deep retractor
Worrall headband
Worrall retractor
Worst intraocular lens
Worst lens
Worst Medallion lens
Worst Medallion sutures
Worst pigtail probe
Worst probe
Wort antral retractor
Worth advancement forceps
Worth chisel
Worth cystitome
Worth forceps
Worth muscle forceps
Worth operation
Worth strabismus forceps
Wötzer operation
wound
wound ballistics
wound care
wound cautery
wound cleaning
wound clip

wound closed
wound closure
wound contraction
wound debrided
wound dehiscence
wound discharge
wound disruption
wound drain
wound drainage
wound dressing
wound edge
wound entrance
wound excision
wound forceps
wound healing
wound irrigated
wound isolation
wound lip
wound margins
wound packed
wound protector
wound tension
wound towels
wound-clip forceps
woven bone
woven bougie
woven catheter
woven Dacron graft
woven elastic bandage
woven Teflon
woven-loop dislodger
woven-loop stone dislodger
woven-silk catheter
woven-tube vascular prosthesis
wrap
wraparound
wraparound dressing
wraparound splint
wrapping of abdominal aortic
    aneurysm
wrapping of aneurysm
Wrattan eye filter
Wreden sign
wrench
        Allen wrench
        Barton tongs wrench
        compression wrench

wrench *continued*
    Fox wrench
    Harrington flat wrench
    hexagonal wrench
    Kurlander orthopedic wrench
    orthopedic wrench
    slotted wrench
    Stader wrench
    T-handle wrench
    Thomas Waldon wrench
    Wilson wrench
wrenching pain
Wright Care-TENS device
Wright Care-TENS unit
Wright fascia needle
Wright knee plate
Wright knee prosthesis
Wright nasal snare
Wright needle
Wright operation
Wright plate
Wright snare
Wright test
Wright Universal brace
Wright version
Wright-Crawford needle
Wrigley forceps
wringer injury
wrinkle
wrinkle line
wrinkling
Wrisberg cartilage
Wrisberg ganglion
Wrisberg ligament
Wrisberg nerve
wrist
wrist bone
wrist excision
wrist flexed
wrist flexion test
wrist fusion
wrist ganglion
wrist joint
wrist prosthesis
wrist restraint
wrist scar

wristdrop
wrist-hand orthosis (WHO)
writhe
writhing
Wullen dislodger
Wullen stone dislodger
Wullstein bur
Wullstein chuck adapter
Wullstein curet
Wullstein drill
Wullstein ear forceps
Wullstein ear knife
Wullstein ear scissors
Wullstein ear self-retaining retractor
Wullstein forceps
Wullstein handpiece
Wullstein high-speed bur
Wullstein knife
Wullstein retractor
Wullstein ring curet
Wullstein scissors
Wullstein spatula
Wullstein transplant spatula
Wullstein tympanoplasty
Wullstein tympanoplasty forceps
Wullstein-House cup-shaped forceps
Wullstein-House forceps
Wullstein-Paparella forceps
Wullstein-Weitlaner retractor
Wullstein-Weitlaner self-retaining retractor
Wullstein-Zollner operation
Wurd catheter
Wurmuth spatula
Wurth crusher
Wurth spur crusher
Wurth vein stripper
Wurzburg plate
Wurzburg plating set
Wurzburg-Walter Lorenz rigid fixation set
Wutzer hernia
Wutzer operation
Wutzler circumcision scissors

Wutzler scissors
Wydase (hyaluronidase)
Wyeth amputation
Wyeth operation
Wyler electrode
Wyler subdural strip electrode
Wylie carotid artery clamp
Wylie clamp
Wylie dilator
Wylie drain
Wylie endarterectomy spatula
Wylie endarterectomy stripper
Wylie forceps
Wylie hypogastric clamp
Wylie operation
Wylie pessary
Wylie retractor

Wylie splanchnic retractor
Wylie stem pessary
Wylie stripper
Wylie uterine dilator
Wylie uterine director
Wylie uterine forceps
Wylie uterine tenaculum
    forceps
Wyllys-Andrews operation
Wynn cleft lip operation
Wynn cleft lip repair
Wynn method
Wynne-Evans tonsil dissector
Wyse pattern for reduction
    mammaplasty
Wyse reduction mammaplasty
Wysler sutures

X-Acto utility knife
X-clamp
x-linked
X-PAK I-A surgical system
x-ray
x-ray absorptiometry
x-ray beam
x-ray burn
x-ray cassette
x-ray dosage
x-ray findings
x-ray generator
x-ray image
x-ray microscope
x-ray pelvimetry
x-ray study
x-ray template
x-ray therapy
x-ray view
X-TEND-O knee flexer
X-Vee surgical system
Xanar 20 Amulase CO2 laser
xanthochromic
xanthoma
xanthoma of joint
xanthomatosis
xanthomatosis of bone
xanthomatous
XECT (xenon-enhanced
    computed tomography)
xenodiagnosis
xenograft
xenograft heart valve
Xenomedica prosthetic valve
xenon
xenon arc photocoagulation
    cautery
xenon arc photocoagulator

xenon photocoagulator
xenon ventilation scan
xenon-133 technique
xenon-enhanced computed
    tomography (XECT)
Xenophor femoral prosthesis
Xenotech graft
Xenotech prosthetic
xenotransplantation
Xeroflo dressing
Xeroform dressing
Xeroform gauze
xerogram
xerography
xeromammogram
xeromammography
xeroradiography
xiphisternal crunching sound
xiphoid
xiphoid angle
xiphoid process
xiphoid to os pubis incision
xiphoid to umbilicus incision
xiphoidectomy
xiphomanubrial junction
Xomed Audiant bone conductor
Xomed Doyle nasal airway
    splint
Xomed endotracheal tube
Xomed Silastic splint
Xylocaine
Xylocaine jelly
Xylocaine with epinephrine
Xyrel pacemaker
xyster
xyster raspatory
Xyticon 5950 bipolar demand
    pacemaker

Y-bandage
Y-bandage dressing
Y-bone plate
Y-connector
Y-double incision
Y-drain
Y-fracture
Y-glass rod
Y-graft
Y-incision
Y-ligament
Y-line
Y-line on x-ray
Y-nailing of arm
Y-osteotomy
Y-plasty procedure
Y-plate
Y-screw
Y-shaped graft
Y-shaped incision
Y-shaped scar
Y-sutures
Y-trough catheter
Y-tube
Y-type incision
Y-type ureteropelvioplasty
Y-V anoplasty
Y-V plasty
Y-V pyeloplasty
Y-V ureteropelvioplasty
Y-view on x-ray
Y-wave
Y-Z plasty
Yaeger lid plate
YAG (yttrium-aluminum-
    garnet)
YAG capsulotomy
YAG laser
YAG laser capsulotomy

Yamanda myelotomy knife
Yankauer antral punch
Yankauer antral trocar
Yankauer antral-punch tip
Yankauer bronchoscope
Yankauer catheter
Yankauer curet
Yankauer ear curet
Yankauer esophagoscope
Yankauer ether inhaler
Yankauer ethmoid forceps
Yankauer ethmoid-cutting
    forceps
Yankauer eustachian instru-
    ments
Yankauer forceps
Yankauer hook
Yankauer laryngoscope
Yankauer ligature passer
Yankauer middle meatus
    cannula
Yankauer multi-orifice tip
Yankauer nasopharyngeal
    speculum
Yankauer nasopharyngoscope
Yankauer needle
Yankauer operation
Yankauer periosteal elevator
Yankauer pharyngeal speculum
Yankauer probe
Yankauer punch
Yankauer salpingeal curet
Yankauer salpingeal knife
Yankauer salpingeal probe
Yankauer scissors
Yankauer septal needle
Yankauer single-orifice tip
Yankauer speculum
Yankauer suction technique

Yankauer suction tip
Yankauer suction tube
Yankauer suture needle
Yankauer tonsillar scissors
Yankauer trocar
Yankauer tube
Yankauer washing tube
Yankauer-Little forceps
Yankauer-Little tube forceps
Yasargil aneurysmal clip
Yasargil arachnoid knife
Yasargil artery forceps
Yasargil bayonet scissors
Yasargil carotid clamp
Yasargil clamp
Yasargil clip
Yasargil curet
Yasargil dissector
Yasargil forceps
Yasargil instrument
Yasargil knife
Yasargil method
Yasargil microclip
Yasargil microinstruments
Yasargil microraspatory
Yasargil microscissors
Yasargil microscope
Yasargil microvascular bayonet
  scissors
Yasargil needle holder
Yasargil neurological instrument
Yasargil pituitary rongeur
Yasargil raspatory
Yasargil retractor
Yasargil scissors
Yasargil scoop
Yasargil suction tube
Yasargil surgical microscope
Yasargil technique
Yazujian bur
Yazujian eye knife
yeast
Yeder tube
Yellen clamp
yellow bone marrow
yellow ligament
yellow marrow

Yellow Springs probe
yellow-eyed dilating bougie
yellowish
yellowness
yellow-tip aspirator
Yeoman biopsy punch
Yeoman forceps
Yeoman probe
Yeoman proctoscope
Yeoman punch
Yeoman rectal biopsy forceps
Yeoman sigmoidoscope
Yeoman uterine forceps
Yeoman-Wittner rectal biopsy
  forceps
Yeoman-Wittner rectal forceps
Yergason sign for subluxation
  of biceps tendon
Ygon tube
yoke
yoke of mandible
yoke of maxilla
yoked muscles
yolk
York-Mason incision
York-Mason repair
Yoshida dissector
Yoshida tonsil dissector
Young approach
Young clamp
Young cystoscope
Young dilator
Young dissector
Young epispadias repair
Young flatfoot procedure
Young forceps
Young intestinal forceps
Young lateral retractor
Young ligature carrier
Young needle holder
Young operation
Young operation for talipes
  valgus
Young prostatectomy
Young prostatic enucleator
Young prostatic retractor
Young prostatic tractor

Young rectal dilator
Young renal pedicle clamp
Young retractor
Young rongeur
Young tongue forceps
Young tongue-seizing forceps
Young tractor
Young urological dissector
Young vasectomy
Young-Dees operation

Younge uterine biopsy curet
Younge uterine biopsy forceps
Younge uterine curet
Younge uterine forceps
Young-Millin holder
Young-Millin needle holder
Yount operation
yttrium pellets
yttrium-aluminum-garnet laser
    (YAG laser)

# Z

Z-cut osteotomy
Z-disk
Z-excision
Z-fixation nail
Z-flap
Z-flap incision
Z-incision
Z-line
Z-marginal tenotomy
Z-plane analysis
Z-plastic relaxing operation
Z-plasty
Z-plasty closure
Z-plasty for ectropion
Z-plasty incision
Z-plasty operation
Z-plasty revision
Z-plasty scar
Z-plate
Z-screw
Z-shaped incision
Z-shaped scar
Z-sutures
Z-technique in laparoscopy
Z-track
Zachary-Cope clamp
Zachary-Cope-DeMartel clamp
Zachary-Cope-DeMartel colon
    clamp
Zachary-Cope-DeMartel triple-
    colon clamp
Zadik ingrown nail proce-
    dure
Zadik procedure
Zahn lines
Zahn ribs
Zahradnicek operation
Zalkind lung retractor
Zalkind-Balfour blade

Zalkind-Balfour self-retaining
    retractor
Zamboni biopsy solution
Zancolli capsulodesis
Zancolli capsuloplasty
Zancolli capsulorrhaphy of
    fingers
Zancolli claw-hand deformity
    repair
Zancolli lasso intrinsicplasty
Zancolli operation
Zander apparatus
Zanelli position
Zang space
Zarins-Rowe procedure
Zaufel bone rongeur
Zaufel sign
Zaufel-Jansen rongeur
Zavod bronchospirometry
    catheter
Zavod catheter
Zeiman herniorrhaphy
Zeir procedure for long thoracic
    nerve palsy
Zeiss aspheric lens
Zeiss beam splitter
Zeiss binocular head magnifier
Zeiss binocular tube
Zeiss camera equipment
Zeiss diploscope microscope
Zeiss eyepiece
Zeiss Formair gonioscope
Zeiss hammer lamp
Zeiss instruments
Zeiss laser
Zeiss lens loupe
Zeiss light coagulation for
    retinal detachment
Zeiss microscope

Zeiss microscope eyepiece
Zeiss operating camera
Zeiss operating microscope
Zeiss ophthalmological instruments
Zeiss OPMI operating microscope
Zeiss OPMI-6 operating microscope
Zeiss photocoagulator
Zeiss slit lamp
Zeiss small-beam splitter
Zeiss stone dislodger
Zeiss unit
Zeiss-Bruening anastigmatic auriscope
Zeiss-Cohan-Barraquer microscope
Zeiss-Opton ophthalmoscope
Zelsmyr Cytobrush cell collector for Pap smear
Zenker dissecting and ligature forceps
Zenker diverticulum
Zenker fixation
Zenker pouch
Zenker raspatory
Zenotech
Zenotech synthetic ligament
Zephiran
Zephiran chloride
Zephiran pack
Zephiran solution
Zephyr rubber elastic dressing
Zervas hypophysectomy kit
Zickel II subtrochanteric system
Zickel intramedullary nail
Zickel nail
Zickel nail fixation
Zickel nailing of femur
Zickel rod
Zickel supracondylar system
Ziegler blade
Ziegler cauterization
Ziegler cautery
Ziegler cautery electrode

Ziegler cilia forceps
Ziegler dilator
Ziegler ectropion repair
Ziegler eye needle-knife
Ziegler eye speculum
Ziegler forceps
Ziegler iridectomy
Ziegler iris knife
Ziegler iris knife-needle
Ziegler knife
Ziegler knife-needle
Ziegler lacrimal probe
Ziegler needle
Ziegler needle probe
Ziegler needle-knife
Ziegler operation
Ziegler probe
Ziegler puncture
Ziegler speculum
Ziegler wash bottle
Ziegler-Furniss clamp
Zielke gouge
Zielke instrument for scoliosis spinal fusion
Zielke rod
Zielke screw
Zieman hernia repair
Zieman operation
ZIFT (zygote intrafallopian tube transfer)
zigzag bilateral cleft lip repair
zigzag incision
zigzag repair
zigzagplasty
Zilkie device
Zim carpal tunnel projection
Zimalate drill
Zimalate twist drill
Zimalate twist drill bit
Zimaloy epiphyseal staple
Zimaloy femoral head prosthesis
Zimaloy hip prosthesis
Zimaloy knee prosthesis
Zimaloy operation
Zimaloy prosthesis
Zimaloy staple

Zerowet Syringe System (per. Dr. Caplin

Zimany bilobed flap
Zimany flap
Zimberg esophageal hiatal
    retractor
Zimcode traction frames tractor
Zim-Flux dressing
Zimfoam finger splint
Zimfoam head halter
Zimfoam head halter traction
Zimfoam padding
Zimfoam pin
Zimfoam splint
Zimmer airplane splint
Zimmer antiembolism support
    stockings
Zimmer arm sling
Zimmer bolt
Zimmer cartilage clamp
Zimmer clamp
Zimmer clavicular cross sling
Zimmer clavicular cross splint
Zimmer compression hip screw
Zimmer drill
Zimmer driver
Zimmer driver-extractor
Zimmer extractor
Zimmer femoral condyle blade
    plate
Zimmer frame
Zimmer Free-Lock hip fixation
    system
Zimmer gouge
Zimmer hand drill
Zimmer head halter
Zimmer hip plate
Zimmer intramedullary knee
    instrumentation
Zimmer intramedullary nail
Zimmer low viscosity cement
Zimmer nail
Zimmer Orthair oscillator
Zimmer Orthair ream driver
Zimmer Orthair reciprocator
Zimmer Orthairtome
Zimmer ototomy
Zimmer pin
Zimmer prosthesis

Zimmer protractor
Zimmer screw
Zimmer screwdriver
Zimmer shoulder prosthesis
Zimmer skin graft mesher
Zimmer sling
Zimmer splint
Zimmer telescoping nail
Zimmer Ti-BAC acetabular
    components
Zimmer tibial bolt
Zimmer tibial nail cap
Zimmer tibial prosthesis
Zimmer total hip prosthesis
Zimmer Universal drill
Zimmer Universal knee
    immobilizer with Zimfoam
    padding
Zimmer-Hoen forceps
Zimmer-Hoff external fixation
    system
Zimmer-Kirschner hand drill
Zimmerman operation
Zimmer-Schlesinger forceps
Zimocel dressing
Zim-Trac traction splint
Zim-Trac traction splint tractor
Zim-Zip rib belt splint
zinc gelatin impregnated gauze
zinc oxide-eugenol dental
    sealant (ZOE dental
    sealant)
Zinco Castaway fixed ankle
    walker
Zinn annulus
Zinn aponeurosis
Zinn artery
Zinn cap
Zinn circle
Zinn circlet
Zinn corona
Zinn ligament
Zinn tendon
Zinn zone
Zinn zonule
zipper scar
Zipser clamp

Zipser penis clamp
Zircate treatment
Zitron pacemaker
Zoalite lamp
Zobec sponge dressing
ZOE dental sealant (zinc oxide
    eugenol dental sealant)
Zoellner hook
Zoellner needle
Zoellner raspatory
Zoellner scissors
Zoellner stapes hook
Zoll NTP pacemaker
Zoll pacemaker
Zollinger multipurpose tissue
    forceps
Zollinger splint
Zollinger-Ellison syndrome
Zollinger-Ellison tumor
Zollinger-Gilmore intraluminal
    vein stripper
Zollinger-Gilmore vein stripper
Zollner suction tube
Zolyse
zonal aberration
zonary placenta
Zonas porous adhesive tape
    dressing
zone
zonogram
zonography
zonula ciliaris
zonular cataract
zonular fibers
zonular placenta
zonular space
zonule fibers
zonule of Zinn
zonule separator
zonulolysis
zonulysis
zoograft
zoografting
Zoroc resin plaster dressing
Zower speculum
Zucker cardiac catheter
Zucker catheter

Zucker splint
Zuelzer awl
Zuelzer hook plate
Zuelzer plate
Zuker bipolar pacing elec-
    trode
Zurich dilatation catheter
Zutt clamp
Zwanck pessary
Zwanck radium pessary
Zweifel angiotribe
Zweifel angiotribe forceps
Zweifel needle holder
Zweifel-DeLee cranioclast
Zweymuller hip prosthesis
Zyclast collagen
Zyderm
Zyderm collagen implant
Zyderm collagen injections
Zyderm implant
Zyderm injection
Zydone analgesic
zygapophyseal joints
zygoma
zygoma elevator
zygoma hook
zygomatic
zygomatic arch
zygomatic bone
zygomatic muscle
zygomatic nerve
zygomatic process
zygomatic reflex
zygomatic region
zygomatic suture line
zygomaticofacial nerve
zygomaticofrontal suture
zygomaticofrontal suture
    lines
zygomaticomaxillary fracture
zygomaticomaxillary suture
zygomaticoorbital artery
zygomaticoorbitalis, arteria
zygomaticotemporal nerve
zygomaticotemporal suture
zygomaticus major, musculus
zygomaticus minor, musculus

zygomaticus, nervus
zygote intrafallopian tube
    transfer (ZIFT)
Zyler tube
Zylik cannula

Zylik operation
Zylik operation for talipes
    equinovarus
Zyplast implant
Zytor sutures

ISBN 0-7216-2128-7

90016